RESOURCE MANUAL TO ACCOMPANY
NURSING RESEARCH
Generating and Assessing Evidence for Nursing Practice, Eighth Edition

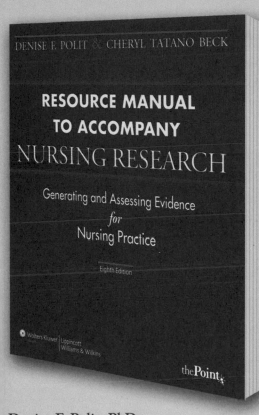

The perfect complement to *Nursing Research: Generating and Assessing Evidence for Nursing Practice, Eighth Edition*, this knowledge-builder will help you develop and reinforce the basic skills essential to today's nursing research.

The Resource Manual includes:

- **11 full research reports** that cover a range of nursing research endeavors, including qualitative and quantitative studies, an instrument development study, and two systematic reviews.

- **Full critiques of two of the research reports** that serve as models for a comprehensive research critique.

- **A never-before-published successful grant application** for a study funded by the *National Institute of Nursing Research*.

The *Resource Manual* also includes *The Toolkit*—a free student resource CD-ROM with methodologic tools. The Toolkit offers ready-to-use research tools, in Word documents that can be downloaded and adapted to fit individual needs—a great timesaver!

Examples of Toolkit resources include:
Templates for wording research questions; informed consent forms; a confidentiality pledge for research staff; literature review protocols; critical appraisal protocols; interviewer training tools; table templates; a demographic form; meta-analysis coding forms; and more!

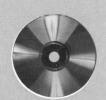

Denise F. Polit, PhD
President, Humanalysis, Inc.,
Saratoga Springs, New York
and
Adjunct Professor,
Griffith University School of Nursing,
Research Centre for Clinical Practice Innovation
Gold Coast, Australia

Cheryl Tatano Beck, DNSc, CNM, FAAN
Professor, School of Nursing,
University of Connecticut
Storrs, Connecticut

Approx. 400 Pages • Softbound
ISBN: 978-0-7817-7052-1

Order Today!

Visit your local health science bookstore or
Call 1-800-399-3110
Visit us on the Web at LWW.com/nursing

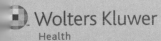
Wolters Kluwer | Lippincott Williams & Wilkins
Health

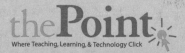
thePoint
Where Teaching, Learning, & Technology Click

Quick Guide to Bivariate Statistical Tests

Level of measurement of dependent variable	Group Comparisons: Number of groups (the independent variable)				Correlational analyses (To examine relationship strength)
	2 Groups		3+ Groups		
	Independent Groups Tests	Dependent Groups Tests	Independent Groups Tests	Dependent Groups Tests	
Nominal (Categorical)	χ^2 pp. 600 to 601 (or Fisher's exact test) p. 601	McNemar"s test p. 601	χ^2 pp. 600 to 601	Cochran's Q	Phi coefficient (dichotomous) or Cramér's V (not restricted to dichotomous) p. 602
Ordinal (Rank)	Mann-Whitney Test (or Median test) p. 596	Wilcoxon signed ranks test p. 596	Kruskal-Wallis H test p. 599	Friedman's test p. 600	Spearman's rho (or Kendall's tau) p. 602
Interval or Ratio (Continuous)*	Independent group t $test$ pp. 593 to 595	Paired t $test$ p. 595	ANOVA pp. 596 to 599	RM-ANOVA p. 599	Pearson's r pp. 601 to 602
	Multifactor ANOVA for 2+ independent variables		p. 599		
	RM-ANOVA for 2+ groups x 2+ measurements over time				

*For distributions that are markedly non-normal or samples that are small, the nonparametric tests in the row above may be needed.

Quick Guide to Designs in an Evidence Hierarchy

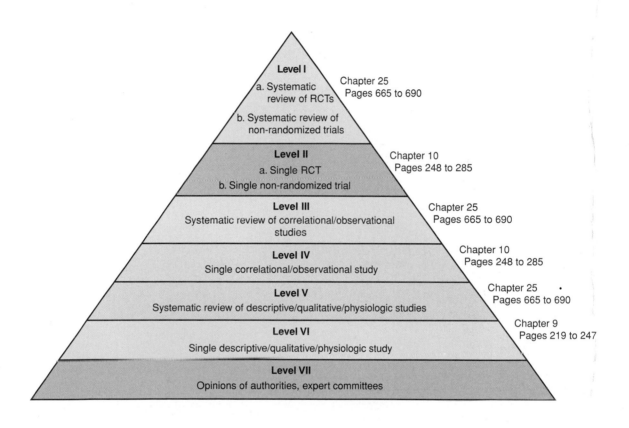

NURSING RESEARCH: GENERATING AND ASSESSING EVIDENCE FOR NURSING PRACTICE

Eighth Edition

Denise F. Polit, PhD

President
Humanalysis, Inc.
Saratoga Springs, New York, *and*
Adjunct Professor
Griffith University School of Nursing,
Research Centre for Clinical Practice Innovation
Gold Coast, Australia
(www.denisepolit.com)

Cheryl Tatano Beck, DNSc, CNM, FAAN

Professor
School of Nursing
University of Connecticut
Storrs, Connecticut

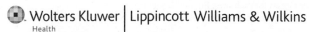

Wolters Kluwer | Lippincott Williams & Wilkins
Health

Philadelphia · Baltimore · New York · London
Buenos Aires · Hong Kong · Sydney · Tokyo

Acquisitions Editor: Hilarie Surrena
Managing Editor: Helen Kogut
Editorial Assistant: Elizabeth Harris
Director of Nursing Production: Helen Ewan
Senior Managing Editor / Production: Erika Kors
Art Director, Design: Joan Wendt
Art Director, Illustration: Brett MacNaughton
Senior Manufacturing Manager: William Alberti
Manufacturing Coordinator: Karen Duffield
Interior Designer: Joan Wendt
Indexer: Greystone Indexing
Compositor: Aptara, Inc.
Printer: R. R. Donnelley, Crawfordsville

8th Edition

Library of Congress Cataloging-in-Publication Data

Polit, Denise F.
   Nursing research : generating and assessing evidence for nursing practice / Denise F. Polit, Cheryl Tatano Beck.—8th ed.
      p. ; cm.
Includes bibliographical references and index.
ISBN 978-0-7817-9468-8 (alk. paper)
1. Nursing—Research—Methodology. I. Beck, Cheryl Tatano. II. Title.
   [DNLM: 1. Nursing Research—methods. WY 20.5 P769n 2008]
   RT81.5.P64 2008
   610.73'072—dc22

                                                                   2007006184

Care has been taken to confirm the accuracy of the information presented and to describe generally accepted practices. However, the authors, editors, and publisher are not responsible for errors or omissions or for any consequences from application of the information in this book and make no warranty, expressed or implied, with respect to the currency, completeness, or accuracy of the contents of the publication. Application of this information in a particular situation remains the professional responsibility of the practitioner; the clinical treatments described and recommended may not be considered absolute and universal recommendations.

The authors, editors, and publisher have exerted every effort to ensure that drug selection and dosage set forth in this text are in accordance with the current recommendations and practice at the time of publication. However, in view of ongoing research, changes in government regulations, and the constant flow of information relating to drug therapy and drug reactions, the reader is urged to check the package insert for each drug for any change in indications and dosage and for added warnings and precautions. This is particularly important when the recommended agent is a new or infrequently employed drug.

Some drugs and medical devices presented in this publication have Food and Drug Administration (FDA) clearance for limited use in restricted research settings. It is the responsibility of the health care provider to ascertain the FDA status of each drug or device planned for use in their clinical practice.

TO NORAH AND RYAN

Whose wedding preparations provided splendid
balance during the writing of this book, and whose
exuberance was contagious

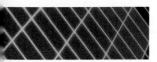 # Reviewers

Mary Bennett, DNSc, APRN, BC, FNP
Assistant Dean, Associate Professor
College of Nursing
Indiana State University
Terre Haute, Indiana

Jeanne Geiger Brown, PhD, RN
Assistant Professor
Work and Health Research Center
University of Maryland School of Nursing
Baltimore, Maryland

Kay Foland, PhD, APRN, BC, CNP
Associate Professor
College of Nursing, West River Department
South Dakota State University
Rapid City, South Dakota

Ann Hilton, RN, PhD
Professor Emerita
School of Nursing
University of British Columbia
Vancouver, British Columbia, Canada

Anne Kearney PhD, RN
Assistant Professor
School of Nursing and Faculty of Medicine
Memorial University of Newfoundland
St. John's, Newfoundland and Labrador, Canada

Elizabeth Petit de Mange, PhD, RN
Assistant Professor
School of Nursing
University of Medicine and Dentistry of New Jersey
Stratford, New Jersey

Janis Seeley, RN, MEd, MScN
Professor of Nursing
Confederation College
Thunder Bay, Ontario, Canada

Sandra L. Siedlecki, PhD, RN, CNS
Senior Nurse Researcher
Department of Nursing Research
Cleveland Clinic Foundation
Adjunct Assistant Professor of Nursing
Frances Payne Bolton School of Nursing
Case Western Reserve University
Cleveland, Ohio

Gail Blair Storr, RN, PhD
Professor
Faculty of Nursing
University of New Brunswick
Fredericton, New Brunswick, Canada

Geri L. Wood, PhD, RN, FAAN
Associate Professor
School of Nursing
University of Texas Health Science Center
Houston, Texas

Patti Rager Zuzelo, EdD, APRN, BC, CNS
Associate Professor & CNS Track Coordinator
La Salle University
Associate Director of Nursing for Research
Albert Einstein Healthcare Network (Joint Position)
Philadelphia, Pennsylvania

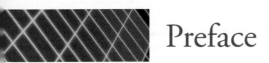

Preface

What a fabulous journey this eighth edition has been! This edition marks the most sweeping revision we have undertaken, as signaled by the book's new title. We have been energized and exhilarated by the new content, the new organizational approach, and the new enrichment opportunities embodied in this book. We see this book as a watershed edition of a classic textbook. We have retained many features that have made this book a classic, but have introduced important innovations that we think will make it easier and more rewarding to embark on a professional pathway that includes research.

NEW TO THIS EDITION

Upfront and Consistent Emphasis on Evidence-Based Practice

We have made several changes to emphasize that research is an evidence-building enterprise that is crucial to nursing practice. We elevated the chapter on evidence-based practice (EBP) to greater prominence by making it the second chapter in the current edition (it was previously the final chapter), and greatly expanded its content. We stress throughout that the decisions researchers make in designing and implementing a study have implications for the quality of evidence the study yields—and that the quality of evidence affects the utility of study findings for nursing practice. We have also added a new chapter on systematic reviews, considered by many to be the cornerstone of EBP. Also, given the need for nurses to evaluate evidence regularly, we have offered critiquing advice in *every* chapter of the book, rather than relegating critiquing guidelines to a chapter at the end.

New Content Reflecting Contributions of Medical Research Methodology

Nurse researchers have historically tended to use methods and jargon based in the social sciences, but the push for EBP in medicine has led to methodologic breakthroughs that have implications for all health care research. Moreover, it is important for nurses to become familiar with medical research terms and approaches so they can stay abreast of new clinical developments. This edition offers a balanced presentation of medical and social science techniques and nomenclature, and features innovative concepts emerging in the medical research literature.

New Organization of Qualitative and Quantitative Materials

Although previous editions endeavored to balance material on qualitative and quantitative methods, this balance may have been obscured by intermingling content on both approaches within chapters. In the previous editions, data collection methods were organized by type of approach (for example, a chapter on self-reports) rather than by the nature of data gathered (structured versus unstructured). Our new organization reflects our revised thinking about how our textbook is used, and how best to convey the spirit of different types of inquiry.

New Chapters

As noted, we have included a new chapter on systematic reviews (Chapter 25). This eighth edition also includes a new chapter on the development of self-report scales (Chapter 18), an area of increasing importance as nurses endeavor to construct high-quality instruments and screening tools to measure clinically important concepts. Finally, we have added a chapter on approaches to enhancing and assessing integrity in qualitative inquiry (Chapter 20). Because qualitative research is not linear—and because strategies for enhancing the quality and integrity of qualitative studies flow throughout the endeavor—we struggled with where in the book it would be best to describe such strategies. In placing this chapter near the end, we do not mean to imply that the strategies are of minor importance, nor that they should be "afterthoughts" to worry about only after data have been collected and analyzed. For those learning to do qualitative research, we consider this one of the most important chapters of the book because it is an all-encompassing topic for qualitative inquiry.

The Toolkit

Our biggest innovation for this edition is included in the accompanying *Resource Manual*. In our technologically advanced environment, it is possi-ble to not only *illustrate* methodologic tools as graphics in the textbook, but to make them directly available for use and adaptation. Thus, we have included dozens upon dozens of documents in Word files that can readily be adapted in research projects, without forcing users to "reinvent the wheel" or tediously retype material from the textbook. Examples include informed consent forms, a demographic questionnaire, content validity forms, templates for tables of statistical results, and a coding sheet for a meta-analysis—to name only a few.

ORGANIZATION OF THE TEXT

The content of this edition is organized into six main parts.

- **Part 1—Foundations of Nursing Research and Evidence-Based Practice** introduces fundamental concepts in nursing research. Chapter 1 summarizes the history and future of nursing research, discusses the philosophical underpinnings of qualitative research versus quantitative research, and describes major purposes of nursing research. Chapter 2 offers guidance on utilizing research to build an evidence-based practice. Chapter 3 introduces readers to key research terms, and presents an overview of steps in the research process for both qualitative and quantitative studies.
- **Part 2—Conceptualizing a Study to Generate Evidence for Nursing** further sets the stage for learning about the research process by discussing issues relating to a study's conceptualization: the formulation of research questions and hypotheses (Chapter 4); the review of relevant research (Chapter 5); the development of theoretical and conceptual contexts (Chapter 6); and the fostering of ethically sound approaches in doing research (Chapter 7).
- **Part 3—Designing a Study to Generate Evidence for Nursing** presents material on the design of qualitative and quantitative nursing research studies. Chapter 8 provides an overview of important issues that must be attended to dur-

ing the planning of any type of study. Chapter 9 is devoted to research designs for qualitative studies, including material on critical theory, feminist, and participatory action research. Chapter 10 describes fundamental principles and applications of quantitative research design, and Chapter 11 focuses on methods to enhance the rigor of a quantitative study, including mechanisms of research control. Chapter 12 examines research with different purposes, including mixed method research in which methods for qualitative and quantitative inquiry are blended. Chapter 13 presents designs and strategies for selecting samples of study participants.

- **Part 4—Collecting Research Data** concerns the gathering of information to address research questions. Chapter 14 discusses the design and implementation of an overall data collection plan. Chapter 15 describes methods of gathering unstructured self-report and observational data for qualitative studies, while Chapter 16 describes the collection of structured data for quantitative studies. Chapter 17 discusses the concept of measurement, and then focuses on methods of assessing the quality of data from formal measuring instruments. Chapter 18 presents new material on how to develop high-quality self-report instruments.
- **Part 5—Analyzing and Interpreting Research Data** discusses analytic methods for qualitative and quantitative research. Chapter 19 discusses methods of doing qualitative analyses, with specific information on grounded theory, phenomenological, and ethnographic analyses. Chapter 20 elaborates on methods qualitative researchers can use to enhance (and assess) integrity and quality throughout their inquiries. Chapters 21, 22, and 23 present an overview of univariate, bivariate, and multivariate statistical analyses, respectively. Chapter 24 describes the development of an overall analytic strategy for quantitative studies, including new material on interpreting results.
- **Part 6—Building an Evidence Base for Nursing Practice** provides additional guidance on linking research and clinical practice. Chapter

25 offers an overview of methods of conducting systematic reviews that support EBP, with an emphasis on meta-analyses and metasyntheses. Chapter 26 discusses dissemination of evidence—how to prepare a research report (including theses and dissertations), and how to disseminate and publish research findings. The concluding chapter (Chapter 27) offers suggestions and guidelines on developing research proposals and getting financial support.

KEY FEATURES

This textbook was designed to be helpful to those who are learning how to do research, as well as to those who are learning to appraise research reports critically and to use research findings in practice. Many of the features successfully used in previous editions have been retained in this eighth edition. Among the basic principles that helped to shape this and earlier editions of this book are (1) an unswerving conviction that the development of research skills is critical to the nursing profession; (2) a fundamental belief that research is an intellectually and professionally rewarding enterprise; and (3) a judgment that learning about research methods need be neither intimidating nor dull. Consistent with these principles, we have tried to present the fundamentals of research methods in a way that both facilitates understanding and arouses curiosity and interest. Key features of our approach include the following:

- **Research examples.** Each chapter concludes with one or two actual research examples designed to highlight critical points made in the chapter and to sharpen the reader's critical thinking skills. In addition, many research examples from around the world are used to illustrate key points in the text and to stimulate students' thinking about a research project.
- **Critiquing guidelines.** Most chapters include a section devoted to guidelines for conducting a critique of each aspect of a research report. These sections provide a list of questions to draw attention to specific aspects of a report that are amenable to appraisal.

- **Clear, "user-friendly" style.** Our writing style is designed to be easily digestible and nonintimidating. Concepts are introduced carefully and systematically, difficult ideas are presented clearly, and readers are assumed to have no prior exposure to technical terms.
- **Specific practical tips on doing research.** The textbook is filled with practical guidance on how to translate the abstract notions of research methods into realistic strategies for conducting research. Every chapter includes several tips for applying the chapter's lessons to real-life situations. The inclusion of these suggestions acknowledges the fact that there is often a large gap between what gets taught in research methods textbooks and what a researcher needs to know in conducting a study.
- **Aids to student learning.** Several features are used to enhance and reinforce learning and to help focus the student's attention on specific areas of text content, including the following: succinct, bulleted summaries at the end of each chapter; tables and figures that provide examples and graphic materials in support of the text discussion; and study suggestions at the end of each chapter.

TEACHING-LEARNING PACKAGE

The eighth edition of *Nursing Research: Generating and Assessing Evidence for Nursing Practice* has an ancillary package designed with both students and instructors in mind.

- **Free CD-ROM** 💿. The textbook also includes a CD-ROM that provides lists of relevant and useful websites for each chapter, which can be "clicked" on directly without having to retype the URL and risk a typographical error. An expanded glossary for the text also appears on this CD-ROM. Finally, statistical tables of significance values for four frequently used statistical tests are also included on the CD-ROM for reference.

- ***Resource Manual to Accompany Nursing Research, Eighth Edition***. The manual augments the textbook in important ways. It provides students with exercises that correspond to each text chapter, with a focus on opportunities to critique actual studies. Answers to most study exercises are included in the appendices. The appendices also include 11 research reports in their entirety, plus a successful grant application for a study funded by the National Institute of Nursing Research. The 11 reports cover a range of nursing research endeavors, including qualitative and quantitative studies, an instrument development study, and two systematic reviews. Full critiques of two of the reports are also included and can serve as models for a comprehensive research critique.
- The Toolkit ✴. This must-have innovation will save considerable time for both students and seasoned researchers. Included on the CD-ROM that accompanies the *Resource Manual to Accompany Nursing Research, Eighth Edition*, the Toolkit offers dozens of research resources in Word documents that can be downloaded and used directly or adapted. The resources, most of which have been pretested and refined in our own research, reflect best-practice research material.
- **The Instructor's Resource CD-ROM.** This includes PowerPoint slides summarizing key points in each chapter, and, in this edition, they are available in a format that permits easy adaptation. An Image Collection that contains all of the figures, boxes, and tables from the book is also included as a resource for instructors. In addition, test questions have been placed into a program that allows instructors to automatically generate tests complete with instructions and an answer key. These tests will help you identify students' areas of strength—as well as those areas needing further attention. Finally, the websites that are included on the free CD-ROM that accompanies the text are also included on the Instructor's Resource CD-ROM for your easy access.
- **ThePoint** ✴ (http://thepoint.lww.com), a trademark of Wolters Kluwer Health, is a web-based

course and content management system providing every resource instructors and students need in one easy-to-use site. Advanced technology and superior content combine at thePoint to allow instructors to design and deliver on-line and off-line courses, maintain grades and class rosters, and communicate with students. Students can visit thePoint to access supplemental multimedia resources to enhance their learning experience, check the course syllabus, download content, upload assignments, and join an on-line study group.

It is our hope that the content, style, and organization of this book continue to meet the needs of a broad spectrum of nursing students and nurse researchers. We also hope that the book will help to foster enthusiasm for the kinds of discoveries that research can produce, and for the knowledge that will help support an evidence-based nursing practice.

DENISE F. POLIT, PHD

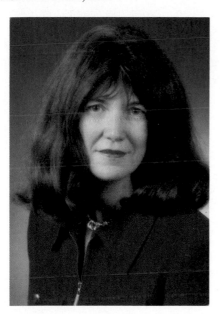

CHERYL TATANO BECK, DNSc, CNM, FAAN

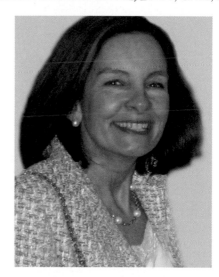

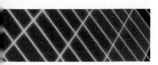

Acknowledgments

This eighth edition, like the previous seven editions, depended on the contribution of many individuals. Many faculty and students who used the text have made invaluable suggestions for its improvement, and to all of you we are very grateful. In addition to all those who assisted us during the past 30 years with the earlier editions, the following individuals deserve special mention.

We would like to acknowledge the comments of reviewers of the previous edition, anonymous to us initially, whose feedback greatly influenced our revisions. Several of the comments, particularly those of Dr. Mary Bennett of Indiana State University, triggered our work on the Toolkit, and for this we are indebted.

Faculty at Griffith University and James Cook University in Australia made important suggestions, and also inspired the inclusion of some new content in this edition. We would also like to acknowledge the valuable contributions of Steve Owen and Tom Knapp who provided advice for improving the data analysis chapters. Jill Livingston, reference librarian at the University of Connecticut, provided ongoing assistance, and Mary Ann Cordeau helped with the section on historical research. We are also grateful for the insights of Robert Gable regarding instrument development in Chapter 18. Deborah Dillon Mac-Donald was extraordinarily generous in giving us access to her NINR grant application and related material for the *Resource Manual*.

We also extend our thanks to those who helped to turn the manuscript into a finished product. The staff at Wolters Kluwer Health has been of great assistance to us over the years. We are indebted to Helen Kogut, Erika Kors, Mary Kinsella, and all the others behind the scenes for their fine contributions. Finally, we thank our family and friends, who provided ongoing support throughout this endeavor, and who were patient when we worked long into the night, over weekends, and during holidays to get this eighth edition finished.

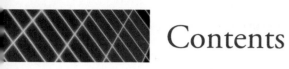

Contents

PART 1

FOUNDATIONS OF NURSING RESEARCH AND EVIDENCE-BASED PRACTICE

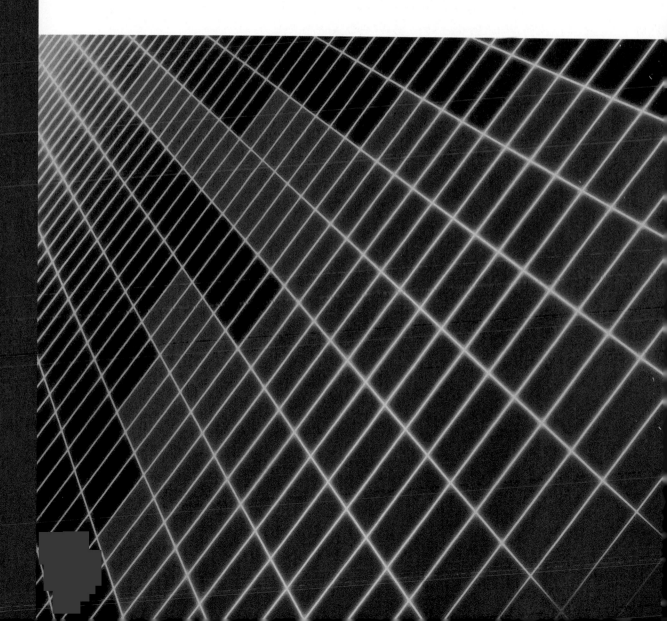

1 | Introduction to Nursing Research in an Evidence-Based Practice Environment

NURSING RESEARCH IN PERSPECTIVE

In all parts of the world, nursing has experienced a profound culture change over the past few decades. Nurses are increasingly expected to understand and conduct research, and to base their professional practice on emerging evidence from research—that is, to adopt an **evidence-based practice (EBP).** EBP is broadly defined as the use of the best clinical evidence in making patient care decisions, and such evidence typically comes from research conducted by nurses and other health care professionals.

What Is Nursing Research?

Research is systematic inquiry that uses disciplined methods to answer questions or solve problems. The ultimate goal of research is to develop, refine, and expand a body of knowledge.

Nurses are increasingly engaged in disciplined studies that benefit the profession and its clients, and that contribute to improvements in the entire health care system. **Nursing research** is systematic inquiry designed to develop trustworthy evidence about issues of importance to the nursing profession, including nursing practice, education, administration, and informatics. In this book, we emphasize **clinical nursing research**, that is, research designed

to guide nursing practice and to improve the health and quality of the life of nurses' clients.

Nursing research has experienced remarkable growth in the past three decades, providing nurses with an increasingly sound evidence base from which to practice. Yet many questions endure, and much remains to be done to incorporate research-based evidence into nursing practice.

> **Examples of nursing research questions:**
> - Does canine visitation (pet) therapy result in decreased pain in hospitalized children? (Sobo, Eng, & Kassity-Krich, 2006)*
> - What is it like to be a family caregiver to relatives with severe and persistent mental illness? (Chang & Horrocks, 2006)

The Importance of Research in Nursing

Because of broad support for evidence-based nursing practice, research has assumed heightened importance for nurses. Although there is not a consensus about what types of "evidence" are appropriate for EBP (Goode, 2000), there is general agreement that research findings from rigorous studies provide especially strong evidence for

---

* Citations to studies such as this are at the end of each chapter, but other citations are at the end of the book, beginning on page 731.

3

informing nurses' decisions and actions. Nurses are accepting the need to base specific nursing actions and decisions on evidence indicating that the actions are clinically appropriate, cost-effective, and result in positive outcomes for clients.

In the United States, research has come to play an important role in nursing in terms of credentialing and status. The American Nurses Credentialing Center—an arm of the American Nurses Association and the largest and most prestigious credentialing organization in the United States—has developed a Magnet Recognition Program to recognize health care organizations that provide very high-quality nursing care, and to elevate the standards and reputation of the nursing profession. As noted by Turkel and her colleagues (2005), "To achieve Magnet status, the Chief Nurse Executive needs to create, foster, and sustain a practice environment where nursing research and evidence-based practice is integrated into both the delivery of nursing care and the framework for nursing administration decision making" (p. 254).

Changes to nursing practice are occurring regularly because of EBP efforts. Often these practice changes are local initiatives, many of which are not publicized, but broader clinical changes are also occurring based on accumulating research evidence about beneficial practice innovations.

Example of evidence-based practice:
Numerous clinical practice changes reflect the impact of research. For example, "kangaroo care" (the holding of diaper-clad preterm infants skin-to-skin, chest-to-chest by parents) is now widely practiced in neonatal intensive care units (NICUs) in the United States (Engler et al., 2002) and elsewhere, but this is a new trend. As recently as the early 1990s, only a minority of NICUs offered kangaroo care options. The adoption of this practice reflects the accumulating evidence that early skin-to-skin contact has clinical benefits without any apparent negative side effects (e.g., Dodd, 2005). Some of that accumulated evidence was developed in rigorous studies by nurse researchers in the United States, Australia, Canada, Taiwan, and other countries (e.g., Chwo et al., 2002; Johnston et al., 2003; Ludington-Hoe et al., 2004).

The Consumer–Producer Continuum in Nursing Research

With the current emphasis on EBP, it has become every nurse's responsibility to engage in one or more roles along a continuum of research participation. At one end of the continuum are those nurses whose involvement in research is indirect. **Consumers of nursing research** read research reports to develop new skills and to search for relevant findings that may affect their practice. Nurses are now expected to maintain this level of involvement with research, at a minimum. EBP depends on well-informed nursing research consumers.

At the other end of the continuum are the **producers of nursing research:** nurses who actively participate in designing and implementing studies. At one time, most nurse researchers were academics who taught in schools of nursing, but research is increasingly being conducted by practicing nurses who want to find what works best for their patients.

Example of research by hospital-based nurses: Huddleston and five other nurses (2005) who worked at Apple Hill Infusion Center and York Hospital in York, Pennsylvania were concerned about drug reactions of patients receiving two chemotherapeutic agents, paclitaxel (Taxol) and carboplatin. They conducted a study that involved reviewing patients' charts at the Infusion Center. Based on their findings, the nursing team collaborated with primary physician providers to develop what they called "rechallenge protocols" for patients who have experienced such reactions.

Between these two end points on the consumer–producer continuum lie a rich variety of research activities in which nurses may engage. These activities include the following:

- Participating in a **journal club** in a practice setting, which involves meetings among nurses to discuss and critique research articles
- Solving clinical problems and making clinical decisions based on rigorous research
- Collaborating in the development of an idea for a clinical research project

- Reviewing a proposed research plan with respect to its feasibility in a clinical setting and offering clinical expertise to improve the plan
- Recruiting potential study participants
- Assisting in the collection of research information (e.g., distributing questionnaires to patients)
- Giving clients information and advice about participation in studies
- Discussing the implications and relevance of research findings with clients

Example of research publicized in the mass media: Here is a headline about a health study that was publicized in newspapers throughout the United States and Canada in September, 2004: "Walking might ward off Alzheimer's." According to the study, which involved thousands of nurses aged 70 to 81 years, even those who walked as little as 1 ½ hours per week did better on tests of mental function that those who were less active.

What would you say if clients asked you about this study? Would you be able to comment on the believability of the findings, based on your assessment of how rigorously the study was conducted? This book should enable you to do this.

In all the possible research-related activities, nurses who have some research skills are better able than those without them to make a contribution to nursing and to EBP. An understanding of nursing research can improve the depth and breadth of *every* nurse's professional practice.

NURSING RESEARCH: PAST, PRESENT, AND FUTURE

Although nursing research has not always had the prominence and importance it enjoys today, its long and interesting history portends a distinguished future. Table 1.1 summarizes some of the key events in the historical evolution of nursing research.

The Early Years: From Nightingale to the 1960s

Most people would agree that research in nursing began with Florence Nightingale. Her landmark publication, *Notes on Nursing* (1859), describes her early interest in environmental factors that promote physical and emotional well-being—an interest that continues among nurses nearly 150 years later. Nightingale's most widely known research contribution involved her analysis of factors affecting soldier mortality and morbidity during the Crimean War. Based on her skillful analyses and presentations, she was successful in effecting some changes in nursing care—and, more generally, in public health.

For many years after Nightingale's work, the nursing literature contained little research. Most studies in the early 1900s concerned nurses' education. For example, in 1923, a group called the Committee for the Study of Nursing Education studied the educational preparation of nurse teachers, administrators, and public health nurses and the clinical experiences of nursing students. The committee issued what has become known as the Goldmark Report, which identified many inadequacies in the educational backgrounds of the groups studied and concluded that advanced educational preparation was essential. As more nurses received university-based education, studies concerning nursing students—their characteristics, problems, and satisfactions—became more numerous.

Funding for independent research was all but nonexistent in the early years. However, signaling its enduring commitment to research, the nursing honor society Sigma Theta Tau (which became Sigma Theta Tau International in 1985) was the first organization to fund nursing research in the United States, awarding a $600 grant to Alice Crist Malone in 1936.

During the 1940s, government-initiated studies of nursing education continued, spurred on by the unprecedented demand for nursing personnel during World War II. For example, Brown (1948) reassessed nursing education in a study initiated at the request of the National Nursing Council for War Service. The findings from the study, like those of

TABLE 1.1 Historical Landmarks Affecting Nursing Research

YEAR	EVENT
1859	Nightingale's *Notes on Nursing* is published
1900	*American Journal of Nursing* begins publication
1923	Columbia University establishes first doctoral program for nurses
	Goldmark Report with recommendations for nursing education is published
1930s	*American Journal of Nursing* publishes clinical cases studies
1936	Sigma Theta Tau awards first nursing research grant in the United States
1948	Brown publishes report on inadequacies of nursing education
1952	The journal *Nursing Research* begins publication
1955	Inception of the American Nurses Foundation to sponsor nursing research
1957	Establishment of nursing research center at Walter Reed Army Institute of Research
1963	*International Journal of Nursing Studies* begins publication
1965	American Nurses Association (ANA) begins sponsoring nursing research conferences
1966	Nursing history archive is established at Mugar Library, Boston University
1969	*Canadian Journal of Nursing Research* begins publication
1971	ANA establishes a Commission on Research
1972	ANA establishes its Council of Nurse Researchers
1976	Stetler and Marram publish guidelines on assessing research for use in practice
1978	The journals *Research in Nursing & Health* and *Advances in Nursing Science* begin publication
1979	*Western Journal of Nursing Research* begins publication
1982	The Conduct and Utilization of Research in Nursing (CURN) project publishes report
1983	*Annual Review of Nursing Research* begins publication
1985	ANA Cabinet on Nursing Research establishes research priorities
1986	National Center for Nursing Research (NCNR) is established within U.S. National Institutes of Health
1987	The journal *Scholarly Inquiry for Nursing Practice* begins publication
1988	The journals *Applied Nursing Research* and *Nursing Science Quarterly* begin publication
	Conference on Research Priorities (CORP #1) is convened by NCNR
1989	U.S. Agency for Health Care Policy and Research (AHCPR) is established
1992	The journal *Clinical Nursing Research* begins publication
1993	NCNR becomes a full institute, the National Institute of Nursing Research (NINR)
	The Cochrane Collaboration is established
	The *Journal of Nursing Measurement* begins publication
1994	The journal *Qualitative Health Research* begins publication
1995	The Joanna Briggs Institute, an international EBP collaborative, is established in Australia
1997	Canadian Health Services Research Foundation is established with federal funding
1999	AHCPR is renamed Agency for Healthcare Research and Quality (AHRQ)
2000	NINR issues funding priorities for 2000–2004; annual funding exceeds $100 million
	The Canadian Institute of Health Research is launched
	The journal *Biological Research for Nursing* begins publication
2004	The journal *Worldviews on Evidence-Based Nursing* begins publication

the Goldmark Report, revealed numerous inadequacies in nursing education. Brown recommended that the education of nurses occur in collegiate settings. Many subsequent studies concerning nurses' roles and attitudes, hospital environments, and nurse–patient interactions stemmed from the Brown report.

A number of forces combined during the 1950s to put nursing research on a rapidly accelerating upswing in the United States. An increase in the number of nurses with advanced educational degrees, the establishment of a nursing research center at the Walter Reed Army Institute of Research, an increase in the availability of funds from the government and private foundations, and the inception of the American Nurses' Foundation—which is devoted exclusively to the promotion of nursing research—provided impetus to nursing research during this period.

Until the 1950s, nurse researchers had few outlets for reporting their studies to the nursing community. The *American Journal of Nursing*, first published in 1900, began on a limited basis to publish some studies in the 1930s. The increasing number of studies being conducted during the 1950s, however, created the need for a journal in which findings could be published; thus, *Nursing Research* came into being in 1952.

Nursing research in the 1950s was not very clinically oriented. Nurses studied themselves: Who is the nurse? What does the nurse do? Why do individuals choose to enter nursing? What are the characteristics of the ideal nurse? How do other groups perceive the nurse?

Knowledge development through research in nursing began in earnest in the 1960s. Nursing leaders began to express concern about the lack of research in nursing practice. Several professional nursing organizations, such as the Western Interstate Council for Higher Education in Nursing, established priorities for research investigations during this period. Practice-oriented research on various clinical topics began to emerge in the literature. The 1960s saw worldwide advances in nursing research. The *International Journal of Nursing Studies* began publication in 1963, and both the

Journal of Nursing Scholarship and the *Canadian Journal of Nursing Research* were first published in the late 1960s.

> **Example of nursing research breakthroughs in the 1960s:** Jeanne Quint Benoliel began a program of research that had a major impact on medicine, medical sociology, and nursing. Quint explored the subjective experiences of patients after diagnosis with a life-threatening illness (1967). Of particular note, physicians in the early 1960s usually did not advise women that they had breast cancer, even after a mastectomy. Quint's (1962, 1963) seminal study of the personal experiences of women after radical mastectomy contributed to changes in communication and information control by physicians and nurses.

Nursing Research in the 1970s

By the 1970s, the growing number of nurses conducting research studies and the discussions of theoretical and contextual issues surrounding nursing research created the need for additional communication outlets. Several journals that focus on nursing research were established in the United States in the 1970s, including *Advances in Nursing Science, Research in Nursing & Health*, and the *Western Journal of Nursing Research*.

During the 1970s, there was a decided change in emphasis in nursing research from areas such as teaching, curriculum, and nurses themselves to the improvement of client care—signifying a growing awareness by nurses of the need for a scientific base from which to practice. Nursing leaders strongly endorsed this direction for nursing research. Lindeman (1975), for example, conducted a study to ascertain the views of nursing leaders concerning the focus of nursing studies; clinical problems were identified as the highest priorities. Nurses also began to pay attention to the utilization of research findings in nursing practice. A seminal article by Stetler and Marram (1976) offered guidance on assessing research for application in practice settings.

In the United States, research skills among nurses continued to improve in the 1970s. The cadre of nurses with earned doctorates steadily increased, especially during the later 1970s. The availability of both predoctoral and postdoctoral research fellowships facilitated the development of advanced research skills.

Nursing research also expanded internationally. The *Journal of Advanced Nursing*, the premier international journal of nursing research, began publication in the United Kingdom in 1976. Nurse researchers in Europe also began efforts at greater collaboration: The Workgroup of European Nurse Researchers was established in 1978 to develop greater communication and opportunities for systematic partnerships among the 25 European National Nurses Associations involved.

Example of nursing research breakthroughs in the 1970s: Kathryn Barnard's research led to breakthroughs in the area of neonatal and young child development. Her research program focused on the identification and assessment of children at risk for developmental and health problems, such as abused and neglected children and failure-to-thrive children (Barnard, 1973, 1976; Barnard & Collar, 1973; Barnard et al., 1977). Her research contributed to early interventions for children with disabilities, and also to the field of developmental psychology.

Nursing Research in the 1980s

The 1980s brought nursing research to a new level of development. An increase in the number of qualified nurse researchers, the widespread availability of computers for the collection and analysis of information, and an ever-growing recognition that research is an integral part of professional nursing led nursing leaders to raise new issues and concerns. More attention was paid to the types of questions being asked, the methods of collecting and analyzing information being used, the linking of research to theory, and the utilization of research findings in practice.

Several events contributed to the momentum in nursing research in this decade. For example, the first volume of the *Annual Review of Nursing Research* was published in 1983. These annual reviews include summaries of current research evidence on selected areas of research practice and encourage utilization of research findings. As another example, the Center for Research for Nursing was created in 1983 by the American Nurses Association. The Center's mission is to develop and coordinate a research program to serve as the source of national information for the profession.

Of particular importance in the United States was the establishment in 1986 of the National Center for Nursing Research (NCNR) at the National Institutes of Health (NIH) by congressional mandate, despite a presidential veto that was overridden largely as a result of nurse-scientists' successful lobbying efforts. The purpose of NCNR was to promote—and financially support—research projects and training relating to patient care. Funding for nursing research also became available in Canada in the 1980s through the National Health Research Development Program (NHRDP) and the Medical Research Council of Canada.

Several nursing groups developed priorities for nursing research during the 1980s. For example, in 1985, the American Nurses Association Cabinet on Nursing Research established priorities that helped focus research more precisely on aspects of nursing practice. Also in the 1980s, nurses began to conduct formal projects specifically designed to increase research utilization, such as the Conduct and Utilization of Research in Nursing (CURN) project.

Dissemination opportunities continued to expand. Many specialty journals (e.g., *Heart & Lung, Cancer Nursing*) increased their coverage of research articles, and several new research-related journals were established: *Applied Nursing Research*, *Scholarly Inquiry for Nursing Practice*, and *Nursing Science Quarterly*. The journal *Applied Nursing Research* is notable for its intended audience: it includes research reports on studies of special relevance to practicing nurses. In Australia, the *Australian Journal Advanced of Nursing* was launched in the 1980s.

Several forces outside of the nursing profession in the late 1980s helped to shape today's nursing research landscape. A group from the McMaster Medical School in Canada designed a clinical learning strategy that was called evidence-based medicine (EBM). EBM, which promulgated the view that research findings were far superior to the opinions of authorities as a basis for clinical decisions, constituted a profound shift for medical education and practice, and has had a major effect on all health care professions.

In 1989, the U.S. government established the Agency for Health Care Policy and Research (AHCPR). AHCPR (which was renamed the Agency for Healthcare Research and Quality, or AHRQ, in 1999) is the federal agency that has been charged with supporting research specifically designed to improve the quality of health care, reduce health costs, and enhance patient safety, and thus plays a pivotal role in the promulgation of EBP.

Example of nursing research breakthroughs in the 1980s: A team of researchers headed by Dorothy Brooten engaged in studies that led to the development and testing of a model of site transitional care. Brooten and her colleagues (1986, 1988, 1989), for example, conducted studies of nurse specialist–managed home follow-up services for very-low-birth-weight infants who were discharged early from the hospital, and demonstrated a significant cost savings—with comparable health outcomes. Brooten and colleagues later expanded their research to other high-risk patients (1994). The site transitional care model, which was developed in anticipation of government cost-cutting measures, has been used as a framework for patients who are at health risk as a result of early discharge from hospitals, and has been recognized by numerous health care disciplines.

Nursing Research in the 1990s

Nursing science came into its maturity in the United States during the 1990s. As but one example, nursing research was strengthened and given more national visibility when NCNR was promoted to full institute status within the NIH: in 1993, the **National Institute of Nursing Research (NINR)** was born. The birth of NINR helped put nursing research more into the mainstream of research activities enjoyed by other health disciplines. Funding for nursing research has also grown. In 1986, the NCNR had a budget of $16 million, whereas in

fiscal year 1999, the budget for NINR had grown to about $70 million. Funding opportunities for nursing research expanded in other countries as well during the 1990s. For example, the Canadian Health Services Research Foundation (CHSRF) was established in 1997 with an endowment from federal funds, and plans for the Canadian Institute for Health Research got underway. Beginning in 1999, the CHSRF allocated $25 million for nursing research through the establishment of a series of research chairs and related programs specific to nursing with a health services orientation.

Several journals were established during the 1990s in response to the growth in clinically oriented research and interest in EBP among nurses, including *Clinical Nursing Research*, *Clinical Effectiveness*, and *Outcomes Management for Nursing Practice*. Another new journal, *Qualitative Health Research*, signaled the emerging importance of in-depth studies using different methodologies than had typically been used in earlier research.

Major contributions to EBP emerged internationally in this decade. Of particular importance, the Cochrane Collaboration was inaugurated in 1993. This collaboration, an international network of institutions and individuals, maintains and updates systematic reviews of hundreds of clinical interventions to facilitate EBP. Another international network devoted to the evaluation of evidence in health disciplines was established in Australia in 1995: The Joanna Briggs Institute has collaborating centers in Europe, Asia, Africa, the Americas, Australia, and New Zealand. International cooperation around the issue of EBP in nursing also began to develop in the 1990s. For example, Sigma Theta Tau International began to focus attention on research utilization, and sponsored the first international research utilization conference, in cooperation with the faculty of the University of Toronto, in 1998.

Some current research in the United States is guided by priorities established by prominent nurse researchers in the 1990s, who were brought together by NCNR for two Conferences on Research Priorities (CORPs). The priorities established by the first CORP for research through 1994 included low birth weight, human immunodeficiency virus (HIV) infection, long-term care, symptom management, nursing informatics, health promotion, and technology dependence. In 1993, the second CORP established the following research emphases for 1995 to 1999: developing and testing community-based nursing models, nursing interventions in HIV/AIDS, approaches to remediating cognitive impairment, testing interventions for coping with chronic illness, and identifying biobehavioral factors and testing interventions to promote immunocompetence.

Example of nursing research breakthroughs in the 1990s: Many studies that Donaldson (2000) identified as *breakthroughs* in nursing research were conducted in the 1990s. This reflects, in part, the growth of **research programs** in which teams of researchers engage in a series of related research on important topics, rather than discrete and unconnected studies. As but one example, several nurse researchers had breakthroughs during the 1990s in the area of psychoneuroimmunology, which has been adopted as the model of mind–body interactions. Barbara Swanson and Janice Zeller, for example, conducted several studies relating to HIV infection and neuropsychological function (Swanson et al., 1993; Swanson, Zeller, & Spear, 1998) that have led to discoveries in environmental management as a means of improving immune system status.

Future Directions for Nursing Research

Nursing research continues to develop at a rapid pace and will undoubtedly flourish in the 21st century. Funding continues to grow—for example, NINR funding in fiscal year 2006 was nearly $140 million. Broadly speaking, the priority for nursing research in the future will be the promotion of excellence in nursing science. Toward this end, nurse researchers and practicing nurses will be sharpening their research skills, and using those skills to address emerging issues of importance to the profession and its clientele.

Certain trends for the early 21st century are evident from developments that were taking shape at the turn of the millennium:

- *Heightened focus on EBP*. Concerted efforts to use research findings in practice are sure to continue, and nurses at all levels will be encouraged to engage in evidence-based patient care. In turn, improvements will be needed both in the quality of nursing studies and in nurses' skills in locating, understanding, critiquing, and using relevant study results. Relatedly, there is an emerging interest in **translational research**—research on how findings from studies can best be translated into nursing practice.

- *Development of a stronger evidence base through more rigorous methods and multiple, confirmatory strategies*. Practicing nurses are unlikely to adopt an innovation based on weakly designed or isolated studies. Strong research designs are essential, and confirmation is usually needed through the **replication** (i.e., the intentional repeating) of studies with different clients, in different clinical settings, and at different times to ensure that the findings are robust. Another confirmatory strategy is the conduct of **multisite studies** by researchers in several locations.

- *Greater emphasis on systematic integrative reviews*. **Systematic reviews** are considered a cornerstone of EBP, and will undoubtedly take on increased importance in nursing and in all health disciplines. The emphasis in a systematic review is on amassing comprehensive research information on the topic, weighing pieces of evidence, and integrating information to draw conclusions about the state of evidence. Best practice clinical guidelines typically rely on such systematic reviews.

- *Expanded local research in health care settings*. In the current evidence-based environment, there is likely to be an increase of small, localized research designed to solve immediate problems. In the United States, this trend will be reinforced as more hospitals apply for (and are recertified for) Magnet Status. Mechanisms will need to be developed to ensure that evidence from these small projects becomes available to others facing similar problems.

- *Strengthening of multidisciplinary collaboration*. Interdisciplinary collaboration of nurses with researchers in related fields (as well as intradisciplinary collaboration among nurse researchers) is likely to continue to expand in the 21st century as researchers address fundamental problems at the biobehavioral and psychobiologic interface. As one example, there are likely to be vast opportunities for nurses and other health care researchers to integrate breakthroughs in human genetics into lifestyle and health care interventions. In turn, such collaborative efforts could lead to nurse researchers playing a more prominent role in national and international health care policies.

- *Expanded dissemination of research findings.* The Internet and other means of electronic communication have a large impact on the dissemination of research information, which in turn helps to promote EBP. Through such technological advances as electronic location and retrieval of research articles, on-line publishing (e.g., the *Online Journal of Knowledge Synthesis for Nursing*, the *Online Journal of Clinical Innovation*), on-line resources such as Lippincott's NursingCenter.com, e-mail, and electronic mailing lists and listservs such as those maintained by the Royal Windsor Society of Nurse Researchers, information about innovations can be communicated more widely and more quickly than ever before.

- *Increasing the visibility of nursing research.* The 21st century is likely to witness efforts to increase the visibility of nursing research. Most people are unaware that nurses are scholars and researchers (Tilden & Potempa, 2003). Nurse researchers internationally must market themselves and their research to professional organizations, consumer organizations, governments, and the corporate world to increase support for their research.

- *Increased focus on cultural issues and health disparities.* The issue of health disparities has emerged as a central concern in nursing and other health disciplines, and this in turn has raised consciousness about the ecological validity and cultural sensitivity of health interventions. **Ecological validity** refers to the extent to which study designs and findings have relevance and meaning in a variety of real-world contexts. There is growing awareness that research must be sensitive to the health beliefs, behaviors, epidemiology, and values of culturally and linguistically diverse populations.

Meeting the health care needs of an increasingly diverse society—and a more globalized world—has become an international concern. For example, in 2002, NINR established a 5-year program specifically designed to address health disparities research, through the creation of 17 Partnership Centers designed to bridge cultural gaps between researchers, service providers, advocates, and community leaders.

Research priorities for the future are under discussion, both by nursing specialty organizations and by broader groups and institutions. In 2005, Sigma Theta Tau International issued a position paper on nursing research priorities that incorporated priorities from nursing organizations internationally, including NINR. The paper also took into consideration the United Nations Millennium Development Goals, which specifically address the complex interaction between socioeconomic factors and health. This synthesis of global nursing priorities identified the following: (1) health promotion and disease prevention, (2) promotion of health of vulnerable and marginalized communities, (3) patient safety and quality of health care, (4) development of EBP and translational research, (5) promotion of the health and well-being of older people, (6) patient-centered care and care coordination, (7) palliative and end-of-life care, (8) care implications of genetic testing and therapeutics, (9) capacity development of nurse researchers, and (10) nurses' working environments (Sigma Theta Tau International, 2005).

⊃ TIP: All websites cited in this chapter, plus additional websites with useful content relating to the foundations of nursing research, are in the "Useful Websites for Chapter 1" file on the accompanying CD-ROM. This will allow you to simply use the "Control/Click" feature to go directly to the website, without having to type in the URL and risk a typographical error. Websites corresponding to the content of most chapters of the book are also in files on the CD-ROM.

SOURCES OF EVIDENCE FOR NURSING PRACTICE

Nurses make clinical decisions based on a large repertoire of knowledge and information (Estabrooks et al., 2005). Nursing students are taught by faculty and textbooks how to practice nursing. Nurses also learn from each other and from interactions with other health care professionals. Some of what students and nurses learn is based on systematic research, but much of it is not. In fact, Millenson (1997) estimated that 85% of health care practice has not been scientifically validated. Although the percentage of validated practices may have increased since 1997, there is widespread support for the notion that nursing practice should rely more heavily on evidence from research.

Information sources for clinical practice vary in dependability and validity. Increasingly there are discussions of **evidence hierarchies** that acknowledge that certain types of evidence and knowledge are superior to others. A brief discussion of some alternative sources of evidence shows how research-based information is different.

Tradition and Authority

Many questions are answered and decisions made based on customs or tradition. Within each culture, certain "truths" are accepted as given. For example, as citizens of democratic societies, most of us accept, without *proof*, that democracy is the highest form of government. This type of knowledge often is so much a part of our heritage that few of us seek verification. Tradition is efficient as an information source: each individual is not required to begin anew in an attempt to understand the world or certain aspects of it. Tradition or custom also facilitates communication by providing a common foundation of accepted truth. Nevertheless, tradition poses some problems because many traditions have never been evaluated for their validity. There is growing concern that many nursing interventions are based on tradition, customs, and "unit culture" rather than on sound evidence.

Another common source of information is an authority, a person with specialized expertise and recognition for that expertise. We are constantly faced with making decisions about matters with which we have had no direct experience; therefore, it seems natural to place our trust in the judgment of people who are authoritative on an issue by virtue of specialized training or experience. As a source of evidence, however, authority has shortcomings. Authorities are not infallible, particularly if their expertise is based primarily on personal experience; yet, like tradition, their knowledge often goes unchallenged.

Clinical Experience, Trial and Error, and Intuition

Clinical experience is a familiar and functional source of knowledge. The ability to generalize, to recognize regularities, and to make predictions based on observations is an important characteristic of the human mind. Nevertheless, personal experience is limited as a knowledge source for practice because each nurse's experience is typically too narrow to be generally useful. A second limitation of experience is that the same objective event is often experienced or perceived differently by two nurses. Getting advice from other nurses based on *their* clinical experience may have similar limitations.

Related to clinical experience is the method of trial and error. In this approach, alternatives are tried successively until a solution to a problem is found. We likely have all used this method in our lives, including in our professional work. For example, many patients dislike the taste of potassium chloride solution. Nurses try to disguise the taste of the medication in various ways until one method meets with the approval of the patient. Trial and error may offer a practical means of securing knowledge, but it is fallible. This method is haphazard, and the solutions may be idiosyncratic. Also, evidence obtained from trial and error is often unrecorded and, hence, inaccessible in subsequent clinical situations.

Finally, intuition is a type of knowledge that cannot be explained on the basis of reasoning or prior instruction. Although intuition and hunches undoubtedly play a role in nursing practice—as they do in the conduct of research—it is difficult to develop policies and practices for nurses on the basis of intuition.

Logical Reasoning

Solutions to many problems are developed by logical thought processes. Logical reasoning as a problem-solving method combines experience, intellectual faculties, and formal systems of thought. **Inductive reasoning** is the process of developing generalizations from specific observations. For example, a nurse may observe the anxious behavior of (specific) hospitalized children and conclude that (in general) children's separation from their parents is stressful. **Deductive reasoning** is the process of developing specific predictions from general principles. For example, if we assume that separation anxiety occurs in hospitalized children (in general), then we might predict that (specific) children in a local hospital whose parents do not room-in will manifest symptoms of stress.

Both systems of reasoning are useful as a means of understanding and organizing phenomena, and both play a role in nursing research. However, reasoning in and of itself is limited because the validity of reasoning depends on the accuracy of the information (or premises) with which one starts.

Assembled Information

In making clinical decisions, health care professionals also rely on information that has been assembled for a variety of purposes. For example, local, national, and international **bench-marking** data provide information on such issues as the rates of using various procedures (e.g., rates of cesarean deliveries) or rates of infection (e.g., nosocomial pneumonia rates), and can serve as a guide in evaluating clinical practices. **Cost data**—that is, information on the costs associated with certain procedures, policies, or practices—are sometimes used as a factor in clinical decision making. **Quality improvement and risk data**, such as medication error reports and evidence on the incidence and prevalence of skin breakdown, can be used to assess practices and determine the need for practice changes.

Such sources, although offering some information that can be used in practice, provide no mechanism for determining whether improvements in patient outcomes result from their use.

Disciplined Research

Research conducted within a disciplined format is the most sophisticated method of acquiring knowledge that humans have developed. Nursing research combines aspects of logical reasoning with other features to create evidence that, although fallible, tends to be more reliable than other methods of knowledge acquisition. Cumulative findings from rigorous, systematically appraised research is at the pinnacle of most evidence hierarchies. The current emphasis on evidence-based health care requires nurses to base their clinical practice to the greatest extent possible on research-based findings rather than on tradition, authority, intuition, or personal experience—although nursing will always remain a rich blend of art and science.

PARADIGMS FOR NURSING RESEARCH

A paradigm is a world view, a general perspective on the complexities of the real world. Paradigms for human inquiry are often characterized in terms of the ways in which they respond to basic philosophical questions:

* *Ontologic*: What is the nature of reality?
* *Epistemologic*: What is the relationship between the inquirer and that being studied?
* *Axiologic*: What is the role of values in the inquiry?
* *Methodologic*: How should the inquirer obtain knowledge?

Disciplined inquiry in the field of nursing is being conducted mainly (although not exclusively, as described in Chapter 9) within two broad paradigms, both of which have legitimacy for nursing research. This section describes the two paradigms and broadly outlines the research methods associated with them.

The Positivist Paradigm

The paradigm that dominated nursing research for decades is known as **positivism** (sometimes referred to as *logical positivism*). Positivism is rooted in 19th century thought, guided by such philosophers as Comte, Mill, Newton, and Locke. Positivism is a reflection of a broader cultural phenomenon that, in the humanities, is referred to as **modernism**, which emphasizes the rational and the scientific.

As shown in Table 1.2, a fundamental assumption of positivists is that there is a reality *out there* that can be studied and known (an **assumption** refers to a basic principle that is believed to be true without proof or verification). Adherents of the positivist approach assume that nature is basically ordered and regular and that an objective reality

TABLE 1.2	Major Assumptions of the Positivist and Naturalistic Paradigms	
ASSUMPTION	**POSITIVIST PARADIGM**	**NATURALISTIC PARADIGM**
Ontologic: What is the nature of reality?	Reality exists; there is a real world driven by real natural causes	Reality is multiple and subjective, mentally constructed by individuals
Epistemologic: How is the inquirer related to those being researched?	The inquirer is independent from those being researched; findings are not influenced by the researcher	The inquirer interacts with those being researched; findings are the creation of the interactive process
Axiologic: What is the role of values in the inquiry?	Values and biases are to be held in check; objectivity is sought	Subjectivity and values are inevitable and desirable
Methodologic: How is evidence best obtained?	Deductive processes Emphasis on discrete, specific concepts Focus on the objective and quantifiable Verification of researchers' predictions Outsider knowledge—researcher is external, separate Fixed, prespecified design Tight controls over context Measured, quantitative information; statistical analysis Seeks generalizations Focus on the product	Inductive processes Emphasis on entirety of some phenomena, holistic Focus on the subjective and nonquantifiable Emerging insight grounded in participants' experiences Insider knowledge—researcher is internal, part of process Flexible, emergent design Context-bound, contextualized Narrative information; qualitative analysis Seeks in-depth understanding Focus on the product and the process

exists independent of human observation. In other words, the world is assumed not to be merely a creation of the human mind. The related assumption of **determinism** refers to the positivists' belief that phenomena are not haphazard or random events, but rather have antecedent causes. If a person has a cerebrovascular accident, the scientist in a positivist tradition assumes that there must be one or more reasons that can be potentially identified. Within the **positivist paradigm**, much research activity is directed at understanding the underlying causes of natural phenomena.

Because of their belief in an objective reality, positivists value objectivity and attempt to hold their personal beliefs and biases in check to avoid contaminating the phenomena under study. The positivists' scientific approach involves the use of orderly, disciplined procedures with tight controls over the research situation to test researchers' hunches about the nature of phenomena being studied and relationships among them.

Strict positivist thinking has been challenged and undermined, and few researchers adhere to the tenets of pure positivism. In the **postpositivist paradigm**, there is still a belief in reality and a desire to understand it, but postpositivists recognize the impossibility of total objectivity. They do, however, see objectivity as a goal and strive to be as neutral as possible. Postpositivists also appreciate the impediments to knowing reality with certainty and therefore seek *probabilistic* evidence—that is, learning what the true state of a phenomenon *probably* is, with a high and ascertainable degree of likelihood. This modified positivist position remains a dominant force in nursing research. For the sake of simplicity, we refer to it as positivism.

The Naturalistic Paradigm

The **naturalistic paradigm** (which is sometimes referred to as the *constructivist paradigm*) began as a countermovement to positivism with writers such as Weber and Kant. Just as positivism reflects the cultural phenomenon of modernism that burgeoned in the wake of the industrial revolution, naturalism

is an outgrowth of the pervasive cultural transformation that is called **postmodernism**. Postmodern thinking emphasizes the value of **deconstruction**—that is, taking apart old ideas and structures—and **reconstruction**—that is, putting ideas and structures together in new ways. The naturalistic paradigm represents a major alternative system for conducting disciplined research in nursing. Table 1.2 compares the major assumptions of the positivist and naturalistic paradigms.

For the naturalistic inquirer, reality is not a fixed entity but rather a construction of the individuals participating in the research; reality exists within a context, and many constructions are possible. Naturalists thus take the position of relativism: if there are always multiple interpretations of reality that exist in people's minds, then there is no process by which the ultimate truth or falsity of the constructions can be determined.

The naturalistic paradigm assumes that knowledge is maximized when the distance between the inquirer and the participants in the study is minimized. The voices and interpretations of those under study are crucial to understanding the phenomenon of interest, and subjective interactions are the primary way to access them. The findings from a naturalistic inquiry are the product of the interaction between the inquirer and the participants.

Paradigms and Methods: Quantitative and Qualitative Research

Broadly speaking, **research methods** are the techniques researchers use to structure a study and to gather and analyze information relevant to the research question. The two alternative paradigms have strong implications for the research methods to be used to develop evidence. The methodologic distinction typically focuses on differences between **quantitative research**, which is most closely allied with the positivist tradition, and **qualitative research**, which is most often associated with naturalistic inquiry—although positivists sometimes undertake qualitative studies, and naturalistic researchers sometimes collect quantitative information. This section provides an overview of the methods associated with the two alternative paradigms.

The Scientific Method and Quantitative Research

The traditional, positivist **scientific method** refers to a general set of orderly, disciplined procedures used to acquire information. Quantitative researchers use deductive reasoning to generate predictions that are tested in the real world. They typically move in an orderly and systematic fashion from the definition of a problem and the selection of concepts on which to focus, to the solution of the problem. By **systematic,** we mean that the investigator progresses logically through a series of steps, according to a prespecified plan of action.

Quantitative researchers use mechanisms designed to control the study. **Control** involves imposing conditions on the research situation so that biases are minimized and precision and validity are maximized. Control mechanisms are discussed at length in this book.

Quantitative researchers gather **empirical evidence**—evidence that is rooted in objective reality and gathered directly or indirectly through the senses. Empirical evidence, then, consists of observations gathered through sight, hearing, taste, touch, or smell. Observations of the presence or absence of skin inflammation, the anxiety level of a patient, or the weight of a newborn infant are all examples of empirical observations. The requirement to use empirical evidence as the basis for knowledge means that findings are grounded in reality rather than in researchers' personal beliefs.

Evidence for a study in the positivist paradigm is gathered according to an established plan, using structured instruments to collect needed information. Usually (but not always) the information gathered in such a study is **quantitative**—that is, numeric information that results from some type of formal measurement and that is analyzed with statistical procedures.

A traditional scientific study strives to go beyond the specifics of the research situation. For example, quantitative researchers are typically not as interested in understanding why a *particular* woman has cervical cancer as in understanding what factors influence its occurrence in women generally. The degree to which research findings can be generalized to individuals other than those who participated in the study (referred to as the **generalizability** of the research) is a widely used criterion for assessing the quality of quantitative studies.

The traditional scientific method used by quantitative researchers has enjoyed considerable stature as a method of inquiry, and it has been used productively by nurse researchers studying a wide range of nursing problems. This is not to say, however, that this approach can solve all nursing problems. One important limitation—common to both quantitative and qualitative research—is that research methods cannot be used to answer moral or ethical questions. Many persistent and intriguing questions about the human experience fall into this area—questions such as whether euthanasia should be practiced or abortion should be legal. Given the many moral issues that are linked to health care, it is inevitable that the nursing process will never rely exclusively on scientific information.

The traditional research approach also must contend with problems of *measurement*. To study a phenomenon, quantitative researchers attempt to measure it, that is, to attach numeric values that express quantity. For example, if the phenomenon of interest is patient morale, researchers might want to assess whether morale is high or low, or higher under certain conditions than under others. Although there are reasonably accurate measures of physiologic phenomena, such as blood pressure and body temperature, comparably accurate measures of such psychological phenomena as hope or self-esteem have not been developed.

Another issue is that nursing research tends to focus on human beings, who are inherently complex and diverse. Traditional quantitative methods typically focus on a relatively small portion of the human experience (e.g., weight gain, depression, chemical dependency) in a single study. Complexities tend to be controlled and, if possible, eliminated, rather than studied directly, and this narrowness of focus can sometimes obscure insights. Finally and relatedly, quantitative research conducted in the positivist paradigm has sometimes been accused of a narrowness and inflexibility of vision, a problem that has been called a *sedimented view* of the world that does not fully capture the reality of human experience.

Naturalistic Methods and Qualitative Research

Naturalistic methods of inquiry attempt to deal with the issue of human complexity by exploring it directly. Researchers in naturalistic traditions emphasize the complexity of humans, their ability to shape and create their own experiences, and the idea that truth is a composite of realities. Consequently, naturalistic investigations place a heavy emphasis on understanding the human experience as it is lived, usually through the careful collection and analysis of **qualitative** materials that are narrative and subjective.

Researchers who reject the traditional scientific method believe that a major limitation of the classical model is that it is *reductionist*—that is, it reduces human experience to only the few concepts under investigation, and those concepts are defined in advance by the researcher rather than emerging from the experiences of those under study. Naturalistic researchers tend to emphasize the dynamic, holistic, and individual aspects of human experience and attempt to capture those aspects in their entirety, within the context of those who are experiencing them.

Flexible, evolving procedures are used to capitalize on findings that emerge in the course of the study. Naturalistic inquiry usually takes place in the **field** (i.e., in naturalistic settings), often over an extended period of time. In naturalistic research, the collection of information and its analysis typically progress concurrently; as researchers sift through information, insights are gained, new questions emerge, and further evidence is sought to amplify or confirm the insights. Through an inductive process, researchers integrate information to develop a theory or description that helps explicate the phenomenon under observation.

Naturalistic studies yield rich, in-depth information that has the potential to elucidate varied dimensions of a complicated phenomenon—for example, the process by which midlife women adapt to menopause. The findings from in-depth qualitative research are typically grounded in the real-life experiences of people with first-hand knowledge of a phenomenon. Nevertheless, the approach has several limitations. Human beings are used directly as the instrument through which information is gathered, and humans are extremely intelligent and sensitive—but fallible—tools. The subjectivity that enriches the analytic insights of skillful researchers can yield trivial and obvious "findings" among less competent ones.

Another potential limitation involves the subjective nature of naturalistic inquiry, which sometimes causes concerns about the idiosyncratic nature of the conclusions. Would two naturalistic researchers studying the same phenomenon in similar settings arrive at similar conclusions? The situation is further complicated by the fact that most naturalistic studies involve a relatively small group of people under study. Thus, the generalizability of findings from naturalistic inquiries is sometimes called into question.

Multiple Paradigms and Nursing Research

Paradigms should be viewed as lenses that help to sharpen our focus on a phenomenon of interest, not as blinders that limit intellectual curiosity. The emergence of alternative paradigms for the study of nursing problems is, in our view, a healthy and desirable trend in the pursuit of new evidence for practice. Although researchers' world view may be paradigmatic, knowledge itself is not. Nursing knowledge would be thin, indeed, if there were not a rich array of methods available within the two paradigms—methods that are often complementary in their strengths and limitations. We believe that intellectual pluralism should be encouraged and fostered.

We have emphasized differences between the two paradigms and their associated methods so that their distinctions will be easy to understand. Subsequent chapters of this book elaborate further on differences in terminology, methods, and research products. It is equally important, however, to note that these two paradigms have many features in common, only some of which are mentioned here:

- *Ultimate goals*. The ultimate aim of disciplined research, regardless of the underlying paradigm, is to gain understanding about phenomena. Both quantitative and qualitative researchers seek to capture the truth with regard to an aspect of the world in which they are interested, and both groups can make significant—and mutually beneficial—contributions to evidence for nursing practice. Moreover, qualitative studies often serve as a crucial starting point for more controlled quantitative studies.

- *External evidence*. Although the word *empiricism* has come to be allied with the classic scientific method, researchers in both traditions gather and analyze evidence empirically, that is, through their senses. Neither qualitative nor quantitative researchers are armchair analysts, relying on their own beliefs and world views to generate knowledge. Information is gathered from others in a deliberate fashion.

- *Reliance on human cooperation*. Because evidence for nursing research comes primarily from humans, human cooperation is essential. To understand people's characteristics and experiences, researchers must persuade them to participate in the investigation *and* to speak and act candidly. For certain topics, the need for candor and cooperation is a challenging requirement—for researchers in either tradition.

- *Ethical constraints*. Research with human beings is guided by ethical principles that sometimes interfere with research goals. For example, if researchers want to test a potentially beneficial intervention, is it ethical to withhold the treatment from some people to see what happens? As discussed in Chapter 7, ethical dilemmas often confront researchers, regardless of paradigms or methods.

- *Fallibility of disciplined research*. Virtually all studies—in either paradigm—have some limitations. Every research question can be addressed in many different ways, and inevitably there are tradeoffs. Financial constraints are often an issue, but limitations may exist even with abundant resources. This does not mean that small, simple studies have no value. *It means that no single study can ever definitively answer a research question.* Each completed study adds to a body of accumulated evidence. If several researchers pose the same question and if each obtains the same or similar results, increased confidence can be placed in the answer to the question. The fallibility of any single study makes it important to understand and critique researchers' methodologic decisions when evaluating the quality of their evidence.

Thus, despite philosophic and methodologic differences, researchers using the traditional scientific method or naturalistic methods often share overall goals and face many similar constraints and challenges. The selection of an appropriate method depends on researchers' personal taste and philosophy, and also on the research question. If a researcher asks, "What are the effects of cryotherapy on nausea and oral mucositis in patients undergoing chemotherapy?" the researcher really needs to express the effects through the careful quantitative assessment of patients. On the other hand, if a researcher asks, "What is the process by which parents learn to cope with the death of a child?" the researcher would be hard pressed to quantify such a process. Personal world views of researchers help to shape their questions.

In reading about the alternative paradigms for nursing research, you likely were more attracted to one of the two paradigms—the one that corresponds most closely to your view of the world and of reality. It is important, however, to learn about and respect both approaches to disciplined inquiry, and to recognize their respective strengths and limitations. In this textbook, we describe methods associated with both qualitative and quantitative research.

THE PURPOSES OF NURSING RESEARCH

The general purpose of nursing research is to answer questions or solve problems of relevance to the nursing profession. Specific purposes can be classified in a number of different ways. We present a few, primarily so that we can illustrate the range of questions that nurse researchers have addressed.

Basic and Applied Research

Sometimes a distinction is made between basic and applied research. As traditionally defined, **basic research** is undertaken to extend the base of knowledge in a discipline, or to formulate or refine a theory. For example, a researcher may perform an in-depth study to better understand normal grieving processes, without having *explicit* nursing applications in mind.

> **Example of basic research:** Cadena (2006) studied the needs and functioning of persons with schizophrenia living in an assisted living facility in relation to the residents' characteristics. The findings had implications for practice, but the research itself did not attempt to solve a particular problem.

Applied research focuses on finding solutions to existing problems and thus tends to be of greater immediate utility for EBP. For example, a study to determine the effectiveness of a nursing intervention to ease grieving would be applied research. Basic research is appropriate for discovering general principles of human behavior and biophysiologic processes; applied research is designed to indicate how these principles can be used to solve problems in nursing practice. In nursing, the findings from applied research may pose questions for basic research, and the results of basic research often suggest clinical applications.

> **Example of applied research:** Smith (2006) conducted a study to determine whether any of three alternative methods of peripheral IV catheter securement could extend the average survival time of such catheters.

Research to Achieve Varying Levels of Explanation

Another way to classify research purposes concerns the extent to which studies are designed to provide explanatory information. Using this framework, the specific purposes of nursing research include identification, description, exploration, explanation, prediction, and control. For each purpose, various types of question are addressed by nurse researchers—some more amenable to qualitative than to quantitative inquiry, and vice versa.

Identification and Description

Qualitative researchers sometimes study phenomena about which little is known. In some cases, so little is known that the phenomenon has yet to be clearly identified or named or has been inadequately defined or conceptualized. The in-depth, probing nature of qualitative research is well suited to the task of answering such questions as, "What is this phenomenon?" and "What is its name?" (Table 1.3). In quantitative research, by contrast, the researcher begins with a phenomenon that has been previously studied or defined—sometimes in a qualitative study. Thus, in quantitative research, identification typically precedes the inquiry.

> **Qualitative example of identification:** Marcinkowski, Wong, and Dignam (2005) studied the experiences of nine adults with osteoarthritis who had undergone a total knee joint arthroplasty. They identified a basic process of adjustment that they called *getting back to the future*.

Description of phenomena is another important purpose of research. Nurse researchers have described a wide variety of phenomena. Examples include patients' stress, pain responses, adaptation processes, and health beliefs. Quantitative description focuses on the prevalence, incidence, size, and measurable attributes of phenomena. Qualitative researchers, on the other hand, describe the dimensions, variations, and importance of phenomena. Table 1.3 compares descriptive questions posed by quantitative and qualitative researchers.

| | TABLE 1.3 | Research Purposes and Research Questions |

PURPOSE	TYPES OF QUESTIONS: QUANTITATIVE RESEARCH	TYPES OF QUESTIONS: QUALITATIVE RESEARCH
Identification		What is this phenomenon? What is its name?
Description	How prevalent is the phenomenon? How often does the phenomenon occur? What are the characteristics of the phenomenon?	What are the dimensions of the phenomenon? What is important about the phenomenon?
Exploration	What factors are related to the phenomenon? What are the antecedents of the phenomenon?	What is the full nature of the phenomenon? What is really going on here? What is the process by which the phenomenon evolves or is experienced?
Explanation	What is the causal pathway through which the phenomenon unfolds? Does the theory explain the phenomenon?	How does the phenomenon work? Why does the phenomenon exist? What does the phenomenon mean? How did the phenomenon occur?
Prediction	What will happen if we alter a phenomenon or introduce an intervention? If phenomenon X occurs, will phenomenon Y follow?	
Control	How can we make the phenomenon happen or alter its prevalence? Can the occurrence of the phenomenon be prevented or controlled?	

Quantitative example of description: Johnson and colleagues (2006) described the prevalence and characteristics of childhood sexual abuse among men incarcerated in Texas.

Qualitative example of description: Rodriguez and Van Cott (2005) undertook an in-depth study to describe the pain experiences of postoperative head and neck cancer patients whose speech impairment prevented them from orally articulating their pain, and to describe nurses' methods of pain assessment.

Exploration

Like descriptive research, exploratory research begins with a phenomenon of interest; but rather than simply observing and describing it, exploratory research investigates the full nature of the phenomenon, the manner in which it is manifested, and the other factors to which it is related. For example, a *descriptive* quantitative study of patients' preoperative stress might seek to document the degree of stress patients experience before surgery and the percentage of patients who actually experience it. An *exploratory* study might ask: What factors diminish or increase a patient's stress? Is a patient's stress related to behaviors of the nursing staff? Is stress related to the patient's cultural background? Qualitative methods are especially useful for exploring the full nature of a little-understood phenomenon. Exploratory qualitative research is designed to shed light on the various ways in which a phenomenon is manifested and on underlying processes.

Quantitative example of exploration:
McCormick, Naimark, and Tate (2006) explored whether the length of time patients spent on a coronary artery bypass graft waiting list influenced their psychosomatic condition.

Qualitative example of exploration: Through in-depth conversations and field writings, Bruce and Davies (2005) explored the experience of *mindfulness* among hospice caregivers who regularly practiced mindfulness meditation at a hospice setting in which Western palliative care and Zen Buddhist philosophy were integrated.

Explanation

The goals of explanatory research are to understand the underpinnings of specific natural phenomena, and to explain systematic relationships among phenomena. Explanatory research is often linked to **theories**, which represent a method of organizing and integrating ideas about phenomena and their interrelationships. Whereas descriptive research provides new information, and exploratory research provides promising insights, explanatory research attempts to offer understanding of the underlying causes or full nature of a phenomenon. In quantitative research, theories or prior findings are used deductively to generate hypothesized explanations that are then tested empirically. In qualitative studies, researchers may search for explanations about how or why a phenomenon exists or what a phenomenon means as a basis for *developing* a theory that is grounded in rich, in-depth, experiential evidence.

Quantitative example of explanation:
Shaughnessy, Resnick, and Macko (2006) tested a theoretical model to explain physical activity among older adults who survived a stroke. The model purported to explain exercise behavior on the basis of theoretically relevant concepts such as self-efficacy and outcome expectations.

Qualitative example of explanation: Weaver, Wuest, and Ciliska (2005) conducted a study to develop an explanatory framework for understanding women's journey of recovery from anorexia nervosa. Interviews with 12 women were used to explain recovery from this eating disorder in the context of family, community, and society.

Prediction and Control

Many phenomena defy explanation. Yet it is frequently possible to make predictions and to control phenomena based on research findings, even in the absence of complete understanding. For example, research has shown that the incidence of Down syndrome in infants increases with the age of the mother. We can predict that a woman aged 40 years is at higher risk for bearing a child with Down syndrome than is a woman aged 25 years. We can partially control the outcome by educating women about the risks and offering amniocentesis to women older than 35 years of age. Note, however, that the ability to predict and control in this example does not depend on an explanation of *why* older women are at a higher risk for having an abnormal child. In many nursing and health-related studies—typically, quantitative ones—prediction and control are key objectives. For example, studies designed to test the effectiveness of nurse-led smoking cessation interventions are ultimately concerned with controlling (improving) patient outcomes and health care costs. Although explanatory studies are powerful in an EBP environment, studies whose purpose is prediction and control are also critical in helping clinicians make decisions.

Quantitative example of prediction: Epstein and Peerless (2006) conducted a study to identify predictors of successful weaning of older adults from mechanical ventilation.

Research Purposes Linked to EBP

Most nursing studies can be described in terms of a purpose on the descriptive-explanatory dimension just described. There are some studies, however, that do not fall neatly into such a system. For example, a study to develop and rigorously test a new method of measuring patient outcomes cannot easily be classified using this categorization.

In both nursing and medicine, several books have been written to facilitate EBP, and these books categorize studies in terms of the types of information needed by clinicians (DiCenso et al., 2005; Guyatt & Rennie, 2002; Melnyk & Fineout-Overholt, 2005; Sackett et al., 2000). These writers focus on several types of clinical concerns: treatment, therapy, or intervention; diagnosis and assessment; prognosis; prevention of harm; etiology; and meaning. Not all nursing studies have these purposes, but many of them do, and such studies have great potential for EBP.

Treatment, Therapy, or Intervention

Nurse researchers are increasingly undertaking studies designed to help nurses make evidence-based treatment decisions. Such studies range from evaluations of highly specific treatments of therapies (e.g., comparing two types of cooling blankets for febrile patients) to complex multi-session or multi-component interventions designed to effect major behavioral changes (e.g., nurse-led smoking cessation interventions). Such **intervention research** plays a critical role in EBP. Before intervening with patients, nurses have a responsibility to determine the benefits and risks of the intervention, and also whether the expenditure of resources for the intervention is justifiable.

Example of a study aimed at treatment/ therapy: Kim and Kim (2005) tested the effectiveness of a relaxation breathing exercise intervention on anxiety, depression, and leukocyte count among patients who had undergone allogenic hemopoietic stem cell transplantation in South Korea. The exercise was found to improve anxiety and depression, but did not affect the number of leukocytes.

Diagnosis and Assessment

A burgeoning number of studies published in the nursing literature concern the rigorous development and evaluation of formal instruments to screen, diagnose, and assess patients and to measure important clinical outcomes. High-quality instruments with documented accuracy are essential both for clinical practice and for further research.

Example of a study aimed at diagnosis/ assessment: England, Tripp-Reimer, and Rubenstein (2005) developed and explored the accuracy of an instrument designed to assess voice-hearing experiences in psychiatric settings, the Inventory of Voice Hearing Experiences.

Prognosis

Studies of prognosis examine the outcomes of a disease or health problem, estimate the probability they will occur, and indicate when (and for which types of people) the outcomes are most likely. Such studies facilitate the development of long-term care plans for patients. They also provide valuable information that can guide patients to make important lifestyle choices or to be vigilant for key symptoms. Prognostic studies can also play a role in resource allocation decisions.

Example of a study aimed at prognosis: McGrath and colleagues (2005) studied the long-term prognosis of infants with risk factors. In particular, they examined the association between low birth weight and indicators of attention deficit–hyperactivity disorder (ADHD) at age 4. Preschool behaviors indicative of a diagnosis of ADHD were more prevalent among children born prematurely and who had had perinatal illness.

Prevention of Harm

Nurses frequently encounter patients who face potentially harmful exposures—some as a result of health care factors, others because of environmental agents, and still others because of personal behaviors or characteristics. Providing useful information to patients about such harms and how best to avoid them, and taking appropriate prophylactic measures with patients in care, depend on the availability of accurate evidence.

Example of a study aimed at identifying and preventing harms: McCullagh, Lewis, and Warlow (2005) tested a health promotion initiative designed to improve men's knowledge of testicular cancer and to promote preventive actions, specifically, regular testicular self-examination.

Etiology or Causation

It is difficult, and sometimes impossible, to prevent harms or treat problems if we do not know what causes them. For example, there would be no smoking cessation programs if research had not provided firm evidence that smoking cigarettes causes or contributes to a wide range of health problems. Thus, determining the factors that affect or cause illness, mortality, or morbidity is an important purpose of many nursing studies.

Example of a study focused on causation: Roberts and Kennedy (2006) studied multi-ethnic college women to investigate why sexually active young women do not use condoms. Factors that were viewed as potentially contributing to low condom use included lower perceived risk, use of drugs and alcohol, and low sexual assertiveness.

Meaning and Processes

Designing effective interventions, motivating people to comply with treatments and to engage in health promotion activities, and providing sensitive advice to patients are among the many health care activities that can greatly benefit from understanding the clients' perspectives. Research that provides evidence about what health and illness mean to clients, what barriers they face to positive health practices, and what processes they experience in a transition through a health care crisis are important to evidence-based nursing practice.

Example of a study focused on meaning: Rahm, Renck, and Ringsberg (2006) explored whether and how women exposed to sexual abuse during childhood expressed unacknowledged overt and covert *shame*, and examined how shame influenced the lives of these women.

ASSISTANCE FOR USERS OF NURSING RESEARCH

This book is designed primarily to help you develop skills for conducting independent research, but in an environment that stresses EBP, it is extremely important to hone your skills in reading, evaluating, and using nursing studies. We provide specific guidance to consumers in most chapters by including guidelines for critiquing aspects of a study covered in the chapter. The questions in Box 1.1 are designed to assist you in using the information in this chapter in an overall preliminary assessment of a research report.

BOX 1.1 Questions for a Preliminary Overview of a Research Report

1. How relevant is the research problem to the actual practice of nursing? Does the study focus on a topic that is considered a priority area for nursing research?
2. Is the research quantitative or qualitative?
3. What is the underlying purpose (or purposes) of the study—identification, description, exploration, explanation, or prediction and control? Does the purpose correspond to an EBP focus such as treatment, diagnosis, prognosis, prevention of harm, etiology, or meaning?
4. What might be some clinical implications of this research? To what type of people and settings is the research most relevant? If the findings are accurate, how might the results of this study be used by *me*?

⚙ The *Resource Manual* that accompanies this book offers particularly rich opportunities to practice your critiquing skills. The Toolkit on the CD-ROM with the *Resource Manual* includes Box 1.1 as a Word document, which will allow you to adapt these questions, if desired, and to answer them directly into a Word document without having to retype the questions.

RESEARCH EXAMPLES

Each chapter of this book concludes with descriptions of actual studies conducted by nurse researchers. The descriptions focus on aspects of the studies emphasized in the chapter. A review of the full journal articles would prove useful for learning more about the studies, their methods, and the findings.

Research Example of a Quantitative Study

Study: "A randomized clinical trial of an HIV-risk reduction intervention among low-income Latina women" (Peragallo et al., 2005)

Study Purpose: The purpose of the study was to evaluate the effectiveness of a culturally tailored nurse-initiated intervention to prevent high–HIV risk sexual behaviors among urban Latina women. The intervention was called SEPA: Salud, Educacion, Prevencion, y Autocuidado (Health, Education, Prevention, and Self-Care).

Study Methods: A total of 657 low-income Mexican and Puerto Rican women aged 18 to 44 years who were sexually active in the previous 3 months and living in Chicago were recruited to participate in the study. Some of the women, at random, were put into a group that received the intervention, whereas those in a control group did not receive it. The intervention, which was facilitated by trained bilingual Latina women, consisted of multiple culturally tailored sessions about a range of topics such as partner communication, violence prevention, and sexually transmitted diseases. (Specific details about the intervention sessions are provided at http://nursing-research-editor.com). Women in the intervention group were expected to attend at least three sessions. The two groups of women were compared at the outset of the study (before the intervention) and then 3 months and 6 months later with regard to seven outcomes:

acculturation, health-protective sexual communication, HIV knowledge, perceptions of peer norms concerning condom use, perceived barriers to condom use, condom use intentions, and actual condom use.

Key Findings: The analysis suggested that the intervention was effective in improving HIV knowledge, partner communication, risk-reduction behavioral intentions, and condom use. Perceived barriers to condom use were lower among women who received the intervention than among those who did not.

Conclusions: Peragallo and her colleagues concluded that culturally sensitive interventions are essential for reducing HIV risk for low-income Latinas.

Research Example of a Qualitative Study

Study: The impact of hyperemesis gravidarum on maternal role assumption (Meighan & Wood, 2005)

Study Purpose: The purpose of this study was to describe women's experiences with hyperemesis gravidarum and to better understand its impact on maternal role assumption during the perinatal period.

Study Methods: Eight pregnant women who had been diagnosed with hyperemesis gravidarum and were being treated for this excessive vomiting participated in the study. Each pregnant woman was privately interviewed about what it is like to have hyperemesis gravidarum.

Key Findings: The main problem women experienced was struggling with the constant nausea and vomiting, which prevented them from carrying out even the simplest activities and led to social isolation. In struggling with this sickness, they sought to find a cause for it and a remedy to end the misery they were experiencing. All eight participants disclosed that none of the remedies they tried worked. The majority of women thought about ending their pregnancy, although none of them did so. Hyperemesis gravidarum robbed women of the joy of pregnancy and interfered with the process of assuming the maternal role. All the women experienced loss of control. Only after their symptoms of nausea and vomiting began to subside were the women able to regain control of their lives and finally start thinking about the baby and the delivery. Women concentrated their efforts then on making up for lost time in becoming attached to their baby.

Conclusions: The researchers concluded that hyperemesis gravidarum can interfere with women's maternal role assumption and that nurses may need to provide additional support to these mothers after delivery as they attach to their infants.

⦾⦾⦾⦾⦾⦾⦾⦾⦾⦾⦾⦾⦾⦾⦾⦾⦾

SUMMARY POINTS

- **Nursing research** is systematic inquiry to develop knowledge about issues of importance to nurses.
- Nurses in various settings are adopting an **evidence-based practice (EBP)** that incorporates research findings into their decisions and their interactions with clients.
- Knowledge of nursing research enhances the professional practice of all nurses—including both **consumers of nursing research** (who read and evaluate studies) and **producers of nursing research** (who design and undertake studies).
- Nursing research began with Florence Nightingale but developed slowly until its rapid acceleration in the 1950s. Since the 1970s, nursing research has focused on problems relating to clinical practice.
- The **National Institute of Nursing Research (NINR)**, established at the U.S. National Institutes of Health in 1993, affirms the stature of nursing research in the United States.
- Future emphases of nursing research are likely to include EBP projects, **replications** of research, research integration through systematic reviews, multi-site and interdisciplinary studies, expanded dissemination efforts, and increased focus on health disparities.
- Disciplined research stands in contrast to other sources of evidence for nursing practice, such as tradition, authority, personal experience, trial and error, intuition, and logical reasoning; rigorous research is at the pinnacle of the **evidence hierarchy** as a basis for making clinical decisions.
- Disciplined inquiry in nursing is conducted within two broad **paradigms**—world views with underlying **assumptions** about the complexities of reality: the positivist paradigm and the naturalistic paradigm.
- In the **positivist paradigm**, it is assumed that there is an objective reality and that natural phenomena are regular and orderly. The related assumption of **determinism** refers to the belief

that phenomena are the result of prior causes and are not haphazard.
- In the **naturalistic paradigm**, it is assumed that reality is not a fixed entity but is rather a construction of human minds—and thus "truth" is a composite of multiple constructions of reality.
- The positivist paradigm is associated with **quantitative research**—the collection and analysis of numeric information. Quantitative research is typically conducted within the traditional **scientific method**, which is a systematic and controlled process. Quantitative researchers base their findings on **empirical evidence** (evidence collected by way of the human senses) and strive for **generalizability** of their findings beyond a single setting or situation.
- Researchers within the naturalistic paradigm emphasize understanding the human experience as it is lived through the collection and analysis of subjective, narrative materials using flexible procedures that evolve in the **field**; this paradigm is associated with **qualitative research**.
- **Basic research** is designed to extend the base of information for the sake of knowledge. **Applied research** focuses on discovering solutions to immediate problems.
- Research purposes for nursing research include identification, description, exploration, explanation, prediction, and control. Many nursing studies can also be classified in terms of a key EBP aim: treatment/therapy/intervention; diagnosis and assessment; prognosis; prevention of harm; etiology and causation; and meaning and process.

⦾⦾⦾⦾⦾⦾⦾⦾⦾⦾⦾⦾⦾⦾⦾⦾⦾

STUDY ACTIVITIES

Chapter 1 of the *Resource Manual to Accompany Nursing Research: Generating and Assessing Evidence for Nursing Practice, 8th edition*, offers some exercises and study suggestions for reinforcing the concepts presented in this chapter. In addition, the following study questions can be addressed:

1. Is your world view closer to the positivist or the naturalistic paradigm? Explore the aspects of the two paradigms that are especially consistent with your world view.

2. Answer the questions in Box 1.1 about the Peragallo and colleagues (2005) study described in the research example section of this chapter. Also address the following: Could this study have been undertaken as a qualitative study? Why or why not?

3. Answer the questions in Box 1.1 about the Meighan and Wood (2005) study described in the research example section of this chapter. Also address the following: Could this study have been undertaken as a quantitative study? Why or why not?

⬤⬤⬤⬤⬤⬤⬤⬤⬤⬤⬤⬤⬤⬤⬤⬤⬤⬤

STUDIES CITED IN CHAPTER 1

Methodologic or theoretical references cited in this chapter can be found in a separate section at the end of the book.

Barnard, K. E. (1973). The effects of stimulation on the sleep behavior of the premature infant. In M. Batey (Ed.), *Communicating nursing research* (Vol. 6, pp. 12–33). Boulder, CO: WICHE.

Barnard, K. E. (1976). The state of the art: Nursing and early intervention with handicapped infants. In T. Tjossem (Ed.), *Proceedings of the 1974 President's Committee on Mental Retardation*. Baltimore: University Park Press.

Barnard, K. E., & Collar, B. S. (1973). Early diagnosis, interpretation, and intervention. *Annals of the New York Academy of Sciences, 205*, 373–382.

Barnard, K. E., Wenner, W., Weber, B., Gray, C., & Peterson, A. (1977). Premature infant refocus. In P. Miller (Ed.), *Research to practice in mental retardation: Vol. 3, Biomedical aspects*. Baltimore: University Park Press.

Brooten, D., Brown, L. P., Munro, B. H., York, R., Cohen, S., Roncoli, M., & Hollingsworth, A. (1988). Early discharge and specialist transitional care. *Image: Journal of Nursing Scholarship, 20*, 64–68.

Brooten, D., Gennaro, S., Knapp, H., Brown, L. P., & York, R. (1989). Clinical specialist pre- and postdischarge teaching of parents of very low birthweight infants. *Journal of Obstetric, Gynecologic, & Neonatal Nursing, 18*, 316–322.

Brooten, D., Kumar, S., Brown, L. P., Butts, P., Finkler, S., Bakewell-Sachs, S., Gibbons, S., & Delivoria-Papadopoulos, M. (1986). A randomized clinical trial of early hospital discharge and home follow-up of very low birthweight infants. *New England Journal of Medicine, 315*, 934–939.

Brooten, D., Roncoli, M., Finkler, S., Arnold, L., Cohen, A., & Mennuti, M. (1994). A randomized clinical trial of early hospital discharge and home follow-up of women having cesarean birth. *Obstetrics and Gynecology, 84*, 832–838.

Bruce, A., & Davies, B. (2005). Mindfulness in hospice care: Practicing meditation-in-action. *Qualitative Health Research, 15*, 1329–1344.

Cadena, S. V. (2006). Living among strangers: The needs and functioning of persons with schizophrenia residing in an assisted living facility. *Issues in Mental Health Nursing, 27*(1), 25–41.

Chang, K. H., & Horrocks, S. (2006). Lived experiences of family caregivers of mentally ill relatives. *Journal of Advanced Nursing, 53*(4), 435–443.

Chwo, M. J., Anderson, G. C., Good, M., Dowling, D. A., Shiau, S. H., & Chu, D. M. (2002). A randomized controlled trial of early kangaroo care for preterm infants: Effects on temperature, weight, behavior, and acuity. *Journal of Nursing Research, 10*, 129–142.

Dodd, V. L. (2005). Implications of kangaroo care for growth and development in preterm infants. *Journal of Obstetric, Gynecologic, & Neonatal Nursing, 34*(2), 218–232.

England, M., Tripp-Reimer, & Rubenstein, L. (2005). Exploration of the psychometric properties of an Inventory of Voice Experiences. *Archives of Psychiatric Nursing, 19*, 58–69.

Engler, A. J., Ludington-Hoe, S. M., Cusson, R. M., Adams, R., Bahnsen, M., Brumbaugh, E., Coates, P., Grieb, J., McHargue, L., Ryan, D. L., Settle, M., & Williams, D. (2002). Kangaroo care: National survey of practice, knowledge, barriers, and perceptions. *MCN: The American Journal of Maternal/Child Nursing, 27*, 146–153.

Epstein, C. D., & Peerless, J. R. (2006). Weaning readiness and fluid balances in older critically ill surgical patients. *American Journal of Critical Care, 15*(1), 54–64.

Estabrooks, C. A., Rutakumwa, W., O'Leary, K., Profetto-McGrath, J., Milner, M., Levers, M. J., & Scott-Findlay, S. (2005). Sources of practice knowledge among nurses. *Qualitative Health Research, 15*(4), 460–476.

Huddleston, R., Berkheimer, C., Landis, S., Houck, D., Proctor, A., & Whiteford, J. (2005). Improving patient outcomes in an ambulatory infusion setting. *Journal of Infusion Nursing, 28*(3), 170–172.

Johnson, R. J., Ross, M. W., Taylor, W. C., Williams, M. L., Carvajal, R. I., & Peters, R. J. (2006). Prevalence of childhood sexual abuse among incarcerated males in county jail. *Child Abuse and Neglect, 30*(1), 75–86.

Johnston, C. C., Stevens, B., Pinelli, J., Gibbins, S., Filion, F., Jack, A., Steele, S., Boyer, K., & Veilleux, A. (2003). Kangaroo care is effective in diminishing pain response in preterm neonates. *Archives of Pediatrics & Adolescent Medicine, 157,* 1084–1088.

Kim, S. D., & Kim, H. S. (2005). Effects of a relaxation breathing exercise on anxiety, depression, and leukocyte in hemopoietic stem cell transplantation patients. *Cancer Nursing, 28,* 79–83.

Lindeman, C. A. (1975). Delphi survey of priorities in clinical nursing research. *Nursing Research, 24,* 434–441.

Ludington-Hoe, S. M., Anderson, G. C., Swinth, J. Y., Thompson, C., & Hadeed, A. J. (2004). Randomized controlled trial of kangaroo care: Cardiorespiratory and thermal effects on healthy preterm infants. *Neonatal Network, 23*(3), 39–48.

Marcinkowski, K., Wong, V. G., & Dignam, D. (2005). Getting back to the future: A grounded theory study of the patient perspective of total knee joint arthroplasty. *Orthopaedic Nursing, 24*(3), 202–209.

McCormick, K. M., Naimark, B. J., & Tate, R. B. (2006). Uncertainty, symptom distress, anxiety, and functional status in patients awaiting coronary artery bypass surgery. *Heart & Lung, 35*(1), 34–45.

McCullagh, J., Lewis, G., & Warlow, C. (2005). Promoting awareness and practice of testicular self-examination. *Nursing Standard, 19*(51), 41–49.

McGrath, M. M., Sullivan, M., Devin, J., Fontes-Murphy, M., Barcelos, S., DePalma, J. L., & Faraone, S. (2005). Early precursors of low attention and hyperactivity in a preterm sample at age four. *Issues in Comprehensive Pediatric Nursing, 28,* 1–15.

Meighan, M., & Wood, A. F. (2005). The impact of hyperemesis gravidarum on maternal role assumption. *Journal of Obstetrics, Gynecologic, & Neonatal Nursing, 34*(2), 172–179.

Quint, J. C. (1962). Delineation of qualitative aspects of nursing care. *Nursing Research, 11,* 204–206.

Quint, J. C. (1963). The impact of mastectomy. *American Journal of Nursing, 63,* 88–91.

Quint, J. C. (1967). *The nurse and the dying patient.* New York: Macmillan.

Peragallo, N., DeForge, B., O'Campo, P., Lee, S. M., Kim, Y. J., Cianelli, R., & Ferrer, L. (2005). A randomized clinical trial of an HIV-risk reduction intervention among low-income Latina women. *Nursing Research, 54,* 108–118.

Rahm, G. B., Renck, B., & Rinsberg, K. C. (2006). "Disgust, disgust beyond description": Shame cues to detect shame in disguise, in interviews with women who were sexually abused during childhood. *Journal of Psychiatric & Mental Health Nursing, 13*(1), 100–109.

Roberts, S. T., & Kennedy, B. L. (2006). Why are young college women not using condoms? Their perceived risk, drug use, and developmental vulnerability may provide important clues to sexual risk. *Archives of Psychiatric Nursing, 20*(1), 32–40.

Rodriguez, C. S., & Van Cott, M. L. (2005). Speech impairment in the postoperative head and neck cancer patient: Nurses' and patients' perceptions. *Qualitative Health Research, 15*(7), 897–911.

Shaugnessey, M., Resnick, B. M., & Macko, R. F. (2006). Testing a model of post-stroke exercise behavior. *Rehabilitation Nursing, 31*(1), 15–21.

Smith, B. (2006). Peripheral intravenous catheter dwell times: A comparison of three securement methods for implementation of a 96-hour scheduled change protocol. *Journal of Infusion Nursing, 29*(1), 14–17.

Sobo, E. J., Eng, B., & Kassity-Krich, N. (2006). Canine visitation (pet) therapy: Pilot data on decreases in child pain perception. *Journal of Holistic Nursing, 24*(1), 51–57.

Swanson, B., Cronin-Stubbs, D., Zeller, J. M., Kessler, H. A., & Bielauskas, L. A. (1993). Characterizing the neuropsychological functioning of persons with human immunodeficiency virus infection. *Archives of Psychiatric Nursing, 7,* 82–90.

Swanson, B., Zeller, J. M., & Spear, G. (1998). Cortisol upregulates HIV p24 antigen in cultured human monocyte-derived macrophages. *Journal of the Association of Nurses in AIDS care, 9,* 78–83.

Weaver, K., Wuest, J., & Ciliska, D. (2005). Understanding women's journey of recovering from anorexia nervosa. *Qualitative Health Research, 15*(2), 188–206.

2 | Translating Research Evidence Into Nursing Practice: Evidence-Based Nursing

T his book will help you to develop the methodologic skills you need for generating and evaluating research evidence for nursing practice. Before we elaborate on methodologic techniques, we discuss key aspects of **evidence-based practice (EBP)** to further clarify the key role that research now plays in nursing.

BACKGROUND OF EVIDENCE-BASED NURSING PRACTICE

This section provides a context for understanding evidence-based nursing practice. Part of this context involves a discussion of a closely related concept, research utilization.

Definition of EBP

EBP is the conscientious use of current best evidence in making clinical decisions about patient care (Sackett et al., 2000). In many areas of clinical decision making, research has demonstrated that "tried and true" methods or practices taught in basic nursing education are not always best. For example, although many nurses were taught to place infants in the prone sleeping position to prevent aspiration, there is now persuasive evidence that the supine (back) sleeping position decreases

the risk for sudden infant death syndrome (SIDS). Because research evidence such as this can provide invaluable insights about human health and illness, nurses and other health care professionals must be lifelong learners who have the skills to search for, understand, and evaluate new information about patient care—as well as the capacity to be flexible and to adapt to change.

A basic feature of EBP as a clinical problem-solving strategy is that it de-emphasizes decisions based on custom, authority, opinion, or ritual; the emphasis is on identifying the best available research evidence and *integrating* it with other factors. Contrary to some misconceptions, advocates of EBP do not minimize the importance of clinical expertise. Rather, evidence-based decision making should integrate best research evidence with clinical expertise, patient preferences and circumstances, and awareness of the clinical setting and resource constraints. A key ingredient in EBP is the effort to personalize the evidence to fit a specific patient's needs and a particular clinical situation.

Research Utilization and EBP

The terms *research utilization* and *evidence-based practice* are sometimes used synonymously. Although there is overlap between the two concepts, they are, in fact, distinct. **Research** utilization (RU), the narrower of the two terms, is the use of findings from a disciplined study or set of studies in a practical application that is unrelated to the original research. In RU, the emphasis is on translating empirically derived knowledge into real-world applications. The genesis of the process is a research-based innovation or new knowledge.

EBP is broader than RU because it incorporates research findings with other factors, as just noted. Also, whereas RU begins with the research itself (how can I put this innovation to good use in my clinical setting?), the start-point in EBP is a clinical question (what does the evidence say is the best approach to solving this problem?).

RU was an important concept in nursing before the EBP movement took hold. This section provides a brief overview of RU in nursing.

The RU Continuum

The start-point of RU is the emergence of new knowledge and new ideas. Research is conducted, and over time, evidence on a topic accumulates. In turn, the evidence works its way into use—to varying degrees and at differing rates.

Theorists who have studied the phenomenon of knowledge development and the diffusion of ideas typically recognize a continuum in terms of the specificity of the use to which research findings are put. At one end of the continuum are discrete, clearly identifiable attempts to base specific actions on research findings (e.g., placing infants in supine instead of prone sleeping position). Research findings can, however, be used in a more diffuse manner—in a way that reflects cumulative awareness, understanding, or enlightenment. Thus, a practicing nurse may read a qualitative research report describing *courage* among individuals with long-term health problems as a dynamic process that includes efforts to fully accept reality and to develop problem-solving skills. The study may make the nurse more observant and sensitive in working with patients with long-term illnesses, but it may not necessarily lead to formal changes in clinical actions.

Estabrooks (1999) studied RU by collecting information from 600 nurses in Canada. She found evidence to support three distinct types of RU: (1)

indirect research utilization, involving changes in nurses' thinking; (2) direct research utilization, involving the direct use of findings in giving patient care; and (3) persuasive utilization, involving the use of findings to persuade others (typically those in decision-making positions) to make changes in policies or practices relevant to nursing care. These varying ways of thinking about RU clearly suggest a role for both qualitative and quantitative research.

The History of RU in Nursing Practice

During the 1980s, *research utilization* emerged as an important buzz word, and several changes in nursing education and nursing research were prompted by the desire to develop a knowledge base for nursing practice. In education, nursing schools increasingly began to include courses on research methods so that students would become skillful research consumers. In the research arena, there was a shift in focus toward clinical nursing problems.

These changes helped to sensitize the nursing community to the desirability of using research as a basis for practice, but concerns about the limited use of research findings in the delivery of nursing care continued to mount. Such concerns were fuelled by some studies suggesting that nurses were often unaware of research results or did not incorporate results into their practice. In one such study, Ketefian (1975) reported on the oral temperature determination practices of 87 registered nurses. The results of several studies in the late 1960s had clearly demonstrated that the optimal placement time for oral temperature determination using glass thermometers is 9 minutes. Ketefian's study was designed to learn what "happens to research findings relative to nursing practice after five or ten years of dissemination in the nursing literature" (p. 90). In Ketefian's study, only 1 of 87 nurses reported the correct placement time, suggesting that these practicing nurses were unaware of or ignored the research findings about optimal placement time. Other studies in the early 1980s (e.g., Kirchhoff, 1982), were similarly discouraging.

The need to reduce the gap between nursing research and nursing practice led to formal attempts to bridge the gap. The best-known of several early nursing RU projects is the **Conduct and Utilization of Research in Nursing (CURN) project**, a 5-year development project awarded to the Michigan Nurses Association by the Division of Nursing in the 1970s. The major objective of CURN was to increase the use of research findings in nurses' daily practice by disseminating current research findings, facilitating organizational changes needed to implement innovations, and encouraging collaborative clinical research. The CURN project staff saw RU as primarily an organizational process, with the commitment of organizations that employ nurses as essential to the RU process (Horsley, Crane, & Bingle, 1978). The CURN project team concluded that RU by practicing nurses was feasible, but only if the research is relevant to practice and if the results are broadly disseminated.

During the 1980s and 1990s, RU projects were undertaken by a growing number of hospitals and organizations, and descriptions of the projects began to appear regularly in the nursing literature. These projects were generally institutional attempts to implement changes in nursing practice on the basis of research findings, and to evaluate the effects of the innovations. Although studies continued to confirm a research–practice gap, the findings suggested some improvements in nurses' utilization of research (e.g., Brett, 1987; Coyle & Sokop, 1990; Rutledge et al., 1996). During the 1990s, however, the call for RU began to be superseded by the push for EBP.

EBP in Nursing

The EBP movement has given rise to considerable debate, with both staunch advocates and critics. Supporters argue that EBP offers a solution to improving health care quality in our current cost-constrained environment. Their position is that a rational approach is needed to provide the best possible care to the most people, with the most cost-effective use of resources. Advocates also note that EBP provides an important framework for self-directed lifelong learning that is essential in an era of rapid clinical advances and the infor-

mation explosion. Critics worry that the advantages of EBP are exaggerated and that individual clinical judgments and patient inputs are being devalued. They are also concerned that, in the current EBP environment, insufficient attention is being paid to the role of qualitative research. Although there is a need for close scrutiny of how the EBP journey unfolds, it seems likely that the EBP path is the one that health care professions will follow in the years ahead.

Overview of the EBP Movement

One of the cornerstones of the EBP movement is the Cochrane Collaboration, which was founded in the United Kingdom based on the work of British epidemiologist Archie Cochrane. Cochrane published an influential book in the early 1970s that drew attention to the dearth of solid evidence about the effects of health care. He called for efforts to make research summaries of clinical trials available to physicians and other health care providers. This eventually led to the development of the Cochrane Center in Oxford in 1993, and an international collaboration called the Cochrane Collaboration, with centers now established in more than a dozen locations throughout the world. The aim of the collaboration is to help providers make good decisions about health care by preparing, maintaining, and disseminating systematic reviews of the effects of health care interventions.

At about the same time that the Cochrane Collaboration got underway, a group from McMaster Medical School in Canada developed a clinical learning strategy they called *evidence-based medicine*. Dr. David Sackett, a pioneer of evidence-based medicine at McMaster, noted that "the practice of evidence-based medicine means integrating individual clinical expertise with the best available external evidence from systematic research" (Sackett et al., 1996, p. 71). The evidence-based medicine movement has shifted over time to a broader conception of using best evidence by all health care practitioners (not just physicians) in a multidisciplinary team.

EBP has been considered a major paradigm shift for health care education and practice. In the EBP environment, a skillful clinician can no longer rely on a repository of memorized information, but rather must be adept in accessing, evaluating, synthesizing, and using new research evidence.

Types of Evidence and Evidence Hierarchies

There is no consensus about what constitutes usable evidence for EBP, but there is general agreement that findings from rigorous research are paramount. There is, however, some debate about what constitutes "*rigorous*" research and what qualifies as "*best*" evidence.

In the initial phases of the EBP movement, there was a definite bias toward reliance on information from a type of study called a *randomized clinical trial* (RCT). This bias stemmed in part from the fact that the Cochrane Collaboration initially focused on evidence about the effectiveness of interventions, rather than about other aspects of health care practice. As we explain in Chapter 10, the methodologic

strategies used in RCTs are especially well suited for drawing conclusions about the effects of health care interventions. The bias in ranking sources of evidence primarily in terms of questions about effective treatments led to some resistance to EBP by nurses who thought that evidence from qualitative and non-RCT studies would be ignored. As Closs and Cheater (1999) noted, "Some antagonism towards EBN (evidence-based nursing) seems to derive from viewing it as an unwelcome extension of the positivist tradition" (p. 13).

Positions about the contribution of various types of evidence are less rigid than previously. Nevertheless, most published **evidence hierarchies,** which rank evidence sources according to the strength of the evidence they provide, look something like the one shown in Figure 2.1. This figure, adapted from schemes presented in several references on EBP

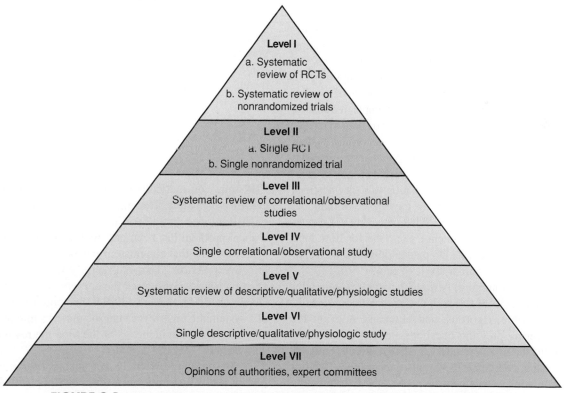

FIGURE 2.1 Evidence hierarchy: levels of evidence regarding effectiveness of an intervention.

(DiCenso et al., 2005; Guyatt & Rennie, 2002; Melnyk & Fineout-Overholt, 2005) shows a 7-level hierarchy that has at its pinnacle systematic reviews of RCTs. That is, the strongest evidence according to this hierarchy comes from **systematic reviews** that integrate findings from multiple RCT studies using rigorous and methodical procedures. Systematic reviews of nonrandomized clinical trials (Level Ib) offer less powerful evidence. The second rung of the hierarchy is individual RCT studies, and so on (the terms in this figure are explained in subsequent chapters of this book). At the bottom of this evidence hierarchy are opinions from experts.

It is important to recognize that *within* any of the levels in an evidence hierarchy, the worth of the evidence can vary considerably. For example, an individual RCT (Level IIa) could be extremely well designed, yielding very persuasive evidence, or it could be so flawed that the evidence would be compromised. We must also emphasize that the evidence hierarchy shown in Figure 2.1 is not universally appropriate—a point that is not always made sufficiently clear. This hierarchy has merit for ranking evidence for certain types of clinical questions, but not others. In particular, this hierarchy is appropriate with regard to questions about the effects of clinical interventions or treatments. For example, a question about the effect of massage therapy on pain in cancer patients would classify evidence according to this hierarchy, but many other important questions would not. The hierarchy in Figure 2.1 would not be relevant for ranking evidence relating to such questions as the following: What is the experience of pain like for patients with cancer? What percentage of cancer patients experience intense pain, and for how long does the pain persist? Do men and women with cancer experience similar levels of pain?

Thus, in nursing, *best evidence* refers generally to findings from research that are methodologically appropriate, rigorous, and clinically relevant for answering pressing questions—questions not only about the efficacy, safety, and cost-effectiveness of nursing interventions, but also about the reliability of nursing assessment measures, the determinants of health and well-being, the meaning of health or illness, and the nature of patients' experiences. Confidence in the evidence is enhanced when the research methods are compelling, when there have been multiple confirmatory replication studies, and when the evidence has been systematically evaluated and synthesized.

Of course, there continue to be clinical practice questions for which there is relatively little research information. In such situations, nursing practice must rely on other sources—for example, benchmarking data, chart review, quality improvement and risk data, and clinical expertise (Goode, 2000). As Sackett and colleagues (2000) have noted, one benefit of the EBP movement is that when clinical questions arise for which there is no satisfactory evidence, a new research agenda can result.

RESOURCES FOR EVIDENCE-BASED PRACTICE

The translation of research evidence into nursing practice is an ongoing challenge, but it is a challenge to which the nursing profession and related health care professions have risen. In this section we describe some of the resources that are available to support evidence-based nursing practice.

Systematic Reviews

EBP relies on meticulous integration of research evidence on a topic. The emphasis on *best evidence* in EBP implies that all (or most) evidence about a clinical problem has been gathered, evaluated, and synthesized so that conclusions can be drawn about effective practices. That is precisely why systematic reviews are considered the cornerstone of EBP (Jennings, 2000; Stevens, 2001): the "bottom line" of a systematic review is a state-of-the-art summary of what the best evidence is at the time the review was written.

A systematic review is not just a literature review, such as reviews we describe in Chapter 5. A systematic review is in itself a methodical, scholarly inquiry that follows many of the same steps as those described in this book for primary studies. Chapter 25 offers some basic guidelines on conducting and critiquing systematic reviews.

Systematic reviews can take various forms. Until fairly recently, the most common type of systematic review was a traditional narrative (qualitative) integration to merge and synthesize research findings. Narrative reviews of quantitative studies increasingly are being replaced by a type of systematic review known as meta-analysis.

Meta-analysis is a technique for integrating quantitative research findings statistically. In essence, meta-analysis treats the findings from a study as one piece of information. The findings from multiple studies on the same topic are combined, and then all the information is analyzed statistically in a manner similar to that in a usual study. Thus, instead of study participants being the **unit of analysis** (the most basic entity on which the analysis focuses), individual studies are the unit of analysis in a meta-analysis. Meta-analysis provides a convenient and objective method of integrating a large body of findings and of observing patterns that might otherwise have gone undetected.

Example of a meta-analysis: Snethen, Broome, and Cashin (2006) conducted a meta-analysis to analyze research on the effectiveness of weight-loss interventions for children. The researchers integrated results from seven intervention studies. The aggregated evidence indicated that such interventions have a positive effect on children's weight loss.

There is also an increasing awareness of the need for integrative reviews of qualitative studies, and efforts are underway to develop techniques for qualitative metasynthesis. A **metasynthesis** involves integrating qualitative research findings on a specific topic that are themselves interpretive syntheses of narrative information (Sandelowski & Barroso, 2003). A metasynthesis is quite distinct from a quantitative meta-analysis: a metasynthesis is less about reducing information and more about amplifying and interpreting it.

Example of a metasynthesis: Goodman (2005) conducted a metasynthesis of seven qualitative studies that focused on the experiences of fatherhood in the early months after the birth of an infant. In all, 134 fathers were represented in the metasynthesis. Goodman identified four overarching phases of becoming a father: entering with expectations and intentions, confronting reality, working to develop a role as an involved father, and reaping the benefits.

Fortunately, systematic reviews on a wide variety of clinical topics are increasingly available and represent a rich resource for EBP. Such reviews are published in professional journals that can be accessed using standard literature search procedures (see Chapter 5), and are also available in databases that are dedicated to such reviews. In particular, the Cochrane Database of Systematic Reviews (CDSR) contains thousands of systematic reviews (mostly meta-analyses) relating to health care interventions. Cochrane reviews have been found to be more rigorous than those published in journals (Jadad et al., 1998), and have the advantage of being checked and updated regularly.

Example of Cochrane review: Ellen Hodnett, a Canadian nurse researcher, and her colleagues (2005) updated an earlier Cochrane review on the effects of maternity care in a homelike birth environment compared with care in conventional hospital settings. Findings from six studies involving more than 8500 women were included in the review. The evidence supported the conclusion that homelike settings for childbirth are associated with modest benefits, including reduced medical interventions and increased maternal satisfaction.

Another critical resource for systematic reviews is the Agency for Healthcare Research and Quality (AHRQ). This agency awarded 12 5-year contracts in 1997 to establish Evidence-Based Practice Centers at institutions in the United States and Canada (e.g., at Johns Hopkins University, McMaster University); new 5-year contracts were awarded in 2002. Each center issues *evidence reports* that are based on rigorous systematic reviews of relevant literature; dozens of these reports are now available to help "improve the quality, effectiveness, and appropriateness of clinical care" (AHRQ website, *http://www.ahrq.gov*).

Many other resources are available for locating systematic reviews. In the United Kingdom, for example, the Centre for Reviews and Dissemination at the University of York produces and commissions systematic reviews focusing on the effectiveness of health care interventions; information about the reviews is available on their Database of Abstracts of Reviews of Effects, or DARE (*http://www.york.ac.uk/inst/crd/index.htm*). The Joanna Briggs Institute at the University of Adelaide in Australia is another useful source for systematic reviews in nursing and other health fields (*http://www.joannabriggs.edu.au*). And in Canada, the Ontario Ministry of Health and Long-Term Care has sponsored the Effective Public Health Practice Project (EPHPP), which undertakes systematic reviews on a broad array of health topics (*http://www.hamilton.ca/phcs/ephpp*).

⊃ TIP: All websites cited in this chapter, plus additional websites with useful content relating to EBP, are in the "Useful Websites for Chapter 2" file on the accompanying CD-ROM.

Clinical Practice Guidelines

Evidence-based **clinical practice guidelines,** like systematic reviews, represent an effort to distill a large body of evidence into a manageable form, but guidelines differ from systematic reviews in a number of respects. First and foremost, clinical practice guidelines, which are usually based on systematic reviews, give specific practice recommendations and prescriptions for evidence-based decision making. Their primary intent is to influence what clinicians do. Second, guidelines also attempt to address all the issues relevant to a clinical decision, including the balancing of benefits and risks. Third, systematic reviews tend to be evidence driven—that is, they are undertaken when a body of evidence has been produced and needs to be synthesized. Guidelines, by contrast, are "necessity driven" (Sackett et al., 2000), meaning that guidelines are developed to

guide clinical practice—even when available evidence is limited or of unexceptional quality. Fourth, whereas systematic reviews are typically done by teams of researchers with strong methodologic skills, guideline development typically involves the consensus of a group of researchers, experts, and clinicians. For this reason, guidelines based on the same evidence may result in different recommendations that take into account contextual factors—for example, guidelines appropriate in the United States may be unsuitable in Taiwan or Sweden.

Guidelines are available for a broad range of diagnostic and therapeutic decisions. Typically, they define a minimum set of services and actions appropriate for certain clinical conditions. Most guidelines allow for a flexible approach in their application to patients who fall outside the scope of their guideline (e.g., those who have significant comorbidities).

It can be challenging to find clinical practice guidelines because there is no single guideline repository. A standard literature search for guidelines in bibliographic databases such as MEDLINE (see Chapter 5) will yield many references—but often a frustrating mixture of citations not only to the actual guidelines but also to commentaries, implementation case studies, and so on. A better approach is to search for guidelines in comprehensive guideline databases, or through specialty organizations that have sponsored guideline development. It would be impossible to list all possible sources, but a few deserve special mention. In the United States, nursing and other health care guidelines are maintained by the National Guideline Clearinghouse (*http://www.guideline.gov*). In Canada, the Registered Nurses Association of Ontario (RNAO) (*http://www.rnao.org/bestpractices*) and the Canadian Medical Association (*http://mdm.ca/cpgsnew/cpgs/index.asp*) maintain information about clinical practice guidelines. In the United Kingdom, two sources for clinical guidelines are the Translating Research Into Practice (TRIP) database (*http://www.tripdatabase.com*) and the National Institute for Clinical Excellence (*http://www.nice.org.uk*). Professional societies and organizations also maintain collections of guidelines of relevance to their area of specialization. In nursing, the Association of Women's Health, Obstetric, and Neonatal Nursing (AWHONN) has provided extraordinary leadership in advocating EBP and has developed a host of clinical practice guidelines (*http://www.awhonn. org*).

Example of a nursing clinical practice guideline: In late 2005, the RNAO released a best practice guideline called "Woman Abuse: Screening, Identification, and Initial Response." Developed by an interdisciplinary panel under the leadership of Daina Mueller, the guideline's purpose is "to facilitate routine universal screening for the abuse of women by nurses in all practice settings" (http://www.rnao. org). The guideline offers a large repertoire of evidence-based strategies, and provides information about the strength of evidence supporting each one.

Although efforts to find, appraise, and implement a clinical practice guideline typically involve a lot of work and collaboration, this is a pathway to EBP that is increasingly being adopted. Fortunately, there is evidence from a systematic review that guideline-driven care in nursing is effective in improving some processes and outcomes of care (Thomas et al., 2000).

There are many topics for which practice guidelines have not yet been developed, but the opposite problem is also true: the dramatic increase in the number of guidelines means that there are sometimes multiple guidelines on the same topic from which clinicians must choose. Worse yet, because of variation in the rigor of guideline development and in the interpretation of the evidence, different guidelines sometimes offer different and even conflicting recommendations (Lewis, 2001). Thus, those who wish to adopt clinical practice guidelines are urged to critically appraise them to identify ones that are based on the strongest evidence, have been meticulously developed, are user friendly, and are appropriate for local use or adaptation. We offer some assistance with these tasks later in this chapter.

Other Preappraised Evidence

Preprocessed or preappraised evidence is research evidence that has been carefully selected from primary studies and evaluated for use by clinicians. We have described two key resources for EBP that offer preprocessed information, namely systematic reviews and clinical practice guidelines. Reviews and guidelines themselves should be critically evaluated before they are used to guide practice decisions, but their availability may eliminate the need to intensely scrutinize the merits and limitations of individual studies. There are several other types of preprocessed evidence that are useful for EBP. We mention only a few to alert you to the possibility of these other resources.

DiCenso and colleagues (2005) have described a hierarchy of preprocessed evidence that puts clinical practice guidelines at the top. On the next rung are synopses of systematic reviews, followed by systematic reviews themselves, and then synopses of single studies. Synopses of systematic reviews and of single studies are available in evidence-based abstract journals such as *Clinical Evidence* (*http://www.-clinicalevidence.com*) and *Evidence-Based Nursing* (*http://www.evidencebasednursing.com*). The *Evidence-Based Nursing* journal, published quarterly by the Royal College of Nursing Publishing Company, presents critical summaries of studies and systematic reviews published in more than 150 journals. The journal only summarizes studies that have met basic standards of methodologic quality. The summaries include commentaries on the clinical implications of each reviewed study. *Evidence-Based Nursing* has been linked to other abstraction journals in the health care field (e.g., *Evidence-Based Mental Health*) into one large electronic resource, *Evidence-Based Medicine Reviews*, available through Ovid Technologies. Another journal-based resource is the "evidence digest" feature in each issue of *Worldviews on Evidence-Based Nursing*. These digests offer concise summaries of methodologically sound and clinically important studies, along with practice implications.

Example of preappraised nursing evidence: The main findings of Beck's (2004) qualitative study of mothers' experiences of posttraumatic stress disorder (PTSD) after traumatic births were summarized in *Evidence-Based Nursing* (Jack, 2005), whose author commented that "Beck provides a compelling description of women's responses to traumatic deliveries. . . . The findings of this study permit privileged access to the emotions and experiences of women with PTSD after childbirth" (p. 59). (Note that Beck's report appears in its entirety in the accompanying *Resource Manual.*)

In some journals and also in some practice settings, tools called **critically appraised topics** (**CATs**) are becoming available. A CAT is a quick summary of a clinical question and an appraisal of the best evidence, and typically begins with a "clinical bottom line"—that is, what the best-practice recommendation is. Sackett and his colleagues (2000) advocate the creation and use of CATs as a teaching and learning tool for EBP, and include software with their book to help generate CATs.

Many websites offer preprocessed evidence designed to guide clinical practice. For example, the Joanna Briggs Institute offers best practice information sheets (*http://www.joannabriggs.edu.au/pubs/best_practice.php*). The Centre for Reviews and Dissemination at the University of York publishes short reports (summaries of systematic reviews) and (until 2004) Effective Health Care bulletins.

Research Findings on EBP and Barriers to Research Utilization

Research about EBP and the process of translating research into practice can be a rich resource in planning an EBP effort. This body of research has been diverse, including both qualitative studies (e.g., a study of the criteria used by nurses to evaluate whether research should be used in practice by French, 2005) and quantitative studies (e.g., a study of how nurses' characteristics affect RU by Margaret-Milner and colleagues, 2005).

The most widely studied topic in this area concerns factors that are barriers to and facilitators of EBP. This is an important area of research because the findings suggest ways in which EBP efforts can be promoted or undermined, and thus raise issues that need to be addressed in advancing evidence-based nursing. Studies that have explored barriers to research use have been done in numerous countries and have yielded remarkably similar results about constraints clinical nurses face (e.g., Gerrish & Clayton, 2004; Glacken & Chaney, 2004; Hutchinson & Johnston, 2004; McCleary & Brown, 2003). Most barriers fall into one of three categories: (1) quality and nature of the research, (2) characteristics of the nurses, and (3) organizational factors.

With regard to the research itself, the main problem is that for some practice areas, high-quality research evidence is limited. There remains an ongoing need for research that directly addresses pressing clinical problems, for replication of studies in a range of settings, for methodologically strong studies that attend to issues of generalizability, and for greater collaboration between researchers and clinicians. Another key issue is that nurse researchers need to improve their ability to communicate their findings (and the clinical implications of their findings) to practicing nurses. Researchers also need to take proactive steps to report their results in a manner that facilitates synthesis—especially meta-analysis (Beck, 1999).

Nurses' attitudes and education consistently have emerged as potential barriers to RU. Studies have found that some nurses do not value research or believe in the benefits of EBP, and others are simply resistant to changing their practices. Fortunately, there is growing evidence from international surveys that many nurses do value nursing research and want to be involved in research-related activities. Additional barriers, however, are that many nurses do not know how to access research information and do not possess the skills to critically evaluate research findings—and even those who do may not know how to effectively incorporate research evidence into clinical decision making. Among nurses in non–English-speaking countries, the lack of English-language skills is another impediment because at the moment most research evidence is reported in English (e.g., Egerod & Hansen, 2005; Oranta, Routasalo, & Hupli, 2002; Patiraki et al., 2004).

Finally, many of the impediments to using research in practice are organizational. "Unit culture" has been found to be a major factor in research use (Pepler et al., 2005), and administrative and other organizational barriers have repeatedly been found to play a role. Although many organizations support the idea of EBP in theory, they do not always provide the necessary supports in terms of staff release time and resources. EBP will become part of organizational norms only if there is a commitment on the part of managers and administrators. Strong leadership in health care organizations is essential to making EBP happen.

Models and Theories for EBP

A number of different models and theories of EBP and RU have been developed. These models offer frameworks for understanding the EBP process and for designing and implementing an EBP project in a practice setting. Some models focus on the use of research from the perspective of individual clinicians (e.g., the Stetler Model), whereas some focus on institutional EBP efforts (e.g., the Iowa Model). Models that offer a framework for launching an EBP or RU effort include the following:

* Advancing Research and Clinical Practice Through Close Collaboration (ARCC) Model (Melnyk & Fineout-Overholt, 2005)
* Center for Advanced Nursing Practice Model (Soukup, 2000)
* Diffusion of Innovations Theory (Rogers, 1995)
* Evidence-Based Multidisciplinary Practice Model (Goode & Piedalue, 1999)
* Framework for Adopting an Evidence-Based Innovation (DiCenso et al., 2005)
* Iowa Model of Research in Practice (Titler et al., 2001)
* Johns Hopkins Nursing EBP Model (Newhouse et al., 2005)
* Model for Change to Evidence-Based Practice (Rosswurm & Larabee, 1999)
* Ottawa Model of Research Use (Logan & Graham, 1998)
* Promoting Action on Research Implementation in Health Services (PARIHS) Model (Rycroft-Malone et al., 2002)
* Stetler Model of Research Utilization (Stetler, 2001)

Although each model offers different perspectives on how to translate research findings into practice, several of the steps and procedures are similar across the models. The most prominent of these models have been the **Diffusion of Innovations Theory,** the **Stetler Model**, and the **Iowa Model**. The latter two, developed by nurses, were originally crafted in an environment that emphasized RU, but they have been updated to incorporate EBP processes. For those wishing to follow a formal EBP model, the cited references should be consulted. Several of the models are also nicely synthesized by Melnyk and Fineout-Overholt (2005). We provide an overview of key activities and processes in EBP efforts, based on a distillation of common elements from the various models, in a subsequent section of this chapter. We rely especially heavily on the Iowa Model, a diagram for which is shown in Figure 2.2.

Example of the application of an EBP model: Thurston and King (2004) described how Rosswurm and Larrabee's 6-step model for EBP was used in an innovative mentorship program between university faculty and nurse clinicians in Canada. The model, which focuses on *planned change*, was used by 10 nursing teams to address clinical practice questions. The mentors concluded that the model was a useful mechanism (albeit one that needed some modification), and deemed the overall project to be successful.

THE PROCESS OF USING RESEARCH IN NURSING PRACTICE

In the years ahead, you are likely to engage in individual and institutional efforts to use research as a basis for clinical decisions. This is almost assuredly going to be the case if you work in a U.S. hospital that is aspiring to or has attained Magnet status. In any EBP activity, you will be well served by having skills in finding, understanding, and critiquing research, and even better served by having the skills to engage in research yourself.

This section, which is based heavily on the various models of EBP and RU, provides an overview

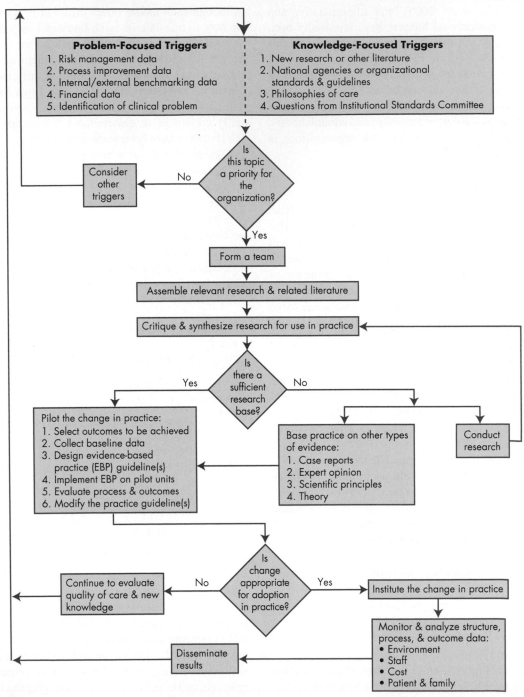

FIGURE 2.2 Iowa Model of Evidence-Based Practice to Promote Quality Care (Adapted from Titler, et al. [2001]. The Iowa Model of Evidence-Based Practice to Promote Quality Care. *Critical Care Nursing Clinics of North America*, *13*, 497–509.)

of how research can be put to use in clinical settings. More extensive guidance is available in textbooks devoted to evidence-based nursing (e.g., DiCenso et al., 2005; Melnyk & Fineout-Overholt, 2005). We have divided this section on the EBP process into two parts, first discussing strategies and steps for individual clinicians and then describing activities used by organizations or teams of nurses.

EBP in Individual Nursing Practice

Individual nurses make many decisions and are called upon to provide health care advice, and so they have ample opportunity to put research into practice. Here are five clinical scenarios that provide examples of such opportunities:

• *Clinical Scenario 1.* You are working on a hemodialysis unit and one of your patients with type 2 diabetes develops severe foot ulceration that ultimately leads to amputation of several toes. You want to know if there is a reliable assessment tool for the earlier detection of foot complications so that the risk for amputation for patients with end-stage renal disease would be reduced.

• *Clinical Scenario 2.* You are an advanced-practice nurse (APRN) working in a rehabilitation hospital, and one of your elderly patients, who had total hip replacement, tells you that she is planning a long airplane trip to visit her daughter after her rehabilitation treatments are completed. You know that a long plane ride will increase the patient's risk for deep vein thrombosis and wonder if compression stockings should be recommended as an effective in-flight treatment. You decide to look for the best possible evidence to answer this question.

• *Clinical Scenario 3.* You are working in an allergy clinic and notice how difficult it is for many children to undergo allergy scratch tests. You wonder if there is an intervention to help allay children's fears about the skin tests.

• *Clinical Scenario 4.* You are caring for a hospitalized patient who, a week before hospitalization, was given a prescription for an SSRI antidepressant. He confides in you that he is ashamed to fill the prescription because he feels it is unmanly. You wonder if there is any evidence about what it feels like for men to begin an SSRI regimen so that you can better understand how to address your patient's concerns.

• *Clinical Scenario 5.* You are caring for a 25-year-old woman who just delivered her first infant by emergency cesarean birth. She is upset, and asks you about the risks of vaginal birth after cesarean (V-BAC). You decide to look for the best possible evidence to answer her question.

In these and thousands of other clinical situations, research evidence can be put to good use to improve the quality of nursing care. Some situations might lead to unit-wide or institution-wide scrutiny of current practices, but in other situations, individual nurses can personally investigate the evidence to help address specific problems.

For individual-level EBP efforts, the major steps in EBP include the following:

1. Asking clinical questions that are answerable with research evidence
2. Searching for and collecting relevant evidence
3. Appraising and synthesizing the evidence
4. Integrating the evidence with your own clinical expertise, patient preferences, and local context
5. Assessing the effectiveness of the decision, intervention, or advice

Asking Well-Worded Clinical Questions

Books on EBP typically devote considerable attention to the first EBP step of asking an answerable clinical question. The authors often distinguish between background and foreground questions. *Background questions* are general, foundational questions about a clinical issue, for example: What is cancer cachexia (progressive body wasting), and what is its pathophysiology? Answers to such background questions are typically found in textbooks. *Foreground questions,* by contrast, are those that can be answered based on current best research evidence on diagnosing, assessing, or treating patients, or on understanding the meaning or prognosis of their health problems. For example, we may wonder, is a fish oil–enhanced nutritional supplement effective in stabilizing weight in patients with advanced cancer? The answer to such a question may provide guidance in how best to treat patients with cachexia—that is, the answer provides an opportunity for EBP.

Textbooks on EBP provide considerable guidance on how to phrase clinical foreground questions in a manner that makes it easier to search for an answer. For example, DiCenso and colleagues (2005) advise that, for questions that call for quantitative information (e.g., about the effectiveness of a treatment), three components should be identified:

1. The *population* (What are the characteristics of the patients or clients?)
2. The *intervention* or *exposure* (What are the treatments or interventions of interest? or, What are the potentially harmful exposures that we are concerned about?)
3. The *outcomes* (What are the outcomes or consequences in which we are interested?)

If we dissected our question about cachexia according to this scheme, we would say that our population is cancer patients with advanced cancer or cachexia; the intervention is fish oil–enhanced nutritional supplements; and the outcome is weight stabilization. As another example, in the first clinical scenario about foot complications cited earlier, the population is diabetic patients undergoing hemodialysis; the intervention is a foot assessment tool; and the outcome is detection of foot problems.

For questions that can best be answered with qualitative information (e.g., about the meaning of an experience or health problem), DiCenso and associates (2005) suggest two components:

1. The *population* (What are the characteristics of the patients or clients?)
2. The *situation* (What conditions, experiences, or circumstances are we interested in understanding?)

For example, suppose our question was, What is it like to suffer from cachexia? In this case, the question

calls for rich qualitative information; the population is patients with advanced cancer, and the situation is the experience of cachexia.

Fineout-Overholt and Johnston (2005) recommended a 5-component scheme for formulating EBP questions and used an acronym (PICOT) as a guide. The five components are population (P), intervention or issue (I), comparison of interest (C), outcome (O), and time (T). Their scheme contrasts an intervention (or issue) with a specific comparison, such as an alternative treatment. For example, we might specifically be interested in learning whether fish oil–enhanced supplements are better than melatonin in stabilizing weight in cancer patients. In some cases, it is important to designate a specific comparison, whereas in others, we might be interested in uncovering evidence about *all* alternatives to the intervention of primary interest. That is, in searching for evidence about the effectiveness of fish oil supplements, we might want to search for studies that compared such supplements to melatonin, placebos, other treatments, or no treatments. The final component in the Fineout-Overholt and Johnston scheme is a timeframe, that is, the timeframe in which the question occurs. Like the "C" component, the "T" is not always needed.

Table 2.1 offers some question templates for asking well-framed clinical questions in selected circumstances. The right-hand panel includes questions with an explicit comparison, whereas the left panel does not. The Toolkit for Chapter 2 of the accompanying *Resource Manual* includes Table 2.1 ⊛ in a word file that can be adapted for your use, so that the template questions can be readily "filled in." Additional EBP resources from this chapter are also in the Toolkit.

Finding Research Evidence

By asking clinical questions in the forms suggested, you should be able to more effectively search the research literature for the information you need. For example, by using the templates in Table 2.1, the information you insert into the blanks constitutes the *keywords* you can use to undertake an electronic search.

For an individual EBP endeavor, the best place to begin is by searching for evidence in a systematic

TABLE 2.1	Question Templates for Selected Clinical Foreground Questions	
TYPE OF QUESTION	**QUESTION TEMPLATE FOR QUESTIONS *WITHOUT* AN EXPLICIT COMPARISON**	**QUESTION TEMPLATE FOR QUESTIONS *WITH* AN EXPLICIT COMPARISON**
Treatment/intervention	In _____ (population), what is the effect of _____ (intervention) on _____ (outcome)?	In _____ (population), what is the effect of _____ (intervention), in comparison to _____ (comparative/ alternative intervention), on _____ (outcome)?
Diagnosis/assessment	For ___ _____ (population), does _____(tool/procedure) yield accurate and appropriate diagnostic/assessment information about _____(outcome)?	For _____ (population), does _____ (tool/procedure) yield more accurate or more appropriate diagnostic/assessment information than _____ (comparative tool/procedure) about _____ (outcome)?
Prognosis	For _____ (population), does _____ (disease or condition) increase the risk for or influence _____ (outcome)?	For _____ (population), does _____ (disease or condition), relative to _____ (comparative disease or condition) increase the risk for or influence _____ (outcome)?
Causation/etiology/harm	Does _____ (exposure or characteristic) increase the risk for ____ _____ (outcome) In _____ (population)?	Does _____ (exposure or characteristic) increase the risk for _____ (outcome) compared with ___ _____ (comparative exposure or condition) in _____ (population)?
Meaning or process	What is it like for _____ (population) to experience _____ (condition, illness, circumstance)? *or* What is the process by which _____ (population) cope with, adapt to, or live with _____ _____ (condition, illness, circumstance)?	(Explicit comparisons not typical in these types of question)

BOX 2.1 Questions for Appraising the Evidence

What is the quality of the evidence—that is, how rigorous and reliable is it?
What *is* the evidence—what is the magnitude of effects?
How precise is the estimate of effects?
What evidence is there of any side effects or side benefits?
What is the financial cost of applying (and not applying) the evidence?
Is the evidence relevant to my particular clinical situation?

review, clinical practice guideline, or other pre-processed source because this approach leads to a much quicker answer—and, if your methodologic skills are not well-honed, potentially a superior answer as well. This is partly because researchers who prepare reviews and clinical guidelines typically are well trained in research methods and use exemplary standards in conducting their evaluation of the evidence. Moreover, preprocessed evidence is usually developed by teams of researchers, which means that the conclusions are presumably cross-validated and fairly objective. Thus, when preprocessed evidence is available to answer a clinical question, you may not need to look any farther, unless the review or guideline is not recent, and so the evidence summary might be outdated.

We offered advice earlier in this chapter on how to track down preprocessed information. When preprocessed evidence cannot be located or is old, you will need to look for best evidence in primary studies, using strategies we describe in Chapter 5.

➲ **TIP:** In Chapter 5, we provide guidance on using the free Internet resource PubMed for searching the bibliographic database MEDLINE. Of special interest to those engaged in an EBP search, PubMed has incorporated a filter that you can use to "screen in" only methodologically sound studies: "Clinical Queries Using Research Methodology Filters."

Appraising the Evidence

After locating appropriate evidence, it should be appraised before taking any clinical action. The critical appraisal of evidence for the purposes of

EBP may involve several types of assessments (Box 2.1). The thoroughness of your appraisal would depend on several factors, the most important of which is the nature of the clinical action for which evidence is being sought. Some clinical actions have strong implications for patient safety, whereas others affect patients' satisfaction. Although using best evidence to guide nursing practice is important for a wide range of outcomes, the appraisal standards would clearly be especially strict for evidence that could affect patient safety and morbidity.

The first appraisal issue is the extent to which the findings are valid. That is, were the methods that were used to generate the evidence sufficiently rigorous that the findings can be believed and accepted? We offer guidance on critiquing studies and evaluating the strength of research evidence from primary studies throughout this book, and a brief critiquing protocol is provided in Chapter 5. If there were several primary studies (and no existing systematic reviews), you would need to draw conclusions about the body of evidence taken as a whole. Clearly, you would need to put most weight on the most rigorous studies. Preappraised evidence is already screened and evaluated, but you may nevertheless need to consider its integrity.

Second, you would need to assess what the results actually are and whether they are clinically important. This criterion considers not whether the results are likely to be "real," but what they are and how powerful the effects are. It is easiest to demonstrate how these first two dimensions (quality of the evidence and strength of effects) might intersect for questions relating to interventions. Effects of an intervention can range from no effects to powerful effects (both positive and negative). To use a concrete example, consider clinical scenario number 2 cited earlier, which suggests the following clinical question: Does the use of compression stockings lower the risk for flight-related deep vein thrombosis in high-risk patients? In our search for evidence, we found a relevant meta-analysis of nine RCTs (Hsieh & Lee, 2005). The conclusion of the meta-analysis is that compression stockings are fairly effective, and the evidence is strong, suggesting that advice about the use of compression stockings may be appropriate, pending an appraisal of other factors.

Determining the magnitude of the effect for quantitative findings is especially important when an intervention is costly or when there are potentially negative side effects. If, for example, there is strong evidence that an intervention is only marginally effective in improving a health problem, it would be important to consider other factors (e.g., evidence on effects on quality of life). There are various ways to quantify the magnitude of effects, several of which are described later in this book. An index known as the *effect size*, for example, can often provide information about the size of effects for outcomes for which average values can be computed (e.g., average length of hospital stay). When the outcomes can be dichotomized (e.g., occurrence versus nonoccurrence of a medical problem), estimates of the magnitude of the effect are often calculated as *absolute risk reduction (ARR)* or *relative risk reduction (RRR)*. We provide further elaboration and methods of calculating these and other related indexes (e.g., *number needed to treat* or NNT) in Chapter 21, but note here that these are important indicators for summarizing the clinical importance of evidence-based interventions. To illustrate with our example, if the RRR for the use of compression stockings were 50%, this would mean that this intervention reduced the risk for deep vein thrombosis by 50% relative to what would occur in the absence of the intervention. An index such as RRR or NNT is especially useful when alternative treatments or interventions are being compared.

Another consideration, relevant when the evidence is quantitative, is how precise the estimate of effect is. This level of appraisal requires some statistical sophistication, and so we postpone our discussion of *confidence intervals* to Chapter 22. Suffice it to say that research results provide only an *estimate* of effects, and it may be useful to understand not only the exact estimate but also the range within which the actual effect probably lies.

If the evidence is judged to be valid and the magnitude of effects suggests that further consideration is warranted, there are situations in which supplementary information is important in guiding decisions. One issue concerns peripheral benefits and costs, evidence for which would typically have emerged during your search. In framing your clinical question, you would have identified the key outcomes in which you were interested—for example, weight stabilization or weight gain for an intervention to address cancer cachexia. Research on this topic, however, would likely have considered other outcomes that would need to be taken into account—for example, quality of life, comfort, side effects, satisfaction, and so on.

Another issue concerns the financial cost of applying the evidence. In some cases, the costs may be small or nonexistent. For example, in clinical scenario 4, in which the question concerned the experience of beginning an SSRI regimen, nursing action would presumably be cost neutral because the evidence would be used primarily to provide information and reassurance to the patient. Some interventions and assessment protocols, however, are costly, and so the amount of time and resources needed to put best evidence into practice would need to be estimated and factored into any decision. Of course, although the cost of a clinical decision needs to be considered, the cost of *not* taking action is equally important.

Finally, it is important to appraise the evidence in terms of whether it has relevance for the clinical situation at hand—that is, for *your* patient in a specific clinical setting. Best practice evidence can most readily be applied to an individual patient in your care if he or she is sufficiently similar to people in the study or studies under review. Would your patient have qualified for participation in the study—or is there some factor such as age, illness severity, mental status, or comorbidity that would have excluded him or her? DiCenso and colleagues (2005), who advised clinicians to ask whether there is some compelling reason to conclude that the results may *not* be applicable in their clinical situation, have written some useful tips (see their Chapter 33) on applying research results to individual patients.

Appraisals of the evidence may lead you to different courses of action. You may reach this point on your EBP path and conclude that the evidence base is not sufficiently sound, or that the likely effect is too small or nonexistent, or that the cost of applying the evidence is too high to merit consideration. The integration of appraisal information may suggest that "usual care" is the simplest and best strategy— or it may suggest the need for a new EBP inquiry. For instance, in the example about cachexia, you likely would have learned that recent best evidence suggests that fish oil–enhanced nutritional supplements may be an ineffective treatment (Jatoi, 2005). However, during your search, you may have come across a Cochrane review that concluded that megestrol acetate improves appetite and weight gain in patients with cancer (Berenstein & Ortiz, 2005). This may lead to a new evidence inquiry and to discussions with other members of your health care team about developing a nutrition-focused protocol for your clinical setting. If, however, the initial appraisal of evidence suggests a promising clinical action, you can proceed to the next step.

Integrating Evidence

As the definition for EBP implies, research evidence needs to be integrated with other types of information, including your own clinical expertise and knowledge about your clinical setting. You may be aware of factors that would make implementation of the evidence, no matter how sound and how promising, inadvisable.

Patient preferences and values are also important. A discussion with the patient may reveal strong negative attitudes toward a potentially beneficial course of action, or contraindications (e.g., previously unsuspected comorbidities), or possible impediments (e.g., lack of health insurance). Another issue concerns the availability of resources in your health care setting. If the resources needed to apply the evidence were not routinely available, you would need to determine the feasibility of reallocation of resources.

One final issue is the importance of integrating evidence from qualitative research for many clinical actions. Qualitative research can provide rich insights about how patients experience a problem, or about barriers to complying with a treatment. A new intervention with strong potential benefits may fail to achieve the desired outcomes if it is not implemented with sensitivity and understanding of the patients' perspectives. As Morse (2005) has so aptly noted, evidence from an RCT may tell us whether a pill is effective, but qualitative research can help you understand why patients may not swallow the pill.

Implementing the Evidence and Evaluating Outcomes

After the first four steps of the EBP process have been completed, you can use the integrated information to make an evidence-based decision or to provide evidence-based advice. Although the steps in the process, as just described, may seem complicated, in reality the process can be quite efficient— *if* there is an adequate evidence base, and especially if it has been skillfully preprocessed. EBP is most challenging when findings from research are contradictory, inconclusive, or "thin"—that is to say, when better-quality evidence is needed.

One last step in an individual EBP effort concerns evaluation. Part of the evaluation process involves following up to determine whether our action or decision was useful and achieved the desired outcome. Another part, however, concerns an evaluation of how well you are performing EBP. Sackett and colleagues (2000, Chapter 9) offer self-evaluation questions to appraise your efforts. The questions relate to the previous EBP steps, such as asking answerable questions (Am I asking any clinical questions at all? Am I asking well-formulated questions?) and finding external evidence (Do I know the best sources of current evidence? Am I becoming more efficient in my searching?). A self-appraisal may lead to the conclusion that at least some of the clinical questions of interest to you are best addressed as a group effort.

EBP in an Organizational Context

Most nurses practice within organizations, such as hospitals or long-term care settings. For some clinical scenarios, individual nurses may have sufficient decision-making autonomy that they can implement an evidence-based strategy on their own (e.g., an APRN providing advice to a patient about using compression stockings on an upcoming flight). However, there are many situations in which decisions must be made at the organizational level, or are best made among a team of nurses working together to solve a recurrent clinical problem. This section describes some additional considerations that are relevant to institutional efforts at EBP—efforts designed to result in a formal policy or protocol affecting the practice of many nurses.

Many of the steps in organizational EBP projects are similar to the ones described in the previous section. For example, gathering and appraising evidence are key activities in both. However, additional issues are relevant at the organizational level.

Selecting a Problem for an EBP Project

An EBP effort within a unit or institution can emerge in response to clinical scenarios such as those presented earlier, but can also arise in other ways. Some EBP projects are "bottoms-up" efforts that originate in deliberations among clinicians who propose problem-solving activities to their supervisors. Others, however, are "top-down" efforts in which administrators take steps to stimulate creative thought and the use of research evidence among clinicians. This latter approach is increasingly likely to occur in U.S. hospitals as part of the Magnet recognition process.

Example of EBP within the Magnet recognition process: Turkel and colleagues (2005) described a model used by Northwest Community Hospital in Illinois to advance EBP as part of the hospital's pursuit of Magnet status. The five steps that were part of this process included establishing a foundation for EBP, identifying areas of concern, creating internal expertise, implementing EBP, and contributing to a research study.

Several models of EBP, such as the Iowa Model, have distinguished two types of stimulus ("triggers")

for an EBP or RU endeavor: (1) *problem-focused triggers*—the identification of a clinical practice problem in need of solution; and (2) *knowledge-focused triggers*—readings in the research literature. Problem-focused triggers may arise in the normal course of clinical practice (as in the case of the clinical scenarios described earlier) or in the context of quality-assessment or quality-improvement efforts. This problem identification approach is likely to have staff support if the selected problem is one that numerous nurses have encountered, and is likely to have considerable clinical relevance because a clinical situation generated interest in the problem in the first place.

Gennaro, Hodnett, and Kearney (2001) advised nurses following this approach to begin by clarifying the practice problem that needs to be solved and framing it as a broad question. The goal can be finding the best way to anticipate a problem (how to *diagnose* it) or how best to solve a problem (how to *intervene*). Initial clinical practice questions may well take the form of "What is the best way to…?"—for example, "What is the best way to stabilize weight in patients with advanced cancer?" These initial questions would have to be transformed to more focused clinical questions capable of being answered through a search for and appraisal of evidence, as previously described.

A second catalyst for an EBP project is the research literature, that is, knowledge-focused triggers. Sometimes this catalyst takes the form of a new clinical guideline, or the impetus could emerge from discussions in a journal club. For EBP projects with knowledge-focused triggers, an assessment might need to be made of the clinical relevance and applicability of the research. The central issue is whether a problem of significance to nurses in that particular setting will be solved by making a change or introducing an innovation. Titler and Everett (2001) offer some suggestions for selecting interventions to test, using concepts from Rogers' Diffusion of Innovations Model.

With both types of triggers, it is important to ensure that there is a consensus about the importance of the problem and the need for improving practice. The first decision point in the Iowa Model (see Fig. 2.2) is the determination of whether the topic is a priority for the organization considering practice changes. Titler and colleagues (2001) advise that the following issues be taken into account when finalizing a topic for EBP: the topic's fit with the organization's strategic plan, the magnitude of the problem, the number of people invested in the problem, support of nurse leaders and of those in other disciplines, costs, and possible barriers to change. Rosenfeld and colleagues (2000) offered a model for prioritizing practice problems as perceived by staff nurses.

Addressing Practical Issues in Organizational EBP Efforts

Many studies have found that the most pervasive barriers to EBP are organizational, and so one upfront issue is that nurse administrators need to create structures and processes that facilitate research translation. Nursing leaders can support EBP as an approach to clinical decision making in many ways, including providing nurses with sufficient time away from their clinical responsibilities to undertake the necessary EBP activities, making available financial and material resources, and developing collaborations with potential mentors who can provide guidance and direction in the search for and appraisal of evidence.

In the early stages of an EBP effort, some other practical matters should be resolved even before a search for evidence begins. One major issue concerns the organization of the team. A motivated and motivational team leader is essential. Another important ingredient is the recruitment and development of EBP team members—which often require an interdisciplinary perspective. Identifying tasks to be undertaken, developing a realistic timetable and budget, assigning members to specific tasks, and scheduling meetings are necessary to ensure that the effort will progress. Finally, it is wise for the team to solicit the support of all key stakeholders who might affect project activities and the eventual implementation of any EBP changes.

Finding and Appraising Evidence: Clinical Practice Guidelines

We focus in this section on clinical practice guidelines because, for an organizational EBP effort, the best possible scenario involves identifying appropriate clinical practice guidelines (or other decision support tools) that have been developed based on rigorous research evidence. Of course, for many problem areas, clinical guidelines will need to be *developed* based on the evidence, and not just implemented or adapted for use.

Some suggestions for locating guidelines were offered earlier, but a few additional tips may be useful. In addition to looking for guidelines in national clearinghouses and in the websites of professional organizations, EBP teams can search bibliographic databases such as MEDLINE or EMBASE. Search terms such as the following can be used: *practice guideline, clinical practice guideline, best practice guideline, evidence-based guideline, standards,* and *consensus statement.* Graham and colleagues (2002) have noted that guidelines are increasingly being posted on the World Wide Web, and these might be missed if you rely exclusively on bibliographic databases. Thus, it is also prudent to do an Internet search for guidelines.

If a relevant guideline is identified, it should be carefully appraised. Several guideline appraisal instruments are available, but the one that appears to have the broadest support is the Appraisal of Guidelines Research and Evaluation (AGREE) Instrument (AGREE Collaboration, 2001). This tool, which was originally developed in the United Kingdom and Europe, has been translated into more than a dozen languages and has been endorsed by the World Health Organization. The AGREE instrument consists of ratings of quality on a 4-point scale (strongly agree, agree, disagree, and strongly disagree) for 23 quality dimensions organized in six domains: Scope and Purpose; Stakeholder Involvement; Rigor of Development; Clarity and Presentation; Application; and Editorial Independence. As examples, one of the statements in the Scope and Purpose domain is: "The patients to whom the guideline is meant to apply are specifically described"; and one of the statements in the Rigor of

Development domain is: "The guideline has been externally reviewed by experts prior to its publication." The AGREE instrument ideally should be applied to the guideline under consideration by a team of two to four appraisers. The instrument and instructions regarding its use are available at *http://www. agreecollaboration.org.*

One final issue is that guidelines typically change more slowly than the evidence. If a high-quality guideline was not recently released, it is advisable to determine whether more up-to-date evidence would alter (or strengthen) the guideline's recommendations. Shekelle and colleagues (2001), who did an analysis of the then-current validity of 17 clinical practice guidelines published by AHRQ, found that 13 needed to be updated and recommended that, to avoid obsolescence, guidelines should be reassessed for validity every 3 years.

Making Decisions Based on Evidence Appraisals

In the Iowa Model, the synthesis and appraisal of research evidence provides the basis for a second major decision. The crux of the decision concerns whether the research base is sufficient to justify an EBP change—for example, whether an existing clinical practice guideline is of sufficient high quality that it can be used or adapted locally, or whether the research evidence is sufficiently rigorous to recommend a practice innovation.

Coming to conclusions about the adequacy of the research evidence can result in several possible outcomes with different pathways for further action. If the research base is weak or inconclusive, the team could either abandon the EBP project or assemble other types of evidence (e.g., through consultation with experts, surveys of clients, and so on) and assess whether that evidence suggests a practice change. Another possibility is to pursue an original clinical study to address the practice question directly, thereby gathering new evidence and contributing to the base of practice knowledge. This last course of action may well be impractical for many and would clearly result in years of delay before any further conclusions could be drawn. If, on the other hand, there is a solid research base or a

high-quality clinical practice guideline, then the team would develop plans for moving forward with implementing a practice innovation.

Assessing Implementation Potential

In some models of the EBP process, the next step after concluding that evidence supports a change in practice is the development and testing of the innovation, followed by an assessment of organizational "fit." Other models recommend steps to assess the appropriateness of innovation within the specific organizational context before implementing it. In some cases, such an assessment (or aspects of it) may be warranted even before embarking on efforts to assemble best evidence. We think a preliminary assessment of the *implementation potential* (or, *environmental readiness*) of a clinical innovation is often sensible, although there may be situations with little need for a formal assessment.

In determining the implementation potential of an innovation in a particular setting, several issues should be considered, particularly the transferability of the innovation, the feasibility of implementing it, and its cost/benefit ratio. Box 2.2 ⊗ presents some relevant assessment questions for these three issues.

- *Transferability*. The main issue with regard to transferability is whether it makes sense to implement the innovation in your practice setting. If there is some aspect of the setting that is fundamentally incongruent with the innovation—in terms of its philosophy, types of client served, personnel, or administrative structure—then it might not be prudent to try to adopt the innovation, even if it has been shown to be clinically effective in other contexts. One possibility, however, is that some organizational changes could be made to make the "fit" better.
- *Feasibility*. The feasibility questions in Box 2.2 address various practical concerns about the availability of staff and resources, the organizational climate, the need for and availability of external assistance, and the potential for clinical evaluation. An important issue is whether nurses will have (or will share) control over the innovation. Hopefully, if nurses will not have full

BOX 2.2 Criteria for Evaluating the Implementation Potential of an Innovation Under Scrutiny

TRANSFERABILITY OF THE FINDINGS

1. Will the innovation "fit" in the proposed setting?
2. How similar are the target population in the research and that in the new setting?
3. Is the philosophy of care underlying the innovation fundamentally different from the philosophy prevailing in the practice setting? How entrenched is the prevailing philosophy?
4. Is there a sufficiently large number of clients in the practice setting who could benefit from the innovation?
5. Will the innovation take too long to implement and evaluate?

FEASIBILITY

1. Will nurses have the freedom to carry out the innovation? Will they have the freedom to terminate the innovation if it is considered undesirable?
2. Will the implementation of the innovation interfere inordinately with current staff functions?
3. Does the administration support the innovation? Is the organizational climate conducive to research utilization?
4. Is there a fair degree of consensus among the staff and among the administrators that the innovation could be beneficial and should be tested? Are there major pockets of resistance or uncooperativeness that could undermine efforts to implement and evaluate the innovation?
5. To what extent will the implementation of the innovation cause friction within the organization? Does the utilization project have the support and cooperation of departments outside the nursing department?
6. Are the skills needed to carry out the utilization project (both the implementation and the clinical evaluation) available in the nursing staff? If not, how difficult will it be to collaborate with or to secure the assistance of others with the necessary skills?
7. Does the organization have the equipment and facilities necessary for the innovation? If not, is there a way to obtain the needed resources?
8. If nursing staff need to be released from other practice activities to learn about and implement the innovation, what is the likelihood that this will happen?
9. Are appropriate measuring tools available for a clinical evaluation of the innovation?

COST/BENEFIT RATIO OF THE INNOVATION

1. What are the risks to which clients would be exposed during the implementation of the innovation?
2. What are the potential benefits that could result from the implementation of the innovation?
3. What are the risks of maintaining current practices (i.e., the risks of *not* trying the innovation)?
4. What are the material costs of implementing the innovation? What are the costs in the short term during testing, and what are the costs in the long run, if the change is to be institutionalized?
5. What are the material costs of *not* implementing the innovation (i.e., could the new procedure result in some efficiencies that could lower the cost of providing service)?
6. What are the potential nonmaterial costs of implementing the innovation to the organization (e.g., lower staff morale, staff turnover, absenteeism)?
7. What are the potential nonmaterial benefits of implementing the innovation (e.g., improved staff morale, improved staff recruitment)?

control over a new procedure, the interdependent nature of the project has been identified early and the EBP team has the necessary interdisciplinary representatives.

- *Cost/benefit ratio.* A critical part of any decision to proceed with an EBP project is a careful assessment of the costs and benefits of the change. The assessment should encompass likely costs and benefits to various groups, including clients, staff, and the overall organization. Clearly, the most important factor is the client. If the degree of risk in introducing a new procedure is high, then the potential benefits must be great and the knowledge base must be extremely sound. A cost/benefit assessment should consider the opposite side of the coin as well: the costs and benefits of *not* instituting an innovation. It is sometimes easy to forget that the status quo bears its own risks and that failure to change—especially when such change is based on a firm evidence base—is costly to clients, to organizations, and to the nursing community.

If the implementation assessment suggests that there might be problems in testing the innovation in that particular practice setting, then the team can either identify a new problem and begin the process anew or consider adopting a plan to improve the implementation potential (e.g., seeking external resources if costs were prohibitive).

➲ **TIP:** Documentation of all steps in the EBP process, including the implementation potential of an innovation, is highly recommended. Committing ideas to writing is useful because such a document can help to resolve ambiguities, serve as a problem-solving tool if problems emerge, and be used to persuade others of the value of the project. All aspects of the EBP project should be transparent and, to the extent possible, reproducible.

Developing Evidence-Based Guidelines or Protocols

If the implementation criteria are met and the evidence base is judged to be adequate, the team can prepare an action plan to move the effort forward,

which would involve laying out strategies for designing and piloting the new clinical practice. In most cases, a key activity will involve developing a local evidence-based clinical practice protocol or guideline, or adapting an existing one.

If a relevant clinical practice guideline has been judged to be of sufficiently high quality, the EBP team needs to decide whether to (1) adopt it in its entirety; (2) adopt only certain recommendations, while disregarding others (e.g., recommendations for which the evidence base is less sound); or (3) adapt the guidelines by making changes deemed necessary based on local circumstances. The risk in modifying guidelines is that the adaptation will not adequately reflect the research evidence. Local adaptations should not involve changing existing evidence-based recommendations unless the evidence itself has changed.

If there is no existing clinical practice guideline (or if existing guidelines are weak), the team will need to develop its own protocol or guideline reflecting the accumulated research evidence. Strategies for developing clinical practice guidelines are suggested by DiCenso and colleagues (2005, Chapter 10), Melnyk and Fineout-Overholt (2005, Chapter 9), and Shekelle and colleagues (1999). Whether a guideline is developed "from scratch" or adapted from an existing one, independent peer review is advisable to ensure that the guidelines are clear, comprehensive, and congruent with best existing evidence.

➲ **TIP:** Guidelines should be clear and user-friendly. Visual devices such as flow charts and decision trees are often useful.

Implementing and Evaluating the Innovation

Once the EBP product has been developed, the next step is to **pilot test** it (give it a trial run) in a clinical setting and to evaluate the outcome. Building on the Iowa Model, this phase of the project likely would involve the following activities:

1. Developing an evaluation plan (e.g., identifying outcomes to be achieved, determining how many clients to involve in the pilot, deciding when and how often to collect outcome information)

2. Collecting information relating to those out-comes before implementing the innovation, to develop a baseline against which the outcomes of the innovation can be compared

3. Training relevant staff in the use of the new guideline and, if necessary, "marketing" the innovation to users so that it is given a fair test

4. Trying the guideline out on one or more units or with a group of clients

5. Evaluating the pilot project, in terms of both process (e.g., How was the innovation received? To what extent were the guidelines actually fol-lowed? What implementation problems were encountered?) and outcomes (e.g., How were client outcomes affected? What were the costs?)

➲ **TIP:** DiCenso and her colleagues (2002) have developed a toolkit designed to facilitate the implementation of clinical practice guidelines. The toolkit is available on the Internet (*http://www.rnao.org*).

A variety of research strategies and designs can be used to evaluate the innovation, as described in our discussion of evaluation research in Chapter 12. In most cases, a fairly informal evaluation will be adequate, for example, comparing outcome information from hospital records before and after the innovation, and gathering information about patient and staff satisfaction. Qualitative informa-tion can also contribute considerably to the evaluation (Sandelowski, 1996, 2004). A qualita-tive perspective can uncover subtleties about the implementation process and help to explain research findings.

Evaluation information should be gathered over a sufficiently long period (typically 6 to 12 months) to allow for a true test of a "mature" innovation. The end result of this process is a decision about whether to adopt the innovation, to modify it for ongoing use, or to revert to prior practices. Another optional step, but one that is highly advisable, is the dissemination of the results of the project so that other practicing nurses can benefit. Finally, the EBP team should develop a plan for when the pro-tocol will be reviewed and, if necessary, updated based on new research evidence or ongoing infor-mation about local costs and outcomes.

➲ **TIP:** Every nurse can play a role in using research evidence. Here are some strategies:

- *Read widely and critically.* Professionally accountable nurses keep abreast of important developments and read journals relating to their specialty, including research reports in them.

- *Attend professional conferences.* Many nursing conferences include presentations of studies that have clinical relevance. Conference attendees get opportunities to meet researchers and to explore practice implications.

- *Learn to expect evidence that a procedure is effective.* Every time nurses or nursing students are told about a standard nursing procedure, they have a right to ask the question: Why? Nurses need to develop expectations that the decisions they make in their clinical practice are based on sound evidence-based rationales.

- *Become involved in a journal club.* Many organizations that employ nurses sponsor journal clubs that review research articles that have potential relevance to practice. The traditional approach for a journal club (nurses coming together as a group to discuss and critique an article) has in some settings been replaced with electronic online journal clubs that acknowledge time constraints and the inability of nurses from all shifts to come together at one time.

- *Pursue and participate in RU/EBP projects.* Several studies have found that nurses who are involved in research-related activities (e.g., a utilization project or data collection activities) develop more positive attitudes toward research and better research skills.

RESEARCH EXAMPLE

Thousands of EBP and RU projects are underway in practice settings worldwide, and many that have been described in the nursing literature offer rich information about planning and implementing such an endeavor. In this section, we summarize a project that was funded by the AHRQ.

Study: "Translation research in long-term care: Improving pain management in nursing homes" (Jones et al., 2004)

Background: In 1999, AHRQ launched an initiative that funded projects designed to close the gap between research evidence and health care practices. The initiative, Translating Research into Practice (TRIP), funded 14 projects initially (TRIP-I) and another 13 in 2000 (TRIP-II). A key feature of the TRIP grants is the development of partnerships between researchers and health care organizations. Several nurse researchers received funding from TRIP grants, including Katherine R. Jones.

Purpose: Jones and her colleagues sought to address a persistent problem in long-term care settings, the suboptimal management of pain. The specific aims of the project were to (1) develop and test a multifaceted, culturally competent intervention to improve nursing home pain practices; (2) improve staff, resident, and physician knowledge about pain and its management; (3) improve pain practices in nursing homes; and (4) improve nursing home policies and procedures relating to pain.

Framework: The intervention strategy was based on Rogers' (1995) Diffusion of Innovation Theory. According to this model, diffusion is the process by which an innovation—such as pain clinical practice guidelines—is communicated and comes to be adopted. In the model, factors influencing adoption success include characteristics of the innovation, characteristics of potential users, characteristics of the overall social system, and the methods of communication. The investigators concluded that the complexity of the pain innovation, the presence of preexisting attitudes about pain management, high staff turnover and low skill mix, and the regulatory environment of the nursing homes imposed severe challenges.

Method: The project team did not develop its own clinical practice guidelines but rather used evidence-based guidelines developed by the American Geriatrics Society and the American Directors Association. The focus of the project involved implementing a structured intervention to encourage adoption of best-practice procedures among nursing home staff. The intervention included both an educational component (e.g., four 30-minute interactive sessions delivered over a 6-month period, a video for residents and family members) and a behavioral component (e.g., formation of a 3-member internal pain team to function as change agents). The project involved the cooperation of 12 nursing homes in Colorado, 6 of which implemented the intervention and 6 of which did not. Jones and her colleagues collected outcome information from all 12 nursing homes before and after the intervention.

Findings: The intervention was partially successful in changing pain practices in the nursing homes that received the intervention. There was no significant reduction in the percentage of residents reporting pain, but there was a significant decrease in the percentage reporting *constant* pain. Staff knowledge about and attitudes toward pain management changed relatively little.

Conclusions: The researchers concluded that the limited success of the intervention was partially attributable to high staff turnover, which resulted in incomplete exposure to the educational components by most staff, and turnover of directors, which influenced constancy of the message. However, the project provided strong evidence of the need for improvements because it documented deficits in knowledge and suboptimal attitudes and beliefs about pain and its management by nursing home staff.

●○●○●○●○●○●○●○●○●○●○●○●○●

SUMMARY POINTS

- **Evidence-based practice (EBP)** is the conscientious use of current best evidence in making clinical decisions about patient care; it is a clinical problem-solving strategy that de-emphasizes decision-making based on custom and emphasizes the integration of research evidence with clinical expertise and patient preferences.

- **Research utilization (RU)** and EBP are overlapping concepts that concern efforts to use research as a basis for clinical decisions, but RU *starts* with a research-based innovation that gets evaluated for possible use in practice.

- RU exists on a continuum, with direct utilization of some specific innovation at one end and more diffuse situations in which users are influenced in their thinking about an issue based on research findings at the other end.

- Nurse researchers have undertaken several major utilization projects (e.g., the **Conduct and Utilization of Research in Nursing [CURN] project**), which demonstrated that RU can be increased but also shed light on barriers to utilization.

- Two underpinnings of the EBP movement are the Cochrane Collaboration (which is based on the work of British epidemiologist Archie Cochrane) and the clinical learning strategy called *evidence-based medicine* developed at the McMaster Medical School.
- EBP involves weighing various types of evidence in an effort to determine *best evidence*; often an **evidence hierarchy** is used to rank study findings and other information according to the strength of evidence provided. Hierarchies for evaluating evidence about health care interventions typically put systematic reviews of *randomized clinical trials* (RCTs) at the pinnacle and expert opinion at the base.
- Resources to support EBP are growing at a rapid pace. Among the resources are systematic reviews (and electronic databases that make them easy to locate); evidence-based clinical practice guidelines; a wealth of other preappraised evidence that makes it possible to practice EBP efficiently; research findings on factors to address in an EBP project; and models of RU and EBP that provide a framework for EBP efforts.
- **Systematic reviews**, a cornerstone of EBP, are rigorous integrations of research evidence from multiple studies on a topic. Systematic reviews can involve either qualitative, narrative approaches to integration (including **metasynthesis** of qualitative studies), or quantitative methods (**meta-analysis**) that integrate findings statistically.
- Evidence-based **clinical practice guidelines** combine a synthesis of research evidence with specific recommendations for clinical decision making. Clinical practice guidelines should be carefully and systematically appraised, for example, using the Appraisal of Guidelines Research and Evaluation (AGREE) instrument.
- Journals and professional organizations are increasingly publishing brief critical synopses of research evidence from high-quality studies and systematic reviews. One type of synopsis has been called a **critically appraised topic** (**CAT**), which typically begins with the "clinical bottom line" or best-practice recommendation on a topic.
- Researchers have found that EBP/RU efforts often face a variety of barriers, including the quality of the evidence base, nurses' characteristics (e.g., limited training in research and EBP), and organizational factors (e.g., lack of organizational support).
- Many models of RU and EBP have been developed, including models that provide a framework for individual clinicians (e.g., the **Stetler Model**) and others for organizations or teams of clinicians (e.g., the **Iowa Model** of Evidence-Based Practice to Promote Quality Care). Another widely used model in RU/EBP efforts is Rogers' **Diffusion of Innovations Theory.**
- Individual nurses have regular opportunity to put research into practice. The 5 basic steps for individual EBP are: (1) framing an answerable clinical question; (2) searching for relevant research-based evidence; (3) appraising and synthesizing the evidence; (4) integrating evidence with other factors; and (5) assessing effectiveness.
- An appraisal of the evidence involves such considerations as the validity of study findings; their clinical importance; the precision of estimates of effects; associated costs and risks; and utility in a particular clinical situation.
- EBP in an organizational context involves many of the same steps as an individual EBP effort, but tends to be more formalized and must take organizational and interpersonal factors into account. "Triggers" for an organizational project include both pressing clinical problems and existing knowledge.
- Team-based or organizational EBP projects typically involve the development or adaptation of clinical practice guidelines or clinical protocols. Before these products can be tested, there should be an assessment of the *implementation potential* of the innovation, which includes the dimensions of transferability of findings, feasibility of using the findings in the new setting, and the cost/benefit ratio of a new practice.

- Once an evidence-based protocol or guideline has been developed and deemed worthy of implementation, the team can move forward with a **pilot test** of the innovation and an assessment of the outcomes before widespread adoption.

●●●●●●●●●●●●●●●●●●●●●●●

STUDY ACTIVITIES

Chapter 2 of the accompanying *Resource Manual to Accompany Nursing Research: Generating and Assessing Evidence for Nursing Practice, 8th edition*, offers exercises and study suggestions for reinforcing the concepts taught in this chapter. In addition, the following study questions can be addressed:

1. Consider your personal situation. What are the barriers that might inhibit your use of research findings in your practice setting? What steps might be taken to address those barriers? What characteristics of your setting promote EBP?

2. With regard to the research example featured at the end of this chapter (Jones et al., 2004), answer the following questions:
   a. What activities could Jones and colleagues have undertaken to assess the implementation potential of the nursing homes before introducing the intervention?
   b. What might Jones and her colleagues have done to develop greater commitment to the intervention among the stakeholders in the nursing homes?

●●●●●●●●●●●●●●●●●●●●●●

STUDIES CITED IN CHAPTER 2

Methodologic or theoretical references cited in this chapter can be found in a separate section at the end of the book.

Beck, C. T. (2004). Post-traumatic stress disorder due to childbirth: The aftermath. *Nursing Research, 53*(4), 216–224.

Berenstein, E. G., & Ortiz, Z. (2005). Megestrol acetate for the treatment of anorexia-cachexia syndrome. *Cochrane Database of Systematic Reviews,* No. CD004310.

Brett, J. L. L. (1987). Use of nursing practice research findings. *Nursing Research, 36,* 344–349.

Coyle, L. A., & Sokop, A. G. (1990). Innovation adoption behavior among nurses. *Nursing Research, 39,* 176–180.

Egerod, I., & Hansen, G. M. (2005). Evidence-based practice among Danish cardiac nurses: A national survey. *Journal of Advanced Nursing, 51*(5), 465–473.

Estabrooks, C. A. (1999). The conceptual structure of research utilization. *Research in Nursing & Health, 22,* 203–216.

French, B. (2005). Evaluating research for use in practice: What criteria do specialist nurses use? *Journal of Advanced Nursing, 50*(3), 235–243.

Gerrish, K., & Clayton, J. (2004). Promoting evidence-based practice: An organizational approach. *Journal of Nursing Management, 12,* 114–123.

Glacken, M., & Chaney, D. (2004). Perceived barriers and facilitators to implementing research findings in the Irish practice setting. *Journal of Clinical Nursing, 13*(6), 731–740.

Goodman, J. H. (2005). Becoming an involved father of an infant. *Journal of Obstetric, Gynecologic, & Neonatal Nursing, 34*(2), 190–200.

Hodnett, E. D., Downe, S., Edwards, N., & Walsh, D. (2005). Home-like versus conventional institutional settings for birth. *Cochrane Database of Systematic Reviews,* No. CD000012.

Hsieh, H. F., & Lee, F. P. (2005). Graduated compression stockings as prophylaxis for flight-related venous thrombosis: Systematic literature review. *Journal of Advanced Nursing, 51*(1), 83–98.

Hutchinson, A. M., & Johnston, L. (2004). Bridging the divide: A survey of nurses' opinions regarding barriers to, and facilitators of, research utilization in the practice setting. *Journal of Clinical Nursing, 13,* 304–315.

Jatoi, A. (2005). Fish oil, lean tissue, and cancer: Is there a role for eicosapentaenoic acid in treating the cancer/anorexia/weight loss syndrome? *Critical Review of Oncology & Hematology, 55,* 37–43.

Jones, K. R., Fink, R., Vojir, C., Pepper, G., Hutt, E., Clark, L., Scott, J., Martinez, R., Vincent, D., & Mellis, B. K. (2004). Translation research in long-term care: Improving pain management in nursing homes. *Worldviews on Evidence-Based Nursing, 1*(S1), S13–S20.

Ketefian, S. (1975). Application of selected nursing research findings into nursing practice. *Nursing Research, 24,* 89–92.

Kirchhoff, K. T. (1982). A diffusion survey of coronary precautions. *Nursing Research, 31,* 196–201.

Margaret-Milner, F., Estabrooks, C. A., & Humphrey, C. (2005). Clinical nurse educators as agents for change: Increasing research utilization. *International Journal of Nursing Studies, 42*(8), 899–914.

McCleary, L., & Brown, G. T. (2003). Barriers to paediatric nurses' research utilization. *Journal of Advanced Nursing, 42,* 364–372.

Oranta, O., Routasalo, P., & Hupli, M. (2002). Barriers to and facilitators of research utilization among Finnish registered nurses. *Journal of Clinical Nursing, 11,* 205–213.

Patiraki, E., Karlou, C., Papadopoulou, D., Spyridou, A., Kouloukoura, C., Bare, E., & Merkouris, A. (2004). Barriers in implementing research findings in cancer care: The Greek registered nurses' perception. *European Journal of Oncology Nursing, 8*(3), 245–256.

Pepler, C. J., Edgar, L., Frisch, S., Rennick, J., Swidzinski, M., White, C., Brown, T. G., & Gross, J. (2005). Unit culture and research-based nursing practice in acute care. *Canadian Journal of Nursing Research, 37*(3), 66–85.

Rutledge, D. N., Greene, P., Mooney, K., Nail, L. M., & Ropka, M. (1996). Use of research-based practices by oncology staff nurses. *Oncology Nursing Forum, 23,* 1235–1244.

Shekelle, P. G., Ortiz, E., Rhodes, S., Morton, S. C., Eccles, M. P., Grimshaw, J. M., & Woolf, S. H. (2001). Validity of the Agency for Healthcare Research and Quality clinical practice guidelines: How quickly do guidelines become outdated? *Journal of the American Medical Association, 286*(12), 1461–1467.

Snethen, J. A., Broome, M. E., & Cashin, S. E. (2006). Effective weight loss for overweight children: A meta-analysis of intervention studies. *Journal of Pediatric Nursing, 21*(1), 45–56.

Thomas, L., Cullum, M., McColl, E., Rousseau, N., Soutter, J., & Steen, N. (2000). Guidelines in professions allied to medicine. *Cochrane Database of Systematic Reviews,* No. CD000349.

Thurston, N. E., & King, K. M. (2004). Implementing evidence-based practice: Walking the talk. *Applied Nursing Research, 17,* 239–247.

3 Generating Evidence: Key Concepts and Steps in Qualitative and Quantitative Research

M ost of the rest of this book concerns the generation of new evidence for use in nursing practice. The intent of most chapters is to provide guidance in designing and conducting studies that yield the best possible evidence for inquiries of relevance to nurses.

This chapter covers a lot of ground—but, for many of you, it is familiar ground. For those who have taken an earlier course on understanding and critiquing research reports, this chapter provides a review of key terms, concepts, and steps in the research process. For those without much previous exposure to research methods, this is an important chapter that offers basic grounding in research terminology.

Research, like any discipline, has its own language—its own *jargon*. Some terms are used by both qualitative and quantitative researchers, whereas others are used predominantly by one or the other group. To make matters even more complex, most research jargon used in nursing research has its roots in the social sciences, but sometimes different terms for the same concepts are used in medical research; we cover both but acknowledge that social scientific jargon predominates.

FUNDAMENTAL RESEARCH TERMS AND CONCEPTS

When researchers address a problem or answer a question through disciplined research—regardless of the underlying paradigm—they are doing a **study** (or an **investigation** or **research project**). Studies involve various people working together in different roles.

The Faces and Places of Research

Studies with humans involve two sets of people: those who do the research and those who provide the information. In a quantitative study, the people being studied are called **subjects** or **study participants**, as shown in Table 3.1. (Subjects who provide information by answering questions—e.g., by filling out a questionnaire—may be called **respondents**.) In a qualitative study, the individuals cooperating in the study play an active rather than a passive role in the research, and are therefore referred to as **informants, key informants**, or study participants. Collectively, both in qualitative and quantitative studies, study participants comprise the **sample**.

The person who conducts the research is the **researcher** or **investigator**. Studies are often undertaken by several people rather than by a single researcher. **Collaborative research** involving a research team with a mixture of clinical, theoretical, and methodologic skills is increasingly common in health care research. When a study is done by a team, the lead person is the **project director** or **principal investigator (PI)**. Two or three researchers collaborating equally are **co-investigators**. **Reviewers** are

TABLE 3.1	Key Terms Used in Quantitative and Qualitative Research	
CONCEPT	**QUANTITATIVE TERM**	**QUALITATIVE TERM**
Person Contributing Information	Subject Study participant Respondent	— Study participant Informant, key informant
Person Undertaking the Study	Researcher Investigator Scientist	Researcher Investigator —
That Which Is Being Investigated	— Concepts Constructs Variables	Phenomena Concepts — —

System of Organizing Concepts	Theory, theoretical framework
	Conceptual framework,
	    conceptual model
		Theory
		Conceptual framework,
		    sensitizing framework

Information Gathered	Data (numeric values)	Data (narrative descriptions)
Connections Between Concepts	Relationships (cause-and-effect, functional)	Patterns of association
Logical Reasoning Processes	Deductive reasoning	Inductive reasoning

sometimes called on to critique various aspects of a study and offer feedback. If these people are at a similar level of experience as the researchers, they may be called **peer reviewers**. When financial assistance is obtained to pay for research costs, the organization providing the money is the **funder** or **sponsor**.

In large-scale projects, dozens of individuals may be involved in planning, managing, and conducting the study. The examples of staffing configurations that follow span the continuum from an extremely large project to a more modest one.

Examples of staffing on a quantitative study: The first author of this book was involved in a complex, multicomponent 6-year study of poor women living in four major cities (Cleveland, Los Angeles, Miami, and Philadelphia). As part of the study, she and two colleagues prepared a book-length report documenting the health problems and health care

concerns of about 4000 welfare mothers who were interviewed in 1998 and again in 2001 (Polit, London, & Martinez, 2001). The total project staff for this research involved over 100 people, including two co-PIs; lead investigators of six project components (Polit was one); more than 50 interviewers and supervisors; and dozens of other senior-level researchers, research assistants, computer programmers, secretaries, editors, and other support staff. Several health consultants, including a prominent nurse researcher (Linda Aiken), were reviewers of the report. The project was funded by a consortium of government agencies and private foundations.

Examples of staffing on a qualitative study: Beck (2002) conducted a qualitative study focusing on the experiences of mothers of twins. The team included Beck as the PI (who gathered and analyzed all the information herself); a childbirth educator (who helped to recruit mothers into the study); an administrative assistant (who handled a variety of administrative tasks, like paying stipends to the mothers); a transcriber (who listened to tape-recorded conversations with the mothers and typed them up verbatim); and a secretary (who handled correspondence). This study had some financial support through Beck's university.

Research can be undertaken in a variety of *settings* (the specific places where information is gathered), and in one or more *sites*. Some studies take place in **naturalistic settings**—in the field, such as in people's homes or places of work. At the other extreme, some studies are done in highly controlled **laboratory settings**. Researchers make decisions about where to conduct a study based on the nature of the research question and the type of information needed to address it. Qualitative researchers are especially likely to engage in **fieldwork** in natural settings because they are interested in the contexts of people's lives and experiences. The *site* is the overall location for the research—it could be an entire community (e.g., a Haitian neighborhood in Miami) or an institution within a community (e.g., a hospital in Toronto). Researchers sometimes engage in **multisite studies** because the use of multiple sites usually offers a larger or more diverse sample of study participants

Example of a multisite study in naturalistic settings: Irvine and colleagues (2006) conducted in-depth interviews with a range of health care professionals in acute and community settings throughout Wales. The interviews focused on language awareness and factors that facilitate or impede language-sensitive health care practice in bilingual settings.

The Building Blocks of Research

Phenomena, Concepts, and Constructs

Research involves abstractions. For example, the terms *pain*, *quality of life*, and *resilience* are all abstractions of particular aspects of human behavior and characteristics. These abstractions are called **concepts** or, in qualitative studies, **phenomena**.

Researchers may also use the term **construct**. Like a concept, a construct refers to an abstraction

or mental representation inferred from situations or behaviors. Kerlinger and Lee (2000) distinguish concepts from constructs by noting that constructs are abstractions that are deliberately and systematically invented (or constructed) by researchers for a specific purpose. For example, *self-care* in Orem's Model of Health Maintenance is a construct. The terms *construct* and *concept* are sometimes used interchangeably, although by convention, a construct often refers to a more complex abstraction than a concept.

Theories and Conceptual Models

A **theory** is a systematic, abstract explanation of some aspect of reality. In a theory, concepts are knitted together into a coherent system to describe or explain some aspect of the world. Theories play a role in both qualitative and quantitative research.

In a quantitative study, researchers often start with a theory, **framework**, or **conceptual model** (the distinctions are discussed in Chapter 6). On the basis of theory, researchers make predictions about how phenomena will behave in the real world *if the theory is true*. The specific predictions deduced from the theory are tested through research, and the results are used to support, reject, or modify the theory.

In qualitative research, theories may be used in various ways (Sandelowski, 1993a). Sometimes conceptual or **sensitizing frameworks**—derived from various qualitative research traditions that we describe later in this chapter—provide an impetus for a study or offer an orienting world view with clear conceptual underpinnings. In such studies, the framework helps to guide the inquiry and to interpret gathered information. In other qualitative studies, theory is the *product* of the research: The investigators use information from study participants inductively to develop a theory firmly rooted in the participants' experiences. The goal is to develop a theory that explains phenomena *as they exist*, not as they are preconceived. Theories generated in qualitative studies are sometimes subjected to controlled testing in quantitative studies.

Variables

In quantitative studies, concepts are usually called **variables**. A variable, as the name implies, is something that varies. Weight, anxiety levels, and body temperature are all variables—each varies from one person to another. In fact, nearly all aspects of human beings are variables. If everyone weighed 150 pounds, weight would not be a variable, it would be a **constant**. But it is precisely because people and conditions *do* vary that most research is conducted. Most quantitative researchers seek to understand how or why things vary, and to learn how differences in one variable are related to differences in another. For example, in lung cancer research, lung cancer is a variable because not everybody has this disease. Researchers have studied factors that might be linked to lung cancer, such as cigarette smoking. Smoking is also a variable because not everyone smokes. A variable, then, is any quality of a person, group, or situation that varies or takes on different values—typically, numeric values. Variables are the central building blocks of quantitative studies.

A term frequently used in connection with variables is *heterogeneity*. When an attribute is extremely varied in the group under investigation, the group is said to be **heterogeneous** with respect to that variable. If the amount of variability is limited, the group is described as relatively **homogeneous**. For example, for the variable height, a group of 2-year-old children is likely to be more homogeneous than a group of 16-year-old adolescents. The degree of **variability** or **heterogeneity** of a group of subjects has implications for study design.

Variables are often inherent characteristics of research subjects, such as their age, blood type, or weight. Variables such as these are *attribute variables*. In many research situations, however, the investigator *creates* a variable. For example, if a researcher tests the effectiveness of patient-controlled analgesia as opposed to intramuscular analgesia in relieving pain after surgery, some patients would be given patient-controlled analgesia and others would receive intramuscular analgesia. In the context of this study, method of pain management is a variable because different patients are given different analgesic methods. Kerlinger and Lee (2000) refer to variables that the researcher creates as *active variables*.

Continuous, Discrete, and Categorical Variables. Some variables take on a wide range of values. A person's age, for instance, can take on values from zero to more than 100, and the values are not restricted to whole numbers. **Continuous variables** have values along a continuum and, in theory, can assume an infinite number of values between two points. For example, consider the continuous variable *weight*: between 1 and 2 pounds, the number of values is limitless: 1.05, 1.7, 1.333, and so on.

By contrast, a **discrete variable** has a finite number of values between any two points, representing discrete quantities. For example, if people were asked how many children they had, they might answer 0, 1, 2, 3, or more. The value for number of children is discrete, because a number such as 1.5 is not meaningful. Between 1 and 3, the only possible value is 2.

Other variables take on a small range of values that do not inherently represent a *quantity*. Blood type, for example, has four values—A, B, AB, and O. Variables that take on a handful of discrete nonquantitative values are **categorical variables**. When categorical variables take on only two values, they may be called **dichotomous variables.** Gender, for example, is dichotomous: male and female.

Dependent and Independent Variables. Many studies are aimed at unraveling and understanding causes of phenomena. Does a nursing intervention *cause* improvements in patient outcomes? Does smoking *cause* lung cancer? The presumed cause is the **independent variable**, and the presumed effect is the **dependent variable**. Some researchers use the term **outcome variable**—the variable capturing the outcome of interest—in lieu of dependent variable.

Variability in the dependent variable is presumed to *depend on* variability in the independent variable. For example, researchers investigate the extent to which lung cancer (the dependent variable) depends on smoking (the independent variable). Or, investigators may be concerned with the extent to which patients' perception of pain (the dependent variable) depends on different nursing actions (the independent variable).

Frequently, the terms *independent variable* and *dependent variable* are used to indicate *direction of influence* rather than causal link. For example, suppose a researcher studied the mental health of caregivers caring for spouses with Alzheimer's disease and found better mental health outcomes for wives than for husbands. The researcher might be unwilling to conclude that caregivers' mental health was *caused* by gender. Yet the direction of influence clearly runs from gender to mental health: it makes *no* sense to suggest that caregivers' mental health influenced their gender! Although in this example the researcher does not infer a cause-and-effect connection, it is appropriate to conceptualize mental health as the dependent variable and gender as the independent variable, because it is the caregivers' mental health that the researcher is interested in understanding, explaining, or predicting.

Many dependent variables studied by nurse researchers have multiple causes or antecedents. If we were interested in studying factors that influence people's weight, for example, we might consider their height, physical activity, and diet as independent variables. Two or more *dependent* variables also may be of interest to researchers. For example, a researcher may compare the effectiveness of two methods of nursing care for children with cystic fibrosis. Several dependent variables could be used to assess treatment effectiveness, such as length of hospital stay, number of recurrent respiratory infections, presence of cough, and so forth. It is common to design studies with multiple independent and dependent variables.

Variables are not *inherently* dependent or independent. A dependent variable in one study could be an independent variable in another. For example, a study might examine the effect of an exercise intervention (the independent variable) on osteoporosis (the dependent variable). Another study might investigate the effect of osteoporosis (the independent variable) on bone fracture incidence (the dependent variable). In short, whether a variable is independent or dependent is a function of the role that it plays in a particular study.

Example of independent and dependent variables: *Research question:* What is the effect of critical care nurses' work schedule on patient safety? (Scott et al., 2006)
Independent variable: Nurses' work schedule
Dependent variable: Patient safety

Conceptual and Operational Definitions

Concepts in a study need to be defined and explicated, and dictionary definitions are almost never adequate. Two types of definitions are of particular relevance in a study—conceptual and operational.

The concepts in which researchers are interested are abstractions of observable phenomena, and researchers' world view shapes how those concepts are defined. A **conceptual definition** presents the abstract or theoretical meaning of the concepts being studied. Even seemingly straightforward terms need to be conceptually defined by researchers. The classic example of this is the concept of *caring*. Morse and her colleagues (1990) scrutinized the works of numerous nurse researchers and theorists to determine how *caring* was defined, and identified five different categories of conceptual definitions: as a human trait; a moral imperative; an affect; an interpersonal relationship; and a therapeutic intervention. Researchers undertaking studies concerned with caring need to make clear which conceptual definition of caring they have adopted—both to themselves and to their audience of readers. In qualitative studies, conceptual definitions of key phenomena may be the major end product of the endeavor, reflecting an intent to have the meaning of concepts defined by those being studied.

In quantitative studies, however, researchers must clarify and define concepts at the outset. This is necessary because quantitative researchers must indicate how the variables will be observed and measured in the study. An **operational definition** of a concept specifies the operations that researchers must perform to collect and measure the required information. Operational definitions should be congruent with conceptual definitions.

Variables differ in the ease with which they can be operationalized. The variable weight, for example, is easy to define and measure. We might operationally define weight as follows: the amount that an object weighs in pounds, to the nearest full pound. Note that this definition designates that weight will be measured using one system (pounds) rather than another (grams); we could also specify that subjects' weight will be measured to the nearest pound using a spring scale with subjects fully undressed after 10 hours of fasting. This operational definition clearly indicates what we mean by the variable *weight*.

Unfortunately, few variables are operationalized as easily as weight. There are multiple methods of measuring most variables, and researchers must choose the one that best captures the variables as they conceptualize them. Take, for example, *anxiety*, which can be defined in terms of both physiologic and psychological functioning. For researchers choosing to emphasize physiologic aspects of anxiety, the operational definition might involve a physiologic measure such as the Palmar Sweat Index. If, on the other hand, researchers conceptualize anxiety as primarily a psychological state, the operational definition might involve a paper-and-pencil measure such as the State Anxiety Scale. Readers of research reports may not agree with how investigators conceptualized and operationalized variables, but definitional precision has the advantage of communicating exactly what terms mean within the context of the study.

Data

Research **data** (singular, datum) are the pieces of information obtained during a study. In quantitative studies, researchers identify the variables of interest, develop conceptual and operational definitions of those variables, and then collect relevant data from subjects. The actual *values* of the study variables constitute the data. Quantitative researchers collect primarily **quantitative data**—information in numeric form. For example, suppose we were conducting a quantitative study in which a key variable was depression; we would need to measure how depressed participants were. We might ask, "Thinking about the past week, how depressed would you say you have been on a scale from 0 to 10, where 0 means 'not at all' and 10 means 'the most possible'?" Box 3.1 presents quantitative data for three fictitious respondents. The subjects provided a number along the 0 to 10 continuum corresponding to their degree of depression—9 for subject 1 (a high level of depression), 0 for subject 2 (no depression), and 4 for subject 3 (little depression). The numeric values for all subjects, collectively, would constitute the data on depression.

In qualitative studies, the researcher collects primarily **qualitative data**, that is, narrative descriptions. Narrative information can be obtained by having conversations with the participants, by making detailed notes about how participants behave in naturalistic settings, or by obtaining narrative records from participants, such as diaries. Suppose we were

Example of conceptual and operational definitions: Doorenbos and colleagues (2005) conceptually defined various aspects of *cultural competence* and described how the definitions were operationalized in an instrument called the Cultural Competence Assessment (CCA). One aspect of cultural competence, for example, is *cultural awareness*, which relates to a care provider's "knowledge about those areas of cultural expression in which groups tend to differ and those in which similarities are noted" (p. 326). Operationally, the CCA captures this dimension by having health care providers indicate their level of agreement with such statements as, "I understand that people from different cultural groups may define the concept of 'healthcare' in different ways."

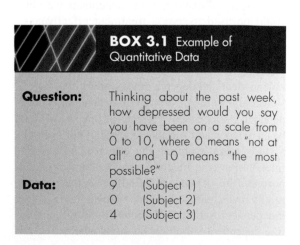

BOX 3.1 Example of Quantitative Data

Question:	Thinking about the past week, how depressed would you say you have been on a scale from 0 to 10, where 0 means "not at all" and 10 means "the most possible?"
Data:	9 (Subject 1)
	0 (Subject 2)
	4 (Subject 3)

BOX 3.2 Example of Qualitative Data

Question: Tell me about how you've been feeling lately—have you felt sad or depressed at all, or have you generally been in good spirits?

Data: Well, actually, I've been pretty depressed lately, to tell you the truth. I wake up each morning and I can't seem to think of anything to look forward to. I mope around the house all day, kind of in despair. I just can't seem to shake the blues, and I've begun to think I need to go see a shrink. (Participant 1)

I can't remember ever feeling better in my life. I just got promoted to a new job that makes me feel like I can really get ahead in my company. And I've just gotten engaged to a really great guy who is very special. (Participant 2)

I've had a few ups and downs the past week, but basically things are on a pretty even keel. I don't have too many complaints. (Participant 3)

---

studying depression qualitatively. Box 3.2 presents qualitative data for three participants responding conversationally to the question, "Tell me about how you've been feeling lately—have you felt sad or depressed at all, or have you generally been in good spirits?" Here, the data consist of rich narrative descriptions of each participant's emotional state.

Relationships

Researchers are rarely interested in a single concept or phenomenon, except in descriptive studies. As an example of a descriptive study, a researcher might do research to determine the percentage of patients receiving intravenous (IV) therapy who experience IV infiltration. In this example, the variable is IV infiltration versus no infiltration. Usually, however, researchers study phenomena in relation to other phenomena—that is, they explore or test relationships. A **relationship** is a bond or a connection between phenomena. For example, researchers repeatedly have found a *relationship* between cigarette smoking and lung cancer. Both qualitative and quantitative studies examine relationships, but in different ways.

In quantitative studies, researchers are primarily interested in the relationship between the independent variables and dependent variables. The research question focuses on whether variation in the dependent variable is systematically related to variation in the independent variable. Relationships are usually expressed in quantitative terms, such as *more than*, *less than*, and so on. For example, let us consider as our dependent variable a person's weight. What variables are related to (associated with) body weight? Some possibilities are height, caloric intake, and exercise. For each of these independent variables, we can make a prediction about its relationship to the dependent variable:

Height: Taller people will weigh more than shorter people.

Caloric intake: People with higher caloric intake will be heavier than those with lower caloric intake.

Exercise: The lower the amount of exercise, the greater will be the person's weight.

Each statement expresses a predicted relationship between weight (the dependent variable) and a measurable independent variable. Terms such as *more than* and *heavier than* imply that as we observe a change in one variable, we are likely to observe a corresponding change in weight. If Nate is taller than Tom, we would predict (in the absence of any other information) that Nate is also heavier than Tom. Most quantitative studies are undertaken to determine whether relationships exist among variables.

Quantitative studies typically address one or more of the following questions about relationships:

- Does a relationship between variables *exist*? (e.g., is cigarette smoking related to lung cancer?)
- What is the *direction* of the relationship between variables? (e.g., are people who smoke *more* likely or *less* likely to get lung cancer than those who do not?)
- How *strong* is the relationship between the variables? (e.g., how powerful is the relationship between smoking and lung cancer? How probable is it that smokers will develop lung cancer?)
- What is the *nature* of the relationship between variables? (e.g., does smoking *cause* lung cancer? Does some other factor *cause* both smoking and lung cancer?)

As this last question suggests, quantitative variables can be related to one another in different ways. One type of relationship is referred to as a **cause-and-effect** (or **causal**) **relationship**. Within the positivist paradigm, natural phenomena are assumed not to be random or haphazard; if phenomena have antecedent causes or determinants, they are presumably discoverable. For instance, in our example about a person's weight, we might speculate that there is a causal relationship between caloric intake and weight: consuming more calories causes weight gain.

Example of a study of causal relationships: Crogan, Velasquez, and Gagan (2005) studied whether giving iron supplements to nursing home residents caused improvements in immune response following an influenza vaccination.

Not all relationships between variables can be interpreted as cause-and-effect relationships. There is a relationship, for example, between a person's pulmonary artery and tympanic temperatures: people with high readings on one tend to have high readings on the other. We cannot say, however, that pulmonary artery temperature *caused* tympanic temperature, nor that tympanic temperature *caused* pulmonary artery temperature,

despite the relationship that exists between the two variables. This type of relationship is sometimes referred to as a **functional relationship** (or an **associative relationship**) rather than as a causal relationship.

Example of a study of functional relationships: Nyamthi and associates (2005) examined the relationship between the perceived health status of tuberculosis-infected homeless people on the one hand and gender on the other.

Qualitative researchers are not concerned with quantifying relationships, nor with testing causal relationships. Rather, qualitative researchers seek patterns of association as a way of illuminating the underlying meaning and dimensionality of phenomena. Patterns of interconnected themes and processes are identified as a means of understanding the whole. In some qualitative studies, theories are generated by identifying relationships between emerging categories. These new connections help to "weave the fractured story back together after the data have been analyzed" (Glaser, 1978, p. 72).

Example of a qualitative study of patterns: Uys and colleagues (2005) conducted group interviews with nurses and people living with HIV or AIDS in five African countries. The interviews probed how participants described the illness and people living with it. An analysis of the descriptions revealed seven distinct categories, with some descriptions used across countries and others unique to a specific country.

MAJOR CLASSES OF QUANTITATIVE AND QUALITATIVE RESEARCH

Researchers usually work within a paradigm that is consistent with their world view, and that gives rise to the types of question that excite their curiosity. The maturity of the concept of interest also may lead to one or the other paradigm: when little is known about a topic, a qualitative approach is often more fruitful than a quantitative one. The progression of activities differs for qualitative and quantitative researchers; we discuss the flow of both in this chapter. First, however, we briefly describe broad categories of quantitative and qualitative research.

Quantitative Research: Experimental and Nonexperimental Studies

A basic distinction in quantitative studies is the difference between experimental and nonexperimental research. In **experimental research**, researchers actively introduce an intervention or treatment. In **nonexperimental research**, on the other hand, researchers are bystanders—they collect data without introducing treatments or making changes. For example, if a researcher gave bran flakes to one group of subjects and prune juice to another to evaluate which method facilitated elimination more effectively, the study would be experimental because the researcher intervened in the normal course of things. In this example, the researcher created an "active variable" involving a dietary intervention. If, on the other hand, a researcher compared elimination patterns of two groups of people whose regular eating patterns differed—for example, some normally took foods that stimulated bowel elimination and others did not—there is no intervention. Such a study focuses on existing attributes and is nonexperimental. In medical and epidemiologic research, an experimental study usually is called a **controlled trial** or **clinical trial**, and a nonexperimental inquiry is called an **observational study.** (As we discuss in Chapter 10, a randomized control trial, or RCT, is a particular type of clinical trial.)

Experimental studies are explicitly designed to test causal relationships—to test whether the intervention *caused* changes in or affected the dependent variable. Sometimes nonexperimental studies also seek to elucidate or detect causal relationships, but doing so is tricky and usually is less conclusive. Experimental studies offer the possibility of greater control over extraneous influences than nonexperimental studies, and therefore causal inferences are more plausible.

Example of experimental research: Cooke and colleagues (2005) tested the effect of music on day surgery patients' level of anxiety. During a preoperative wait, some patients received the intervention—the opportunity to listen to patient-preferred music—and others did not.

In this example, the researcher intervened by designating that some patients would have the opportunity to listen to music while others were not given this opportunity. In other words, the researcher *controlled* the independent variable, which in this case was the music intervention.

Example of nonexperimental research: Taxis and co-authors (2004) studied coping skills and perceptions of stress in white and Hispanic school-aged children in Texas. The primary stressor was "feeling sick" and one of the children's most frequently identified coping strategies was "watching TV or listening to music." Greater use of coping strategies was associated with lower stress.

In this nonexperimental study, the researchers did not intervene in any way. They were interested in similar variables as in the previously described experimental study (music listening and stress/anxiety), but their intent was to describe the status quo and explore existing relationships rather than to test a potential solution to a problem.

Qualitative Research: Disciplinary Traditions

Qualitative studies are often rooted in research traditions that originated in the disciplines of anthropology, sociology, and psychology. Three such traditions have had especially strong influences on qualitative nursing research and are briefly described here. Chapter 9 provides a fuller discussion of qualitative research traditions and the methods associated with them.

The **grounded theory** tradition, which has its roots in sociology, seeks to describe and understand the key social psychological and structural processes that occur in a social setting. Grounded theory was developed in the 1960s by two sociologists, Glaser and Strauss (1967). The focus of most grounded theory studies is on a developing social experience—the social and psychological stages and phases that characterize a particular event or episode. A major component of grounded theory is the discovery of a *core variable* that is central in explaining what is going on in that social scene. Grounded theory researchers strive to generate comprehensive explanations of phenomena that are grounded in reality.

Example of a grounded theory study:
King and colleagues (2006) conducted a series of grounded theory studies with men and women from five ethnocultural groups in Canada who had been diagnosed with coronary artery disease (CAD). The analysis focused on the process through which patients met the challenge of managing CAD risk.

Phenomenology, rooted in a philosophical tradition developed by Husserl and Heidegger, is concerned with the lived experiences of humans. Phenomenology is an approach to thinking about what life experiences of people are like and what they mean. The phenomenological researcher asks the questions: What is the *essence* of this phenomenon as experienced by these people? Or, What is the meaning of the phenomenon to those who experience it?

Example of a phenomenological study:
O'Dell and Jacelon (2005) conducted in-depth interviews to explore the experiences of women who had undergone vaginal closure surgery to correct severe vaginal prolapse.

Ethnography is the primary research tradition within anthropology, and provides a framework for studying the patterns, lifeways, and experiences of a cultural group in a holistic fashion. Ethnographers typically engage in extensive fieldwork, often participating to the extent possible in the life of the culture under study. Ethnographic research is in some cases concerned with broadly defined cultures (e.g., Hmong refugee communities), but sometimes focuses on more narrowly defined cultures (e.g., the culture of an emergency department). The aim of ethnographers is to learn from

(rather than to study) members of a cultural group, to understand their world view as they perceive and live it, and to describe their customs and norms.

Example of an ethnographic study:
Schoenfeld and Juarbe (2005) conducted ethnographic fieldwork in two rural Ecuadorian communities and studied the burdens of women's roles, the women's perceived health needs, and their health care resources.

MAJOR STEPS IN A QUANTITATIVE STUDY

In quantitative studies, researchers move from the beginning point of a study (the posing of a question) to the end point (the obtaining of an answer) in a reasonably linear sequence of steps that is broadly similar across studies. In some studies, the steps overlap, whereas in others, certain steps are unnecessary. Still, there is a general flow of activities that is typical of a quantitative study (Fig. 3.1). This section describes that flow, and the next section describes how qualitative studies differ.

Phase 1: The Conceptual Phase

The early steps in a quantitative research project typically involve activities with a strong conceptual or intellectual element. These activities include reading, conceptualizing, theorizing, reconceptualizing, and reviewing ideas with colleagues or advisers. During this phase, researchers call on such skills as creativity, deductive reasoning, insight, and a firm grounding in previous research on the topic of interest.

Step 1: Formulating and Delimiting the Problem
One of the first things a researcher must do is identify an interesting, significant research problem and good **research questions**. Good research depends to a great degree on good questions. In developing a research question to be studied, nurse researchers must pay close attention to substantive issues (Is this research question important, given the existing

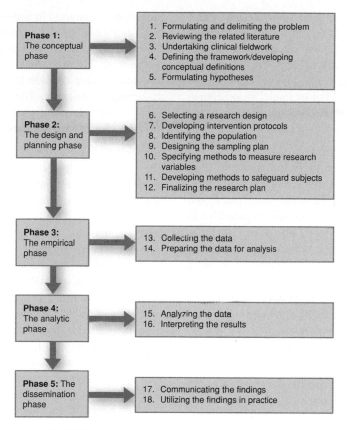

Phase 1:
The conceptual phase

1. Formulating and delimiting the problem
2. Reviewing the related literature
3. Undertaking clinical fieldwork
4. Defining the framework/developing conceptual definitions
5. Formulating hypotheses

Phase 2:
The design and planning phase

6. Selecting a research design
7. Developing intervention protocols
8. Identifying the population
9. Designing the sampling plan
10. Specifying methods to measure research variables
11. Developing methods to safeguard subjects
12. Finalizing the research plan

Phase 3:
The empirical phase

13. Collecting the data
14. Preparing the data for analysis

Phase 4:
The analytic phase

15. Analyzing the data
16. Interpreting the results

Phase 5: The dissemination phase

17. Communicating the findings
18. Utilizing the findings in practice

FIGURE 3.1 Flow of steps in a quantitative study.

evidence base?); theoretical issues (Is there a broader conceptual context for enhancing understanding of this problem?); clinical issues (Could findings from this research be useful in clinical practice?); methodologic issues (How can this question best be studied to yield high-quality evidence?); and ethical issues (Can this question be rigorously addressed without committing ethical transgressions?)

➲ TIP: A critical ingredient in developing good research questions is personal interest. Begin with topics that fascinate you or about which you have a passionate interest or curiosity.

Step 2: Reviewing the Related Literature
Quantitative research is typically conducted within the context of previous knowledge. To contribute to the evidence base, quantitative researchers strive to understand what is already known about a research problem. A thorough **literature review** provides a foundation on which to base new evidence and usually is conducted well before any data are collected. For clinical problems, it may also be necessary to learn as much as possible about the "status quo" of current procedures relating to the topic, and to review existing practice guidelines or protocols.

Step 3: Undertaking Clinical Fieldwork
In addition to refreshing or updating clinical knowledge based on written work, researchers embarking on a clinical nursing study benefit from spending time in clinical settings, discussing the topic with clinicians and health care administrators, and observing current practices. Such **clinical fieldwork** can provide perspectives on recent clinical trends,

current diagnostic procedures, and relevant health care delivery models; it can also help researchers better understand affected clients and the settings in which care is provided. Such fieldwork can also be valuable in developing methodologic strategies for strengthening the study. For example, in the course of clinical fieldwork, researchers might discover the need for research assistants who are bilingual.

Step 4: Defining the Framework and Developing Conceptual Definitions

Theory is the ultimate aim of science in that it transcends the specifics of a particular time, place, and group of people and aims to identify regularities in the relationships among variables. When quantitative research is performed within the context of a theoretical framework, the findings may have broader significance and utility. Even when the research question is not embedded in a theory, researchers must have a conceptual rationale and a clear sense of the concepts under study. Thus, an important task in the initial phase of a project is the development of conceptual definitions.

Step 5: Formulating Hypotheses

A **hypothesis** is a statement of the researcher's expectations about relationships between study variables. Hypotheses, in other words, are predictions of expected outcomes; they state the relationships researchers expect to find as a result of the study. The research question asks how the concepts under investigation might be related; a hypothesis is the predicted answer. For example, the research question might be as follows: Is preeclamptic toxemia related to stress factors during pregnancy? This might be translated into the following hypothesis: Women with a higher incidence of stressful events during pregnancy will be more likely than women with a lower incidence of stress to experience preeclamptic toxemia. Most quantitative studies are designed to test hypotheses through statistical analysis.

Phase 2: The Design and Planning Phase

In the second major phase of a quantitative study, researchers make decisions about the methods and procedures to be used to address the research question, and plan for the actual collection of data. Sometimes the nature of the question dictates the methods to be used, but more often than not, researchers have considerable flexibility and must make many decisions. These methodologic decisions usually have crucial implications for the integrity of the study findings.

Step 6: Selecting a Research Design

The **research design** is the overall plan for obtaining answers to the questions being studied and for handling some of the difficulties encountered during the research process. A wide variety of research designs are available for quantitative studies, including numerous experimental and nonexperimental designs. In designing the study, researchers specify which specific design will be adopted and what will be done to minimize bias and enhance the interpretability of results. In quantitative studies, research designs tend to be highly structured and controlled. Research designs also indicate other aspects of the research—for example, how often data will be collected, what types of comparisons will be made, and where the study will take place. The research design is the architectural backbone of the study.

Step 7: Developing Protocols for the Intervention

In experimental research, researchers actively intervene and create the independent variable, which means that participants are exposed to different treatments or conditions. For example, if we were interested in testing the effect of biofeedback in treating hypertension, the independent variable would be biofeedback compared with either an alternative treatment (e.g., relaxation therapy), or no treatment. The **intervention protocol** for the study would need to be developed, specifying exactly what the biofeedback treatment would entail (e.g., who would administer it, how frequently and over how long a period the treatment would last, and so on) *and* what the alternative condition would be. The goal of well-articulated protocols is to have all subjects in each group treated in the same way. (In nonexperimental research, of course, this step is not necessary.)

Step 8: Identifying the Population

Quantitative researchers need to know what characteristics the study participants should possess, and clarify the group to whom study results can be generalized—that is, they must identify the population to be studied. A **population** is *all* the individuals or objects with common, defining characteristics. For example, the population of interest might be all patients undergoing chemotherapy in California.

Step 9: Designing the Sampling Plan

Researchers typically collect data from a sample, which is a subset of the population. Using samples is clearly more practical and less costly than collecting data from an entire population, but the risk is that the sample might not adequately reflect the population's traits. In a quantitative study, a sample's adequacy is assessed by the criterion of **representativeness.** That is, the quality of the sample depends on how typical, or representative, the sample is of the population. Sophisticated sampling procedures can produce samples that have a high likelihood of being representative. The **sampling plan** specifies in advance how the sample will be selected and recruited, and how many subjects there will be.

Step 10: Specifying Methods to Measure the Research Variables

Quantitative researchers must develop or borrow methods to measure the research variables as accurately as possible. Based on the conceptual definitions, the researcher identifies or designs appropriate methods to operationalize the variables and collect the data. A variety of quantitative data collection approaches exist; the primary methods are *self-reports* (e.g., interviews), *observations* (e.g., observing the sleep–wake state of infants), and *biophysiologic measurements*. The task of measuring research variables and developing a **data collection plan** is a complex and challenging process.

Step 11: Developing Methods to Safeguard Human or Animal Rights

Most nursing research involves human subjects, although some studies involve animals. In either case, procedures need to be developed to ensure that the study adheres to ethical principles. Each aspect of the study plan needs to be scrutinized to determine whether the rights of subjects have been adequately protected. Often that review involves a formal presentation to an external review committee.

Step 12: Reviewing and Finalizing the Research Plan

Before actually collecting research data, researchers often perform a number of "tests" to ensure that plans will work smoothly. For example, they may evaluate the *readability* of any written materials to determine whether participants with low reading skills can comprehend them, or they may *pretest* their measuring instruments to assess their adequacy. Normally, researchers also have their research plan critiqued by peers, consultants, or other reviewers to obtain substantive, clinical, or methodologic feedback before implementing the plan. Researchers seeking financial support for their study submit a **proposal** to a funding source, and reviewers usually suggest improvements.

Phase 3: The Empirical Phase

The empirical portion of quantitative studies involves collecting research data and preparing those data for analysis. In many studies, the empirical phase is one of the most time-consuming parts of the investigation. Data collection typically requires several weeks, or even months, of work.

Step 13: Collecting the Data

The actual collection of data in a quantitative study often proceeds according to a preestablished plan. The researcher's plan typically specifies procedures for the actual collection of data (e.g., where and when the data will be gathered); for describing the study to participants; and for recording information. Technological advances in the past few decades have expanded possibilities for automating data collection.

Step 14: Preparing the Data for Analysis

Data collected in a quantitative study are rarely amenable to direct analysis—preliminary steps are needed. One such step is **coding**, which is the process of translating verbal data into numeric form.

For example, patients' responses to a question about their gender might be coded "1" for female and "2" for male (or vice versa). Another preliminary step involves transferring the data from written documents onto computer files for subsequent analysis.

Phase 4: The Analytic Phase

Quantitative data gathered in the empirical phase are subjected to analysis and interpretation, which occurs in the fourth major phase of a project.

Step 15: Analyzing the Data

To answer research questions and test hypotheses. researchers need to process and analyze their data in an orderly, coherent fashion. Quantitative information is analyzed through statistical procedures. **Statistical analyses** cover a broad range of techniques, from simple procedures that we all use regularly (e.g., computing an average) to complex and sophisticated methods. Although some methods are computationally formidable, the underlying logic of statistical tests is relatively easy to grasp, and computers have eliminated the need to get bogged down with detailed mathematic operations.

Step 16: Interpreting the Results

Interpretation is the process of making sense of study results and of examining their implications. Researchers attempt to explain the findings in light of prior evidence, theory, and their own clinical experience—and in light of the adequacy of the methods they used in the study. Interpretation also involves determining how the findings can best be used in clinical practice, or what further research is needed before utilization can be recommended.

Phase 5: The Dissemination Phase

In the analytic phase, the researcher comes full circle: the questions posed at the outset are answered. The researchers' responsibilities are not completed, however, until the study results are disseminated.

Step 17: Communicating the Findings

Another—and often final—task of a research project is the preparation of a **research report** that can be shared with others. Research reports can take various forms: term papers, dissertations, journal articles, presentations at conferences, and so on. Journal articles—reports appearing in such professional journals as *Nursing Research*—usually are the most useful because they are available to a broad, international audience. We discuss the content of journal articles later in this chapter.

Step 18: Utilizing the Findings in Practice

Ideally, the concluding step of a high-quality study is to plan for its use in practice settings. Although nurse researchers may not themselves be in a position to implement a plan for utilizing research findings, they can contribute to the process by including in their research reports recommendations regarding how the evidence from the study could be incorporated into the practice of nursing, by ensuring that adequate information has been provided for a meta-analysis, and by vigorously pursuing opportunities to disseminate the findings to practicing nurses.

ACTIVITIES IN A QUALITATIVE STUDY

Quantitative research involves a fairly linear progression of tasks—researchers plan in advance the steps to be taken to maximize study integrity and then follow those steps as faithfully as possible. In qualitative studies, by contrast, the progression is closer to a circle than to a straight line—qualitative researchers are continually examining and interpreting data and making decisions about how to proceed based on what has already been discovered (Fig. 3.2).

Because qualitative researchers have a flexible approach to the collection and analysis of data, it is impossible to define the flow of activities precisely—the flow varies from one study to another, and researchers themselves do not know ahead of time exactly how the study will proceed. We try to provide a sense of how qualitative studies are conducted, however, by describing some major activities and indicating how and when they might be performed.

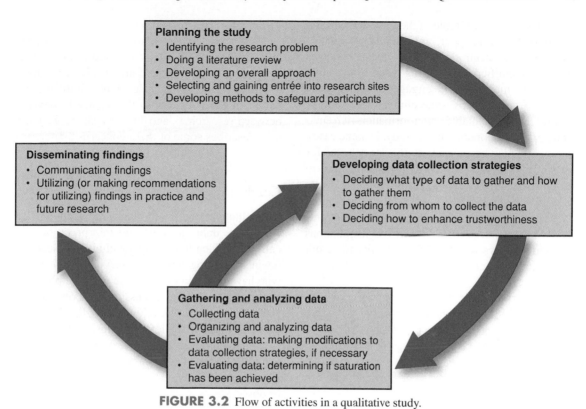

FIGURE 3.2 Flow of activities in a qualitative study.

Conceptualizing and Planning a Qualitative Study

Identifying the Research Problem

Qualitative researchers usually begin with a broad topic area, focusing on an aspect of a topic that is poorly understood and about which little is known. They therefore may not develop hypotheses or pose refined research questions at the outset. The general topic area may be narrowed and clarified on the basis of self-reflection and discussion with colleagues (or clients), but researchers may proceed initially with a fairly broad research question that allows the focus to be sharpened and delineated more clearly once the study is underway.

Doing a Literature Review

Qualitative researchers do not all agree about the value of doing an upfront literature review. Some believe that researchers should not consult the liter- ature before collecting data. Their concern is that prior studies might influence their conceptualiza- tion of the phenomena under study. According to this view, the phenomena should be elucidated based on participants' viewpoints rather than on any prior information. Those sharing this viewpoint often do a literature review at the end of the study rather than at the beginning. Others feel that researchers should conduct at least a preliminary up-front literature review to obtain a general grounding. Still others believe that a full up-front literature review is appropriate. In any case, quali- tative researchers typically find a relatively small body of relevant previous work because of the types of question they ask.

Selecting and Gaining Entrée Into Research Sites

Before going into the field, qualitative researchers must identify a site that is consistent with the research topic. For example, if the topic is the health beliefs of the urban poor, an inner-city neighborhood with a concentration of low-income residents must be identified. In making such a decision, researchers may need to engage in anticipatory fieldwork (and perhaps some clinical fieldwork) to identify the most suitable and information-rich environment for the conduct of the study. In some cases, researchers may have access to the site selected for the study. In others, however, researchers need to **gain entrée** into the site or settings within it. A site may be well suited to the needs of the research, but if researchers cannot "get in," the study cannot proceed. Gaining entrée typically involves negotiations with **gatekeepers** who have the authority to permit entry into their world.

⟳ **TIP:** The process of gaining entrée is usually associated with doing fieldwork in a qualitative study, but quantitative researchers often need to gain entrée into sites for collecting their data as well.

Developing an Overall Approach

Quantitative researchers do not collect data until the research design has been finalized. In a qualitative study, by contrast, the research design is often referred to as an **emergent design**—a design that emerges during the course of data collection. Certain design features are guided by the qualitative research tradition within which the researcher is working, but nevertheless few qualitative studies have rigidly structured designs that prohibit changes while in the field.

Although qualitative researchers do not always know in advance exactly how the study will progress in the field, they nevertheless must have some sense of how much time is available for fieldwork and must also arrange for and test needed equipment, such as tape recorders or laptop computers. Other planning activities include such tasks as hiring and training interviewers to assist in the collection of data; securing interpreters if the informants speak a different language; and hiring appropriate consultants, transcribers, and support staff.

Addressing Ethical Issues

Qualitative researchers, like quantitative researchers, must also develop plans for addressing ethical issues—and, indeed, there are special concerns in qualitative studies because of the more intimate nature of the relationship that typically develops between researchers and study participants. Chapter 7 describes some of these concerns.

Conducting the Qualitative Study

In qualitative studies, the tasks of sampling, data collection, data analysis, and interpretation typically take place iteratively. Qualitative researchers begin by talking with or observing a few people who have first-hand experience with the phenomenon under study. The discussions and observations are loosely structured, allowing for the expression of a full range of beliefs, feelings, and behaviors. Analysis and interpretation are ongoing, concurrent activities that guide choices about the kinds of people to sample next and the types of questions to ask or observations to make.

The actual process of data analysis involves clustering together related types of narrative information into a coherent scheme. As analysis and interpretation progress, researchers begin to identify **themes** and categories, which are used to build a rich description or theory of the phenomenon. The kinds of data obtained and the people selected as participants tend to become increasingly focused and purposeful as the conceptualization is developed and refined. Concept development and verification shape the sampling process—as a conceptualization or theory develops, the researcher seeks participants who can confirm and enrich the theoretical understandings, as well as participants who can potentially challenge them and lead to further theoretical development.

Quantitative researchers decide in advance how many subjects to include in the study, but qualitative researchers' sampling decisions are guided by the data themselves. Many qualitative researchers use the principle of **data saturation**, which occurs when themes and categories in the data become repetitive and redundant, such that no new information can be gleaned by further data collection.

In quantitative studies, researchers seek to collect high-quality data by using measuring instruments that have been demonstrated to be accurate and valid. Qualitative researchers, by contrast, must take steps to demonstrate the *trustworthiness* of the data while in the field. The central feature of these efforts is to confirm that the findings accurately reflect the experiences and viewpoints of participants, rather than perceptions of the researchers. One confirmatory activity, for example, involves going back to participants and sharing preliminary interpretations with them so that they can evaluate whether the researcher's thematic analysis is consistent with their experiences.

An issue that qualitative researchers sometimes need to address is the development of appropriate strategies for leaving the field. Because qualitative researchers may develop strong relationships with study participants and entire communities, they need to be sensitive to the fact that their departure from the field might seem like a form of rejection or abandonment. Graceful departures and methods of achieving closure are important.

Disseminating Qualitative Findings

Qualitative nursing researchers also strive to share their findings with others at conferences and in journal articles. Qualitative findings, because of their depth and richness, also lend themselves more readily to book-length manuscripts than do quantitative findings. Regardless of researchers' position about *when* a literature review should be conducted, they usually include a summary of prior research in their reports as a means of providing context for the study.

Quantitative reports almost never contain any **raw data**—that is, data in the form they were collected, which are numeric values. Qualitative reports, by contrast, are usually filled with rich verbatim passages directly from participants. The excerpts are used in an evidentiary fashion to support or illustrate researchers' interpretations and thematic construction.

Example of raw data in a qualitative report: Zengerle-Levy (2006) studied the experiences of nurses caring for families of critically burned children. In-depth interviews with 16 pediatric nurses on a burn ICU revealed that while helping burned children cope holistically, nurses also grieved with the families, as illustrated by the following quote: *"I had a 17-year-old female who was real sick. I took care of her pretty much for 2½ weeks straight. She was very septic, she was in traction, she had a cultured fungus, and the room was terribly hot always because she couldn't keep her temperature because she was septic. She had a profound odor about her. She was much like in a comatose state, but I got to know her through the mother. I had a real bond with the mother. A lot of people say you're not supposed to get so close to the family, but how can you not? You are human and you can't block yourself off from that."*

Like quantitative researchers, qualitative nurse researchers want their findings used by others. Qualitative findings often are the basis for formulating hypotheses that are tested by quantitative researchers, for developing measuring instruments for both research and clinical purposes, and for designing effective nursing interventions. Qualitative studies help to shape nurses' perceptions of a problem or situation, their conceptualizations of potential solutions, and their understanding of patients' concerns and experiences.

RESEARCH JOURNAL ARTICLES

Research **journal articles**, which summarize the context, design, and results of a study, are the primary method of disseminating research evidence. This section reviews the content and style of research journal articles to ensure that you will be equipped to delve into the research literature. A more detailed discussion of the structure of journal articles is presented in Chapter 26, which provides guidance on writing research reports.

Content of Journal Articles

Quantitative journal articles—and many qualitative ones—typically follow a conventional organizational format called the **IMRAD format**. This format, which loosely follows the steps of quantitative studies, involves organizing material into four main sections—Introduction, Methods, Results, and Discussion. The main text of the report is usually preceded by an abstract and followed by references.

The Abstract

The **abstract** is a brief description of the study placed at the beginning of the article. The abstract answers, in about 100 to 200 words, the following questions: What were the research questions? What methods did the researcher use to address those questions? What did the researcher find? and What are the implications for nursing practice? Readers can review an abstract to assess whether the entire report is of interest. Some journals have moved from having traditional abstracts—which are single paragraphs summarizing the main features of the study—to slightly longer, more structured abstracts with specific headings. For example, abstracts in *Nursing Research* after 1997 present information about the study organized under the following headings: Background, Objectives, Method, Results, and Conclusions.

The Introduction

The introduction acquaints readers with the research problem and its context. The introduction, which usually is not specifically labeled "Introduction," follows immediately after the abstract. This section usually describes the following:

* The central phenomena, concepts, or variables under study
* The statement of purpose, and research questions or hypotheses to be tested
* A review of the related literature
* The theoretical or conceptual framework
* The significance of and need for the study

Thus, the introduction sets the stage for a description of what the researcher did and what was learned. The introduction corresponds roughly to the conceptual phase (Phase 1) of a study.

The Method Section

The method section describes the methods used to answer the research questions. The method section tells readers about major methodologic decisions made in the design and planning phase (Phase 2), and may offer rationales for those decisions. In a quantitative study, the method section usually describes the following, which may be presented as labeled subsections:

* The research design
* The sampling design and description of study participants
* Methods of data collection, and specific instruments used
* Study procedures
* Analytic procedures and methods (sometimes)

Qualitative researchers discuss many of the same issues, but with different emphases. For example, a qualitative study often provides more information about the research setting and the context of the study, and less information on sampling. Also, because formal instruments are not used to collect qualitative data, there is little discussion about data collection methods, but there may be more information on data collection procedures. Increasingly, reports of qualitative studies are including descriptions of the researchers' efforts to enhance the rigor of the study. Qualitative reports may also have a detailed subsection on data analysis.

The Results Section

The results section presents the **research findings**—that is, the results obtained during the analytic phase of the study. The text summarizes key findings, often accompanied by more detailed tables or figures. Virtually all results sections contain basic descriptive information, including a description of the participants (e.g., average age, percentage male or female). In quantitative studies, the researcher provides basic descriptive information for the key variables, using simple statistics. For example, in a study of the effect of a nursing intervention on smoking cessation, the results section might begin by describing the average number of cigarettes smoked weekly before the intervention, or the percentage of subjects who smoked two packs or more daily.

In quantitative studies, the results section also reports the following information relating to any statistical tests performed:

- *The names of statistical tests used.* **Statistical tests** are used to test hypotheses and evaluate the believability of the findings. For example, if the percentage of smokers who smoke two packs or more daily is computed to be 40%, how probable is it that the percentage is accurate? If the researcher finds that the average number of cigarettes smoked weekly is lower among those in an intervention group than among those not getting the intervention, how probable is it that the same would be true for other smokers not in the study? That is, is the relationship between the intervention and smoking behavior *real* and likely to be replicated with a new sample of smokers—or does the result reflect a peculiarity of the sample? Statistical tests help to answer such questions. Statistical tests are based on common principles; you do not have to know the names of all statistical tests—there are dozens of them –to comprehend the findings.

- *The value of the calculated statistic.* Computers are used to calculate a numeric value for the particular statistical test used. The value allows researchers to draw conclusions about the meaning of the results. The *actual* numeric value of the statistic, however, is not inherently meaningful and need not concern you.

- *The significance.* The most important information is whether the results of the statistical tests were significant (not to be confused with important or clinically relevant). If a researcher reports that the results are **statistically significant**, it means the findings are probably valid and replicable with a new sample. Research reports also indicate the **level of significance**, which is an index of how probable it is that the findings are reliable. For example, if a report indicates that a finding was significant at the .05 level, this means that only 5 times out of 100 $(5 \div 100 = .05)$ would the obtained result be spurious. In other words, 95 times out of 100, similar results would be obtained with a new sample. Readers can therefore have a high degree of confidence—but not total assurance—that the findings are reliable.

> **Example from the results section of a quantitative study:** "The total FIM (Functional Independence Measure) score was 84.9 . . . on admission, indicating functional dependency, compared with 101.6 . . . on discharge, indicating modified functional independence. A paired *t*-test revealed that mean total FIM scores were significantly higher on discharge [$t(39) = -6.517$, $p = 0.0001$] than on admission to the GRU (Geriatric Rehabilitation Unit)" (McCloskey, 2004, p. 190).

In this excerpt, McCloskey indicated that the elders' average score on the measure of functional ability was *significantly* better at discharge than on admission. The average improvement of nearly 17 points on the scale was not likely to have been a haphazard change, and would probably be replicated with a new sample of elders. This finding is highly reliable: only one time in 10,000 ($p = 0.0001$) would an improvement this great have occurred as a fluke. Note that to comprehend this finding, you do not need to understand what the t statistic is, nor do you need to concern yourself with the actual value of the statistic, -6.517.

In qualitative reports, the researcher often organizes findings according to the major themes, processes, or categories that were identified in the data. The results section of qualitative reports sometimes has several subsections, the headings of which correspond to the researcher's labels for the themes. Excerpts from the raw data are presented to support and provide a rich description of the thematic analysis.

The Discussion Section

In the discussion section, the researcher draws conclusions about the meaning and implications of the findings. This section tries to unravel what the results mean, why things turned out the way they did, and how the results can be used in practice. The discussion in both qualitative and quantitative reports may incorporate the following elements:

- An interpretation of the results
- Clinical and research implications
- Study limitations and ramifications for the believability of the results

With regard to a discussion of limitations, the researcher is in the best position possible to point out sample deficiencies, design problems, weaknesses in data collection, and so forth. A discussion section that presents these limitations demonstrates to readers that the author was aware of these limitations and probably took them into account in interpreting the findings.

The Style of Research Journal Articles

Research reports tell a story. However, the style in which many research journal articles are written—especially reports of quantitative studies—makes it difficult for many readers to figure out or become interested in the story. To unaccustomed audiences, research reports may seem pedantic and bewildering. Four factors contribute to this impression:

1. *Compactness*. Journal space is limited, so authors try to compress a lot of information into a short space. Interesting, personalized aspects of the investigation cannot be reported, and, in qualitative studies, only a handful of supporting quotes can be included.
2. *Jargon*. The authors of both qualitative and quantitative reports use research terms that are assumed to be part of readers' vocabulary, but that may seem esoteric.
3. *Objectivity*. Quantitative researchers tend to avoid any impression of subjectivity, and so they tell their research stories in a way that makes them sound impersonal. For example, most quantitative research reports are written in the passive voice (i.e., personal pronouns are avoided), which tends to make a report less inviting and lively than use of the active voice. (Qualitative reports, by contrast, are more subjective and personal, and are written in a more conversational style.)
4. *Statistical information*. The majority of nursing studies are quantitative, and thus most research reports summarize the results of statistical analyses. In fact, nurse researchers have become increasingly sophisticated and have begun to use more powerful and complex statistical tools. Numbers and statistical symbols may intimidate readers who do not have strong mathematic interest or training.

In this textbook, we try to assist you in dealing with these issues and also strive to encourage you to tell *your* research stories in a manner that makes them accessible to practicing nurses.

Tips on Reading Research Reports

As you progress through this textbook, you will acquire skills for evaluating various aspects of research reports critically. Some preliminary hints on digesting research reports and dealing with the issues previously described follow.

* Grow accustomed to the style of research reports by reading them frequently, even though you may not yet understand all the technical points.
* Read from a report that has been photocopied (or downloaded and printed) so that you can highlight or underline portions of the article and write questions or notes in the margins.
* Read journal articles slowly. It may be useful to skim the article first to get the major points and then read the article more carefully a second time.
* On the second reading of a journal article, train yourself to become an *active* reader. Reading actively means that you are constantly monitoring yourself to determine whether you understand what you are reading. If you have comprehension problems, go back and reread difficult passages or make notes about your confusion so that you can ask someone for clarification. In most cases, that "someone" will be your research instructor, but also consider contacting the researchers themselves. The postal and e-mail addresses of the researchers are usually included in the journal article, and researchers often are more than willing to discuss their research with others.
* Keep this textbook with you as a reference while you are reading articles so that you can look up unfamiliar terms in the glossary at the end of the book, or in the index.
* Try not to get bogged down in (or scared away by) statistical information. Try to grasp the gist of the story without letting symbols and numbers frustrate you.

BOX 3.3 Additional Questions for a Preliminary Review of a Study

1. What is the study all about? What are the main phenomena, concepts, or constructs under investigation?
2. If the study is quantitative, what are the independent and dependent variables?
3. Do the researchers examine relationships or patterns of association among variables or concepts? Does the report imply the possibility of a causal relationship?
4. Are key concepts clearly defined, both conceptually and operationally?
5. What type of study does it appear to be, in terms of types described in this chapter—experimental/nonexperimental? grounded theory? phenomenology? ethnography?
6. Does the report provide any information to suggest how long the study took to complete?
7. Does the format of the report conform to the traditional IMRAD format? If not, in what ways does it differ?

- Until you become accustomed to the style and jargon of research journal articles, you may want to "translate" them mentally or in writing. You can do this by expanding compact paragraphs into looser constructions, by translating jargon into more familiar terms, by recasting the report into an active voice, and by summarizing the findings with words rather than numbers. (Chapter 3 in the accompanying *Resource Manual* has an example of such a translation.)
- Although it is certainly important to read research reports with understanding, it is also important to read them critically. A critical reading involves an evaluation of the researcher's major conceptual and methodologic decisions. It may be difficult to criticize these decisions at this point, but your conceptual and methodologic skills will be strengthened as you progress through this book. Guidelines for critiquing various aspects of a research report are included in most chapters of this book, and key critiquing questions are suggested in Chapter 5.

GENERAL QUESTIONS IN REVIEWING A STUDY

Most of the remaining chapters of this book contain guidelines to help you evaluate different aspects of a research report critically, focusing pri-marily on the methodologic decisions that the researcher made in conducting the study. Box 3.3 presents some further suggestions for performing a preliminary review of a research report, drawing on concepts explained in this chapter. These guidelines supplement those presented in Box 1.1, Chapter 1.

RESEARCH EXAMPLES

In this section, we illustrate the progression of activities and discuss the time schedule of two studies (one quantitative and the other qualitative) conducted by the second author of this book.

Project Schedule for a Quantitative Study

Beck and Gable (2001) undertook a study to evaluate the accuracy and utility of a scale they developed, the Postpartum Depression Screening Scale (PDSS), in screening new mothers for this mood disorder.

Phase 1. Conceptual Phase: 1 Month
This phase was the shortest, in large part because much of the conceptual work had been done in Beck and Gable's (2000) first study, in which they actually developed the screening scale. The literature had already been reviewed, so they only needed to update it. The same framework and conceptual definitions that had been used in the first study were used in the new study.

Phase 2. Design and Planning Phase: 6 Months

The second phase was time-consuming. It included not only fine-tuning the research design but also gaining entrée into the hospital where subjects were recruited and obtaining approval of the hospital's human subjects review committee. During this period, Beck met with statistical consultants and an instrument development consultant (Gable) numerous times to finalize the study design.

Phase 3. Empirical Phase: 11 Months

Data collection took almost a year to complete. The design called for administering the PDSS to 150 mothers who were 6 weeks postpartum, and then scheduling a psychiatric diagnostic interview to determine whether they were suffering from postpartum depression. Women were recruited into the study during prepared childbirth classes. Recruitment began 4 months before data collection, and then the researchers had to wait until 6 weeks after delivery to gather data. The nurse psychotherapist, who had her own clinical practice, was able to come to the hospital (a 2-hour drive for her) only 1 day a week to conduct the diagnostic interviews; this contributed to the time required to achieve the desired sample size.

Phase 4. Analytic Phase: 3 Months

Statistical tests were performed to determine a cut-off score on the PDSS above which mothers would be identified as having screened positive for postpartum depression. Data analysis also was undertaken to determine the accuracy of the PDSS in predicting diagnosed postpartum depression. During this phase, Beck met with Gable and with statisticians to interpret results.

Phase 5. Dissemination Phase: 18 Months

The researchers prepared and submitted their report to the journal *Nursing Research* for possible publication. It was accepted within 4 months, but it was "in press" (awaiting publication) for 14 months before being published. During this period, the authors presented their findings at regional and international conferences. The researchers also had to prepare a summary report for submission to the agency that funded the research.

Project Schedule for a Qualitative Study

Beck (2004) conducted a phenomenological study of women's experiences of birth trauma. Total time from start to finish was approximately 3 years.

Phase 1. Conceptual Phase: 3 Months

Beck, who was renowned for her program of research on postpartum depression, became interested in birth trauma when she was invited to deliver the keynote address at the September 2001 Australasian Marcé Society Biennial Scientific Meeting in New Zealand. She was asked to speak on perinatal anxiety disorders. In reviewing the literature to prepare for her address, Beck located only a handful of articles that had been published describing birth trauma and its resulting posttraumatic stress disorder (PTSD). Following her keynote speech, a mother made a riveting and heartbreaking presentation about her experience of PTSD due to a traumatic childbirth. The mother, Sue Watson, was one of the founders of Trauma and Birth Stress (TABS), a charitable trust located in New Zealand. Before Watson had finished her presentation, Beck knew that she wanted to do research on birth trauma. At lunch that day, Watson and Beck discussed the possibility of Beck conducting a qualitative study with the mothers who were members of TABS. Gaining entrée into TABS was facilitated by Watson, who, with four other founders of TABS, approved the study.

Phase 2. Design and Planning Phase: 3 Months

Beck selected a phenomenological design for this research, which was designed to describe the experience of a traumatic birth to mothers who participated. She corresponded by e-mail with Watson to plan for the best approach for recruiting mothers. Plans were made for Beck to write an introductory letter explaining the study, and Watson, the chairperson of TABS, would also write a letter endorsing the study. Both letters would be sent to the mothers who were members of TABS, asking for their cooperation. Once the basic design was developed, the research proposal was submitted to and approved by the human subjects committee at Beck's university.

Phase 3. Empirical/Analytic Phase: 24 Months

Data for the study were collected over an 18-month period. During that period, 40 mothers sent their stories of birth trauma to Beck via e-mail attachments. For an additional 6 months, Beck analyzed the mothers' stories. Four themes emerged from data analysis: To care for me: Was that too much to ask? To communicate with me: Why was this neglected? To provide safe care: You betrayed my trust and I felt powerless, and The end justifies the means: At whose expense? At what price?

Phase 4 Dissemination Phase: 5+ Months

A manuscript describing this study was submitted for publication to the journal *Nursing Research* in April 2003. In June, Beck received a letter from the journal's editor indicating that the reviewers of her manuscript recommended she revise and resubmit it. Six weeks later, Beck resubmitted her revised manuscript that incorporated the reviewers' recommendations. In September 2003, Beck received notification that her revised manuscript had been accepted for publication in *Nursing Research*. The article was published in the January/February 2004 issue. In addition to disseminating the results as a journal article, Beck has presented the findings at numerous national and international research conferences.

SUMMARY POINTS

- The people who provide information to the **researchers** (**investigators**) in a study are referred to as **subjects, study participants**, or **respondents** (in quantitative research) or study participants or **informants** in qualitative research; collectively, they make up the **sample**.
- The *site* is the overall location for the research; researchers sometimes engage in **multisite studies**. *Settings* are the more specific places where data collection will occur. Settings for nursing research can range from totally naturalistic environments to formal laboratories.
- Researchers investigate **concepts** and **phenomena** (or **constructs**), which are abstractions or mental representations inferred from behavior or characteristics.
- Concepts are the building blocks of **theories**, which are systematic explanations of some aspect of the real world.
- In quantitative studies, concepts are called *variables*. A **variable** is a characteristic or quality that takes on different values (i.e., varies from one person or object to another).
- Groups that are highly varied with respect to some attribute are described as **heterogeneous**; groups with limited variability are **homogeneous**.

- **Continuous variables** can take on an infinite range of values along a continuum (e.g., weight). **Discrete variables** have a finite number of values between two points (e.g., number of children). **Categorical variables** have distinct categories that do not represent a quantity (e.g., gender).
- The **dependent** (or **outcome**) **variable** is the behavior, characteristic, or outcome the researcher is interested in understanding, explaining, or affecting. The **independent variable** is the presumed cause of, antecedent to, or influence on the dependent variable.
- A **conceptual definition** describes the abstract or theoretical meaning of the concepts being studied. An **operational definition** specifies the procedures required to measure a variable.
- **Data**—the information collected during the course of a study—may take the form of narrative information (**qualitative data**) or numeric values (**quantitative data**).
- A **relationship** is a bond or connection (or pattern of association) between two variables. Quantitative researchers examine the relationship between the independent variables and dependent variables.
- When the independent variable causes or affects the dependent variable, the relationship is a **cause-and-effect** (or **causal**) **relationship**. In a **functional** or **associative relationship**, variables are related in a noncausal way.
- A basic distinction in quantitative studies is between **experimental research**, in which researchers actively intervene, and **nonexperimental** (or **observational**) **research,** in which researchers make observations of existing phenomena without intervening.
- Qualitative research often is rooted in research traditions that originate in other disciplines. Three such traditions are grounded theory, phenomenology, and ethnography.
- **Grounded theory** seeks to describe and understand key social psychological and structural processes that occur in a social setting.
- **Phenomenology** focuses on the lived experiences of humans and is an approach to learning

about what the life experiences of people are like and what they mean.

- **Ethnography** provides a framework for studying the meanings, patterns, and lifeways of a culture in a holistic fashion.

- In a quantitative study, researchers usually progress in a linear fashion from asking research questions to answering them. The main phases in a quantitative study are the conceptual, planning, empirical, analytic, and dissemination phases.

- The *conceptual phase* involves (1) defining the problem to be studied; (2) doing a **literature review**; (3) engaging in **clinical fieldwork** for clinical studies; (4) developing a framework and conceptual definitions; and (5) formulating **hypotheses** to be tested.

- The *planning phase* entails (6) selecting a **research design**; (7) developing **intervention protocols** if the study is experimental; (8) specifying the **population**; (9) developing a **sampling plan**; (10) specifying methods to measure the research variables; (11) developing strategies to safeguard the rights of subjects; and (12) finalizing the research plan (e.g., conferring with colleagues, *pretesting* instruments).

- The *empirical phase* involves (13) collecting data; and (14) preparing data for analysis.

- The *analytic phase* involves (15) analyzing data through **statistical analysis**; and (16) interpreting the results.

- The *dissemination phase* entails (17) communicating the findings through the preparation of **research reports**; and (18) promoting the use of the study evidence in nursing practice.

- The flow of activities in a qualitative study is more flexible and less linear. Qualitative studies typically involve an **emergent design** that evolves during fieldwork.

- Qualitative researchers begin with a broad question regarding a phenomenon of interest, often focusing on a little-studied aspect. In the early phase of a qualitative study, researchers select a site and seek to **gain entrée** into it, which typically involves enlisting the cooperation of **gatekeepers** within the site.

- Once in the field, researchers select informants, collect data, and then analyze and interpret the data in an iterative fashion; field experiences help to shape the design of the study.

- Early analysis in qualitative research leads to refinements in sampling and data collection, until **data saturation** (redundancy of information) is achieved.

- Both qualitative and quantitative researchers disseminate their findings, most often by publishing reports of their research as **journal articles**, which concisely communicate what the researcher did and what was found.

- Journal articles often consist of an **abstract** (a brief synopsis of the study) and four major sections that typically follow the **IMRAD format**: an **I**ntroduction (explanation of the study problem and its context); **M**ethod section (the strategies used to address the problem); **R**esults section (study findings); **and D**iscussion (interpretation of the findings).

- Research reports are often difficult to read because they are dense, concise, and contain a lot of jargon. Quantitative research reports may be intimidating at first because, compared with qualitative reports, they are more impersonal and report on statistical tests.

- **Statistical tests** are procedures for testing research hypotheses and evaluating the believability of the findings. Findings that are **statistically significant** are ones that have a high probability of being "real."

STUDY ACTIVITIES

Chapter 3 of the *Resource Manual to Accompany Nursing Research: Generating and Assessing Evidence for Practice, 8th edition*, offers various exercises and study suggestions for reinforcing concepts presented in this chapter. In addition, the following study questions can be addressed:

1. Suggest ways of conceptually and operationally defining the following concepts: nursing

competency, aggressive behavior, pain, home health hazards, postsurgical recovery, and body image.

2. In the following research problems, identify the independent and dependent variables:
   a. Does problem-oriented recording lead to more effective patient care than other recording methods?
   b. Do elderly patients have lower pain thresholds than younger patients?
   c.. Are the sleeping patterns of infants affected by different forms of stimulation?
   d. Can home visits by nurses to released psychiatric patients reduce readmission rates?
3. Which type of research do you think is easier to conduct—qualitative or quantitative research? Defend your response.

STUDIES CITED IN CHAPTER 3

Methodologic or theoretical references cited in this chapter can be found in a separate section at the end of the book.

Beck, C. T. (2002). Releasing the pause button: Mothering twins during the first year of life. *Qualitative Health Research, 12*, 593–608.

Beck, C. T. (2004). Birth trauma: In the eye of the beholder. *Nursing Research, 53*(1), 28–35.

Beck, C. T., & Gable, R. K. (2000). Postpartum Depression Screening Scale: Development and psychometric testing. *Nursing Research, 49*, 272–282.

Beck, C. T., & Gable, R. K. (2001). Further validation of the Postpartum Depression Screening Scale. *Nursing Research, 50*, 155–164.

Cooke, M., Chaboyer, W., Schluter, P., & Hiratos, M. (2005). The effect of music on preoperative anxiety in day surgery. *Journal of Advanced Nursing, 52*(1), 47–55.

Crogan, N. L., Velasquez, D., & Gagan, M. J. (2005). Testing the feasibility and initial effects of iron and vitamin C to enhance nursing home residents' immune status following an influenza vaccine. *Geriatric Nursing, 26*(3), 188–194.

Doorenbos, A. Z., Schim, S. M., Benkert, R., & Borse, N. N. (2005). Psychometric evaluation of the Cultural Competence Assessment instrument among healthcare providers. *Nursing Research, 54*(5), 324–331.

Irvine, F. E., Roberts, G. W., Jones, P., Spencer, L. H., Baker, C. R., & Williams, C. (2006). Communicative sensitivity in the bilingual healthcare setting: A qualitative study of language awareness. *Journal of Advanced Nursing, 53*(4), 422–434.

King, K. M., Thomlinson, E., Sanguins, J., & Leblanc, P. (2006). Men and women managing coronary artery disease risk. *Social Science and Medicine, 62*(5), 1091–1102.

McCloskey, R. (2004). Functional and self-efficacy changes of patients admitted to a Geriatric Rehabilitation Unit. *Journal of Advanced Nursing, 46*, 186–193.

Nyamathi, A., Berg, J., Jones, T., & Leake, B. (2005). Predictors of perceived health status of tuberculosis-infected homeless. *Western Journal of Nursing Research, 27*(7), 896–910.

O'Dell, K. K., & Jacelon, C. S. (2005). Not the surgery for a young person: Women's experience with vaginal closure surgery for severe prolapse. *Urologic Nursing, 25*(5), 345–351.

Polit, D. F., London, A., & Martinez, J. (2001). *The health of poor urban women.* New York: Manpower Demonstration Research Corporation. Retrieved October 2, 2006, from http://www.mdrc.org

Schoenfeld, N., & Juarbe, T. C. (2005). From sunrise to sunset: An ethnography of rural Ecuadorian women's perceived health needs and resources. *Health Care for Women International, 26*(10), 957–977.

Scott, L. D., Rogers, A. E., Hwang, W. T., & Zhang, Y. (2006). Effects of critical care nurses' work hours on vigilance and patients' safety. *American Journal of Critical Care, 15*(1), 30–37.

Taxis, JC., Rew, L., Jackson, K., & Kouzekanani, K. (2004). Protective resources and perceptions of stress in a multi-ethnic sample of school-aged children. *Pediatric Nursing, 30*(6), 477–482.

Uys, L., Chirwa, M., Diamini, P., Greeff, M., Kobi, T., Holzemer, W., Makoae, L., Naidoo, J. R., & Phetlhu, R. (2005). "Eating plastic," "winning the lotto," "joining the www".... Descriptions of HIV/AIDS in Africa. *Journal of the Association of Nurses in AIDS Care, 16*(3), 11–21.

Zengerle-Levy, K. (2006). The inextricable link in caring for families of critically burned children. *Qualitative Health Research, 16*(1), 5–26.

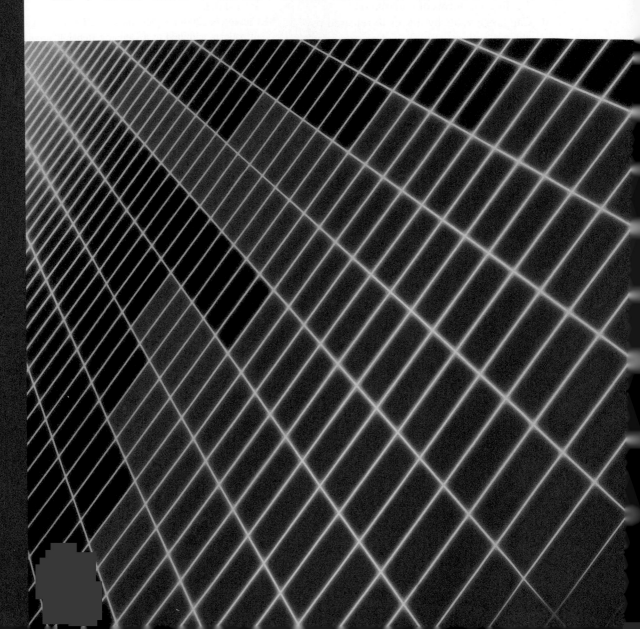

PART 2

CONCEPTUALIZING A STUDY TO GENERATE EVIDENCE FOR NURSING

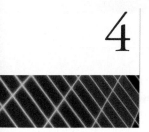

4 Conceptualizing Research Problems, Research Questions, and Hypotheses

OVERVIEW OF RESEARCH PROBLEMS

Studies to generate new research evidence begin in much the same fashion as an EBP effort—as problems that need to be solved or as questions that need be answered. This chapter discusses the formulation and development of research problems. We begin by clarifying some relevant terms.

Basic Terminology

At the most general level, a researcher selects a **topic** or a phenomenon on which to focus. Examples of research topics are claustrophobia during MRI tests, pain management for sickle cell disease, and nutrition during pregnancy. Within each of these broad topic areas are many potential research problems. In this section, we illustrate various terms using the topic *side effects of chemotherapy*.

A **research problem** is an enigmatic, perplexing, or troubling condition. Both qualitative and quantitative researchers identify a research problem within a broad topic area of interest. The purpose of research is to "solve" the problem—or to contribute to its solution—by accumulating relevant information. A **problem statement** articulates the problem to be addressed and indicates the need for a study through the development of an *argument*. Table 4.1

presents a simplified problem statement related to the topic of side effects of chemotherapy.

Research questions are the specific queries researchers want to answer in addressing the research problem. Research questions guide the types of data to be collected in a study. Researchers who make specific predictions about answers to research questions pose **hypotheses** that are tested empirically.

Many reports include a **statement of purpose** (or purpose statement), which is the researcher's summary of the overall goal of a study. A researcher might also identify several **research aims** or **objectives**—the specific accomplishments the researcher hopes to achieve by conducting the study. The objectives include answering research questions or testing research hypotheses but may also encompass some broader aims (e.g., developing recommendations for changes to nursing practice based on the study results).

These terms are not always consistently defined in research methods textbooks, and differences between the terms are often subtle. Table 4.1 illustrates the interrelationships among terms as we define them.

Research Problems and Paradigms

Some research problems are better suited to qualitative versus quantitative methods. Quantitative studies usually involve concepts that are fairly well

TABLE 4.1	Example of Terms Relating to Research Problems

TERM	EXAMPLE
Topic/focus	Side effects of chemotherapy
Research problem (problem statement)	Nausea and vomiting are common side effects among patients on chemotherapy, and interventions to date have been only moderately successful in reducing these effects. New interventions that can reduce or prevent these side effects need to be identified.
Statement of purpose	The purpose of the study is to test an intervention to reduce chemotherapy-induced side effects—specifically, to compare the effectiveness of patient-controlled and nurse-administered antiemetic therapy for controlling nausea and vomiting in patients on chemotherapy.
Research question	What is the relative effectiveness of patient-controlled antiemetic therapy versus nurse-controlled antiemetic therapy with regard to (a) medication consumption and (b) control of nausea and vomiting in patients on chemotherapy?
Hypotheses	Subjects receiving antiemetic therapy by a patient-controlled pump will (1) be less nauseated (2) vomit less, and (3) consume less medication than subjects receiving the therapy by nurse administration.
Aims/objectives	This study has as its aim the following objectives: (1) to develop and implement two alternative procedures for administering antiemetic therapy for patients receiving moderate emetogenic chemotherapy (patient controlled versus nurse controlled); (2) to test three hypotheses concerning the relative effectiveness of the alternative procedures on medication consumption and control of side effects; and (3) to use the findings to develop recommendations for possible changes to clinical procedures.

developed, about which there is an existing body of literature, and for which reliable methods of measurement have been (or can be) developed. For example, a quantitative study might be undertaken to determine whether seniors with chronic illness who continue working are less (or more) depressed than those who retire. There are relatively accurate measures of depression that would yield quantitative information about the level of depression in a sample of employed and retired chronically ill seniors.

Qualitative studies are often undertaken because some aspect of a phenomenon is poorly understood, and the researcher wants to develop a rich, comprehensive, and context-bound understanding of it. Qualitative studies are often initiated to heighten awareness and create a dialogue about a phenomenon. Qualitative methods would not be well suited

to comparing levels of depression among employed and retired seniors, but they would be ideal for exploring, for example, the *meaning* of depression among chronically ill retirees. Thus, the nature of the research question is closely allied to paradigms and research traditions within paradigms.

Sources of Research Problems

Where do ideas for research problems come from? How do researchers select topic areas and develop research questions? At the most basic level, research topics originate with researchers' interests. Because research is a time-consuming enterprise, curiosity about and interest in a topic are essential to a project's success. Explicit sources that might fuel researchers' curiosity include clinical experience, the nursing literature, social issues, theories, and suggestions from others.

Experience and Clinical Fieldwork

Nurses' everyday clinical experience is a rich source of ideas for research problems. As you are performing your nursing duties, you are bound to find a wealth of research ideas if you are curious about why things are the way they are or about how things could be improved. You may be on the way to developing a research idea if you have ever asked such questions as: Why are things done this way? What caused this situation? What would happen if....? For beginning researchers in particular, clinical experience is often the most compelling source for topics. Immediate problems that need a solution—analogous to problem-focused triggers discussed in Chapter 2—are meaningful and may generate more enthusiasm than abstract or distant problems inferred from a theory.

➔ **TIP:** Personal experiences in clinical settings are a provocative source of research ideas. Here are some hints on how to proceed:

- Watch for recurring problems and see if you can discern a pattern in situations that lead to the problem.
  Example: Why do many patients complain of being tired after being transferred from a coronary care unit to a progressive care unit?
- Think about aspects of your work that are irksome, are frustrating, or do not result in the intended outcome — then try to identify factors contributing to the problem that could be changed.Example: Why is suppertime so frustrating in a nursing home?
- Critically examine some decisions you make in performing your functions. Are these decisions based on tradition, or are they based on systematic evidence that supports their efficacy?
  Example: What would happen if you used the return of flatus to assess the return of GI motility after abdominal surgery, rather than listening to bowel sounds?

Nursing Literature

Ideas for studies often come from reading the nursing literature (knowledge-focused triggers). Beginning nurse researchers can profit from regularly reading nursing journals, either clinical specialty journals or research journals such as *Nursing Research* or the *Journal of Advanced Nursing*. Nonresearch articles can be helpful in alerting researchers to clinical trends and issues of importance in clinical settings. Published research reports may suggest problem areas indirectly by stimulating the imagination and directly by explicitly recommending additional research.

Inconsistencies in research findings sometimes generate ideas for studies. For example, there are inconsistencies regarding which type of tactile stimulation or touch (e.g., gentle touch, stroking, rubbing) has the most beneficial physiologic and behavioral effects on preterm infants. Such discrepancies can lead to the design of a study to help resolve the matter.

Researchers may also wonder whether a study similar to one reported in a journal article would yield comparable results if applied in a different setting or with a different population. Replications are needed to establish the validity and generalizability of previous findings.

In summary, a familiarity with existing research, or with emerging nursing issues that have yet to be understood and investigated systematically, is an important route to developing a research topic. In Chapter 5, we discuss how to locate and review research literature.

➔ **TIP:** If you are struggling for an idea, do not hesitate to replicate an earlier study. Replications are a valuable learning experience and can make important contributions to the base of evidence on a topic.

Social Issues

Sometimes, topics are suggested by more global contemporary social or political issues of relevance to the health care community. For example, the feminist movement has raised questions about such topics as sexual harassment, domestic violence, and gender equity in health care. The civil rights movement has led to research on minority health problems, access to health care, and culturally sensitive interventions. Thus, an idea for a study may stem from a familiarity with social concerns or controversial social problems.

Theory

The fourth major source of research problems lies in the theories and conceptual schemes that have been developed in nursing and related disciplines. To be useful, theories must be tested through research for their applicability to hospitals, clinics, and other nursing environments.

When basing a study on an existing theory, researchers use a deductive process. Essentially, they must ask the following questions: If this theory is correct, what kind of behavior would I expect to find in certain situations or under certain conditions? What kind of evidence would support this theory? This process, which is described more fully in Chapter 6, would eventually result in a problem that could be subjected to systematic study.

Ideas From External Sources

External sources sometimes provide the impetus for a research idea. In some cases, a research topic may be given as a direct suggestion. For example, a faculty member may give students a list of topics from which to choose or may actually assign a specific topic to be studied. Organizations that sponsor funded research, such as government agencies, often identify topics on which research proposals are encouraged. Research ideas sometimes represent a response to priorities that are established within the nursing profession, examples of which were discussed in Chapter 1.

Often, ideas for studies emerge as a result of a brainstorming session. By discussing possible research topics with peers, advisers, or researchers with advanced skills, ideas often become clarified and sharpened or enriched and more fully developed. Professional conferences provide an excellent opportunity for such discussions.

DEVELOPING AND REFINING RESEARCH PROBLEMS

Unless a research problem is formulated on the basis of theory or an explicit suggestion from an external source, the actual procedures for developing a research idea are difficult to describe. The process is rarely a smooth and orderly one; there are likely to be false starts, inspirations, and setbacks. The few suggestions offered here are not intended to imply that there are techniques for making this first step easy but rather to encourage beginning researchers to persevere in the absence of instant success.

Selecting a Topic

The development of a research problem is a creative process that depends on imagination and ingenuity. In the early stages when you are generating research ideas, it is unwise to be overly self-critical. It is better to relax and jot down general areas of interest as they come to mind. At this point, it matters little if the terms used to remind you of your ideas are broad or specific, technical or colloquial—the important point is to put some ideas on paper.

After this first step, the ideas can be sorted in terms of interest, knowledge about the topics, and the perceived feasibility of turning the topics into a research project. When the most fruitful idea has been selected, the list should not be discarded; it may be necessary to return to it.

➲ **TIP:** The process of selecting and refining a research problem usually takes longer than you might think. The process involves starting with some preliminary ideas, having discussions with colleagues and advisers, looking at the research literature, looking at what is happening in clinical settings, and engaging in a lot of reflection.

Narrowing the Topic

Once you have identified a topic of interest, you can begin to ask some broad questions that can lead you to a researchable problem. Examples of question stems that may help to focus an inquiry include the following:

- What is going on with...?
- What is the process by which...?
- What is the meaning of...?
- What is the extent of...?
- What influences or causes...?
- What differences exist between...?
- What are the consequences of...?
- What is the relationship between...?
- What factors contribute to...?
- What conditions prevail before...?
- How effective is...?

Here again, early criticism of ideas is often counterproductive. Try not to jump to the conclusion that an idea sounds trivial or uninspired without giving it more careful consideration or exploring it with others.

Beginning researchers often develop problems that are too broad in scope or too complex and unwieldy for their level of methodologic expertise. The transformation of the general topic into a workable problem is typically accomplished in a number of steps, involving a series of successive approximations. Each step should result in progress toward the goals of narrowing the scope of the problem and sharpening and defining the concepts.

As researchers move from general topics to more specific researchable problems, more than one potential problem area can emerge. Let us consider the following example. Suppose you were working on a medical unit and were puzzled by the fact that some patients always complained about having to wait for pain medication when certain nurses were assigned to them and, yet, these same patients offered no complaints with other nurses. The general problem area is discrepancy in complaints from patients regarding pain medications administered by different nurses. You might ask the following: What accounts for this discrepancy? How can I improve the situation? Such questions are not actual research questions; they are too broad and vague. They may, however, lead you to ask other questions, such as the following: How do the two groups of nurses differ? What characteristics

are unique to each group of nurses? What characteristics do the complaining patients share? At this point, you may observe that the ethnic background of the patients and nurses may be a relevant factor. This may lead you to search the literature for studies concerning ethnicity in relation to nursing care, or it may provoke you to discuss the observations with others. The result of these efforts may be several researchable questions, such as the following:

- What is the essence of patient complaints among patients of different ethnic backgrounds?
- How do complaints by patients of different ethnic backgrounds get expressed by patients and perceived by nurses?
- Is the ethnic background of nurses related to the frequency with which they dispense pain medication?
- Do nurses' dispensing behaviors change as a function of the similarity between their own ethnic background and that of patients?

All these questions stem from the same general problem, yet each would be studied differently—for example, some suggest a qualitative approach, and others suggest a quantitative one. A quantitative researcher might become curious about ethnic differences in nurses' dispensing behaviors. Both ethnicity and nurses' dispensing behaviors are variables that can be measured reliably A qualitative researcher who noticed differences in patient complaints would likely be more interested in understanding the *essence* of the complaints, the patients' *experience* of frustration, or the *process* by which the problem got resolved. These are aspects of the research problem that would be difficult to quantify.

Researchers finalize the problem to be studied based on several factors, including its inherent interest to them and its compatibility with a paradigm of preference. In addition, tentative problems usually vary in their feasibility and worth. It is at this point that a critical evaluation of ideas is appropriate.

Evaluating Research Problems

There are no rules for making a final selection of a research problem, but some criteria should be kept in mind. Four important considerations are the significance, researchability, and feasibility of the problem, and its interest to you.

Significance of the Problem

A crucial factor in selecting a problem to be studied is its significance to nursing. Evidence from the study should have the potential of contributing meaningfully to nursing practice. Within the context of the existing body of evidence, the new study should be the right "next step." The right next step could involve an original idea for a line of inquiry, but it could also involve a replication or a study to answer previously asked questions with greater rigor or with different types of people.

In evaluating the significance of an idea, you should pose the following kinds of questions: Is the problem an important one? Will patients, nurses, or the broader health care community benefit from the evidence that will be produced? Will the results lead to practical applications? Will the findings challenge (or lend support to) untested assumptions? Will the study help to formulate or alter nursing practices? If the answer to all these questions is "no," then the problem should be abandoned.

Researchability of the Problem

Not all problems are amenable to research inquiry. Questions of a moral or ethical nature, although provocative, are incapable of being researched. Take, for example, the following: Should assisted suicide be legalized? The answer to such a question is based on a person's values. There are no *right* or *wrong* answers, only points of view. The problem is suitable to debate, not to research. To be sure, it is possible to ask related questions that could be researched, such as the following:

- What are nurses' attitudes toward assisted suicide?
- What moral dilemmas are perceived by nurses who might be involved in assisted suicide?
- Do terminally ill patients living with high levels of pain hold more favorable attitudes toward assisted suicide than those with less pain?
- How do family members experience the loss of a loved one through assisted suicide?

The findings from studies addressing such questions would have no bearing, of course, on whether assisted suicide should be legalized, but the information could be useful in developing a better understanding of the issues.

Feasibility of Addressing the Problem

A third consideration in evaluating a problem concerns feasibility, which encompasses several issues. Not all of the following factors are relevant for every problem, but they should be kept in mind in making a final decision.

Time and Timing. Most studies have deadlines or at least goals for completion. Therefore, the problem must be one that can be adequately studied within the time allotted. This means that the scope of the problem should be sufficiently restricted that enough time will be available for the various steps and activities reviewed in Chapter 3. It is wise to be conservative in estimating time for various tasks because research activities usually require more time to complete than anticipated. Qualitative studies may be especially time-consuming.

A related consideration concerns timing. Some of the research steps—especially data collection—may be more readily performed at certain times than at others. For example, if the problem focused on patients with peptic ulcers, the research might be more easily conducted in the fall and spring because of the increase in the number of patients with peptic ulcers during these seasons. When the timing requirements of the tasks do not match the time available for their performance, the feasibility of the project may be jeopardized.

Availability of Study Participants. In any study involving humans, researchers need to consider whether individuals with the desired characteristics will be available and willing to cooperate. Securing people's cooperation may in some cases be easy (e.g., getting nursing students to complete a questionnaire in a classroom), but other situations may pose more difficulties. Some people may not have the time, others may have no interest in a study that has little personal benefit, and others may not feel well enough to participate. Fortunately, people usually *are* willing to cooperate if research demands are minimal. If the research is time-consuming or demanding, however, researchers may need to exert extra effort in recruiting participants—or may have to offer a monetary incentive.

An additional problem may be that of identifying and locating people with needed characteristics. For example, if we were interested in studying the coping strategies of people who had lost a family member through suicide, we would have to develop a plan for identifying prospective participants from this distinct and inconspicuous population.

Cooperation of Others. Often, it is insufficient to obtain the cooperation of prospective study participants alone. If the sample included children, mentally incompetent people, or senile individuals, it would be necessary to secure the permission of parents or guardians, an issue discussed in the chapter on ethics (see Chapter 7). In institutional or organizational settings (e.g., hospitals), access to clients, members, personnel, or records requires authorization. Most health care facilities require that any project be presented to a panel of reviewers for approval. As noted in Chapter 3, a critical requirement in many studies is gaining entrée into an appropriate community, setting, or group, and developing the trust of gatekeepers.

Facilities and Equipment. All studies have resource requirements, although needs may in some cases be modest. It is prudent to consider what facilities and equipment will be needed and whether they will be available before embarking on a project. The following is a partial list of considerations:

- Will assistants be needed, and are such assistants available?
- If technical equipment and apparatus are needed, can they be secured, and are they functioning properly? Will audiotaping or videotaping equipment be required, and is it of sufficient sensitivity? Will laboratory facilities be required, and are they available?
- Will space be required, and can it be obtained?
- Will telephones, office equipment, or other supplies be required?

Money. Monetary requirements for research projects vary widely, ranging from $100 to $200 for small student projects to hundreds of thousands (or even millions) of dollars for large-scale, government-sponsored research. The investigator on a limited budget should think carefully about projected expenses before making the final selection of a problem. Some major categories of research-related expenditures are the following:

- Literature costs—computerized literature search and retrieval service charges, Internet access charges, reproduction costs, books and journals
- Personnel costs—payment to individuals hired to help with the data collection (e.g., for conducting interviews, coding, data entry, transcribing, word processing)
- Study participant costs—payment to participants as an incentive for their cooperation or to offset their own expenses (e.g., transportation or baby-sitting costs)
- Supplies—paper, envelopes, computer disks, postage, audiotapes, and so forth
- Printing and duplication costs—expenditures for printing forms, questionnaires, participant recruitment notices, and so on
- Equipment—laboratory apparatus, computers and software, audio or video recorders, calculators, and the like
- Laboratory fees for the analysis of biophysiologic data
- Transportation costs

Researcher Experience. The problem should be chosen from a field about which investigators have some prior knowledge or experience. Researchers may struggle in undertaking a study on a topic that is totally new and unfamiliar—although upfront clinical fieldwork may make up for certain deficiencies. In addition to substantive knowledge, the issue of technical expertise should not be overlooked. Beginning researchers with limited methodologic skills should avoid research problems that might require the development of sophisticated measuring instruments or that involve complex data analyses.

Ethical Considerations. A research problem may not be feasible because the investigation of the problem would pose unfair or unethical demands on participants. Researchers need to be thoroughly knowledgeable about the rights of human or animal subjects. An overview of major ethical considerations concerning human study participants is presented in Chapter 7 and should be reviewed when considering the feasibility of a project.

Researcher Interest

Even if the tentative problem is researchable, significant, and feasible, there is one more criterion: your own interest in the problem. Genuine interest in and curiosity about the chosen research problem are critical prerequisites to a successful study. A great deal of time and energy are expended in a study; there is little sense devoting these personal resources to a project that does not generate enthusiasm.

➡ **TIP:** Beginning researchers often seek out suggestions on topic areas, and such assistance may be helpful in getting started. Nevertheless, it is rarely wise to be talked into a topic toward which you are not personally inclined. If you do not find a problem attractive or stimulating during the beginning phases of a study—when opportunities for creativity and intellectual enjoyment are at their highest—then you are bound to regret your choice later.

COMMUNICATING RESEARCH PROBLEMS

Every study needs to have a problem statement—the articulation of what it is that is problematic and that is the impetus for the research. Most research reports also present either a statement of purpose, research questions, or hypotheses, and often combinations of these three elements are included.

Many beginning researchers do not really understand problem statements and may even have trouble identifying them in a research article—not to mention developing one. A problem statement is presented early in a research report and often begins with the very first sentence after the abstract. Specific research questions, purposes, or hypotheses appear later in the introduction. Typically, however, the order is reversed in the actual progression of the project. Researchers usually start their inquiry by framing a research question or a purpose, and then they develop an argument in the form of a problem statement to lay out the rationale for the new research. This section discusses the wording for statements of purpose, research questions, and problem statements; the following major section discusses hypotheses.

Statements of Purpose

Many researchers articulate their research goals as a statement of purpose, worded in the declarative form. The purpose statement establishes the general direction of the inquiry and captures—usually in one or two clear sentences—the essence of the study. It is usually easy to identify a purpose statement because the word *purpose* is explicitly stated: "The purpose of this study was . . ."—although sometimes the words *aim*, *goal*, *intent*, or *objective* are used instead, as in "The aim of this study was. . . ."

In a quantitative study, a statement of purpose identifies the key study variables and their possible interrelationships, as well as the nature of the population of interest.

Example of a statement of purpose from a quantitative study: "The purpose of this study was to examine the incidence and prevalence of lipodystrophy-related symptoms in persons with HIV and to determine the impact of these symptoms on health-related quality of life" (Nicholas et al., 2005, p. 55).

This purpose statement identifies the population of interest, persons with HIV, and indicates two interrelated goals. The first is descriptive, that is, to determine the incidence and prevalence of lipodystrophy-related symptoms within the population. In the second, the researchers plan to examine the effects of these symptoms (the independent variables) on health-related quality of life (the dependent variable).

In qualitative studies, the statement of purpose indicates the nature of the inquiry, the key concept or phenomenon, and the group, community, or setting under study.

Example of a statement of purpose from a qualitative study: "The purpose of this study was to explore the memories of patients who had a short-term admission to the ICU, with particular focus on dreams, nightmares, and confusion" (Magarey & McCutcheon, 2005, p. 344).

This statement indicates that the central phenomenon of interest is patients' memories of dreams, nightmares, and confusion and that the group under study is patients with a short-term ICU admission.

The statement of purpose communicates more than just the nature of the problem. Through researchers' selection of verbs, a statement of purpose suggests the manner in which they sought to solve the problem, or the state of knowledge on the topic. That is, a study whose purpose is to *explore* or *describe* some phenomenon is likely to be an investigation of a little-researched topic, often involving a qualitative approach such as a phenomenology or ethnography. A statement of purpose for a qualitative study—especially a grounded theory study—may also use verbs such as *understand, discover, develop,* or *generate.* Creswell (1998) noted that the statements of purpose in qualitative studies often "encode" the tradition of inquiry not only through the researcher's choice of verbs but also through the use of certain terms or "buzz words" associated with those traditions, as follows:

- *Grounded theory:* processes; social structures; social interactions
- *Phenomenological studies:* experience; lived experience; meaning; essence
- *Ethnographic studies:* culture; roles; lifeways; cultural behavior

Quantitative researchers also suggest the nature of the inquiry through their selection of verbs. A purpose statement indicating that the purpose of the study is to *test* or *evaluate* the effectiveness of an intervention suggests an experimental design, for example. A study whose purpose is to *examine* or *assess* the relationship between two variables is more likely to involve a nonexperimental quantita-

tive design. In some cases, the verb is ambiguous: a purpose statement indicating that the researcher's intent is to *compare* could be referring to a comparison of alternative treatments (using an experimental approach) or a comparison of two preexisting groups (using a nonexperimental approach). In any event, verbs such as *test, evaluate,* and *compare* suggest an existing knowledge base, quantifiable variables, and designs with scientific controls.

Note that the choice of verbs in a statement of purpose should connote objectivity. A statement of purpose indicating that the intent of the study was to *prove, demonstrate,* or *show* something suggests a bias.

➲ **TIP:** In wording your statement of purpose, it may be useful to look at published research articles for models. Unfortunately, some reports fail to state unambiguously the study purpose, leaving readers to infer the purpose from such sources as the title of the report. In other reports, the purpose is clearly stated but may be difficult to find. Researchers most often state their purpose at the end of the report's introduction.

Research Questions

Research questions are, in some cases, direct rewordings of statements of purpose, phrased interrogatively rather than declaratively, as in the following example:

- The purpose of this study is to assess the relationship between the dependency level of renal transplant recipients and their rate of recovery.
- What is the relationship between the dependency level of renal transplant recipients and their rate of recovery?

The question form has the advantage of simplicity and directness. Questions invite an answer and help to focus attention on the kinds of data that would have to be collected to provide that answer. Some research reports thus omit a statement of purpose and state only research questions. Other researchers use a set of research questions to clarify or lend greater specificity to a global purpose statement.

Research Questions in Quantitative Studies

In Chapter 2, we discussed the framing of clinical "foreground" questions to guide an EBP inquiry. Many of the EBP question templates in Table 2.1 could yield questions to guide a research project as well, but *researchers* tend to conceptualize their questions in terms of their *variables*. Take, for example, the first question in Table 2.1, which states, "In (population), what is the effect of (intervention) on (outcome)? A researcher would be more likely to think of the question in these terms: "In (population), what is the effect of (independent variable) on (dependent variable)? The advantage of thinking in terms of variables is that researchers must consciously make decisions about how to operationalize their variables and how to guide an analysis strategy with their variables. Thus, we can say that in quantitative studies, research questions identify the key study variables, the relationships among them, and the population under study. The variables are all measurable concepts, and the questions suggest quantification.

Most research questions concern relationships among variables, and thus many quantitative research questions could be articulated using a general question template: "In (population), what is the relationship between (independent variable or IV) and (dependent variable or DV)?" Examples of minor variations include the following:

- *Treatment, intervention:* In (population), what is the effect of (IV: intervention) on (DV)?
- *Prognosis:* In (population), does (IV: disease, condition) affect or increase risk for (DV)?
- *Causation, etiology:* In (population), does (IV: exposure, characteristic) cause or increase risk for (DV)?

Thus, questions are sometimes phrased in terms of the *effects* of an independent variable on the dependent variable—but this still involves a *relationship* between the two.

There is one important distinction between the clinical foreground questions for an EBP-focused evidence search as described in Chapter 2 and a research question for an original study. As shown in Table 2.1, sometimes clinicians ask questions about explicit comparisons (e.g., they want to compare intervention A to intervention B) and sometimes they do not (e.g., they want to learn the effects of intervention A, compared with any other intervention that has been studied or to the absence of another intervention). In a research question, there must *always* be a designated comparison because the independent variable must be operationally defined; this definition would articulate exactly what is being studied. As we discuss in subsequent chapters, the nature of the comparison has implications for the strength of the study and the interpretability of the findings.

Another distinction between EBP and research questions is that research questions sometimes are more complex than typical clinical foreground questions for EBP. As an example, suppose that we began with a general interest in nurses' use of humor with cancer patients, and the effects that humor has on these patients. One research question might be, "What is the effect of nurses' use of humor (the IV, versus absence of humor) on stress (the DV) in hospitalized cancer patients (the population)? But we might also be interested in whether the relationship between the IV and DV, once established, is influenced by or *moderated* by a third variable. For example: Does nurses' use of humor have a different effect on stress in male versus female patients? In this example, gender is a moderator variable. A **moderator variable** is a variable that affects the strength or direction of an association between the independent and dependent variable (Bennett, 2000). Therefore, identifying key moderators may be important in understanding *when* to expect a relationship between the IV and DV and can often have clinical relevance. Moderator (or *moderating*) variables can be characteristics of the population (e.g., male versus female patients) or of the circumstances (e.g., rural versus urban settings). Here are examples of question templates that involve moderator variables (MVs):

- *Treatment, intervention:* In (population), does the effect of (IV: intervention) on (DV) vary by (MV)?
- *Prognosis:* In (population), does the effect of (IV: disease, condition) on (DV) vary by (MV)?

• *Causation, etiology:* In (population), does (IV: exposure, characteristic) cause or increase risk for (DV) differentially by (MV)?

When the researcher's intent is to understand causal pathways, research questions may involve a **mediating variable**—a variable that intervenes between the IV and the DV and helps to explain why the relationship exists. In our hypothetical example, we might ask the following: Does nurses' use of humor have a direct effect on the stress of hospitalized patients with cancer, or is the effect *mediated by* humor's effect on natural killer cell activity? In questions involving mediators, researchers may be as interested in the mediator as they are in the independent variable because mediators are key explanatory mechanisms.

Some research questions are primarily descriptive. As examples, here are some descriptive questions that could be answered in a quantitative study on nurses' use of humor:

• What is the frequency with which nurses use humor as a complementary therapy with hospitalized cancer patients?
• What type of humor do nurses most often use with hospitalized cancer patients?
• What are the characteristics of nurses who use humor as a complementary therapy with hospitalized cancer patients?
• Is my Use of Humor Scale an accurate and valid measure of nurses' use of humor with patients in clinical settings?

Answers to such questions might, if addressed in a methodologically sound study, be useful in developing effective strategies for reducing stress in patients with cancer.

Example of a research question from a quantitative study: Lee, Miles, and Holditch-Davis (2006) conducted a study about fathers' support of mothers of medically fragile infants. Their primary research question was about the existence and strength of a relationship: *To what extent do factors in the mother–father system (marital status) and the child system (amount of technology dependence, birth weight, and gender) affect maternal perceptions of paternal support over time?*

The Toolkit for Chapter 4 of the accompanying *Resource Manual* includes question templates in a Word document that can be "filled in" to generate many types of research questions. ✲

Research Questions in Qualitative Studies

Research questions in qualitative statements include the phenomenon of interest and the group or population of interest. Researchers in the various qualitative traditions vary in their conceptualization of what types of questions are important. Grounded theory researchers are likely to ask *process* questions, phenomenologists tend to ask *meaning* questions, and ethnographers generally ask *descriptive* questions about cultures. The terms associated with the various traditions, discussed previously in connection with purpose statements, are likely to be incorporated into the research questions.

Example of a research question from a phenomenological study: What is the structure of the lived experience of feeling respected? (Parse, 2006)

It is important to note, however, that not all qualitative studies are rooted in a specific research tradition. Many researchers use naturalistic methods to describe or explore phenomena without focusing on cultures, meaning, or social processes.

Example of a research question from a descriptive qualitative study: Bottorff and her colleagues (2005) explored couple dynamics and interactions related to tobacco use before pregnancy. Their two research questions were: (a) *What are the couple routines that accommodate tobacco use by one or both individuals in intimate relationships?* and (b) *How do couple interpersonal dynamics influence tobacco use—and how are these dynamics influenced by tobacco use?*

In qualitative studies, research questions sometimes evolve over the course of the study. The researcher begins with a *focus* that defines the general boundaries of the inquiry. However, the boundaries are not cast in stone; the boundaries "can be altered and, in the typical naturalistic inquiry, will be" (Lincoln & Guba, 1985, p. 228).

The naturalist begins with a research question that provides a general starting point but does not prohibit discovery; qualitative researchers are often sufficiently flexible that the question can be modified as new information makes it relevant to do so.

Problem Statements

Problem statements express the dilemma or disturbing situation that needs investigation and develop a rationale for a new inquiry. A problem statement identifies the nature of the problem that is being addressed in the study and its context and significance. A problem statement is *not* merely a statement of the purpose of the study; it is a well-structured formulation of what it is that is problematic, what it is that "needs fixing," or what it is that is poorly understood. Problem statements, especially for quantitative studies, often have most of the following six components:

1. *Problem identification:* What is wrong with the current situation?
2. *Background:* What is the nature of the problem, the context of the situation that readers need to understand?
3. *Scope of the problem:* How big a problem is it; how many people are affected?
4. *Consequences of the problem:* What is the cost of *not* fixing the problem?
5. *Knowledge gaps:* What information about the problem is lacking?

6. *Proposed solution:* What is the basis for believing that the proposed study would contribute to the solution of the problem?

The Toolkit for Chapter 4 of the accompanying *Resource Manual* includes these questions in a Word document that can be "filled in" and reorganized as needed, as an aid to developing a problem statement.

To pursue our earlier example, suppose our topic was humor as a complementary therapy for reducing stress in hospitalized patients with cancer. Our research question might be, "What is the effect of nurses' use of humor on stress and natural killer cell activity in hospitalized cancer patients?" Box 4.1 presents a rough draft of a problem statement for such a study. This problem statement is a reasonable first draft—although it is missing the relevant citations needed to support the assertions. The draft has several, but not all, of the six components and could be strengthened.

Box 4.2 illustrates how the problem statement could be made more powerful by adding information about scope (component 3), long-term consequences (component 4), and possible solutions (component 6). This second draft builds a stronger and more compelling argument for new research: millions of people are affected by cancer, and the disease has adverse consequences not only for those diagnosed and their families but also for society. The revised problem statement also suggests a basis for the new study by describing a

---

BOX 4.1 Draft Problem Statement on Humor and Stress

A diagnosis of cancer is associated with high levels of stress. Sizeable numbers of patients who receive a cancer diagnosis describe feelings of uncertainty, fear, anger, and loss of control. Interpersonal relationships, psychological functioning, and role performance have all been found to suffer following cancer diagnosis and treatment.

A variety of alternative/complementary therapies have been developed in an effort to decrease the harmful effects of stress on psychological and physiologic functioning, and resources devoted to these therapies (money and staff) have increased in recent years. However, many of these therapies have not been carefully evaluated to determine their efficacy, safety, or cost-effectiveness. For example, the use of humor has been recommended as a therapeutic device to improve quality of life, decrease stress, and perhaps improve immune functioning, but the evidence to justify its popularity is scant.

BOX 4.2 Some Possible Improvements to Problem Statement on Humor and Stress

Each year, more than 1 million people are diagnosed with cancer, which remains one of the top causes of death among both men and women (citations). Numerous studies have documented that a diagnosis of cancer is associated with high levels of stress. Sizeable numbers of patients who receive a cancer diagnosis describe feelings of uncertainty, fear, anger, and loss of control (citations). Interpersonal relationships, psychological functioning, and role performance have all been found to suffer following cancer diagnosis and treatment (citations). These stressful outcomes can, in turn, adversely affect health, long-term prognosis, and medical costs among cancer survivors (citations).

A variety of alternative/complementary therapies have been developed in an effort to decrease the harmful effects of stress on psychological and physiologic functioning, and resources devoted to these therapies (money and staff) have increased in recent years (citations). However, many of these therapies have not been carefully evaluated to determine their efficacy, safety, or cost-effectiveness. For example, the use of humor has been recommended as a therapeutic device to improve quality of life, decrease stress, and perhaps improve immune functioning (citations), but the evidence to justify its popularity is scant. Preliminary findings from a recent small-scale endocrinology study with a healthy sample exposed to a humorous intervention (citation), however, hold promise for further inquiry with immunocompromised populations.

possible solution on which the new study might build.

As this example suggests, the problem statement is usually interwoven with findings from the research literature. The findings provide the evidence backing up assertions in the problem statement and suggest gaps in knowledge. In many research articles, it is difficult to disentangle the problem statement from the literature review, unless there is a subsection specifically labeled "Literature Review" or something similar.

Problem statements for a qualitative study similarly express the nature of the problem, its context, its scope, and information needed to address it, as in the following example:

Example of a problem statement from a qualitative study: "Hospitalization is a common experience for elderly people in the United States. More than four out of every ten people 75 years or older are hospitalized each year, with an average stay of almost 7 days. . . . While hospitalized, elders and hospital staff are concerned about maintaining the elders' dignity. . . . Gaylin (1984) commented that dignity is often talked about but rarely examined. Almost 20 years later, this statement continues to be true; the few reports on the nature of dignity vary widely in their findings. To support elderly patients'

dignity, health care providers must understand the nature of dignity and the strategies employed by patients to maintain it" (Jacelon, 2003).

Qualitative studies that are embedded in a particular research tradition usually incorporate terms and concepts in their problem statements that foreshadow their tradition of inquiry (Creswell, 1998). For example, the problem statement in a grounded theory study might refer to the need to generate a theory relating to social processes. A problem statement for a phenomenological study might note the need to know more about people's experiences (as in the preceding example) or the meanings they attribute to those experiences. And an ethnographer might indicate the desire to describe how cultural forces affect people's behavior.

RESEARCH HYPOTHESES

A hypothesis is a prediction about the relationship between two or more variables. A hypothesis thus translates a quantitative research question into a precise prediction of expected outcomes. In qualitative studies, researchers do not begin with a hypothesis, in part because there is usually too little known about the topic to justify a hypothesis, and in part because qualitative researchers want the inquiry to be guided by participants' viewpoints rather than by their own *a priori* hunches. Thus, our discussion here focuses on hypotheses in quantitative research.

Function of Hypotheses in Quantitative Research

Research questions, as we have seen, are usually queries about relationships between variables. Hypotheses are predicted answers to these queries. For instance, the research question might ask: Does sexual abuse in childhood affect the development of irritable bowel syndrome in women? The researcher might predict the following: Women who were sexually abused in childhood have a higher incidence of irritable bowel syndrome than women who were not.

Hypotheses sometimes follow directly from a theoretical framework. Scientists reason from theories to hypotheses and test those hypotheses in the real world. The validity of a theory is never examined directly. It is through hypothesis testing that the worth of a theory can be evaluated. Let us take as an example the theory of reinforcement. This theory maintains that behavior that is positively reinforced (rewarded) tends to be learned or repeated. The theory itself is too abstract to be put to an empirical test, but if the theory is valid, it should be possible to make predictions about certain kinds of behavior. For example, the following hypotheses have been deduced from reinforcement theory:

- Nursing home residents who are praised (reinforced) by nursing personnel for self-feeding require less assistance in feeding than those who are not praised.
- Pediatric patients who are given a reward (e.g., a balloon or permission to watch television) when they cooperate during nursing procedures tend to be more cooperative during those procedures than unrewarded peers.

Both of these propositions can be put to a test in the real world. The theory gains support if the hypotheses are confirmed.

Not all hypotheses are derived from theory. Even in the absence of a theory, well-conceived hypotheses offer direction and suggest explanations. Perhaps an example will clarify this point. Suppose we hypothesized that the incidence of desaturation and bradycardia in extremely low-birth-weight infants undergoing intubation and ventilation would be lower using the closed tracheal suction system (CTSS) than using the partially ventilated endotracheal suction method (PVETS). We could justify our speculation based on theory, earlier studies, clinical observations, or some combination of these. *The development of predictions in and of itself forces researchers to think logically, to exercise critical judgment, and to tie together earlier research findings.*

Now let us suppose the preceding hypothesis is not confirmed by the evidence collected; that is, we find that rates of bradycardia and desaturation are similar for both the PVETS and CTSS methods. *The failure of data to support a prediction forces researchers to analyze theory or previous research critically, to carefully review the limitations of the study's methods, and to explore alternative explanations for the findings.* The use of hypotheses in quantitative studies tends to induce critical thinking and to facilitate understanding and interpretation of the data.

To illustrate further the utility of hypotheses, suppose we conducted the study guided only by the research question, Is there a relationship between suction method and rates of desaturation and bradycardia? The investigator without a hypothesis is, apparently, prepared to accept any results. The problem is that it is almost always possible to explain something superficially after the fact, no matter what the findings are. Hypotheses guard against superficiality and minimize the possibility that spurious results will be misconstrued.

Characteristics of Testable Hypotheses

Testable research hypotheses state expected relationships between the independent variable (the presumed cause or antecedent) and the dependent variable (the presumed effect or outcome) within a population.

Example of a research hypothesis: Among women who have had a breast cancer diagnosis, those who initially used an avoidance coping strategy will have poorer psychological adjustment 3 years later than women low on avoidance (Hack & Degner, 2004).

In this example, the population is women with a breast cancer diagnosis, the independent variable is the women's coping strategy (high versus low on avoidance), and the dependent variable is long-term psychological adjustment. The hypothesis predicts that these two variables are related within the population—poorer adjustment is expected among those with higher avoidance.

Researchers occasionally present hypotheses that do not make a relational statement, as in the following example: *Pregnant women who receive prenatal instruction regarding postpartum experiences are not likely to experience postpartum depression.* This statement expresses no anticipated relationship; in fact, there is only one variable (postpartum depression), and a relationship by definition requires at least two variables.

The problem is that without a prediction about an anticipated relationship, the hypothesis is difficult to test using standard statistical procedures. In our example, how would we know whether the hypothesis was supported—what absolute standard could be used to decide whether to accept or reject the hypothesis? To illustrate the problem more concretely, suppose we asked a group of mothers who had been given prenatal instruction on postpartum experiences the following question 1 month after delivery: On the whole, how depressed have you been since you gave birth? Would you say (1) extremely depressed, (2) moderately depressed, (3) a little depressed, or (4) not at all depressed?

Based on responses to this question, how could we compare the actual outcome with the predicted outcome? Would *all* the women have to say they were "not at all depressed?" Would the prediction be supported if 51% of the women said they were "not at all depressed" *or* "a little depressed?" It is difficult to test the accuracy of the prediction.

A test is simple, however, if we modify the prediction to the following: *Pregnant women who receive prenatal instruction are less likely to experience postpartum depression than those with no prenatal instruction.* Here, the dependent variable is the women's depression, and the independent variable is their receipt versus nonreceipt of prenatal instruction. The relational aspect of the prediction is embodied in the phrase *less than.* If a hypothesis lacks a phrase such as *more than, less than, greater than, different from, related to, associated with,* or something similar, it is usually not amenable to testing in a quantitative study. To test this revised hypothesis, we could ask two groups of women with different prenatal instruction experiences to respond to the question on depression and then compare the groups' responses. The absolute degree of depression of either group would not be at issue.

Hypotheses should be based on sound, justifiable rationales. Hypotheses often follow from previous research findings or are deduced from a theory. When a relatively new area is being investigated, the researcher may have to turn to logical reasoning or clinical experience to justify the predictions.

The Derivation of Hypotheses

Many students ask the question, How do I go about developing hypotheses? Two basic processes—induction and deduction—constitute the intellectual machinery involved in deriving hypotheses.

An **inductive hypothesis** is a generalization inferred from observed relationships. Researchers observe certain patterns, trends, or associations among phenomena and then use the observations as a basis for predictions. Related literature should be examined to learn what is already known on a topic, but an important source for inductive hypotheses is clinical experiences, combined with critical analysis. For example, a nurse might notice that presurgical patients who ask a lot of questions relating to pain or who express many pain-related apprehensions have a more difficult time in learning appropriate postoperative procedures. The nurse could then formulate a testable hypothesis, such as the following: Patients who are stressed by fear of pain will have more difficulty in deep breathing and coughing after their surgery than patients who are not stressed. Qualitative studies are an important source of inspiration for inductive hypotheses.

Example of deriving an inductive hypothesis: In Beck's (2004) qualitative study of posttraumatic stress disorder (PTSD) due to childbirth, one of her findings was that mothers suffering from PTSD were bombarded with terrifying flashbacks in which they relived their traumatic births. A hypothesis that can be derived from this qualitative finding might be as follows: Women who experience PTSD due to birth trauma experience more flashbacks of their labor and delivery than women who do not experience a traumatic birth. (Beck's study appears in its entirety in the accompanying *Resource Manual*.)

The other mechanism for deriving hypotheses is through deduction. Theories of how phenomena behave and interrelate cannot be tested directly. Through deductive reasoning, a researcher can develop hypotheses based on general theoretical principles. Inductive hypotheses begin with specific observations and move toward generalizations; **deductive hypotheses** have as a starting point theories that are applied to particular situations. The following syllogism illustrates the reasoning process involved:

- All human beings have red and white blood cells.
- John Doe is a human being.
- Therefore, John Doe has red and white blood cells.

In this simple example, the hypothesis is that John Doe does, in fact, have red and white blood cells, a deduction that could be verified.

Theories thus can serve as a valuable point of departure for hypothesis development. Researchers must ask: If this theory is valid, what are the implications for a phenomenon of interest? In other words, researchers deduce that if the general theory is true, then certain outcomes or consequences can be expected. Specific predictions derived from general principles must then be subjected to testing through the collection of empirical data. If these data are congruent with hypothesized outcomes, then the theory is strengthened.

The advancement of nursing knowledge depends on both inductive and deductive hypotheses. Ideally, an iterative process is set in motion wherein observations are made (e.g., in a qualitative study); inductive hypotheses are formulated; systematic observations are made to test the hypotheses; theories are developed on the basis of the results; deductive hypotheses are formulated from the theory; new data are gathered; theories are modified; and so forth. Researchers need to be organizers of concepts (think inductively), logicians (think deductively), and, above all, critics and skeptics of resulting formulations, constantly demanding evidence.

Wording of Hypotheses

A good hypothesis is worded in clear and concise language. In general, hypotheses should be worded in the present tense. Researchers make predictions about relationships that exist in the population, and not just about a relationship that will be revealed in a particular sample. As we discuss in this section, there are various types of hypotheses.

Simple Versus Complex Hypotheses

For the purpose of this book, we define a **simple hypothesis** as a hypothesis that expresses an expected relationship between *one* independent and *one* dependent variable. A **complex hypothesis** is a prediction of a relationship between two (or more) independent variables and/or two (or more) dependent variables.

We give some concrete examples of both types of hypotheses, but let us first explain the differences in abstract terms. Simple hypotheses state a relationship between a single independent variable, which we will call X, and a single dependent variable, which we will label Y. Y is the predicted effect, outcome, or consequence of X, which is the presumed cause, antecedent, or precondition. The nature of this relationship is presented in Figure 4.1**A**. The circles represent variables X and Y, and the hatched area designates the strength of the relationship between them. If there were a one-to-one correspondence between variables X and Y, the two

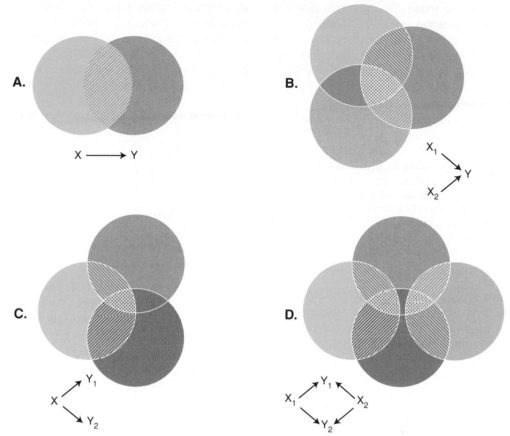

FIGURE 4.1 Schematic representation of various hypothetical relationships.

circles would overlap completely, and the entire area would be hatched. If the variables were totally unrelated, the circles would not overlap at all.

> **Example of a simple hypothesis:** Children whose mothers participate in a nurse case management intervention for women exposed to intimate partner violence [X] will have fewer behavioral problems [Y] than children whose mothers receive routine screening and information only (McFarlane et al., 2005).

Most phenomena are the result not of one variable but of a complex array of variables. A person's weight, for example, is affected simultaneously by such factors as his or her height, diet, bone structure, activity level, and metabolism. If Y in Figure

4.1**A** was weight, and X was a person's caloric intake, we would not be able to explain or understand individual variation in weight completely. For example, knowing that Nate O'Hara's daily caloric intake averaged 2500 calories would not permit a good prediction of his weight. Knowledge of other factors, such as his height, would improve the accuracy with which his weight could be predicted.

Figure 4.1**B** presents a schematic representation of the effect of two independent variables on one dependent variable. The complex hypothesis would state the nature of the relationship between Y on the one hand and X_1 and X_2 on the other. To pursue the preceding example, the hypothesis might be: Taller people (X_1) and people with higher caloric intake (X_2) weigh more (Y) than shorter people and those with lower caloric intake. As the figure shows, a larger proportion of the area of Y is hatched when there are two independent variables than when there is only one. This means that caloric intake *and* height do a better job in helping us explain variations in weight (Y) than caloric intake alone. Complex hypotheses have the advantage of allowing researchers to capture some of the complexity of the real world.

Example of a complex hypothesis—multiple independent variables: Among women with multiple sclerosis, functional limitations [Y] are influenced by the women's external resources, such as their education [X_1], marital status [X_2], social support [X_3], employment status [X_4], and perceived economic adequacy [X_5] (Clingerman, Stuifbergen, & Becker, 2004).

Just as a phenomenon can result from more than one independent variable, a single independent variable can affect or influence more than one phenomenon, as illustrated in Figure 4.1C. A number of studies have found, for example, that cigarette smoking (the independent variable, X), can lead to both lung cancer (Y_1) and coronary disorders (Y_2). Complex hypotheses are common in studies that try to assess the impact of a nursing intervention on multiple outcomes.

Example of a complex hypothesis—multiple dependent variables: Among nurses working in psychiatric wards, a 5-day training course in aggression management [X] will positively influence nurses' tolerance towards patient aggression (Y_1) and their feelings toward aggressive patients [Y_2] (Needham et al., 2005).

A more complex type of hypothesis, which links two or more independent variables to two or more dependent variables, is shown in Figure 4.1D. An example might be a hypothesis that smoking *and* the consumption of alcohol during pregnancy might lead to lower birth weights *and* lower Apgar scores in infants.

Finally, hypotheses are also complex if mediating or moderator variables are included in the prediction. For example, it might be hypothesized that

the effect of caloric intake (X) on weight (Y) is moderated by gender (Z)—that is, the relationship between height and weight is different for men and women. Or, we might predict that the effect of ephedra (X) on weight (Y) is indirect, mediated by its effect on metabolism (Z).

Example of a complex hypothesis with moderator: The effect of postural change from upright to supine [X] on the systolic amplitude [Y] of patients is moderated by their left ventricular systolic function (LVSF), that is, whether their LVSF is normal or depressed [Z] (DeMarzo et al., 2005).

Directional Versus Nondirectional Hypotheses

Hypotheses can be stated in a number of ways, as in the following examples:

1. Older patients are more at risk for experiencing a fall than younger patients.
2. There is a relationship between the age of a patient and the risk for falling.
3. The older the patient, the greater the risk that she or he will fall.
4. Older patients differ from younger ones with respect to their risk for falling.
5. Younger patients tend to be less at risk for a fall than older patients.
6. The risk for falling increases with the age of the patient.

In all these examples, the hypotheses indicate the population (patients), the independent variable (patients' age), the dependent variable (risk for falling), and the anticipated relationship between them.

Hypotheses can be either directional or nondirectional. A **directional hypothesis** is one that specifies not only the existence but also the expected direction of the relationship between variables. In the six versions of the hypothesis, versions 1, 3, 5, and 6 are directional because there is an explicit prediction that older patients are at greater risk for falling than younger ones.

A **nondirectional hypothesis**, by contrast, does not stipulate the direction of the relationship. Versions 2 and 4 in the example illustrate nondirectional hypotheses. These hypotheses state the prediction that a patient's age and the risk for falling are related; they do not stipulate, however, whether the researcher thinks that *older* patients or *younger* ones are at greater risk.

Hypotheses derived from theory are almost always directional because theories explain phenomena, thus providing a rationale for expecting variables to be related in certain ways. Existing studies also offer a basis for directional hypotheses. When there is no theory or related research, when the findings of related studies are contradictory, or when researchers' own experience leads to ambivalence, nondirectional hypotheses may be appropriate. Some people argue, in fact, that nondirectional hypotheses are preferable because they connote a degree of impartiality. Directional hypotheses, it is said, imply that researchers are intellectually committed to certain outcomes, and such a commitment might lead to bias. This argument fails to recognize that researchers typically *do* have hunches about outcomes, whether they state those expectations explicitly or not. We prefer directional hypotheses—when there is a reasonable basis for them—because they clarify the study's framework and demonstrate that researchers have thought critically about the phenomena under study. Directional hypotheses may also permit a more sensitive statistical test through the use of a *one-tailed test*—a rather fine point that is discussed in Chapter 22.

Research Versus Null Hypotheses

Hypotheses are sometimes described as being either research hypotheses or null hypotheses. **Research hypotheses** (also referred to as *substantive, declarative,* or *scientific* hypotheses) are statements of expected relationships between variables. All the hypotheses presented thus far are research hypotheses that indicate actual expectations.

The logic of statistical inference operates on principles that may be somewhat confusing. This logic requires that hypotheses be expressed as an expected *absence* of a relationship. **Null hypotheses** (or *statistical hypotheses*) state that there is no relationship between the independent and dependent variables. The null form of the hypothesis used earlier might be: "Patients' age is unrelated to their risk for falling" or "Older patients are just as likely as younger patients to fall." The null hypothesis might be compared with the assumption of innocence of an accused criminal in English-based systems of justice: the variables are assumed to be "innocent" of any relationship until they can be shown "guilty" through appropriate statistical procedures. The null hypothesis represents the formal statement of this assumption of innocence.

➲ **TIP:** Avoid stating hypotheses in null form in a proposal or a report because this gives an amateurish impression. When statistical tests are performed, the underlying null hypothesis is assumed without being explicitly stated.

Hypothesis Testing

Hypotheses are formally tested through statistical procedures; researchers seek to determine through statistics whether their hypotheses have a high probability of being correct. However, hypotheses are never *proved* through hypothesis testing; rather, they are *accepted* or *supported*. Findings are always tentative. Certainly, if the same results are replicated in numerous investigations, then greater confidence can be placed in the conclusions. Hypotheses come to be increasingly supported with mounting evidence.

Let us look more closely at why this is so. Suppose we hypothesized that height and weight are related. We predict that, on average, tall people weigh more than short people. We then obtain height and weight measurements from a sample and analyze the data. Now suppose we happened by chance to get a sample that consisted of short, heavy people, and tall, thin people. Our results might indicate that there is no relationship between a person's height and weight. Would we then be justified in stating that this study *proved* or *demonstrated* that height and weight in humans are unrelated?

As another example, suppose we hypothesized that tall nurses are more effective than short ones.

This hypothesis is used here only to illustrate a point because, in reality, we would expect no relationship between height and a nurse's job performance. Now suppose that, by chance again, we drew a sample of nurses in which tall nurses received better job evaluations than short ones. Could we conclude definitively that height is related to a nurse's performance? These two examples illustrate the difficulty of using observations from a sample to generalize to a population. Other issues, such as the accuracy of the measures, the effects of uncontrolled variables, and the validity of underlying assumptions prevent researchers from concluding with finality that hypotheses are proved.

TIP: If a researcher uses any statistical tests (as is true in most quantitative studies), it means that there are underlying hypotheses—regardless of whether the researcher explicitly states them—because statistical tests are designed to test hypotheses. In planning a quantitative study of your own, do not be afraid to make predictions, that is, to state hypotheses.

CRITIQUING RESEARCH PROBLEMS, RESEARCH QUESTIONS, AND HYPOTHESES

In critiquing research reports, you will need to evaluate whether researchers have adequately communicated their research problem. The delineation of the problem, statement of purpose, research questions, and hypotheses set the stage for the description of what was done and what was learned. Ideally, you should not have to dig too deeply to decipher the research problem or to discover the questions.

A critique of the research problem involves multiple dimensions. Substantively, you need to consider whether the problem has significance for nursing and has the potential to produce evidence to improve nursing practice. Studies that build in a meaningful way on existing knowledge are well poised to make contributions to evidence-based nursing practice. Researchers who develop a systematic *program of research*, building on their own earlier findings, are

especially likely to make significant contributions (Conn, 2004). For example, Beck's series of studies relating to postpartum depression (Beck, 1993, 1996, 2001; Beck & Gable, 2002, 2003) have influenced women's health care worldwide. Also, research problems stemming from established research priorities (see Chapter 1) have a high likelihood of yielding important new evidence for nurses because they reflect expert opinion about areas of needed research.

Another dimension in critiquing the research problem concerns methodologic issues—in particular, whether the research problem is compatible with the chosen research paradigm and its associated methods. You should also evaluate whether the statement of purpose or research questions have been properly worded and lend themselves to empirical inquiry.

In a quantitative study, if the research report does not contain explicit hypotheses, you need to consider whether their absence is justified. If there are hypotheses, you should evaluate whether the hypotheses are logically connected to the research problem and whether they are consistent with available knowledge or relevant theory. The wording of the hypothesis should also be assessed. The hypothesis is a valid guidepost to scientific inquiry only if it is testable. To be testable, the hypothesis must contain a prediction about the relationship between two or more measurable variables.

Specific guidelines for critiquing research problems, research questions, and hypotheses are presented in Box 4.3. ✖

●●●●●●●●●●●●●●●●●●●●●●

RESEARCH EXAMPLES

This section describes how the research problem and research questions were communicated in two nursing studies, one quantitative and one qualitative.

Research Example of a Quantitative Study

Study: "Changing the tide: An Internet/video exercise and low-fat diet intervention with middle-school students" (Frenn et al., 2005)

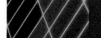

BOX 4.3 Guidelines for Critiquing Reasearch Problems, Research Questions, and Hypotheses

1. What is the research problem? Is the problem statement easy to locate and is it clearly stated? Does the problem statement build a cogent and persuasive argument for the new study?
2. Does the problem have significance for nursing? How might the research contribute to nursing practice, administration, education, or policy?
3. Is there a good fit between the research problem and the paradigm within which the research was conducted? Is there a good fit with the qualitative research tradition?
4. Does the report formally present a statement of purpose, research question, and/or hypotheses? Is this information communicated clearly and concisely, and is it placed in a logical and useful location?
5. Are purpose statements or questions worded appropriately? (e.g., are key concepts/variables identified and the population of interest specified? Are verbs used appropriately to suggest the nature of the inquiry and/or the research tradition?)
6. If there are no formal hypotheses, is their absence justified? Are statistical tests used in analyzing the data despite the absence of stated hypotheses?
7. Do hypotheses (if any) flow from a theory or previous research? Is there a justifiable basis for the predictions?
8. Are hypotheses (if any) properly worded—do they state a predicted relationship between two or more variables? Are they directional or nondirectional, and is there a rationale for how they were stated? Are they presented as research or as null hypotheses?

Problem Statement: "Poor diet, obesity, and inactivity result in more than 300,000 preventable deaths per year and chronic disease accounts for 60% of medical care expenditures in the United States.... When compared with early adolescents in other countries, those in the U.S. exercise less frequently and have less healthy diets.... Patterns established during middle-school years are important in the development of adult health-related habits.... Extensive reviews of research ... on the effectiveness of nutrition education revealed many studies in which nutrition knowledge and attitudes of children were improved. School-based interventions were more effective than interventions conducted outside the school setting ..." (p. 13). (Citations were omitted to streamline the presentation.)

Statement of Purpose: The purpose of this investigation was to examine the effectiveness of a tailored 8-session health promotion Internet/video-delivered intervention to increase physical activity and reduce dietary fat among low-income, culturally diverse 7th-grade students. The intervention was based on a widely used model of health promotion, the Transtheoretical Model. (This model is described in Chapter 6.)

Hypotheses: It was hypothesized that students participating in more than half of the intervention sessions would have (1) higher physical activity and (2) lower dietary fat intake compared with students not in the intervention group.

Study Methods: The study was conducted in an urban public middle school. Students in certain classrooms were invited to be in the intervention group that received the special intervention, whereas students in other classrooms were in a control group that had the usual curriculum. Data relating to the students' physical activities and food consumption were collected both before and after the intervention from students in both groups. The analyses testing the study hypotheses were completed with 60 control group students and 31 students in the intervention group who completed at least 5 of the 8 sessions.

Key Findings: Intervention students who completed more than half of the sessions increased moderate/vigorous exercise by an average of 22 minutes, compared with an average *decrease* of 46 minutes for students in the control group. Those in the intervention group also had a significant reduction in the percentage of dietary fat, whereas those in the control group had dietary fat intake that was virtually unchanged during the study period. The study findings thus suggested that computer-tailored interventions can be effective in improving health behaviors in middle-school students.

Research Example of a Qualitative Study

Study: "Interaction patterns of adolescents with depression and the important adults in their lives" (Draucker, 2005)

Problem Statement: "Adolescent depression is a prevalent, serious mental health problem that often goes untreated. . . . Estimates of the 1-year prevalence of MDD (major depressive disorder) in adolescents are as high as 8.3%, compared to 5.3% in the adult population. . . . Depression in adolescents is associated with many negative outcomes, including increased risk for suicide, interpersonal problems, and missed education and job opportunities. . . . Adolescents who are depressed rely on adult family members and other important adults in their lives (e.g., school personnel, community- and faith-based youth workers) to detect the depression, provide support and guidance, and, if needed, facilitate mental health treatment. Experts believe that relationships among depressed children and their family members significantly influence the expression and course of depression. . ." (pp. 942–943). (Citations were omitted to streamline the presentation.)

Statement of Purpose: The purpose of this study was to describe common interaction patterns between adolescents who are depressed and the important adults in their lives, with special attention given to interactions that influence the course of the teens' depression.

Research Questions: Draucker identified three specific research questions: (1) What are the common interaction patterns between adolescents who are depressed and the important adults in their lives? (2) What interaction patterns negatively influence the course of the depression? and (3) What interaction patterns positively influence the course of the depression?

Method: Grounded theory methods were used to generate in-depth qualitative data to address the questions. The sample included 52 young adults between the ages of 18 and 21 who experienced depressive symptoms as adolescents, 4 of their parents, and 8 professionals who worked with youth. Each participant was interviewed once in a safe, accessible location (e.g., churches, community agencies).

Key Findings: All participants discussed how both the adolescents and adults ignored, hid, or minimized the teens' distress by putting up a façade. The three interaction patterns that were identified—maintaining the façade, poking holes in the façade, and breaking down the façade—were responses to the façade.

SUMMARY POINTS

- A **research problem** is a perplexing or enigmatic situation that a researcher wants to address through disciplined inquiry.
- Researchers usually identify a broad **topic**, narrow the scope of the problem, and then identify questions consistent with a paradigm of choice.
- The most common sources of ideas for nursing research problems are clinical experience, relevant literature, social issues, theory, and external suggestions.
- Various criteria should be considered in assessing the value of a research problem. The problem should be clinically significant; researchable (questions of a moral or ethical nature are inappropriate); feasible; and of personal interest.
- Feasibility involves the issues of time, cooperation of study participants and other people, availability of facilities and equipment, researcher experience, and ethical considerations.
- Researchers communicate their aims in research reports as problem statements, statements of purpose, research questions, or hypotheses.
- A **statement of purpose**, which summarizes the overall study goal and identifies the key concepts (variables) and the study group or population. Purpose statements often communicate, through the use of verbs and other key terms, the underlying research tradition of qualitative studies, or whether the study is experimental or nonexperimental in quantitative ones.
- A **research question** is the specific query researchers want to answer in addressing the research problem. In quantitative studies, research questions usually are about the existence, nature, strength, and direction of relationships.
- Some research questions are about **moderator variables** that affect the strength or direction of a relationship between the independent and dependent variables; others are about **mediating variables** that intervene between

the independent and dependent variable and help to explain why the relationship exists.

- The **problem statement** articulates the nature, context, and significance of a problem to be studied. Problem statements include several components: problem identification; background, scope, and consequences of the problem; knowledge gaps; and possible solutions to the problem.

- In quantitative studies, a **hypothesis** is a statement of predicted relationships between two or more variables. A testable hypothesis states the anticipated association between one or more independent and one or more dependent variables.

- **Simple hypotheses** express a predicted relationship between one independent variable and one dependent variable, whereas **complex hypotheses** state an anticipated relationship between two or more independent variables and two or more dependent variables (or state predictions about mediating or moderator variables).

- **Directional hypotheses** predict the direction of a relationship; **nondirectional hypotheses** predict the existence of relationships, not their direction.

- **Research hypotheses** predict the existence of relationships; **null hypotheses** express the absence of a relationship.

- Hypotheses are never proved or disproved in an ultimate sense—they are accepted or rejected, supported or not supported by the data.

● ● ● ● ● ● ● ● ● ● ● ● ● ● ● ● ● ● ●

STUDY ACTIVITIES

Chapter 4 of the *Resource Manual to Accompany Nursing Research: Generating and Assessing Research Evidence, 8th edition*, offers various exercises and study suggestions for reinforcing the concepts presented in this chapter. In addition, the following study questions can be addressed:

1. Think of a frustrating experience you have had as a nursing student or as a practicing nurse. Identify the problem area. Ask yourself a series of questions until you have one that you think is researchable. Evaluate the problem in terms of the evaluation criteria discussed in this chapter.

2. Examine a recent issue of a nursing research journal. Find an article that does not present a formal, well-articulated statement of purpose. Write a statement of purpose (or research questions) for that study.

3. To the extent possible, use the critiquing questions in Box 4.3 to appraise the research problems for the two studies used as research examples at the end of this chapter.

● ● ● ● ● ● ● ● ● ● ● ● ● ● ● ● ● ● ●

STUDIES CITED IN CHAPTER 4

Methodologic or theoretical references cited in this chapter can be found in a separate section at the end of the book.

Beck, C. T. (1993). "Teetering on the edge": A substantive theory of postpartum depression. *Nursing Research, 42,* 42–48.

Beck, C. T. (1996). Postpartum depressed mothers' experiences interacting with their children. *Nursing Research, 45,* 98–104.

Beck, C. T. (2001). Predictors of postpartum depression: An update. *Nursing Research, 50,* 275–285.

Beck, C. T. (2004). Post-traumatic stress disorder due to childbirth: The aftermath. *Nursing Research, 53,* 216–224.

Beck, C. T., & Gable, R. K. (2002). Postpartum Depression Screening Scale manual. Los Angeles: Western Psychological Services.

Beck, C. T., & Gable, R. K. (2003). Postpartum Depression Screening Scale—Spanish version. *Nursing Research, 52,* 296–306

Beck, C. T., & Gable, R. K. (2005). Screening performance of the Postpartum Depression Screening Scale—Spanish version. *Journal of Transcultural Nursing, 16,* 331–338.

Bottorff, J. L., Kalaw, C., Johnson, J. L., Chambers, N., Stewart, M., Greaves, L., & Kelly, M. (2005). Unraveling smoking ties: How tobacco use is embedded in couple interactions. *Research in Nursing & Health, 28,* 316–328.

Clingerman, E., Stuifbergen, A., & Becker, H. (2004). The influence of resources on perceived functional limitations among women with multiple sclerosis. *Journal of Neuroscience Nursing, 36*(6), 312–321.

DeMarzo, A. P., Calvin, J. E., Kelly, R. F., & Stamos, T. D. (2005). Using impedence cardiography to assess left ventricular systolic function via postural change in patients with heart failure. *Progress in Cardiovascular Nursing, 20*(4), 163–167.

Draucker, C. B. (2005). Interaction patterns of adolescents with depression and the important adults in their lives. *Qualitative Health Research, 15*(7), 942–963.

Frenn, M., Malin, S., Brown, R. L., Greer, Y., Fox, J., Greer, J., & Smyczek, S. (2005). Changing the tide: An Internet/video exercise and low-fat diet intervention with middle-school students. *Applied Nursing Research, 18*(1), 13–21.

Hack, T. F., & Degner, L. F. (2004). Coping responses following breast cancer diagnosis predict psychological adjustment three years later. *Psycho-Oncology, 13*, 235–247.

Jacelon, C. S. (2003). The dignity of elders in an acute care hospital. *Qualitative Health Research, 13*, 543–556.

Lee, T., Miles, M. S., & Holditch-Davis, D. (2006). Fathers' support to mothers of medically fragile infants. *Journal of Obstetric, Gynecologic, & Neonatal Nursing, 35*(1), 46–55.

Magarey, J. M., & McCutcheon, H. H. (2005). "Fishing with the dead"—Recall of memories from the ICU. *Intensive Critical Care Nursing, 21*(6), 344–354.

McFarlane, J. M., Groff, J. Y., O'Brien, J., & Watson, K. (2005). Behaviors of children exposed to intimate partner violence before and 1 year after a treatment program for their mother. *Applied Nursing Research, 18*(1), 7–12.

Needham, I., Abderhalden, C., Halfens, R. J., Dassen, T., Haug, H. J., & Fischer, J. E. (2005). The effects of a training course in aggression management on mental health nurses' perceptions of aggression: A cluster randomized trial. *International Journal of Nursing Studies, 42*(6), 649–655.

Nicholas, P. K., Kirksey, K. M., Corless, I. B., & Kemppainen, J. (2005). Lipodystrophy and quality of life in HIV: Symptom management issues. *Applied Nursing Research, 18*(1), 55–58.

Parse, R. R. (2006). Feeling respected: A Parse method study. *Nursing Science Quarterly, 19*(1), 51–56.

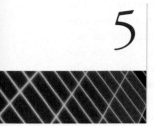

5 | Finding and Critiquing Evidence: Research Literature Reviews

Researchers rarely conduct research in an intellectual vacuum; their studies are undertaken within the context of an existing base of knowledge. Researchers usually undertake a thorough **literature review** to familiarize themselves with that knowledge base. This chapter describes a range of activities associated with conducting a literature search and preparing a written review, including locating and critiquing studies and drawing conclusions about existing evidence. Many of these activities overlap with early steps in an evidence-based practice (EBP) project, as described in Chapter 2.

GETTING STARTED ON A LITERATURE REVIEW

Before discussing the activities involved in undertaking a research-based literature review, we briefly discuss some general issues. The first concerns the viewpoint of qualitative researchers.

Literature Reviews in Qualitative Research Traditions

As indicated in Chapter 3, qualitative researchers have differing opinions about reviewing the litera-

ture before doing a new study. Some of the differences reflect viewpoints associated with qualitative research traditions.

In grounded theory studies, researchers often collect data in the field before reviewing the literature. As the data are analyzed, the grounded theory begins to take shape. Once the theory appears to be sufficiently developed, researchers then turn to the literature, seeking to relate prior findings to the theory. Glaser (1978) warns that "It's hard enough to generate one's own ideas without the 'rich' detailment provided by literature in the same field" (p. 31). Thus, grounded theory researchers may defer a literature review, but then determine how previous research fits with or extends the emerging theory.

Phenomenologists often undertake a search for relevant materials at the outset of a study. In reviewing the literature for a phenomenological study, researchers look for experiential descriptions of the phenomenon being studied (Munhall, 2007). The purpose is to expand the researcher's understanding of the phenomenon from multiple perspectives. Van Manen (1990) suggests that, in addition to past research studies, artistic sources of experiential descriptions should be located, such as poetry, novels, plays, films, and art. These artistic sources can offer powerful examples and images of the experience under study.

Even though "ethnography starts with a conscious attitude of almost complete ignorance" (Spradley, 1979, p. 4), a review of the literature that led to the choice of the cultural problem to be studied is often done before data collection. Munhall (2007) points out that this literature review may be more conceptual than data based. A second, more thorough literature review is often done during data analysis and interpretation so that findings can be compared with previous literature.

It might be noted, however, that if funding is sought for a qualitative project—regardless of tradition—an upfront literature review will almost surely be needed to provide context for the proposed study and to persuade reviewers that the study should be undertaken.

Purposes and Scope of Research Literature Reviews

Written literature reviews are undertaken for many different purposes, and the length of the written product varies considerably depending on its purpose. Nevertheless, a good literature review, regardless of length, requires thorough familiarity with available evidence. As Garrard (2004) advises, you must strive to *own* the literature on a topic to be confident of preparing a comprehensive, state-of-the-art review. The major types of written research review include the following:

- *A review included in a research report.* As discussed in Chapter 3, the introduction to research reports typically includes a brief literature review that has two major goals: to provide readers with an overview of existing evidence on the problem being addressed and to develop an argument that demonstrates the need for the new study. These reviews are usually only two to four double-spaced pages. This means that only key studies can be cited, and it also means that not much space can be devoted to a critical evaluation of individual studies: the emphasis is on evaluating the overall body of research.
- *A review included in a proposal.* Research proposals designed to persuade funders (or advi-

sors) about the merits of a proposed study include a literature review section. As with a review in a research report, a review in a proposal provides a knowledge context and confirms the need for and significance of new research. In a proposal, however, a review also demonstrates the writer's "ownership" of the literature. The length of such reviews is typically established in proposal guidelines, but they are often limited to less than 10 pages, which means that although the literature review must reflect expertise on the topic, not much space can be devoted to critiquing individual studies.

- *A review in a thesis or dissertation.* Doctoral dissertations in the traditional format (see Chapter 26) often include a thorough, critical review of the research on the problem area. An entire chapter often is devoted to a literature review, and such chapters are frequently 15 to 25 pages (or more) in length. Such reviews typically include an evaluation of the overall body of literature as well as critiques of key individual studies.
- *Free-standing literature reviews.* Nurses also prepare literature reviews that critically appraise and summarize a body of research, even when they are not intending to pursue primary research on the topic. For example, students are sometimes asked to prepare a critical research review for a course, and clinical nurses sometimes do literature reviews as part of an EBP project. Researchers who are experts in a field also may do systematic reviews that are published in journals, as discussed in greater detail in Chapter 25. Free-standing literature reviews designed to appraise a body of research critically are usually at least 15 to 20 pages long.

This chapter focuses on the preparation of written reviews as a critical component of an original research study, although most of the activities are similar for other types of review. A literature review helps to lay the foundation and provide context for a new study. By doing a thorough review, researchers can determine how best to make a contribution to the existing base of evidence—for example, whether there are gaps or inconsistencies in a body of research, or whether a replication with a new study population is the right next step. Reviewing the literature also can help to identify relevant conceptual frameworks or appropriate research methods. A literature review also plays a role at the end of the study as researchers try to make sense of their findings.

Types of Information to Seek for a Research Review

Written materials vary in their quality, their intended audience, and the kind of information they contain. In performing a review of the literature, you will have to decide what to read or what to include in a written review. We offer some suggestions that may help in making such decisions.

The most important type of information for a research review includes findings from prior studies. For a literature review used as the basis for a new study, you should rely mostly on **primary source** research reports, which are descriptions of studies written by the researchers who conducted them.

Secondary source research documents are descriptions of studies prepared by someone other than the original researcher. Literature reviews, then, are secondary sources. Such reviews, if they are recent, are often a good place to start because they provide a quick overview of the literature and a valuable bibliography. However, secondary descriptions of studies should not be considered substitutes for primary sources for a new literature review. Secondary sources typically fail to provide much detail about studies, and they are seldom completely objective.

➲ TIP: For an EBP project, a recent, high-quality systematic review may be sufficient to provide the needed information about the evidence base, although it is usually wise to search for recent studies not covered by the review.

Examples of primary and secondary sources:

• Secondary source, a review of the literature on nurses' role in the care of community-dwelling

incontinent patients: DuMoulin, M., Hamers, J., Paulus, A., Berendsen, C., & Halfens, R. (2005). The role of the nurse in community continence care: A systematic review. *International Journal of Nursing Studies, 42*(4), 479–492.

• Primary source, an original experimental study of the effects of a nurse-initiated intervention for urinary incontinence: Liao, Y., Dougherty, M., Liou, Y., & Tseng, I. (2006). Pelvic floor muscle training effect on urinary incontinence knowledge, attitudes, and severity. *International Journal of Nursing Studies, 43*(1), 29–37.

In addition to empirical references, your search may yield various nonresearch references, including opinion articles, case reports, anecdotes, and clinical descriptions. Such nonresearch materials may serve to broaden understanding of a research problem, illustrate a point, demonstrate a need for research, or describe aspects of clinical practice. These writings may thus may play an important role in formulating research ideas—or may even suggest ways to broaden or focus the literature search—but they usually have limited utility in written research reviews because they are subjective and do not address the central question of written reviews: What is the current state of *evidence* on this research problem?

Major Steps and Strategies in Doing a Literature Review

Conducting a literature review is a little bit like doing a full-fledged study, in the sense that a reviewer must start with a question, formulate and implement a plan for gathering information, and analyze and interpret the information. Then the "findings" must be summarized in a written product.

Figure 5.1 summarizes the literature review process. As the figure suggests, there are several potential feedback loops, with opportunities to go back to earlier steps in search of more information. This chapter discusses each of these steps, although considerably more information about some of the steps is presented in Chapter 25 in our discussion of systematic reviews.

Conducting a high-quality literature review is more than a mechanical exercise—it is an art and a

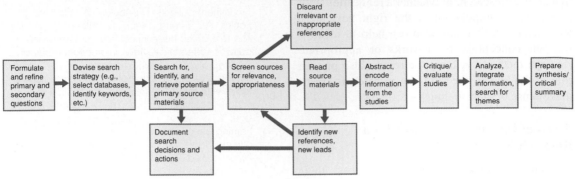

FIGURE 5.1 Flow of tasks in a literature review.

science. Several qualities characterize a high-quality review. First, the review must be comprehensive and thorough, and must incorporate up-to-date references. To "own" the literature (Garrard, 2004), you must be determined to become an expert on your topic, which in turn means that you will need to be creative and diligent—especially in hunting down "leads" for possible sources of information.

➲ TIP: Locating all relevant information on a research question is a bit like being a detective. The various literature retrieval tools we discuss in this chapter are a tremendous aid, but there inevitably needs to be some digging for, and a lot of sifting and sorting of, the clues to evidence on a topic. Be prepared for sleuthing!

Second, a high-quality review is systematic. Decision rules need to be clear, and the criteria for including or excluding a study from the review need to be explicit. In part this is because a third characteristic of a good review is that it is reproducible. This means that another diligent reviewer would be able to apply the same decision rules and criteria and come to similar conclusions about the state of evidence on your topic.

Another desirable attribute of a literature review is balance and the absence of bias. This is more easily achieved when systematic rules for evaluating and analyzing the information are followed—although reviewers cannot totally elude their personal judgments. For this reason, free-standing systematic

reviews are typically conducted by teams of researchers who can evaluate each other's conclusions. Finally, in addition to making an effort to achieve a written product that is well-organized and clearly written, reviewers should strive for a review that is insightful and scholarly, and that is more than "the sum of its parts." Reviewers have an opportunity to contribute to knowledge through an astute and incisive synthesis of the evidence.

A viewpoint that we recommend in doing a literature review is to think of it as doing a qualitative study. This means having a flexible approach to "data collection" and thinking creatively about opportunities for new sources of information. It means pursuing leads until "saturation" is achieved—that is, until your search strategies yield redundant information about studies to include. And it also means that the analysis of your "data" will typically involve a search for important themes.

Primary and Secondary Questions for a Review

For free-standing literature reviews and EBP projects, the reviewer may seek to summarize research evidence on a single focused question, such as those described in Chapter 2 (see Table 2.1 for question templates). For those who are undertaking a literature review as part of a new study, the *primary question* for the literature review is typically the same as the actual research question for the new study. The researcher wants to know, What is the current state of knowledge on the question that I will be addressing in *my* study? The process of developing and refining research questions for a study was described in Chapter 4.

If you are doing a review for a new study, you inevitably will need to search for existing evidence on several *secondary questions* as well. This is because you will need to develop an argument for the new study in the problem statement—that is, you will need to provide a rationale with supporting evidence to justify the new research. An example (which we will use throughout this chapter) will clarify this point.

Suppose that we were conducting a study to address the following research question: What characteristics of nurses are associated with effective pain management for hospitalized pediatric patients? In other words, our primary question is about whether there are characteristics of nurses that are associated with appropriate responses to children's pain. Such a question would arise within the context of a perceived problem, such as a concern that nurses' treatment of children's pain is not always optimal. A simplified statement of the problem might be as follows:

• • •

Many children are hospitalized annually, and many hospitalized children experience high levels of pain. There are long-lasting, harmful effects to the nervous system when severe or persistent pain in children is untreated. Although effective analgesic and nonpharmacologic methods of controlling children's pain exist, and although there are reliable methods of assessing children's pain, nurses do not always manage children's pain effectively. *What characteristics distinguish nurses who are effective and those who are not?*

• • •

This simplified problem statement suggests a number of *secondary questions* for which research evidence from the literature will need to be located and evaluated. Examples of such secondary questions in this example include the following:

• How many children are hospitalized annually?
• What types and levels of pain do hospitalized children experience?

• What are the consequences of untreated pain in children?
• How can pain be reliably assessed in children?
• How can pain in hospitalized children be effectively treated?
• How adequately do nurses manage pain in hospitalized pediatric patients?

Thus, conducting a literature review tends to be a multi-pronged endeavor when it is done as part of a new study. Although most of the "detective work" in searching the literature (and most of the detailed analysis) that we describe in this chapter applies principally to the primary question, it is important to keep in mind the other questions for which information from the research literature needs to be retrieved.

LOCATING RELEVANT LITERATURE FOR A RESEARCH REVIEW

As shown in Figure 5.1, an early step in the literature review process is devising a strategy to locate relevant studies. The ability to identify and locate documents on a research topic is an important skill that requires adaptability—rapid technological changes, such as the expanding use of the Internet, are making manual methods of finding information from print resources obsolete, and more sophisticated methods of searching the literature are being introduced continuously. We urge you to consult with librarians, colleagues, or faculty at your institution for updated suggestions.

Formulating a Search Strategy

There are many ways to go about searching for research evidence, and it is wise to begin a search with some strategies in mind. Cooper (1998) has identified several approaches, the first of which is one to which we devote considerable attention in this chapter: searching for references through the use of bibliographic databases. A second approach, called the *ancestry approach* (or "footnote chasing"), is to use the citations from relevant studies to track down earlier research upon which the studies are based (the "ancestors"). A third method, called the *descendancy approach*, is to find a pivotal early study and to search forward in citation indexes to find more recent studies ("descendants") that cited the key study. Other strategies involve methods for tracking down what is sometimes referred to as the *grey literature*, which refers to studies with more limited distribution, such as conference papers, unpublished reports, dissertations, and so on. We describe these strategies in Chapter 25, which discusses systematic reviews. If your intent is to totally "own" the literature, then you will likely want to adopt all of these strategies, but in some cases, the first two or three might suffice.

➲ **TIP:** You may be tempted to begin a literature search through an Internet search engine, such as Google or Yahoo. Such a search is likely to provide you with a lot of "hits" on your topic, including information about support groups, advocacy organizations, interest groups, clinical services, commercial products, and the like. However, such Internet searches are not likely to give you comprehensive bibliographic information on the *research* literature on your topic—and you might become frustrated with searching through the vast number of websites now available.

Another part of a search plan concerns decisions about delimiting the search. These decisions need to be explicit to ensure the reproducibility of your efforts. If you are multilingual, you may not need to constrain your search to studies written in your own language, but many reviewers will need to do this. You may also want to limit your search to studies conducted within a certain time frame (e.g., within the past 15 years). In some cases, you may want to exclude studies with certain types of study participants. For instance, in our example of a literature search about nurses' characteristics and treatment of children's pain, we might want to exclude studies in which the "children" were neonates. Finally, you may choose to limit your search in terms of the definition of your key variables. For instance, in our example, you may (or may not) wish to exclude studies in which the focus was on nurses' *attitudes* toward children's pain.

➲ **TIP:** Constraining your search might help you to avoid irrelevant or nonuseful material, but you should be quite cautious about putting too many restrictions on your search, especially initially. You can always make decisions to exclude studies at a later point (provided you have a defensible rationale and clear criteria). In particular, be sure not to limit your search to only very recent studies or to studies exclusively in the nursing literature. It is also unwise to adopt too narrow a view about the operationalization of key constructs.

Searching Bibliographic Databases

Print-based literature search resources that must be searched manually are becoming outmoded. Reviewers typically begin by searching bibliographic databases that can be accessed by computer.

Several commercial vendors (e.g., Aries Knowledge Finder, Ovid, EbscoHost, ProQuest) offer information retrieval services for bibliographic databases. Their programs are user-friendly, offering menu-driven systems with on-screen support so that retrieval can usually proceed with minimal instruction. Some providers offer discount rates for students and trial services that allow you to test them before subscribing. In most cases, however, your university or hospital library is already a subscriber.

Before undertaking a search of an electronic database, you should become familiar with the features of the software you are using to access the database. The software will give you options for restricting your search, for combining the results of two searches, for saving your search, and so on. Most of the available programs have tutorials that offer useful information to improve the efficiency and effectiveness of your search.

You will also need to learn how to get from "point A" (the constructs in which you are interested) to "point B" (the way that the program stores and organizes information about the constructs). Most software you are likely to use has mapping capabilities. *Mapping* is a feature that allows you to search for topics using your own **keywords**, rather than needing to enter a term that is exactly the same as a **subject heading** (subject codes) in the database. The vendor's software translates ("maps") the keywords you enter into the most plausible subject heading. In addition to mapping your term onto a database-specific subject heading, most programs will also search in the *text fields* of records (usually the title and abstract) for the keyword entered.

➔ TIP: The keywords you begin with are usually your key independent or dependent variables, and perhaps your population. If you have used the question templates in Table 2.1 or in the Toolkit for Chapter 4, the words you entered in the blanks would be keywords.

Even when there are mapping capabilities, you should learn the relevant subject headings of the database you are using because keyword searches and subject heading searches yield overlapping but nonidentical search results. Subject headings for databases can be located in the database's thesaurus or other reference tools. Another strategy is to use the keywords that researchers themselves identify to classify their studies. A good place to find such keywords is in a journal article once you have found a relevant reference.

➔ TIP: If you want to identify all major research reports on a topic, you need to be flexible and to think broadly about the keywords that could be related to your topic. For example, if you are interested in anorexia nervosa, you might look under *anorexia, eating disorders,* and *weight loss,* and perhaps under *appetite, eating behavior, food habits, bulimia,* and *body weight changes.*

Key Electronic Databases for Nurse Researchers

Three especially useful electronic databases for nurse researchers are CINAHL (**C**umulative **I**ndex to **N**ursing and **A**llied **H**ealth **L**iterature), MEDLINE (**Med**ical **Lit**erature On-**Line**), and the Institute for Scientific Information (ISI) Web of Knowledge, which we discuss in greater detail in the next sections. Other potentially useful bibliographic databases for nurse researchers include the following:

- AIDSEARCH (includes more than 20 AIDS research databases)
- CancerLit (**Cancer Lit**erature)
- Cochrane Database of Systematic Reviews
- Dissertation Abstracts online
- EMBASE (the **E**xcerpta **M**edica data**base**)
- ERIC (**E**ducation **R**esources **I**nformation **C**enter database)
- HAPI (**H**ealth **a**nd **P**sychosocial **I**nstruments database)
- PsycINFO (**Psyc**hology **Info**rmation)

Note that a search strategy that works well in one database does not necessarily produce satisfactory results in another. Thus, it is important to explore strategies in each relevant database, and to understand how each database is structured (e.g., what subject headings are used and how they are organized in a larger hierarchy). Each database and software program also has certain peculiarities. For example, using PubMed (to be discussed later) to search the Medline database, you could restrict your search, if this were appropriate, to nursing journals. However, if you did this you would be excluding studies that appear in several journals in which nurses routinely publish, such as *Birth, Qualitative Health Research,* and *Pain Management Nursing,* because these journals are not coded for the nursing subset.

The CINAHL Database

The **CINAHL database** is an extremely important electronic database for nurses. It covers references to virtually all English-language nursing and allied health journals, as well as to books, book chapters, nursing dissertations, and selected conference proceedings in nursing and allied health fields.

The CINAHL database includes materials dating from 1982 to the present and contains more than 1 million records. In addition to providing bibliographic information for locating references (i.e., the author, title, journal, year of publication, volume, and page numbers), CINAHL provides abstracts of most citations. Supplementary information, such as names of data collection instruments, is available for many records in the database. Documents of interest can typically be ordered electronically. CINAHL can be accessed online or by CD-ROM, either directly through CINAHL (*http://www.cinahl.com*) or through a commercial vendor. We illustrate some of the features of the CINAHL database using Ovid software, but note that some of the features discussed may be unavailable or labeled differently if you are using different software to access CINAHL.

At the outset, you might begin with a "basic search" by simply entering keywords or phrases relevant to your primary question (or the name of a known researcher/author). You may want to restrict your search in a number of ways, for example, by limiting the records retrieved to a certain type of document (e.g., only research reports); to records with certain features (e.g., only ones with abstracts); to specific publication dates (e.g., only those after 1999); or to those written in English. A few simple clicks in the field labeled "Limits" can accomplish this, and clicking on "More Limits" offers more options.

To illustrate how searches can be delimited with a concrete example related to the problem discussed earlier, suppose we were interested in recent research on nurses' pain management for children. Here is an example of how many "hits" there were on successive restrictions to the search, using one of many possible keyword search strategies, and using the CINAHL database through October 18, 2006:

SEARCH TOPIC/RESTRICTION	HITS
Pain	48,699
Pain AND child$ AND nurs$	1430
Limit to research reports	562
Limit to English	515
Limit to entries with abstracts	467
Limit to nursing journals	337
Limit to 2000 through 2006 publications	178

This narrowing of the search—from more than 48,000 initial references on pain to 178 references for recent research reports in nursing journals with content on pain, nurses, and children—took less than 1 minute to perform. Two things about this search should be noted. First, we used the *Boolean operator* AND to search only for records that had *all three* keywords in which we were interested. (Another example of a Boolean operator is OR, which would retrieve records with *any* of the three keywords; in our example, if we had used OR we would have *broadened* the search, and 490,257 records would have been identified.) And second, we used a "**wildcard**" **character**, which in Ovid is "$." This instructed the computer to search for any word that begins with "child" such as children or childhood, and for any word beginning with "nurs" such as nurse or nursing.

The 178 references from the search would be displayed on the monitor, and we could then print full bibliographic information for the ones that appeared especially promising. An example of an abridged CINAHL record entry for a study identified through this search on children's pain is presented in Figure 5.2. Each entry shows an accession number that is the unique identifier for each record in the database, as well as other identifying numbers. Then, the authors and title of the reference are displayed, followed by source information. The source indicates the following:

- Name of the journal (*Journal of Pediatric Nursing*)
- Year and month of publication (2004 Feb)
- Volume (19)
- Issue (1)
- Page numbers (40–50)
- Number of cited references (64)

The printout also shows the CINAHL subject headings that were coded for this particular study. Any of these headings could have been used in the search process to retrieve this reference. Note that the subject headings include substantive/topical headings such as *Nurse Attitudes* and *Pain*, and also include methodologic (e.g., *Questionnaires*), theoretical (*Orem Self-Care Model*), and sample characteristic headings (e.g., *Child*). Next, when formal, named instruments are used in a study, these are printed under Instrumentation. The abstract for the study is then presented. Additional information, not shown here, includes any funding for the study and the full list of citations.

Based on the abstract, we would then decide whether this reference was pertinent to our inquiry. Documents referenced in the database usually can

ACCESSION NUMBER
2005021272 NLM Unique Identifier: 14963869.

AUTHORS
Vincent CV. Denyes MJ.

INSTITUTION
School of Nursing, Oakland University, Rochester, MI 48309-4401; vincent@oakland.edu.

TITLE
Relieving children's pain: nurses' abilities and analgesic administration practices.

SOURCE
Journal of Pediatric Nursing: Nursing Care of Children and Families. 2004 Feb; 19(1): 40–50. (64 ref)

ABBREVIATED SOURCE
J PEDIATR NUR. 2004 Feb; 19(1): 40–50. (64 ref)

CINAHL SUBJECT HEADINGS

Adolescence	*Nursing Knowledge/ev [Evaluation]
Analgesics/tu {Therapeutic use}	Orem Self-Care Model
Child	Pain Measurement
Child, Preschool	*Pain/pc [Prevention and Control]
Clinical Assessment Tools	Pearson's Correlation Coefficient
Convenience Sample	*Pediatric Nursing
Descriptive Statistics	Questionnaires
Midwestern United States	Regression
*Nurse Attitudes	Scales

INSTRUMENTATION
Nurses' Knowledge and Attitudes Survey Regarding Pain [modified].

ABSTRACT
A primary purpose of this study was to examine relationships among nurses' knowledge and attitudes about children's pain relief, nurses' abilities to overcome barriers to optimal pain management, nurses' analgesic practices, and pain levels of hospitalized children. Significant positive relationships were found between nurses' ($N = 67$) analgesic administration and children's pain, and between nurses' years of practice with children and nurses' abilities to overcome barriers to optimal pain management. The children's ($N = 132$) mean pain level was 1.63 (scale of 0 to 5), with one half of the children reporting moderate to severe pain. Of the 117 children who reported pain, 74% received analgesia. Nurses administered a mean of 37.9% of available morphine and means of 36% to 54% of recommended amounts of morphine, acetaminophen, and codeine.

FIGURE 5.2 Example of a printout from a CINAHL search.

be ordered or directly downloaded, so it is not necessary for your library to subscribe to the referenced journal.

➲ **TIP:** Each bibliographic database (or search software for the database) has special features that you should learn about to search more productively. For example, *focus* and *explode* are commands available in Ovid for narrowing or broadening a search. You can sometimes get additional clues by learning about the structuring of the database. For example, Ovid's database tools can be accessed by clicking on "Search Tools" from the advanced mode search page. After entering a basic keyword (e.g., "pain"), you can click on several options. One option is *Tree*, which is the hierarchical vocabulary structure of the CINAHL database (e.g., the tree for the subject heading "pain" would show us that "pain" is a subheading of "Nervous system diseases"). Another search tool option is *Subheadings*, which in our case would display major subheadings of pain. Examples include "etiology" and "symptoms." A search can be launched from within any of these search tool options by clicking an appropriate entry (e.g., from the subheadings display we could click "etiology" to get a list of the more than 1700 references classified in this category).

The MEDLINE Database

The MEDLINE database was developed by the U.S. National Library of Medicine (NLM), and is widely recognized as the premier source for bibliographic coverage of the biomedical literature. MEDLINE covers about 5000 medical, nursing, and health journals published in about 70 countries and contains more than 15 million records dating back to the mid-1960s. In 1999, abstracts of reviews from the Cochrane Collaboration became available through MEDLINE.

The MEDLINE database can be accessed online through a commercial vendor for a fee, but this database can be accessed for free on the Internet through the PubMed website (*http://www.ncbi.nlm.nih.gov/PubMed*). ●This means that anyone, anywhere in the world with Internet access can search for journal articles, and thus PubMed is a lifelong resource regardless of your institutional affiliation. PubMed has an excellent tutorial.

MEDLINE/PubMed uses a controlled vocabulary called MeSH (Medical Subject Headings) to index articles. MeSH terminology provides a consistent way to retrieve information that may use different terminology for the same concepts. You can search for references using the MeSH database by clicking on "MeSH database" in the left blue panel of the PubMed home page, listed under PubMed services. If, for example, we searched the MeSH database for "pain," we would find that Pain is a MeSH subject heading (a definition is provided) and that there are 37 additional categories listed—for example, "pain measurement" and "somatoform disorders." Note that MeSH subject headings may overlap with, but are not identical to, the subject headings used in the CINAHL database.

You can also search by doing a keyword search that looks for your keyword in text fields of the record. If you begin with your own keyword, you can click on the "Display" tab near the top right of the screen to see how the term you entered mapped onto MeSH terms, which might lead you to pursue other leads. For example, if we entered the keyword "pain" in the search field of the initial screen, the Display would show us that PubMed searched for all references that have "pain" in any text fields of the database record, *and* it also searched for any references for which "pain" has been coded as a subject heading because "pain" is a MeSH subject heading.

If we did a PubMed search of MEDLINE similar to the one we described earlier for CINAHL, this is what we would find:

SEARCH TOPIC/RESTRICTION	HITS
Pain	335,949
Pain AND child* AND nurs*	2054
Limit to research reports (NA)	
Limit to English	1834
Limit to entries with abstracts	1430
Limit to nursing journals	794
Limit to 2000 through 2006 publications	399

This search yielded more references than was the case in CINAHL, but we were not able to limit the search to research reports because the publication types in this database are categorized differently than in the case of Ovid's version of CINAHL. For example, we could limit the search to several *types* of research (e.g., clinical trials), but it is risky to use this restriction criterion. Note that in PubMed, the wildcard code used to extend truncated words is * rather than $.

Figure 5.3 shows the full citation for the same reference we located earlier in the CINAHL database (see Fig. 5.2). To get this full citation, you would need to use a pull-down menu near the top that offers alternative Displays—in this case, you would designate "Citation." The citation display presents all of the MeSH terms that were used for this particular reference, and as you can see, the MeSH terms are quite different from the subject headings for the same reference in CINAHL.

➔ **TIP:** Many database search programs have an extremely useful feature that allows you to find references to other similar studies. That is, once you have found a study that is a good exemplar of what you are looking for, you can search for other similar studies. In PubMed, for example, after identifying a key study, you could click on "Related Articles" on the right of the screen to search for other similar studies. In CINAHL via Ovid, you would click on "Find Similar."

The ISI Web of Knowledge

The Institute for Scientific Information (ISI) maintains a multidisciplinary resource called the Web of Knowledge, which offers integrated searching opportunities in several bibliographic databases. The Web of Knowledge covers most fields of the social, pure, and applied sciences, including medicine and nursing. Available databases include Current Contents Connect, the Science Citation Index, and the Social Sciences Citation Index. The citation indexes, together, are known as the Web of Science. From the Web of Science home page you can access an excellent tutorial, and you can also click on "Information for New Users."

Within the Web of Knowledge, you can conduct a general search by topic or author for articles published from 1992 to the present. An example of the results of a search similar to the one we undertook earlier is as follows:

SEARCH TOPIC/RESTRICTION	HITS
Pain	>100,000
Pain AND child* AND nurs*	479
Limit to research reports (NA)	
Limit to English	436
Limit to entries with abstracts (NA)	
Limit to nursing journals (NA)	
Limit to 2000 through 2006 publications	279

As this and the previous displays suggest, the three searches of different databases using similar search instructions yielded a different number of references. The searches are not totally overlapping, and so it is wise to search in multiple databases. For example, even though the Web of Knowledge search yielded more references than the Ovid/CINAHL search, the retrieved citation presented in Figures 5.2 and 5.3 was not identified in the Web of Knowledge databases.

A particularly useful component of the Web of Knowledge is its citation indexes, which can be used in applying a descendancy strategy—that is, tracking down articles that cite an earlier relevant one. For example, an early study that looked at nurse characteristics in relation to their response to children's pain was published by Hamers and colleagues ("Factors influencing nurses' pain assessment and intervention in children") in the *Journal of Advanced Nursing* in 1994. Using a "Cited Reference" search, the Web of Science indicated that the Hamers study had been cited 29 times, and provided full bibliographic information for these 29 articles.

Note that Ovid/CINAHL can also be used to pursue descendancy searches by clicking on a "Find Citing Articles" field that appears with each located reference. However, because the databases overlap but are not identical, you could not expect to find the same list of citations in Ovid/CINAHL and Web of Science. For example, within Ovid/CINAHL, a citation search for the Hamers study yielded only 16 results.

1: J. Pediatr Nurs. 2004 Feb; 19(1): 40–50.   Related Articles.   Links

Relieving children's pain: nurses' abilities and analgesic administration practices.

Vincent CV, Denyes MJ.

School of Nursing, Oakland University, Rochester, Michigan 48309-4401, USA. vincent@oakland.edu

A primary purpose of this study was to examine relationships among nurses' knowledge and attitudes about children' pain relief, nurses' abilities to overcome barriers to optimal pain management, nurses' analgesic practices, and pain levels of hospitalized children. Significant positive relationships were found between nurses' ($N = 67$) analgesic administration and children's pain, and between nurses' years of practice with children and nurses' abilities to overcome barriers to optimal pain management. The children's ($N = 132$) mean pain level was 1.63 (scale of 0 to 5), with one half of the children reporting moderate to severe pain. Of the 117 children who reported pain, 74% received analgesia. Nurses administered a mean of 37.9% of available morphine and means of 36% to 54% of recommended amounts of morphine, acetaminophen, and codeine.

MeSH Terms:
- Adolescent
- Adult
- Analgesia/nursing*
- Analgesics/administration & dosage
- Child
- Child Welfare*
- Child, Preschool
- Clinical Competence
- Evaluation Studies
- Health Knowledge, Attitudes, Practice*
- Humans

Male
Midwestern United States
Nurse's Role*
Nursing Assessment/methods
Nursing Evaluation Research
Pain/nursing*
Pediatric Nursing/methods
Pediatric Nursing/standards*
Quality Assurance/Health Care
Research Support, Non-U.S. Gov't
Research Support, U.S. Gov't, P.H.S

Substances:
- Analgesics

Grant Support:
- T32NR07068/NR/NINR

PMID: 14963869 [PubMed - indexed for MEDLINE]

FIGURE 5.3 Example of a printout from a PubMed search.

→ **TIP:** Searching for qualitative studies can pose special challenges. Walters, Wilczynski, and Haynes (2006) describe how they developed optimal search strategies for qualitative studies in the EMBASE database.

Screening and Gathering References

References that have been identified through the literature search need to be screened. One screen is totally practical—is the reference readily accessible? For example, although abstracts of dissertations may be easy to retrieve, full dissertations may not be; some references may be written in a language you do not read. A second screen is the relevance of the reference, which you can usually (but not always) surmise by reading the abstract. If abstracts are not available in the bibliographic database, you will need to take a guess about relevance based on the title. When you are screening an article, keep in mind that some of the articles judged to be not relevant for your primary question may be right on target for some of your secondary questions. A third criterion may include the study's methodologic quality—that is, the quality of evidence the study yields, a topic discussed in a later section.

We strongly urge you to obtain full copies of relevant studies rather than simply taking notes. It is often necessary to re-read a report or to get further details about an aspect of a study, which can easily be done if you have a copy of the article. Furthermore, as discussed later in this chapter, we recommend using a coding scheme to index information in the reports, to provide you with easier access to key pieces of information. Online retrieval of full text articles has increasingly become possible—a tremendous advantage in terms of efficiency. Articles that are not directly available online through your institution can be retrieved in a number of ways, including through a commercial vendor, by photocopying an article from a hardcopy journal, or by directly communicating with the authors of the report by e-mail or mail and requesting a copy.

Each obtained article should be stored in a manner that permits easy access. Some authors (Garrard, 2004) advocate a chronological filing method (e.g., by date of publication), but we think that alphabetical filing (using last name of the first author) is easier.

Documentation in Literature Retrieval

If your goal is to "own" the literature, you will be using a variety of databases, keywords, subject headings, and strategies in your endeavor to pursue every possible lead. As you meander through the complex world of research information, you will likely lose track of your efforts if you do not document your actions from the outset.

It is highly advisable to maintain a notebook (or computer database program) to record your search strategies and your search results. You should make note of information such as the following: databases searched; exclusion and inclusion criteria applied (i.e., limits put on your search); specific keywords, subject headings, and authors used to direct the search; combining strategies adopted; studies used to inaugurate a "Related Articles" or descendancy search; websites visited; links pursued; authors contacted to request further information or copies of articles not readily available; and any other information that would help you keep track of what you have done. Part of your strategy usually can be documented by printing your search history from your exploration of electronic databases.

By documenting your actions, you will be able to conduct a more efficient search—that is, you will not inadvertently duplicate a strategy you have already pursued. Documentation will also help you to assess what else needs to be tried—where to go next in your search. Finally, documenting your efforts is a step in ensuring that your literature review is reproducible.

⊗ The Toolkit of the accompanying *Resource Manual* offers a template for documenting certain types of information during a literature search. The template, as a Word document, can easily be augmented and adapted.

ABSTRACTING AND RECORDING INFORMATION

Tracking down relevant research on a topic is only the beginning of doing a literature review. Once you have a stack of useful articles, you need to develop a strategy for making sense of the mass of information contained in the articles. If a literature review is fairly simple, it may be sufficient to jot down notes about key features of the studies under review, and to use these notes as the basis for your analysis. However, literature reviews are often complex—for example, there may be numerous studies in the review, or the studies may vary extensively in terms of operationalizing key constructs. In such situations, it is useful to adopt a formal system of recording key pieces of information from each study. We describe two mechanisms for doing this, a formal protocol and matrices. First, though, we discuss the advantages of developing a coding scheme.

Coding the Studies

Reviewers who undertake a free-standing systematic review often develop intricate coding systems to support a computer analysis of their information. Although coding may not always be necessary in less formal reviews, we do think that coding of the research findings can be quite useful, and so we offer some simple suggestions and an example.

To develop a coding scheme, you will need to read at least a subset of your studies and look for opportunities to categorize findings. Let us take the example we have been using throughout this chapter, the relationship between nurses' characteristics (the independent variable) and nurses' responses to children's pain (the dependent variable). By perusing the articles we retrieved, we find that several nurse characteristics have been studied—for example, their age, gender, educational background, and so on. We can assign codes to each characteristic. Then let us consider the dependent variable, nurses' responses to children's pain. We find that some studies have focused on nurses' perceptions of children's pain, others have examined nurses' use of analgesia, and so on. These different outcomes can also be coded. An example of a coding scheme is presented in Box 5.1.

The codes can then be applied to the studies. You can use these codes to record information about the

---

BOX 5.1 Codes for Results Matrix/Coding in Margins

CODES FOR NURSE CHARACTERISTICS (INDEPENDENT VARIABLES)

1. Age
2. Gender
3. Education
4. Years of clinical experience
5. Race/ethnicity
6. Personal experience with pain
7. Nurse practitioner status

CODES FOR RESPONSES TO CHILDREN'S PAIN (DEPENDENT VARIABLES)

a. Perceptions of children's pain
b. Pain treatment (use of analgesia)
c. Pain treatment (use of nonpharmacologic methods)
d. Other (e.g., perceived barriers to optimal pain management)

study's research variables in the protocol or matrices (which we discuss next), but you can also use the codes in the margins of the articles themselves, so that you can easily locate important information. Figure 5.4, which presents an excerpt from the Results section of the pain study by Vincent and Denyes (2004), shows marginal coding of key variables.

Coding is flexible and can be a useful organizational tool even when a review is highly focused. For example, if our research question was about nurses' use of nonpharmacologic methods of pain treatment only (i.e., not about use of analgesics nor about pain perceptions), our outcome categories could be specific nonpharmacologic approaches, such as distraction, guided imagery, massage, and so on. The point is to organize information in a way that makes it easy to retrieve and analyze.

Literature Review Protocols

One method of systematically recording and organizing information from research articles is to use a formal protocol. Protocols are a means of recording various aspects of a study systematically, including the full citation, theoretical foundations, methodologic features, findings, and conclusions. Evaluative information (e.g., your assessment of the study's strengths and weaknesses) can also be noted.

There is no fixed format for such a protocol. You must decide what elements are important to *consistently* record across studies to help you organize and analyze information. We present an example in Figure 5.5, ✷ which can be adapted to fit your needs. (Although many of the terms on this protocol may not be familiar to you at this point—especially with regard to methodologic aspects—you will learn their meaning in subsequent chapters.) Note that if you have developed a coding scheme, as suggested in the previous section, you can use the codes to enter information about the study variables rather than writing out their names. Once you have developed a draft protocol, you should pilot test it with several studies to make sure it is sufficiently comprehensive and well structured. A literature review protocol such as the one in Figure 5.5 can easily be used for inputting information into a computer, should you wish to undertake a computerized analysis.

Literature Review Matrices

For traditional narrative reviews of the literature, we prefer the use of two-dimensional matrices as a means of organizing information from research articles because matrices directly support a thematic analysis of information. As with the protocol, the content of the matrices (and the number of matrices)

For research question 2, the only significant relationship found between nurse characteristics (basic conditioning factors) and either the two nursing agency variables of knowledge and attitude, and ability to overcome barriers, or the nursing action/system variable of analgesic administration was a positive correlation between nurses' years of practice and nurses' abilities to overcome barriers to optimal pain management, r = .41, p = .001. Nurses who had longer practice experience with children also reported greater ability to overcome barriers to optimal pain management.

1b 1d

3b 3d

4b 4d

5b 5d

6b 6d

FIGURE 5.4 Coded excerpt from Results section. From Vincent, C. V., & Denyes, M. J. [2004]. Relieving children's pain: Nurses' abilities and analgesic administration practices. *Journal of Pediatric Nursing, 19*[1], 40–50.

Citation: Authors: _____
                Title: _____
                Journal: _____
                Year: _____ Volume: _____ Issue: _____ Pages: _____

Type of Study: ☐ Quantitative   ☐ Qualitative   ☐ Mixed Method

Location/Setting: _____

Key concepts/   Concepts: _____
Variables: Intervention/Independent Variable: _____
                Dependent Variable: _____
                Controlled Variable: _____

Framework/Theory: _____
Design Type: ☐ Experimental   ☐ Quasi-experimental   ☐ Nonexperimental
                Specific Design: _____
                Blinding? ☐ None   ☐ Single:_____   ☐ Double _____
                Descrip. of Intervention: _____
                _____
                _____
                Comparison group(s): _____
                ☐ Cross-sectional ☐ Longitudinal/Prospective No. of data collection points: __

Qual. Tradition: ☐ Grounded theory ☐ Phenomenology ☐ Ethnography ☐ Other: _____

Sample: Size:_____ Sampling method: _____
                Sample characteristics: _____

Data Sources: Type: ☐ Self-report ☐ Observational ☐ Biophysiologic ☐ Other _____
                Description of measures: _____
                _____
                Data Quality: _____

Statistical Tests: Bivariate: ☐ T test ☐ ANOVA ☐ Chi-square ☐ Pearson's r ☐ Other: ___
                Multivar: ☐ Multiple regression ☐ MANOVA ☐ Logistic regression ☐ Other: __

Findings/   _____
Effect Sizes/   _____
Themes   _____
                _____
                _____
                _____

Recommendations: _____

Strengths: _____

Weaknesses: _____

FIGURE 5.5 ✳ Example of a literature review protocol.

can vary. A matrix can be constructed in handwritten form, in a word processing file (e.g., as a Word table), or in a spreadsheet. One advantage of computerizing the effort is that the information in the matrices can then be easily manipulated and sorted (e.g., the matrix entries can be sorted chronologically, by authors' last name, etc.). We present some basic ideas, but there is considerable flexibility in designing matrices to organize information.

We think three types of matrix are useful:

- A Methodologic Matrix, which organizes information to answer: How have researchers studied this research question?
- Results Matrixes, which addresses: What have researchers *found*?
- An Evaluation Matrix, designed to answer: How much confidence do we have in the evidence?

We discuss the first two types of matrix here, and the third type in a later section.

A Methodologic Matrix is used to record key features of the study design. The columns are used for the types of information you want to systematically capture across studies, and the rows represent each study. An abbreviated example of such a matrix for the question about nurses' characteristics in relation to their treatment of children's pain is presented in Figure 5.6, ✸ which, again, can be adapted as needed. This matrix only has five entries (other relevant studies were not included because of space constraints), but nevertheless it is clear that the information arrayed in this fashion allows us to see patterns that might otherwise have gone unnoticed. For example, we can readily discern the following by looking down the columns: the broad research question has attracted international interest; samples of convenience have predominated; and few studies have been linked to a formal theoretical framework. When the matrix is completed with entries from all relevant studies, it will be fairly easy to draw conclusions about how the research question has been addressed.

To discern themes in the pattern of *results*, we recommend developing multiple Results Matrices to record information about the findings. We find it useful to have as many separate matrices as there are codes (assuming a coding scheme has been developed) for either the independent or dependent variables—whichever is greater. In our example of a coding scheme shown in Box 5.1, there are seven independent variables and four dependent variables, and so we would set up seven separate Results Matrixes. Each matrix would correspond to a single independent variable. For example, the matrix in Figure 5.7 ✸ is for recording information about studies that examined nurses' education in relation to the management of children's pain. Other matrices would focus on nurses' age, years of experience, and so on. In each matrix, columns are used for the dependent variables, and rows are used for separate studies. Findings about the relationship between a particular independent variable and a particular dependent variable would be noted in the cells. As shown in Figure 5.7, cell entries can indicate more precisely how dependent variables were operationalized, the direction of any relationships, and level of significance. More information could be entered if deemed necessary, such as average values, and so on. Although there are only four studies included in this abbreviated Results Matrix, here again we can begin to detect some patterns: the evidence, although not consistent, mostly suggests that nurses' level of education is unrelated to their responses to children's pain. However, it appears that older studies were more likely than recent ones to find that more education was associated with better pain management by nurses.

Great care should be taken in abstracting results information. Researchers sometimes note explicitly only the findings that are statistically significant. Take, for example, the coded paragraph in Figure 5.4. The researchers (Vincent & Denyes, 2004) only fully elaborated results about the relationship between the nurses' years of experience and their ability to overcome barriers to optimal pain management. However, as indicated in the entry in the Methodologic Matrix (see Fig. 5.6), this study gathered and analyzed data about five characteristics of nurses in relation to two pain management outcomes, and so there are 10 codes in the margin. Consequently, 10 entries are needed in cells of Results Matrixes. Thus, although nothing in the

Authors	Pub Yr	Country	Theory	Dependent Variables	Independent Variables	Study Design	Sample Size	Sampling Method	How Data Collected?	Age of Children
Griffin et al.	2007	USA	—	Perception of child's pain, use of analgesic & nonpharmaco-logic methods	Nurses' age, clin exper, ed., nurse pract. status, pain experience	Cross-sectional, correlational	332 nurses, national sample	Random	Self-report questionnaire vignette	8–10
Vincent & Denyes	2004	USA	Orem	Use of analgesics, perceived barriers to optimal pain management	Nurses' age, race, clinical experience, education, pain experience	Cross-sectional, correlational	67 nurses from 7 hospital units	Convenience	Observation, self-report questionnaire	3–17
Polkki et al.	2001	Finland	—	Nurses' use of nonpharmacol-ogic methods of pain relief	Nurses' age, education, clincl exper, # own children	Cross-sectional, correlational	162 nurses from 5 hospitals	Convenience	Self-report questionnaire	8–12
Hamers et al.	1997	Netherlands	—	Assessments of child's pain, confidence in assessment, use of analgesics	Level of experience in pediatric nursing	Cross-sectional, correlational	695 nurses	Convenience	Video, vignette, self-report questionnaire	5–10
Margolius et al.	1995	USA	—	Perceptions of pain, perceptions of adequacy of pain management	Nurses' education, age, years of nursing experience	Cross-sectional, correlational	228 nurses in one pediatric setting	Convenience	Self-report questionnaire	NA

FIGURE 5.6 Example of a methodologic matrix for recording key methodologic features of studies for a literature review: nurse characteristics and management of children's pain.

Independent Variable: *Nurses Education* (Code 3)

Authors	Pub Year	DV.a Pain Perceptions	DV.b Use of Analgesics	DV.c Use of Non-Pharmacologics	DV.d Other
Griffin et al.	2007	Rating of child's pain: no significant relationship	Amount used within PRN: no significant relationship	Number of nonpharm strategies used: no significant relationship	—
Vincent & Denyes	2004	—	% of prescribed medications administered: no significant relation	—	Perceived barriers to optimal pain management: no significant relationship
Polkki et al.	2001	—	—	Use of nonpharmacologic methods higher in those with more education ($p < .05$)	—
Margolius et al.	1995	Perception of children's pain: higher with more education ($p < .05$)	—	—	—

FIGURE 5.7 ⊗ Example of a results matrix for recording key findings for a literature review: nurses' education and management of children's pain.

paragraph mentions nurses' education, we have entered "no significant relationship" in two cells of Figure 5.7 because the paragraph implies that all but one relationship studied was nonsignificant.

➤ **TIP:** Results matrices can also be made for qualitative studies. Instead of columns for independent or dependent variables, columns can be used to record themes, concepts, or categories.

CRITIQUING STUDIES AND EVALUATING THE EVIDENCE

In drawing conclusions about a body of research, reviewers must not only record factual information about studies—their methodologic features and findings—but also make judgments about the worth of the studies' evidence. This section discusses issues relating to research critiques and recording evaluative information.

Research Critiques of Individual Studies

A research **critique** is a careful appraisal of the strengths and weaknesses of a study. A good critique objectively identifies areas of adequacy and inadequacy, virtues as well as faults. Although our emphasis in this chapter is on the evaluation of research evidence within the context of a literature review, we must pause to offer advice about other types of critiques.

Many research critiques focus on a single study rather than on a whole body of research. For example, most nursing journals that publish research articles have a policy of independent, anonymous critiques by two or more peer reviewers who prepare written critiques and make a recommendation about whether or not to publish the report. Peer reviewers' critiques can address a wide array of concerns, but they typically are brief and focus primarily on key substantive and methodologic issues.

Students taking a research methods course also may be asked to critique a study, to provide evidence of their mastery of methodologic concepts. Such critiques are usually expected to be comprehensive; students are expected to critique various dimensions of a report, including substantive and theoretical aspects, ethical issues, methodologic decisions, interpretation, and the report's organization, thoroughness, and presentation. The purpose of such a thorough critique is to cultivate critical thinking, to induce students to use newly acquired skills in research methods, to obtain documentation of those skills, and to prepare students for a professional nursing career in which evaluating research will almost surely play a role. Writing research critiques is an important first step on the path to developing an EBP.

➲ **TIP:** As you embark on a research critique, we suggest that you read the article you are critiquing at least twice, and you may need to read parts of it several times. Obviously, the first step in preparing a critique is to understand what the report is saying. We encourage you to write in the margins of the article, and to circle keywords.

In this textbook, we provide support for such comprehensive critiques of individual studies in several ways. First, detailed critiquing suggestions that correspond to chapter content are included in most chapters of the book. Second, we offer an abbreviated set of key critiquing guidelines for quantitative and qualitative reports here in this chapter, in Boxes 5.2 ✪ and 5.3, ✪ respectively. Finally, it is always illuminating to have a good model, and so Appendices G and H of the accompanying *Resource Manual* include completed comprehensive research critiques of a quantitative and qualitative study (the studies themselves are printed in their entirety as well).

The guidelines in Boxes 5.2 and 5.3 are organized according to the structure of most research reports—Abstract, Introduction, Method, Results, and Discussion. The second column lists some key critiquing questions that have broad applicability to quantitative and qualitative studies, and the third column provides cross-references to the more detailed guidelines in the various chapters of the book. (We recognize that many of the critiquing questions may be too difficult for you to answer at this point, but your methodologic and critiquing skills will develop as you progress through this book.)

A few comments about these guidelines are in order. First, the wording of the questions calls for a yes or no answer (although for some, it may well be that the answer will be "Yes, *but . . .*"). In all cases, the desirable answer is "yes," that is, a "no" suggests a possible limitation and a "yes" suggests a strength. Therefore, the more "yeses" a study gets, the stronger it is likely to be. Thus, these guidelines can cumulatively suggest a global assessment: a report with 25 "yeses" is likely to be superior to one with only 10. However, it is also important to realize that not all "yeses" and "nos" are equal. Some elements are far more important in drawing conclusions about the rigor of a study than others. For example, the inadequacy of a literature review is far less damaging to the worth of the study's *evidence* than the use of a faulty design. In general, the questions addressing the researchers' methodologic decisions (i.e., the questions under "Method"), as well as questions relating to the analysis, are especially important in evaluating the integrity of a study's evidence.

Although the questions in these boxes elicit yes or no responses, a comprehensive written critique would obviously need to do more than point out what the study did and did not do. Each relevant issue would need to be discussed and your criticism justified. For example, if you answered "no" to the question about whether the problem was easy to identify, you would need to describe your concern and perhaps offer an improved problem statement.

We must acknowledge that our simplified critiquing guidelines have a number of shortcomings. In particular, they are generic despite the fact that critiquing cannot really use a one-size-fits-all list of questions. Critiquing questions that are relevant to certain types of studies (e.g., experiments) do not fit into a set of general questions for all quantitative studies. Furthermore, many supplementary questions would be needed to thoroughly assess certain types of research—for example, grounded theory

BOX 5.2 Guide to an Overall Critique of a Quantitative Research Report

Aspect of the Report	Basic Questions for a Critique of Individual Studies	Detailed Critiquing Guidelines
Title	• Is the title a good one, succinctly suggesting key variables and the study population?	
Abstract	• Does the abstract clearly and concisely summarize the main features of the report (problem, methods, results, conclusions)?	
Introduction		
Statement of the problem	• Is the problem stated unambiguously, and is it easy to identify? • Does the problem statement build a cogent and persuasive argument for the new study? • Does the problem have significance for nursing? • Is there a good match between the research problem and the paradigm and methods used? Is a quantitative approach appropriate?	Box 4.3, page 101
Hypotheses or research questions	• Are research questions and/or hypotheses explicitly stated? If not, is their absence justified? • Are questions and hypotheses appropriately worded, with clear specification of key variables and the study population? • Are the questions/hypotheses consistent with the literature review and the conceptual framework?	Box 4.3, page 101
Literature review	• Is the literature review up to date and based mainly on primary sources? • Does the review provide a state-of-the-art synthesis of evidence on the research problem? • Does the literature review provide a solid basis for the new study?	Box 5.4, page 135
Conceptual/theoretical framework	• Are key concepts adequately defined conceptually? • Is there a conceptual/theoretical framework, rationale, and/or map, and (if so) is it appropriate? If not, is the absence of one justified?	Box 6.3, page 161
Method		
Protection of participants' rights	• Were appropriate procedures used to safeguard the rights of study participants? Was the study subject to external review? • Was the study designed to minimize risks and maximize benefits to participants?	Box 7.3, page 187
Research design	• Was the most rigorous possible design used, given the purpose of the research? • Were appropriate comparisons made to enhance interpretability of the findings? • Was the number of data collection points appropriate?	Box 10.1, page 280

BOX 5.2 Guide to an Overall Critique of a Quantitative Research Report (continued)

	• Did the design minimize biases and threats to the internal and external validity of the study (e.g., was blinding used, was attrition minimized)?	
Population and sample	• Was the population identified and described? Was the sample described in sufficient detail? • Was the best possible sampling design used to enhance the sample's representativeness? Were sample biases minimized? • Was the sample size adequate? Was a power analysis used to estimate sample size needs?	Box 13.1, page 360
Data collection and measurement	• Are the operational and conceptual definitions congruent? • Were key variables operationalized using the best possible method (e.g., interviews, observations, and so on) and with adequate justification? • Are the specific instruments adequately described and were they good choices, given the study purpose and study population? • Does the report provide evidence that the data collection methods yielded data that were high on reliability and validity?	Box 14.1, page 388; Box 16.4, page 443; Box 17.1, page 470
Procedures	• If there was an intervention, is it adequately described, and was it properly implemented? Did most participants allocated to the intervention group actually receive the intervention? • Were data collected in a manner that minimized bias? Were the staff who collected data appropriately trained?	Box 10.1, page 280; Box 14.1, page 388
Results Data analysis	• Were analyses undertaken to address each research question or test each hypothesis? • Were appropriate statistical methods used, given the level of measurement of the variables, number of groups being compared, and so on? • Was the most powerful analytic method used? (e.g., did the analysis help to control for confounding variables)? • In intervention studies, were analyses performed using the intention-to-treat approach? • Were Type I and Type II errors avoided or minimized?	Box 21.1, page 578; Box 22.1, page 610
Findings	• Are the findings adequately summarized, with good use of tables and figures? • Are findings reported in a manner that facilitates a meta-analysis, and with sufficient information needed for evidence-based practice?	Box 21.1, page 578 Box 22.1, page 610 Box 24.1, page 660

BOX 5.2 Guide to an Overall Critique of a Quantitative Research Report (continued)

Discussion Interpretation of the findings	• Are all major findings interpreted and discussed within the context of prior research and/or the study's conceptual framework? • Are the interpretations consistent with the results and with the study's limitations? • Does the report address the issue of the generalizability of the findings?	Box 24.1, page 660
Implications/ recomendations	• Do the researchers discuss the implications of the study for clinical practice or further research—and are those implications reasonable and complete?	
Global Issues Presentation	• Is the report well written, well organized, and sufficiently detailed for critical analysis? • Was the report written in a manner that makes the findings accessible to practicing nurses?	Box 26.2, page 709
Researcher credibility	• Do the researchers' clinical, substantive, or methodologic qualifications and experience enhance confidence in the findings and their interpretation?	
Summary assessment	• Despite any identified limitations, do the study findings appear to be valid—do you have confidence in the *truth* value of the results? • Does the study contribute any meaningful evidence that can be used in nursing practice or that is useful to the nursing discipline?	

studies. Thus, you would need to use some judgment about whether the guidelines are sufficiently comprehensive for the type of study you are critiquing.

➡ **TIP:** The critiquing guidelines are available as Word documents in the Toolkit of the accompanying *Resource Manual*; the question list can be adapted, as appropriate.

Another word of caution is that we developed these guidelines based on our years of experience as researchers and research methodologists. They do not represent a formal, rigorously developed set of questions that can be used for a formal systematic review. They should, however, facilitate beginning efforts to critically appraise nursing studies.

Finally, there are questions in these guidelines for which there are no totally objective answers. Even experts sometimes disagree about what are

the best methodologic strategies for a study. Thus, you should not be afraid to "stick out your neck" to express an evaluative opinion—but do be sure that your comments have some basis in methodologic principles discussed in this book.

➡ **TIP:** An important thing to remember is that it is appropriate to assume the posture of a skeptic when you are critiquing a report. Just as a careful clinician seeks evidence from research findings that certain practices are or are not effective, you as a reviewer should demand evidence from the report that the researchers' substantive and methodologic decisions were sound.

Evaluating a Body of Research

In reviewing the literature, you typically would not undertake a comprehensive critique of *each* study—although you would need to make judgments about the quality of evidence in each study so that you

BOX 5.3 Guide to an Overall Critique of a Qualitative Research Report

Aspect of the Report	Basic Questions for a Critique	Detailed Critiquing Guidelines
Title	• Was the title a good one, suggesting the key phenomenon and the group or community under study?	
Abstract	• Does the abstract clearly and concisely summarize the main features of the report?	
Introduction Statement of the problem	• Is the problem stated unambiguously and is it easy to identify? • Does the problem statement build a cogent and persuasive argument for the new study? • Does the problem have significance for nursing? • Is there a good match between the research problem on the one hand and the paradigm, tradition, and methods on the other?	Box 4.3, page 101
Research questions	• Are research questions explicitly stated? If not, is their absence justified? • Are the questions consistent with the study's philosophical basis, underlying tradition, conceptual framework, or ideological orientation?	Box 4.3, page 101
Literature review	• Does the report adequately summarize the existing body of knowledge related to the problem or phenomenon of interest? • Does the literature review provide a solid basis for the new study?	Box 5.4, page 135
Conceptual underpinnings	• Are key concepts adequately defined conceptually? • Is the philosophical basis, underlying tradition, conceptual framework, or ideological orientation made explicit and is it appropriate for the problem?	Box 6.3, page 161
Method Protection of participants' rights	• Were appropriate procedures used to safeguard the rights of study participants? Was the study subject to external review? • Was the study designed to minimize risks and maximize benefits to participants?	Box 7.3, page 187
Research design and research tradition	• Is the identified research tradition (if any) congruent with the methods used to collect and analyze data? • Was an adequate amount of time spent in the field or with study participants? • Did the design unfold in the field, giving researchers opportunities to capitalize on early understandings?	Box 9.1, page 242

BOX 5.3 Guide to an Overall Critique of a Qualitative Research Report (continued)

	• Was there evidence of reflexivity in the design?	
	• Was there an adequate number of contacts with study participants?	
Sample and setting	• Was the group or population of interest adequately described? Were the setting and sample described in sufficient detail?	Box 13.2, page 361
	• Was the approach used to gain access to the site or to recruit participants appropriate?	
	• Was the best possible method of sampling used to enhance information richness and address the needs of the study?	
	• Was the sample size adequate? Was saturation achieved?	
Data collection	• Were the methods of gathering data appropriate? Were data gathered through two or more methods to achieve triangulation?	Box 14.1, page 388; Box 15.3, page 410
	• Did the researcher ask the right questions or make the right observations, and were they recorded in an appropriate fashion?	
	• Was a sufficient amount of data gathered? Was the data of sufficient depth and richness?	
Procedures	• Were data collection and recording procedures adequately described and do they appear appropriate?	Box 14.1, page 388; Box 15.3, page 410
	• Were data collected in a manner that minimized bias or behavioral distortions? Were the staff who collected data appropriately trained?	
Enhancement of rigor	• Were methods used to enhance the trustworthiness of the data (and analysis), and was the description of those methods adequate?	Box 20.1, page 552
	• Were the methods used to enhance credibility appropriate and sufficient?	
	• Did the researcher document research procedures and decision processes sufficiently that findings are auditable and confirmable?	
Results Data analysis	• Were the data management (e.g., coding) and data analysis methods sufficiently described?	Box 19.3, page 531
	• Was the data analysis strategy compatible with the research tradition and with the nature and type of data gathered?	
	• Did the analysis yield an appropriate "product" (e.g., a theory, taxonomy, thematic pattern, etc.)?	
	• Did the analytic procedures suggest the possibility of biases?	

BOX 5.3 Guide to an Overall Critique of a Qualitative Research Report (continued)

Findings	• Were the findings effectively summarized, with good use of excerpts and supporting arguments? • Do the themes adequately capture the meaning of the data? Does it appear that the researcher satisfactorily conceptualized the themes or patterns in the data? • Did the analysis yield an insightful, provocative, and meaningful picture of the phenomenon under investigation?	Box 19.3, page 531
Theoretical integration	• Are the themes or patterns logically connected to each other to form a convincing and integrated whole? • Were figures, maps, or models used effectively to summarize conceptualizations? • If a conceptual framework or ideological orientation guided the study, are the themes or patterns linked to it in a cogent manner?	Box 19.3, p. 531
Discussion Interpretation of the findings	• Are the findings interpreted within an appropriate frame of reference? • Are major findings interpreted and discussed within the context of prior studies? • Are the interpretations consistent with the study's limitations? • Does the report address the issue of the transferability of the findings?	Box 19.3, page 531 Box 20.1, page 552
Implications/ recommendations	• Do the researchers discuss the implications of the study for clinical practice or further inquiry—and are those implications reasonable and complete?	
Global Issues Presentation	• Was the report well written, well organized, and sufficiently detailed for critical analysis? • Was the description of the methods, findings, and interpretations sufficiently rich and vivid?	Box 26.2, page 709
Researcher credibility	• Do the researchers' clinical, substantive, or methodologic qualifications and experience enhance confidence in the findings and their interpretation?	
Summary assessment	• Do the study findings appear to be trustworthy—do you have confidence in the *truth* value of the results? • Does the study contribute any meaningful evidence that can be used in nursing practice or that is useful to the nursing discipline?	

could draw conclusions about the overall body of evidence. Critiques for a literature review tend to focus on methodologic aspects.

In free-standing systematic reviews, methodologic quality often plays a role right at the outset

of the review because studies judged to be of low quality may be screened out from further consideration. Using methodologic quality as a screening criterion is somewhat controversial, however. Systematic reviews are also especially likely to involve the use of a formal evaluation instrument that gives quantitative ratings to different aspects of the study, so that appraisals across studies ("scores") can be compared and summarized. Methodologic screening issues and formal scoring instruments are described in Chapter 25.

In literature reviews undertaken to develop a context for a new primary study, methodologic features of the studies under review need to be assessed with an eye to answering a very broad question: To what extent do the findings reflect the *truth* (the true state of affairs) or, conversely, to what extent do biases undermine the believability of the findings? The "truth" is most likely to be discovered when researchers use powerful designs, good sampling plans, strong data collection instruments and procedures, and appropriate analyses.

Judgments about the rigor of each study can be entered in an Evaluation Matrix—or, alternatively, additional columns for evaluative information can be added to the Methodologic Matrix. The advantage of combining information into one matrix is that methodologic features and assessments about those features would be in a single table. The disadvantage

is that the matrix would have so many columns that it might be cumbersome. A simple Evaluation Matrix is presented in Figure 5.8, ✪ which provides space in the columns for noting major strengths and weaknesses for each study (the rows). More fine-grained column headings are likely to be useful when there are numerous studies under review. For example, there could be separate strengths/weaknesses columns for major methodologic features, such as design, sample, measurement, and analysis. If a "score" for overall quality is derived from a formal scoring instrument (e.g., counting all the "yeses" from Boxes 5.2 or 5.3), this information can also be added to the evaluation matrix.

ANALYZING AND SYNTHESIZING INFORMATION

Once all the relevant studies have been retrieved, read, abstracted, and critiqued, the information has to be analyzed and synthesized. As previously noted, we find the analogy between doing a literature review and doing a qualitative study useful,

Authors	Year of Publication	Major Strengths	Major Weaknesses	Quality Score*
Vincent & Denyes	2004	• Measured actual use of analgesics, not self-report • Linkage to Orem's theory • Good descriptive info on knowledge, attitudes, and use of analgesics	• Small and unrepresentative sample ($N = 67$), strong likelihood of Type II error (questionable power analysis) • Weak design for studying Q1 (effect of knowledge on analgesic use, effect of analgesic use on actual pain); several internal validity threats • Possibility that nurses' behavior in administering analgesics was affected by knowing they were in a study	12
Study 2				
Study 3				

*The quality score is fictitious and is shown here to indicate that information of this type could be recorded in the evaluation matrix.

FIGURE 5.8 ✪ Example of an evaluation matrix for recording strengths and weaknesses of studies for a literature review: nurse characteristics and management of children's pain.

and this is particularly true with respect to the analysis of the "data" (i.e., the information from the retrieved studies): in both, the focus is on the identification of important *themes*.

A thematic analysis essentially involves the detection of patterns and regularities—as well as inconsistencies. A number of different types of themes can be identified, including the following:

- *Substantive themes*: What is the pattern of evidence? How much evidence is there? How consistent is the body of evidence? How powerful are the observed effects? How persuasive is the evidence? What gaps are there in the body of evidence?
- *Theoretical themes*: What theoretical or conceptual frameworks have been used to address the primary question—or has most research been atheoretical? How congruent are the theoretical underpinnings? Do findings vary in relation to differences in underlying frameworks?
- *Methodologic themes*: What designs and methods have been used to address the question? What methodologic strategies have *not* been used? What are the predominant methodologic deficiencies and strengths? What methodologic features do the most rigorous studies have in common? Do findings vary in relation to differences in methodologic approaches?
- *Generalizability/transferability themes*: To what types of people or settings do the findings apply? Do the findings vary for different types of people (e.g., men versus women) or setting (e.g., urban versus rural)?
- *Historical themes*: Have there been substantive, theoretical, or methodologic trends over time? Is the evidence getting better? When was most of the research conducted?
- *"Researcher" themes*: Who has been doing the research, in terms of discipline, specialty area, nationality, prominence, and so on? Has the research been developed within a systematic program of research?

The reason we have recommended using various matrices should be clear from reading this list of possible themes: it is easier to discern patterns by reading down the columns of the matrices than by flipping through a stack of literature review protocols. However, it should be noted that some of the suggested themes could only be addressed by integrating information from multiple matrices; for example, to detect whether findings varied depending on methodologic approach, it would be necessary to assemble information from Methodologic and Results matrices.

Clearly, it is not possible—even in lengthy freestanding reviews—to analyze all the themes we have identified. Reviewers have to make decisions about which patterns to pursue. In preparing a review as part of a new study, you would need to determine which pattern is of greatest relevance for developing an argument and providing readers with a context for the new research.

PREPARING A WRITTEN LITERATURE REVIEW

Writing literature reviews can be quite challenging, especially when voluminous information and intricate thematic analyses must be condensed into a small number of pages, as is typically the case for a journal article or research proposal. We offer a few suggestions, but readily acknowledge that skills in writing literature reviews develop over time.

Organizing the Review

Organization of information is a critical task in preparing a written review. It is almost always essential to develop an outline to structure the flow of presentation. If the review is complex, a written outline is recommended; a mental outline may be sufficient for simpler reviews. The outline should list the main topics or themes (and subtopics) to be discussed, and indicate the order of presentation. The important point is to have a plan before starting to write so that the review has a meaningful and understandable flow. Lack of organization is a common weakness in first attempts at writing a research literature review. Although the specifics of the organization differ from topic to topic, the overall goal is to structure the review in such a way that the presentation is logical, demonstrates meaningful thematic integration, and leads to a conclusion about the state of evidence on the topic.

Writing a Literature Review

Although it is beyond the scope of this textbook to offer detailed guidance on writing research reviews, we offer a few comments on their content and style. Additional assistance is provided in books such as those by Fink (2005) and Galvan (2003).

Content of the Written Literature Review

A written research review should provide readers with an objective, well-organized synthesis of the current state of evidence on a topic. A literature review should be neither a series of quotes nor a series of abstracts. The central tasks are to summarize and critically evaluate the overall evidence so as to reveal the current state of knowledge on a topic with regard to themes deemed to be important—not simply to describe what researchers have done.

Although key studies may be described in some detail, it is not necessary to provide particulars for every reference (especially when there are page constraints). Studies with comparable findings often can be summarized together.

Example of grouped studies: Cottrell (2006, pp. 24–25) summarized several studies as follows: "Vaginal douching is associated with adverse reproductive and gynecologic outcomes that include a high risk for pelvic inflammatory disease, tubal pregnancy, possibly bacterial vaginitis (BV) infection-induced stillbirths, chlamydial infection, higher rates of HIV transmission, cervical cancer, preterm birth, low birthweight infants, and BV (CDC, 2003, 2004; Cottrell, 2003; Fiscella et al., 1998; Goldenberg and Thompson, 2003; Leitich et al., 2003; Zhang et al., 1997)."

The literature should be summarized in your own words. The review should demonstrate that consideration has been given to the cumulative worth of the body of research. Stringing together quotes from various documents fails to show that previous research has been assimilated and understood.

The review should be objective, to the extent possible. Studies that are at odds with your hypotheses obviously should not be omitted. The review also should not ignore a study because its findings contradict other studies. Inconsistent results should be analyzed and the supporting evidence evaluated objectively.

A literature review typically concludes with a concise summary of current evidence on the topic. The summary should recap key findings and indicate how credible they are and should also make note of gaps in the evidence. If the literature review is conducted as part of a new study, this critical summary should demonstrate the need for the research and should clarify the context within which any hypotheses were developed.

As you progress through this book, you will become increasingly proficient in critically evaluating the research literature. We hope you will understand the mechanics of doing a research review once you have completed this chapter, but we do not expect that you will be in a position to write a state-of-the-art review until you have acquired more skills in research methods.

Style of a Research Review

Students preparing a written research review often have trouble adjusting to the standard style of such reviews. In particular, students sometimes accept research results without criticism or reservation, perhaps reflecting a common misunderstanding about the conclusiveness of research. You should keep in mind that hypotheses cannot be proved or disproved by empirical testing, and no research question can be definitely answered in a single study. Every study has at least some methodologic limitations. The fact that hypotheses cannot be ultimately proved or disproved does not, of course, mean that we must disregard research evidence—especially if findings have been replicated. The problem is partly semantic: hypotheses are not proved, they are *supported* by research findings.

➲ **TIP:** When describing study findings, you should generally use phrases indicating tentativeness of the results, such as the following:

- Several researchers have *found* …
- Findings thus far *suggest*…
- Results from a landmark study *indicated*…
- The data *supported* the hypothesis …
- There *appears* to be strong evidence that …

A related stylistic problem is the interjection of opinions into the review. The review should include opinions sparingly, if at all, and should be explicit about their source. Reviewers' own opinions do not belong in a review, with the exception of assessments of study quality.

The left-hand column of Table 5.1 presents several examples of stylistic flaws. The right-hand column offers recommendations for rewording the sentences to conform to a more acceptable form for a research literature review. Many alternative wordings are possible.

CRITIQUING RESEARCH LITERATURE REVIEWS

It is often difficult to critique a research review because the author is almost invariably more knowledgeable about the topic than the readers. It is thus not usually possible to judge whether the author has included all relevant literature and has adequately summarized evidence on that topic. Many aspects of a research review, however, are amenable to evaluation by readers who are not experts on the topic. Some suggestions for critiquing written research reviews are presented in Box 5.4. ✪ Additionally, when a review is published as a stand-alone article, it should include information to help readers evaluate its thoroughness, as discussed in Chapter 25.

TABLE 5.1	Examples of Stylistic Difficulties for Research Literature Reviews
PROBLEMATIC STYLE OR WORDING	**IMPROVED STYLE OR WORDING***
Women who do not participate in childbirth preparation classes manifest a high degree of anxiety during labor.	*Researchers have found that* women who participate in childbirth preparation classes *tend to* manifest less anxiety than those who do not (Keehn, 2006; Kim, 2007; Yepsen, 2006).
Studies have proved that doctors and nurses do not fully understand the psychobiologic dynamics of recovery from a myocardial infarction.	Studies by Fortune (2006) and Crampton (2007) *suggest that many* doctors and nurses do not fully understand the psychobiologic dynamics of recovery from a myocardial infarction.
Attitudes cannot be changed quickly.	Attitudes *have been found to be* relatively stable, enduring attributes that do not change quickly (Nicolet & Ryan, 2007; Walsh, 2005).
It is known that uncertainty engenders stress.	*According to* Dr. A. Cassard (2006), an expert on stress and anxiety, uncertainty is a stressor.

*Italicized words in the improved version indicate key alterations.

BOX 5.4 Guidelines for Critiquing Literature Reviews

1. Does the review seem thorough—does it include all or most of the major studies on the topic? Does it include recent research? Are studies from other related disciplines included, if appropriate?
2. Does the review rely on appropriate materials (e.g., mainly on research reports, using primary sources)?
3. Is the review merely a summary of existing work, or does it critically appraise and compare key studies? Does the review identify important gaps in the literature?
4. Is the review well organized? Is the development of ideas clear?
5. Does the review use appropriate language, suggesting the tentativeness of prior findings? Is the review objective? Does the author paraphrase, or is there an over-reliance on quotes from original sources?
6. If the review is part of a research report for a new study, does the review support the need for the study?
7. If it is a review designed to summarize evidence for clinical practice, does the review draw appropriate conclusions about practice implications?

In assessing a literature review, the overarching question is whether it summarizes the current state of research evidence. If the review is written as part of an original research report, an equally important question is whether the review lays a solid foundation for the new study.

RESEARCH EXAMPLES OF LITERATURE REVIEWS

The best way to learn about the style, content, and organization of a research literature review is to read reviews that appear in the nursing literature. We present excerpts from two reviews here and urge you to read other reviews on a topic of interest to you.

Literature Review From a Quantitative Research Report

Study: "Testing videotape education for heart failure" (Smith et al., 2005)

Statement of Purpose: The purpose of this study was to test a videotape educational intervention that was designed to improve patient knowledge and self-management of heart failure and ultimately improve functional status.

Literature Review (Excerpt): "Heart failure (HF) is a debilitating chronic illness that affects an estimated 5 million Americans (American Heart Association, 2004)* and 350,000 Canadians (Canadian Cardiovascular Society, 2001) and is increasing rapidly with the aging of the population (Heart Failure Society of American, 2004). HF is one of the most common reasons for hospitalizations in older Americans and Canadians, accounting for nearly a million hospitalizations annually in the United States (Kozak et al., 2004) and more than 100,000 in Canada (Tsuyuki et al., 2003). Despite the existence of effective treatments, readmission rates of 30% to 50% are reported (Rich, 2002; Tsuyuki et al., 2003). Most rehospitalizations can be traced to patients' lack of information, understanding, or compliance with the complex regimen of HF home care (Bennett et al., 2003; Evangelista et al., 2003; Jaarsma et al., 1999; Tsuyuki et al., 2003). Researchers have found that HF patients lack even the basic knowledge necessary for dietary or symptom management (Horowitz et al., 2004), have little continuity or education for home care (Naylor et al., 2004), and infrequently attend posthospital educational sessions (Dougherty et al., 2002).

Evidence indicates that HF discharge or posthospital education can significantly reduce rehospitalization

---

*Consult the full research report for references cited in this excerpted literature review.

(Ahmed, 2002; Blue et al., 2001; Philbin, 1999; Stewart & Blue, 2001; Wright et al., 2003). The recommended multidisciplinary education programs are expensive and rarely available outside major cities, and even rudimentary HF information is not consistently taught at discharge (Ekman et al., 1998; Phillips et al., 2004; Rich, 2003). A study of 85,000 patients hospitalized across the United States showed that only 31% received the basic HF discharge instructions recommended by the Joint Commission on the Accreditation of Healthcare Organizations (JCAHO, 2004; see also Fonarow, 2003 . . .).

Short instructional videotapes that can be viewed repeatedly at home can present the large amounts of information necessary to adequately learn to manage HF home care (Krumholz et al, 2002; Smith et al., 2003). Videotapes depicting patients successfully managing their chronic conditions have been found to have greater outcomes than written instruction materials, lectures, and even in-person teaching (Bull et al., 2001; Koehler et al., 2001; Krouse, 2001; Smith & Curtas, 1999). In an American Heart Association study with an ethnically diverse group of 657 high-risk adults, a 12-minute videotape directed participants to monitor and report stroke symptoms (Stern et al., 1999). Regardless of ethnicity, gender, age, or education level, participants had significant knowledge gain and, during the subsequent 3-month follow-up, used the symptom reporting illustrated in the videotape. Videotape education has been especially effective in older adults and those with decreased cognition, depression, or poor literacy (Chelf et al., 2001; Given et al., 2003; Nielsen-Bohlman et al., 2004; Reznik et al., 2004)" (pp. 192–193).

Literature Review From a Qualitative Research Report

Study: "Disability in everyday life" (Lutz & Bowers, 2005)

Statement of Purpose: The purpose of this study was to describe how persons with disabilities perceived the experience of disability in their everyday lives.

Literature Review (Excerpt): "In the past 10 years, disability has become a priority in health care research and delivery. The Institute of Medicine, Centers for Disease Control, *Healthy People 2010*, and the World Health Organization (WHO) have all identified disability and services for persons with disability as important areas for research and targeted interventions (Brandt & Pope, 1997;

Pope & Tarlov, 1991; DHHS, 2000; WHO, 2002).* Data from the U.S. National Health Interview Survey indicate that disability is present in at least 13% of the noninstitutionalized population (Brandt & Pope, 1997; Fujiura, 2001). In 1997, direct costs of disability were estimated to be approximately US $200 billion and indirect costs 'may be as high as $155 billion' (Brandt & Pope, 1997, p. 61).

In addition, persons with physical disabling conditions . . . face many individual 'costs' of disability. They are twice as likely to be unemployed as persons without disabilities, and they are three times as likely to live in poverty (National Organization on Disability, 2004). Also, because of their disabling conditions, persons with disabilities have a 'thinner margin of health' (DeJong et al., 2002); that is, they are likely to become more ill more quickly from common illnesses such as colds and influenza, and they are more likely to be hospitalized as a result of these illnesses. They are also susceptible to secondary conditions such as decubiti, pneumonia, urinary tract infections, fractured bones, contractures, and arthritis (Burns et al., 1990), and they experience the effects of aging at a quicker rate than persons without disabilities (DeJong & Brannon, 1998; DeJong et al., 2002).

Persons with disabilities often require services from many different sources, both private and public. Researchers have suggested developing comprehensive integrated systems of care that include health care, and supportive services, such as transportation, personal care, assistive devices, vocational services, and assistance for housing for persons with disabilities (Brandt & Pope, 1997; Chermak, 1990; DeJong & Brannon, 1998; Leutz et al., 1997). However, not much is known about how these systems should be designed to serve the self-defined needs of persons with disabilities best" (pp. 1037–1038).

SUMMARY POINTS

- A research **literature review** is a written summary of the state of evidence on a research problem.
- The major steps in preparing a written research review include formulating a question, devising a search strategy, conducting a search, retrieving

---

*Consult the full research report for references cited in this excerpted literature review.

relevant sources, abstracting and encoding information, critiquing studies, analyzing the aggregated information, and preparing a written synthesis.

- Written literature reviews vary in purpose and length, ranging from brief reviews in the introduction of a research report to establish a context for a new study to lengthier stand-alone reviews that critically appraise the state of research evidence.

- For a research review, study findings (which are usually published in journal articles) are the key ingredients. Information in nonresearch references—including opinion articles, case reports, anecdotes, and clinical descriptions—may serve to broaden understanding of a research problem or demonstrate a need for research, but in general has limited utility in written research reviews.

- A **primary source** in a research review is the original description of a study prepared by the researcher who conducted it; a **secondary source** is a description of the study by a person unconnected with it. Literature reviews should be based on primary source material.

- Strategies for finding studies on a topic include the use of bibliographic tools, but also include the **ancestry approach** (tracking down earlier studies cited in a reference list of a report) and the **descendancy approach** (using a pivotal study to search forward to subsequent studies that cited it).

- An important development for locating references for a research review is the widespread availability of various bibliographic databases that can be searched electronically. For nurses, the **CINAHL** and **MEDLINE** databases are especially useful, and the **Web of Knowledge** includes citation indexes that support a descendancy strategy.

- In searching a bibliographic database, users can perform a **keyword** search that looks for searcher-specified terms in text fields of a database record (or that maps keywords onto the database's subject codes) or can search according to the **subject heading** codes themselves. Author searches are also available.

- References that have been identified must be screened for relevance and read, and then pertinent information must be abstracted and encoded for subsequent analysis. Tools to facilitate the encoding process include formal review protocols and matrices.

- Matrices (two-dimensional arrays) are a convenient means of abstracting and organizing information for a literature review. A Methodologic Matrix can be used to record methodologic features of a set of studies; methodologic strengths and weaknesses can also be recorded, or can be noted in a separate Evaluation Matrix. Research findings can be recorded in a series of Results Matrices—one corresponding to each independent or dependent variable. The use of such matrices facilitates thematic analysis of the retrieved information.

- A research **critique** is a careful appraisal of the strengths and weaknesses of a study. Critiques of studies for the purpose of a research review tend to focus on the methodologic aspects of a set of studies. Critiques of individual studies (e.g., by students in a research methods class) tend to be more comprehensive.

- The analysis of information from a literature search essentially involves the identification of important themes—regularities and patterns (and inconsistencies and omissions) in the information. The themes can take many forms, including substantive, methodologic, and theoretic themes.

- In preparing a written review, it is important to organize materials in a logical, coherent fashion. The preparation of an outline is recommended. The written review should not be a succession of quotes or abstracts. The reviewers' role is to point out what has been studied, how adequate and dependable the studies are, what gaps exist in the body of research, and (in the context of a new study), what contribution the study would make.

STUDY ACTIVITIES

Chapter 5 of the *Resource Manual to Accompany Nursing Research: Generating and Assessing*

Evidence for Nursing Practice, 8th edition, offers various exercises and study suggestions for reinforcing the concepts presented in this chapter. In addition, the following study questions can be addressed:

1. Suppose you were planning to study the relationship between chronic transfusion therapy and quality of life in adolescents with sickle cell disease. Identify 5 to 10 keywords that could be used to search for relevant prior research.

2. Suppose you were studying factors affecting the discharge of chronic psychiatric patients. Obtain references for five studies for this topic, and compare them with those of other students.

3. Carefully examine Figures 5.6 and 5.7 and see how many themes you can identify. Also see how many incongruities there are among studies in the matrixes (i.e., the absence of consistent themes).

4. To the extent possible, use the critiquing questions in Box 5.4 to appraise the literature review excerpts of the two studies used as examples at the end of this chapter.

STUDIES CITED IN CHAPTER 5

Methodologic or theoretical references cited in this chapter can be found in a separate section at the end of the book.

Cottrell, B. H. (2006). Vaginal douching practices of women in eight Florida panhandle counties. *Journal of Obstetric, Gynecologic, & Neonatal Nursing, 35*(1), 24–33.

DuMoulin, M., Hamers, J., Paulus, A., Berendsen, C., & Halfens, R. (2005). The role of the nurse in community continence care: A systematic review. *International Journal of Nursing Studies, 42*(4), 479–492.

Griffin, R. A., Polit, D. F., & Byrne, M. W. (2007). *Nurse characteristics and inferences about children's pain.* Manuscript submitted for publication.

Hamers, J. P., Abu-Saad, H. H., Halfens, R. J., & Schumacher, J. N. (1994). Factors influencing nurses' pain assessment and interventions in children. *Journal of Advanced Nursing, 20*, 853–860.

Hamers, J. P., van den Hout, M. A., Halfens, R. J., Abu-Saad, H. H., & Heijlties, A. E. (1997). Differences in pain assessment and decisions regarding the administration of analgesics between novices, intermediates and experts in pediatric nursing. *International Journal of Nursing Studies, 34*(5), 325–334.

Liao, Y., Dougherty, M., Liou, Y., & Tseng, I. (2006). Pelvic floor muscle training effect on urinary incontinence knowledge, attitudes, and severity. *International Journal of Nursing Studies, 43*(1), 29–37.

Lutz, B. J., & Bowers, B. J. (2005). Disability in everyday life. *Qualitative Health Research, 15*(8), 1037–1054.

Margolius, F. R., Hudson, K. A., & Miche, Y. (1995). Beliefs and perceptions about children in pain: A survey. *Pediatric Nursing, 21*, 111–115.

Polkki, T., Vehvilainen-Julkunen, K., & Pietila, A. M. (2001). Nonpharmacological methods in relieving children's postoperative pain: A survey on hospital nurses in Finland. *Journal of Advanced Nursing, 34*(4), 483–492.

Smith, C. E., Koehler, J., Moore, J. M., Blanchard, E., & Ellerbeck, E. (2005). Testing videotape education for heart failure. *Clinical Nursing Research, 14*(2), 191–205.

Vincent, C. V., & Denyes, M. J. (2004). Relieving children's pain: Nurses' abilities and analgesic administration practices. *Journal of Pediatric Nursing, 19*(1), 40–50.

6

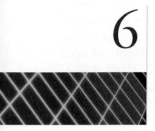

Developing a Theoretical or Conceptual Context

H igh-quality studies typically achieve a high level of *conceptual integration*. This means, for example, that the research questions are appropriate for the chosen methods and strategies, that the questions are consistent with the existing body of research evidence, and that there is a plausible conceptual rationale for the way in which things are expected to unfold—including a rationale for any hypotheses to be tested or for designing an intervention in a certain way. For example, suppose we hypothesized that a nurse-led smoking cessation intervention would reduce rates of smoking among patients with cardiovascular disease. Why would we make this prediction? That is, what is our "theory" (our theoretical rationale) about how the intervention might have beneficial effects? What is it about the intervention (and the population under study) that could bring about behavior change—do we predict that the intervention will change patients' knowledge? attitudes? motivation? social supports? sense of control over their own decision making? Our view of how the intervention would "work" would have implications for the design of both the intervention and the study. To use a nonexperimental example, suppose we hypothesized gender differences in coping with the loss of a child. What is our "theory" for why men and women would differ—do we suspect innate biologic gender differences? role socialization differences?

social expectation differences? differences in social capital?

Design decisions and data collection strategies cannot be developed in a vacuum—there must be an underlying conceptualization of people's behaviors and characteristics, and how these affect and are affected by interpersonal and environmental forces. In some studies, the underlying conceptualization is fuzzy or unstated, but in good research, a clear and defensible conceptualization is made explicit. This chapter discusses theoretical and conceptual contexts for nursing research problems.

THEORIES, MODELS, AND FRAMEWORKS

Many terms have been used in connection with conceptual contexts for research, including theories, models, frameworks, schemes, and maps. There is some overlap in how these terms are used, partly because they are used differently by different writers, and partly because they are interrelated. We offer guidance in distinguishing these terms, but note that our definitions are not universal.

Theories

The term *theory* is used in many ways. For example, nursing instructors and students frequently use the term to refer to the content covered in classrooms, as opposed to the actual practice of performing nursing activities. In both lay and scientific usage, the term theory connotes an *abstraction*.

In research circles, the term theory is used in various ways by different authors. Classically, scientists have used **theory** to refer to an abstract generalization that offers a systematic explanation about how phenomena are interrelated. The traditional definition requires a theory to embody at least two concepts that are related in a manner that the theory purports to explain.

Others, however, use the term *theory* less restrictively to refer to a broad characterization of a phenomenon. According to this less restrictive definition, a theory can account for (i.e., thoroughly describe) a single phenomenon. Some authors specifically refer to this type of theory as **descriptive theory**. For example, Fawcett (1999) defines descriptive theories as empirically driven theories that "describe or classify specific dimensions or characteristics of individuals, groups, situations, or events by summarizing commonalities found in discrete observations" (p. 15). Descriptive theory plays an especially important role in qualitative studies. Qualitative researchers often strive to develop a conceptualization of the phenomena under study that is grounded in actual observations.

Components of a Traditional Theory

As traditionally defined, scientific theories involve a series of propositions regarding interrelationships among concepts. The writings on scientific theory include a variety of terms such as *proposition*, *postulate*, *premise*, *axiom*, *law*, *principle*, and so forth, some of which are used interchangeably, and others of which introduce subtleties that are too complex for our discussion. Here, we present a simplified analysis of the components of a theory.

Concepts are the basic building blocks of a theory. Classical theories comprise a set of propositions that indicate relationships among the concepts. Relationships are denoted by such terms as "is associated with," "varies directly with," or "is contingent on." The propositions form a logically interrelated deductive system. This means that the

theory provides a mechanism for logically arriving at new statements from the original propositions.

Let us consider the following example, which illustrates these points. The **Theory of Planned Behavior** (TPB; Ajzen, 2005), which is an extension of an earlier theory called the Theory of Reasoned Action or TRA (Ajzen & Fishbein, 1980), provides a framework for understanding people's behavior and its psychological determinants. A greatly simplified construction of the TPB consists of the following propositions:

1. Behavior that is volitional is determined by people's intention to perform that behavior.
2. Intention to perform or not perform a behavior is determined by three factors:
   - Attitudes toward the behavior (i.e., the overall evaluation of performing the behavior)
   - Subjective norms (i.e., perceived social pressure to perform or not perform the behavior)
   - Perceived behavioral control (i.e., anticipated ease or difficulty of engaging in the behavior)
3. The relative importance of the three factors in influencing intention varies across behaviors and situations.

⊃ **TIP:** There are websites devoted to many of the theories and conceptual models mentioned in this chapter, including the TPB. A number of specific websites are listed in the "Useful Websites for Chapter 6" file on the accompanying CD-ROM, for you to click on directly. An excellent Internet resource on nursing theory has been developed by the Hahn School of Nursing and Health Science at the University of San Diego: *http://www.sandiego.edu/nursing/theory*. Also, two good websites for dozens of theories relating to behavior change (a key construct in nursing intervention studies) are maintained by The Communication Initiative:
http://www.comminit.com/changetheories.html
and by the University of South Florida:
http://hsc.usf.edu/~kmbrown/hlth_beh_models.htm

The concepts that form the basis of the TPB include behaviors, intentions, attitudes, subjective norms, and perceived self-control. The theory, which specifies the nature of the relationship among these concepts, provides a framework for generating many hypotheses relating to health behaviors. We might hypothesize on the basis of the TPB, for example, that compliance with a medical regimen (the behavior) could be enhanced by influencing people's attitudes toward compliance, or by increasing their sense of control. The TPB has been used as the underlying theory in studying a wide range of health decision-making behaviors (e.g., contraceptive choice, condom use, preventive health screening) as well as in developing health-promoting interventions.

Example of the TPB: Steele and Porche (2005) used the Theory of Planned Behavior to predict the intention of rural women from southeastern Louisiana to have a mammogram. Perceived behavioral control was the strongest predictor of mammography intention.

Types of Traditional Theories

Theories differ in their level of generality and abstraction. So-called **grand theories** or *macrotheories* purport to describe and explain large segments of the human experience. Some learning theorists, such as Clark Hull, or sociologists, such as Talcott Parsons, developed general theoretical systems to account for broad classes of behavior. Sometimes general theories about the nursing process are referred to as grand theories.

Many theories are more restricted in scope, focusing on a narrow range of experience. Such **middle-range theories** attempt to explain such phenomena as decision making, stress, self-care, health promotion, and infant attachment. Smith and Liehr (2003) describe eight specific middle-range theories that are especially relevant in nursing, several of which will be briefly described in this chapter. Tomey and Alligood (2006) provide additional examples of middle-range theories, including the theory of postpartum depression of Beck, one of this book's authors.

Conceptual Models

Conceptual models, conceptual frameworks, or **conceptual schemes** (we use the terms interchangeably) represent a less formal attempt at organizing phenomena than theories. Conceptual models, like theories, deal with abstractions (concepts) that are assembled by virtue of their relevance to a common theme. What is absent from conceptual models is the deductive system of propositions that assert and explain relationships among concepts. Conceptual models provide a perspective regarding interrelated phenomena, but are more loosely structured than theories. A conceptual model broadly presents an understanding of the phenomenon of interest and reflects the assumptions and philosophic views of the model's designer. Conceptual models can serve as springboards for generating research hypotheses.

Much of the conceptual work that has been done in connection with nursing practice falls into the category we call conceptual models. These models represent conceptualizations of the nursing process and the nature of nurse–client relationships. A subsequent section of this chapter describes some conceptual models in nursing and illustrates how they have been used in nursing research.

Schematic Models

The term *model* is often used in connection with symbolic representations of a conceptualization. There are many references in the research literature to **schematic models**. Schematic models are visual representations of some aspect of reality; like conceptual models and theories, they use concepts as building blocks, but with a minimal use of words. A visual or symbolic representation of a theory or conceptual framework often helps to express abstract ideas in a concise and readily understandable form.

Schematic models, which are common in both qualitative and quantitative research, represent phenomena graphically. Concepts and the linkages between them are represented through the use of boxes, arrows, or other symbols. An example of a schematic model (also referred to as a **conceptual map**) is presented in Figure 6.1. This model, known as **Pender's Health Promotion Model**, is a model for explaining and predicting the health-promotion component of lifestyle (Pender, Murdaugh, & Parsons, 2006). Schematic models of this type can be useful in clarifying and succinctly communicating linkages among concepts.

INDIVIDUAL
CHARACTERISTICS
AND EXPERIENCES

BEHAVIOR-SPECIFIC
COGNITIONS
AND AFFECT

BEHAVIORAL
OUTCOME

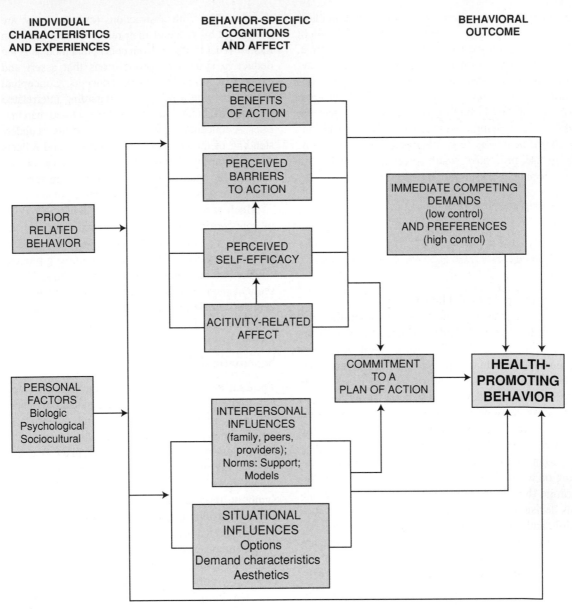

FIGURE 6.1 The Health Promotion Model (From Pender's website, *http://www.nursing.umich.edu/faculty/pender/chart.gif*. Retrieved January 13, 2006.)

Frameworks

A **framework** is the overall conceptual underpinnings of a study. Not every study is based on a formal theory or conceptual model, but every study has a framework—a theoretical rationale. In a study based on a theory, the framework is referred to as the **theoretical framework**; in a study that has its roots in a specified conceptual model, the framework is often called the **conceptual framework** (although the terms conceptual framework and theoretical framework are frequently used interchangeably).

In most nursing studies, the framework is not an explicit theory or conceptual model, and often the underlying theoretical rationale for the inquiry is not explained. Rather, the framework is often implicit, without being formally acknowledged or described. In studies that fail to articulate a conceptual framework, it may be difficult to figure out what the researchers thought was "going on"—and why.

Sometimes researchers fail even to adequately describe key concepts at the conceptual level. The concepts in which researchers are interested are by definition abstractions of observable phenomena, and our world view (and views on nursing) shapes how those concepts are defined and operationalized. When researchers fail to clarify the conceptual underpinnings of their research variables, it becomes difficult to integrate research findings. Researchers undertaking a study should make clear the conceptual definition of their key variables, thereby providing information about the study's framework.

Waltz, Strickland, and Lenz (2005) described a five-step process for developing conceptual (theoretical) definitions. These steps include (1) developing a preliminary definition, (2) reviewing relevant literature, (3) developing or identifying exemplars, (4) mapping the concept's meaning, and (5) stating the developed conceptual definition.

Example of developing a conceptual definition: Lee and colleagues (2004) provided an example of developing a conceptual definition of the concept of *family resilience* in the context of Korean families with a chronically ill child.

1. *Preliminary definition*: Family resilience "is a character (property or driving force) that causes changes in family functioning according to a family's own belief or value system, when a family faces an internal or external stressor" (p. 639).
2. *Literature review*: Theoretical and empirical research literature from authors in Western countries and South Korea for the past two decades was reviewed.
3. *Developing a model case*: The family of a sick male child consisted of the father, mother, a daughter, and the sick child. When the child was first diagnosed with leukemia, the doctor assessed the chance of 5-year survival at lower than 30%.

The family initially fell into despair, but soon they decided to do the best for their son (making meaning of adversity, i.e., bouncing back), believing that family efforts would cure him in the end (positive outlook). The sick child's parents came increasingly to rely on their religion after the diagnosis (transcendence and spirituality). Whenever the parents made a decision, they had long and straightforward discussions about it (openness in expression). The daughter moved in with her grandmother, as her parents did not have time to care for her. She adapted to these new circumstances well (flexibility). When the patient's condition was good enough for him to go out, the family went on picnics to spend time together (connectedness). The parents had insufficient funds to care for the child, so their relatives offered financial assistance. The husband's co-workers raised money to help finance the child's bone marrow transplantation (social and economic resources). Although family members were not fully satisfied with their lifestyle, they thought that they should be strongly united (cohesion) and tolerate discomforts to overcome the adversities (sense of control). They had pride in themselves for coping well with this challenge to their family situation (family self-esteem). They adapted well to their new roles (adaptation) and hoped that the existing situation would not deteriorate.

4. *Mapping the concept's meaning*: By integrating literature with interview with 11 Korean parents with a chronically ill child a conceptual map was developed that organized 21 conceptual attributes of family resilience.
5. *Stating the revised conceptual definition*: "Family resilience is an enduring force that leads a family to change its dynamics of functioning in order to solve problems associated with stresses encountered. It comprises 21 attributes that can be divided into 4 dimensions: (i) intrinsic family characteristics, (ii) family member orientation, (iii) responsiveness to stress, and (iv) external orientation" (p. 644).

Quantitative researchers are guiltier of failing to identify their frameworks than qualitative researchers. In most qualitative studies, the frameworks are part of the research tradition in which the study is embedded. For example, ethnographers usually begin their work within a theory of culture. Grounded theory researchers incorporate sociologic principles into their framework and their approach to looking at phenomena. The questions that most qualitative researchers ask and the methods they use to address those questions inherently reflect certain theoretical formulations.

THE NATURE OF THEORIES AND CONCEPTUAL MODELS

Theories and conceptual models have much in common, including their origin, general nature, purposes, and role in research. In this section, we examine some general characteristics of theories and conceptual models. We use the term *theory* in its broadest sense, inclusive of conceptual models.

Origin of Theories and Models

Theories, conceptual frameworks, and models are not *discovered*; they are created and invented. Theory building depends not only on facts and observable evidence, but also on the originator's ingenuity in pulling facts together and making sense of them. Thus, theory construction is a creative and intellectual enterprise that can be engaged in by anyone who is insightful, has a firm grounding in existing evidence, and has the ability to knit together observations and evidence into an intelligible pattern.

Tentative Nature of Theories and Models

Theories and conceptual models cannot be proved. A theory is a scientist's best effort to describe and explain phenomena; today's successful theory may be discredited or revised tomorrow. This may happen if new evidence or observations undermine a previously accepted theory. Or, a new theory might integrate new observations with an existing theory to yield a more parsimonious or accurate explanation of a phenomenon. For example, the Theory of Reasoned Action was modified and renamed the Theory of Planned Behavior as evidence supporting modifications accrued.

Theories and models that are not congruent with a culture's values and philosophic orientation also may fall into disfavor over time. It is not unusual for a theory to lose supporters because some aspects of it are no longer in vogue. For example, certain psychoanalytic and structural social theories, which had broad support for decades, have come to be challenged as a result of changes in views about women's roles. This link between theory and values may surprise you if you think of science as being completely objective. Remember, though, that theories are deliberately invented by humans; they are not totally free from human values and ideals, which can change over time.

Thus, theories and models are never considered final and verified. There always remains the possibility that a theory will be modified or discarded. Many theories in the physical sciences have received considerable empirical support, and their well-accepted propositions are often referred to as **laws**, such as Boyle's law of gases. Nevertheless, we have no way of knowing the ultimate accuracy and utility of any theory and should, therefore, treat all theories as tentative. This caveat is nowhere more relevant than in sciences that focus on human beings, such as nursing.

Purposes of Theories and Conceptual Models

Theoretical and conceptual frameworks play several interrelated roles in the progress of a science. Their overall purpose is to make research findings meaningful and generalizable. Theories allow researchers to knit together observations and facts into an orderly scheme. They are efficient mechanisms for drawing together accumulated facts, sometimes from separate and isolated investigations. The linkage of findings into a coherent structure can make the body of accumulated evidence more accessible and, thus, more useful.

In addition to summarizing, theories and models can guide a researcher's understanding of not only the *what* of natural phenomena but also the *why* of their occurrence. Theories often provide a basis for predicting the occurrence of phenomena. Prediction, in turn, has implications for the control of those phenomena. A utilitarian theory has potential to bring about desirable changes in people's behavior or health. Thus, theories are an important resource for the development of nursing interventions.

Theories and conceptual models help to stimulate research and the extension of knowledge by providing both direction and impetus. Many studies have been designed explicitly to examine aspects of a conceptual model of nursing. Thus, theories may serve as a springboard for advances in knowledge and the accumulation of evidence for practice.

Relationship Between Theory and Research

The relationship between theory and research is reciprocal and mutually beneficial. Theories and models are built inductively from observations, and an excellent source for those observations is prior research, including in-depth qualitative studies. Concepts and relationships that are validated empirically through research become the foundation for theory development. The theory, in turn, must be tested by subjecting deductions from it (hypotheses) to further systematic inquiry. Thus, research plays a dual and continuing role in theory building and testing. Theory guides and generates ideas for research; research assesses the worth of the theory and provides a foundation for new theories.

Example of theory development: Jean Johnson (1999) developed a middle-range theory called Self-Regulation Theory that explicates relationships between health care experiences, coping, and health outcomes. Here is how she described theory development: "The theory was developed in a cyclic process. Research was conducted using the self-regulation theory of coping with illness. Propositions supported by data were retained, other propositions were altered when they were not supported, and new theoretical propositions were added when research produced unexpected findings. This cycle has been repeated many times over three decades leading to the present stage of development of the theory" (pp. 435–436). As an example, LaMontagne and colleagues (2005) developed and tested interventions for adolescents undergoing scoliosis that were based on Self-Regulation Theory.

CONCEPTUAL MODELS USED IN NURSING RESEARCH

Nurse researchers have used both nursing and non-nursing frameworks to provide a conceptual context for their studies. This section briefly discusses several frameworks that have been found useful by nurse researchers.

Conceptual Models of Nursing

In the past few decades, several nurses have formulated conceptual models of nursing practice. These models constitute formal explanations of what the nursing discipline is and what the nursing process entails, according to the model developer's point of view. As Fawcett (2005) has noted, four concepts are central to models of nursing: *human beings*, *environment*, *health*, and *nursing*. The various conceptual models, however, define these concepts differently, link them in diverse ways, and give different emphases to relationships among them. Moreover, different models emphasize different processes as being central to nursing. For example, Sister Callista Roy's Adaptation Model identifies adaptation of patients as a critical phenomenon (Roy & Andrews, 1999). Martha Rogers (1986), by contrast, emphasized the centrality of the individual as a unified whole, and her model views nursing as a process in which clients are aided in achieving maximum well-being within their potential.

The conceptual models were not developed primarily as a base for nursing research. Indeed, most models have had more impact on nursing education and clinical practice than on nursing research. Nevertheless, nurse researchers have turned to these conceptual frameworks for inspiration in formulating research questions and hypotheses. Table 6.1 lists 10 prominent conceptual models in nursing that have been used by researchers. The table briefly describes the model's key feature and identifies a study that has claimed the model as its framework. Two nursing models that have generated particular interest as a basis for research are described in greater detail.

TABLE 6.1 Conceptual Models of Nursing Used by Nurse Researchers

THEORIST AND REFERENCE	NAME OF MODEL/THEORY	KEY THESIS OF THE MODEL	RESEARCH EXAMPLE
F. Moyra Allen, 2002	McGill Model of Nursing	Nursing is the science of health-promoting interactions. Health promotion is a process of helping people cope and develop; the goal of nursing is to actively promote patient and family strengths and the achievement of life goals.	Cossette and colleagues (2002) included elements of the McGill Model in their study to document the types of nursing approaches that were associated with reductions in psychological distress among patients after myocardial infarction.
Madeline Leininger, 2006	Theory of Culture Care Diversity and Universality	Caring is a universal phenomenon but varies transculturally.	Guided by Leininger's theory, Plowden and colleagues (2005) explored cultural and social factors that influence high-risk behaviors among inner-city HIV-positive African Americans.
Myra Levine, 1973	Conservation Model	Conservation of integrity contributes to maintenance of a person's wholeness.	Melancon and Miller (2005) used Levine's model to guide their study on the effect of massage therapy versus traditional therapy for relief of lower back pain.
Betty Neuman, 2001	Health Care Systems Model	Each person is a complete system; the goal of nursing is to assist in maintaining client system stability.	Jones-Cannon and Davis (2005) used Neuman's model as the framework in their study on the coping strategies of African-American daughters who functioned as caregivers.
Margaret Newman, 1994, 1997	Health as Expanding Consciousness	Health is viewed as an expansion of consciousness with health and disease parts of the same whole; health is seen in an evolving pattern of the whole in time, space, and movement.	Berry (2004) used Newman's theory to study behavior changes and personal self-discovery in women who maintained weight loss for 1 year or more.
Dorothea Orem, 2003	Self-Care Deficit Nursing Theory	Self-care activities are what people do on their own	Kreulen & Braden (2004) developed a model of

TABLE 6.1 (continued)			
THEORIST AND REFERENCE	**NAME OF MODEL/THEORY**	**KEY THESIS OF THE MODEL**	**RESEARCH EXAMPLE**
		behalf to maintain health and well-being; the goal of nursing is to help people meet their own therapeutic self-care demands.	relationships between self-help–promoting nursing interventions and health status outcomes, using concepts from Orem's model.
Rosemarie Rizzo Parse, 1999	Theory of Human Becoming	Health and meaning are co-created by indivisible humans and their environment; nursing involves having clients share views about meanings.	Jonas-Simpson and colleagues (2006) studied the experience of being listened to among older adults in long-term care settings.
Martha Rogers, 1970, 1986	Science of Unitary Human Beings	The individual is a unified whole in constant interaction with the environment; nursing helps individuals achieve maximum well-being within their potential.	Wright (2004) studied the relationship between trust and power in adults as a way of illuminating nurse–client relationships, using Rogers's theory.
Sr. Callista Roy, 1999	Adaptation Model	Humans are adaptive systems that cope with change through adaptation; nursing helps to promote client adaptation during health and illness.	Shyu and associates (2004) tested Roy's model in their study of environmental barriers and mobility among elders in Taiwan.
Jean Watson, 2005	Theory of Caring	Caring is the moral ideal, and entails mind–body–soul engagement with one another.	Hemsley and colleagues (2006) used Watson's model in a phenomenological study of the transformational experiences of nurse healers.

Roy's Adaptation Model

In **Roy's Adaptation Model**, humans are viewed as biopsychosocial adaptive systems who cope with environmental change through the process of adaptation (Roy & Andrews, 1999; Roy & Zhan, 2006). Within the human system, there are four subsystems: physiologic/physical, self-concept/group iden-

tity, role function, and interdependence. These subsystems constitute adaptive modes that provide mechanisms for coping with environmental stimuli and change. Health is viewed as both a state and a process of being and becoming integrated and whole that reflects the mutuality of persons and environment. The goal of nursing, according to this model, is to promote client adaptation; nursing also regulates stimuli affecting adaptation. Nursing interventions usually take the form of increasing, decreasing, modifying, removing, or maintaining internal and external stimuli that affect adaptation.

Example using Roy's Adaptation Model:
Fawcett and several colleagues (2005) conducted an international multi-site study (in the United States, Finland, and Australia) of women's perceptions of and responses to cesarean birth using concepts from Roy's Adaptation Model. The researchers studied the influence of the contextual stimuli of culture and geography on women's adaptation to cesarean birth.

Rogers's Science of Unitary Human Beings

The building blocks of **Rogers's Science of Unitary Human Beings** (Rogers, 1970, 1986) are five assumptions relating to humans and their life process: wholeness (a human as a unified whole, more than the sum of the parts); openness (humans and the environment continuously exchanging matter and energy); unidirectionality (life processes existing along an irreversible space/time continuum); pattern and organization (which identify humans and reflect their wholeness); and sentience and thought (a human as capable of abstraction, imagery, language, and sensation). Four critical elements are basic to Rogers's proposed system. First, *energy fields* are the fundamental unit of the living (human energy fields) and the nonliving (environmental energy field). Second, *open systems* describe the open nature of the fields, which allow for an interchange of energy. Third, *pattern* is the distinguishing characteristic of energy fields, and human behavior can be regarded as manifestations of changing pattern. And fourth, *pandimensionality* describes a nonlinear domain without temporal or spatial attributes. The keys to Rogers's conceptual framework are her principles of homeodynamics, which represent a way of viewing unitary human beings and provide guidance to the practice of nursing. The three principles include integrality, helicy, and resonancy. *Integrality* concerns the continuous and mutual processes between human and environmental fields—changes in one field will bring about changes in the other. *Helicy* refers to the continuous

and innovative diversity of human and environmental field patterns. Finally, *resonancy* describes the continuous change from lower to higher frequency wave patterns in human and environmental energy fields. Rogerian science continues to be developed by theorists and researchers, and specific research methods have been developed based on Rogerian principles (e.g., Cowling, 2004).

Example using a Rogerian framework:
Yarcheski, Mahon, and Yarcheski (2004) studied the relationship of perceived field motion and human field rhythms to adolescents' perceived health status and well-being. Their aim was to explore which health-related variables are most compatible with Rogers's Science of Unitary Human Beings.

Other Models and Middle Range Theories Developed by Nurses

In addition to conceptual models that are designed to describe and characterize the entire nursing process, nurses have developed other middle-range theories and models that focus on more specific phenomena of interest to nurses. Examples of middle-range theories developed by nurses that have been used in research include the Theory of Unpleasant Symptoms (Lenz et al., 1997), Johnson's (1999) Self-Regulation Theory, Kolcaba's (2003) Comfort Theory, Reed's Self-Transcendence Theory (1991), the Theory of Transitions (Meleis et al., 2000), the Symptom Management Model (Dodd et al., 2001), Pender's Health Promotion Model (Pender et al., 2006), and Mishel's Uncertainty in Illness Theory (1990). The latter two are briefly described here.

The Health Promotion Model

Nola Pender's (2006) Health Promotion Model (HPM) focuses on explaining health-promoting behaviors, using a wellness orientation. According to the recently revised model (see Fig. 6.1), *health promotion* entails activities directed toward developing resources that maintain or enhance a person's well-being. The model embodies a number of theoretical propositions that can be used in developing and testing interventions and understanding health behaviors. For example, one HPM proposition is that people commit to engaging in behaviors from which they anticipate deriving valued benefits, and another is that perceived competence or self-efficacy relating to a given behavior increases the likelihood of commitment to action and actual performance of the behavior. Greater perceived self-efficacy is also viewed as resulting in fewer perceived barriers to a specific health behavior. The model also incorporates interpersonal and situational influences on a person's commitment to health-promoting actions.

Example using the HPM: Ronis, Hong, and Lusk (2006) tested the revised HPM to explain the decisions of 703 construction workers to use hearing protection devices. Results supported the revised model and suggested the new model was more successful in predicting hearing protection than the original HPM.

Uncertainty in Illness Theory
Mishel's Uncertainty in Illness Theory (Mishel, 1990) focuses on the concept of uncertainty—the inability of a person to determine the meaning of illness-related events. According to this theory, people develop subjective appraisals to assist them in interpreting the experience of illness and treatment. Uncertainty occurs when people are unable to recognize and categorize stimuli. Uncertainty results in the inability to obtain a clear conception of the situation, but a situation appraised as uncertain will mobilize individuals to use their resources to adapt to the situation. Mishel's theory as originally conceptualized was most relevant to patients in an acute phase of illness or in a downward illness trajectory, but it has been reconceptualized to include constant uncertainty in a chronic or recurrent illness. Mishel's conceptualization of uncertainty (and her Uncertainty in Illness Scale) have been used in many nursing studies.

Example using Uncertainty in Illness Theory: Clayton, Mishel, and Belyea (2006) tested a model of symptoms, communication with providers, and uncertainty in affecting the well-being of older breast cancer survivors. In their model, communication was conceptualized as a factor influencing uncertainty, which in turn was seen as influencing emotional and cognitive well-being.

Other Models Used by Nurse Researchers

Many concepts in which nurse researchers are interested are not unique to nursing, and therefore their studies are sometimes linked to frameworks that are not models from the nursing profession. Several of these alternative models have gained special prominence in the development of multifaceted nursing interventions to promote health-enhancing behaviors and life choices. In addition to the previously described Theory of Planned Behavior, four nonnursing models or theories have frequently been used in nursing studies: Bandura's Social Cognitive Theory, Prochaska's Transtheoretical (Stages of Change) Model, the Health Belief Model, and Lazarus and Folkman's Theory of Stress and Coping.

Bandura's Social Cognitive Theory
Social Cognitive Theory (Bandura, 1985, 1997) offers an explanation of human behavior using the concepts of self-efficacy, outcome expectations, and incentives. Self-efficacy expectations are focused on people's belief in their own capacity to carry out particular behaviors (e.g., smoking cessation). Self-efficacy expectations, which are context specific, determine the behaviors people choose to perform, their degree of perseverance, and the quality of the performance. Bandura identified four factors that influence people's cognitive appraisal of self-efficacy: (1) their own mastery experience; (2) verbal persuasion; (3) vicarious experience; and (4) physiologic and affective cues, such as pain and anxiety. The role of self-efficacy has been studied in relation to numerous health behaviors such as weight control, self-management of chronic illness, and smoking.

➔ **TIP:** Bandura's self-efficacy construct is a key mediating variable in several models and theories discussed in this chapter. Self-efficacy has repeatedly been found to explain a significant amount of variation in people's behaviors and to be amenable to change, and so self-efficacy enhancement is often a goal in interventions designed to change people's health-related actions and behaviors (Conn et al., 2001).

Example using Social Cognitive Theory:
Using social cognitive constructs, Gates, Fitzwater, and Succop (2005) developed and tested the effectiveness of a violence-prevention intervention for nursing assistants working in long-term care settings. The intervention was designed to increase knowledge, self-efficacy, and skills.

The Transtheoretical (Stages of Change) Model

There are several dimensions in the **Transtheoretical Model** (Prochaska & Velicer, 1997; Prochaska, Redding, & Evers, 2002), a model that has been used in numerous interventions to change people's behavior—especially smoking cessation. The core construct around which the other dimensions are organized is the *stages of change,* which conceptualizes a continuum of motivational readiness to change problem behavior. The five stages of change are precontemplation, contemplation, preparation, action, and maintenance. Transitions from one stage to the next are affected by processes of change. Studies have shown that successful self-changers use different processes at each particular stage, thus suggesting the desirability of interventions that are individualized to the person's stage of readiness for change. The model also incorporates a series of intervening variables, one of which is self-efficacy.

Example using the Transtheoretical Model:
Chouinard and Robichaud-Ekstrand (2005) developed and tested a nurse-delivered inpatient smoking cessation program for patients with cardiovascular disease based on the Transtheoretical Model. Telephone follow-up was tailored to levels of readiness to quit smoking.

The Health Belief Model

The **Health Belief Model** (HBM; Becker, 1976, 1978) has become a popular conceptual framework in nursing studies focused on patient compliance and preventive health care practices. The model postulates that health-seeking behavior is influenced by a person's perception of a threat posed by a health problem and the value associated with actions aimed at reducing the threat. The major components of the HBM include perceived suscepti-

bility, perceived severity, perceived benefits and costs, motivation, and enabling or modifying factors. Perceived susceptibility is a person's perception that a health problem is personally relevant or that a diagnosis is accurate. Even when one recognizes personal susceptibility, action will not occur unless the individual perceives the severity to be high enough to have serious organic or social implications. Perceived benefits are the patients' beliefs that a given treatment will cure the illness or help prevent it, and perceived costs are the complexity, duration, and accessibility of the treatment. Motivation is the desire to comply with a treatment. Among the modifying factors that have been identified are personality variables, patient satisfaction, and sociodemographic factors.

Example using the HBM: Sethares and Elliott (2004) developed and tested a tailored message intervention for persons with heart failure, using the Health Belief Model as a guiding framework. The intervention was found to change the patients' beliefs about the benefits and barriers of taking medications and following a sodium-restricted diet.

Lazarus and Folkman's Theory of Stress and Coping

The **Theory of Stress and Coping** (Lazarus, 1966; Lazarus & Folkman, 1984) is an effort to explain people's methods of dealing with stress, that is, environmental and internal demands that tax or exceed a person's resources and endanger his or her well-being. The model posits that coping strategies are learned, deliberate responses used to adapt to or change stressors. According to this model, a person's perception of mental and physical health is related to the ways he or she evaluates and copes with the stresses of living.

Example using the Theory of Stress and Coping: Skybo (2005) studied the stresses and appraisal processes of school-aged children from low-income areas who witnessed violence in their environments. The appraisals of violent encounters were consistent with Lazarus' appraisal category of harm/loss and threat. Children who witnessed more violent encounters tended to exhibit more stress symptoms.

Theoretical Contexts and Nursing Research

As previously noted, theory and research have reciprocal, beneficial ties. Theory can serve as the impetus of scientific investigations, and findings from research can shape the development of theory. However, this relationship has not always characterized the progress of nursing science. Many have criticized nurse researchers for producing isolated studies that are not placed in a theoretical context.

This criticism was more justified a decade ago than it is today. Many researchers are developing studies (and interventions) on the basis of conceptual models of nursing processes and human behavior. Nursing science is still struggling, however, to integrate accumulated knowledge within theoretical systems. This struggle is reflected, in part, in the number of controversies surrounding the issue of theoretical frameworks in nursing.

One of these controversies concerns whether there should be one single, unified model of nursing or multiple, competing models. We believe that research can play a critical role in testing the utility and validity of alternative nursing models.

Another controversy involves the desirability and utility of developing theories unique to nursing. Some commentators argue that theories relating to humans developed in other disciplines, such as physiology, psychology, and sociology (so-called **borrowed theories**), can and should be applied to nursing problems. In fact, some have argued that theories that make specific predictions about how to change people's behavior are more useful in developing nursing interventions than global models of nursing processes (Conn et al., 2001). Others, however, advocate the development of unique nursing theories, claiming that only through such development can knowledge to guide nursing practice be produced. When a borrowed theory is tested and found to be empirically adequate in health-relevant situations of interest to nurses, it becomes **shared theory**.

We think that nurse researchers are likely to continue on their current path of conducting studies within a multidisciplinary and multitheoretical perspective—and further developing and refining

theories on the basis of their research. We are inclined to see the use of multiple frameworks as a healthy part of the development of nursing science.

TESTING, USING, AND DEVELOPING A THEORY OR FRAMEWORK

The manner in which theory and conceptual frameworks are used by qualitative and quantitative researchers is elaborated on in the following section. In the discussion, the term *theory* is used in its broadest sense to include both conceptual models, formal theories, and frameworks.

Theories and Qualitative Research

Theory is almost always present in studies that are embedded in a qualitative research tradition such as ethnography or phenomenology. As previously noted, these research traditions inherently provide an overarching framework that gives qualitative studies a theoretical grounding. However, different traditions involve theory in different ways.

Sandelowski (1993) made a useful distinction between **substantive theory** (conceptualizations of the target phenomenon that is being studied) and theory that reflects a conceptualization of human inquiry. Some qualitative researchers insist on an atheoretical stance *vis-à-vis* the phenomenon of interest, with the goal of suspending *a priori* conceptualizations (substantive theories) that might bias their collection and analysis of data. For example, phenomenologists are in general committed to theoretical naiveté, and explicitly try to hold preconceived views of the phenomenon in check. Nevertheless, phenomenologists are guided in their inquiries by a framework or philosophy that focuses their analysis on certain aspects of a person's lifeworld. That framework is based on the premise that human experience is an inherent property of the experience itself, not constructed by an outside observer.

Ethnographers typically bring a strong cultural perspective to their studies, and this perspective shapes their initial fieldwork. Fetterman (1997) has observed that most ethnographers adopt one of two cultural theories: **ideational theories**, which suggest that cultural conditions and adaptation stem from mental activity and ideas, or **materialistic theories**, which view material conditions (e.g., resources, money, production) as the source of cultural developments.

The theoretical underpinning of grounded theory studies is a melding of sociologic formulations (Glaser, 2003). The most noteworthy theoretical system in grounded theory is **symbolic interaction** (or *interactionism*), which has three underlying premises (Blumer, 1986). First, humans act toward things based on the meanings that the things have for them. Second, the meaning of things is derived from (or arises out of) the interaction humans have with other fellow humans. And third, meanings are handled in, and modified through, an interpretive process in dealing with the things humans encounter.

> **Example of a grounded theory study:**
> St. John, Cameron, and McVeigh (2005) conducted a grounded theory study based on a symbolic interactionist framework to explore the social reality and symbolic meanings that words, gestures, activities, and experiences had for new fathers during the early works after childbirth as they interacted with their partners, the newborn, family, friends, and others.

Despite this theoretical perspective, grounded theory researchers, like phenomenologists, attempt to hold prior substantive theory (existing knowledge and conceptualizations about the phenomenon) in abeyance until their own substantive theory begins to emerge. Grounded theory methods are designed to facilitate the generation of theory that is *conceptually dense*, that is, with many conceptual patterns and relationships. The goal of grounded theory researchers is to develop a conceptualization of a phenomenon that is *grounded* in actual observations—that is, to explicate an empirically based conceptualization for integrating and making sense of a process or phenomenon. Theory development in a grounded theory study is an inductive process. Grounded theory researchers seek to identify patterns, commonalities, and relationships through the scrutiny of specific instances and events. During the ongoing analysis of data, the researchers move from specific pieces of data to abstract generalizations that synthesize and give structure to the observed phenomenon. The goal is to use the data, grounded in reality, to provide a description or an explanation of events as they occur in reality—not as they have been conceptualized in preexisting theories. Once the grounded theory starts to take shape, however, grounded theorists do not ignore the literature and prior theory; rather, previous literature is used for comparison with the emerging and developing categories of the theory. Sandelowski (1993) has noted that previous substantive theories or conceptualizations, when used in this manner, are essentially data themselves, and can be taken into consideration, along with study data, as part of an inductively driven new conceptualization.

> **⬤ TIP:** The use of theory in qualitative studies has been the topic of some debate in recent years. Morse (2002a) called for qualitative researchers to not be "theory ignorant but theory smart" (p. 296) and to "get over" their theory phobia. Morse elaborated (2004a) by noting that qualitative research does not necessarily begin with holding in check all prior knowledge of the phenomenon under study. She suggested that if the boundaries of the concept of interest can be identified, a qualitative researcher can use these boundaries as a scaffold to inductively explore the attributes of the concept.

In recent years, a growing number of qualitative nurse researchers have been adopting a perspective know as **critical theory** as a framework in their research. Critical theory is a paradigm that involves a critique of society and societal processes and structures, as we discuss in greater detail in Chapter 9.

Qualitative researchers sometimes use conceptual models of nursing as an interpretive framework. For example, a number of qualitative nurse researchers acknowledge that the philosophic roots of their studies lie in conceptual models of nursing such as those developed by Newman, Parse, and Rogers. Silva and Sorrell (1992) refer to such linkages as a means of testing nursing theory through the description of personal experiences.

> **Example of using nursing theory in a qualitative study:** Neill (2005) conducted a qualitative study of recognizing patterns in the lives of women with multiple sclerosis. She used relevant concepts from Margaret Newman's theory of health as expanding consciousness to help reveal the life patterns from the detailed narratives of seven women with multiple sclerosis.

Finally, a systematic review of qualitative studies on a specific topic is another strategy that can lead to theory development. In such metasyntheses, qualitative studies are combined to identify their essential elements. The findings from different sources are then used for theory building. Paterson (2001), for example, used the results of 292 qualitative studies that described the experiences of adults with chronic illness to develop the shifting perspectives model of chronic illness. This model depicts living with chronic illness as an ongoing, constantly shifting process in which individuals' perspectives change in the amount to which illness is in the foreground or background in their lives.

Theories in Quantitative Research

Quantitative researchers, like qualitative researchers, link research to theory or models in several ways. The classic approach is to test hypotheses deduced from a previously proposed theory.

Testing a Theory

Theories sometimes stimulate new studies. For example, a nurse might read about Pender's Health Promotion Model (see Fig. 6.1), and as reading progresses, conjectures such as the following might arise: "If the HPM is valid, then I would expect that patients with osteoporosis who perceived the benefit of a calcium-enriched diet would be more likely to alter their eating patterns than those who perceived no benefits." Such a conjecture, derived from a theory or conceptual framework, can serve as a starting point for testing the theory's adequacy.

In testing a theory, quantitative researchers deduce implications (as in the preceding example) and develop research hypotheses, which are predictions about the manner in which variables would be interrelated if the theory were correct. The hypotheses are then subjected to empirical testing through systematic data collection and analysis.

➲ **TIP:** If you are testing a specific theory or model, be sure to read about it from a primary source, and rely on the most up-to-date reference because models are often revised as research accumulates.

The focus of the testing process involves a comparison between observed outcomes and those predicted in the hypotheses. Through this process, a theory is continually subjected to potential disconfirmation. If studies repeatedly fail to disconfirm a theory, the theory gains support and acceptance (e.g., the Theory of Planned Behavior). The testing process continues until pieces of evidence cannot be interpreted within the context of the theory but *can* be explained by a new theory that also accounts for previous findings. Theory-testing studies are most useful when researchers devise logically sound deductions from the theory, design a study that reduces the plausibility of alternative explanations for observed relationships, and use methods that assess the theory's validity under maximally heterogeneous situations so that potentially competing theories can be ruled out.

Researchers sometimes base a new study on a theory in an effort to explain earlier descriptive findings. For example, suppose several researchers had found that nursing home patients demonstrate greater levels of anxiety and noncompliance with nursing staff around bedtime than at other times. These findings shed no light on underlying causes of the problem, and consequently suggest no way to improve it. Several explanations, rooted in models such as Lazarus and Folkman's Stress and Coping Model or Neuman's Health Care Systems Model, may be relevant in explaining nursing home patients' behavior. By directly testing the theory in a new study (i.e., deducing hypotheses derived from the theory), a researcher might learn *why* bedtime is a vulnerable period for the elderly in nursing homes.

⮕ TIP: It is useful to read research reports of other studies that were based on a theory in which you are interested — even if the research problem is not similar to your own. By reading other studies, you will be better able to judge how much empirical support the theory has received, how key variables were measured, and perhaps how the theory should be adapted.

Researchers sometimes combine elements from more than one theory as a basis for generating hypotheses. In doing this, researchers need to be thoroughly knowledgeable about *both* theories to see if there is an adequate conceptual and empirical basis for conjoining them. If underlying assumptions or conceptual definitions of key concepts are not compatible, the theories should not be combined (although perhaps elements of the two can be used to create a new conceptual framework with its own assumptions and definitions). Two theories that have given rise to combinatory efforts are the HBM and the Theory of Reasoned Action (TRA).

Example of testing two combined models:
Poss (2001) combined the HBM and the TRA to examine the factors associated with Mexican migrant farm workers' participation in a tuberculosis screening program. Figure 6.2 illustrates how Poss integrated these two models/theories in her study. More recently, Ham (2006) combined elements of the TRA and HPM to study Korean women's intention to receive a mammogram.

⮕ TIP: It is often suggested that theories first be evaluated before being used as a basis for a study — an enterprise that may be difficult for beginning researchers. For advanced students, Chinn and Kramer (2004) and Fawcett (2005) present criteria for assessing conceptual frameworks. Box 6.1, also included in the Toolkit, presents some basic questions that can be asked in a preliminary assessment of a theory or model.

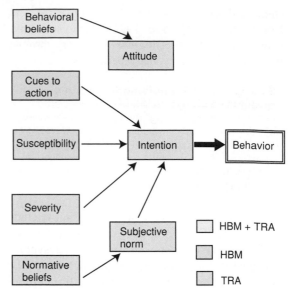

FIGURE 6.2 Combined Health Belief Model (HBM) and Theory of Reasoned Action (TRA). (Adapted with permission from Poss, J. E. [2001]. Developing a new model for cross-cultural research: Synthesizing the health belief model and the theory of reasoned action. *Advances in Nursing Science, 23*, 12.)

Testing Two Competing Theories

Researchers who directly test two competing theories that purport to explain a phenomenon may be in a particularly good position to advance knowledge. Almost all phenomena can be explained in alternative ways, as suggested by the various conceptual models of nursing. There are also competing theories for such phenomena as stress, child development, behavior change, and grieving, all of which are important to nursing. Each competing theory suggests alternative approaches to facilitating a positive outcome or minimizing a negative one. In designing effective nursing interventions, it is important to know which explanation has more validity.

Theory-testing research most often tests a single theory or model, and so to evaluate the worth of competing theories, nurses must compare the results of different studies. Such comparisons are difficult because each study design is unique. For example, one study of stress might use a sample of nursing students taking an examination, another

BOX 6.1 Some Questions for a Preliminary Assessment of a Model or Theory

ISSUE	QUESTIONS
Theoretical clarity	• Are key concepts defined and are the definitions sufficiently clear? • Do all concepts "fit" within the theory? Are concepts used in the theory in a manner compatible with conceptual definitions? • Are basic assumptions consistent with one another? • Are schematic models helpful, and are they compatible with the text? Are schematic models needed but not presented? • Can the theory be followed—is it adequately explained? Are there ambiguities?
Theoretical complexity	• Is the theory sufficiently rich and detailed to explain phenomena of interest? • Is the theory overly complex? • Can the theory be used to explain or predict, or only to describe phenomena?
Theoretical grounding	• Are the concepts identifiable in reality? • Is there an empirical basis for the theory and is the empirical basis solid? • Can the theoretical concepts be adequately operationalized?
Appropriateness of the theory	• Does the theory suggest possibilities for influencing nursing practice? • Are the tenets of the theory compatible with nursing's philosophy? • Are key concepts within the domain of nursing?
Importance of the theory	• Will research based on this theory answer critical questions? • How will testing the theory contribute to nursing's evidence base?
General issues	• Are there theories or models that do a better job of explaining phenomena of interest? • Is the theory compatible with your world view?

might use military personnel in a combat situation, and yet another might use terminally ill patients with cancer. Each study might, in addition to having divergent samples, measure stress differently. If the results of these studies support alternative theories of stress to different degrees, it would be difficult to know the extent to which the results reflected differences in study design rather than differences in the validity of the theories.

Researchers who openly test two or more competing theories, using a single sample of subjects and identical measures of key constructs, may be able to make powerful and meaningful comparisons directly. Such a study requires considerable advance planning and the inclusion of a wider array of measures than would otherwise be the case, but such efforts are important. In recent years, several nurse researchers have used this approach to refine understanding and to provide promising new leads for research.

Example of a test of competing theories:
Mahon and Yarcheski (2002) tested two alternative models of happiness in early adolescents: a theory relating happiness to enabling mechanisms and a theory of happiness based on adolescents' personality traits. The findings suggested that enabling mechanisms had more explanatory power than personality characteristics in predicting happiness.

Testing Theory-Based Interventions
Tests of a theory increasingly are taking the form of testing theory-based interventions. If a theory is correct, it has implications for strategies to influence people's health-related attitudes or behavior, and hence their health outcomes. And, if an intervention is developed on the basis of an explicit conceptualization of human behavior and thought, then it likely has a greater chance of being effective than if it is developed in a conceptual vacuum.

Several issues relating to theory-driven interventions deserve special mention. The first relates to a concept known as **construct validity**. As we will see in Chapter 17, construct validity is most often defined as the conceptual adequacy of instruments that measure abstract human traits. When instrument developers design new instruments, they typically devote considerable effort to ensuring that the instruments capture the theoretically meaningful concepts (variables) of interest. For example, if an intervention is designed to reduce despair in patients with HIV/AIDS, we would want to measure the outcome variable (despair) using an instrument with good construct validity to be sure that it is really patient despair that is being measured. There has been less recognition of the fact that interventions should have compelling construct validity as well (Shadish, Cook, & Campbell, 2002). There needs to be a strong match between the *idea* behind the intervention and its operationalization, and this match can most readily occur within the context of a theory of how the intervention would have desired effects on the targeted outcomes. In other words, good intervention research requires construct validity for both the dependent variables (the outcomes) and the independent variable (the intervention). The research example at the end of this chapter illustrates an intervention with good construct validity.

Interventions rarely affect outcomes directly—there are mediating factors that play a role in the causal pathway between the intervention and the outcomes. For example, interventions based on Social Cognitive Theory posit that improvements to a person's self-efficacy will result in positive changes in health behavior—in other words, the theory stipulates self-efficacy as a key mediator variable that must be addressed through the intervention. In health promotion interventions, the most common theory-based mediator variables include decisional balance, goal-setting, outcome expectations, self-determination, self-efficacy, social support, and stress (Ory, Jordan, & Bazarre, 2002).

It should be noted that interventions need not be based on formal theories or conceptual models, such as the HPM. The impetus for a nursing intervention may be a theory developed within the context of qualitative studies (Gamel et al., 2001; Morse, 2002b).

➲ **TIP:** If your research involves an intervention, you should unquestionably develop a theoretical rationale for how the intervention is expected to have intended effects. Without a theoretical rationale, your intervention might be insufficiently powerful (e.g., it might miss key components or features), and the research could be seriously flawed in terms of design, measurement of key mediator variables, and analytic strategies.

Example of theory testing in an intervention study: Kolanowski, Litaker, and Buettner (2005) used a middle-range theory called the Need-driven Dementia-compromised Behavior (NDB) model in developing a recreational intervention designed to improve affect and behavior in long-term care residents with dementia. The NDB-derived activities, which were tailored to meet individual needs (skill levels and interests) resulted in greater participation, more positive affect, and less passivity.

Using a Model or Theory as an Organizing Structure

Many researchers who cite a theory or model as their framework are not directly testing the theory. Silva (1986), in her analysis of 62 studies that claimed their roots in five nursing models, found that only 9 were direct and explicit tests of the models cited by the researchers. She found that the most common use of the nursing models was to provide an organizing structure for the studies. In such an approach, researchers begin with a broad conceptualization of nursing (or stress, health beliefs, and so on) that is consistent with that of the model developers. The researchers *assume* that the models they espouse are valid, and then use the models' constructs or proposed schemas to provide a broad organizational or interpretive context. Some use data collection instruments that are allied with the models. Silva pointed out that using models in this fashion can serve a valuable organizing purpose, but noted that such studies offer little evidence about the validity of the theory itself.

BOX 6.2 Criteria to Determine Whether a Theory/Model Is Being Tested

1. Is the purpose of the study to determine the validity of a theory's assumptions or propositions?
2. Does the report explicitly note that the theory is the framework for the research?
3. Is the theory discussed in sufficient detail that the relationship between the theory on the one hand and the study hypotheses or research questions on the other is clear?
4. Are study hypotheses directly deduced from the theory?
5. Are study hypotheses empirically tested in an appropriate manner, so as to shed light on the validity of the theory?
6. Is the validity of the theory's assumptions or propositions supported (or challenged) based on evidence from the empirical tests?
7. Does the report discuss how evidence from empirical tests supports or refutes the theory, or how the theory explains relevant aspects of the findings?

Adapted from Silva M. C. (1986). Research testing nursing theory: State of the art. *Advances in Nursing Science, 9,* 1–11.

Example of using a model as organizing structure: Kirchhoff, Conradt, and Anumandia (2003) studied ICU nurses' preparation of families for death of patients following withdrawal of ventilator support. Their descriptive study used Self-Regulation Theory (SRT) as a framework. SRT was used as the basis for asking about the types of activities in which the nurses engaged, but the validity of the SRT was not tested.

To our knowledge, Silva's study has not been replicated with a more recent sample of studies—although Taylor and colleagues (2000) also found that most studies of Orem's Self-Care Deficit Theory were primarily descriptive rather than theory testing. We suspect that, even today, most quantitative studies that offer models and theories as their conceptual frameworks are using them primarily as organizational or interpretive tools. Silva (1986) offered seven evaluation criteria for determining whether a study was actually testing a theory, rather than simply identifying an organizational context. Box 6.2, broadly adapted from Silva's criteria, presents a set of evaluative questions to determine whether a study was actually testing a theory.

Example of a study meeting Silva's theory-testing criteria: Woods and Isenberg (2001) tested one aspect of a middle-range theory based on

the Roy Adaptation Model. Their purpose was to test the efficacy of *adaptation* as a mediator of intimate abuse and traumatic stress in battered women. They tested the following two relational statements: "(1) physical abuse, emotional abuse, and risk of homicide are focal stimuli that elicit the response of post traumatic stress disorder (PTSD) in battered women and (2) adaptation in the physiologic, self-concept, role, and interdependence modes acts as a mediator between the focal stimuli of intimate physical abuse, emotional abuse, and risk of homicide and the response of PTSD in women" (p. 215). As a result of empirical testing, Woods and Isenberg reported that adaptation in three of the four modes partially mediated the relationship among intimate abuse, the focal stimuli, and the response of PTSD.

Fitting a Problem to a Theory

The preceding sections described situations in which a researcher *begins* with a specific theory or model and uses it either as the basis for developing hypotheses or for organizational or interpretive purposes. Circumstances sometimes arise in which the problem is formulated before consideration is given to a conceptual framework. Even in such situations, researchers sometimes try to devise a theoretical context. In some situations such an approach may be appropriate, but we caution that an after-the-fact linkage of theory to a problem may not enhance the study's worth. An exception is when the researcher is struggling to make sense of findings, and calls on an existing theory to help explain or interpret them.

If it is necessary to find a relevant theory after selecting a problem, the search for such a theory must begin by first conceptualizing the problem on an abstract level. For example, take the research question: "Do daily telephone conversations between a psychiatric nurse and a patient for 2 weeks after discharge from the hospital result in lower rates of readmission by short-term psychiatric patients?" This is a relatively concrete research problem, but it might profitably be viewed within the context of Orem's Self-Care Model, a theory of reinforcement, a theory of social influence, or a theory of crisis resolution. Part of the difficulty in finding a theory is that a single phenomenon of interest can be conceptualized in a number of ways and, depending on the manner chosen, may refer the researcher to conceptual schemes from a wide range of disciplines.

➲ **TIP:** If you begin with a research problem and are trying to identify a suitable framework, it is probably wise to confer with others—especially with people who may be familiar with a broad range of theoretical perspectives. By having an open discussion, you are more likely to become aware of your own conceptual perspectives and are thus in a better position to identify an appropriate framework.

Textbooks, handbooks, and encyclopedias (and perhaps certain websites) in the chosen discipline usually are a good starting point for the identification of a framework. These sources usually summarize the status of a theoretical position and document the efforts to confirm and disconfirm it. Journal articles contain more current information but are usually restricted to descriptions of specific studies rather than to broad expositions or evaluations of theories.

Fitting a problem to a theory after the fact should be done with circumspection. It is true that having a theoretical context can enhance the meaningfulness of a study, but artificially "cramming" a problem into a theory is not the route to scientific utility, nor to enhancing nursing's evidence base.

There are many published studies that purport to have a conceptual framework when, in fact, the tenuous *post hoc* linkage is all too evident. In Silva's (1986) previously mentioned analysis of 62 studies that claimed a nursing model as their underpinnings, approximately one third essentially paid only lip service to a model. If a conceptual framework is really linked to a research problem, then the design of the study, the selection of data collection methods, the data analysis, and (especially) the interpretation of the findings *flow* from that conceptualization.

➲ **TIP:** If you begin with a research question and then subsequently identify a theory or model, be willing to adapt or augment your original research problem as you gain greater understanding of the theory. The linking of theory and research question may involve an iterative approach.

Developing a Framework in a Quantitative Study

Novice researchers may think of themselves as unqualified to develop a conceptual scheme of their own. But theory development depends much less on research experience than on powers of observation, grasp of a problem, and knowledge of prior research. There is nothing to prevent an imaginative and sensible person from formulating an original conceptual framework for a study. The conceptual scheme may not be a full-fledged formal theory, but it should place the issues of the study into some broader perspective.

The basic intellectual process underlying theory development is induction—that is, reasoning from particular observations and facts to broader generalizations. The inductive process involves integrating what one has experienced or learned into some organized scheme. For quantitative research, the observations used in the inductive process usually are findings from other studies. When patterns of relationships among variables are derived in this fashion, one has the makings of a theory that can be put to a more rigorous test. The first step in the development of a framework, then, is to formulate a generalized scheme of relevant concepts that is firmly grounded in the research literature.

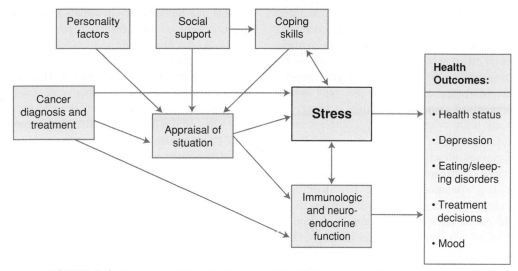

FIGURE 6.3 Conceptual Model of Stress and Health Outcomes in Patients with Cancer.

Let us use as an example a hypothetical study question that we described in Chapter 4, namely, What is the effect of humor on stress in patients with cancer? (See the problem statement in Box 4.2). In undertaking a literature review, we find that researchers and reviewers (e.g., Christie & Moore, 2005) have suggested a myriad of complex relationships among such concepts as humor, social support, stress, coping, appraisal, immune function, and neuroendocrine function on the one hand and various health outcomes (pain tolerance, mood, depression, health status, and eating and sleeping disturbances) on the other. Although there is a fair amount of research evidence for the existence of these relationships, it is not clear how they all fit together. Without some kind of "map" or conceptualization of what might be going on, it would be difficult to design a strong study—we might, for example, not measure all the key variables, or we might not undertake an appropriate analysis. And, if our plan is to test an innovative humor therapy, we might also struggle in developing a strong intervention in the absence of a framework.

The conceptual map in Figure 6.3 represents an attempt to put the pieces of the puzzle together for a study involving a test of a humor intervention to improve health outcomes for patients with cancer.

Many other conceptualizations are possible based on the same research findings from our review, but this is a conceptualization that could be put to a test and can guide us in designing the study. According to this map, stress is affected by a cancer diagnosis and treatment both directly and indirectly, through the person's appraisal of the situation. That appraisal, in turn, is affected by the patient's coping skills, personality factors, and available social supports (factors which themselves are interrelated). Stress and physiologic function (neuroendocrine and immunologic) have reciprocal relationships.

Note that we have not yet put in a "box" for humor. How do we think humor might operate? If we see humor as having primarily a direct effect on physiologic response, we would place humor near the bottom and draw an arrow from the box to immune and neuroendocrine function. But perhaps humor reduces stress because it helps a person cope (i.e., its effects are primarily psychological). Or maybe humor will affect the person's appraisal of the situation. Alternatively, nurse-initiated humor therapy might have its effect primarily because it is a form of social support. All these conceptualizations have implications for study design. To give but one example, if the humor therapy is viewed primarily as a form of social support, then we might want to compare our intervention to an alternative intervention that involves the presence of a comforting nurse (another form of social support), without any special effort at including humor. The conceptualization could also affect the intervention—for example, what *type* of humor to use, how intense the intervention must be, whether it should be reinforced with other types of complementary therapies, and so on.

This type of inductive conceptualization process on the basis of research findings is a useful means of providing guidance and a theoretical rationale for a study. Of course, our research question in this example could have been addressed within the context of an existing conceptualization, such as Lazarus and Folkman's Theory of Stress and Coping or the psychoneuroimmunology (PNI) framework (McCain et al., 2005), but hopefully our example illustrates how developing an original framework can inform researchers' decisions and strengthen the study.

➲ **TIP:** We strongly encourage you to draw a conceptual map before launching an investigation based on either a formal theory or your own inductive conceptualization—even if you do not plan to formally test the entire model or present the model in a report. Such maps are extremely valuable heuristic devices in planning a study.

Example of model development: Horowitz and her colleagues (2005) conducted a study based on their own conceptual model of the predictors of postpartum depression. Their model represented a synthesis of findings from the literature and from several theoretical writings about depression.

CRITIQUING FRAMEWORKS IN RESEARCH REPORTS

You will find references to theories and conceptual frameworks in some (but not all) of the studies you read. It is often challenging to critique the theoretical context of a published research report—or its absence—but we offer a few suggestions.

In a qualitative study in which a grounded theory is developed and presented, you probably will not be given enough information to refute the proposed descriptive theory because only evidence supporting the theory is presented. However, you can determine whether the theory seems logical, whether the conceptualization is truly insightful, and whether the evidence is solid and convincing. In a phenomenological study, you should look to see if the researcher addresses the philosophical underpinnings of the study. The researcher should briefly discuss the philosophy of phenomenology upon which the study was based.

Critiquing a theoretical framework in a quantitative report is also difficult, especially because you are not likely to be familiar with the range of relevant theories and models. Some suggestions for evaluating the conceptual basis of a quantitative study are offered in the following discussion and in Box 6.3. ✷

The first task is to determine whether the study does, in fact, have a theoretical or conceptual framework. If there is no mention of a theory, model, or framework, you should consider whether the study's contribution is diminished by the absence of a conceptual context. Nursing has been criticized for producing many pieces of isolated research that are difficult to integrate because of the absence of a theoretical foundation, but in some cases, the research may be so pragmatic that it does not really need a theory to enhance its usefulness. For example, research designed to determine the optimal frequency of turning patients has a utilitarian goal; a theory might not enhance the value of the findings. If, however, the study involves the test of an intervention or hypotheses, the absence of a formally stated framework or rationale suggests conceptual fuzziness and perhaps ensuing methodologic problems.

If the study does involve an explicit framework, you must then ask whether the particular framework is appropriate. You may not be in a position to challenge the researcher's use of a particular theory or model or to recommend an alternative, but you can evaluate the logic of using a particular framework and assess whether the link between

BOX 6.3 Guidelines for Critiquing Theoretical and Conceptual Frameworks

1. Does the report describe an explicit theoretical or conceptual framework for the study? If not, does the absence of a framework detract from the usefulness or significance of the research?
2. Does the report adequately describe the major features of the theory or model so that readers can understand the conceptual basis of the study?
3. Is the theory or model appropriate for the research problem? Would a different framework have been more fitting?
4. If there is an intervention, was there a cogent theoretical basis or rationale for the intervention?
5. Is the theory or model used as the basis for generating hypotheses that were tested, or is it used as an organizational or interpretive framework? Was this appropriate?
6. Do the research problem and hypotheses (if any) naturally flow from the framework, or does the purported link between the problem and the framework seem contrived? Are deductions from the theory logical?
7. Are the concepts adequately defined in a way that is consistent with the theory? If there is an intervention, are intervention components consistent with the theory?
8. Is the framework based on a conceptual model of nursing or on a model developed by nurses? If it is borrowed from another discipline, is there adequate justification for its use?
9. Did the framework guide the study methods? For example, was the appropriate research tradition used if the study was qualitative? If quantitative, do the operational definitions correspond to the conceptual definitions? Were hypotheses tested statistically?
10. Does the researcher tie the findings of the study back to the framework at the end of the report? How do the findings support or undermine the framework? Are the findings interpreted within the context of the framework?

the problem and the theory is genuine. Does the researcher present a convincing rationale for the framework used? Do the hypotheses flow from the theory? Will the findings contribute to the validation of the theory? Does the researcher interpret the findings within the context of the framework? If the answer to such questions is no, you may have grounds for criticizing the study's framework, even though you may not be able to articulate how the conceptual basis of the study could be improved.

RESEARCH EXAMPLES

Throughout this chapter, we have mentioned studies that were based on various conceptual and theoretical models. This section presents more detailed examples of the linkages between theory and research from the nursing research literature—one from a quantitative study and the other from a qualitative study.

Research Example From a Quantitative Study: Social Cognitive Theory

Study: "Effectiveness of a behavioral change intervention in Thai elders after knee replacement" (Harnirattisai & Johnson, 2005)

Statement of Purpose: The purpose of the study was to evaluate the effects of a theory-based behavioral change intervention (BCI) on self-efficacy and outcome expectations for exercise and functional activity, physical activity participation, and physical performance of older adults in Thailand.

Theoretical Framework: Social Cognitive Theory guided the development of the BCI, as shown in Figure 6.4. Nurse–patient interactions were designed to increase patients' self-efficacy and outcome expectations. Each component of the intervention corresponded to an explicit aspect of the theory. For example, three intervention strategies were linked to the patients' mastery experience, which was considered a source of self-efficacy information: *patient–nurse interaction* (nurse–patient discussions regarding success and failure of exercise and

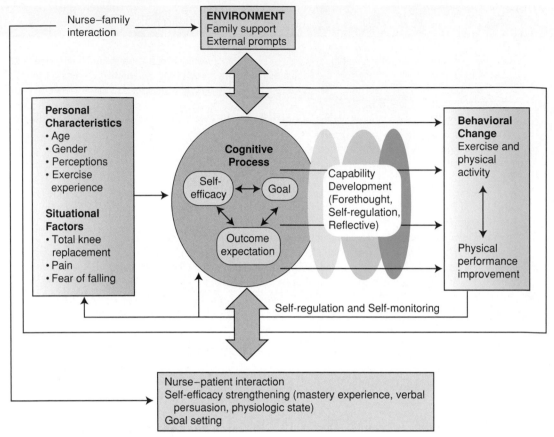

FIGURE 6.4 Model for a behavioral change intervention to improve physical performance after knee replacement surgery, based on Social Cognitive Theory. (From Harnirattisai, T., & Johnson, R. A. [2005]. Effectiveness of a behavioral change intervention in Thai elders after knee replacement. *Nursing Research, 54*[2] 98.)

physical activity); *self-monitoring* (instruction on how to observe and record their performance in a physical activity diary and how to identify their barriers); and *goal setting* (discussions with patients about appropriate goals for exercise and physical activity in different postoperative phases).

Method: A sample of sixty-three older adults undergoing total knee replacement surgery were allocated by chance to either an intervention group that received the BCI or to another group that received usual nursing care. The intervention began 4 days after surgery and occurred again at a follow-up session 2 weeks postoperatively (PO). Most outcome variables were measured at PO day 4 and at PO weeks 2 and 6. Participants also maintained an activity diary for several weeks.

Key Findings: Elders in the intervention group had significantly greater improvements in self-efficacy for exercise, outcome expectations for exercise, and functional activity than those in the other group. Intervention elders also participated in more exercise and showed significantly greater improvement in physical performance.

Research Example From a Qualitative Study: A Grounded Theory

Study: "Abuse experiences, perceptions, and associated decisions during the childbearing cycle" (Lutz, 2005)

Statement of Purpose: The purpose of the study was to generate a theoretical understanding of women's experiences and perceptions of intimate partner abuse during the childbearing cycle.

Method: Grounded theory methods were used in this study. Data were collected through 21 in-depth, personal interviews with 12 women who were either pregnant and being abused or who had been abused during a prior childbearing cycle. The women were diverse demographically and in their abuse experiences. Interviews, which were audiotaped, lasted between 1 and 4 hours. All but three participants were interviewed twice.

Theoretical Framework: Lutz directly acknowledged the theoretical links between her grounded theory study and symbolic interactionism. As she indicated, central to the methods she used was "the symbolic interactionist understanding that the process of thinking is governed by and reflective of one's interaction with others" (p. 804). Within this broad framework, Lutz developed a rich descriptive theory of women's experience of intimate partner abuse during pregnancy that was grounded in the women's reports.

Key Findings: Based on in-depth interviews, Lutz identified an underlying social process that she labeled "Living Two Lives." The theory involves the linkage in the women's lives between two seemingly incongruent phenomena—abuse and childbearing. Two conditions occurred simultaneously—guarding and revealing the intersection between their public and private lives and pregnancy. The women engaged in five different strategies in their effort to negotiate these conditions. Lutz's theory, summarized in an elaborate conceptual map (Figure 1, p. 810), revealed the context of the process, the intervening conditions and crystallizing events, the women's actions and strategies, and the consequences.

SUMMARY POINTS

- High-quality research requires *conceptual integration*, one aspect of which is having a defensible theoretical rationale for undertaking the study in a given manner or for testing specific hypotheses. Researchers demonstrate their conceptual clarity through the delineation of a theory, model, or framework on which the study is based.

- A **theory** is a broad abstract characterization of phenomena. As classically defined, a theory is an abstract generalization that systematically explains relationships among phenomena.

Descriptive theory thoroughly describes a phenomenon.

- The basic components of a theory are concepts; classically defined theories consist of a set of propositions about the interrelationships among concepts, arranged in a logically interrelated system that permits new statements to be derived from them.

- **Grand theories** (or *macrotheories*) attempt to describe large segments of the human experience. **Middle-range theories** are more specific to certain phenomena.

- Concepts are also the basic elements of **conceptual models**, but concepts are not linked in a logically ordered, deductive system. Conceptual models, like theories, provide context for nursing studies.

- In research, the overall objectives of theories and models are to make findings meaningful, to summarize existing knowledge into coherent systems, to stimulate new research, and to explain phenomena and relationships among them.

- **Schematic models** (or **conceptual maps**) are graphic representations of phenomena and their interrelationships using symbols or diagrams and a minimal use of words.

- A **conceptual framework** is the conceptual underpinning of a study, including an overall rationale and conceptual definitions of key concepts. In qualitative studies, the framework usually springs from distinct research traditions.

- Several conceptual models of nursing have been developed and have been used in nursing research. The concepts central to models of nursing are human beings, environment, health, and nursing.

- Two major conceptual models of nursing used by nurse researchers are Roy's Adaptation Model and Rogers's Science of Unitary Human Beings.

- Nonnursing models used by nurse researchers (e.g., Bandura's Social Cognitive Theory) are referred to as **borrowed theories**; when the appropriateness of borrowed theories for nursing inquiry is confirmed, the theories become **shared theories**.

- In some qualitative research traditions (e.g., phenomenology), the researcher strives to suspend previously held **substantive theories** of the phenomena under study; nevertheless, there is a rich theoretical underpinning associated with the tradition itself.

- Some qualitative researchers specifically seek to develop *grounded theories*, data-driven explanations to account for phenomena under study through inductive processes.
- In the classical use of theory, researchers test hypotheses deduced from an existing theory. An emerging trend is the testing of theory-based interventions, in which an objective is to develop an intervention with strong **construct validity**.
- In both qualitative and quantitative studies, researchers sometimes use a theory or model as an organizing framework, or as an interpretive tool.
- Researchers sometimes develop a problem, design a study, and *then* look for a conceptual framework; such an after-the-fact selection of a framework is less compelling than the systematic testing of a particular theory.
- Even in the absence of a formal theory, quantitative researchers can inductively weave together the findings from prior studies into a conceptual scheme that provides methodologic and conceptual direction to the inquiry.

STUDY ACTIVITIES

Chapter 6 of the *Resource Manual to Accompany Nursing Research: Generating and Assessing Evidence for Nursing Practice*, *8th edition*, offers various exercises and study suggestions for reinforcing concepts presented in this chapter. In addition, the following study questions can be addressed:

1. Select one of the conceptual models or theories described in this chapter. Formulate a research question and one or two hypotheses that could be used empirically to test the utility of the conceptual framework or model in nursing practice.

2. Answer appropriate questions from Box 6.3 regarding Harnirattisai and Johnson's intervention study for Thai elders described at the end of the chapter. Also, consider what the implications of the study are in terms of the cross-cultural utility of Social Cognitive Theory.

3. Answer appropriate questions from Box 6.3 regarding Lutz's grounded theory study of intimate partner abuse described at the end of the chapter. Also, consider the following additional questions: (a) Was Lutz directly testing the theory of symbolic interactionism? (b) In what way was the use of theory different in Lutz's study than in the previous study by Harnirattisai and Johnson?

STUDIES CITED IN CHAPTER 6

Methodologic or theoretical references cited in this chapter can be found in a separate section at the end of the book.

Berry, D. (2004). An emerging model of behavior change in women maintaining weight loss. *Nursing Science Quarterly, 17*(3), 242–252.

Chouinard, M., & Robichad-Ekstrand, S. (2005). The effectiveness of a nursing inpatient smoking cessation program in individuals with cardiovascular disease. *Nursing Research, 54*(4), 243–254.

Christie, W., & Moore, C. (2005). The impact of humor on patients with cancer. *Clinical Journal of Oncology Nursing, 9*(2), 211–218.

Clayton, M. F., Mishel, M. H., & Belyea, M. (2006). Testing a model of symptoms, communication, uncertainty, and well-being, in older breast cancer survivors. *Research in Nursing & Health, 29*(1), 18–29.

Cossette, S., Frasure-Smith, N., & Lespérance, F. (2002). Nursing approaches to reducing psychological distress in men and women recovering from myocardial infarction. *International Journal of Nursing Studies, 39*, 479–494.

Fawcett, J., Aber, C., Weiss, M., Haussler, S., Myers, S. T., King, C., Newton, J., & Silva, V. (2005). Adaptation to cesarean birth: Implementation of an international multisite study. *Nursing Science Quarterly, 18*(3), 204–210.

Gates, D., Fitzwater, E., & Succop, P. (2005). Reducing assaults against nursing home caregivers. *Nursing Research, 54*(2), 119–127.

Ham, O. K. (2006). Factors affecting mammography behavior and intention among Korean women, *Oncology Nursing Forum, 33*(1), 113–119.

Harnirattisai, T., & Johnson, R. A. (2005). Effectiveness of a behavioral change intervention in Thai elders after knee replacement surgery. *Nursing Research, 54*(2), 97–107.

Hemsley, M., Glass, N., & Watson, J. (2006). Taking the eagle's view: Using Watson's conceptual model to investigate the extraordinary and transformative experiences of nurse healers. *Holistic Nursing Practice, 20*(2), 85–94.

Horowitz, J. A., Damato, E. G., Duffy, M. E., & Solon, L. (2005). The relationship of maternal attributes, resources, and perceptions of postpartum experiences to depression. *Research in Nursing & Health, 28,* 159–171.

Jonas-Simpson, C., Mitchell, G. J., Fisher, A., Jones, G., & Linscott, J. (2006). The experience of being listened to: A qualitative study of older adults in long-term care settings. *Journal of Gerontological Nursing, 32*(1), 46–53.

Jones-Cannon, S., & Davis, B. L. (2005). Coping among African-American daughters caring for aging parents. *ABNF Journal, 16*(6), 118–123.

Kirchhoff, K. T., Conradt, K. L., & Anumandia, P. R. (2003). ICU nurses' preparation of families for death of patients following withdrawal of ventilator support. *Applied Nursing Research, 16,* 85–92.

Kolanowski, A. M., Litaker, M., & Buettner, L. (2005). Efficacy of theory-based activities for behavioral symptoms of dementia. *Nursing Research, 54,* 219–228.

Kreulen, G. J., & Braden, C. J. (2004). Model test of the relationship between self-help promoting nursing interventions and self-care and health status outcomes. *Research in Nursing & Health, 27,* 97–109.

LaMontagne, L. L., Hepworth, J. T., Cohen, F., & Salisbury, M. H. (2005). Adolescent scoliosis: Effects of corrective surgery, cognitive behavioral interventions, and age on activity outcomes. *Applied Nursing Research, 17*(3), 168–177.

Lee, I., Le, E. O., Kim, H. S., Park, Y. S., Song, M., & Park, Y. T. H. (2004). Concept development of family resilience: A study of Korean families with a chronically ill child. *Journal of Clinical Nursing, 13,* 636–645.

Lutz, K. F. (2005). Abuse experiences, perceptions, and associated decisions during the childbearing cycle. *Western Journal of Nursing Research, 27*(7), 802–824.

Mahon, N. E., & Yarcheski, A. (2002). Alternative theories of happiness in early adolescents. *Clinical Nursing Research, 11,* 306–323.

Melancon, B., & Miller, L. H. (2005). Massage therapy versus traditional therapy for low back pain relief. *Holistic Nursing Practice, 19*(3), 116–121.

Neill, J. (2005). Recognizing patterns in the lives of women with multiple sclerosis. In C. Picard & D. Jones (Eds.), *Giving voice to what we know: Margaret Newman's theory of health as expanding consciousness in nursing practice, research, and education* (pp. 153–165). Sudbury, MA: Jones & Bartlett.

Paterson, B. L. (2001). The shifting perspectives model of chronic illness. *Journal of Nursing Scholarship, 33,* 21–26.

Plowden, K. O., Fletcher, A., & Miller, J. L. (2005). Factors influencing HIV-risk behaviors among HIV-positive urban African Americans. *Journal of the Association of Nurses in AIDS Care, 16*(1), 21–28.

Poss, J. E. (2001). Developing a new model for cross-cultural research: Synthesizing the Health Belief Model and the Theory of Reasoned Action. *Advances in Nursing Science, 23,* 1–15.

Ronis, D. L., Hong, O., & Lusk, S. L. (2006). Comparison of the original and revised structures of the Health Promotion Model in predicting construction workers' use of hearing protection. *Research in Nursing & Health, 29*(1), 3–17.

Sethares, K. A., & Elliott, K. (2004). The effect of a tailored message intervention on heart failure readmission rates, quality of life, and benefit and barrier beliefs in persons with heart failure. *Heart & Lung, 22*(4), 249–260.

Shyu, Y., Liang, J., Lu, J., & Wu, C. (2004). Environmental barriers and mobility in Taiwan: Is the Roy Adaptation Model applicable? *Nursing Science Quarterly, 17,* 165–170.

Skybo, T. (2005). Witnessing violence: Biopsychosocial impact on children. *Pediatric Nursing, 31*(4), 263–270.

St. John, W., Cameron, C., & McVeigh, C. (2005). Meeting the challenge of new fatherhood during the early weeks. *Journal of Obstetric, Gynecologic, & Neonatal Nursing, 34*(2), 180–189.

Steele, S. K., & Porche, D. J. (2005). Testing the theory of planned behavior to predict mammography intention. *Nursing Research, 54* (5), 332–338.

Taylor, S. G., Geden, E., Isaramalai, S., & Wongvatunyu, S. (2000). Orem's Self-Care Deficit Nursing Theory: Its philosophic foundation and the state of the science. *Nursing Science Quarterly, 13*(2), 104–110.

Woods, S. J., & Isenberg, M. A. (2001). Adaptation as a mediator of intimate abuse and traumatic stress in battered women. *Nursing Science Quarterly, 14,* 215–221.

Wright, B. W. (2004). Trust and power in adults: An investigation using Rogers' Science of Unitary Human Beings. *Nursing Science Quarterly, 17,* 139–146.

Yarcheski, A., Mahon, N. E., & Yarcheski, T. J. (2004). Health and well-being in early adolescents using Rogers' science of unitary human beings. *Nursing Science Quarterly, 17* (1), 72–77.

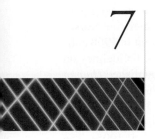

7

Generating Research Evidence Ethically

I n any discipline that involves research with human beings or animals, researchers must address a range of ethical issues. Ethical concerns are especially prominent in nursing research because the line of demarcation between what constitutes the expected practice of nursing and the collection of research information can sometimes get blurred. Furthermore, ethics can create particular challenges because ethical requirements sometimes conflict with the need to produce evidence of the highest possible quality for practice. This chapter discusses major ethical principles that must be considered in designing research.

ETHICS AND RESEARCH

When humans are used as study participants—as they usually are in nursing research—care must be exercised in ensuring that the rights of those humans are protected. The requirement for ethical conduct may strike you as so self-evident as to require no further comment, but the fact is that ethical considerations have not always been given adequate attention. In this section, we consider some of the reasons that ethical guidelines became imperative.

Historical Background

As modern, civilized people, we might like to think that systematic violations of moral principles within a research context occurred centuries ago rather than in recent times, but this is not the case. The Nazi medical experiments of the 1930s and 1940s are the most famous example of recent disregard for ethical conduct. The Nazi program of research involved the use of prisoners of war and racial "enemies" in numerous experiments designed to test the limits of human endurance and human reaction to diseases and untested drugs. The studies were unethical not only because they exposed these people to permanent physical harm and even death but also because subjects could not refuse participation. Wartime experiments that raised ethical concerns were also conducted in Japan and Australia (McNeill, 1993).

There are more recent examples from the United States and other Western countries. For instance, between 1932 and 1972, a study known as the Tuskegee Syphilis Study, sponsored by the U.S. Public Health Service, investigated the effects of syphilis among 400 men from a poor African-American community. Medical treatment was deliberately withheld to study the course of the untreated disease. A public health nurse, Eunice Rivers, is credited with much of the recruitment of participants in that study (Vessey & Gennarao, 1994). Similarly, Dr. Herbert Green of the National Women's Hospital in Auckland, New Zealand studied women with cervical cancer in the 1980s; patients with carcinoma *in situ* were not given treatment so that researchers could study the natural progression of the disease. Another well-known case of unethical research involved the injection of live cancer cells into elderly patients at the Jewish Chronic Disease Hospital in Brooklyn in the 1960s without the consent of those patients. At about the same time, Dr. Saul Krugman was conducting research on hepatitis in the Willowbrook Study in nearby Staten Island. At Willowbrook, an institution for the mentally retarded, children were deliberately infected with the hepatitis virus. Even more recently, it was revealed in 1993 that U.S. federal agencies had sponsored radiation experiments since the 1940s on hundreds of people, many of them prisoners or elderly hospital patients. Many other examples of studies with ethical transgressions—often much more subtle than these examples—have emerged to give ethical concerns the high visibility they have today.

Codes of Ethics

In response to human rights violations, various **codes of ethics** have been developed. One of the first internationally recognized efforts to establish ethical standards is referred to as the Nuremberg Code, developed after the Nazi atrocities were made public in the Nuremberg trials. Several other international standards have subsequently been developed, the most notable of which is the Declaration of Helsinki, which was adopted in 1964 by the World Medical Association and most recently revised in 2000.

Most disciplines have established their own code of ethics. For example, guidelines for psychologists were published by the American Psychological Association (2002) in *Ethical Principles of Psychologists and Code of Conduct*. The American Sociological Association published the most recent version of its *Code of Ethics* in 1999. The

American Medical Association regularly updates its *Code of Medical Ethics*.

Nurses have developed their own ethical guidelines. In the United States, the American Nurses Association (ANA) issued a statement in 1968 entitled "The Nurse in Research: ANA Guidelines on Ethical Values," and then in 1975 published *Human Rights Guidelines for Nurses in Clinical and Other Research*. In 1995, the ANA issued *Ethical Guidelines in the Conduct, Dissemination, and Implementation of Nursing Research* (Silva, 1995). The ANA also published in 2001 a revised *Code of Ethics for Nurses With Interpretive Statements*, a document that covers primarily ethical issues for practicing nurses but that also includes principles that apply to nurse researchers. In Canada, the Canadian Nurses Association first published a document entitled *Ethical Guidelines for Nurses in Research Involving Human Participants* in 1983, which was revised most recently in 2002.

Some nurse ethicists have called for an international code of ethics for nursing research, but nurses in most countries have developed their own professional codes or follow the codes established by their governments. The International Council of Nurses (ICN), however, has developed the *ICN Code of Ethics for Nurses*, which was most recently updated in 2000.

➔ **TIP:** There are many useful websites devoted to ethical principles, only some of which are mentioned in this chapter. Several websites are listed in the "Useful Websites for Chapter 7" file on the accompanying CD-ROM, for you to click on directly.

Government Regulations for Protecting Study Participants

Governments throughout the world fund research and establish rules for how such research must adhere to ethical principles. For example, Health Canada specified the *Tri-Council Policy Statement: Ethical Conduct for Research Involving Humans* as the guidelines to protect human subjects in all types of research. In Australia, the National Health and

Medical Research Council issued the *National Statement on Ethical Conduct in Research Involving Humans* in 1999 and also issued a special statement on research with Aboriginal peoples in 2003.

In the United States, an important code of ethics was adopted by the National Commission for the Protection of Human Subjects of Biomedical and Behavioral Research (1978). The commission, established by the National Research Act (Public Law 93–348), issued a report in 1978 that is referred to as the **Belmont Report**, which provided a model for many of the guidelines adopted by disciplinary organizations in the United States. The *Belmont Report* also served as the basis for regulations affecting research sponsored by the U.S. government, including studies supported by the National Institute of Nursing Research (NINR). The U.S. Department of Health and Human Services (DHHS) has issued ethical regulations that have been codified at Title 45, Part 46 of the Code of Federal Regulations (45CFR46). These regulations, revised most recently in 2005, are among the most widely used guidelines in the United States for evaluating the ethical aspects of studies in most disciplines.

Ethical Dilemmas in Conducting Research

Research that violates ethical principles is rarely done specifically to be cruel or immoral, but more typically occurs out of a conviction that knowledge is important and potentially life-saving or beneficial to others in the long run. There are research problems in which participants' rights and study demands are put in direct conflict, posing **ethical dilemmas** for researchers. Here are examples of research problems in which the desire for rigor conflicts with ethical considerations:

1. *Research question:* Are nurses equally empathic in their treatment of male and female patients in the ICU?
   Ethical dilemma: Ethics require that participants be cognizant of their role in a study. Yet if the researcher informs nurses participating in this study that their degree of empathy in treating male and female ICU patients will be scrutinized, will their behavior be "normal?" If the nurses' usual behavior is altered because of the known presence of research observers, then the findings will not be valid.

2. *Research question:* What are the coping mechanisms of parents whose children have a terminal illness?
   Ethical dilemma: To answer this question, the researcher may need to probe into the psychological state of the parents at a vulnerable time in their lives; such probing could be painful and even traumatic. Yet knowledge of the parents' coping mechanisms might help to design more effective ways of dealing with parents' grief and stress.

3. *Research question:* Does a new medication prolong life in patients with cancer?
   Ethical dilemma: The best way to test the effectiveness of an intervention is to administer the intervention to some participants but withhold it from others to see if differences between the groups emerge. However, if the intervention is untested (e.g., a new drug), the group receiving the intervention may be exposed to potentially hazardous side effects. On the other hand, the group *not* receiving the drug may be denied a beneficial treatment.

4. *Research question:* What is the process by which adult children adapt to the day-to-day stresses of caring for a parent with Alzheimer's disease?
   Ethical dilemma: In a qualitative study, which would be appropriate for this research question, a researcher may become so closely involved with participants that they become willing to share "secrets" and privileged information. Interviews can become confessions—sometimes of unseemly or even illegal or immoral behavior. In this example, suppose a woman admitted to physically abusing her mother—how does the researcher respond to that information without undermining a pledge of confidentiality? And, if the researcher divulges the information to appropriate authorities, how can a pledge of confidentiality be given in good faith to other participants?

As these examples suggest, researchers are sometimes in a bind. Their goal is to advance knowledge and develop the highest-quality evidence for practice, using the best methods available; however, they must also adhere to the dictates of ethical rules that have been developed to protect human rights. Another type of dilemma arises from the fact that nurse researchers may be confronted with conflict-of-interest situations, in which their expected behavior as nurses comes into conflict with the expected behavior of researchers (e.g., deviating from a standard research protocol to give needed assistance to a patient). It is precisely because of such conflicts and dilemmas that codes of ethics have been developed to guide the efforts of researchers.

ETHICAL PRINCIPLES FOR PROTECTING STUDY PARTICIPANTS

The *Belmont Report* articulated three primary ethical principles on which standards of ethical conduct in research are based: beneficence, respect for human dignity, and justice. We briefly discuss these principles and then describe procedures researchers adopt to comply with these principles.

Beneficence

One of the most fundamental ethical principles in research is that of **beneficence**, which imposes a duty on researchers to minimize harm and to maximize benefits. Human research should be intended to produce benefits for participants themselves or—a situation that is more common—for other individuals or society as a whole. This principle covers multiple dimensions.

The Right to Freedom From Harm and Discomfort

Researchers have an obligation to avoid, prevent, or minimize harm (*nonmaleficence*) in studies with humans. Participants must not be subjected to unnecessary risks for harm or discomfort, and their participation in research must be essential to achieving scientifically and societally important aims that could not otherwise be realized. In research with humans, *harm* and *discomfort* can take many forms: they can be physical (e.g., injury, fatigue), emotional (e.g., stress, fear), social (e.g., loss of social support), or financial (e.g., loss of wages). Ethical researchers must use strategies to minimize all types of harms and discomforts, even ones that are temporary. Such strategies are especially important when the research involves a test of an innovative intervention or therapy.

Research should be conducted only by qualified people, especially if potentially dangerous technical equipment or specialized procedures are used. Ethical researchers must be prepared to terminate the research if there is reason to suspect that continuation would result in injury, death, disability, or undue distress to study participants. When a new medical procedure or drug is being tested, it is almost always advisable to experiment with animals or tissue cultures before proceeding to tests with humans. (Ethical guidelines relating to the treatment of animal subjects are discussed later in this chapter.)

Although protecting human beings from physical harm may be straightforward, the psychological consequences of participating in a study are usually subtle and thus require close attention and sensitivity. For example, participants may be asked questions about their personal views, weaknesses, or fears. Such queries might lead people to reveal sensitive personal information. The point is not that researchers should refrain from asking questions but rather that they need to be aware of the nature of the intrusion on people's psyches.

The need for sensitivity may be greater in qualitative studies, which often involve in-depth exploration into highly personal areas. In-depth probing may expose deep-seated fears and anxieties that study participants had previously repressed. Qualitative researchers, regardless of the underlying research tradition, must thus be especially vigilant in anticipating such problems.

Example of intense self-scrutiny in a qualitative study: Caelli (2001) conducted a phenomenological study to illuminate nurses' understandings of health, and how such understandings translated into nursing practice. One participant, having explored her experience of health with the researcher over several interview sessions, resigned from her city hospital job as a result of gaining a new recognition of the role health played in her life.

The Right to Protection From Exploitation

Involvement in a research study should not place participants at a disadvantage or expose them to situations for which they have not been prepared. Participants need to be assured that their participation, or information they might provide, will not be used against them in any way. For example, a person describing his or her economic circumstances to a researcher should not be exposed to the risk of losing public health care benefits; a person reporting illegal drug use should not fear exposure to criminal authorities.

Study participants enter into a special relationship with researchers, and it is crucial that this relationship not be exploited. Exploitation may be overt and malicious (e.g., sexual exploitation, use of subjects' identifying information to create a mailing list, and use of donated blood for the development of a commercial product), but it might also be more subtle. For example, suppose subjects agreed to participate in a study requiring 30 minutes of their time and that the researcher decided 1 year later to go back to them, to follow their progress or circumstances. Unless the researcher had previously explained to participants that there might be a follow-up study, the researcher might be accused of not adhering to the agreement previously reached and of exploiting the researcher–participant relationship.

Because nurse researchers may have a nurse–patient (in addition to a researcher–participant) relationship, special care may need to be exercised to avoid exploiting that bond. Patients' consent to participate in a study may result from their understanding of the researcher's role as *nurse*, not as *researcher*.

In qualitative research, the risk for exploitation may become especially acute because the psychological distance between investigators and participants typically declines as the study progresses. The emergence of a pseudotherapeutic relationship is not uncommon, which imposes additional responsibilities on researchers—and additional risks that exploitation could inadvertently occur. On the other hand, qualitative researchers typically are in a better position than quantitative researchers to *do good*, rather than just to avoid doing harm, because of the close relationships they often develop with participants. Munhall (2001) has argued that qualitative nurse researchers have the responsibility of ensuring that the "therapeutic imperative of nursing (advocacy) takes precedent over the research imperative (advancing knowledge) if conflict develops" (p. 538).

Example of therapeutic research experiences: Beck (2005) documented that participants in one of her studies on birth trauma and posttraumatic stress disorder (PTSD) expressed a range of benefits they derived from e-mail exchanges with Beck during the study. Here is what one informant voluntarily shared: "You thanked me for everything in your e-mail, and I want to THANK YOU for caring. For me, it means a lot that you have taken an interest in this subject and are taking the time and effort to find out more about PTSD. For someone to even acknowledge this condition means a lot for someone who has suffered from it" (p. 417). (Beck's PTSD report is included in its entirety in the accompanying Resource Manual.)

Respect for Human Dignity

Respect for human dignity is the second ethical principle articulated in the *Belmont Report*. This principle includes the right to self-determination and the right to full disclosure.

The Right to Self-Determination

Humans should be treated as autonomous agents, capable of controlling their own activities. The principle of **self-determination** means that prospective participants have the right to decide voluntarily whether to participate in a study, without risking any penalty or prejudicial treatment. It also means that people have the right to ask questions, to refuse to give information, or to withdraw from the study.

A person's right to self-determination includes freedom from coercion of any type. **Coercion** involves explicit or implicit threats of penalty from failing to participate in a study or excessive rewards from agreeing to participate. The obligation to protect people from coercion requires careful thought when the researcher is in a position of authority, control, or influence over potential participants, as might often be the case in a nurse–patient relationship. The issue of coercion may require scrutiny even when there is not a preestablished relationship. For example, a generous monetary incentive (or **stipend**) offered to encourage the participation of an economically disadvantaged group (e.g., the homeless) might be considered mildly coercive because such incentives may place undue pressure on prospective participants.

The Right to Full Disclosure

The principle of respect for human dignity encompasses people's right to make informed, voluntary decisions about study participation, which requires full disclosure. **Full disclosure** means that the researcher has fully described the nature of the study, the person's right to refuse participation, the researcher's responsibilities, and likely risks and benefits. The right to self-determination and the right to full disclosure are the two major elements on which informed consent—discussed later in this chapter—is based.

Adherence to the guideline for full disclosure is not always straightforward. Full disclosure can sometimes create two types of bias: first, biases resulting from inaccurate data, and second, a bias resulting from sample recruitment problems. Suppose we were testing the hypothesis that high school students with a high rate of absenteeism are more likely to be substance abusers than students with good attendance. If we approached potential participants and fully explained the purpose of the study, some students likely would refuse to partici-

pate, and nonparticipation would be selective; those least likely to volunteer for such a study might well be students who are substance abusers—the very group of primary interest. Moreover, by knowing the research question, those who do participate might not give candid responses. In such a situation, full disclosure could undermine the study.

One technique that researchers sometimes use in such situations is **covert data collection** or **concealment**—the collection of information without participants' knowledge and thus without their consent. This might happen, for example, if a researcher wanted to observe people's behavior in a real-world setting and was concerned that doing so openly would result in changes in the very behavior of interest. Researchers might choose to obtain the information through concealed methods, such as by observing through a one-way mirror, videotaping with hidden equipment, or observing while pretending to be engaged in other activities. In general, covert data collection may be acceptable as long as risks are negligible and participants' right to privacy has not been violated. Covert data collection is least likely to be ethically acceptable if the research is focused on sensitive aspects of people's behavior, such as drug use, sexual conduct, or illegal acts.

A more controversial technique is the use of deception. **Deception** can involve deliberately withholding information about the study, or providing participants with false information. For example, in studying high school students' use of drugs, we might describe the research as a study of students' health practices, which is a mild form of misinformation.

Deception and concealment are problematic ethically because they interfere with participants' right to make truly informed decisions about personal costs and benefits of participation. Some people argue that deception is never justified. Others, however, believe that if the study involves minimal risk to subjects and if there are anticipated benefits to the profession and society, then deception may be justified to enhance the validity of the findings. ANA guidelines offer this advice about deception and concealment:

• • •

The investigator understands that concealment or deception in research is controversial, depending on the type of research. Some investigators believe that concealment or deception in research can never be morally justified. The investigator further understands that before concealment or deception is used, certain criteria must be met: (1) The study must be of such small risk to the research participant and of such great significance to the advancement of the public good that concealment or deception can be morally justified.... (2) The acceptability of concealment or deception is related to the degree of risks to research participants.... (3) Concealment or deception are used only as last resorts, when no other approach can ensure the validity of the study's findings.... (4) The investigator has a moral responsibility to inform research participants of any concealment or deception as soon as possible and to explain the rationale for its use (Silva, 1995, p. 10, Section 4.2).

• • •

Another issue relating to the principle of respect that has emerged in this new era of electronic communications concerns the collection of data from people over the Internet. For example, some researchers are analyzing the content of messages posted to chat rooms or on listserves. The issue is whether such messages can be used as data without the authors' permission and their informed consent. Some researchers believe that anything posted electronically is in the public domain and therefore can be used without consent for purposes of research. Others, however, feel that the same ethical standards must apply in cyberspace research and that electronic researchers must carefully protect the rights of individuals who are participants in "virtual" communities. Schrum (1995) has offered some ethical guidelines for use by such researchers. As one example, she advocated that researchers, before collecting electronic data, negotiate their entry into an electronic community (e.g., a chat room) with the list owner. Sixsmith and Murray (2001) also warn researchers that obtaining consent from list moderators does not necessarily mean that every member of the listserve or chat room has pro-

vided consent. Researchers should periodically remind members of the online group of their presence at the site. Additional guidance for the ethical conduct of health-related research on the Internet has been developed by Im and Chee (2002) and Flicker, Haans, and Skinner (2004).

Justice

The third broad principle articulated in the *Belmont Report* concerns justice, which includes participants' right to fair treatment and their right to privacy.

The Right to Fair Treatment

Justice connotes fairness and equity, and so one aspect of the justice principle concerns the equitable distribution of benefits and burdens of research. The selection of study participants should be based on research requirements and not on the vulnerability or compromised position of certain people. Historically, subject selection has been a key ethical concern, with many researchers selecting groups deemed to have lower social standing (e.g., poor people, prisoners, slaves, the mentally retarded) as study participants. The principle of justice imposes particular obligations toward individuals who are unable to protect their own interests (e.g., dying patients) to ensure that they are not exploited for the advancement of knowledge.

Distributive justice also imposes duties to neither neglect nor discriminate against individuals and groups who may benefit from advances in research. During the 1980s and early 1990s, there was growing evidence that women and minorities were being unfairly *excluded* from many clinical studies in the United States. This led to the promulgation of regulations (updated in 2001) requiring that researchers who seek funding from the National Institutes of Health (NIH; including NINR) include women and minorities as study participants. The regulations also require researchers to examine whether clinical interventions had any differential effects (e.g., whether benefits were different for men than for women).

The principle of fair treatment covers issues other than subject selection. For example, the right to fair treatment means that researchers must treat people who decline to participate in a study (or who withdraw from the study after agreeing to participate) in a nonprejudicial manner; that they must honor all agreements made with participants (including the payment of any promised stipends); that they demonstrate sensitivity to and respect for the beliefs, habits, and lifestyles of people from different backgrounds or cultures; that they give participants access to research personnel for any desired clarification; and that they afford participants courteous and tactful treatment at all times.

The Right to Privacy

Virtually all research with humans involves intruding into personal lives. Researchers should ensure that their research is not more intrusive than it needs to be and that participants' privacy is maintained throughout the study. Participants have the right to expect that any data they provide will be kept in strictest confidence.

Privacy issues have become even more salient in the U.S. health care community since the passage of the Health Insurance Portability and Accountability Act of 1996 (HIPAA), which articulates federal standards to protect patients' medical records and other health information. In response to the congressional mandate in the HIPAA legislation, the U.S. Department of Health and Human Services issued the regulations *Standards for Privacy of Individually Identifiable Health Information.* For most covered entities (health care providers who transmit health information electronically), compliance with these regulations, known as the Privacy Rule, was required as of April 14, 2003.

➲ **TIP:** Some information relevant to researchers' compliance with HIPAA is presented in this chapter, but you should confer with any organizations that are involved in the research (if they are covered entities) regarding their practices and policies relating to HIPAA provisions. Also, there are websites that provide extensive information about the implications of HIPAA for health research: *http://privacyruleandresearch.nih.gov* and *http://www.hhs.gov/ocr/hipaa/guidelines/research.pdf*

PROCEDURES FOR PROTECTING STUDY PARTICIPANTS

Now that you are familiar with fundamental ethical principles for conducting research, you need to understand the procedures researchers follow to adhere to them.

Risk/Benefit Assessments

One of the strategies that researchers use to protect study participants is to conduct a **risk/benefit assessment**. Such an assessment is designed to determine whether the benefits of participating in a study are in line with the costs, be they financial, physical, emotional, or social—that is, whether the *risk/benefit ratio* is acceptable. The assessment of risks and benefits that individual participants might experience should be shared with them so that they can evaluate whether it is in their best interest to participate. Box 7.1 summarizes major costs and benefits of research participation.

➲ **TIP:** The Toolkit with the accompanying *Resource Manual* includes a Word document with the factors in Box 7.1 arranged in worksheet form for you to complete in doing a risk/benefit assessment. By completing the worksheet, it may be easier for you to envision opportunities for "doing good" and to avoid possibilities of doing harm.

The risk/benefit ratio should also be considered in terms of whether the risks to participants are commensurate with the benefit to society and the nursing profession in terms of the quality of evidence produced. The general guideline is that the degree of risk to be taken by those participating in the research should never exceed the potential humanitarian benefits of the knowledge to be gained. Thus, the selection of a significant topic that has the potential to improve patient care is the first step in ensuring that research is ethical.

BOX 7.1 Potential Benefits and Risks of Research to Participants

MAJOR POTENTIAL BENEFITS TO PARTICIPANTS

- Access to a potentially beneficial intervention that might otherwise be unavailable to them
- Comfort in being able to discuss their situation or problem with a friendly, objective person
- Increased knowledge about themselves or their condition, either through opportunity for introspection and self-reflection or through direct interaction with researchers
- Escape from normal routine, excitement of being part of a study
- Satisfaction that information they provide may help others with similar problems or conditions
- Direct monetary or material gains through stipends or other incentives

MAJOR POTENTIAL RISKS TO PARTICIPANTS

- Physical harm, including unanticipated side effects
- Physical discomfort, fatigue, or boredom
- Psychological or emotional distress resulting from self-disclosure, introspection, fear of the unknown, discomfort with strangers, fear of eventual repercussions, anger or embarrassment at the type of questions being asked
- Social risks, such as the risk for stigma, adverse effects on personal relationships, loss of status
- Loss of privacy
- Loss of time
- Monetary costs (e.g., for transportation, child care, time lost from work)

All research involves some risks, but in many cases, the risk is minimal. **Minimal risk** is defined as risks anticipated to be no greater than those ordinarily encountered in daily life or during routine physical or psychological tests or procedures. When the risks are not minimal, researchers must proceed with caution, taking every step possible to reduce risks and maximize benefits. If the perceived risks and costs to participants outweigh the anticipated benefits of the study, the research should either be abandoned or redesigned.

In quantitative studies, most of the details of the study are usually spelled out in advance, and therefore a reasonably accurate risk/benefit ratio assessment can be developed. Qualitative studies, however, usually evolve as data are gathered, and it may therefore be more difficult to assess all risks at the outset of a study. Qualitative researchers thus must remain sensitive to potential risks throughout the research process.

Example of risk/benefit assessment: Hentz (2002) studied the phenomenon of *body memory* following the loss of a loved one. Here is how she described risks and benefits: "One of the benefits for the participants was the ability to share experiences with someone interested and concerned. The other benefit was in knowing that the participants' stories may help others facing similar experiences. The actual interview often evoked strong emotions; however, many of the participants commented that they felt better having told their stories. Having their stories heard and acknowledged was experienced by participants as therapeutic." (p. 165).

Box 7.1 ⊗ indicates that one potential benefit to participants is monetary. Stipends offered to prospective participants are rarely viewed as an opportunity for financial gain, but there is considerable evidence that stipends are useful as an incentive to participation. Stipends used as a financial incentive appear to be especially effective when the group under study is difficult to recruit, when the study is time-consuming or tedious, or when there are study-related costs to participants such as for transportation. Stipends range from $1 to hundreds of dollars, but most are in the $20 to $30 range.

➲ **TIP:** In evaluating the anticipated risk/benefit ratio of a study design, you might want to consider how comfortable *you* would feel about being a study participant.

Informed Consent and Participant Authorization

One particularly important procedure for safeguarding participants and protecting their right to self-determination involves obtaining their informed consent. **Informed consent** means that participants have adequate information regarding the research, are capable of comprehending the information, and have the power of free choice, enabling them to consent to or decline participation voluntarily. This section discusses procedures for obtaining informed consent and for complying with HIPAA rules regarding accessing patients' health information.

The Content of Informed Consent

Fully informed consent involves communicating the following pieces of information to participants:

1. *Participant status.* Prospective participants need to understand clearly the distinction between *research* and *treatment.* They should be told which health care activities are routine and which are implemented specifically for the study. They also should be informed that data they provide will be used for research purposes.
2. *Study goals.* The overall goals of the research should be stated, in lay rather than technical terms. The use to which the data will be put should be described.
3. *Type of data.* Prospective participants should be told the type of data that will be collected.
4. *Procedures.* Prospective participants should be given a description of the data collection procedures, and of the procedures to be used in any innovative treatment.

5. *Nature of the commitment.* Information should be provided regarding participants' estimated time commitment at each point of contact, and the number of contacts within specified timeframes.
6. *Sponsorship.* Information on who is sponsoring or funding the study should be noted; if the research is part of an academic requirement, this information should be shared.
7. *Participant selection.* Researchers should explain how prospective participants were selected for recruitment, and how many people will be participating.
8. *Potential risks.* Prospective participants should be informed of any foreseeable risks (physical, psychological, social, or economic) or discomforts that might be incurred as a result of participation, and any efforts that will be taken to minimize risks. The possibility of unforeseeable risks should also be discussed, if appropriate. If injury or damage is possible, treatments that will be made available to participants should be described. When risks are more than minimal, prospective participants should be encouraged to seek the advice of others before consenting.
9. *Potential benefits.* Specific benefits to participants, if any, should be described, as well as possible benefits to others.
10. *Alternatives.* If appropriate, researchers should provide information about alternative procedures or treatments that might be advantageous to participants.
11. *Compensation.* If stipends or reimbursements are to be paid (or if treatments are offered without fee), these arrangements should be discussed.
12. *Confidentiality pledge.* Prospective participants should be assured that their privacy will at all times be protected. If anonymity can be guaranteed, this should be noted.
13. *Voluntary consent.* Researchers should indicate that participation is strictly voluntary and that failure to volunteer will not result in any penalty or loss of benefits.
14. *Right to withdraw and withhold information.* Prospective participants should be told that even after consenting, they have the right to

withdraw from the study and to refuse to provide any specific piece of information. Researchers may, in some cases, need to provide participants with a description of circumstances under which researchers would terminate the overall study.

15. *Contact information.* The researcher should provide information on whom participants could contact in the event of further questions, comments, or complaints.

In qualitative studies, especially those requiring repeated contact with the same participants, it may be difficult to obtain meaningful informed consent at the outset. Qualitative researchers do not always know in advance how the study will evolve. Because the research design emerges during the data collection and analysis process, researchers may not know the exact nature of the data to be collected, what the risks and benefits to participants will be, or how much of a time commitment they will be expected to make. Thus, in a qualitative study, consent is often viewed as an ongoing, transactional process, referred to as **process consent**. In process consent, the researcher continually renegotiates the consent, allowing participants to play a collaborative role in the decision-making process regarding ongoing participation.

Example of process consent: Wuest and colleagues (2003) studied the health promotion processes of single-parent families after leaving abusive partners or fathers. Tape-recorded interviews were conducted with 36 mothers in a location of their choice; each woman gave informed consent before participation. As data analysis proceeded, the researchers conducted second interviews with each family. On repeat interviews, consent was reconfirmed.

Comprehension of Informed Consent
Consent information is normally presented to prospective participants while they are being recruited, either orally or in writing. A written notice should not, however, take the place of spoken explanations. Oral presentations provide opportunities for greater elaboration and for participant questioning.

Because informed consent is based on a person's evaluation of the potential risks and benefits of participation, it is important that the critical information be not only communicated but also understood. Researchers must assume the role of teacher in communicating consent information. They should be careful to use simple language and to avoid jargon and technical terms whenever possible; they should also avoid biased language that might unduly influence the person's decision to participate. Written statements should be consistent with the participants' reading levels and educational attainment. For participants from a general population (e.g., patients in a hospital), the statement should be written at about the seventh- or eighth-grade reading level.

For studies involving more than minimal risk, researchers need to make special efforts to ensure that prospective participants understand what participation will involve. In some cases, this might involve testing participants for their comprehension of the informed consent material before deeming them eligible for participation.

Documentation of Informed Consent
Researchers usually document the informed consent process by having participants sign a **consent form**. In the United States, federal regulations covering studies funded by government agencies require written consent of human subjects, except under certain circumstances. In particular, when the study does not involve an intervention and data are collected anonymously—or when existing data from records or specimens are used and identifying information is not linked to the data—regulations requiring written informed consent do not apply. HIPAA legislation is explicit about the type of information that must be eliminated from patient records for the data to be considered **de-identified**.

The consent form should contain all the information essential to informed consent. Prospective participants (or their legally authorized representative) should have ample time to review the written document before signing it. The document should also be signed by the researcher, and a copy should be retained by both parties.

An example of a written consent form used in a study of one of the authors is presented in Figure 7.1. ✖ The numbers in the margins of this figure correspond to the types of information for informed consent outlined earlier. (Note that the form does not indicate how subjects were selected, because this is implied in the study purpose, and prospective participants knew they were recruited from a support group for mothers of multiples.)

➡ **TIP:** In developing a consent form, the following suggestions might prove helpful:

1. Organize the form coherently so that prospective participants can follow the logic of what is being communicated. If the form is complex, use headings as an organizational aid.
2. Use a large enough font so that the form can be easily read, and use spacing that avoids making the document appear too dense. Make the form as attractive and inviting as possible.
3. In general, simplify. Use clear and consistent terminology, and avoid technical terms if possible. If technical terms are needed, include definitions.
4. If possible, use a **readability formula** to estimate the form's reading level, and make revisions to ensure an appropriate reading level for the group under study. There are several such formulas, the most widely used being the FOG Index (Gunning, 1968), the SMOG index (McLaughlin, 1969), and the Flesch Reading Ease score and Flesch-Kincaid grade level score (Flesch, 1948). Specialized software (e.g., RightWriter) is available, and some word-processing software (e.g., Microsoft Word) also provides readability information.
5. Test the form with people similar to those who will be recruited, and ask for feedback.

If the informed consent information is lengthy, researchers whose studies are funded by U.S. government agencies have the option of presenting the full information orally and then summarizing essential information in a **short form**. If a short form is used, however, the oral presentation must be witnessed by a third party, and the signature of the witness must appear on the short consent form. The signature of a third-party witness is also advisable in studies involving more than minimal risk, even when a long and comprehensive consent form is used.

For studies that are not government sponsored, researchers should err on the side of being conservative. They should implement consent procedures that fully adhere to the principle that prospective participants can make good decisions about participation only if they are fully informed about the study's risks and benefits.

One additional note is that when the primary means of data collection is through a self-administered questionnaire, some researchers opt not to obtain written informed consent because they assume **implied consent** (i.e., that the return of the completed questionnaire reflects voluntary consent to participate). This assumption, however, may not always be warranted (e.g., if patients feel that their treatment might be affected by failure to cooperate with the researcher).

➡ **TIP:** The Toolkit with the accompanying *Resource Manual* includes the informed consent form in Figure 7.1, and an additional informed consent form, in a Word document so that the forms can easily be adapted for your use. The Toolkit also includes several other resources designed to help you with the ethical aspects of a study.

Authorization to Access Private Health Information

Under HIPAA regulations, a covered entity such as a hospital can disclose individually identifiable health information (IIHI) from its records if the patient signs an authorization granting access. The authorization can be incorporated into the consent form, or it can be a separate document. ✖ Using a separate authorization form may be advantageous to protect the patients' confidentiality because the authorization form does not need to provide detailed information about the purpose of the

Informed Consent Form

1 2 3,5 4 12 11 8	I understand that I am being asked to participate in a research study at Saint Francis Hospital and Medical Center. This research study will evaluate: What it is like being a mother of multiples during the first year of the infants' lives. If I agree to participate in the study, I will be interviewed for approximately 30 to 60 minutes about my experience as a mother of multiple infants. The interview will be tape-recorded and take place in a private office at Saint Francis Hospital. No identifying information will be included when the interview is transcribed. I understand I will receive $25.00 for participating in the study. There are no known risks associated with this study.
7	I realize that I may not participate in the study if I am younger than 18 years of age or I cannot speak English.
10	I realize that the knowledge gained from this study may help either me or other mothers of multiple infants in the future.
13 14	I realize that my participation in this study is entirely voluntary, and I may withdraw from the study at any time I wish. If I decide to discontinue my participation in this study, I will continue to be treated in the usual and customary fashion.
12	I understand that all study data will be kept confidential. However, this information may be used in nursing publications or presentations.
8	I understand that if I sustain injuries from my participation in this research project, I will not be automatically compensated by Saint Francis Hospital and Medical Center.
15	If I need to, I can contact Dr. Cheryl Beck, University of Connecticut, School of Nursing, any time during the study.
1,2	The study has been explained to me. I have read and understand this consent form, all of my questions have been answered, and I agree to participate. I understand that I will be given a copy of this signed consent form.

_____   _____
Signature of Subject   Date

_____   _____
Signature of Witness   Date

_____   _____
Signature of Investigator   Date

FIGURE 7.1 ⊗ Example of an informed consent form.

research. If the research purpose is not sensitive, or if the hospital or entity is already cognizant of the study purpose, an integrated authorization and consent form should suffice.

The authorization, whether obtained separately or included in the consent form, must include the following information: (1) who will receive the information; (2) what type of information will be disclosed; and (3) what further disclosures the researcher anticipates. The need for patient authorization to access IIHI can be waived only under certain circumstances. It is important to note that patient authorization usually must be obtained for data that are *created* as part of the research, as well as for information already maintained in institutional records (Olsen, 2003).

Confidentiality Procedures

Study participants have the right to expect that any data they provide will be kept in the strictest confidence. Participants' right to privacy is protected through various confidentiality procedures.

Anonymity

Anonymity, the most secure means of protecting confidentiality, occurs when even the researcher cannot link participants to their data. For example, if questionnaires were distributed to a group of nursing home residents and were returned without any identifying information on them, responses would be anonymous. As another example, if a researcher reviewed hospital records from which all identifying information (e.g., name, address, social security number, and so forth) had been expunged, anonymity would again protect participants' right to privacy. Whenever it is possible to achieve anonymity, researchers should strive to do so. Distributed questionnaires through the mail, to groups of participants, or over the Internet are especially conducive to anonymity.

> **Example of anonymity:** Suzuki and colleagues (2005) distributed an anonymous questionnaire to more than 4000 nurses in eight large hospitals in Japan to investigate the nurses' sleep patterns, daytime sleepiness, and experience of occupational accidents and medical error.

Confidentiality in the Absence of Anonymity

When anonymity is impossible, appropriate confidentiality procedures need to be implemented. A promise of **confidentiality** is a pledge that any information participants provide will not be publicly reported in a manner that identifies them and will not be made accessible to others. This means that research information should not be shared with strangers, nor with people known to the participants (e.g., family members, physicians, other nurses), unless the participant gives the researcher explicit permission to do so.

Researchers can take a number of steps to ensure that a *breach of confidentiality* does not occur, including the following:

- Obtain identifying information (e.g., name, address) from participants only when essential.
- Assign an **identification** (ID) **number** to each participant and attach the ID number rather than other identifiers to the actual data.
- Maintain identifying information in a locked file.
- Restrict access to identifying information to a small number of people on a need-to-know basis.
- Enter no identifying information onto computer files.
- Destroy identifying information as quickly as practical.
- Make research personnel sign confidentiality pledges if they have access to data or identifying information. ✪
- Report research information in the aggregate; if information for a specific participant is reported, take steps to disguise the person's identity, such as through the use of a fictitious name.

➲ **TIP:** Researchers who plan to collect data from study participants on multiple occasions (or who use multiple data forms that need to be linked) might think that anonymity is not possible because of the need to link information from different sources. However, a technique that has been successfully used is to have participants themselves generate an ID number. They might be instructed, for example, to use their birth year and the first three letters of their mother's maiden names as their ID code (e.g., 1946CRU). This code would be put on every form participants complete, but researchers would not know participants' identities.

Qualitative researchers may need to take extra steps to safeguard the privacy of their participants. Anonymity is almost never possible in qualitative studies because researchers typically become closely involved with participants. Moreover, because of the in-depth nature of qualitative studies, there may be a greater invasion of privacy than is true in quantitative research. Researchers who spend time in the home of a participant may, for example, have difficulty segregating the public behaviors that the participant is willing to share from the private behaviors that unfold unwittingly during the course of data collection. A final issue is adequately disguising participants in research reports. Because the number of respondents is small, qualitative researchers may need to take considerable precautions to safeguard identities. This may mean more than simply using a fictitious name. Qualitative researchers may have to slightly distort identifying information in their reports, or provide only general descriptions. For example, a 49-year-old antique dealer with ovarian cancer might be described as "a middle-aged cancer patient who worked in retail sales" to avoid identification that could occur with the more detailed description.

⊃ **TIP:** As a means of enhancing both individual and institutional privacy, research reports frequently avoid giving explicit information about the locale of the study. For example, the report might say that data were collected in a 200-bed, private, for-profit nursing home, without mentioning its name or location.

Example of confidentiality procedures in a qualitative study: Spiers (2002) described interpersonal contexts in which care was negotiated between home care nurses and their patients. Her qualitative study was based on an analysis of 31 videotaped home visits. The video portion of the tapes was not altered, inasmuch as the researcher wanted to analyze facial expressions. However, any audio containing names or other identifying information was removed in dubbed tapes. Pseudonyms were used in the transcripts.

Certificates of Confidentiality

There are situations in which confidentiality can create tensions between researchers and legal or other authorities, especially if study participants are involved in criminal or dangerous activity (e.g., substance abuse, unprotected sexual intercourse). To avoid the possibility of forced, involuntary disclosure of sensitive research information (e.g., through a court order or subpoena), researchers in the United States can apply for a **Certificate of Confidentiality** from the NIH (Lutz et al., 2000). Any research that involves the collection of personally identifiable, sensitive information is potentially eligible for a Certificate, even if the study is not receiving federal funding. Information is considered sensitive if its release might damage the person's financial standing, employability, or reputation or might lead to discrimination; information about a person's mental health, as well as genetic information, is also considered sensitive.

A Certificate of Confidentiality protects the forced disclosure of research information in a wide range of situations. A Certificate allows researchers and others who have access to research data to refuse to disclose identifying information on study participants in any civil, criminal, administrative, or legislative proceeding at the federal, state, or local level.

A Certificate of Confidentiality helps researchers to achieve their research objectives without threat of involuntary disclosure and thus can be helpful in recruiting study participants. Researchers who obtain a Certificate of Confidentiality should alert prospective participants about this valuable protection in the consent form, and should also note any planned exceptions to those protections. For example, a researcher might decide to voluntarily comply with state child abuse reporting laws even though the Certificate would prevent authorities from punishing researchers who chose not to comply.

Example of obtaining a Certificate of Confidentiality: Hatton and Kaiser (2004) described a range of ethical issues that arose in a study that tested an intervention with homeless women living in a transitional shelter. The researchers obtained a Certificate of Confidentiality because they recognized that many participants would have histories of illegal activities. Nevertheless, they voluntarily complied with California's statutes that required reporting harm to self and others and abuse, and informed participants of this fact during the informed consent process. (This study is described in greater detail in Chapter 8).

Example of referrals: Neufeld and Harrison (2003) studied appraisals of support among women caring for a family member with dementia. The research involved a series of interviews over an 18-month period with the women caregivers. Referrals to mental health or other support services were available to study participants who expressed a need.

Debriefings and Referrals

Researchers can often show their respect for study participants—and proactively minimize emotional risks—by carefully attending to the nature of the interactions they have with them. For example, researchers should always be gracious and polite, should phrase questions tactfully, and should be sensitive to cultural and linguistic diversity.

There are also more formal strategies that researchers can use to communicate their respect and concern for participants' well-being. For example, it is sometimes advisable to offer **debriefing** sessions after data collection is completed to permit participants to ask questions or air complaints. Debriefing is especially important when the data collection has been stressful or when ethical guidelines had to be "bent" (e.g., if any deception was used in explaining the study).

Example of debriefing: Sandgren and colleagues (2006) studied the strategies that palliative cancer nurses used to avoid being emotionally overloaded. They conducted in-depth interviews with 46 nurses, and after each interview "we made sure that the participants were doing well, and we assessed possible needs for emotional support" (p. 81).

Researchers can also demonstrate their interest in study participants by offering to share study findings with them once the data have been analyzed (e.g., by mailing them a summary or advising them of an appropriate website). Finally, in some situations, researchers may need to assist study participants by making referrals to appropriate health, social, or psychological services.

Treatment of Vulnerable Groups

Adherence to ethical standards is often straightforward. However, the rights of special vulnerable groups may need to be protected through additional procedures and heightened sensitivity. **Vulnerable subjects** (the term used in U.S. federal guidelines) may be incapable of giving fully informed consent (e.g., mentally retarded people) or may be at high risk for unintended side effects because of their circumstances (e.g., pregnant women). Researchers interested in studying high-risk groups should become acquainted with guidelines governing informed consent, risk/benefit assessments, and acceptable research procedures for such groups. In general, research with vulnerable subjects should be undertaken only when the risk/benefit ratio is low or when there is no alternative (e.g., studies of childhood development require child participants).

Among the groups that nurse researchers should consider as being vulnerable are the following:

- *Children.* Legally and ethically, children do not have the competence to give informed consent, and so the informed consent of children's parents or legal guardians should be obtained. However, it is appropriate—especially if the child is at least 7 years of age—to obtain the child's assent as well. **Assent** refers to the child's affirmative agreement to participate. If the child is developmentally mature enough to understand the basic information involved in informed consent (e.g., a 12-year-old), it is advisable to obtain written assent from the child as well, as evidence of respect for the child's right to self-determination. ✹ Lindeke, Hauck, and Tanner (2000) and Broome (1999) provide guidance regarding children's assent and consent to participate in research. The U.S. government has issued special regulations (Subpart D of the Code of Federal Regulations, 2005) for the additional protection of children as study participants.

- *Mentally or emotionally disabled people.* Individuals whose disability makes it impossible for them to weigh the risks and benefits of participation and make an informed decision (e.g., people affected by cognitive impairment, mental illness, coma, and so on) also cannot legally or ethically provide informed consent. In such cases, researchers should obtain the written consent of a legal guardian. Researchers should, however, be aware of the fact that a legal guardian may not necessarily have the person's best interests in mind. In such cases, informed consent should also be obtained from someone whose primary interest is the person's welfare. To the extent possible, informed consent or assent from prospective participants themselves should be sought as a supplement to consent by a guardian.

- *Severely ill or physically disabled people.* For patients who are very ill or undergoing certain treatments, it might be necessary to assess their ability to make reasoned decisions about study participation. For example, Higgins and Daly (1999) described a process they used to assess the decisional capacity of mechanically ventilated patients. Another issue is that for certain disabilities, special procedures for obtaining consent may be required. For example, with deaf participants, the entire consent process may need to be in writing. For people whose physical impairment prevents them from writing or for participants who cannot read and write, alternative procedures for documenting informed consent (such as audiotaping or videotaping consent proceedings) should be used.

- *The terminally ill.* Terminally ill people who participate in the study can seldom expect to benefit personally from the research, and thus the risk/benefit ratio needs to be carefully assessed. Researchers must also take steps to ensure that if the terminally ill participate in the study, the health care and comfort of these individuals are not compromised. Special procedures may be required for obtaining informed consent if they are physically or mentally incapacitated.

- *Institutionalized people.* Nurses often conduct studies with institutionalized people. Particular care may be required in recruiting such people because they often depend on health care personnel and may feel pressured into participating or may feel that their treatment would be jeopardized by their failure to cooperate. Inmates of prisons and other correctional facilities, who have lost their autonomy in many spheres of activity, may similarly feel constrained in their ability to give free consent. The U.S. government has issued specific regulations for the protection of prisoners as study participants (see Code of Federal Regulations, 2005, Subpart C). Researchers studying institutionalized groups need to emphasize the voluntary nature of participation.

- *Pregnant women.* The U.S. government has issued stringent additional requirements governing research with pregnant women and fetuses (Code of Federal Regulations, 2005, Subpart B). These requirements reflect a desire to safeguard both the pregnant woman, who may be at heightened physical and psychological risk, and the fetus, who cannot give informed consent. The regulations stipulate that a pregnant woman cannot be involved in a study unless the purpose of the research is to meet the health needs of the pregnant woman and risks to her and the fetus are minimized or there is only a minimal risk to the fetus.

Example of research with a vulnerable group: Anderson and colleagues (2001) conducted a study to explore perceptions of risk for HIV/AIDS among adolescents in juvenile detention. The researchers obtained approval to conduct the study from the presiding judge, the detention facility, and a human subjects committee at their own institution. The consent forms assured teens that their participation would be voluntary and would influence neither the duration of their detention nor their adjudication process. The data were collected in spaces that provided privacy for sound and afforded visual surveillance by probation staff.

It should go without saying that researchers need to proceed with extreme caution in conducting research with people who might fall into two or more vulnerable categories, as was the case in this example.

TIP: Jacobson (2005) has astutely pointed out the need to be vigilant on behalf of persons not traditionally identified as vulnerable, and therefore not covered in standard protocols regarding vulnerable participants. *Anybody* may be vulnerable at any given time due to acute illness or special circumstances that challenge the capacity to provide truly informed consent.

External Reviews and the Protection of Human Rights

Researchers may not be objective in assessing risk/benefit ratios or in developing procedures to protect participants' rights. Biases may arise as a result of the researchers' commitment to an area of knowledge and their desire to conduct a study with as much rigor as possible. Because of the risk of a biased evaluation, the ethical dimensions of a study should normally be subjected to external review.

Most hospitals, universities, and other institutions where research is conducted have established formal committees and protocols for reviewing proposed research plans before they are implemented. These committees are sometimes called *human subjects committees*, *ethical advisory boards*, or *research ethics committees*. In the United States, the committee likely will be called an **Institutional Review Board (IRB)**, whereas in Canada, the committees are called **Research Ethics Boards (REBs)**. In the United States, some institutions have established separate **Privacy Boards** to review researchers' compliance with provisions in HIPAA, including review of authorization forms and requests for waivers.

TIP: If the research is being conducted within an institution or with its help (e.g., assistance in recruiting subjects), you should find out early what the institution's requirements are regarding ethical issues, in terms of its forms, procedures, and review schedules. Many institutions, especially universities, offer free online tutorials on research ethics and review procedures.

In the United States, federally sponsored studies (including fellowships) are subject to strict guidelines for evaluating the treatment of human participants. Before undertaking such a study, researchers must submit research plans to the IRB, and must also go through a formal human subjects training and certification process that can be completed online. (The website to access training is included in the list of websites on the accompanying CD-ROM, and many universities provide direct links).

The duty of the IRB is to ensure that the proposed plans meet the federal requirements for ethical research. An IRB can approve the proposed plans, require modifications, or disapprove the plans. The main requirements governing IRB decisions may be summarized as follows (Code of Federal Regulations, 2005, §46.111):

- Risks to participants are minimized.
- Risks to participants are reasonable in relation to anticipated benefits, if any, and the importance of the knowledge that may reasonably be expected to result.
- Selection of participants is equitable.
- Informed consent will be sought, as required.
- Informed consent will be appropriately documented.
- Adequate provision is made for monitoring the research to ensure participants' safety.
- Appropriate provisions are made to protect participants' privacy and confidentiality of the data.
- When vulnerable groups are involved, appropriate additional safeguards are included to protect their rights and welfare.

Example of IRB approval: Long and her colleagues (2006) tested the effectiveness of a school-based nutrition education website specifically designed for minority adolescents genetically at risk for type 2 diabetes. The procedures and protocols for the study were approved by the IRB of the researchers' university and by the IRB of the Independent School District of the city where the school was located.

Many research projects require a full IRB review. For a full review, the IRB convenes meetings at which most IRB members are present. An IRB must have five or more members, at least one of whom is not a researcher (e.g., a member of the clergy or a lawyer may be appropriate). One IRB member must be a person who is not affiliated with the institution and is not a family member of a person who is affiliated. To protect against potential biases, the IRB cannot comprise entirely men, women, or members from a single profession.

For certain kinds of research involving no more than minimal risk, the IRB can use expedited review procedures, which do not require a meeting. In an **expedited review**, a single IRB member (usually the IRB chairperson or a member designated by the chairperson) carries out the review. An example of research that qualifies for an expedited IRB review is minimal-risk research "…employing survey, interview, focus group, program evaluation, human factors evaluation, or quality assurance methodologies" (Code of Federal Regulations, 2005, §46.110).

The federal regulations also allow certain types of research to be totally exempt from IRB review. These are studies in which there are no apparent risks to human participants. The website of the Office of Human Research Protections, in its policy guidance section, includes decision charts designed to clarify whether a study is exempt from the federal regulations.

➲ TIP: In the United States, when researchers apply for a Certificate of Confidentiality, they must first obtain IRB approval for their research because IRB approval is a prerequisite for the Certificate. Applications for the Certificate should be submitted at least 3 months before participants are expected to enroll in the study.

It might be noted that there has been some concern among qualitative researchers in various countries that the standard ethical review procedures and regulations established by government agencies are not sensitive to special issues and circumstances faced in qualitative research. There is concern that the regulations were "…created for quantitative work, and can actually impede or interrupt work that is not hypothesis-driven 'hard science'" (Van de Hoonaard, 2002, p. i). Thus, qualitative researchers may need to take extra care to explain their methods, rationales, and approaches to ethical conduct to review board members unfamiliar with qualitative research.

➲ TIP: It is sometimes suggested that qualitative researchers make a conscious effort to avoid using terms in the IRB proposal that members of the IRB, who typically are not qualitative researchers themselves, may not know. For example, instead of using the phenomenological term "lived experience," it may be preferable to just use the term "experience."

Not all research is subject to government guidelines, and so not all studies are reviewed by formal committees. Nevertheless, researchers must ensure that their research plans are ethically sound and are encouraged to seek outside advice on the ethical dimensions of a study before it gets underway. Advisors might include faculty members, the clergy, representatives from the group being asked to participate, or advocates for that group.

Building Ethics Into the Design of the Study

Researchers need to give careful thought to ethical requirements during the planning of a research project and should ask themselves continually whether planned safeguards for protecting humans are sufficient. They must persist in being vigilant throughout the implementation of the research plans as well because unforeseen ethical dilemmas may arise during the study. Of course, first steps in doing ethical research include scrutinizing the research question to determine whether it is clinically significant and designing the study in a manner that yields sound evidence—it can be construed as unethical to do poorly conceived or weakly designed research because it would be a poor use of people's time.

The remaining chapters of the book offer advice on how to design studies that yield high-quality evidence for practice. Methodologic decisions about rigor, however, must factor in ethical considerations. Box 7.2 lists some examples of the kinds of questions that might be posed in thinking about various aspects of study design.

TIP: Once the study procedures have been developed, researchers should undertake a self-evaluation of those procedures to determine whether they meet ethical requirements. Box 7.3, later in this chapter, provides some guidelines that can be used for such a self-evaluation.

OTHER ETHICAL ISSUES

In discussing ethical issues relating to the conduct of nursing research, we have given primary consideration to the protection of human study participants. Two other ethical issues also deserve mention: the treatment of animals in research and research misconduct.

Ethical Issues in Using Animals in Research

A small but growing number of nurse researchers use animals rather than human beings as their subjects, typically focusing on biophysiologic phenomena. Despite some opposition to such research by animal rights activists, it seems likely that researchers in health fields will continue to use animals to explore basic physiologic mechanisms and to test experimental interventions that could pose risks (as well as offer benefits) to humans.

Ethical considerations are clearly different for animals and humans; for example, the concept of *informed consent* is not relevant for animal subjects. Specific guidelines have been developed gov-

---

BOX 7.2 Examples of Questions for Building Ethics Into a Study Design

RESEARCH DESIGN

- Will participants be allocated to different treatment groups fairly?
- Will steps to reduce bias or enhance integrity add to the risks participants will incur?
- Will the setting for the study protect against participant discomfort?

INTERVENTION

- Is the intervention designed to maximize good and minimize harm?
- Under what conditions might a treatment be withdrawn or altered?

SAMPLE

- Is the population defined so as to unwittingly and unnecessarily exclude important segments of people (e.g., women, minorities)?
- Will potential participants be recruited into the study equitably?

DATA COLLECTION

- Will data be collected in such a way as to minimize respondent burden?
- Will procedures for ensuring confidentiality of data be adequate?
- Will data collection staff be appropriately trained to be sensitive and courteous?

REPORTING

- Will participants' identities be adequately protected?

BOX 7.3 Questions for Critiquing the Ethical Aspects of a Study

1. Was the study approved and monitored by an Institutional Review Board, Research Ethics Board, or other similar ethics review committee?
2. Were study participants subjected to any physical harm, discomfort, or psychological distress? Did the researchers take appropriate steps to remove or prevent harm?
3. Did the benefits to participants outweigh any potential risks or actual discomfort they experienced? Did the benefits to society outweigh the costs to participants?
4. Was any type of coercion or undue influence used to recruit participants? Did they have the right to refuse to participate or to withdraw without penalty?
5. Were participants deceived in any way? Were they fully aware of participating in a study, and did they understand the purpose and nature of the research?
6. Were appropriate informed consent procedures used with all participants? If not, were there valid and justifiable reasons?
7. Were adequate steps taken to safeguard the privacy of participants? How were data kept anonymous or confidential? Were Privacy Rule procedures followed (if applicable)? Was a Certificate of Confidentiality obtained?
8. Were vulnerable groups involved in the research? If yes, were special precautions instituted because of their vulnerable status?
9. Were groups omitted from the inquiry without a justifiable rationale (e.g., women, minorities)?

erning treatment of animal subjects. In the United States, the Public Health Service issued a policy statement on the humane care and use of animals, most recently amended in 2002. The guidelines articulate nine principles for the proper care and treatment of animals used in biomedical and behavioral research. These principles cover such issues as the transport of research animals, alternatives to using animals, pain and distress in animal subjects, researcher qualifications, use of appropriate anesthesia, and euthanizing animals under certain conditions during or after the study. In Canada, researchers who use animals in their studies must adhere to the policies and guidelines of the Canadian Council on Animal Care (CCAC) as articulated in the two-volume *Guide to the Care and Use of Experimental Animals.*

Holtzclaw and Hanneman (2002), in discussing the use of animals in nursing research, noted several important considerations. First, there must be a compelling reason to use an animal model—not simply convenience or novelty. Second, the study procedures should be humane, well planned, and well funded. They noted that animal studies are not necessarily less costly than those with human participants, and they require serious ethical and scientific consideration to justify their use.

Example of research with animals: Briones and her colleagues (2005) studied the effects of behavioral rehabilitation training following transient global cerebral ischemia on dentate gyrus neurogenesis using 72 adult male rats. They reported that "all efforts were made to minimize animal distress and to reduce the number of animals used" (p. 169). The experimental protocols were approved by an institutional animal care committee and were in accordance with federal guidelines on the use of animals in research.

Research Misconduct

Millions of movie-goers watched breathlessly as Dr. Richard Kimble (Harrison Ford) exposed the fraudulent scheme of a medical researcher in the film *The Fugitive*. The film reminds us that ethics in research involves not only the protection of the rights of human and animal subjects, but also protection of the public trust.

The issue of **research misconduct** (also referred to as *scientific misconduct*) has received increasing attention in recent years as incidents of researcher fraud and misrepresentation have come to light. Currently, the federal agency responsible for overseeing efforts to improve research integrity in the United States and for handling allegations of research misconduct is the Office of Research Integrity (ORI) within the Department of Health and Human Services, established in 1992.

Research misconduct, as defined by a U.S. Public Health Service regulation that was revised in 2005 (42 CFR Part 93, Subpart A), is "fabrication, falsification, or plagiarism in proposing, performing, or reviewing research, or in reporting research results...Research misconduct does not include honest error or differences of opinion." *Fabrication* involves making up data or study results and reporting them. *Falsification* involves manipulating research materials, equipment, or processes; it also involves changing or omitting data, or distorting results such that the research is not accurately represented in research reports. *Plagiarism* involves the appropriation of someone's ideas, results, or words without giving due credit, including information obtained through the confidential review of research proposals or manuscripts. Although the official definition focuses on only these three types of misconduct, there is widespread agreement that research misconduct covers many other issues, including improprieties of authorship, poor data management, conflicts of interest, inappropriate financial arrangements, failure to comply with governmental regulations, and unauthorized use of confidential information. Conflicts of interest may be a particularly salient issue in health-related research funded by for-profit organizations.

Example of research misconduct: In 1999, the U.S. Office of Research Integrity ruled that a nurse who had been the data manager for the National Surgical Adjuvant Breast and Bowel Project at a cancer center affiliated with Northwestern University engaged in scientific misconduct by intentionally falsifying or fabricating follow-up data on three patients enrolled in clinical trials for breast cancer (ORI Newsletter, March, 1999).

Although examples of publicly exposed misconduct by nurse researchers are not common, research dishonesty and fraud are major concerns in nursing. Rankin and Esteves (1997) asked a sample of nursing research coordinators and deans about their experience with research misconduct; nearly half perceived that plagiarism occasionally occurred among faculty in their institutions, and about one third perceived that other offenses such as misrepresentation of findings or protocol violations sometimes occurred. Interest in the issue has not subsided. For example, Jeffers (2005) engaged in work to identify and describe research environments that promote integrity. In a study that focused on ethical issues faced by editors of nursing journals, Freda and Kearney (2005) found that 64% of the 88 participating editors reported some type of ethical dilemma, such as duplicate publication, plagiarism, or conflicts of interest. And, since 2001, NINR and other institutes within NIH have teamed with ORI to offer grants for researchers to conduct "Research on Research Integrity"—that is, to study the factors that affect, both positively and negatively, integrity in research.

Example of research on research integrity: In 2004, Sheila Santacroce of Yale University was awarded a 2-year grant through NINR under the Research on Research Integrity initiative. Her study is exploring *intervention fidelity* (the consistent delivery of an intervention according to a research plan and professional standards) in two federally funded nursing intervention studies. The premise is that lack of attention to fidelity can lead to false statements about the implementation and effects of an intervention.

CRITIQUING THE ETHICS OF RESEARCH STUDIES

Guidelines for critiquing the ethical aspects of a study are presented in Box 7.3 on page 187. Members of an IRB or human subjects committee should be provided with sufficient information to answer all these questions. Research reports, however, do not always include detailed information about ethical procedures because of space constraints in journals. Thus, it may not always be possible to critique researchers' adherence to ethical guidelines. Nevertheless, we offer a few suggestions for considering the ethical aspects of a study.

Many research reports do acknowledge that the study procedures were reviewed by an IRB or human subjects committee of the institution with which the researchers are affiliated. When a research report specifically mentions a formal external review, it is generally safe to assume that a panel of concerned people thoroughly reviewed the ethical issues raised by the study.

You can also come to some conclusions based on a description of the study methods. There may be sufficient information to judge, for example, whether study participants were subjected to physical or psychological harm or discomfort. Reports do not always specifically state whether informed consent was secured, but you should be alert to situations in which the data could not have been gathered as described if participation were purely voluntary (e.g., if data were gathered unobtrusively).

In thinking about the ethical aspects of a study, you should also consider who the study participants were. For example, if the study involves vulnerable groups, there should be more information about protective procedures. You might also need to attend to who the study participants were *not*. For example, there has been considerable concern about the omission of certain groups (e.g., minorities) from clinical research.

It is often especially difficult to determine by reading research reports whether the privacy of the participants was safeguarded unless the researcher specifically mentions pledges of confidentiality or anonymity. A situation requiring special scrutiny arises when data are collected from two people simultaneously (e.g., a husband and wife who are jointly interviewed); in such situations, the absence of privacy raises not only ethical concerns but also questions regarding participants' candor. As noted by Forbat and Henderson (2003), ethical issues arise when two people in an intimate relationship are interviewed about a common issue, even when they are interviewed privately. They described the

potential for being "stuck in the middle" when trying to get two sides of a story, and facing the dilemma of how to ask one person probing questions after having been given confidential information about the topic by the other.

RESEARCH EXAMPLES

Because researchers usually attempt to report research results as succinctly as possible, they rarely describe in much detail the efforts they have made to safeguard participants' rights. (The absence of any mention of such safeguards does not, of course, imply that no precautions were taken.) Researchers are especially likely to discuss their adherence to ethical guidelines for studies that involve more than minimal risk or when the people being studied are a vulnerable group. Two research examples that highlight ethical issues are presented in the following sections.

Research Example from a Quantitative Study

Study: "Prevalence and correlates of chlamydia infection in Canadian street youth" (Shields et al., 2004)

Study purpose: The purpose of the study was to document the prevalence of chlamydia infection among Canadian street youth and to identify background factors associated with increased risk for infection.

Research methods: Nurses who had experience working with street youth recruited a total of 1355 youth aged 15 to 24 years in seven large urban centers throughout Canada. Information was collected through nurse-administered questionnaires. Participants also provided a urine sample to test for chlamydia trachomatis.

Ethics-related procedures: Recruitment of participants occurred through drop-in centers, which provided an environment suitable for confidential discussions. Youth who were intoxicated (on drugs or alcohol) were excluded from the study. Informed consent was obtained from each youth before participation in the study. The youth were advised that they could withdraw from the study at any point and that, if they so desired, their questionnaire would be destroyed. Questionnaires were assigned an identification number—names were never attached to them. Test results for the urine sample were linked to the questionnaires by this ID number. Youth were strongly encouraged to return to the drop-in center to learn their test results, and those who tested positive were given a dose of azithromycin. A food voucher was offered to each youth as an incentive to participate in the study. The study design, procedures, and questionnaire were approved by local universities or hospital Research Ethics Boards in each city where the study took place.

Key Findings: The prevalence rate of chlamydia was 8.6%, a high prevalence rate compared with the general population of youth. Higher prevalence rates were found in females (10.9%) than in males (7.3%). Among females, factors associated with higher risk for infection included being Aboriginal and having been in foster care.

Research Example from a Qualitative Study

Study: "Perinatal violence assessment: Teenagers' rationale for denying violence when asked" (Renker, 2006)

Study purpose: The purpose of the study was to describe teenagers' experiences with violence assessments from health care and social service providers, and to explore their reasons for failing to disclose violence.

Study methods: Renker recruited 20 teenagers (18- and 19-year-olds) who were no longer pregnant but who had experienced physical or sexual abuse in the year before or during a pregnancy. All women were interviewed in person and asked in-depth questions about their experiences relating to violence.

Ethics-related procedures: Renker recruited teenagers primarily at two outpatient gynecologic clinics. Teenagers who were deemed eligible for the study were invited to schedule an interview at a location of their choice. All but one of the young women who volunteered chose a public library or a university office rather than their own homes. Teens were offered a $50 stipend to partially compensate them for the time spent in the interview (30 to 90 minutes). Before beginning the interview, informed consent issues were discussed, including the researcher's responsibility to report child abuse and harm to third parties. Study participants were told that no specific questions would be asked about either of these reportable issues, but that the researcher would assist them in reporting any abuse situations if they so desired. To protect their confidentiality, Renker encouraged each teenager to make up a name for herself, the perpetrator, and other family members. Each interview was assigned an ID number,

and the data files contained no information that could identify participants or the locale of their recruitment. Interviews were conducted in a private setting without the presence of the teenagers' partners, parents, or children aged 2 years or older. At the end of the interview, Renker provided the teenagers with information designed to promote their safety (e.g., danger assessments, review of legal options, information about local community resources). Renker received IRB approval from her university and from the medical systems of the two clinics from which participants were recruited.

Key Findings: The teenagers reported a range of violence experiences from their current and previous intimate partners, their parents, and gangs. Their reasons for not disclosing violence to health care providers fell into categories that corresponded to four continua: Power/ Powerlessness; Fear/Hope; Trust/Mistrust; and Action/ Inertia.

SUMMARY POINTS

- Because research has not always been conducted ethically, and because of genuine **ethical dilemmas** that researchers often face in designing studies that are both ethical and methodologically rigorous, **codes of ethics** have been developed to guide researchers.

- Three major ethical principles from the *Belmont Report* are incorporated into most guidelines: beneficence, respect for human dignity, and justice.

- **Beneficence** involves the performance of some good and the protection of participants from physical and psychological harm and exploitation (*nonmaleficence*).

- Respect for human dignity involves the participants' right to **self-determination**, which means participants have the freedom to control their own activities, including their voluntary participation in the study.

- **Full disclosure** means that researchers have fully described to prospective participants their rights and the risks and benefits of the study. When full disclosure poses the risk of biased results, researchers sometimes use **covert data collection** or **concealment** (the collection of information without the participants' knowledge or consent) or **deception** (either withholding information from participants' or providing false information).

- Justice includes the right to fair treatment (and equitable treatment) and the right to privacy. In the United States, privacy has become a major issue because of the Privacy Rule regulations that resulted from the Health Insurance Portability and Accountability Act (HIPAA).

- Various procedures have been developed to safeguard study participants' rights, including the performance of a risk/benefit assessment, the implementation of informed consent procedures, and taking steps to safeguard participants' confidentiality.

- In a **risk/benefit assessment**, the potential benefits of the study to individual participants and to society are weighed against the costs to individuals.

- **Informed consent** procedures, which provide prospective participants with information needed to make a reasoned decision about participation, normally involve signing a **consent form** to document voluntary and informed participation. Because of the Privacy Rule, a separate authorization form regarding the use of health data may also be needed.

- In qualitative studies, consent may need to be continually renegotiated with participants as the study evolves, through **process consent** procedures.

- Privacy can be maintained through **anonymity** (wherein not even researchers know participants' identities) or through formal confidentiality procedures that safeguard the information participants provide.

- In some studies, it may be advantageous for U.S. researchers to obtain a **Certificate of Confidentiality** that protects them against the forced disclosure of confidential information through a court order or other legal or administrative process.

- Researchers sometimes offer **debriefing** sessions after data collection to provide participants with more information or an opportunity to air complaints.

- **Vulnerable subjects** require additional protection. These people may be vulnerable because they are not able to make a truly informed decision about study participation (e.g., children); because of diminished autonomy (e.g., prisoners); or because their circumstances heighten the risk for physical or psychological harm (e.g., pregnant women, the terminally ill).

- External review of the ethical aspects of a study by a human subjects committee, **Research Ethics Board (REB)**, or **Institutional Review Board (IRB)** is highly desirable and may be required by either the agency funding the research or the organization from which participants are recruited.

- In studies in which risks to participants are minimal, an **expedited review** (review by a single member of the IRB) may be substituted for a full board review; in cases in which there are no anticipated risks, the research may be exempted from review.

- Researchers are always advised, even in the absence of a mandated external review, to consult with at least one advisor whose perspective allows an objective evaluation of the ethics of a proposed study.

- Researchers need to give careful thought to ethical requirements throughout the study's planning and implementation and to ask themselves continually whether safeguards for protecting humans are sufficient.

- Ethical conduct in research involves not only protection of the rights of human and animal subjects, but also efforts to maintain high standards of integrity and avoid such forms of **research misconduct** as plagiarism, fabrication of results, or falsification of data.

STUDY ACTIVITIES

Chapter 7 of the *Resource Manual to Accompany Nursing Research: Generating and Assessing Evidence for Nursing Practice, 8th edition*, offers various exercises and study suggestions for reinforcing concepts presented in this chapter. In addition, the following study questions can be addressed:

1. For the study described in the research example section (Shields et al., 2004), prepare a consent form that includes required information, as described in the section on informed consent.

2. Answer the relevant questions in Box 7.3 regarding the Shields et al. (2004) study. Also consider the following questions: (a) Parental consent was apparently not obtained in this study—should it have been? (b) Could the data for this study have been collected anonymously? Why or why not?

3. Answer the relevant questions in Box 7.3 regarding the Renker (2006) study. Also consider the following questions: (a) Renker paid participants a $50 stipend—was this ethically appropriate? (b) Did the teenagers' creation of a pseudonym result in anonymity? (c) Might Renker have benefited from obtaining a Certificate of Confidentiality for this research?

STUDIES CITED IN CHAPTER 7

Methodologic or theoretical references cited in this chapter can be found in a separate section at the end of the book.

Anderson, N. L. R., Nyamathi, A., McAvoy, J. A., Conde, F., & Casey, C. (2001). Perceptions about risk for HIV/AIDS among adolescents in juvenile detention. Western Journal of Nursing Research, 23, 336–359.

Briones, T. L., Suh, E., Hattar, H., & Wadowska, M. (2005). Dentate gyrus neurogenesis after cerebral ischemia and behavioral training. Biological Research for Nursing, 6, 167–179.

Caelli, K. (2001). Engaging with phenomenology: Is it more of a challenge than it needs to be? Qualitative Health Research, 11, 273–281.

Freda, M. C., & Kearney, M. (2005). Ethical issues faced by nursing editors. Western Journal of Nursing Research, 27(4), 487–499.

Hatton, D. C., & Kaiser, L. (2004). Methodological and ethical issues emerging from pilot testing an intervention with women in a transitional shelter. Western Journal of Nursing Research, 26(1), 129–136.

Hentz, P. (2002). The body remembers: Grieving and a circle of time. Qualitative Health Research, 12, 161–172.

Long, J. D., Armstrong, M. L., Amos, E., Shriver, B., et al. (2006). Pilot using World Wide Web to prevent diabetes in adolescents. Clinical Nursing Research, 15(1), 67–79.

Neufeld, A., & Harrison, M. J. (2003). Unfulfilled expectations and negative interactions: Nonsupport in the relationships of women caregivers. Journal of Advanced Nursing, 41, 323–331.

Rankin, M., & Esteves, M.D. (1997). Perceptions of scientific misconduct in nursing. Nursing Research, 46, 270–275.

Renker, P. R. (2006). Perinatal violence assessment: Teenagers' rationale for denying violence when asked. Journal of Obstetric, Gynecologic, & Neonatal Nursing, 35(1), 56–67.

Sandgren, A., Thulesius, H., Fridlund, B., & Petersson, K. (2006). Striving for emotional survival in palliative cancer nursing. Qualitative Health Research, 16(1), 79–96.

Shields, S. A., Wong, T., Mann, J., Jolly, A. M., Haase, D., Mahaffey, S., Moses, S., Morin, M., Patrick, D. M., Predy, G., Rossi, M., & Sutherland, D. (2004). Prevalence and correlates of chlamydia infection in Canadian street youth. Journal of Adolescent Health, 34, 384–390.

Spiers, J. A. (2002). The interpersonal contexts of negotiating care in home care nurse-patient interactions. Qualitative Health Research, 12, 1033–1057.

Suzuki, K., Ohida, T., Kaneita, Y., Yokoyama, E., & Uchiyama, M. (2005). Daytime sleepiness, sleep habits, and occupational accidents among hospital nurses. Journal of Advanced Nursing, 52(4), 445–453.

Wuest, J., Ford-Gilboe, M., Merritt-Gray, M., & Berman, H. (2003). Intrusion: The central problem for family health promotion among children and single mothers after leaving an abusive partner. Qualitative Health Research, 13, 597–622.

PART 3

DESIGNING A STUDY TO GENERATE EVIDENCE FOR NURSING

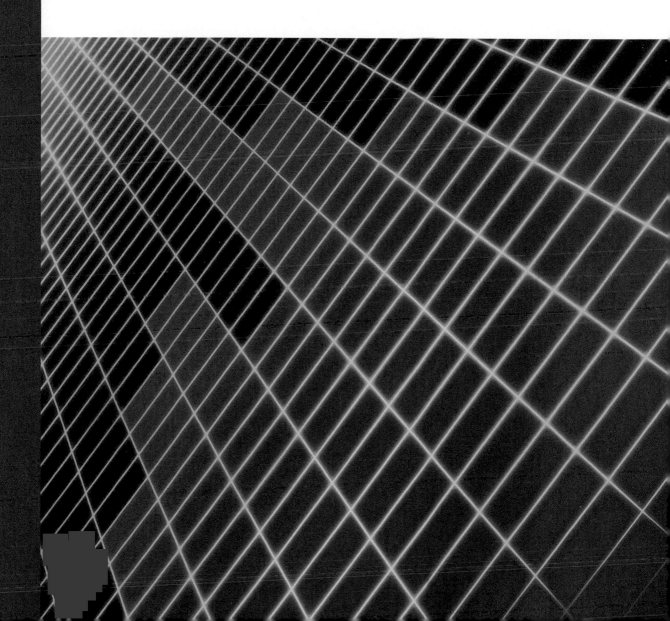

8

Planning a Nursing Study

A dvance planning is required for all research, and is especially important for quantitative studies because typically the study design and methods must be finalized before the study can proceed. This chapter provides some guidance for planning qualitative and quantitative studies.

After developing a research problem, articulating research questions or hypotheses, and developing a theoretical rationale in the conceptual phase of a study, researchers face numerous challenges, including the following:

- Financial challenges (How will the study be paid for? Will available resources be adequate?)
- Administrative challenges (Is there sufficient time to complete the study? Can needed research personnel be recruited and adequately trained and monitored?)
- Practical challenges (Will I be able to gain entrée into a good study site? Will there be enough study participants?)
- Ethical challenges (Can the study be designed rigorously to yield high-quality evidence without infringing on human or animal rights?)
- Clinical challenges (Will the research goals conflict with clinical goals? What difficulties will be encountered in doing research with vulnerable or frail patients?)

- Methodologic challenges (Will the methods used to address the research question yield accurate and valid results?)

Most of this book provides guidance relating to the methodologic challenges, but other challenges impinge on researchers' ability to design methodologically sound studies and will require consideration during the planning phase of a project.

TOOLS AND CONCEPTS FOR PLANNING RIGOROUS RESEARCH

In planning a study, it is important to keep in mind not only the challenges of doing rigorous research but also options for addressing them. This section discusses key methodologic concepts and tools in meeting those challenges.

Reliability, Validity, and Trustworthiness

Researchers want their findings to reflect the *truth*. Research cannot contribute evidence to guide clinical practice if the findings are inaccurate, biased, fail to represent the experiences of the target group adequately, or are based on a misinterpretation of the data. Consumers of research need to assess the quality of evidence offered in a study by evaluating the conceptual and methodologic decisions the researchers made, and producers of research need to strive to make good decisions to produce evidence of the highest possible quality.

Quantitative researchers use several criteria to assess the quality of a study, sometimes referred to as its **scientific merit.** Two especially important criteria are reliability and validity. **Reliability** refers to the accuracy and consistency of information obtained in a study. The term is most often associated with the methods used to measure research variables. For example, if a thermometer measured Alan's temperature as 98.1°F one minute and as 102.5°F the next minute, the reliability of the thermometer would be highly suspect. The concept of reliability is also important in interpreting the results of statistical analyses. *Statistical reliability* refers to the probability that the same results would be obtained with a completely new sample of subjects—that is, that the results are an accurate reflection of a wider group than just the particular people who participated in the study.

Validity is a more complex concept that broadly concerns the *soundness* of the study's evidence—that is, whether the findings are unbiased, cogent, and well grounded. Like reliability, validity is an important criterion for evaluating methods to measure research variables. In this context, the validity question is whether there is evidence to support the assertion that the methods are really measuring the abstract concepts that they purport to measure. Is a paper-and-pencil measure of depression *really* measuring depression? Or is it measuring something else, such as loneliness, low self-esteem, or stress? Researchers strive for solid conceptual definitions of research variables and valid methods to operationalize them.

Another aspect of validity concerns the quality of the researcher's evidence regarding the effect of the independent variable on the dependent variable. Did a nursing intervention *really* bring about improvements in patients' outcomes—or were other factors responsible for patients' progress? Researchers make numerous methodologic decisions that can influence this type of study validity.

Qualitative researchers use somewhat different criteria (and different terminology) in evaluating a study's quality. In general, qualitative researchers discuss methods of enhancing the **trustworthiness** of the study's data (Lincoln & Guba, 1985). Trustworthiness encompasses several different dimensions—credibility, transferability (discussed later in the chapter), confirmability, and dependability. **Dependability** refers to evidence that is consistent and stable. **Confirmability** is similar to objectivity; it is the degree to which study results are derived from characteristics of participants and the study context, not from researcher biases.

Credibility, an especially important aspect of trustworthiness, is achieved to the extent that the research methods engender confidence in the truth of the data and in the researchers' interpretations of the data. Credibility in a qualitative study can be enhanced through various approaches (see Chapter 20), but one strategy in particular merits early discussion because it has implications for the design of all studies, including quantitative ones. **Triangulation** is the use of multiple sources or referents to draw conclusions about what constitutes the truth. In a quantitative study, this might mean having multiple operational definitions of a dependent variable to determine whether predicted effects are consistent. In a qualitative study, triangulation might involve trying to understand the full complexity of a poorly understood phenomenon by using multiple means of data collection to converge on the truth (e.g., having in-depth discussions with study participants, as well as watching their behavior in natural settings). Or, it might involve triangulating the ideas and interpretations of multiple researchers working together as a team. Nurse researchers are also beginning to triangulate across paradigms—that is, to integrate both qualitative and quantitative data in a single study to offset the shortcomings of each approach and enhance the validity of the conclusions.

Example of triangulation: Wheatley (2006) explored how nurses make assessments of hospitalized patients to detect indicators of patient deterioration. This ethnographic study triangulated information from in-depth interviews with nursing staff and observations of nurses' behavior.

Nurse researchers need to design their studies in such a way that the reliability, validity, and trustworthiness of their studies are maximized. This book offers advice on how to do this.

Bias

Bias is a major concern in designing a study because it can threaten the study's ability to reveal the truth. In general, a **bias** is an influence that produces a distortion or error in the study results. Biases can affect the quality of evidence in both qualitative and quantitative studies.

Bias can result from a number of factors that need to be considered in planning a study. These include the following:

- *Participants' lack of candor.* Sometimes people distort their behavior or their self-disclosures—consciously or subconsciously—in an effort to present themselves in the best possible light.
- *Researcher subjectivity.* Investigators may distort information in the direction of their expectations or hypotheses, or in line with their own experiences—or they may (perhaps unintentionally) communicate their expectations to participants and thereby induce biased revelations or behavior.
- *Sample imbalances.* The sample itself may be biased; for example, if a researcher studies abortion attitudes but includes only members of right-to-life (or pro-choice) groups in the sample, the results would be distorted. Sample biases can result from a faulty sampling approach, as well as biases from poor retention of study participants.
- *Faulty methods of data collection.* An inadequate method of capturing key concepts can lead to biases; for example, a flawed paper-and-pencil measure of patient satisfaction with nursing care may exaggerate or underestimate patients' concerns.
- *Inadequate study design.* A researcher may have structured the study in such a way that an

unbiased answer to the research question cannot be achieved.
- *Flawed implementation.* Even a well-designed study can sustain biases if the design (or the intervention, if any) is not carefully implemented. Monitoring for bias throughout the study is important.

Example of respondent bias: Collins, Shattell, and Thomas (2005) studied 316 pages of interview transcripts from three separate phenomenological studies and searched for instances in which participants may have distorted their responses in a manner that would make them "look good," or that would flatter or spare offending the interviewers. Although they identified only six potential instances of what they called "problematic interviewee behavior," they concluded, based on these instances, that "it is probably not a good idea for nurses to interview patients to whom they have personally delivered (or will deliver) care" (p. 197).

It is the job of researchers to reduce or eliminate bias to the extent possible, to establish mechanisms to detect or measure it when it exists, and to take known biases into account in interpreting the study findings. And it is the job of consumers to carefully scrutinize methodologic decisions to establish whether biases undermined the study evidence.

Unfortunately, bias can seldom be avoided totally because the potential for its occurrence is so pervasive. Some bias is haphazard and affects only small segments of the data. As an example of such **random bias**, a handful of study participants might fail to provide accurate information as a result of extreme fatigue at the time the data were collected. **Systematic bias**, on the other hand, results when the bias is consistent or uniform. For example, if a spring scale consistently measured people's weights as being 2 pounds heavier than their true weight, there would be systematic bias in the data on weight.

Researchers adopt a variety or strategies and methods to eliminate or minimize systematic bias and thereby strengthen the rigor of their studies. Triangulation is one such approach, the idea being that multiple sources of information or points of view can help counterbalance biases and offer avenues to identify them. The methods that quantitative researchers use to combat the effects of bias often involve research control.

Research Control

One of the central features of quantitative studies is that they typically involve efforts to tightly control various aspects of the research. **Research control** most typically involves holding constant other influences on the dependent variable so that the true relationship between the independent and dependent variables can be understood. In other words, research control attempts to eliminate contaminating factors that might cloud the relationship between the variables that are of central interest.

The issue of contaminating factors—or **extraneous** (or **confounding) variables**, as they are called—can best be illustrated with an example. Suppose we were interested in studying whether teenage women are at higher risk for having low-birth-weight infants than are older mothers *because of their age*. In other words, we want to test whether there is something about women's maturational development that causes differences in birth weight. Existing studies have shown that, in fact, teenagers have a higher rate of low-birth-weight babies than women in their 20s. The question here is whether maternal age itself (the independent variable) causes differences in birth weight (the dependent variable), or whether there are other mechanisms that account for the relationship between age and birth weight. We need to design a study so as to control other determinants of the dependent variable—determinants that are also related to the independent variable.

Two extraneous variables in our hypothetical study are the mother's nutritional habits and her prenatal care. Teenagers tend to be less careful than older women about nutrition during pregnancy, and are also less likely to obtain adequate prenatal care. Both nutrition and the amount of care could, in turn, affect the baby's birth weight. Thus, if these two factors are not controlled, then any observed relationship between a mother's age and her baby's weight at birth could be caused by the mother's age itself, her diet, or her prenatal care.

These three possible explanations might be portrayed schematically as follows:

1. Mother's age → infant birth weight
2. Mother's age → prenatal care → infant birth weight
3. Mother's age → nutrition → infant birth weight

The arrows here symbolize a causal mechanism or an influence. In models 2 and 3, the effect of maternal age on infant birth weight is *mediated* by prenatal care and nutrition, respectively. Some research is specifically designed to test paths of mediation, but in the present example, these variables are extraneous to the research question. Our task is to design a study so that the first explanation can be tested. Both nutrition and prenatal care must be controlled if our goal is to learn whether explanation 1 is valid.

How can we impose such control? There are a number of ways, as discussed in Chapter 11, but the general principle underlying each alternative is that the extraneous variables must be **held constant**. The extraneous variables must somehow be handled so that, *in the context of the study*, they are not related to the independent or dependent variable. As an example, let us say we want to compare the birth weights of infants born to two groups of women: those aged 15 to 19 years and those aged 25 to 29 years. We must then design a study in such a way that the nutritional and prenatal health care practices of the two groups are comparable, even though, in general, the two groups are not comparable in these respects.

Table 8.1 illustrates one control method—not an especially strong one, as we shall see in later chapters, but one that provides an easily understood demonstration. This **matching** approach involves deliberately selecting study participants in such a way that both older and younger mothers have similar eating habits and amounts of prenatal attention. The two groups are matched in terms of the two extraneous variables; one third of both groups have the same nutrition ratings and amount of prenatal care. By building in this comparability, nutrition and prenatal care have been held constant in the two groups. If the two groups differed in birth

TABLE 8.1	Fictitious Example: Control of Two Extraneous Variables		
AGE OF MOTHER (YEARS)	**NUTRITIONAL PRACTICES**	**NO. OF PRENATAL VISITS**	**INFANT BIRTH WEIGHT**
15–19	33% rated "good" 33% rated "fair" 33% rated "poor"	33% 1–3 visits 33% 4–6 visits 33% > 6 visits	20% ≤ 2500 g; 80% > 2500 g
25–29	33% rated "good" 33% rated "fair" 33% rated "poor"	33% 1–3 visits 33% 4–6 visits 33% > 6 visits	9% ≤ 2500 g; 91% > 2500 g

weight (as they, in fact, do in Table 8.1), then we might infer that age (and not diet or prenatal care) influenced the infants' birth weights. If the groups did not differ, however, we might tentatively conclude that it is not mother's age *per se* that causes young women to have a higher percentage of low-birth-weight babies, but rather some other variable, such as nutrition or prenatal care. It is important to note that although we have designated prenatal care and nutrition as extraneous variables in this particular study, they are not at all extraneous to a full understanding of the factors that influence birth weight; in other studies, nutritional practices and frequency of prenatal care might be key independent variables.

By exercising control in this example, we have taken a step toward explaining the relationship between variables. The world is complex, and many variables are interrelated in complicated ways. When studying a particular problem within the positivist paradigm, it is difficult to examine this complexity directly; researchers must usually analyze a couple of relationships at a time and put pieces together like a jigsaw puzzle. That is why even modest studies can make contributions to knowledge. The extent of the contribution in a quantitative study, however, is often directly related to how well researchers control extraneous influences.

In the present example, we identified three variables that could affect birth weight, but dozens of others might be relevant, such as maternal stress,

mothers' use of drugs or alcohol during pregnancy, and so on. Researchers need to isolate the independent and dependent variables in which they are interested and then identify the confounding variables that need to be controlled.

Example of control through matching: Mateo and colleagues (2005) compared psychiatric inpatients with and without mild traumatic brain injury to explore whether the brain injury was related to patient outcomes, such as length of hospital stay and functional ability. To control extraneous variables, the two groups were matched in terms of age, gender, and diagnostic category—all factors that could have affected the outcomes, independent of brain injury status.

It is often impossible to control all variables that affect the dependent variable, and not even necessary to do so. Extraneous variables need to be controlled only if they simultaneously are related to both the dependent and independent variables. This notion is illustrated in Figure 8.1, which has the following elements:

- Each circle represents all the variability associated with a particular variable.
- The large circle in the center stands for the dependent variable, infant birth weight.
- Smaller circles stand for factors affecting infant birth weight.
- Overlapping circles indicate the degree to which the variables are related to each other.

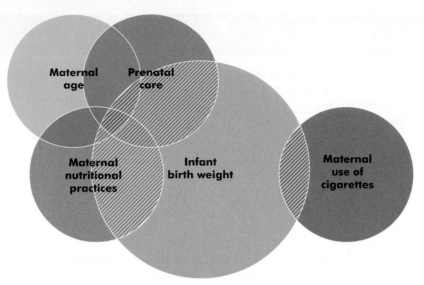

FIGURE 8.1 Hypothetical representation of factors affecting infant birth weight.

In this hypothetical example, four variables are related to infant birth weight: mother's age, amount of prenatal care, nutritional practices, and smoking during pregnancy. The first three of these variables are also interrelated; this is shown by the fact that these three circles overlap not only with infant birth weight but also with each other. That is, younger mothers tend to have different patterns of prenatal care and nutrition than older mothers. The mother's prenatal use of cigarettes, however, is unrelated to these three variables. In other words, women who smoke during their pregnancies (according to this fictitious representation) are as likely to be young as old, to eat properly as not, and to get adequate prenatal care as not. If this representation were accurate, then maternal smoking would not need to be controlled to study the effect of maternal age on infant birth weight. If this scheme is incorrect—if teenage mothers smoke more or less than older mothers—then maternal smoking practices should be controlled.

Figure 8.1 does not show infant birth weight as being totally determined by the four other variables. The middle area of the birth weight circle represents "unexplained" variability in infant birth weight. That is, other determinants of birth weight are needed for us to understand fully what causes babies to be born weighing different amounts. Genetic characteristics, events occurring during the pregnancy, and medical treatments administered to pregnant women are examples of other factors that contribute to an infant's weight at birth. Dozens of circles would need to be sketched onto Figure 8.1 for us to understand factors affecting infant birth weight. In designing a study, quantitative researchers should attempt to control those variables that overlap with both independent and dependent variables to understand fully the relationship between the main variables of interest.

Research control in quantitative studies is viewed as a critical tool for managing bias and for enhancing the validity of researchers' conclusions. There are situations, however, in which too much control can introduce bias. For example, if researchers tightly control the ways in which key study variables are manifested, it is possible that the true nature of those variables will be obscured. When the key concepts are phenomena that are poorly understood or the dimensions of which have not been clarified, then an approach that allows some flexibility is better suited to the study aims—such as in a qualitative study. Research rooted in the naturalistic paradigm does not impose controls.

With their emphasis on holism and the individuality of human experience, qualitative researchers typically adhere to the view that to impose controls on a research setting is to remove irrevocably some of the meaning of reality.

Randomness

For quantitative researchers, a powerful tool for eliminating bias involves the concept of **randomness**—having certain features of the study established by chance rather than by design or researcher preference. When people are selected at random to participate in the study, for example, each person in the initial pool has an equal probability of being selected. This in turn means that there are no systematic biases in the make-up of the sample. Men and women have an equal chance of being selected, for example. Similarly, if study participants are allocated at random to groups that will be compared (e.g., an intervention and "usual care" group), then there can be no systematic biases in the composition of the groups. Randomness is a compelling method of controlling confounding variables and reducing bias.

Qualitative researchers almost never consider randomness a desirable tool for fully understanding a phenomenon. Qualitative researchers tend to use information obtained early in the study in a purposive (nonrandom) fashion to guide their inquiry and to pursue information-rich sources that can help them expand or refine their conceptualizations. Researchers' judgments are viewed as indispensable vehicles for uncovering the complexities of the phenomena of interest.

Masking or Blinding

A rather charming (but problematic) quality of people is that they usually want things to turn out well. Researchers want their ideas to work, and they want their hypotheses about how to improve patient care supported. And study participants want to be cooperative and helpful, and they also want to present themselves in the best light. These tendencies can lead to biases because they can affect what participants do and say (and what researchers ask and perceive) in ways that distort the truth.

A procedure known as **masking** is used in many quantitative studies to prevent biases stemming from *awareness*. Masking involves concealing information from participants, research agents such as data collectors, care providers, or data analysts to enhance objectivity. For example, if study participants are not aware of whether they are getting an experimental drug or a sham drug (a *placebo*), then their outcomes cannot be influenced by their expectations of its efficacy. Masking typically involves disguising or withholding information about participants' status in the study (e.g., whether they are in a certain group or whether they are in the study because of certain characteristics or conditions) or about the study hypotheses.

It should be noted that the term **blinding** is widely used in lieu of masking to describe concealment strategies. This term has fallen into some disfavor, however, because of possible pejorative connotations, and some professional organizations (e.g., the American Psychological Association) have recommended that the term masking be used instead. Medical researchers, however, appear to prefer *blinding* unless the people in the study have vision impairments (e.g., Schultz, Chalmers, & Altman, 2002).

When it proves to be unfeasible or undesirable to use masking, the study is sometimes called an **open study**, in contrast to a **closed study** that results from masking. When masking is used with only some of the people involved in the study (e.g., the study participants), it is often called a **single-blind study**, but when it is possible to mask with two groups (e.g., those delivering an intervention and those receiving it), it is called a **double-blind study.**

Reflexivity

Qualitative researchers do not use methods such as research control, randomness, or masking, but they are nevertheless as interested as quantitative researchers in discovering the true state of human experience. Qualitative researchers often rely on reflexivity to guard against personal bias in making judgments. **Reflexivity** is the process of reflecting critically on the self, and of analyzing and making note of personal values that could affect data collection and interpretation.

Schwandt (1997) has described reflexivity as having two aspects. The first concerns the acknowledgement that the researcher is part of the setting, context, or social phenomenon under study. The second involves the process of self-reflection about one's own biases, preferences, stakes in the research, and theoretical inclinations. Qualitative researchers are encouraged to explore these issues, to be reflexive about every decision made during the inquiry, and to record their reflexive thoughts in personal diaries and memos.

Reflexivity is typically discussed as an individual activity, engaged in by researchers working "solo" on a project. Barry and colleagues (1999) have argued that when researchers collaborate in a qualitative study, both individual and group reflexivity are needed. They suggested mechanisms to promote reflexivity in studies conducted by teams of researchers, and implementation of their suggestions has been described by a Canadian nurse researcher (Hall et al., 2005).

Example of reflexivity: Myrick and Yonge (2004) studied the process used in the preceptorship experience to enhance critical thinking in graduate nursing education. Their study involved interviews with graduate students and preceptors. During the study, both researchers maintained a journal of personal reflections.

⮕ **TIP:** Reflexivity can be a useful tool in quantitative as well as qualitative research—self awareness and introspection can enhance the quality of any study.

Generalizability and Transferability

Nurses increasingly rely on evidence from disciplined research as a guide in their clinical practice. Evidence-based practice is based on the assumption that study findings are not unique to the people, places, or circumstances of the original research.

As noted in Chapter 1, **generalizability** is the criterion used in quantitative studies to assess the extent to which the findings can be applied to other groups and settings. How do researchers enhance the generalizability of a study? First and foremost, they must design studies strong in reliability and validity. There is little point in wondering whether results are generalizable if they are not accurate or valid. In selecting participants, researchers must also give thought to the types of people to whom the results might be generalized—and then select subjects in such a way that a nonbiased sample is obtained. If a study is intended to have implications for male and female patients, then men and women should be included as participants. If an intervention is intended to benefit patients in urban and rural hospitals, then perhaps a multisite study is warranted. Chapter 11 describes other issues to consider in enhancing generalizability.

Qualitative researchers do not specifically seek to make their findings generalizable. Nevertheless, qualitative researchers often seek understandings that might prove useful in other situations. Lincoln and Guba (1985), in their highly influential book on naturalistic inquiry, discuss the concept of **transferability**, the extent to which qualitative findings can be transferred to other settings, as another aspect of a study's trustworthiness. An important mechanism for promoting transferability is the amount of information qualitative researchers provide about the contexts of their studies. **Thick description**, a widely used term among qualitative researchers, refers to a rich and thorough description of the research setting and of observed transactions and processes. Quantitative researchers, like qualitative researchers, need to describe their study participants and their research settings thoroughly so that the utility of the evidence for others can be assessed.

⮕ **TIP:** When planning a study, it is wise to keep a sharp focus on the potential your study could have for evidence-based nursing practice—it may play a role in some of the methodologic decisions you make. Make an effort to think about generalizability and transferability because these are critical concerns in EBP efforts.

OVERVIEW OF RESEARCH DESIGN FEATURES

The research design of a study spells out the basic strategies that researchers adopt to develop evidence that is accurate and interpretable. The research design incorporates some of the most important methodologic decisions that researchers make, particularly in quantitative studies. Thus, it is important to understand design options when planning a research project.

Table 8.2 describes six key design features that typically need to be considered in planning a quantitative study. Many of these features are also pertinent in qualitative studies. These features include the following:

- Whether or not there is an *intervention*
- How extraneous variables will be *controlled*
- Whether *masking* will be used to avoid biases
- What types of *comparisons* will be made to enhance interpretability
- The *location* where the study will take place
- What the *timeframes* of the study are

This section provides additional information about the last three of these features because they are relevant in planning both qualitative and quantitative studies, and Chapters 10 and 11 elaborate on the first three.

➔ **TIP:** In planning a study, you will need to make many important design decisions that will affect the overall believability of your findings. In some cases, the decisions will influence whether you receive funding (if you are seeking financial support) or whether you are able to publish your findings (if you plan to submit to a journal). Therefore, a great deal of care and thought should go into these decisions.

TABLE 8.2	Key Design Features	
FEATURE	**KEY QUESTIONS**	**DESIGN OPTIONS**
Intervention	Will there be an intervention? (What will the intervention entail? What specific design will be used?)	Experimental, quasi-experimental, nonexperimental design (see Chapter 10)
Control over extraneous variables	How will extraneous variables be controlled? (Which extraneous variables will be controlled?)	Matching, homogeneity, blocking, crossover, randomization, statistical control (see Chapter 11)
Masking	From whom will critical information be withheld to avert bias?	Open versus closed study; single-blind, double-blind studies
Comparisons	What type of comparisons will be made to illuminate key processes or relationships?	Within-subjects design, between-subjects design, external comparisons
Location	Where will the study take place?	Single site versus multi-site; in the field versus controlled setting
Timeframes	How often will data be collected? (When, relative to other events, will data be collected? When will information on independent and dependent variables be collected—looking backward or forward?)	Cross-sectional, longitudinal design Retrospective, prospective design

Comparisons

In most studies, especially quantitative ones, researchers incorporate comparisons into their designs to provide a context for interpreting results. Indeed, as noted in Chapter 4, most research questions are phrased in terms of a comparison because the comparison typically embodies the independent variable. For example, if our research question was, what is the effect of massage on anxiety in hospitalized children, the implied comparison is massage versus no massage—that is, the independent variable.

Researchers can structure their studies to examine various types of comparison, the most common of which are as follows:

1. *Comparison between two or more groups.* For example, if we were studying the emotional consequences of having an abortion, we might compare the emotional status of women who had an abortion with that of women with an unintended pregnancy who delivered the baby. In an intervention study, we might want to compare those receiving the special intervention with those receiving "usual care." Or, in a qualitative study, we might want to compare men and women with respect to their experience of having a child diagnosed with schizophrenia.

2. *Comparison of one group's status at two or more points in time.* For example, we might want to compare patients' levels of stress before and after introducing a new procedure to reduce preoperative stress. Or we might want to compare coping processes among caregivers of patients with AIDS early and later in the caregiving experience.

3. *Comparison of one group's status under different circumstances.* For example, we might compare people's heart rates during two different types of exercise.

4. *Comparison based on relative rankings.* If, for example, we hypothesized a relationship between the pain level of cancer patients and their degree of hopefulness, we would be asking whether patients with high levels of pain felt less hopeful than patients with low levels

of pain. This research question involves a comparison of those with different rankings—higher versus lower—on both variables.

5. *Comparison with other studies.* Researchers may directly compare their results with results from other studies, sometimes using statistical procedures. This type of comparison typically supplements rather than replaces other types of comparisons. In quantitative studies, this approach is useful primarily when the dependent variable is measured with a widely accepted approach (e.g., blood pressure measures or scores on a standard measure of depression).

> **Example of using comparative data from other studies:** Beckie, Beckstead, and Webb (2001) studied quality of life and health of women who had suffered a cardiac event. Women in their sample were administered standard scales for which there were national comparison data, enabling the researchers to evaluate their sample's outcomes relative to national norms in the United States.

Research designs are sometimes categorized on the basis of the type of comparisons that are made. Studies that compare two or more groups of different people (as in examples 1 and 4) are referred to as **between-subjects designs**. Sometimes, however, it is preferable to make comparisons for the *same* study participants at different times or under difference circumstances, as in examples 2 and 3. Such designs are referred to as **within-subjects designs**.

Comparisons are often the central focus of a study, but even when they are not, they provide a context for understanding the findings. In the example of studying the emotional status of women who had an abortion, it would be difficult to know whether their emotional state was troubling without comparing it to that of others—or without comparing it to their emotional state earlier (e.g., before their pregnancy).

In some studies, a natural comparison group suggests itself. For example, if we were testing the effectiveness of a new nursing procedure for nursing home residents, an obvious comparison group would be nursing home residents who were exposed to the standard procedure rather than to the innovation. In other cases, however, the choice of a comparison group is less clearcut, and the researcher's decision about a comparison group can affect the interpretability of the findings. In the example about the emotional consequences of an abortion, we proposed using women who had delivered a baby as the comparison group. This reflects a comparison focusing on pregnancy *outcome* (i.e., pregnancy termination versus live birth). An alternative comparison group might be women who had a miscarriage. In this case, the comparison focuses not on the outcome (in both groups, the outcome is pregnancy loss) but rather on the *determinant* of the outcome. Thus, in designing a study, researchers must choose comparisons that will best illuminate the central issue under investigation.

TIP: Try not to make design decisions single-handedly. Seek the advice of professors, colleagues, or research consultants. Once you have made design decisions, it may be useful to write out a rationale for your choices, and share it with those you have consulted to see if they can find any flaws in your reasoning or if they can make suggestions for further improvements. A worksheet for documenting design decisions and rationales is available as a Word document in the Toolkit of the accompanying *Resource Manual*.

Research Location

An important task during the planning phase is to identify the sites (and settings) for the study. There are some research situations in which a site for the study is a "given," as might be the case for a clinical study conducted in a hospital or institution with which the researchers are affiliated, but in many studies, the identification of an appropriate site involves considerable effort.

Planning for this aspect of the study involves two types of activities—selecting the site or sites, and gaining access to them. Although some of the issues we discuss here are of particular relevance to qualitative researchers working in the field, many quantitative studies also need to attend to these matters in planning a project.

Site Selection

The primary consideration in site selection is whether the site is appropriate for the research question—that is, whether it is likely to have people with the behaviors, experiences, or characteristics of interest. Relatedly, the site must have a sufficient *number* of these kinds of people and adequate *diversity* or mix of people to achieve research goals. In addition, the site must be one in which entry is possible or plausible, and access to study participants can be granted. The site should also be one that matches other requirements, such as space needs, personnel, laboratory facilities, and so forth. The ideal site is one in which methodologic goals (e.g., ability to exert needed controls) and ethical requirements (e.g., ability to ensure privacy and confidentiality) can be achieved. Finally, the site should be one in which the researcher will be allowed to maintain an appropriate role *vis-à-vis* study participants (and clinical staff) for the duration of the study.

TIP: Before searching for a suitable site, it might be helpful to jot down the site characteristics that you would ideally like to have, so that you can more clearly assess the degree to which the reality matches the ideal. Once you have compiled a list, it might be profitable to brainstorm with colleagues, advisors, or other professionals about your needs to see if they can help you to identify potential sites.

In some cases, researchers may have to decide *how many* study sites to include. Having multiple sites is advantageous in terms of enhancing the generalizability of the study findings, but multi-site studies are complex and pose management, financial, and logistical challenges. Multiple sites are a good strategy when several co-investigators are working together on a project or when researchers explicitly want to test an intervention or explore experiences in divergent settings.

Site visits to potential sites and some clinical fieldwork are almost always needed to determine the "fit" between what the researcher needs and what the site has to offer. In essence, site visits involve "prior ethnography" (Erlandson et al., 1993), in which the researcher must make and record observations and converse with key gate-keepers or stakeholders in the site to better understand its characteristics and constraints.

Gaining Access

Researchers must gain access to (gain entrée into) those sites deemed suitable for the inquiry. If the site is an entire community, a multi-tiered effort of gaining acceptance from gatekeepers may be needed. For example, it may be necessary to enlist the cooperation first of community leaders and subsequently of administrators and staff in specific institutions (e.g., domestic violence organizations) or leaders of specific groups (e.g., support groups).

Because the establishment of *trust* is a central issue, gaining entrée requires strong interpersonal skills, as well as familiarity with the customs and language of the site. Researchers' ability to gain the gatekeepers' trust can only occur if researchers are congenial, persuasive, forthright about research requirements, and—perhaps most important—express genuine interest in and concern for the situations of the people in the site. Certain strategies are more likely to succeed than others. For example, gatekeepers might be persuaded to be cooperative if it can be demonstrated that there will be direct benefits to them or their constituents—or if a great humanitarian purpose will be served.

No matter how congenial the researcher may be, gatekeepers need information on which to base their decision about granting access, and this information usually should be put in writing, even if the negotiation takes place in person. The letter or information sheet should cover the following points: (1) the purpose of the research, and who the beneficiaries would be; (2) why the site was chosen or is considered desirable; (3) what the research would entail, including when the study would start, how long research staff would be at the site, how much disruption there likely would be, and what the resource requirements are; (4) how ethical guidelines would be maintained, including how results would be reported; and (5) what the gatekeeper or others at the site have to gain from cooperating in the study. Figure 8.2 ⊗ presents an example of a letter of inquiry for gaining entrée into a facility.

Gaining entrée is likely to be an ongoing process of establishing relationships and rapport with gatekeepers and others at the site, including prospective informants. The process might involve *progressive entry*, in which certain privileges are negotiated at first and then are subsequently expanded (Erlandson et al., 1993). Morse and Field (1995) advise ongoing communication with gatekeepers between the time that access is granted and the start-up of the study, which may be lengthy if funding is being sought or if study preparations (e.g., instrument development) are time-consuming. Not only is it courteous to keep people informed, but it also may prove critical to the success of the project because circumstances (and leadership) at the site can change.

Timeframes

The research design also designates when, and how often, data will be collected. In most studies, data are collected from participants at a single point in time. For example, patients might be asked on a single occasion to describe their health-promoting behaviors. Some designs, however, call for multiple contacts with participants, often to determine how things have changed over time. Thus, in planning a study, researchers must decide on the number of data collection points needed to address the research question properly. The research design also designates *when*, relative to other events, data will be collected. For example, the design might call for measurement of cholesterol levels 4 weeks and 8 weeks after a dietary intervention for patients with hypertension.

Designs are often categorized in terms of how they deal with time. The major distinction, for both qualitative and quantitative researchers, is between cross-sectional and longitudinal designs, but we will also discuss designs called retrospective and prospective because they also involve time-related issues.

Cross-Sectional Designs

Cross-sectional designs involve the collection of data once: the phenomena under study are captured

Ms. Wendy Smith, R.N.
Family Birth Place
General Hospital
Hartford, CT

Dear Ms. Smith:

I am the Principal Investigator of a study whose primary goal is to improve the detection of post-partum depression in Hispanic mothers. The study will involve testing a standard Spanish version of the Postpartum Depression Screening Sale (PDSS). Postpartum depression is a cross-cultural mental illness that can have devastating effects for 10%–15% of new mothers and their families. It has been estimated that up to 50% of all cases go undetected. Non–English-speaking women in this country may be even more dis-advantaged and isolated in their environments and may thus be at even higher risk for depression than English-speaking women, and thus effective screening with a valid instrument may be especially important.

Your hospital would be a desirable site for this research because of the high percentage of Hispanic women who deliver at your Family Birth Place. The research would require a sample of 75 Hispanic mothers 18 years of age or older who have given birth within the past 3 months. Each mother would complete the PDSS-Spanish Version and would participate in a diagnostic interview for *DSM-IV* depressive disorders, conducted by a female Hispanic psychologist. If a woman is diagnosed with postpartum depression, she would be referred for psychiatric follow-up. Each mother would be given a gift certificate for $25.00 for participating in the study.

If feasible, I would like to approach the 75 Hispanic women to invite them to participate in the study soon after delivery, while they are on the postpartum unit. The mothers would be recruited by a Hispanic research assistant who is an RN. Prospective participants will be asked to sign an informed consent form, which will be available in both English and Spanish (whichever language version participants prefer). Confidentiality will be strictly maintained. No name or identifying information will be written on any of the data collection forms. All data will be kept in a locked file cabinet in my office at the University of Connecticut.

Results of the study will be presented at research conferences and in a nursing research journal. The study findings will provide you with a more complete picture of your own Hispanic population and the percentage suffering from postpartum depression. A Spanish version of the PDSS will be made available for your use for screening Hispanic mothers at your hospital.

If it is possible, I would like to schedule an appointment with you so that we can discuss the possibility of my conducting this research on your unit.

Sincerely,
Cheryl Tatano Beck, DNSc, CNM, FAAN
Professor

FIGURE 8.2 Sample letter of inquiry for gaining entrée into a research site (fictitious).

during one period of data collection. Cross-sectional studies are appropriate for describing the status of phenomena or for describing relationships among phenomena at a fixed point in time. For example, we might be interested in determining whether psychological symptoms in menopausal women are correlated contemporaneously with physiologic symptoms.

Cross-sectional designs are sometimes used for time-related purposes, but the results may be misleading or ambiguous. For example, we might test the hypothesis, using cross-sectional data, that a determinant of excessive alcohol consumption is low impulse control, as measured by a psychological test. When both alcohol consumption and impulse control are measured concurrently, however, it is difficult to know which variable influenced the other, if either. Cross-sectional data can most appropriately be used to infer a time sequence under two circumstances: (1) when there is evidence or logical reasoning indicating that one variable preceded the other (e.g., in a study of the effects of low birth weight on morbidity in school-aged children, there would be no confusion over whether birth weight came first); and (2) when a cogent theoretical rationale guides the analysis.

Cross-sectional studies can also be designed to permit inferences about processes evolving over time, such as when measurements capture a process at different points in its evolution with different people. As an example, suppose we wanted to study changes in nursing students' professionalism as they progress through a 4-year baccalaureate program. One way to investigate this would be to gather data from students every year until they graduate and then examine changes over time; this would be a longitudinal design. On the other hand, we could use a cross-sectional design by gathering data at a single point from members of the four classes, and then comparing the four groups. If seniors had higher scores on a measure of professionalism than freshmen, it might be inferred that nursing students become increasingly socialized professionally by their educational experiences. To make this kind of inference, we would need to assume that the seniors would have responded as the freshmen responded had they been questioned 3 years earlier, or, conversely, that freshmen students would demonstrate increased professionalism if they were questioned 3 years later. Such a design, which involves a comparison of multiple age cohorts, is sometimes referred to as a **cohort comparison design**.

The main advantage of cross-sectional designs is that they are relatively economical. There are, however, problems in inferring changes over time using a cross-sectional design. In our example, seniors and freshmen may have different attitudes toward the nursing profession, independent of experiences during their 4 years of education. The large number of social and technological changes in our society frequently makes it questionable to assume that differences in the behaviors or characteristics of different age groups are the result of time passing rather than a reflection of cohort or generational differences. In cross-sectional studies designed to study change, there are frequently several alternative explanations for the findings—and that is precisely what good research design tries to avoid.

> **Example of a cross-sectional study:** Chen and Kennedy (2005) used a cross-sectional design to study age and other factors associated with obesity in Chinese-American children. Older children were more likely than younger ones to have a higher body mass index.

Longitudinal Designs

A study in which data are collected at more than one point in time *over an extended period* uses a **longitudinal design**. (A study involving the collection of postoperative patient data on vital signs eight times over a 2-day period would not be described as longitudinal.) Four situations call for a longitudinal design:

1. *Studying time-related processes.* Some research problems specifically concern phenomena that evolve over time (e.g., healing, learning, recidivism, and physical growth).
2. *Determining time sequences.* It is sometimes important to determine the sequencing of phenomena. For example, if it is hypothesized that

infertility results in depression, then it would be important to determine that the depression did not precede the fertility problem.

3. *Making comparisons over time.* Some studies are undertaken to examine whether changes have occurred over time. For example, an experimental study might examine whether an intervention had both short-term and long-term benefits. A qualitative study might explore the evolution of grieving among parents of infants who died of SIDS.

4. *Enhancing research control.* Quantitative researchers sometimes collect data at multiple points to enhance the interpretability of the results. For example, when two groups are being compared with regard to the effects of alternative interventions, the collection of data before any intervention occurs allows the researcher to detect—and control—any initial differences between groups.

There are several types of longitudinal designs. Most involve collecting data from one group of study participants multiple times, but others involve different samples. **Trend studies**, for example, are investigations in which samples from a population are studied over time with respect to some phenomenon. Different samples are selected at repeated intervals, but the samples are always drawn from the same population. Trend studies permit researchers to examine patterns and rates of change over time and to predict future developments. For example, trend studies have been conducted to analyze the number of students entering nursing programs to forecast future supplies of nurses. There are also many trend studies that document trends in public health problems, such as smoking, obesity, child abuse, and so on.

Example of a trend study: Edwards and colleagues (2005) conducted a trend study to determine whether gender differences associated with coronary artery revascularization changed over time. Data from 1993 and then 2003 were analyzed.

In **panel studies**, the *same* people are used to supply data at two or more points in time. The term panel refers to the sample of subjects providing data. Because the same people are studied over time, researchers can identify individuals who did and did not change and then examine characteristics that differentiate the two groups. As an example, a panel study could be designed to explore the antecedent characteristics of smokers who were later able to quit. Panel studies also allow researchers to examine how conditions and characteristics at time 1 influence characteristics and conditions at time 2. For example, health outcomes at time 2 could be studied among individuals with different health-related behaviors at time 1. Panel studies are intuitively appealing as an approach to studying change but are expensive to manage and face problems of **attrition**—the loss of participants over time. Attrition is problematic because those who drop out of the study often differ in important ways from those who continue to participate, resulting in potential biases and difficulty with generalizability.

Example of a panel study: Wu and Pender (2005) tested Pender's Health Promotion model using data from a two-wave panel study of Taiwanese adolescents. Data for a number of variables measured in the first wave (e.g., social support, self-efficacy, barriers to physical activity) were used to predict amount of physical activity in the second wave.

Follow-up studies are similar to panel studies, but are usually undertaken to determine the subsequent development of individuals who have a specified condition or who have received a specific intervention—unlike panel studies, which have samples drawn from more general populations. For example, patients who have received a particular nursing intervention or clinical treatment may be followed to ascertain the long-term effects of the treatment. As another example, samples of premature infants may be followed to assess their later cognitive and motor development. Like panel studies, a major challenge of conducting follow-up studies is to retain study participants.

Example of a follow-up study: Lukkarinen and Henteninen (2006) conducted a follow-up study of 280 patients who had undergone various treatments for coronary artery disease. Data relating to the patients' quality of life were gathered 1 year and 8 years after their treatment.

In sum, longitudinal designs are appropriate for studying the dynamics of a phenomenon over time. Researchers must make decisions about the number of data collection points and the intervals between them based on the nature of study and available resources. When change or development is rapid, numerous time points at short intervals may be needed to document it. Researchers interested in outcomes that may occur years after the original data collection must use longer-term follow-up. However, the longer the interval, the greater the risk for attrition and resulting biases.

➲ **TIP:** In planning your study and making design decisions, you will often need to balance various considerations, such as time, cost, ethical issues, and study integrity. Try to get a firm understanding of your "upper limits" before making final design decisions. That is, what is the *most* money that can be spent on the project? What is the *maximal amount* of time available for conducting the study? What is the limit of acceptability with regard to deception or other ethical issues, given the risk/benefit ratio of the study? These limits often eliminate some design options. With these constraints in mind, the central focus should be on designing a study that maximizes the validity or trustworthiness of the study.

Retrospective and Prospective Designs

Time is also relevant to designs that are either retrospective or prospective, but these terms refer to the timing of the independent and dependent variables, not to the timing of data collection. A study with a **retrospective design** involves collecting data on an outcome occurring in the present, and then linking it retrospectively to antecedents or determinants occurring in the past. Retrospective studies are typically cross-sectional—that is, data about both present outcomes, and past events and occurrences are collected at a single point in time. This involves having participants give retrospective accounts about the past, which is sometimes problematic. Asking people if they had a headache at any time in the previ-

ous 12 months might not be difficult to answer, but asking them to report how many times they had a headache, or what it felt like to have a headache 6 months ago, is likely to result in unreliable answers.

Example of a retrospective study: Colville and Gracey (2006) retrospectively gathered information about mothers' experiences and distress during their child's stay on a pediatric intensive care unit. They measured parental stress 8 months after the child's discharge and examined whether current stress was related to the mothers' recollections of stress during the hospitalization.

In **prospective studies,** information is first collected about a presumed cause or antecedent, and then subsequently the effect or outcome is measured. This sounds like a longitudinal design, but in fact, not all prospective studies are longitudinal, and *vice versa*. For example, intervention studies are prospective, in the sense that the researcher introduces the intervention and then determines its effect. A study that collected data 1 day after the intervention would be prospective, but not longitudinal. As we discuss in Chapter 10, prospective designs usually yield better-quality evidence than retrospective designs.

Example of a prospective study: Parsons, Bidewell, and Nagy (2006) used a prospective design to study the effect of pregnant women's natural eating behavior during the latent phase of labor on outcomes in active labor. Women who voluntarily ate food were compared with women who consumed only clear fluids in terms of duration of labor, need for medical intervention, vomiting, and adverse birth outcomes.

➲ **TIP:** Although qualitative studies would not be characterized as having retrospective designs, many qualitative studies involve obtaining retrospective accounts about a person's past and ongoing experiences or processes.

ORGANIZATION OF A RESEARCH PROJECT

Studies typically take many months to complete and, if the study is longitudinal, it may require years of work. During the planning phase, it is important to develop at least preliminary estimates of how long various research tasks will require. This may be easier to accomplish for quantitative studies than for qualitative ones because the former tend to have a more linear progression of prespecified activities and strategies, but even qualitative studies profit from a tentative schedule.

Almost all studies are conducted under some time pressure. Students in research courses have end-of-term deadlines; government-sponsored research involves funds granted for a specified time. Those who do not have formal time constraints (e.g., graduate students working on dissertations) have their own goals for project completion. Setting up a timetable in advance may be an important means of meeting such goals. Having deadlines for tasks—even tentative ones—helps to impose order and delimits tasks that might otherwise continue indefinitely, such as problem selection and literature reviews.

Chapter 3 presented a sequence of steps that quantitative researchers follow in doing a study. The steps represented an idealized conception of what researchers do. The research process rarely follows a neatly prescribed pattern of sequential procedures, even in quantitative studies. Developments in one step, for example, may require alterations in a previously completed activity. Iteration and backtracking are the norm—for example, decisions about sample size may require revised thinking about how many sites are needed. Selection of methods to measure key research variables might require changes to how the population is defined, and so on. Nevertheless, especially for quantitative researchers, preliminary time estimates are very important. In particular, it is important to have a sense of how much total time the study will require and when it will begin.

➲ **TIP:** It is not possible to give even approximate figures for the relative percentage of time that should be spent on each task. Some projects require many months to develop and test new measuring instruments, whereas other studies use previously existing ones, for example. Clearly, not all steps are equally time-consuming. It would not make sense simply to divide the available time by the number of tasks.

Researchers sometimes develop visual timelines or charts to help them organize a study, and such timelines are especially useful if external funding is sought because the schedule helps researchers to understand when and for how long staff support (e.g., for data collection) is needed. This can best be illustrated with an example, in this case of a hypothetical quantitative study.

Suppose a researcher was studying the following problem: Is a woman's decision to have an annual mammogram related to her perceived susceptibility to breast cancer? Using the organization of steps outlined in Chapter 3, here are some of the tasks that might be undertaken*:

1. The researcher, who lost her mother to breast cancer, is concerned that many older women do not get mammograms regularly. Her specific *research question* is whether mammogram practices are different for women who have different views about their susceptibility to breast cancer.
2. The researcher *reviews the research literature* on breast cancer, mammography use, and factors affecting mammography decisions.
3. The researcher does *clinical fieldwork* by discussing the problem with nurses and other health care professionals in various clinical settings (health clinics, private obstetrics and gynecology practices) and by informally discussing the problem with women in a support group for breast cancer victims.
4. The researcher examines *theoretical frameworks* for conceptualizing the problem. She finds that the Health Belief Model is relevant, and this helps her to develop a theoretical rationale for her study and a conceptual definition of susceptibility to breast cancer.
5. Based on what the researcher has learned, the following *hypothesis is developed:* Women who perceive themselves as not susceptible to breast cancer are less likely than other women to get an annual mammogram.

*This is, of course, only a partial list of tasks and is designed to illustrate the flow of activities; the flow in this example is more orderly than would ordinarily be true.

6. The researcher adopts a nonexperimental, cross-sectional, between-subjects *research design*. Her comparison strategy will be to compare women with different rankings on susceptibility to breast cancer. She designs the study to control the extraneous variables of age, marital status, and general health status. Her research site will be Los Angeles.

7. There is no *intervention* in this study (the design is nonexperimental), and so this step does not need to be undertaken.

8. The researcher designates that the *population* of interest is women between the ages of 50 and 65 years living in Los Angeles who have not been previously diagnosed as having any form of cancer.

9. The researcher will recruit 250 women living in Los Angeles as her *research sample*; they are identified at random using a telephone procedure known as random-digit dialing and so she does not need to gain entrée into any institution or organization.

10. *Research variables will be measured* by self-report; that is, the independent variable (perceived susceptibility), dependent variable (mammogram history), and extraneous variables will be measured by asking participants a series of questions. The researcher will use existing measuring instruments, rather than developing new ones.

11. The Institutional Review Board (IRB) at the researcher's institution is asked to review the research plans to determine whether the study *adheres to ethical standards.*

12. *Plans for the study are finalized:* the methods are reviewed and refined by colleagues with clinical and methodologic expertise and by the IRB; the data collection instruments are pretested; and interviewers who will collect the data are trained.

13. *Data are collected* by conducting telephone interviews with the research sample.

14. *Data are prepared for analysis* by coding them and entering them onto a computer file.

15. *Data are analyzed* using a statistical software package.

16. The results indicate that the hypothesis is supported; however, the researcher's *interpretation* must take into consideration that many women who were asked to participate in the study declined to do so.

17. The researcher presents an early report on her findings and interpretations at a conference of Sigma Theta Tau International. She subsequently publishes the report in the *Western Journal of Nursing Research.*

18. The researcher seeks out clinicians to discuss how the study findings can be *utilized in practice.*

The researcher in this study is planning to conduct this study over a 2-year period. Figure 8.3 presents a hypothetical schedule for the research tasks to be completed. Note that many steps overlap or are undertaken concurrently. Some steps are projected to involve little time, whereas others require months of work. ❷

In developing a time schedule of this sort, a number of considerations should be kept in mind, including researchers' level of knowledge and methodologic competence. Resources available to researchers, in terms of research funds and personnel, greatly influence time estimates. In the present example, if the researcher needed funding to help pay for the cost of hiring interviewers, the timeline would need to be expanded to accommodate the time period required to prepare a proposal and await the funding decision.

It is also important to consider the practical aspects of performing the study, which were not enumerated in the preceding section. Obtaining supplies, securing permissions, getting approval for using forms or instruments, hiring staff, and holding meetings are all time-consuming, but necessary, activities.

Individuals differ in the kinds of tasks that appeal to them. Some people enjoy the preliminary phase, which has a strong intellectual component, whereas others are more eager to collect the data, a task that is more interpersonal. Researchers should, however, allocate a reasonable amount of time to do justice to each activity.

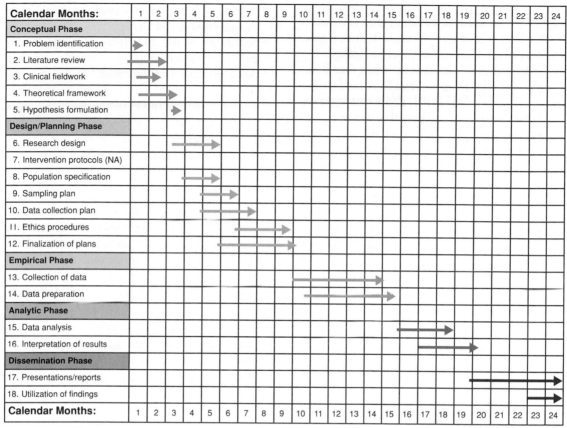

Calendar Months:	1	2	3	4	5	6	7	8	9	10	11	12	13	14	15	16	17	18	19	20	21	22	23	24
Conceptual Phase																								
1. Problem identification																								
2. Literature review																								
3. Clinical fieldwork																								
4. Theoretical framework																								
5. Hypothesis formulation																								
Design/Planning Phase																								
6. Research design																								
7. Intervention protocols (NA)																								
8. Population specification																								
9. Sampling plan																								
10. Data collection plan																								
11. Ethics procedures																								
12. Finalization of plans																								
Empirical Phase																								
13. Collection of data																								
14. Data preparation																								
Analytic Phase																								
15. Data analysis																								
16. Interpretation of results																								
Dissemination Phase																								
17. Presentations/reports																								
18. Utilization of findings																								
Calendar Months:	1	2	3	4	5	6	7	8	9	10	11	12	13	14	15	16	17	18	19	20	21	22	23	24

FIGURE 8.3⊗   Project timeline, in calendar months: hypothetical study of mammography decisions and perceived susceptibility to breast cancer.

The Toolkit with the accompanying *Resource Manual* includes the timeline in Figure 8.3 as well as other material in this chapter for you to adapt for your study. ⊗

PILOT STUDIES

A consistent conclusion in systematic reviews is that the quality of evidence on problems of relevance to nursing, and health care in general, is less than optimal. This means that "best evidence" currently available for nursing practice is seldom the best evidence possible. There is a growing recognition that it takes a lot of skill and effort to undertake research that has strong scientific merit.

In developing research plans, researchers intent on conducting a study that will yield high-quality evidence sometimes incorporate a pilot study into their plans. A **pilot study** is a small-scale version or trial run designed to test the methods to be used in a larger, more rigorous study, which is sometimes referred to as the **parent study.** Pilot studies are not just studies with a small number of participants, nor are they small, exploratory studies such as may be conducted by graduate students. The focus of pilot studies is not substantive—that is, their purpose is not to answer a research question. The purpose of a pilot study is to prevent an expensive fiasco—the misfortune of undertaking a costly but flawed large-scale study. For this reason, pilot studies are sometimes referred to as *feasibility studies.*

→ TIP: Many studies in the nursing research literature are called pilots when, in fact, they appear to be small-scale exploratory efforts, often with numerous methodologic flaws. Calling a study a "pilot" does not remove those flaws or absolve researchers for having those flaws. Avoid using the term pilot study unless you truly plan to use information from the pilot to assess the possibility of developing a stronger, larger investigation on the same topic.

Pilot studies can serve a number of important functions in planning a rigorous parent study, including evaluation of the following:

* Adequacy of study methods and procedures
* Likely success of a participant recruitment strategy
* Appropriateness and quality of instruments
* Strength of relationships between key variables so that the number of needed study participants can be estimated
* Identification of confounding variables that need to be controlled
* Adequacy of training materials for research staff
* Potential problems, such as loss of participants during the course of the study
* Extent to which the preliminary evidence justifies subsequent, more rigorous research

Pilot studies play an especially important role in research involving new interventions—and, indeed, we would argue that it is almost *essential* to pilot the intervention before a full test of its effectiveness. In intervention research, the pilot is a test of not only the methods of conducting the research but also the intervention itself, providing opportunities for refining and improving it. The pilot can also offer insights into the feasibility of implementing the intervention in real-world settings. Data from the pilot testing of an intervention can shed light on a number of things, including the following:

* Acceptability of the intervention to intended beneficiaries (e.g., patients), intervention agents (e.g., nurses), and administrators

* Adequacy, comprehensiveness, and clarity of the intervention protocols
* Suitability of the underlying theoretical rationale for the intervention
* Appropriateness of the "dose" of the intervention
* Extent to which **intervention fidelity** can be maintained (i.e., the faithfulness with which the protocols are actually adhered to)
* Rate of retention in the intervention
* Safety of the intervention, and any unforeseen side effects it might yield

In summary, the outcomes of a pilot study are "lessons" that can inform subsequent efforts to generate strong evidence for nursing practice. Pilots can help researchers minimize the "if-only-I-had" laments that plague most efforts. Thus, in planning a study, it is wise to consider the many possible benefits of undertaking a pilot.

→ TIP: Researchers usually should not seek funding for a full-fledged intervention study until they have completed pilot work and can report on the lessons they learned in their proposals.

CRITIQUING PLANNING ASPECTS OF A STUDY

Except in articles designed to specifically illuminate the research process, such as in the example of a pilot study described in the next section, researchers typically do not reveal much about the planning process or about problems that arose during the course of the study. Thus, there is typically little that a consumer can do to critique the researcher's efficiency or effectiveness during the planning phase of a study. What *can* be critiqued, of course, are the outcomes of the planning—that is, the actual methodologic decisions themselves. Guidelines for critiquing those decisions will be provided in subsequent chapters of this book.

There are, however, a few things that readers can be alert to relating to the planning of a study. First, it is likely that a researcher was more careful in planning if there is evidence in a report that the study was carefully conceptualized. If a conceptual map is presented (or implied) in the report, it means that the researcher had a "road map" that could serve as a planning aid for the research.

Second, readers can consider whether the researcher's plans reflect adequate attention to concerns about EBP. For example, was the comparison group strategy designed to reflect a realistic practice concern? Was the setting one that maximizes potential for the generalizability of the findings? Did the timeframes for data collection correspond to clinically important milestones? Was the intervention sensitive to the constraints of a typical practice environment?

Finally, confidence in the efficacy of study planning can be strengthened by evidence that the researcher devoted sufficient time and resources in preparing for the study. For example, if the report indicates that the study was preceded by a pilot test, this suggests that some of the "bugs" were probably worked out. If the report indicates that the study grew out of earlier research on a similar topic, or that the researcher had previously used the same instruments, or had completed other studies in the same setting, this also suggests that the researcher was not plunging into completely unfamiliar waters. Unrealistic planning can sometimes be inferred from a discussion about the sample and sample recruitment. If the report indicates that the researcher was unable to recruit the originally hoped-for number of study participants, or if recruitment took months longer than anticipated, this suggests that the researcher may not have done adequate homework during the planning phase.

●●●●●●●●●●●●●●●●●●●●●●●●

RESEARCH EXAMPLE

In this section, we describe the outcomes of a pilot study for a larger intervention study. A report for another pilot study appears in its entirety in the *Resource Manual* that accompanies this book.

Research Example of a Pilot Study

Study: "Methodological and ethical issues emerging from pilot testing an intervention with women in a transitional shelter" (Hatton & Kaiser, 2004)

Purpose: The purpose of the article was to describe some of the lessons that were learned during the pilot test of a social support intervention with women who had experienced homelessness and were living in a transitional shelter.

Pilot study methods: The pilot involved a preliminary test of an intervention designed to help sheltered women to improve their health and health maintenance behaviors. An intervention nurse met with women in groups for four to eight sessions at a transitional shelter, and then with each woman individually on a monthly basis for 12 months. The intervention used a set of modules with specific objectives and activities for each session. A total of 58 women (27 in the intervention group and 31 in a nonintervention group) participated in the pilot, which took 2 years to complete.

Pilot study findings: The researchers identified several ethical and methodologic challenges that emerged during the pilot, leading to concrete recommendations for subsequent research. First, there was considerable staff turnover at the shelter, and this required ongoing time on the researchers' part to cultivate and maintain relationships. The researchers noted that this type of effort should be anticipated in working with community agencies and urged that time and resources be budgeted for this. Second, they found that the interviews with study participants sometimes served as an intervention in and of themselves (e.g., triggering women to get a Pap test), and this led them to conclude that it might have been better to compare two nursing interventions rather than having one group merely get treatment as usual. Third, sensitive and troubling information was revealed during data collection (e.g., sexual assaults at the workplace), which suggested the need for training research assistants to effectively address such problems. Fourth, they learned that a particular challenge was managing participant attrition. Although they had gathered "locator" information from participants at the outset, they recommended updating this information every 2 weeks and offering incentives for completing the updated forms. And fifth, they discovered that many of the women, even though they did not drop out of the study, failed to keep appointments. The researchers had several suggestions to address this, including having early, explicit discussions during the group sessions about missing appointments.

Conclusions: The researchers felt it was important to share these lessons from their pilot study with the research community so that strategies for conducting research with marginalized groups could be improved.

○○○○○○○○○○○○○○○○○○○○○

SUMMARY POINTS

- Researchers face numerous conceptual, practical, ethical, and methodologic challenges that must be considered in planning a study. The major methodologic challenge is designing studies that are reliable and valid (quantitative studies) or trustworthy (qualitative studies).

- **Reliability** refers to the accuracy and consistency of information obtained in a study. **Validity** is a more complex concept that broadly concerns the *soundness* of the study's evidence—that is, whether the findings are cogent, convincing, and well grounded.

- **Trustworthiness** in qualitative research encompasses several different dimensions. **Dependability** refers to evidence that is believable, consistent, and stable over time. **Confirmability** refers to evidence of the researcher's objectivity. **Credibility** is achieved to the extent that the research methods engender confidence in the truth of the data and in the researchers' interpretations of the data.

- **Triangulation**, the use of multiple sources or referents to draw conclusions about what constitutes the truth, is one approach to establishing credibility.

- A **bias** is an influence that produces a distortion in the study results. **Systematic bias** results when a bias is consistent across participants or situations.

- In quantitative studies, **research control** is used to hold constant outside influences on the dependent variable so that the relationship between the independent and dependent variables can be better understood.

- The external influences researchers seek to control are **extraneous (confounding) variables**—extraneous to the purpose of a specific study. There are a number of ways to control such influences, but the general principle is that the extraneous variables must be **held constant**.

- For a quantitative researcher, a powerful tool to eliminate bias concerns **randomness**—having certain features of the study established by chance rather than by design or personal preference.

- **Masking** (or **blinding**) is sometimes used to avoid biases stemming from participants' or research agents' awareness of study hypotheses or research status. **Single-blind studies** involve masking for one group (e.g., participants), and **double-blind studies** involve masking of two groups.

- **Reflexivity**, the process of reflecting critically on the self and of scrutinizing personal values that could affect data collection and interpretation, is an important tool in qualitative research.

- **Generalizability** in a quantitative study concerns the extent to which the findings can be applied to other groups and settings. A similar concept in qualitative studies is **transferability**, the extent to which qualitative findings can be transferred to other settings. An important mechanism for promoting transferability is **thick description**, the rich and thorough description of the research setting or context so that others can make inferences about contextual similarities.

- In planning a study, researchers make many design decisions, including whether to have an intervention, how to control extraneous variables, whether masking will be used, what type of comparisons will be made, where the study will take place, and what the timeframes of the study will be.

- Researchers often incorporate comparisons into their designs to enhance interpretability. **Between-subjects designs**, in which different groups of people are compared, contrast with **within-subjects designs** that involve comparisons of the same subjects.

- Site selection for a study is based on several substantive and practical issues and often involves **site visits** to evaluate suitability and feasibility. Gaining entrée into a site usually involves developing and maintaining trust with the gatekeepers.

- **Cross-sectional designs** involve the collection of data at one point in time, whereas **longitudinal designs** involve data collection at two or more points over an extended period.
- Longitudinal studies, which are used to study trends, changes, or development over time, include **trend studies** (multiple points of data collection with different samples from the same population), and **panel studies** and **follow-up studies** (which gather data from the *same* subjects more than once).
- Longitudinal studies are typically expensive, time-consuming, and subject to the risk for **attrition** (loss of participants over time), but can produce extremely valuable information.
- Another design decision concerns timing *vis-à-vis* the independent and dependent variables in a quantitative study. A **retrospective design** involves the collection of data about an outcome in the present and about possible causes or antecedents in the past. A **prospective design** involves having information about a cause or antecedent first, and then the subsequent collection of information about outcomes.
- A **pilot study** (or *feasibility study*) is a small-scale version or trial run designed to test methods to be used in a larger, more rigorous study (the **parent study**). Pilot studies provide invaluable information that can enhance the quality of evidence a study can yield and should be considered in planning a project, especially one involving an intervention.

STUDY ACTIVITIES

Chapter 8 of the *Resource Manual to Accompany Nursing Research: Generating and Assessing Evidence for Nursing Practice, 8th edition*, offers various exercises and study suggestions for reinforcing concepts presented in this chapter. In addition, the following study questions can be addressed:

1. Find a study published in a nursing journal in 2000 or earlier that is described as a pilot study. Do you think the study really is a pilot study, or do you think this label was used inappropriately? Justify your response.

2. Suppose you wanted to study how children's attitudes toward smoking change over time. Design a cross-sectional study to research this question, specifying the samples that you would want to include. Now design a longitudinal study to research the same problem. Identify the strengths and weaknesses of each approach.

STUDIES CITED IN CHAPTER 8

Methodologic or theoretical references cited in this chapter can be found in a separate section at the end of the book.

Beckie, T. M., Beckstead, J. W., & Webb, M. S. (2001). Modeling women's quality of life after cardiac events. *Western Journal of Nursing Research, 23*, 179–194.

Chen, J. L., & Kennedy, C. (2005). Factors associated with obesity in Chinese-American children. *Pediatric Nursing, 31*(2), 110–115.

Collins, M., Shattell, M., & Thomas, S. P. (2005). Problematic interviewee behaviors in qualitative research. *Western Journal of Nursing Research, 27*(2), 188–199

Colville, G. A., & Gracey, D. (2006). Mothers' recollections of the paediatric intensive care unit: Associations with psychopathology and views on follow-up. *Intensive and Critical Care Nursing, 22*(1), 49–55.

Edwards, M. L., Albert, N. M., Wang, C., & Apperson-Hansen, C. (2005). 1993–2003 gender differences in coronary artery revascularization: Has anything changed? *Journal of Cardiovascular Nursing, 20*(6), 461–467.

Hatton, D. C., & Kaiser, L. (2004). Methodological and ethical issues emerging from pilot testing an intervention with women in a transitional shelter. *Western Journal of Nursing Research, 26*(1), 129–136.

Lukkarinen, H., & Hentinen, M. (2006). Treatments of coronary artery disease improve quality of life in the long term. *Nursing Research, 55*(1), 26–33.

Mateo, M. A., Glod, C. A., Hennen, J., Price, B. H., & Merrill, N. (2005). Mild traumatic brain injury in psychiatric inpatients. *Journal of Neuroscience Nursing, 37*(1), 28–33.

Myrick, F., & Yonge, O. (2004). Enhancing critical thinking in the preceptorship experience in nursing education. *Journal of Advanced Nursing, 45,* 371–380.

Parsons, M., Bidewell, J., & Nagy, S. (2006). Natural eating behavior in latent labor and its effect on outcomes in active labor. *Journal of Midwifery & Women's Health, 51*(1), 1–6.

Wheatley, I. (2006). The nursing practice of taking level 1 patient observations. *Intensive and Critical Care Nursing,22*(2), 115–121.

Wu, T. Y., & Pender, N. (2005). A panel study of physical activity in Taiwanese youth. *Family & Community Health, 28*(2), 113–124.

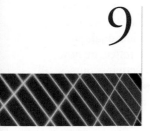

9

Developing an Approach for a Qualitative Study

THE DESIGN OF QUALITATIVE STUDIES

Quantitative researchers carefully specify a research design before collecting even one piece of data, and rarely depart from that design once the study is underway. In qualitative research, by contrast, the study design typically evolves over the course of the project. Decisions about how best to obtain data, from whom to obtain data, how to schedule data collection, and how long each data collection session should last are made in the field as the study unfolds. Qualitative studies use an **emergent design**—a design that emerges as researchers make ongoing decisions reflecting what has already been learned. As noted by Lincoln and Guba (1985), an emergent design in qualitative studies is not the result of sloppiness or laziness on the part of researchers, but rather a reflection of their desire to have the inquiry based on the realities and viewpoints of those under study—realities and viewpoints that are not known or understood at the outset.

Characteristics of Qualitative Research Design

Qualitative inquiry has been guided by different disciplines, and each has developed methods for addressing questions of particular interest. However,

some general characteristics of qualitative research design tend to apply across disciplines. In general, qualitative design:

- Often involves a merging together of various data collection strategies (i.e., triangulation);
- Is flexible and elastic, capable of adjusting to what is being learned during the course of data collection;
- Tends to be holistic, striving for an understanding of the whole;
- Requires researchers to become intensely involved, often remaining in the field for lengthy periods of time;
- Requires the researcher to become the research instrument; and
- Requires ongoing analysis of the data to formulate subsequent strategies and to determine when fieldwork is done.

With regard to the first characteristic, qualitative researchers tend to put together a complex array of data, derived from a variety of sources and using a variety of methods. This tendency has sometimes been described as **bricolage**, and the qualitative researcher has been referred to as a **bricoleur**, a person who "is adept at performing a large number of diverse tasks, ranging from interviewing to intensive reflection and introspection" (Denzin & Lincoln, 2000, p. 6).

Qualitative Design and Planning

Although design decisions are not specified in advance, qualitative researchers typically do considerable advance planning that supports their flexibility in developing an emergent design. In the total absence of planning, design choices might actually be constrained. For example, researchers initially might anticipate a 6-month period for data collection, but may need to be prepared (financially and emotionally) to spend even longer periods of time in the field to pursue data collection opportunities that could not have been foreseen. In other words, qualitative researchers plan for broad contingencies that may be expected to pose decision opportunities once the study has begun. In addition to the planning activities described in Chapter 8, advance planning is especially useful with regard to the following:

- Selecting a broad framework or tradition (described in the next section) to guide certain design decisions
- Determining the maximum amount of time available for the study, given costs and other constraints
- Developing a broad data collection strategy (e.g., will interviews be conducted?) and identifying opportunities for enhancing trustworthiness (e.g., through triangulation) and documenting it
- Collecting relevant written or photographic materials about the site (e.g., maps, organizational charts, resource directories)
- Identifying the types of equipment that could aid in the collection and analysis of data in the field (e.g., audio and video recording equipment, laptop computers) and the type of assistance needed (if any) to complete the project
- Identifying personal biases, views, and presuppositions *vis-à-vis* the phenomenon or the study site, as well as ideological stances (reflexivity)

Thus, qualitative researchers need to plan for a variety of potential circumstances, but decisions about how to deal with them must be resolved when the social context of time, place, and human interactions is better understood. By both allowing for and anticipating an evolution of strategies, qualitative researchers seek to make their research design responsive to the situation and to the phenomenon under study. In planning their qualitative studies, nurse researchers should also reflect on how the findings might be useful to practicing nurses and, if possible, seek opportunities to enhance the evidenced-based practice potential of the research.

Qualitative Design Features

Some of the design features discussed in Chapter 8 apply to qualitative studies. However, qualitative design features are often *post hoc* characterizations of what happened in the field rather than features specifically planned in advance. To further contrast qualitative and quantitative research design, we refer you to the design elements identified in Table 8.2.

Intervention, Control, and Masking

Qualitative research is almost always nonexperimental—although, as discussed in Chapter 12, qualitative research sometimes is embedded in an experimental project. Researchers conducting a study within the naturalistic paradigm do not normally conceptualize their studies as having independent and dependent variables, and they rarely control or manipulate any aspect of the people or environment under study. Masking is also not a strategy used by qualitative researchers because there is no intervention or hypothesis to conceal. The goal of most qualitative studies is to develop a rich understanding of a phenomenon as it exists in the real world and as it is constructed by individuals in the context of that world.

Comparisons

Qualitative researchers typically do not plan in advance to make comparisons because the intent of most qualitative studies is to thoroughly describe and explain a phenomenon. Nevertheless, patterns emerging in the data often suggest that certain comparisons are relevant and illuminating. Indeed, as Morse (2004b) has noted in an editorial about qualitative comparisons that appeared in *Qualitative Health Research*, "All description requires comparisons"

(p. 1323). Inevitably in coding qualitative information and in determining whether categories are saturated, there is a need to compare "this" to "that." Morse noted that qualitative comparisons are often not dichotomous: "life is usually on a continuum" (p. 1324). Of course, group comparisons sometimes *are* planned in qualitative studies (e.g., a comparison of nurses' and patients' perspectives about a phenomenon).

> **Example of qualitative comparisons:** Hilden and Honkasalo (2006) explored how nurses interpret patient autonomy in end-of-life decision making. Based on interviews with 17 nurses, they discovered that there were three distinct patterns, which they called the "supporter," the "analyst," and the "practical," each of which characterized a certain position for patients and relatives and a certain identity for nurses in end-of-life decision making.

Research Settings

Qualitative researchers usually collect their data in real-world, naturalistic settings. And, whereas a quantitative researcher usually strives to collect data in one type of setting to maintain control over the environment (e.g., conducting all interviews in study participants' homes), qualitative researchers may deliberately strive to study phenomena in a variety of natural contexts. Qualitative researchers may also conduct their studies in multiple sites.

> **Example of variation in settings and sites:** Sterling and Peterson (2005) conducted a qualitative study to examine treatment decision making among African-American families of children with asthma. Their study was conducted in two sites, Seattle and New Orleans. Data were collected in multiple settings where families spent their time, including home, workplace, sports venues, church, and community festivals.

Timeframes

Qualitative research, like quantitative research, can be either cross-sectional, with one data collection point, or longitudinal, with multiple data collection points over an extended time period, to observe the evolution of some phenomenon. Sometimes qualitative researchers plan in advance for a longitudinal design, but in other cases, the decision to study a phenomenon longitudinally may be made in the field after preliminary data have been collected and analyzed.

> **Examples of the time dimension in qualitative studies:**
> - *Cross-sectional:* Daff and colleagues (2006) studied the experiences of family carers in moving a relative from an acute hospital admission into a residential care placement. The data were gathered at a fixed point in time, relying on retrospective accounts of the transitional process, rather than gathering the data as the transition occurred.
> - *Longitudinal:* Connell, Patterson, and Newman (2006) conducted a longitudinal study of the experiences of young women with breast cancer. Data were collected in three phases, and issues relating to the women's concerns about fertility, pregnancy, and breastfeeding were explored. The researchers found that the women's perceptions of fertility changed over time.

QUALITATIVE RESEARCH TRADITIONS

Despite the fact that there are some features common to many qualitative research designs, there is nevertheless a wide variety of overall approaches. Unfortunately, there is no readily agreed-upon classification system or taxonomy for the various approaches. Some authors have categorized qualitative studies in terms of analysis styles; others have classified them according to their broad focus. One useful system, as noted in Chapter 3, is to describe qualitative research according to disciplinary traditions. These traditions vary in their conceptualization of what types of questions are important to ask and in the methods they consider appropriate for answering those questions. The section that follows provides an overview of several qualitative research traditions (some of which we have previously introduced), and subsequent sections describe in greater detail traditions that have been especially prominent in nursing research.

Overview of Qualitative Research Traditions

The research traditions that have provided a theoretical underpinning for qualitative studies come primarily from the disciplines of anthropology, psychology, and sociology. As shown in Table 9.1, each discipline has tended to focus on one or two broad domains of inquiry.

The discipline of anthropology is concerned with human cultures. **Ethnography** (discussed more fully later in this chapter) is the primary research tradition in anthropology. Ethnographers study cultural patterns and experiences in a holistic fashion. **Ethnoscience** (sometimes referred to as **cognitive anthropology**) focuses on the cognitive world of a culture, with particular emphasis on the semantic rules and shared meanings that shape behavior. Cognitive anthropologists assume that a group's cultural knowledge is reflected in its language.

Example of an ethnoscientific study: Hirst (2002) used ethnoscientific methods to articulate a definition of resident abuse as perceived by nurses working in long-term care settings. She focused on the linguistic symbols and "folk terms" of the culture in long-term care institutions.

TABLE 9.1	Overview of Qualitative Research Traditions		
DISCIPLINE	**DOMAIN**	**RESEARCH TRADITION**	**AREA OF INQUIRY**
Anthropology	Culture	Ethnography	Holistic view of a culture
		Ethnoscience (cognitive anthropology)	Mapping of the cognitive world of a culture; a culture's shared meanings, semantic rules
Psychology/ philosophy	Lived experience	Phenomenology	Experiences of individuals within their lifeworld
		Hermeneutics	Interpretations and meanings of individuals' experiences
Psychology	Behavior and events	Ethology	Behavior observed over time in natural context
		Ecologic psychology	Behavior as influenced by the environment
Sociology	Social settings	Grounded theory	Social structural process within a social setting
		Ethnomethodology	Manner by which shared agreement is achieved in social settings
		Semiotics	Manner by which people make sense of social interactions
Sociolinguistics	Human communication	Discourse analysis	Forms and rules of conversation
History	Past behavior, events, and conditions	Historical analysis	Description and interpretation of historical events

Phenomenology has its disciplinary roots in both philosophy and psychology. As noted in Chapter 3, phenomenology focuses on the meaning of lived experiences of humans. A closely related research tradition is **hermeneutics**, which uses lived experiences as a tool for better understanding the social, cultural, political, or historical context in which those experiences occur. Hermeneutic inquiry almost always focuses on meaning and interpretation—how socially and historically conditioned individuals interpret their world within their given context.

The discipline of psychology has several other qualitative research traditions that focus on *behavior*. Human **ethology**, which is sometimes described as the biology of human behavior, studies behavior as it evolves in its natural context. Human ethologists use primarily observational methods in an attempt to discover universal behavioral structures. Warnock and Allen (2003) have urged nurse researchers to consider using ethological methods, and used neonatal pain to illustrate how ethology can be used to develop descriptive nursing knowledge and middle-range theory.

Example of an ethological study: Morse and Pooler (2002) used ethological methods to study the interactions of patients' family members with the patients and with nurses in the trauma-resuscitation room of an emergency department. The analysis was based on 193 videotapes of trauma room care.

Ecological psychology focuses more specifically on the influence of the environment on human behavior, and attempts to identify principles that explain the interdependence of humans and their environmental context. Viewed from an ecological context, people are affected by (and affect) a multilayered set of systems, including family, peer group, and neighborhood, as well as the more indirect effects of health care and social services systems, and the larger cultural belief and value systems of the society in which individuals live.

Example of an ecological study: Salazar and colleagues (2004) used an ecological framework in their study of perceptions of occupational hazards associated with pesticide exposure among Hispanic adolescent farmworkers in Oregon. The adolescents' risk perceptions were examined on four levels of environmental influence: microenvironment, organizational environment, social/community environment, and macroenvironment.

Sociologists study the social world in which we live and have developed several research traditions of importance to qualitative researchers. The **grounded theory** tradition (elaborated upon later in this chapter) seeks to describe and understand key social psychological and structural processes in social settings.

Ethnomethodology seeks to discover how people make sense of their everyday activities and interpret their social worlds so as to behave in socially acceptable ways. Within this tradition, researchers attempt to understand a social group's norms and assumptions that are so deeply ingrained that the members no longer think about the underlying reasons for their behaviors.

Example of an ethnomethodologic study: French (2005) used an ethnomethodologic approach in studying the practical reasoning process of specialist nurses in the United Kingdom during their use of research.

Unlike most other qualitative researchers, ethnomethodologists occasionally engage in **ethnomethodologic experiments**. During such experiments, researchers disrupt ordinary activity by doing something that violates the group's norms and assumptions. They then observe what group members do and how they try to make sense of what is happening. An example is observing what happens when a nurse violates expectations of appropriate behavior at nurses' change of shift report on a medical intensive care unit. For example, a nurse might be enlisted to start her day shift by deliberately taking out a novel and reading it while the charge nurse from nights is reporting on the status of critically ill patients. The researcher would then observe how the rest of the unit staff deals with this departure from expected behavior.

Symbolic interaction (or *interactionism*) is a sociological and social-psychological tradition with roots in American pragmatism and is sometimes associated with grounded theory research. As noted in Chapter 6, symbolic interaction focuses on the manner in which people make sense of social interactions and the interpretations they attach to social symbols, such as language. Symbolic interactionists sometimes use **semiotics**, which refers to the study of signs and their meanings. A sign is any entity or object that carries information (e.g., a diagram, map, or picture).

Example of a semiotic analysis: Giarelli (2006) did a semiotic analysis of the manifest and latent meanings in editorial cartoons published in the United States between 2001 and 2004 relating to cloning and stem cell research.

The domain of inquiry for sociolinguists is human communication. The tradition often referred to as **discourse analysis** (sometimes called *conversation analysis*) seeks to understand the rules, mechanisms, and structure of conversations. Discourse analysts are interested in understanding the action that a given kind of talk "performs." The data for discourse analysis typically are transcripts from naturally occurring conversations, such as those between nurses and their patients. In discourse analysis, the texts are situated in their social, cultural, political, and historical context.

Example of a discourse analysis: Li and Arber (2006) explored how nurses constructed dying patients' moral identities and how they used *emotion talk* to interpret patients' behavior. The researchers used discourse analysis to study interactive discourse between nurses and patients and among nurses.

Finally, **historical research**—the systematic collection and critical evaluation of data relating to past occurrences—is also a tradition that relies primarily on qualitative data. Nurses have used historical research methods to examine a wide range of phenomena in both the recent and more distant past.

Researchers in each of these traditions have developed methodologic strategies for the design and conduct of relevant studies. Thus, once a researcher has identified what aspect of the human experience is of greatest interest, there is typically a wealth of advice available about methods likely to be productive and design issues that need to be handled in the field.

➲ **TIP:** Sometimes a research report identifies more than one tradition as having provided the framework for a qualitative inquiry (e.g., a phenomenological study using the grounded theory method). However, such "method slurring" (Baker, Wuest, & Stern, 1992) has been criticized because each research tradition has different intellectual assumptions and methodologic prescriptions.

Ethnography

Ethnography is a type of qualitative inquiry that involves the description and interpretation of cultural behavior. Ethnographies are a blend of a process and a product, fieldwork, and a written text. Fieldwork is the process by which the ethnographer inevitably comes to understand a culture, and the ethnographic text is how that culture is communicated and portrayed. Because culture is, in itself, not visible or tangible, it must be constructed through ethnographic writing. Culture is inferred from the words, actions, and products of members of a group.

Ethnographic research is in some cases concerned with broadly defined cultures (e.g., a Samoan village culture), in what is sometimes referred to as a **macroethnography.** However, ethnographies sometimes focus on more narrowly defined cultures in a **microethnography** or **focused ethnography**. Microethnographies are exhaustive, fine-grained studies of either small units in a group or culture (e.g., the culture of homeless shelters) or specific activities in an organizational unit (e.g., how nurses communicate with children in an emergency department). An underlying assumption of the ethnographer is that every human group eventually evolves a culture that guides the members' view of the world and the way they structure their experiences.

Example of a focused ethnography: Ensign and Bell (2004) used a focused ethnographic approach to study the illness experiences of clinic- and street-based homeless youth aged 15 to 23 years living in the Seattle area.

Ethnographers seek to learn from (rather than to study) members of a cultural group—to understand their world view. Ethnographic researchers sometimes refer to "emic" and "etic" perspectives (terms that originate in linguistics, i.e., phon*emic* versus phon*etic*). An **emic perspective** refers to the way the members of the culture envision their world—it is the insiders' view. The emic is the local language, concepts, and means of expression that are used by the members of the group under study to characterize their experiences. The **etic perspective**, by contrast, is the outsiders' interpretation of the experiences of that culture; it is the language used by those doing the research to refer to the same phenomena. Ethnographers strive to acquire an emic perspective of a culture under study. Moreover, they strive to reveal what has been referred to as **tacit knowledge**, information about the culture that is so deeply embedded in cultural experiences that members do not talk about it or may not even be consciously aware of it.

Ethnographers almost invariably undertake extensive fieldwork to learn about a cultural group. Ethnographic research typically is a labor-intensive endeavor that requires long periods of time in the field—years of fieldwork may be required. In most cases, researchers strive to participate actively in cultural events and activities. The study of a culture requires a certain level of intimacy with members of the cultural group, and such intimacy can be developed only over time and by working directly with those members as active participants. The concept of **researcher as instrument** is frequently used by anthropologists to describe the significant role ethnographers play in analyzing and interpreting a culture.

Three broad types of information are usually sought by ethnographers: cultural behavior (what members of the culture do), cultural artifacts (what members of the culture make and use), and cultural speech (what people say). This implies that ethnographers rely on a wide variety of data sources, including observations, in-depth interviews, records, charts, and other types of physical evidence (e.g., photographs, diaries, letters). Ethnographers typically use a strategy known as **participant observation** in which they make observations of the culture under study while participating in its activities. Ethnographers observe people day after day in their natural environments to observe behavior in a wide array of circumstances. Ethnographers also enlist the help of **key informants** to help them understand and interpret the events and activities being observed.

Some ethnographers undertake an **egocentric network analysis**, which focuses on the pattern of relationships and networks of individuals. Each person has his or her own network of relationships that cut across many groups and that are presumed to contribute to the person's behaviors and attitudes. In studying these networks, researchers develop lists of a person's network members (called *alters*) and seek to understand the scope and nature of interrelationships and social supports. Network data from such efforts are often quantified and analyzed statistically. Egocentric network analysis attempts to understand features of personal networks and has been used to explain such phenomena as longevity, coping with crisis, and risk taking.

The product of ethnographic research usually is a rich and holistic description of the culture under study. Ethnographers also make interpretations of the culture, describing normative behavioral and social patterns. Among health care researchers, ethnography provides access to the health beliefs and health practices of a culture or subculture. Ethnographic inquiry can thus help to facilitate understanding of behaviors affecting health and illness.

In addition to written reports about ethnographic findings, ethnographers have recently used their research as the basis for performance ethnographies. A **performance ethnography** has been described as a scripted and staged re-enactment of ethnographically derived notes that reflect an interpretation of the culture. Denzin (2000) noted that "we inhabit a performance-based, dramaturgical culture. The dividing line between performance and audience blurs, and culture itself becomes a dramatic performance" (p. 903).

A rich array of ethnographic methods have been developed and cannot be fully explicated in this general textbook, but more information may be found in Hammersley and Atkinson (1995), Spradley and McCurdy (1972), Fetterman (1997), and Brewer (2000). Three variants of ethnographic research (ethnonursing research, institutional ethnography, and auto-ethnography) are described here, and a fourth (critical ethnography) is described later in this chapter.

Ethnonursing Research

Many nurse researchers have undertaken ethnographic studies. Indeed, Leininger has coined the phrase **ethnonursing research**, which she defines as "the study and analysis of the local or indigenous people's viewpoints, beliefs, and practices about nursing care behavior and processes of designated cultures" (1985, p. 38). In conducting an ethnonursing study, the investigator uses a broad theoretical framework to guide the research, such as the Theory of Culture Care (Leininger & McFarland, 2006).

Leininger and McFarland (2006) have described a number of enablers to guide researchers in conducting ethnonursing research. *Enablers* are ways to help discover complex phenomena like human care. Some of her enablers include her Stranger–Friend Model, Observation–Participation–Reflection Model, and Acculturation Enabler Guide. The stranger–friend enabler serves as a guide for researchers to use to map their progress and to be more aware of their feelings, behaviors, and responses as they transition from stranger to trusted friend. The phases of Leininger's observation–participation–reflection enabler include (1) primary observation and active listening, (2) primary observation with limited participation, (3) primary participation with continuing observations, and (4) primary reflection and reconfirmation of results with informants. The acculturation enabler guide was designed to aid researchers in assessing the degree of acculturation

of a person or group with regard to the specific culture under study.

> **Example of an ethnonursing study:** Hubbert (2005) conducted an ethnonursing study focusing on the subculture of homeless adults living in an urban homeless shelter. The focus was on the participants' meanings and experiences of care, or lack of care.

Institutional Ethnography

A type of ethnographic approach called **institutional ethnography** was pioneered by Dorothy Smith, a Canadian sociologist (1999). Institutional ethnography has been used in such fields as nursing, social work, community health, and occupational therapy to study the organization of professional services, examined from the perspective of those who are clients or front-line workers. Institutional ethnography seeks to understand the social determinants of people's everyday experiences, especially the institutional work processes that form the ground of people's lived experiences. The focus in institutional ethnography is on social organization and institutional work processes, and so research findings have the potential to play a role in organizational change.

> **Example of institutional ethnography:** Vukic and Keddy (2002) conducted an institutional ethnography designed to shed light on the nature of outpost nursing work and the day-to-day realities of nursing practice in a remote northern primary health care setting in Canada.

Auto-Ethnography

Ethnographers are often, but not always, "outsiders" to the culture under study. A type of ethnography that involves self-scrutiny (including scrutiny of groups or cultures to which researchers themselves belong) usually is referred to as **auto-ethnography,** but other terms such as *insider research*, *peer research*, and *complete member research* also have been used. There are numerous advantages to doing an auto-ethnography, the most obvious being ease of access, ease of recruitment, and the ability to get particularly candid, in-depth data based on preestablished trust and rapport. Another potential advantage is the researcher's ability to detect subtle nuances that an outsider might miss or take months to uncover. Lipson (2001), in her study of multiple chemical sensitivity sufferers, described how benefits can also accrue to the researcher personally and to study participants in an auto-ethnographic study. A potential limitation, however, is the researcher's inability to be objective about group (or self) processes, which can result in unconscious myopia about important but sensitive issues. Auto-ethnography demands that researchers maintain consciousness of their role and monitor their internal state and their interactions with others during the study. Various methodologic strategies have been developed for auto-ethnographic work and are summarized by Ellis and Bochner (2000).

Example of a performance auto-ethnography: Schneider (2005) described an auto-ethnography that explored how mothers of adults with schizophrenia talk about their children. Schneider herself was the mother of a schizophrenic person. Her report presented the script for a performance auto-ethnography based on her research.

Phenomenology

Phenomenology, rooted in a philosophical tradition developed by Husserl and Heidegger, is an approach to exploring and understanding people's everyday life experiences.

Phenomenological researchers ask: What is the *essence* of this phenomenon as experienced by these people and what does it *mean?* Phenomenologists assume there is an *essence*—an essential invariant structure—that can be understood, in much the same way that ethnographers assume that cultures exist. Essence is what makes a phenomenon what it is, and without which it would not be what it is. Phenomenologists investigate subjective phenomena in the belief that critical truths about reality are grounded in people's lived experiences. The phenomenological approach is especially useful when a phenomenon has been poorly defined or conceptualized. The topics appropriate to phenomenology are ones that are fundamental to the life experiences of humans; for health researchers, these include such topics as the meaning of suffering, the experience of domestic violence, and the quality of life with chronic pain.

Phenomenologists believe that lived experience gives meaning to each person's perception of a particular phenomenon. The goal of phenomenological inquiry is to understand fully lived experience and the perceptions to which it gives rise. Four aspects of lived experience that are of interest to phenomenologists are *lived space*, or spatiality; *lived body*, or corporeality; *lived time*, or temporality; and *lived human relation*, or relationality.

Phenomenologists view human existence as meaningful and interesting because of people's consciousness of that existence. The phrase **being-in-the-world** (or *embodiment*) is a concept that acknowledges people's physical ties to their world—they think, see, hear, feel, and are conscious through their bodies' interaction with the world.

In phenomenological studies, the main data source typically is in-depth conversations, with researchers and informants as co-participants. Researchers help informants to describe lived experiences without leading the discussion. Through in-depth conversations, researchers strive to gain entrance into the informants' world, to have full access to their experiences as lived. Two or more separate interviews or conversations are sometimes needed. Typically, phenomenological studies involve a small number of study participants—often 10 or fewer. For some phenomenological researchers, the inquiry includes not only gathering information from informants but also making efforts to experience the phenomenon in the same way, typically through participation, observation, and introspective reflection.

Phenomenologists share their insights in rich, vivid reports. A phenomenological text that describes the results of a study should help the readers "see" something in a different way that enriches their understanding of experiences. Van Manen (1997a) warns that if a phenomenological text is flat and boring, it "loses power to break through the taken-for-granted dimensions of everyday life" (p. 346).

A wealth of resources are available on phenomenological methods. Interested readers may wish to consult Spiegelberg (1975), Giorgi (1985, 2005), Colaizzi (1973, 1978), or Van Manen (1997b).

There are a number of variants and methodologic interpretations of phenomenology. The two main schools of thought are descriptive phenomenology and interpretive phenomenology (hermeneutics). Lopez and Willis (2004) provide a useful discussion about the need to differentiate the two and lay out underlying philosophical assumptions in nursing studies.

Descriptive Phenomenology

Descriptive phenomenology was developed first by Husserl (1962), who was primarily interested in the question: What do we know as persons? His philosophy emphasized descriptions of human experience. Descriptive phenomenologists insist on the careful description of ordinary conscious experience of everyday life—a description of "things" as people experience them. These "things" include hearing, seeing, believing, feeling, remembering, deciding, evaluating, acting, and so forth.

Descriptive phenomenological studies often involve the following four steps: bracketing, intuiting, analyzing, and describing. **Bracketing** refers to the process of identifying and holding in abeyance preconceived beliefs and opinions about the phenomenon under study. Although bracketing can never be achieved totally, researchers strive to bracket out the world and any presuppositions in an effort to confront the data in pure form. Bracketing is an iterative process that involves preparing, evaluating, and providing systematic ongoing feedback about the effectiveness of the bracketing. Phenomenological researchers (as well as other qualitative researchers) often maintain a *reflexive journal* in their efforts to bracket. Ahern (1999) provides 10 tips to help qualitative researchers with bracketing through notes in a reflexive journal:

1. Identify interests that, as a researcher, you may take for granted.
2. Clarify your personal values and identify areas in which you know you are biased.
3. Identify areas of possible role conflict.
4. Recognize gatekeepers' interests and make note of the degree to which they are favorably or unfavorably disposed toward your research.
5. Identify any feelings you have that may indicate a lack of neutrality.
6. Describe new or surprising findings in collecting and analyzing data.
7. Reflect on and profit from methodologic problems that occur during your research.
8. After data analysis is complete, reflect on how you write up your findings.
9. Reflect on whether the literature review is truly supporting your findings, or whether it is expressing the similar cultural background that you have.
10. Consider whether you can address any bias in your data collection or analysis by interviewing a participant a second time or reanalyzing the transcript in question.

Further guidance on bracketing has been offered by Gearing (2004), who suggests that there are six different types of bracketing, some of which are associated with qualitative traditions other then phenomenology. In each type, there are three general but distinct phases in the bracketing process, but the temporal structure varies from type to type.

Intuiting, the second step in descriptive phenomenology, occurs when researchers remain open to the meanings attributed to the phenomenon by those who have experienced it. Phenomenological researchers then proceed to the analysis phase (i.e., extracting significant statements, categorizing, and making sense of the essential meanings of the phenomenon). Chapter 19 provides further information regarding the analysis of data collected in phenomenological studies. Finally, the descriptive phase occurs when researchers come to understand and define the phenomenon.

Example of a descriptive phenomenological study: Fu (2005) used descriptive phenomenological methods to describe the experience of managing lymphedema in breast cancer survivors. Data were collected in three interviews with 12 women who described how they managed lymphedema in their daily lives.

Interpretive Phenomenology

Heidegger, a student of Husserl, moved away from his professor's philosophy into **interpretive phenomenology**, or hermeneutics. To Heidegger (1962), the critical question is: What is Being? He stressed interpreting and understanding—not just describing—human experience. His premise is that the lived experience is inherently an interpretive process, and argued that hermeneutics ("understanding") is a basic characteristic of human existence. Indeed, the term hermeneutics refers to the art and philosophy of interpreting the meaning of an object (such as a *text*, work of art, and so on). The goals of interpretive phenomenological research are to enter another's world and to discover the practical wisdom, possibilities, and understandings found there.

Gadamer (1976), another influential interpretive phenomenologist, described the interpretive process as a circular relationship, known as the **hermeneutic circle**, in which one understands the whole of a text (e.g., a transcribed interview) in terms of its parts and the parts in terms of the whole. In his view, researchers enter into a dialogue with the text, during which the researcher continually questions its meaning.

One distinction between descriptive and interpretive phenomenology is that in an interpretive phenomenological study, bracketing does not necessarily occur. For Heidegger, it was not possible to bracket one's being-in-the-world. Hermeneutics presupposes prior understanding on the part of the researcher. In Gearing's (2004) typology of bracketing, *reflexive bracketing*—in which researchers attempt to identify internal suppositions to facilitate greater transparency, but without bracketing them out—is described as a tool for hermeneutical inquiry. Interpretive phenomenologists ideally approach each interview text with openness—they must be open to hearing what it is the text is saying. As Heidegger (1971) stated, "We never come to thoughts. They come to us" (p. 6).

Example of an interpretive phenomenological study: Phinney (2006) studied involvement in meaningful activity among persons with dementia, as interpreted by family members caring for their relatives. Repeated interviews were conducted with persons with dementia and family members to explore strategies the families used to support activity involvement and to examine the meaning of such involvement to families.

Interpretive phenomenologists, like descriptive phenomenologists, rely primarily on in-depth interviews with individuals who have experienced the phenomenon of interest, but they may go beyond a traditional approach to gathering and analyzing data. For example, interpretive phenomenologists sometimes augment their understandings of the phenomenon through an analysis of supplementary texts, such as novels, poetry, or other artistic expressions—or they use such materials in their conversations with study participants.

Example of a hermeneutic study using artistic expression: Lauterbach (2001) studied the phenomenon of maternal mourning over the death of a wished-for baby. She increased her "attentive listening" to this phenomenon by turning to examples of infant death experiences illustrated in the arts, literature, and poetry. For example, she included a poem written by Shakespeare as he mourned his son's death. She also described the painting "Rachel Weeping" by Charles Wilson Peale, which depicts the artist's daughter, who had died of smallpox, laid out in her burial dress. Lauterbach also visited cemeteries to discover memorial art in babies' grave stones. She used the examples of memorial art and of literature to validate the themes of mothers' experiences in her research.

> **TIP:** As Mackey (2005) has pointed out, nurse researchers undertaking interpretive phenomenological studies should fully understand the philosophical and methodologic underpinnings of this tradition so that the results will be coherent. The same caution is true for other qualitative traditions, and we urge you to read original sources before undertaking a study.

Grounded Theory

Grounded theory has become an important research method for the study of nursing phenomena, and has contributed to the development of many middle-range theories of phenomena relevant to nurses. Grounded theory began more as a systematic method of qualitative research than as a philosophy. Grounded theory was developed in the 1960s by two sociologists, Glaser and Strauss (1967), one of whom (Strauss) had strong theoretical training in symbolic interaction. One of their earliest studies (Glaser & Strauss, 1965) was a grounded theory study on dying in hospitals, in which the "prime controllable" variable was characterized as *awareness context* (i.e., who knows what about the patient's dying).

Grounded theory tries to account for actions in a substantive area from the perspective of those involved. Grounded theory researchers seek to understand the actions by focusing on the main concern or problem that the individuals' behavior is designed to resolve (Glaser, 1998). The manner in which people resolve this main concern is called the **core variable**. One type of core variable is called a **basic social process (BSP)**. The goal of grounded theory is to discover this main concern and the BSP that explains how people continually resolve it. The main concern or problem must be discovered from the data.

Grounded theory is a general inductive method that is not inextricably linked to a particular theoretical perspective or type of data (Glaser, 2005). Although the perspective of symbolic interaction has been used in many grounded theory studies, there are other theoretical perspectives that can be used in grounded theory research.

Conceptualization is essential for grounded theory (Glaser, 2003). Grounded theory researchers generate emergent conceptual categories and their properties and integrate them into a substantive theory grounded in the data. Through this conceptual process, the grounded theory that is generated represents an abstraction based on the participants' actions and their meanings. The grounded theorist uncovers and names latent patterns (categories) from the participants' accounts. Glaser (2003) emphasizes that concepts transcend time, place, and person. "In grounded theory behavior is a pattern that a person engages in; it is not the person. People are not categorized, behavior is" (p. 53).

Grounded theory methods constitute an entire approach to the conduct of field research. For exam-

ple, a study that truly follows Glaser and Strauss's precepts does not begin with a highly focused research problem; the problem emerges from the data. In grounded theory, both the research problem and the process used to resolve it are discovered during the study. A fundamental feature of grounded theory research is that data collection, data analysis, and sampling of participants occur simultaneously. The grounded theory process is recursive: researchers collect data, categorize them, describe the emerging central phenomenon, and then recycle earlier steps.

A procedure referred to as **constant comparison** is used to develop and refine theoretically relevant categories. Categories elicited from the data are constantly compared with data obtained earlier in the data collection process so that commonalities and variations can be determined. As data collection proceeds, the inquiry becomes increasingly focused on emerging theoretical concerns. Data analysis in a grounded theory framework is described in greater depth in Chapter 19.

In-depth interviews and observation are the most common data source in grounded theory studies, but existing documents and other data sources may also be used. Grounded theory research can involve the analysis of quantitative as well as qualitative data (Glaser & Strauss, 1967), but this rarely happens in practice.

➲ **TIP:** Beginning qualitative researchers should be aware that if they have constraints in the amount of time they can devote to conducting a study, a grounded theory study is a much lengthier and more complex process than a phenomenological study.

Example of a grounded theory study: Levy (2006) sought to develop a substantive theory of the process by which midwives in the United Kingdom facilitate informed decision making by pregnant women. The basic social process identified in the study was *protective steering*, whereby midwives protected the women in their care, as well as themselves, when choices were being made.

Like most theories (see Chapter 6), a grounded theory is conceptually modifiable as the researcher (or other researchers) collect new data. Modification is an ongoing process in grounded theory research, and is the method by which theoretical completeness is enhanced (Glaser, 2001). As more data are found and more qualitative studies are published in the substantive area, the grounded theory can be modified to accommodate these new or different dimensions.

Example of a grounded theory study: Beck (2007) modified her 1993 grounded theory study, "Teetering on the Edge," which was a substantive theory of postpartum depression. Since Beck's original study had been conducted, 10 qualitative studies of postpartum depression in women from other cultures had been published. The results from these 10 transcultural studies were compared with the findings from the original grounded theory. Maximizing differences among comparative groups is a powerful method for enhancing the generation of theoretical properties and extending the theory.

Alternate Views of Grounded Theory

In 1990, Strauss and Corbin published what was to become a controversial book, *Basics of Qualitative Research: Grounded Theory Procedures and Techniques*. Strauss and Corbin stated that the purpose of the book was to provide beginning grounded theory researchers with basic knowledge and procedures involved in building theory at the substantive level.

Glaser, however, disagreed with some of the procedures advocated by Strauss (his original co-author) and Corbin (a nurse researcher). Glaser published a rebuttal in 1992, *Emergence Versus Forcing: Basics of Grounded Theory Analysis*. Glaser believed that Strauss and Corbin developed a method that is not grounded theory but rather what he calls "full conceptual description." According to Glaser, the purpose of grounded theory is to generate concepts and theories about their relationships that explain, account for, and interpret variation in behavior in the substantive area under study. *Conceptual description*, in contrast, is aimed at describing the full range of behavior of what is occurring in the substantive area, "irrespective of relevance and accounting for variation in behavior" (Glaser, 1992, p. 19).

Nurse researchers have conducted grounded theory studies using both the original Glaser and Strauss and the Strauss and Corbin (1998) approaches.

Example of grounded theory alternatives: Kendall (1999) provided an excellent comparison of the two approaches to grounded theory from her own research on families with a child with attention deficit–hyperactivity disorder. She described study results two ways—first, results obtained using Strauss and Corbin's approach, and second, the findings that emerged using Glaser and Strauss's original grounded theory approach. Kendall thought that Strauss and Corbin's coding procedure was a distraction that hindered her ability to reach the higher level of abstract thinking needed in grounded theory analysis.

Formal Grounded Theory

Glaser and Strauss (1967) distinguished two types of grounded theory: substantive and formal. **Substantive theory** is grounded in data on a specific substantive area, such as postpartum depression. It can serve as a springboard for **formal grounded theory**, which involves developing a higher, more abstract level of theory from a compilation of substantive grounded theory studies regarding a particular phenomenon. Glaser and Strauss's (1971) theory of status passage is an example of a formal grounded theory.

Kearney (1998) used an interesting analogy to differentiate substantive theories (custom-tailored clothing) and formal theory (ready-to-wear clothing). Formal grounded theories were likened to clothing sold in department stores that can fit a variety of users. Formal grounded theory is not personally tailored like substantive theory, but rather provides a conceptualization that applies to a broader population experiencing a common phenomenon. Formal grounded theories are not situation specific. The best data for constructing formal grounded theories are substantive grounded theories.

Example of a formal grounded theory: Kearney and O'Sullivan (2003) used a formal grounded theory approach to synthesize the findings of 14 studies, with the goal of identifying common elements of individuals' efforts to change a variety of unhealthy behaviors. The concept of *identity shift* was discovered as a core process.

➲ **TIP:** The terminology for qualitative integration approaches can be confusing. Researchers use different terms to label qualitative synthesis, such as qualitative meta-analysis, metaethnography, or metainterpretation. Kearney's (2001) "meta family" helps to clear up some of the confusion by placing current approaches to qualitative synthesis on a continuum from most theorizing to most interpretive. Starting with the theorizing end of the continuum and going to the interpretive end, Kearney orders these approaches as follows: formal grounded theory, metainterpretation, aggregated analysis, metastudy, metasynthesis, and metaethnography.

Historical Research

Historical research is the systematic collection, critical evaluation, and interpretation of historical evidence (i.e., data relating to past occurrences). In general, historical research is undertaken to answer questions about causes, effects, or trends relating to past events that may shed light on present behaviors or practices. Historians seek to explain why events happen. An understanding of contemporary nursing theories, practices, or issues can often be enhanced by an investigation of a specified segment of the past. Historical data are usually qualitative, but quantitative data are sometimes used (e.g., historical census data).

Historical research can take many forms. For example, nurse researchers have undertaken *biographical histories* that study the experiences or contributions of individuals, such as nursing leaders. Currently, some historians are focusing on the history and experience of the ordinary person, often studying such issues as gender, race, and class. Other historical researchers undertake *social histories* that focus on a particular period in attempts to understand prevailing values and beliefs that may have helped to shape subsequent developments. Still others undertake what might be called *intellectual histories*, in which historical ideas or ways of thinking are scrutinized. *Technological histories* are another form of historical research that has emerged recently in nursing (Sandelowski, 1997).

Historical research should not be confused with a review of the literature about historical events. Like other types of research, historical inquiry has as its goal the discovery of *new* knowledge, not the summary of existing knowledge. One important difference between historical research and a literature review is that historical researchers, in addition to being guided by specific questions focused on explaining and interpreting past events or conditions, are often guided by a theoretical orientation or ideology (e.g., feminism).

Example of a theoretical framework in historical research: Cordeau (2004) used Leininger's Sunrise Model as a framework to explain how the Medical Department of the Union Army, the U.S. Sanitary Commission, and the U.S. Christian Commission produced the experience of nurse-caring by Northern women during the Civil War.

After research questions are developed, researchers must determine what types of data are available. Historical researchers typically need to devote considerable effort to identifying and evaluating data sources on events and situations that occurred in the past.

Collecting Historical Data

Data for historical research are usually in the form of written records: diaries, letters, notes, newspapers, minutes of meetings, medical or legal documents, and so forth. However, nonwritten materials may also be of interest. For example, physical remains and objects are potential sources of information. Visual materials, such as photographs and films, are forms of data, as are audio materials, such as records and tapes. In some cases, it is possible to conduct interviews with people who participated in historical events (e.g., nurses who served in the Vietnam War).

Many historical materials may be difficult to obtain and, in many cases, have been discarded. Historically significant materials are not always conveniently indexed by subject, author, or title. The identification of appropriate historical materials usually requires a considerable amount of time, effort, and detective work. Fortunately, there are several archives of historical nursing documents, such as the collections at several universities. The website of the American Association for the History of Nursing provides information about archives in the United States and several other countries (*http://www.aahn.org*). ⊖ Useful sources for identifying other archives in the United States include the *National Inventory of Documentary Sources in the United States* and the *Directory of Archives and Manuscript Repositories in the United States*.

➔ TIP: Archives are different from libraries. Archives contain unpublished materials that are accessed through **finding aids** rather than card catalogues. A finding aid is a resource that tells researchers what is in the archive. Archival materials do not circulate; researchers are almost always required to use the material on site (although sometimes microfiches are available). Typically, because of the fragile nature of the material, it cannot be photocopied, so researchers must take detailed notes (laptop computers are invaluable). Sometimes gloves are required when touching original materials. Access to archives may be limited to researchers who present a description of a proposed project to archivists.

Historical materials usually are classified as either primary or secondary sources. A **primary source** is first-hand information, such as original documents, or artifacts. Examples are diaries and writings of historically important nurses, minutes of American Nurses Association meetings, and so forth. Primary source documents are authored by people directly *involved* in a described event. Primary sources represent the most direct link with historical events or situations: Only the narrator (in the case of written materials) intrudes between original events and the historical researcher. Multiple primary sources are usually needed for comparison.

Secondary sources are second- or third-hand accounts of historical events or experiences. For example, textbooks, other reference books, and newspaper articles are secondary sources. Secondary sources, in other words, are discussions of events written by individuals who did not participate in them, but are often summarizing or interpreting primary source materials. Secondary sources may be historical (e.g., newspaper accounts contemporaneous with the events under study), or more modern interpretations of past events. Primary

sources should be used whenever possible in historical research. The further removed from the historical event the information is, the less reliable, objective, and comprehensive the data are likely to be. However, secondary sources can be useful in identifying primary sources. It is particularly important in reading secondary source material to pay careful attention to footnotes, which often provide important clues about primary sources. Secondary sources are also needed to provide context for evaluating events.

Example of primary and secondary sources:
Sandelowski (1997), in describing her research on technology in American nursing between 1870 and 1940, wrote: "The primary sources I used included advice and instructional literature for nurses (i.e., textbooks and professional journal articles), hospital and training school procedure manuals, medical trade and advertising ephemera, photographs and drawings, and a miscellaneous collection of materials, such as hospital correspondence and student lecture notes. I also had the opportunity to see and handle in museum collections certain implements used in practice in the late nineteenth and early twentieth centuries, such as glass cups and metal scarifiers for wet cupping. Many of the devices used then (e.g., glass thermometers, enema cans with rubber tubing, manually operated beds) were still in use when I began to practice as a nurse in the late 1960s. The secondary sources I used were in the history of nursing and medical technology. Together, these sources offer a basis for understanding continuity and change in the history of technology in nursing, a story that remains largely untold" (p. 5).

HIPAA's Impact on Historical Research

The Health Insurance Portability and Accountability Act of 1996 (HIPAA) has resulted in the creation of new barriers between nurse historians and archival resources (Lusk & Sacharski, 2005). Historians face potential restrictions to accessing collections. These access restrictions vary from archive to archive. In addition to problems of access, nurse historians may lose some of the context for their historical analysis because individual identities may be protected. Nurse historians may also face constraints on their ability to use photographs, such as images of patients. Researchers conducting historical research will have to gain permission to access patient records from, for example, the 18th century, in the same way as those attempting to gain access from current records in the beginning of the 21st century. Waivers of authorization are options that may be obtained from Institutional Review Boards (IRBs). Lusk and Sacharski bring to our attention that HIPAA's privacy rule was not developed with historical research in mind, and so areas of confusion need to be clarified.

Evaluating Historical Data

Historical evidence is subjected to two types of evaluation, which historians refer to as external and internal criticism. **External criticism** is concerned with the data's authenticity. For example, a nurse historian might have a diary presumed to be written by Dorothea Dix. External criticism would involve asking such questions as: Is this the handwriting of Ms. Dix? Is the diary's paper of the right age? Are the writing style and ideas expressed consistent with her other writings? There are various scientific techniques available to determine the age of materials, such as x-ray and radioactive procedures. Other flaws, however, may be less easy to detect. For example, there is the possibility that material of interest may have been written by a ghost writer, that is, by someone other than the person of interest. There are also potential problems of mechanical errors associated with transcriptions, translations, or typed versions of historical materials.

Internal criticism of historical data refers to an evaluation of the worth of the evidence. The focus of internal criticism is not on the physical aspects of the materials but on their content. The key issue is the accuracy or truth of the data. For example, researchers must question whether a writer's representations of historical events are unbiased. It may also be appropriate to ask if the author of a document was in a position to make a valid report of an event or occurrence, or whether the writer was competent as a recorder of fact. Evidence bearing on the accuracy of historical data often includes comparisons with other people's accounts of the same event to determine the degree of agreement,

knowledge of the time at which the document was produced (reports of events or situations tend to be more accurate if they are written immediately after the event), and knowledge of the writers' point of view or biases and their competence to record events authoritatively and accurately.

➔ **TIP:** Tuchman (1994) offers this useful advice: "Ask questions of all data, primary and secondary sources. Do not assume anything about the data is 'natural,' inevitable, or even true. To be sure, a datum has a physical presence: One may touch the page . . . one has located. But that physical truth may be radically different from the interpretive truth . . ." (p. 321).

Analyzing and Interpreting Historical Data

In historical research, data analysis and data collection are usually ongoing, concurrent activities. The analysis of historical data is broadly similar to other approaches to qualitative analysis (see Chapter 19), in that researchers search for themes. In historical research, however, the thematic analysis is often guided by underlying theoretical frameworks. Within the selected framework, researchers concentrate on particular issues present in the data.

Historical research is usually interpretive. Historical researchers try to describe what happened, and also how and why it happened. Relationships between events and ideas, between people and organizations, are explored and interpreted within both their historical context and the context of new viewpoints about what is historically significant.

Resources available for those interested in undertaking historical nursing research include Lewenson (2003), Fitzpatrick (2001), and Lusk (1997).

Example of historical research: Benedict's (2006) historical study of Maria Stromberger, a nurse in the resistance in Auschwitz, is riveting. During World War II, Stromberger risked her life on numerous occasions to save the lives of Polish inmates. Benedict used excellent primary sources in her research, including an interview with Helen Spitzer Tichauer, a survivor of Auschwitz-Birkenau.

OTHER TYPES OF QUALITATIVE RESEARCH

Qualitative studies typically can be characterized and described in terms of the disciplinary research traditions discussed in the previous section. However, several other important types of qualitative research also deserve mention. This section discusses qualitative research that is not associated with any particular discipline.

Case Studies

Case studies are in-depth investigations of a single entity or a small number of entities. The entity may be an individual, family, group, institution, community, or other social unit. In a case study, researchers obtain a wealth of descriptive information and may examine relationships among different phenomena, or may examine trends over time. Case study researchers attempt to analyze and understand issues that are important to the history, development, or circumstances of the entity under study.

One way to think of a case study is to consider what is at center stage. In most studies, whether qualitative or quantitative, a certain phenomenon or variable (or set of variables) is the core of the inquiry. In a case study, the *case* itself is central. As befits an intensive analysis, the focus of case studies is typically on determining the dynamics of *why* an individual thinks, behaves, or develops in a particular manner rather than on *what* his or her status, progress, or actions are. It is not unusual for probing research of this type to require detailed study over a considerable period. Data are often collected that relate not only to the person's present state but also to past experiences and situational factors relevant to the problem being examined.

There are four basic types of designs for case studies: single case, holistic; single case, embedded; multiple case, holistic; and multiple case, embedded (Yin, 2003). A **single case study** is an appropriate design when (1) it is a critical case in testing a well-formulated theory, (2) it represents an extreme or unique case, (3) it is a representative or typical case,

(4) it is the revelatory case, and (5) it is a longitudinal case (Yin, 2003). A **multiple case design** is a study that involves more than a single case. Single and multiple case studies can be either holistic or embedded. In a **holistic design,** the global nature of a case—be it an individual, program, community, or organization—is examined. An **embedded design** involves more than one unit of analysis. Attention is given to subunits. As in most qualitative inquiry, a wide variety of data can be used in case studies, including data from interviews, observations, documents, records, and artifacts.

A distinction is sometimes drawn between an intrinsic and instrumental case study. In an *intrinsic case study,* researchers do not have to select the case. For instance, an evaluation of the process of implementing an innovation is often a case study of a particular institution; the "case" is a given. In an *instrumental case study*, researchers begin with a research question or perplexity, and seek out a case that offers illumination. The aim of such a case study is to use the case to understand something else, some phenomenon of interest. In such a situation, a case is usually selected not because it is typical, but rather because it can maximize what can be learned about the phenomenon (Stake, 1995). Case studies can also be layered, which involves having a large case study built out of smaller ones (Patton, 2002).

Although the foremost concern of a case study is to understand the particular case, case studies are sometimes a useful way to explore phenomena that have not been rigorously researched. The information obtained in case studies can be used to develop hypotheses to be tested more rigorously in subsequent research. The intensive probing that characterizes case studies often leads to insights concerning previously unsuspected relationships. Furthermore, case studies may serve the important role of clarifying concepts or of elucidating ways to capture them.

➲ **TIP:** Sometimes thematic maps or models are created in case study research as a method of understanding and interpreting the case's experiences. For example, in Donna Zucker's case study of two men with coronary heart disease (CHD), creating a map "contributed to my ability to visualize the *aha* necessary to make meaning of Bernie's and Ed's experiences. It became evident that these two gentlemen experienced more variation in their patterns of living with chronic CHD than previously reported in the literature" (Hunter et al., 2002, p. 392).

The greatest strength of case studies is the depth that is possible when a limited number of individuals, institutions, or groups is being investigated. Case studies provide researchers with opportunities for having an intimate knowledge of a person's condition, thoughts, feelings, actions (past and present), intentions, and environment. On the other hand, this same strength is a potential weakness because researchers' familiarity with the person or group may make objectivity more difficult—especially if the data are collected by observational techniques for which the researchers are the main (or only) observers. Perhaps the biggest criticism of case studies concerns generalizability: If researchers discover important relationships, it is difficult to know whether the same relationships would occur with others. However, case studies can often play a critical role in challenging generalizations based on other types of research.

It is important to recognize that case study *research* is not simply anecdotal descriptions of a particular incident or patient, such as a case report. Case study research is a disciplined process and typically requires an extended period of systematic data collection. Excellent resources for further reading on case study methods are the books by Yin (2003) and Stake (1995, 2005).

> **Example of a multiple case study:** Carlsson, Ehrenberg, and Ehnfors (2004) conducted in-depth case studies of three people who had had a stroke 2 years earlier and were experiencing eating difficulties. Repeated interviews were conducted, and observations were made of the three cases.

➲ **TIP:** Although most case studies involve the collection of qualitative data, some use statistical methods to analyze quantitative data. As an example, Normann and

colleagues (2005) did a case study to explore the presence of lucidity in a woman with severe dementia. Data from more than 20 hours of conversation with the woman and her daughter were analyzed statistically.

Narrative Analyses

Narrative analysis focuses on *story* as the object of inquiry, to determine how individuals make sense of events in their lives. Narratives are viewed as a type of "cultural envelope" into which people pour their experiences and relate their importance to others (Riessman, 1991). What distinguishes narrative analysis from other types of qualitative research designs is its focus on the broad contours of a narrative; stories are not fractured and dissected. The broad underlying premise of narrative research is that people most effectively make sense of their world—and communicate these meanings—by constructing, reconstructing, and narrating stories. Individuals construct stories when they wish to understand specific events and situations that require linking an inner world of desire and motive to an external world of observable actions. Analyzing stories opens up *forms* of telling about experience, and is more than just content. Narrative analysts ask, "Why was the story told that way?" (Riessman, 1993, p. 2).

There are a number of structural approaches that researchers can use to analyze stories. The choice should be made on the basis of the fit between the structural approach and the types of narratives to be analyzed. Three of the more popular structural approaches include those of Gee (1991, 1996), Labov and Waletzky (1967), and Burke (1969). Gee offers a linguistic approach for narrative analysis that moves from the part to the whole. His method draws on oral rather than text-based tradition and attends to how the story is told. First he pays attention to changes in pitch, loudness, stress, and length of various syllables, as well as to hesitations and pauses. He also examines the cohesion of each sentence or line, how they form larger units (stanzas). His analysis examines the rhetorical function of each stanza in relation to every other stanza. Stanzas are then organized into larger units (strophes), which are analyzed to see how the themes of the text are organized.

Example of a narrative analysis using Gee's approach: Crepeau (2000) analyzed the stories that a geropsychiatric team, which included nurses, social workers, a psychiatrist, and a dietitian, told about "Gloria" in the construction of an image of the patient during team meetings. Crepeau based her methods on Gee's approach, and presented numerous stanzas in her report.

Labov and Waletzky (1967) view narratives as a social phenomenon. Their structural approach proposes that a complete narrative consists of the following six components: the abstract (summary), orientation (time, place, individuals), complicating action (sequence of events), evaluation (significance of the action), result or resolution (what occurred at the end), and coda (perspective returned back to the present). As a social phenomenon, narratives vary by social context (hospital, home, and so on), and evaluative data extracted from the narratives will vary by the social context in which they were collected.

Example of a narrative analysis using Labov and Waletzky's approach: Bailey (2004) conducted a narrative analysis of chronic obstructive pulmonary disease patients' stories of breathlessness during an acute exacerbation. Ten patients, 10 nurses, and 15 family caregivers were interviewed. As a first step in her analysis, Bailey partitioned their stories into Labov and Waletzky's six elements.

Burke's (1969) **pentadic dramatism** is yet another approach for analysis of narratives. For Burke, there are five key elements of a story: act, scene, agent, agency, and purpose. Analysis of a story "will offer some kind of answers to these five questions: what was done (act), when or where it was done (scene), who did it (agent), how he did it (agency), and why (purpose)" (Burke, 1969, p. xv). The five terms of Burke's pentad are meant to be understood paired together as ratios, such as, act: agent, act: scene, agent: agency, purpose: agent. The analysis focuses on the internal relationships and tensions of these five terms to each other. Each pairing of terms in the pentad provides a different way of directing the researcher's attention, or, as Burke calls it, a different "terministic screen" for viewing the story. What drives the narrative analysis is not just the interaction of the pentadic terms but also an imbalance between two or more of these terms. Bruner (1991) modified Burke's pentad with the addition of a sixth term that he called Trouble with a capital T. Bruner included this sixth element to provide more focus in narrative analysis on Burke's imbalance between the terms in his pentad.

Example of a narrative analysis using Burke's approach: One of the authors of this textbook (Beck, 2006) conducted a narrative analysis of birth trauma. Eleven mothers sent their stories of traumatic childbirth to the researcher via the Internet. Burke's pentad of terms was used to analyze these narratives. The most problematic ratio imbalance that appeared prominently in the data was between act and agency. Frequently in the mothers' narratives, it was "How" an act was carried out by the labor and delivery staff that led to the women perceiving their childbirth as traumatic.

Descriptive Qualitative Studies

Most qualitative researchers acknowledge a link to one of the research traditions or types of studies discussed in this chapter. Some qualitative studies, however, claim no particular disciplinary or methodologic roots. The researchers may simply indicate that they have conducted a qualitative study or a naturalistic inquiry, or they may say that they have done a *content analysis* of their qualitative data (i.e., an analysis of themes and patterns that emerge in the narrative content). Thus, some qualitative studies do not have a formal name or do not fit into the typology we have presented in this chapter. We refer to these as **descriptive qualitative studies**.

Sandelowski (2000a) notes that in doing such descriptive qualitative studies, researchers tend not to penetrate their data in any interpretive depth. These studies present comprehensive summaries of a phenomenon or of events in everyday language. Qualitative descriptive designs tend to be eclectic and are based on the general premises of naturalistic inquiry. Sandelowski stresses that researchers should not be ashamed to "just" use qualitative description as their research design. It is the method of choice if what they want is straight description of an event or phenomenon.

> **Example of a descriptive qualitative study:** D'Auria and colleagues (2006) undertook a descriptive qualitative study to explore and describe the early responses of HIV-positive mothers to the birth of their HIV-exposed infants during the first few months of the infants' life.

RESEARCH WITH IDEOLOGICAL PERSPECTIVES

Some qualitative researchers conduct inquiries within an ideological framework, typically to draw attention to certain social problems or the needs of certain groups and to effect change. These approaches represent important investigative avenues and are briefly described in this section.

Critical Theory

Critical theory originated with a group of Marxist-oriented German scholars in the 1920s, collectively referred to as the Frankfurt School. Variants of critical theory abound in the social sciences. Essentially, a critical researcher is concerned with a critique of society and with envisioning new possibilities.

Critical social science is typically action oriented. Its broad aim is to integrate theory and practice such that people become aware of contradictions and disparities in their beliefs and social practices, and become inspired to change them. Critical researchers reject the idea of an objective and disinterested inquirer and are oriented toward a transformation process. An important feature of critical theory is that it calls for inquiries that foster enlightened self-knowledge and sociopolitical action. Moreover, critical theory involves a self-reflective aspect. To prevent a critical theory of society from becoming yet another self-serving ideology, critical theorists must account for their own transformative effects.

The design of research in critical theory often begins with a thorough analysis of certain aspects of the problem. For example, critical researchers might analyze and critique taken-for-granted assumptions that underlie the problem, the language used to depict the situation, and the biases of prior researchers investigating the problem. Critical researchers often triangulate multiple methodologies, and emphasize multiple perspectives (e.g., alternative racial or social class perspectives) on problems. Critical researchers typically interact with study participants in ways that emphasize participants' expertise. Some of the features that distinguish more traditional qualitative research and critical research are summarized in Table 9.2.

Critical theory has been applied in a number of disciplines, and has played an especially important role in ethnography. **Critical ethnography** focuses on raising consciousness and aiding emancipatory goals in the hope of effecting social change. Critical ethnographers address the historical, social, political, and economic dimensions of cultures and their value-laden agendas. An assumption in critical ethnographic research is that actions and thoughts are mediated by power relationships (Hammersley, 1992). Critical ethnographers attempt to increase the political dimensions of cultural research and undermine oppressive systems—there is always an explicit political purpose. Cook (2005) has argued that critical ethnography is especially well suited to health promotion research because both are concerned with enabling people to take control over their own situation.

Carspecken (1996) developed a widely acclaimed 5-stage approach to critical ethnography that has been found useful in nursing studies (e.g., Hardcastle, Usher, & Holmes, 2006) and in health promotion research. Morrow and Brown (1994) also provide guidance about critical theory methodology.

> **Example of a critical ethnography:** Caldwell, Arthur, and Rideout (2005) examined the influences of rurality on the lives of women after myocardial infarction, using data from in-depth interviews with 12 women from southwestern Ontario. The researchers chose a critical ethnographic approach so that they could move beyond description and invite reflection on the social, political, and cultural forces associated with rurality and generate possibilities for change.

TABLE 9.2	Comparison of Traditional Qualitative Research and Critical Research	

ISSUE	TRADITIONAL QUALITATIVE RESEARCH	CRITICAL RESEARCH
Research aims	Understanding; reconstruction of multiple constructions	Critique; transformation; consciousness raising; advocacy
View of knowledge	Transactional/subjective; knowledge is created in interaction between investigator and participants	Transactional/subjective; value-mediated and value-dependent; importance of historical insights
Methods	Dialectic: truth is arrived at logically through conversations	Dialectic and didactic: dialogue designed to transform naivety and misinformation
Evaluative criteria for inquiry quality	Authenticity; trustworthiness	Historical situatedness of the inquiry; erosion of ignorance; stimulus for change
Researcher's role	Facilitator of multivoice reconstruction	Transformative agent; advocate; activist

→ **TIP:** Denzin (1997) has described ethnography as having passed through five "historical moments": (1) traditional ethnography (1900 to World War II), (2) modernist ethnography (World War II to middle of 1970s), (3) blurred genres (1970 to 1986), (4) crisis of representation (1986 to present), and (5) the present. For example, in the traditional period, ethnographers wrote objective accounts of their fieldwork, whereas in the second, modernist phase, researchers focused on formalizing qualitative methods based in the language of positivism. By the middle of the 1980s, ethnographers' writings became more reflexive, and gender, social class, and ethnicity became key concerns. Denzin described ethnography at the beginning of the 21st century as starting its sixth moment — a time of intense reflection, experiments with auto-ethnography, performance-texts, ethnographic poetics, and narratives of self.

Feminist Research

Feminist research approaches are similar to critical theory research, but the focus is sharply on gender domination and discrimination within patriarchal societies. Similar to critical researchers, feminist researchers seek to establish collaborative and nonexploitative relationships with their informants, to place themselves within the study to avoid objectification, and to conduct research that is transformative.

Gender is the organizing principle in feminist research, and investigators seek to understand how gender and a gendered social order have shaped women's lives and their consciousness. The aim is to ameliorate the "invisibility and distortion of female experience in ways relevant to ending women's unequal social position" (Lather, 1991, p. 71).

Although feminist researchers generally agree that it is important to focus on women's diverse situations and the institutions and relationships that frame those situations, there are many variants of feminist inquiry. Three broad models (within each of which there is diversity) have been identified: (1) *feminist empiricism*, whose adherents usually work within fairly standard norms of qualitative inquiry but seek to portray more accurate pictures of the social realities of women's lives; (2) *feminist standpoint research*, which holds that inquiry ought to begin in and be tested against the lived everyday sociopolitical experiences of women, and that women's views are particular and privileged; and (3) *feminist postmodernism*, which stresses that "truth" is a destructive illusion, and views the world as endless stories, texts, and narratives. In nursing and health care, feminist empiricism and feminist standpoint research have been most prevalent.

The scope of feminist research ranges from studies of the particular and subjective views of individual women, to studies of social movements, structures, and broad policies that affect (and often exclude) women. Olesen (2000), a sociologist who studied nurses' career patterns and definitions of success, has noted that some of the best feminist research on women's subjective experiences has been done in the area of women's health.

Feminist research methods typically include in-depth, interactive, and collaborative individual interviews or group interviews that offer the possibility of reciprocal educational encounters. Feminists usually seek to negotiate the meanings of the results with those participating in the study, and to be self-reflective about what they themselves are experiencing and learning.

Feminist research, like other research that has an ideological perspective, has raised the bar for the conduct of ethical research. With the emphasis on trust, empathy, and nonexploitative relationships, proponents of these newer modes of inquiry view any type of deception or manipulation as abhorrent. As Punch (1994) has noted in speaking about ethics and feminist research, "you do not rip off your sisters" (p. 89).

Those interested in feminist methodologies may wish to consult such writers as Lather (1991), Reinharz (1992), and Romazanoglu and Holland (2002).

Example of feminist research: Giddings (2005) conducted a cross-cultural study to explore nurses' experiences of institutionalized social injustices that lead to health disparities. Her study, informed by feminist theory and critical theory, involved life history interviews (two to three each) with 26 women nurses in the United States and New Zealand. Giddings' study appears in its entirety in the accompanying *Resource Manual*.

Participatory Action Research

A type of research known as participatory action research is closely allied to both critical research and feminist research. **Participatory action research (PAR)**, one of several types of *action*

research that originated in the 1940s with social psychologist Kurt Lewin, is based on a recognition that the production of knowledge can be political and can be used to exert power. Researchers in this approach typically work with groups or communities that are vulnerable to the control or oppression of a dominant group or culture.

Participatory action research is, as the name implies, participatory. There is collaboration between researchers and study participants in the definition of the problem, the selection of an approach and research methods, the analysis of the data, and the use to which findings are put. The aim of PAR is to produce not only knowledge but also action and consciousness raising. Researchers specifically seek to empower people through the process of constructing and using knowledge. The PAR tradition has as its starting point a concern for the powerlessness of the group under study. Thus, a key objective is to produce an impetus that is used to make improvements through education and sociopolitical action.

In PAR, the research methods take second place to emergent processes of collaboration and dialogue that can motivate, increase self-esteem, and generate community solidarity. Thus, the "data-gathering" strategies used are not only the traditional methods of interview and observation (including both qualitative and quantitative approaches) but also may include storytelling, sociodrama, drawing and painting, plays and skits, and other activities designed to encourage people to find creative ways to explore their lives, tell their stories, and recognize their own strengths. Useful resources for learning more about PAR include Whyte (1990) and Morrison and Lilford (2001).

Example of PAR: Strickland, Walsh, and Cooper (2006) conducted a PAR project to obtain parents' and elders' perspectives on the impact of colonization and community needs in a Pacific Northwest American Indian tribe. The researchers sought to identify strengths on which the community could build to reduce the risk for youth suicide. Members of this community provided consultation in the study design and its implementation, data collection, and analysis of the data.

CRITIQUING QUALITATIVE DESIGNS

Evaluating a qualitative design is often difficult. Qualitative researchers do not always document design decisions and are even less likely to describe the process by which such decisions were made. Researchers often do, however, indicate whether the study was conducted within a specific qualitative tradition. This information can be used to come to some conclusions about the study design. For example, if a report indicated that the researcher conducted 1 month of fieldwork for an ethnographic study, there would be reason to suspect that insufficient time had been spent in the field to obtain a true emic perspective of the culture under study. Ethnographic studies may also be critiqued if their only source of information was from interviews, rather than from a broader range of data sources, particularly observations.

In a grounded theory study, you might also be concerned if the researcher relied exclusively on data from interviews; a stronger design might have been obtained by including participant observations. Also, look for evidence about when the data were collected and analyzed. If the researcher collected all the data before analyzing any of it, you might question whether the constant comparative method was used correctly.

Glaser and Strauss (1967) offered four properties on which a grounded theory should be evaluated: fitness, understanding, generality, and control. The theory should fit the substantive area for which the data were collected. A grounded theory should increase the understanding of those working in that substantive area. Also, the categories in the grounded theory should be abstract enough to allow the theory to be a general guide to changing situations—but not so abstract to decrease their sensitizing features. Lastly, the substantive theory must allow individuals who apply it to have some control in daily situations.

In critiquing a phenomenological study, you should first determine whether the study is descriptive or interpretive. This will help you to assess how closely the researcher kept to the basic tenets of that qualitative research tradition, For example, in a descriptive phenomenological study, did the researcher bracket? When critiquing phenomenological studies, in addition to critiquing the methodology, you should look at the power of the studies to show and present the meaning of the phenomena being studied. Van Manen (1997a) calls for phenomenological researchers to address five textual features in their reports: lived thoroughness (placing the phenomenon concretely in the lifeworld), evocation (phenomenon is vividly brought into presence), intensification (give key phrases their full value), tone (let the text speak to the reader), and epiphany (sudden grasp of the meaning).

No matter what qualitative design is identified in a study, look to see whether the researchers stayed true to a single qualitative tradition throughout the study or mixed qualitative traditions and weakened the rigor of the study. For example, did the researcher state that a grounded theory design was used, but then present results that described themes instead of generating a substantive theory?

The guidelines in Box 9.1 ⊗ are intended to assist you in critiquing the designs of qualitative studies.

⊙⊙⊙⊙⊙⊙⊙⊙⊙⊙⊙⊙⊙⊙⊙⊙⊙⊙⊙

RESEARCH EXAMPLES

Nurse researchers have conducted studies in all the qualitative research traditions described in this chapter, and several actual examples have been cited. In the following sections, we present more detailed descriptions of three qualitative nursing studies.

Research Example of an Ethnography

Study: "Gendered elder care exchanges in a Caribbean village" (Kelley, 2005a) and "Minor children and adult care exchanges with community-dwelling frail elders in a St. Lucian village" (Kelley, 2005b)

Statement of Purpose: The purpose of the study was to describe the involvement of adults and children living in a small village on a Caribbean island in naturally occurring elder care networks.

BOX 9.1 Guidelines for Critiquing Qualitative Designs

1. Is the research tradition for the qualitative study identified? If none was identified, can one be inferred? If more than one was identified, is this justifiable, or does it suggest "method slurring"?
2. Is the research question congruent with a qualitative approach and with the specific research tradition (i.e., is the domain of inquiry for the study congruent with the domain encompassed by the tradition)? Are the data sources, research methods, and analytic approach congruent with the research tradition?
3. How well is the research design described? Are design decisions explained and justified? Does it appear that the researcher made all design decisions up-front, or did the design emerge during data collection, allowing researchers to capitalize on early information?
4. Is the design appropriate, given the research question? Does the design lend itself to a thorough, in-depth, intensive examination of the phenomenon of interest? What design elements might have strengthened the study (e.g., a longitudinal perspective rather than a cross-sectional one)?
5. Was there appropriate evidence of reflexivity in the design?
6. Was the study undertaken with an ideological perspective? If so, is there evidence that ideological methods and goals were achieved? (e.g., Was there evidence of full collaboration between researchers and participants? Did the research have the power to be transformative, or is there evidence that a transformative process occurred?)

Setting and Socioeconomic Context: The research was conducted in the village of Hillside (a pseudonym), a semirural village of approximately 4000 people on St. Lucia, an English-speaking island. The village was chosen because of its limited governmental or formal paid services for elder care. Unemployment there is high, and about 25% of the people on the island live in poverty. There is an expectation that elders should be cared for by family members, particularly their children. Young men are encouraged to pursue a good job in urban areas or to migrate to the United States or the United Kingdom and send back money, especially to support their mothers.

Method: The study was a 4-phase ethnographic field study that was conducted between May, 1998 and June, 2003. The first phase was a community context study to describe the island and village context and expectations for elder care. This phase used data from formal and informal interviews, group interviews, participant observation, a review of documents, and a survey of school children. Phase 2 was an egocentric network study of 14 elder households that built on findings from Phase 1. Phase 3 was a validation and extension of the findings through review with key elder and village informants. Phase 4 involved dissemination of study findings to village informants and the Ministry of Health. Elders selected for the

Phase 2 work (reported here) were all older than 65 years, were homebound, and had functional impairment (e.g., blindness, weakness). Data were gathered from the 14 elder families and their network members by conducting interviews at all times of the day, making observations, and journaling all care exchanges for a minimum of 1 week for each key informant. The ethnographic analysis involved both qualitative approaches (using a thematic analysis of the content of narrative materials) and quantitative ones (counts of network elements and care activities and benefits to caregivers).

Key Findings: There were 143 adults and 45 children in the elders' care networks; the majority of adults were women. Male care activities included primarily food, money, visits, and supplies. Women provided visits and food, but also personal and domestic tasks. Benefits derived by the caregivers included exchange of services (e.g., child care), commodities (housing), and future expectations (e.g., expectations about land). Men and women differed in the motivational mechanisms that influenced their involvement in elder care. Kelley also found that children younger than 7 years provided nearly one third of all care activities. The report (2005b) provided rich descriptions of the situations in which young children were and were not used as part of the elders' care networks.

Research Example of a Phenomenological Study

Study: "The phenomenology of deciding about hemodialysis among Taiwanese" (Lin, Lee, & Hicks, 2005)

Statement of Purpose: The purpose of this phenomenological study was to describe the experiences of making a decision about hemodialysis among a group of Taiwanese with end-stage renal disease (ESRD).

Setting and Sample: Study participants were recruited from hemodialysis centers in district hospitals, medical centers, and community hospitals in Southern Taiwan. A total of 12 people (6 men and 6 women) who had begun receiving hemodialysis in the previous 6 months participated.

Method: A 5-month pilot study was first undertaken to develop and refine study procedures, which led to the decision to interview patients retrospectively (i.e., *after* the dialysis decision was made) rather than as the decision making was unfolding, because the stress of the new diagnosis made it difficult for patients to reflect on the meaning of the experience. In the parent study, in-depth interviews that lasted between 50 minutes and 2½ hours were conducted either in the participants' homes or at the hemodialysis center, whichever the participant preferred. The interviews were tape-recorded for subsequent transcription. Participants were encouraged to talk about their early decision-making experiences following the ESRD diagnosis. Examples of the interview questions include: How did you feel when the physician told you that you had to receive hemodialysis? and What were the factors influencing your decision about receiving hemodialysis?

Key Findings: The data analysis revealed 3 broad categories and 10 themes. The first category, for example, was *confronting the dialysis treatment,* which encompassed 4 themes: *fear caused by false beliefs, a sense of threat to life, concern about impaired self-concept,* and *fear of physical limitations.* The study's themes revealed the difficulties that ESRD patients dealt with and the influence these difficulties had on treatment choices.

Research Example of a Feminist Grounded Theory Study

Study: "Strengthening capacity to limit intrusion: Theorizing family health promotion in the aftermath of woman abuse" (Ford-Gilboe, Wuest, & Merritt-Gray, 2005)

Statement of Purpose: The purpose of this study was to develop a substantive theory to explain variation in health promotion processes in mother-headed single-parent families with a history of woman abuse.

Feminist and Participatory Perspective: The researchers noted that a feminist perspective in a grounded theory study increased the emphasis on capturing women's diversity and strength in their experiences. This perspective also reinforced for them the importance of attending to broader social contexts in their theory development. The researchers' commitment to an agenda of positive change and shared power led them to adopt purposefully participatory strategies.

Method: The researchers recruited 40 single mothers living in the aftermath of intimate partner violence from New Brunswick and Ontario, Canada. Children older than 12 years also participated in interviews, either alone or with their mothers, if both agreed. The in-depth interviews involved broad questions, and participants were encouraged to set the pace in discussing health promotion after leaving their partners. As the theory developed, the researchers went back to participants for further discussion and refinement. Constant comparison was used in the analysis. Consistent with a feminist orientation, the researchers paid careful attention in their analysis to ways in which structural factors (e.g., access to income and employment) intersected with family efforts to promote health.

Key Findings: The researchers found that the central problem faced by these families is *intrusion*—unwanted interference in everyday life that stems from abuse and its fallout. Over time, the families promoted their health through the basic social process of *strengthening capacity to limit intrusion.* They accomplished this through four subprocesses: *providing, regenerating family, renewing self,* and *rebuilding security.*

SUMMARY POINTS

- Qualitative research involves an **emergent design**—a design that emerges in the field as the study unfolds.
- As **bricoleurs**, qualitative researchers tend to be creative and intuitive, putting together an array of data drawn from many sources to arrive at a holistic understanding of a phenomenon.
- Although qualitative design is elastic and flexible, qualitative researchers nevertheless plan for broad

contingencies that can be expected to pose decision opportunities for study design in the field.

- Qualitative research traditions have their roots in anthropology (e.g., **ethnography** and **ethnoscience**); philosophy (**phenomenology** and **hermeneutics**); psychology (**etology** and **ecological psychology**); sociology (**grounded theory, ethnomethodology,** and **semiotics**); sociolinguistics (**discourse analysis**); and history (**historical research**).

- Ethnography focuses on the culture of a group of people and relies on extensive fieldwork that usually includes **participant observation** and in-depth interviews with **key informants**. Ethnographers strive to acquire an **emic** (insider's) **perspective** of a culture rather than an **etic** (outsider's) **perspective**.

- The concept of **researcher as instrument** is frequently used by ethnographers to describe the significant role researchers play in analyzing and interpreting a culture. The product of ethnographic research is typically a rich, holistic description of the culture, but sometimes the products are **performance ethnographies**, which involve the development of interpretive scripts that are performed.

- Nurses sometimes refer to their ethnographic studies as **ethnonursing research**. Other types of ethnographic work include **institutional ethnographics** (which focus on the organization of professional services from the perspective of the front-line workers or clients) and **auto-ethnographies** or *insider research* (which involves an ethnography of a group or culture to which the researcher belongs).

- Phenomenology seeks to discover the *essence* and *meaning* of a phenomenon as it is experienced by people, mainly through in-depth interviews with people who have had the relevant experience.

- In **descriptive phenomenology**, which seeks to describe lived experiences, researchers strive to **bracket** out preconceived views and to **intuit** the essence of the phenomenon by remaining open to meanings attributed to it by those who have experienced it.

- **Interpretive phenomenology (hermeneutics)** focuses on interpreting the meaning of experiences, rather than just describing them.

- **Grounded theory** aims to discover theoretical precepts grounded in the data. Grounded theory researchers try to account for people's actions by focusing on the main concern that the individuals' behavior is designed to resolve. The manner in which people resolve this main concern is the **core variable**. The goal of grounded theory is to discover this main concern and the **basic social process (BSP)** that explains how people continually resolve it.

- Grounded theory uses **constant comparison**: categories elicited from the data are constantly compared with data obtained earlier.

- There are two types of grounded theory: **substantive theory**, which is grounded in data on a specific substantive area, and **formal grounded theory** (often using data from substantive theory studies), which is at a higher level of abstraction.

- A major controversy among grounded theory researchers concerns whether to follow the original Glaser and Strauss procedures or to use the adapted procedures of Strauss and Corbin; Glaser has argued that the latter approach does not result in *grounded theories* but rather in *conceptual descriptions*.

- **Historical research** is the systematic attempt to establish facts and relationships about past events. Historical data are normally subjected to **external criticism**, which concerns the authenticity of the source, and **internal criticism**, which assesses the worth of the evidence.

- **Case studies** are intensive investigations of a single entity or a small number of entities, such as individuals, groups, organizations, families, or communities; such studies usually involve collecting data over an extended period. Case study designs can be **single** or **multiple**, and **holistic** or **embedded**.

- **Narrative analysis** focuses on *story* in studies in which the purpose is to determine how individuals make sense of events in their lives. Several different structural approaches can be used to analyze narrative data, including, for example, Burke's **pentadic dramatism**.

- **Descriptive qualitative studies** have no formal name or do not fit into any disciplinary tradition. Such studies may simply be referred to as qualitative studies, naturalistic inquiries, or as qualitative content analyses.
- Research is sometimes conducted within an ideological perspective, and such research tends to rely primarily on qualitative research.
- **Critical theory** is concerned with a critique of existing social structures; critical researchers strive to conduct inquiries that involve collaboration with participants and foster enlightened self-knowledge and transformation. **Critical ethnography** uses the principles of critical theory in the study of cultures.
- **Feminist research**, like critical research, is designed to be transformative, but the focus is sharply on how gender domination and discrimination shape women's lives and their consciousness.
- **Participatory action research (PAR)** produces knowledge through close collaboration with groups or communities that are vulnerable to control or oppression by a dominant culture; in PAR research, methods take second place to emergent processes that can motivate people and generate community solidarity.

STUDY ACTIVITIES

Chapter 9 of the *Resource Manual to Accompany Nursing Research: Generating and Assessing Evidence for Nursing Practice, 8th edition*, offers various exercises and study suggestions for reinforcing concepts presented in this chapter. In addition, the following study questions can be addressed:

1. Which of the following topics is best suited to a phenomenological inquiry? To an ethnography? To a grounded theory study? Provide a rationale for each response.
   a. The passage through menarche among Haitian refugees
   b. The process of coping among AIDS patients
   c. The experience of having a child with leukemia
   d. Rituals relating to dying among nursing home residents
   e. The experience of waiting for service in a hospital emergency department
   f. The decision-making process among nurses regarding do-not-resuscitate orders

2. Apply the questions in Box 9.1 to one of the three studies described at the end of the chapter, referring as necessary to the full research reports for additional information.

STUDIES CITED IN CHAPTER 9

Methodologic or theoretical references cited in this chapter can be found in a separate section at the end of the book.

Bailey, P. H. (2004). The dyspnea-anxiety-dyspnea cycle—COPD patients' stories of breathlessness: "It's scary/when you can't breathe." *Qualitative Health Research, 14,* 760–778.

Beck, C. T. (2006). Pentadic cartography: Mapping birth trauma narratives. *Qualitative Health Research, 16,* 453–466.

Beck, C. T. (2007). Exemplar: Teetering on the edge. A continually emerging theory of postpartum depression (pp 273-292). In P. Munhall (Ed.), *Nursing research: A qualitative perspective* (4th ed., pp. 273–292). Sudbury, MA: Jones & Bartlett.

Benedict, S. (2006). Maria Stromberger: A nurse in the resistance in Auschwitz. *Nursing History Review, 14,* 189–202.

Caldwell, P., Arthur, H. M., & Rideout, E. (2005). Lives of rural women after myocardial infarction. *Canadian Journal of Nursing Research, 37*(1), 54–67.

Carlsson, E., Ehrenberg, A., & Ehnfors, M. (2004). Stroke and eating difficulties: Long-term experiences. *Journal of Clinical Nursing, 13*(7), 825–834.

Connell, S., Patterson, C., & Newman, B. (2006). A qualitative analysis of reproductive issues raised by young Australian women with breast cancer. *Health Care for Women International, 27*(1), 94–110.

Cordeau, M. A. (2004). *Acts of caring: A history of the lived experience of nurse-caring by Northern women during the American Civil War.* Unpublished dissertation, University of Connecticut, Storrs.

Crepeau, E. B. (2000). Reconstructing Gloria: A narrative analysis of team meetings. *Qualitative Health Research, 10*(6), 766–787.

Daff, D., Stepien, J. M., Wundke, R., Paterson, J., Whitehead, C. H., & Crotty, M. (2006). Perspectives of carers on the move from a hospital to a transitional care unit. *Qualitative Health Research, 16*(2), 189–205.

D'Auria, J. P., Christian, B. J., & Miles, M. S. (2006). Being there for my baby: Early responses of HIV-infected mothers with an HIV-exposed infant. *Journal of Pediatric Health Care, 20*(1), 11–18.

Ensign, J., & Bell, M. (2004). Illness experiences of homeless youth. *Qualitative Health Research, 14*(9), 1239–1254.

Ford-Gilboe, M., Wuest, J., & Merritt-Gray, M. (2005). Strengthening capacity to limit intrusion: Theorizing family health promotion in the aftermath of woman abuse. *Qualitative Health Research, 15*(4), 477–501.

French, B. (2005). The process of research use in nursing. *Journal of Advanced Nursing, 49*(2), 125–134.

Fu, M. R. (2005). Breast cancer survivors' intentions of managing lymphedema. *Cancer Nursing, 28*(6), 446–457.

Giarelli, E. (2006). Images of cloning and stem cell research in editorial cartoons in the United States. *Qualitative Health Research, 16*(1), 61–78.

Giddings, L. S. (2005). Health disparities, social injustices, and the culture of nursing. *Nursing Research, 54*(5), 304–312.

Glaser, B., & Strauss, A. (1965). *Awareness of dying.* Chicago: Aldine.

Hardcastle, M., Usher, K., & Holmes, C. (2006). Carspecken's five-stage critical qualitative research method: An application to nursing research. *Qualitative Health Research, 16*(1), 151–161.

Hilden, H. M., & Honkasalo, M. L. (2006). Finnish nurses' interpretations of patient autonomy in the context of end-of-life decision making. *Nursing Ethics, 13*(1), 41–51.

Hirst, S. P. (2002). Defining resident abuse within the culture of long-term care institutions. *Clinical Nursing Research, 11,* 267–284.

Hubbert, A. O. (2005). An ethnonursing research study: Adults residing in a Midwestern Christian philosophy urban homeless shelter. *Journal of Transcultural Nursing, 16*(3), 236–244.

Kearney, M. H., & O'Sullivan, J. (2003). Identity shifts as turning points in health behavior change. *Western Journal of Nursing Research, 25,* 134–152.

Kelley, L. S. (2005a). Gendered elder care exchanges in a Caribbean village. *Western Journal of Nursing Research, 27*(1), 73–92.

Kelley, L. S. (2005b). Minor children and adult care exchanges with community-dwelling frail elders in a St. Lucian village. *Journal of Gerontology: Social Sciences, 60B*(2), S62–73.

Kendall, J. (1999). Axial coding and the grounded theory controversy. *Western Journal of Nursing Research, 21,* 743–757.

Lauterbach, S. S. (2001). Longitudinal phenomenology: An example of "doing" phenomenology over time. Phenomenology of maternal mourning: Being-a-mother in another world (1992) and five years later (1997). In P. L. Munhall (Ed.), *Nursing research: A qualitative perspective* (pp. 185–208). Sudbury, MA: Jones & Bartlett.

Levy, V. (2006). Protective steering: A grounded theory study of the processes by which midwives facilitate informed choices during pregnancy. *Journal of Advanced Nursing, 53*(1), 114–122.

Li, S., & Arber, A. (2006). The construction of troubled and credible patients: A study of emotion talk in palliative care settings. *Qualitative Health Research, 16*(1), 27–46.

Lin, C., Lee, B., & Hicks, F. D. (2005). The phenomenology of deciding about hemodialysis among Taiwanese. *Western Journal of Nursing Research, 27*(7), 915–929.

Lipson, J. G. (2001). We are the canaries: Multiple chemical sensitivity sufferers. *Qualitative Health Research, 11,* 103–116.

Morse, J. M., & Pooler, C. (2002). Patient-family-nurse interactions in the trauma-resuscitation room. *American Journal of Critical Care, 11,* 240–249.

Normann, H. K., Henriksen, N., Norberg, A., & Asplund, K. (2005). Lucidity in a woman with severe dementia: A case study. *Journal of Clinical Nursing, 14*(7), 891–896.

Phinney, A. (2006). Family strategies for supporting involvement in meaningful activity by persons with dementia. *Journal of Family Nursing, 12*(1), 80–101.

Salazar, M. K., Napolitano, M., Scherer, J. A., & McCauley, L. A. (2004). Hispanic adolescent farmworkers' perceptions associated with pesticide exposure. *Western Journal of Nursing Research, 26*(2), 146–166.

Sandelowski, M. (1997). "Making the best of things": Technology in American nursing 1870–1940. *Nursing History Review, 8,* 3–22.

Schneider, B. (2005). Mothers talk about their children with schizophrenia: A performance autoethnography. *Journal of Psychiatric & Mental Health Nursing, 12*(3), 333–340.

Sterling, Y. M., & Peterson, J. W. (2005). Lessons learned from a longitudinal qualitative family systems study. *Applied Nursing Research, 18*(1), 44–49.

Strickland, C. J., Walsh, E., & Cooper, M. (2006). Healing fractured families: Parents' and elders' perspectives on the impact of colonization and youth suicide prevention in a Pacific Northwest American Indian tribe. *Journal of Transcultural Nursing, 17*(1), 5–12.

Vukic, A., & Keddy, B. (2002). Northern nursing practice in a primary health care setting. *Journal of Advanced Nursing, 40*(5), 542–548.

10

Designing Quantitative Studies

CAUSALITY

In designing a quantitative study, researchers have to take into consideration a number of things, including various practical, ethical, and theoretical challenges. The methodologic challenge is to design a study that will yield the strongest possible evidence to answer the research question, given the other challenges.

As we have seen in Chapters 2 and 4, there are several broad categories of research questions that are relevant to evidence-based nursing practice—questions about interventions; diagnosis and assessment; prognosis; etiology and harm; and meaning or process (see Table 2.1). Descriptive questions about meaning or process call for a qualitative study, approaches to which were described in the previous chapter. Questions about diagnosis or assessment, as well as other types of questions about the status quo of health-related situations, are also typically descriptive. Many research questions, however, are about *causes* and *effects:*

- Does a telephone therapy intervention for patients with prostate cancer *cause* improvements in their psychological distress and coping skills? (intervention question)
- Do birthweights under 1500 grams *cause* developmental delays in children? (prognosis question)

- Does cigarette smoking *cause* lung cancer? (etiology/harm question)

Although causality is a hotly debated philosophical issue, we all understand the general concept of a **cause**. For example, we understand that failure to sleep *causes* fatigue and that high caloric intake *causes* weight gain.

In thinking about causality, it is important to recognize that most phenomena are multiply determined. Weight gain, for example, can be the effect of consuming too many calories, but other factors cause weight gain as well. Most causes in which health researchers are interested are not *deterministic*, they only increase the probability that an effect will occur. For example, there is ample evidence that smoking is a cause of lung cancer, but not everyone who smokes develops lung cancer, and not everyone with lung cancer was a smoker.

The Counterfactual Model

Although it might be easy to grasp what researchers have in mind when they talk about a *cause,* what exactly is an **effect**? Shadish, Cook, and Campbell (2002), who wrote a widely acclaimed book on research design and causal inference, explained that a good way to grasp the meaning of an effect is through the conceptualization of a counterfactual.

In a research context, a **counterfactual** is what would have happened *to the same people* exposed to a causal factor if they *simultaneously* were *not* exposed to the causal factor. An effect represents the difference between what actually did happen with the exposure and what would have happened without it. This counterfactual model clearly represents an ideal that cannot ever be realized, but it is a good model to keep in mind in designing a study to provide evidence about causes and effects. As Shadish and colleagues (2002) have noted, "A central task for all cause-probing research is to create reasonable approximations to this physically impossible counterfactual" (p. 5).

Criteria for Causality

Several writers have proposed criteria for establishing a cause-and-effect relationship. Lazarsfeld (1955), whose thinking reflects the ideas of John Stuart Mill, identified three criteria for causality. The first criterion is *temporal*: a cause must precede an effect in time. If we were testing the hypothesis that aspartame causes fetal abnormalities, it would be necessary to demonstrate that the abnormalities did not develop before the mothers' exposure to aspartame. The second requirement is that there be an *empirical relationship* between the presumed cause and the presumed effect. In the aspartame example, we would have to demonstrate an association between aspartame consumption and the presence of a fetal abnormality, that is, that a higher percentage of aspartame users than nonusers had infants with fetal abnormalities. The final criterion for establishing a causal relationship is that the relationship cannot be explained as being *caused by a third variable*. Suppose, for instance, that people who used aspartame tended also to drink more coffee than nonusers of aspartame. There would then be a possibility that any relationship between maternal aspartame use and fetal abnormalities reflects an underlying causal relationship between a substance in coffee and the abnormalities.

Additional criteria, first articulated in 1968, were proposed by Bradford-Hill (1971) as part of the discussion about the causal connection between smoking and lung cancer—these are sometimes referred to as the Surgeon General's criteria for that reason. Two of Bradford-Hill's criteria foreshadow the importance of meta-analyses, the techniques for which had not yet been fully developed when the criteria were first proposed. The criterion of *coherence* involves similar evidence from multiple sources, and the criterion of *consistency* involves having similar levels of statistical relationship in several studies. Another important criterion in health research is *biologic plausibility*, that is, evidence from laboratory or basic physiologic studies that a causal pathway is credible.

Researchers investigating casual relationships must provide persuasive evidence regarding these criteria through their study design. Some research designs are better at revealing cause-and-effect relationships than others, as suggested by the evidence hierarchy in Figure 2.1 in Chapter 2. Most of this chapter is devoted to identifying designs that have been used to illuminate causal relationships.

DESIGN TERMINOLOGY

It is easy to get confused about the terms used to refer to a research design because there is a lot of inconsistency among writers. Moreover, the design terms used by medical and epidemiologic researchers are usually different than the terms used by social scientists. Many early nurse researchers got their research training in social science fields such as psychology or sociology before doctoral-level training became available in schools of nursing, and so social scientific design terms have predominated in the nursing research literature.

Among those interested in establishing an evidence-based practice, it is imperative to be able to understand studies published in nursing, medical, epidemiologic, and social science journals. We use both medical and social science terms in this book, although the latter predominate. Table 10.1 provides a list of several important design terms used by social scientists and the corresponding terms used by medical researchers.

| TABLE 10.1 | Research Design Terminology in the Social Scientific and Medical Literature |

SOCIAL SCIENTIFIC TERM	MEDICAL RESEARCH TERM
Experiment, true experiment, experimental study	Randomized controlled trial, randomized clinical trial, RCT
Quasi-experiment, quasi-experimental study	Controlled trial, controlled trial without randomization
Nonexperimental study; correlational study	Observational study
Retrospective study	Case-control study
Prospective nonexperimental study	Cohort study
Group, condition (e.g., experimental or control group/condition)	Arm (e.g., intervention or control arm)

EXPERIMENTAL DESIGN

A basic distinction in quantitative research design is that between experimental and nonexperimental research. In an **experiment** (or **randomized controlled trial, RCT**), researchers are active agents, not passive observers. Early physical scientists learned that although pure observation of phenomena is valuable, complexities occurring in nature often make it difficult to understand important relationships. This problem was handled by isolating phenomena in a laboratory and controlling the conditions under which they occurred. The procedures developed by physical scientists were profitably adopted by biologists during the 19th century, resulting in many achievements in physiology and medicine. The 20th century has witnessed the use of experimental methods by researchers interested in human behavior.

The controlled experiment is considered by many to be the gold standard for yielding reliable evidence about causes and effects. The strength of true experiments lies in the fact that experimenters can achieve greater confidence in the genuineness of causal relationships because they are observed under controlled conditions and because they typically meet the previously discussed criteria for establishing causality. As we pointed out in Chapter 4, hypotheses are never proved or disproved by scientific methods, but true experiments offer the most convincing evidence about the effect one variable has on another.

A true experimental or RCT design is characterized by the following properties:

- *Manipulation*—the experimenter *does* something to at least some subjects—that is, there is some type of intervention.
- *Control*—the experimenter introduces controls over the experimental situation, including devising a good approximation of a counterfactual—usually a control group that does not receive the intervention.
- *Randomization*—the experimenter assigns subjects to a control or experimental condition on a random basis.

➜ **TIP:** All experimental studies are inherently prospective because the researcher institutes the intervention (manipulates the independent variable) and subsequently determines its effect. Thus, it is not necessary to describe an RCT as prospective.

Design Features of True Experiments

Researchers have many options in designing an experiment. We begin by discussing several features of experimental designs.

Manipulation: The Experimental Intervention

Manipulation involves *doing* something to study participants. The experimenter manipulates the independent variable by administering a **treatment** (**intervention**) to some subjects and withholding it from others, or by administering some other treatment. The experimenter thus deliberately *varies* the independent variable and observes the effect on the dependent variable.

For example, suppose we hypothesized that gentle massage is effective as a pain relief measure for elderly nursing home residents. The independent variable (the presumed cause) in this example is receipt of gentle massage, which could be manipulated by giving some patients the massage intervention and withholding it from others. We would then compare patients' pain level (the dependent variable) in the two groups to see if differences in receipt of the intervention resulted in differences in average pain levels.

In designing experimental studies, researchers make many decisions about what the experimental condition entails, and these decisions can affect the researchers' conclusions. To give an experimental intervention a fair test, researchers need to carefully design an intervention that is appropriate to the problem, consistent with a theoretical rationale, and of sufficient intensity and duration that effects might reasonably be expected. The full nature of the intervention must be clearly delineated in formal protocols that spell out exactly what the treatment is. Among the questions researchers need to address are the following:

- What *is* the intervention, and how does it differ from usual methods of care?
- If there are two alternative interventions, how exactly do they differ?
- What are the specific procedures to be used with those receiving the intervention?
- What is the dosage or intensity of the intervention?
- Over how long a period will the intervention be administered, how frequently will it be administered, and when will the treatment begin (e.g., 2 hours after surgery)?

- Who will administer the intervention? What are their credentials, and what type of special training will they receive?
- Under what conditions will the intervention be withdrawn or altered?

The goal in most experimental studies is to have an identical intervention for all subjects in the treatment group. For example, in most drug studies, subjects in the experimental group are given the exact same ingredient, in the same dose, administered in exactly the same manner—all according to well-articulated protocols. There is, however, a growing interest in **patient-centered interventions**, or **PCIs** (Lauver et al., 2002). The purpose of patient-centered interventions is to enhance the efficacy of the treatment by taking people's characteristics or needs into account. Interventions based on the Transtheoretical (stages of change) Model, discussed in Chapter 6, are PCIs because the intervention is tailored to fit people's readiness to change their behavior. In such tailored interventions, each person receives an intervention customized to certain characteristics, including demographic characteristics (e.g., gender, age), cognitive factors (e.g., reading level), or affective factors (e.g., values or attitudes). There is some evidence that tailored interventions are more effective than standardized interventions (e.g., Lauver et al., 2003). There is, however, a need for more research in this area, and such research is likely to play an important role in our current evidence-based practice environment in which there is a strong interest in understanding not only *what* works, but also what works for *whom*.

Example of a patient-centered intervention: Giesler and colleagues (2005) developed a nurse-driven cancer care intervention for patients with prostate cancer, and tested its effectiveness using an experimental design. Patients in the intervention group met once a month for 6 months with an oncology nurse, who helped patients identify their quality-of-life needs and provided education and support tailored to meet those needs.

⊃ **T I P :** Although PCIs are not universally standardized, they are nevertheless typically administered according to well-defined procedures and guidelines, and the intervention agents are carefully trained in making decisions about who should get what type of treatment.

Manipulation: The Control Condition

Obtaining evidence about relationships requires making at least one comparison. If we were to supplement the diet of premature infants with a particular nutrient for 2 weeks, their weight at the end of 2 weeks would tell us nothing about treatment effectiveness. At a bare minimum, we would need to compare their posttreatment weight with their pretreatment weight to determine whether, at least, their weight had increased. But let us assume that we find an average weight gain of 1 pound. Does this gain support the conclusion that the nutritional supplement (the independent variable) caused weight gain (the dependent variable)? No, it does not. Babies normally gain weight as they mature. Without a control group—a group that does *not* receive the nutritional supplements—it is impossible to separate the effects of maturation from those of the treatment. As noted earlier, one of the criteria for establishing causality is that the relationship between the independent and dependent variables cannot be explained as being caused by something else.

The term **control group** refers to a group of subjects whose performance on a dependent variable is used to evaluate the performance of the treatment group on the same dependent variable. As noted in Table 10.1, researchers with training from a social science tradition use the term "group" or "condition" (e.g., the experimental group or the control condition), but medical researchers often use the term "arm," as in the intervention arm or the control arm of the study.

The control group condition used as a basis of comparison in a study represents a proxy for the ideal counterfactual as previously described, and is sometimes referred to as the counterfactual. Researchers have choices about what to use as the counterfactual. Their decision is sometimes based on theoretical or substantive grounds, but may also be driven by practical or ethical concerns. In some research, control group subjects receive no treatment at all—they are merely observed with respect to performance on the dependent variable. This kind of situation is seldom feasible in nursing research. For example, if we wanted to evaluate the effectiveness of a nursing intervention on hospital patients, we would not devise an experiment in which patients in the control group received no nursing care at all. Among the other possibilities for the counterfactual are the following:

1. An alternative intervention; for example, subjects could receive two different types of distraction as alternative therapies for pain.
2. A **placebo** or pseudointervention presumed to have no therapeutic value; for example, in studies of the effectiveness of drugs, some patients get the experimental drug, and others get an innocuous substance. Placebos are used to control for the nonpharmaceutical effects of drugs, such as the attention being paid to subjects. (There can, however, be **placebo effects**—changes in the dependent variable attributable to the placebo condition—because of subjects' expectations of benefits or harms).

Example of a placebo control group:
Anderson and Gross (2004) randomly assigned ambulatory surgery patients who complained of nausea to one of three aromatherapy treatments to examine effects on nausea: isopropyl alcohol, oil of peppermint, and placebo (saline).

3. Standard methods of care—the usual procedures used to treat patients. This is the most typical control condition in nursing studies.
4. Different doses or intensities of treatment wherein all subjects get some type of intervention, but the experimental group gets an intervention that is richer, more intense, or longer. This approach is often used when there is a desire to analyze **dose-response effects**, that is, to test whether larger doses are associated with larger benefits, or whether a smaller (and perhaps less costly or burdensome) dose would suffice.

Example of a dose-response analysis: Keller, Robinson, and Pickens (2004) used an experimental design to test the efficacy and dose-response effects of two different "doses" of walking frequency (3 versus 5 days a week) on cardiovascular risk factors in sedentary, postmenopausal African-American women.

5. **Wait-list control group**, with delayed treatment; the control group eventually receives the full experimental treatment, but treatment is deferred.

Example of a wait-list control group: Ross, Davis, and MacDonald (2005) tested the efficacy of an 8-week group treatment program for asthmatic adults suffering from coexisting panic disorder. Study participants were assigned at random to the treatment condition or to a wait-list control condition.

Methodologically, the best possible test is between two conditions that are as different as possible, as when the experimental group receives a strong treatment and the control group gets no treatment at all. Ethically, however, the most appealing counterfactual is probably the wait-list/delay-of-treatment approach (number 5), which may be difficult to do pragmatically. Testing two competing interventions (number 1) also has ethical appeal, but the risk is that the results will be inconclusive because it is difficult to detect differential effects, especially if both interventions are at least moderately effective.

Some researchers elect to combine two or more comparison strategies. For example, they might test two alternative treatments (option 1) against usual methods of care (option 3). Another alternative is to compare an intervention, a placebo, and no treatment. Clearly, the control group decision should be based on the underlying conceptualization of how the intervention might *cause* the intended effect.

Example of a three-group design: Nikoletti and colleagues (2005) assigned patients receiving chemotherapy to one of three groups—a plain ice group, a flavored ice group, and a usual care group—to determine the effects of two alternative forms of oral cryotherapy versus a control condition on oral mucositis.

Sometimes researchers include an **attention control group**, especially if the primary control group receives no treatment or treatment as usual. An attention control group typically is used when researchers want to rule out the possibility that intervention effects are caused by the special attention given to the people receiving the intervention, rather than by the actual content of the treatment. The idea is to try to separate the "active ingredients" of the treatment from the "inactive ingredients" of special attention. The use of multiple comparison groups is often attractive but, of course, adds to the cost and complexity of the study.

Example of an attention control group: Movaffaghi and colleagues (2006) studied the effects of therapeutic touch (TT) on hemoglobin and hematocrit levels in healthy individuals. The design involved three groups—a group that received TT, an attention control group that received mimic TT, and a no-treatment control group.

The decision about a control group strategy should entail careful reflection on what it is that needs to be controlled. For example, if attention control groups are being considered, there should be an underlying conceptualization of the construct of "attention" (Gross, 2005).

Whatever decision is made about a control group strategy, researchers need to be as careful in spelling out the counterfactual as they are in delineating the intervention. In research reports, researchers sometimes say that the control group got the "usual methods of care" without explaining what that condition was and how different it was from the intervention being tested. In drawing on an evidence base for practice, nurses need to understand exactly what happened to study participants in different conditions. Barkauskas, Lusk, and Eakin (2005) and Shadish and associates (2002) offer some useful advice about developing a control group strategy.

Randomization

Randomization (also called **random assignment** or **random allocation**) involves placing subjects into treatment conditions at random. *Random* means that every subject has an equal chance of being assigned to any group. If subjects are placed in groups randomly, there is no systematic bias in the groups with respect to attributes that could affect the dependent variable.

Randomization Principles. The overall purpose of random assignment is to approximate the ideal—but impossible—counterfactual of having the same people in multiple treatment groups simultaneously. As an illustration, suppose we wanted to study the effectiveness of a contraceptive counseling program for multiparous women who have just given birth. Two groups of subjects are included—one will be counseled and the other will not. The women in the sample are likely to differ from one another in many ways, such as age, marital status, financial situation, religion, and the like. Any of these characteristics could affect a woman's diligence in practicing contraception, independent of whether she receives counseling. We need to have the "counsel" and "no counsel" groups equal with respect to these extraneous characteristics to assess the impact of the experimental counseling program on subsequent pregnancies. That is, we need to create a counterfactual group that is equivalent, to the fullest extent possible, to the intervention group. The random assignment of subjects to one group or the other is designed to perform this equalization function. One method might be to flip a coin for each woman (more elaborate procedures are discussed later). If the coin comes up "heads," the woman would be assigned to one group; if the coin comes up "tails," she would be assigned to the other group.

Although randomization is the preferred scientific method for equalizing groups, there is no *guarantee* that the groups will, in fact, be equal. As an extreme example, suppose the study sample involves 10 women who have given birth to 4 or more children. Five of the 10 women are aged 35 years or older, and the remaining 5 are younger than age 35. We would expect random assignment to result in two or three women from the two age ranges in each group. But suppose that, by chance, the older five women all ended up in the experi-

mental group. Because these women are nearing the end of their childbearing years, the likelihood of their conceiving is diminished. Thus, follow-up of their subsequent childbearing (the dependent variable) might suggest that the counseling program was effective in reducing subsequent pregnancies; however, a higher birth rate for the control group may reflect only age and fecundity differences, not lack of exposure to counseling.

Despite this possibility, randomization remains the most trustworthy and acceptable method of equalizing groups. Unusual or deviant assignments such as this one are rare, and the likelihood of obtaining markedly unequal groups is reduced as the number of subjects increases.

You may wonder why we do not consciously control those subject characteristics that are likely to affect the outcome. As described in an earlier chapter, the procedure known as *matching* is sometimes used to accomplish this. For example, if matching were used in the contraceptive counseling study, we might want to ensure that if there were a married, 38-year-old woman with six children in the experimental group, there would be a married, 38-year-old woman with six children in the control group. There are two serious problems with matching, however. First, to match effectively, we must know (and measure) the characteristics that are likely to affect the dependent variable, but this information is not always known. Second, even if we knew the relevant traits, the complications of matching on more than two or three characteristics simultaneously are prohibitive. With random assignment, on the other hand, *all* possible distinguishing characteristics—age, gender, intelligence, blood type, religious affiliation, and so on—are likely to be equally distributed in all groups. Over the long run, the groups tend to be counterbalanced with respect to an infinite number of biologic, psychological, economic, and social traits.

Basic Randomization. To demonstrate how random assignment is performed, we turn to another example. Suppose we were testing two alternative interventions to lower the preoperative anxiety of children who are about to undergo tonsillectomy. One intervention involves giving structured information about the surgical team's activities (procedural information); the other involves structured information about what the child will feel (sensation information). A third control group receives no special intervention. With a sample of 15 subjects, 5 children will be in each of the three groups. With three groups, we cannot use a coin flip to determine group assignments. We could, however, write the children's names on slips of paper, put the slips into a hat, and then draw names. The first five individuals whose names were drawn would be assigned to group I, the second five would be assigned to group II, and so on.

Pulling names from a hat involves a lot of work if the sample is large. Researchers can use a **table of random numbers** in the randomization process. A portion of such a table is reproduced in Table 10.2. In a table of random numbers, any digit from 0 to 9 is equally likely to follow any other digit. Going in any direction from any point in the table produces a random sequence.

In our example, we would number the 15 subjects from 1 to 15, as shown in the second column of Table 10.3, and then draw numbers between 01 and 15 from the random number table. A simple procedure for finding a starting point is to close your eyes and let your finger fall at some point on the table. For the sake of following the example, let us assume that our starting point is at number 52, bolded in Table 10.2. We can move in any direction in the table from that point, selecting numbers that fall between 01 and 15. Let us move to the right, looking at two-digit combinations (to get numbers greater than 9, i.e., from 10 to 15). The number to the right of 52 is 06. The person whose number is 06, Nathan O., is assigned to group I. Moving along in the table, the next number within the range of 01 to 15 is 11. (To find numbers in the required range, we have to bypass numbers between 16 and 99.) Alaine J., whose number is 11, is also assigned to group I. When we get to the end of the row, we move down to the next row, and so forth. The next three numbers are 01, 15, and 14. Thus, Kristina N., Ryan W., and Paul M. are all put into group I. The next five numbers between 01 and 15 that emerge in

the random number table are used to assign five individuals to group II in the same fashion, as shown in the third column of Table 10.3. The remaining five people in the sample are put into group III. Note that numbers that have already been used often reappear in the table before the task is completed. For example, the number 15 appeared four times during the randomization procedure. This is perfectly normal because the numbers are random. After the first time a number appears and is used, subsequent appearances can be ignored.

It might be useful to look at the three groups to see if they are about equal with respect to one readily discernible characteristic, that is, the subjects' gender. We started out with eight girls and seven boys in all. As Table 10.4 shows, randomization did a good job of allocating boys and girls about equally across the three research groups. We must accept on faith the probability that other characteristics (e.g., family income, age, race, preoperative anxiety) are fairly well distributed in the randomized groups as well. The larger the sample, the stronger the likelihood that the groups will be comparable across all confounding factors that could affect the outcomes.

Researchers usually assign subjects to groups in proportion to the number of groups being compared. For example, a sample of 300 subjects in a two-group design would generally aim to have 150 people in the experimental group and 150 in the control group. If there were three groups being compared, there would be 100 per group. However, it is also possible (and sometimes desirable ethically) to have a different allocation. For example, if an especially promising treatment for a serious illness were developed, we could assign 200 to the treatment group and 100 to the control group. Such an allocation does, however, make it more difficult to detect treatment effects at statistically significant levels—or, to put it another way, the overall sample size must be larger to attain the same level of statistical reliability.

Tables of random numbers and manual methods of randomization are becoming obsolete in our technologically advanced age. We used a simple example of a random number table here to

TABLE 10.2			Small Table of Random Digits												

46	85	05	23	26		34	67	75	83	00		74	91	06	43	45
69	24	89	34	60		45	30	50	75	21		61	31	83	18	55
14	01	33	17	92		59	74	76	72	77		76	50	33	45	13
56	30	38	73	15		16	**52**	06	96	76		11	65	49	98	93
81	30	44	85	85		68	65	22	73	76		92	85	25	58	66
70	28	42	43	26		79	37	59	52	20		01	15	96	32	67
90	41	59	36	14		33	52	12	66	65		55	82	34	76	41
39	90	40	21	15		59	58	94	90	67		66	82	14	15	75
88	15	20	00	80		20	55	49	14	09		96	27	74	82	57
45	13	46	35	45		59	40	47	20	59		43	94	75	16	80
70	01	41	50	21		41	29	06	73	12		71	85	71	59	57
37	23	93	32	95		05	87	00	11	19		92	78	42	63	40
18	63	73	75	09		82	44	49	90	05		04	92	17	37	01
05	32	78	21	62		20	24	78	17	59		45	19	72	53	32
95	09	66	79	46		48	46	08	55	58		15	19	11	87	82
43	25	38	41	45		60	83	32	59	83		01	29	14	13	49
80	85	40	92	79		43	52	90	63	18		38	38	47	47	61
80	08	87	70	74		88	72	25	67	36		66	16	44	94	31
80	89	07	80	02		94	81	33	19	00		54	15	58	34	36
93	12	81	84	64		74	45	79	05	61		72	84	81	18	34
82	47	42	55	93		48	54	53	52	47		18	61	91	36	74
53	34	24	42	76		75	12	21	17	24		74	62	77	37	07
82	64	12	28	20		92	90	41	31	41		32	39	21	97	63
13	57	41	72	00		69	90	26	37	42		78	46	42	25	01
29	59	38	86	27		94	97	21	15	98		62	09	53	67	87
86	88	75	50	87		19	15	20	00	23		12	30	28	07	83
44	98	91	68	22		36	02	40	08	67		76	37	84	16	05
93	39	94	55	47		94	45	87	42	84		05	04	14	98	07
52	16	29	02	86		54	15	83	42	43		46	97	83	54	82
04	73	72	10	31		75	05	19	30	29		47	66	56	43	82

Reprinted from *A Million Random Digits With 100,000 Normal Deviates*. New York: The Free Press, 1955. Used with permission of the Rand Corporation, Santa Monica, CA.

illustrate the process. There are resources available for free on the Internet to help with the randomization process. One such website is *http://www.randomizer.org*, which has a useful tutorial. ☻ Standard statistical software packages (e.g., SPSS or SAS) can also be used (see Shadish et al., 2002, p. 311).

➲ **TIP:** There is considerable confusion—even in other nursing research methods textbooks—about random assignment versus random sampling. Randomization (random assignment) is a *signature* of an experimental design. If there is no random allocation of subjects to treatment conditions, then the design is not a true experiment. Random *sampling*, by contrast, refers to a

TABLE 10.3	Example of Random Assignment Procedure

NAME OF SUBJECT	NUMBER	GROUP ASSIGNMENT
Kristina N.	1	I
Derek A.	2	III
Trinity A.	3	III
Lauren J.	4	II
Grace S.	5	II
Nathan O.	6	I
Norah J.	7	III
Thomas N.	8	III
Daniel B.	9	II
Rita T.	10	III
Alaine J.	11	I
Katie B.	12	II
Vadim B.	13	II
Paul M.	14	I
Ryan W.	15	I

TABLE 10.4	Breakdown of the Gender Composition of the Three Groups

GENDER	GROUP I	GROUP II	GROUP III
Boys	3	2	2
Girls	2	3	3

method of selecting subjects for a study, as we discuss in Chapter 13. Random sampling (also called random selection) is *not* a signature of an experimental design. In fact, most experiments or RCTs do *not* involve random sampling.

Randomization Procedures. The success of randomization depends on two factors. First, the allocation process should be truly random and unbiased, for example, by using a table of random numbers. And second, there must be strict adherence to the resulting randomization schedule. The latter can best be achieved if the allocation is unpredictable (for both study participants and those enrolling them) and tamperproof. Random assignment should, in other words, involve **allocation concealment** that prevents those who enroll subjects from knowing the upcoming assignments.

Several methods have been devised to ensure allocation concealment, many of which involve developing a randomization schedule before the study begins. This is often advantageous when

subjects do not enter a study at the same time, but rather on a *rolling enrollment* basis. In such situations, the sequence of allocation can be predetermined before enrollment (e.g., the first person is allocated randomly to group III, the second is allocated randomly to group I). One widely used method is to have a sequence of sealed, opaque envelopes containing assignment information. As each participant enters the study, he or she receives the next envelope in the sequence. There is evidence, however, that envelope systems can be subject to errors (Friedman, Furberg, & DeMets, 1998). The preferred method is to have those enrolling subjects obtain treatment allocation information, by telephone or e-mail, from a person unconnected with recruitment, enrollment, or treatment. This person is trained to strictly follow the randomization. In multi-site trials, a centralized randomization process is strongly recommended.

The timing of randomization is also important. Eligibility for the study—whether a person meets the criteria for inclusion—should be ascertained before randomization. If **baseline data** are collected at the outset of the study (e.g., to measure preintervention levels on key outcomes), this should occur before randomization to rule out any possibility that group assignment in and of itself affected the outcomes. Randomization should occur as closely as possible to the start of the intervention to maximize the likelihood that all randomized subjects will actually receive the condition to which they have been assigned. Figure 10.1 illustrates the sequence of steps that occurs in most

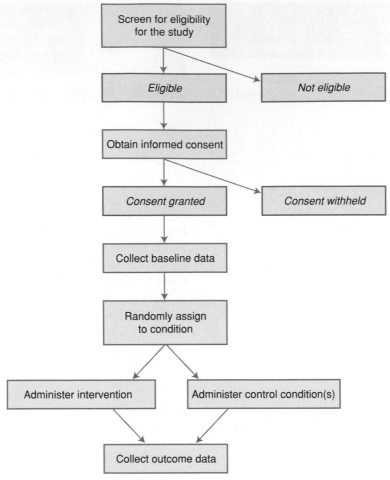

FIGURE 10.1 Sequence of steps in a conventional randomization design.

experimental studies, including the timing for obtaining informed consent.

Randomization Variants. In most cases, randomization involves the random assignment of individual subjects to different conditions. However, an alternative is **cluster randomization**, which involves randomly assigning clusters of individuals to different treatment groups (Hauck et al., 1991). Cluster randomization may sometimes enhance the feasibility of conducting a true experiment. Groups of patients who enter a hospital unit at the same time, or groups of patients from different sites, can be randomly

assigned to a treatment condition as a unit—thus ruling out, in some situations, some practical impediments to randomization. This approach also reduces the possibility of **contamination of treatments**, that is, the mingling of subjects in the groups, which could cloud the results if they exchange information. The main disadvantages of cluster randomization are that the statistical analysis of data obtained through this approach is more complex, and sample size requirements are usually greater for a given level of accuracy. Moreover, the number of units being randomized must be fairly large for the randomization to be successful in equalizing across units. Cluster randomization can also complicate efforts at research synthesis through meta-analysis. Donner and Klar (2004) offer a useful discussion about planning a study using cluster randomization.

> **Example of cluster randomization:** DiIorio and colleagues (2006) tested the efficacy of two alternative HIV-prevention interventions for adolescents and their mothers. The study was conducted at 11 sites (Boys and Girls Clubs), and the sites were randomly assigned to either a life skills program (3 sites), a program based on social cognitive theory (4 sites), or a control condition that received no special intervention (4 sites).

Although simple randomization is usually adequate for creating groups with comparable characteristics, sometimes researchers take steps to ensure that subgroups of study participants are allocated equally to treatment conditions. This is sometimes referred to as **stratification**. For example, if a researcher stratified on the basis of gender, men and women would be randomly assigned to conditions separately, thus ensuring that both men and women received the intervention in the right proportions. In multi-site studies, randomization is usually stratified by site.

Sometimes subjects are randomly assigned within blocks, in what has been called **permuted block randomization**. In such a system, rather than having a randomization schedule for the entire sample, randomization occurs for blocks of subjects of even size—for example, 6 or 8 at a time. If the entire sample is randomly allocated to conditions, by chance alone, the first 5 or 6 subjects could be allocated to one or another condition. But if allocation is done in blocks, random assignment within the small block would guarantee an appropriate distribution across conditions. Such a system is especially appropriate when enrollment occurs over a long period of time because in such situations there is a possibility that the type of people enrolling might change—or the intervention itself might change as a result of improved proficiency in implementing it.

> **Example of stratified, permuted block randomization:** Lai and colleagues (2006) studied the effect of music during kangaroo care on maternal anxiety and infant response. Mother–infant dyads were randomly assigned to the treatment or control group using permuted block randomization, stratified on infant gender.

One controversial randomization variant is called **randomized consent** or a **Zelen design** after its originator (Zelen, 1979). Study participants often have a preference about which condition they would like to be in, and so if randomization occurs *after* fully informed consent is obtained (as in Fig. 10.1), people may choose not to participate if they are not allocated to their preferred condition. Zelen proposed a simple solution: randomize first and *then* obtain consent, thereby eliminating the possibility that the consent process will generate preferences. Those in the intervention group are then approached and offered the intervention, which they can accept or decline. If the control group condition is standard care, control group subjects may not even be asked for their consent because they would not be getting anything new or different. The ethical controversies surrounding this form of randomization, as well as its merits and other limitations, have been well described by Homer (2002).

> **Example of the Zelen design:** Steiner and colleagues (2001) compared postacute intermediate care in an inpatient nurse-led unit and conventional postacute care on general medical wards in terms of such outcomes as patients' length of stay, functional status, and mortality. The investigators, who used the Zelen design to randomize their subjects, argued that conventional randomization was found to be distressful and confusing to many older patients.

Another method of addressing subject preferences has been called the **partially randomized patient preference (PRPP)** approach, wherein all study participants are asked preferences about treatment conditions. Only those without a strong preference are randomized, but all subjects are followed up. Lambert and Wood (2000) outline the benefits and problems of this approach.

Masking or Blinding

Allocation concealment is intended to prevent biases that could stem from foreknowledge of allocations before the assignment actually occurs. To use an exaggerated example, if the person in charge of enrollment knew that the next person enrolled would be assigned to a promising intervention, he or she might defer enrollment until a particularly needy patient came along. Allocation concealment can always be implemented, regardless of the intervention.

Masking (or blinding), as noted in Chapter 8, addresses *awareness* or *expectancy bias*, the bias that can result from subjects' awareness of their treatment condition or the study hypotheses, or researchers' awareness of who is in which treatment condition. Unlike allocation concealment, masking is not always possible. Drug studies often lend themselves to masking, but many nursing interventions do not. For example, if the intervention were a smoking cessation program, the subjects would be aware that they were receiving the intervention, and the intervener would be aware of who was in the program. However, it is often possible, and desirable, to at least mask the subjects' treatment status from the people collecting outcome data.

Example of a single-blind experiment: Scott and her colleagues (2005) compared the efficacy of two diets before bowel cleansing with sodium phosphates oral solution in preparation for a colonoscopy. The standard liquid diet was compared to a liberalized diet that included a normal breakfast and a low-residue lunch the day before the colonoscopy. Patients knew what group they were in, but the colonoscopists, who reported on overall cleansing efficacy, did not.

➲ **TIP:** When masking is possible, it is a good idea to assess the effectiveness of the masking. This can easily be accomplished by asking participants what intervention group they thought they were in, or asking members of the research team to guess participants' allocation. If masking was successful, then people should do no better than chance with their guesses.

Specific Experimental Designs

There are numerous experimental designs, including many that are not discussed in this book, such as *nested designs* and the *Solomon four-group design*. The most widely used designs in nursing research are described in this section and summarized in Table 10.5.

Basic Experimental Designs

At the beginning of this chapter, we described a study that tested the effect of gentle massage on the pain levels of elderly nursing home residents. This example illustrates a simple design that is sometimes referred to as an **after-only design** or a **posttest-only design** because data on the dependent variable are collected only once—after random assignment is completed and the experimental treatment has been introduced.

A second basic design—the most widely used experimental design by nurse researchers—involves the collection of baseline data, as illustrated in Figure 10.1. Suppose we hypothesized that convective airflow blankets are more effective than conductive water-flow blankets in cooling critically ill patients with fever. Our design involves assigning patients to the two different types of blankets (the independent variable) and measuring the dependent variable (body temperature) twice, before and after the intervention. This scheme permits us to examine whether one blanket type is more effective that the other in *reducing* fever—that is, with this design researchers can examine *change*. This design is referred to as a **before–after design** or a **pretest–posttest design**. Many before–after designs include data collection at multiple postintervention points.

Example of a before–after experimental design: Shin and colleagues (2006) conducted an experiment to compare the relative effectiveness of hand acupuncture and moxibustion (an ancient form of heat therapy) in decreasing pain and "coldness" in Korean women who had a hysterectomy. Pain levels and digital infrared thermographic imaging measurements were obtained from all subjects both before and after the intervention.

Factorial Design

The two designs described thus far are ones in which the experimenter manipulates only one

| TABLE 10.5 | Experimental Designs | | |

NAME OF DESIGN	PREINTERVENTION DATA?	WITHIN- OR BETWEEN-GROUPS	FEATURES
Posttest-only (after-only)	No	Between	One data collection point after the intervention; not appropriate for measuring *change*
Pretest–posttest (before–after)	Yes	Between	Data collection both before and after the intervention; appropriate for measuring change; can determine differences between groups (experimental) and change within groups (quasi-experimental)
Factorial	Optional	Between	Experimental manipulation of more than one independent variable; permits a test of *main effects* for each manipulated variable and *interaction effects* for combinations of manipulated variables
Randomized block	Optional	Between	Random assignment to groups within different levels of a blocking variable that is not under experimental control (e.g., gender)
Crossover	Optional	Within	Subjects are exposed to all treatments but are randomly assigned to different orderings of treatments; subjects serve us their own controls

independent variable. It is possible, however, to manipulate two or more variables simultaneously. Suppose we were interested in comparing two therapies for premature infants: tactile stimulation versus auditory stimulation. At the same time, we want to learn if the daily *amount* of stimulation (15, 30, or 45 minutes) affects infants' progress. The dependent variables for the study are measures of infant development (e.g., weight gain and cardiac responsiveness). Figure 10.2 illustrates the structure of this experiment.

This **factorial design** allows us to address three research questions:

1. Does auditory stimulation have a more beneficial effect on the development of premature infants than tactile stimulation, or *vice versa*?
2. Does the duration of stimulation (independent of type) affect infant development?
3. Is auditory stimulation most effective when linked to a certain dose and tactile stimulation most effective when coupled with a different dose?

The third question demonstrates the strength of factorial designs: they permit us to evaluate not only **main effects** (effects resulting from experimentally manipulated variables, as exemplified in questions 1 and 2) but also **interaction effects** (effects resulting from combining treatments). We may feel that it is insufficient to say that auditory stimulation is preferable to tactile stimulation (or *vice versa*) and that 45 minutes of stimulation per day is more effective than 15 or 30 minutes per day. How these two variables interact (how they behave in combination) is also of interest. Our results may indicate that 45 minutes of auditory stimulation is the most beneficial treatment. We could not have learned this by conducting two separate experiments that manipulated only one independent variable and held the second one constant.

In factorial experiments, subjects are assigned at random to a specific combination of conditions. In the example that Figure 10.2 illustrates, premature infants would be assigned randomly to one of six **cells**—that is, six treatment conditions or boxes in the schematic diagram. The two independent variables in a factorial design are the **factors**. Type of stimulation is factor A and amount of daily exposure is factor B. Level 1 of factor A is auditory, and level 2 of factor A is tactile. When describing the dimensions of the design, researchers refer to the number of **levels**. The design in Figure 10.2 is a 2 × 3 design: two levels in factor A times three levels in factor B. Factorial experiments can be performed with three or more independent variables (factors), but designs with more than three factors are rare.

Example of a factorial design: McDonald, Wiczorek, and Walker (2004) used a 2 × 2 factorial design to study the effect of background noise (noise versus no noise) and interruption (interruption versus no interruption) on learning health information in a sample of college students.

Randomized Block Design

A design that looks similar to a factorial design in structure is the **randomized block design.*** In such a design, there are two factors (independent variables), but one factor is *not* experimentally manipulated—the second factor is a stratifying variable. If we were interested in comparing the effects of tactile versus auditory stimulation for male versus female infants, we might stratify on gender before randomization. We could structure this as a 2 × 2 experiment, with type of stimulation as one factor and gender as the other. The variable gender, which we cannot manipulate, is the *blocking* or *stratifying* variable. We obviously could not randomly assign subjects to one of four cells, as in a factorial experiment, because infants' gender is a given. We could, however, randomly assign male and female subjects separately to the two stimulation methods. In randomized block designs, as in factorial designs, interaction effects can be examined.

The design can be extended to include more than one blocking variable. It is also possible to include more than one manipulated variable, thereby creating a design that is both a randomized block and a factorial design. In theory, the number of blocking and manipulated variables is unlimited, but practical concerns usually dictate a relatively small number of each. As a general rule of thumb, a minimum of 20 subjects per cell is recommended to achieve stability within cells. This means that, whereas a minimum of 80 subjects would be needed for a 2 × 2 design, 160 subjects would be needed for a 2 × 2 × 2 design.

Example of a combined randomized block and factorial design: Metzger, Jarosz, and Noureddine (2000) studied the effects of two experimentally manipulated factors (high-fat versus

Type of stimulation

		Auditory A1		Tactile A2	
Daily exposure	15 Min. B1	A1	B1	A2	B1
	30 Min. B2	A1	B2	A2	B2
	45 Min. B3	A1	B3	A2	B3

FIGURE 10.2 Example of a factorial design.

---

*The terminology for this design varies from text to text. Some authors refer to this as a *factorial design;* others call it a *levels by treatment design.*

low-fat diet and forced exercise versus sedentary condition) on obesity in rats. The blocking variable in this study was the genetic obesity of the rats: both genetically obese and lean rats were randomly assigned to the four treatment conditions, yielding a $2 \times 2 \times 2$ design.

Crossover Design

Thus far, we have described experimental studies in which subjects who are randomly assigned to different treatments are different people. For instance, in the previous example, the infants exposed to auditory stimulation were not the same infants as those exposed to tactile stimulation. A **crossover design** involves the exposure of the same subjects to more than one experimental treatment. This type of within-subjects design has the advantage of ensuring the highest possible equivalence among subjects exposed to different conditions—the groups being compared are equal with respect to age, weight, health, and so on because they are composed of the same people.

Because randomization is a signature characteristic of an experiment, subjects in a crossover experimental design must be randomly assigned to different orderings of treatments. For example, if a crossover design were used to compare the effects of auditory and tactile stimulation on infant development, some infants would be randomly assigned to receive auditory stimulation first, and others would be assigned to receive tactile stimulation first. When there are three or more conditions to which each subject will be exposed, the procedure of **counterbalancing** can be used to rule out ordering effects. For example, if there were three conditions (A, B, C), subjects would be randomly assigned to six different orderings in a counterbalanced scheme:

A,	B,	C	A,	C,	B
B,	C,	A	B,	A,	C
C,	A,	B	C,	B,	A

Although crossover designs are extremely powerful, they are inappropriate for certain research questions because of the problem of **carry-over effects**. When subjects are exposed to two different treatments or conditions, they may be influenced in the second condition by their experience in the first condition. As one example, drug studies rarely use a crossover design because drug B administered *after* drug A is not necessarily the same treatment as drug B administered *before* drug A.

> **Example of a crossover design:** Axelin, Salantera, and Lehtonen (2006) used a randomized crossover design to examine the effect of facilitated tucking (holding the infant in a flexed position) by parents in the management of pain during endotracheal suctioning in preterm infants. Scores on the Neonatal Infant Pain Scale were obtained during suctioning both with and without parent facilitated tucking, the order of which was randomized.

Strengths and Limitations of Experiments

Controlled experiments are often considered the ideal of science. In this section, we explore the reasons why experimental methods are held in high esteem and examine some of their limitations.

Experimental Strengths

True experiments are the most powerful method available for testing hypotheses of cause-and-effect relationships between variables. An experimental design is considered the gold standard for intervention studies because it yields the highest-quality evidence regarding intervention effects. Through randomization and the use of a comparison condition, experimenters come as close as possible to attaining the "ideal" counterfactual. Experiments offer greater corroboration than any other research approach that, *if* the independent variable (e.g., diet, drug dosage, teaching approach) is manipulated, *then* certain consequences in the dependent variable (e.g., weight loss, recovery of health, learning) may be expected to ensue. The great strength of experiments, then, lies in the confidence with which causal relationships can be inferred. Through the controls imposed by manipulation, comparison, and—especially—randomization, alternative explanations to a causal interpretation can often be ruled out or discredited. This is especially likely to be the case if the intervention was developed on the basis of a sound theoretical rationale. It is because of these strengths that meta-analyses of RCTs, which integrate evidence from multiple studies using an experimental design, are at the pinnacle of almost all evidence hierarchies for questions relating to causes (see Fig. 2.1 of Chapter 2).

Experimental Limitations

Despite the benefits of experimental research, this type of design also has limitations. First of all, there are often constraints that make an experimental approach impractical or impossible. These constraints are discussed later in this chapter.

⮕ **TIP :** Shadish, Cook, and Campbell (2002) provide guidance about 10 situations that are especially conducive to randomized experiments (pp. 269–275).

Experiments are sometimes criticized for their artificiality. Part of the difficulty lies in the requirements for randomization and then (for most experiments) comparable treatment within groups. In ordinary life, the way we interact with people is not random. For example, certain aspects of a patient (e.g., age, physical appearance, or severity of illness) may cause us to modify our behavior and our care. The differences may be subtle, but they undoubtedly are not random.

Another aspect of experiments that is sometimes considered artificial is the focus on only a handful of variables while holding all else constant. This requirement has been criticized as being reductionist and as artificially constraining human experience. Experiments that are undertaken without a guiding theoretical framework are sometimes criticized for being able to establish a causal connection between an independent and dependent variable without providing any causal explanation for *why* the intervention resulted in the observed outcomes.

A problem with experiments conducted in clinical settings is that it is often clinical staff, rather than researchers, who administer an intervention, and therefore it can sometimes be difficult to determine whether subjects in the experimental group actually received the treatment, and if those in the control group did not. It may be especially difficult to maintain the integrity of the intervention and control conditions if the study period extends over time. Moreover, clinical studies are usually conducted in environments over which researchers have little control—and control is a critical factor in experimental research. McGuire and her colleagues (2000) describe some issues relating to the challenges of testing interventions in clinical settings.

Sometimes a problem emerges if subjects themselves have discretion about participation in the treatment. Suppose, for example, that we randomly assigned patients with HIV infection to a special support group intervention or to a control group. Experimental subjects who elect not to participate in the support groups, or who participate infrequently, actually are in a "condition" that looks more like the control condition than the experimental one. The treatment is diluted through nonparticipation, and it may become difficult to detect any effects of the treatment, no matter how effective it might otherwise have been. Such issues need to be taken into consideration in designing the study. We discuss this at greater length in the next chapter.

Another potential problem is the **Hawthorne effect**, which is a kind of placebo effect that is caused by people's expectations. The term is derived from a series of experiments conducted at the Hawthorne plant of the Western Electric Corporation in which various environmental conditions, such as light and working hours, were varied to determine their effects on worker productivity. Regardless of what change was introduced, that is, whether the light was made better or worse, productivity increased. Knowledge of being included in the study appears to have affected people's behavior, thereby obscuring the effect of the variable of interest. In a hospital situation, researchers might have to contend with a double Hawthorne effect. For example, if an experiment to investigate the effect of a new postoperative patient routine were conducted, nurses and hospital staff, as well as patients, might be aware of their participation in a study, and both groups might alter their actions accordingly. It is precisely for this reason that double-blind RCTs, in which neither subjects nor those who administer the treatment know who is in the experimental or control group, are so powerful.

In sum, despite the superiority of experiments in terms of their ability to test causal hypotheses, they are subject to a number of limitations, some of which may make them difficult to apply to real-world problems. Nevertheless, with the growing demand for evidence-based practice, true experimental designs are increasingly being used to test the effects of nursing interventions.

➲ TIP: There are several commercial vendors who offer support services for managing clinical trials. We offer links to two of them for you to investigate, should you need this type of assistance: Velos eResearch (*http://www.veloseresearch.com*) and Clinical Trials Net, Inc. (*http://www.clinicaltrialsnet.com*).

QUASI-EXPERIMENTS

Quasi-experiments, like true experiments, involve an intervention. However, quasi-experimental designs lack randomization, the signature of a true experiment. Some quasi-experiments, which are referred to as controlled trials without randomization in the medical literature, even lack a control group. The signature of a quasi-experimental design, then, is an intervention in the absence of randomization.

Quasi-Experimental Designs

Quasi-experiments are not as powerful as experiments in establishing causal connections between interventions and outcomes. Before showing why this is so, it is useful to introduce some notation based on Campbell and Stanley's (1963) classic monograph. Figure 10.3 presents a symbolic representation of a before–after experimental design. In this figure, R means random assignment to groups; O represents an observation (i.e., the collection of data on the dependent variable); and X stands for exposure to an intervention. Thus, the top line in this figure represents the experimental group that

R	O_1	X	O_2
R	O_1		O_2

R = Randomization
O = Observation or measurement
X = Treatment or intervention

FIGURE 10.3 Symbolic representation of a pretest–posttest (before–after) experimental design.

had subjects randomly assigned to it (R), had both a pretest (O_1) and a posttest (O_2), and has been exposed to an experimental intervention (X). The second row represents the control group, which differs from the experimental group only by absence of the treatment (X). We are now equipped to examine some quasi-experimental designs and to better understand their limitations relative to experimental designs.

Nonequivalent Control Group Designs

The most frequently used quasi-experimental design is the **nonequivalent control group before–after design**, which involves an experimental treatment and two groups of subjects observed before and after its implementation. Suppose, for example, we wished to study the effect of introducing a new hospital-wide model of care that involved having a patient care facilitator (PCF) be the primary point person for all patients during their stay. Our main outcome is patient satisfaction. Because the new system is being implemented throughout the hospital, randomization is not possible. Therefore, we decide to collect data in another similar hospital that is not instituting the PCF model. Data on patient satisfaction are collected in both hospitals at baseline, before the change is made, and again after its implementation.

Figure 10.4 depicts this study symbolically. The top row is our experimental (PCF) hospital, and the second row is the comparison hospital. This diagram is identical to the one in Figure 10.3, *except* that subjects have not been randomly assigned to

O_1		X		O_2
O_1				O_2

FIGURE 10.4 Nonequivalent control group before–after design.

treatment groups in the second diagram. The design in Figure 10.4 is weaker because *it can no longer be assumed that the experimental and comparison groups are equivalent at the outset.* Without randomization, this study is quasi-experimental rather than experimental. Quasi-experimental comparisons are much farther from an ideal counterfactual than experimental comparisons. The design is nevertheless strong because the baseline data allow us to determine whether patients in the two hospitals had similar satisfaction initially. If the comparison and experimental groups are similar at baseline, we could be relatively confident inferring that any posttest difference in satisfaction was the result of the new model of care. If patient satisfaction is different initially, however, it will be difficult to interpret any posttest differences, although there are statistical procedures that can help. Note that in quasi-experiments, the term **comparison group** is sometimes used in lieu of *control group* to refer to the group against which outcomes in the treatment group are evaluated.

Now suppose we had been unable to collect baseline data. This design, diagramed in Figure 10.5, has a flaw that is difficult to remedy. We no longer have information about the initial equivalence of the two hospitals. If we find that patient satisfaction in the experimental hospital is higher than that in the control hospital at the posttest, can we conclude that the new method of delivering care *caused* improved satisfaction? There could be alternative explanations for the posttest differences. In particular, it might be that patient satisfaction in the two hospitals differed initially. Campbell and Stanley (1963) called the *nonequivalent control group after-only design* in Figure 10.5 *preexperimental* rather than quasi-experimental because of its fundamental weakness—although Shadish, Cook, and Campbell (2002), in their more recent book on causal inference, did not use this label, but simply called this a weaker quasi-experimental design.

X   O
O

FIGURE 10.5 Nonequivalent control group after-only design.

> **Example of a nonequivalent control group before–after design:** Gates, Fitzwater, and Succop (2005) evaluated the effectiveness of a violence-prevention intervention for nursing assistants working in long-term care. The intervention was implemented in three nursing homes, and three other nursing homes served as the comparison. Data on anxiety, self-efficacy, and violence-prevention skills were collected before and after the intervention and 6 months later.

An improvement upon the standard before–after nonequivalent control group, in which groups thought to be similar are compared, is to use *matching* to ensure that the groups are, in fact, equivalent on at least some key variables related to the outcomes. For example, if an intervention was designed to reduce patient anxiety, then it would be desirable not only to *measure* preintervention anxiety in the intervention and comparison group but also to take steps to ensure that the anxiety levels of both groups were comparable by matching subjects' initial anxiety. Because matching on more than a couple of variables is unwieldy, a more sophisticated method of matching, called **propensity matching**, can be used by researchers with sufficient statistical sophistication. This method involves the creation of a single **propensity score** that captures the conditional probability of exposure to a treatment given various preintervention characteristics. Experimental and comparison group members can then be matched on this score (Joffe & Rosenbaum, 1999). Both conventional and propensity matching are most easily implemented when there is a large pool of potential comparison group subjects from which good matches to treatment group subjects can be selected.

In lieu of using a contemporaneous nonrandomized comparison group, researchers sometimes use a **historical comparison group**. That is, comparison data are gathered from or about a group of people before the implementation of the intervention. Even when the subjects are from the same institutional setting, however, it is risky to assume that the two groups are comparable, or that the environments are comparable in every respect except for the new intervention. There remains the possibility that something other than the intervention could account for any observed differences in outcomes.

> **Example of a historical comparison group:** McNulty, Katz, and Kim (2005) studied the effects of argatroban therapy on patients who developed heparin-induced thrombocytopenia following exposure to heparin due to intravascular catheter or heparin flush. Outcomes (e.g., platelet count) of those who received the therapy were compared with historical controls, for whom baseline data were also available so that comparability could be assessed.

Time Series Designs

In the designs just described, a control group was used but randomization was not, but some quasi-experiments have neither. Let us suppose that a hospital is adopting a new requirement that all its nurses accrue a certain number of continuing education units before being eligible for a promotion or raise. The nursing administrators want to assess the consequences of this mandate on turnover rate, absentee rate, number of raises and promotions awarded, and so on. For the purposes of this example, assume there is no other hospital that can serve as a good comparison for this study. In such a case, the only kind of comparison that can be made is a before–after contrast. If the requirement were inaugurated in January, one could compare the turnover rate, for example, for the 3-month period before the new rule with the turnover rate for the subsequent 3-month period. The schematic representation of such a study is shown in Figure 10.6.

This one-group pretest–posttest design seems straightforward, but it has weaknesses. What if either of the 3-month periods is atypical, apart from the new regulation? What about the effects of any other hospital rules inaugurated during the same period? What about the effects of external factors that influence employment decisions, such as changes in the local economy? This design (also

referred to as preexperimental by Campbell and Stanley) cannot control these factors.*

This one-group pretest–posttest design could be modified so that at least some alternative explanations for change in nurses' turnover rate could be ruled out. One such design is the **time series design** (sometimes referred to as the *interrupted time series design*) and is diagrammed in Figure 10.7. In a time series design, information is collected over an extended period, and an intervention is introduced during that period. In the figure, O_1 through O_4 represent four separate instances of data collection on a dependent variable before treatment; X represents the treatment (the introduction of the independent variable); and O_5 through O_8 represent four post-treatment observations. In our present example, O_1 might be the number of nurses who left the hospital in January through March in the year before the new continuing education rule, O_2 the number of resignations in April through June, and so forth. After the rule is implemented, data on turnover are similarly collected for four consecutive 3-month periods, giving us observations O_5 through O_8.

Even though the time series design does not eliminate all problems of interpreting changes in turnover rate, the extended time period strengthens the ability to attribute change to the intervention. Figure 10.8 demonstrates why this is so. The two diagrams (A and B) in the figure show two possible outcome patterns for eight turnover observations. The vertical dotted line in the center represents the timing of the continuing education rule. Patterns A and B both reflect a feature common to most time series studies—fluctuation from one data point to another. These fluctuations are normal. One would not expect that, if 48 nurses resigned from a hospital in a year, the resignations would be spaced evenly with four resignations per month. It is

$$O_1 \qquad\qquad X \qquad\qquad O_2$$

FIGURE 10.6 One group before–after design.

---

*One-group before–after designs are not always unproductive. For example, if the intervention involved a brief teaching intervention, with baseline knowledge data obtained immediately before the intervention and posttest knowledge data collected immediately after it, it may be reasonable to conclude that the intervention is the most plausible—and perhaps the only—explanation for knowledge gains.

$$O_1 \qquad O_2 \qquad O_3 \qquad O_4 \qquad X \qquad O_5 \qquad O_6 \qquad O_7 \qquad O_8$$

FIGURE 10.7 Time series design.

precisely because of these fluctuations that the design shown in Figure 10.6, with only one observation before and after the experimental treatment, is so weak.

Let us compare the kind of interpretations that can be made for the outcomes reflected in Figure 10.8, patterns A and B. In both cases, the number of resignations increased between O_4 and O_5, that is, immediately after the new continuing education requirement. In B, however, the number of resignations fell at O_6 and continued to fall at O_7. The increase at O_5 looks similar to other apparently haphazard fluctuations in the turnover rate at other periods. Therefore, it probably would be erroneous to conclude that the new rule affected resignations. In A, on the other hand, the number of resignations increases at O_5 and remains relatively high for all subsequent observations. Of course, there may be other explanations for a change in turnover rate from one year to the next. The time series design, however, does permit us to rule out the possibility

that the data reflect unstable measurements of resignations at only two points in time. If we had used the design in Figure 10.6, it would have been analogous to obtaining the measurements at O_4 and O_5 of Figure 10.8 only. The outcomes in both A and B look similar at these two points in time. Yet the broader time perspective leads us to draw different conclusions about two patterns of outcomes. Nevertheless, the absence of a comparison group means that the situation is far from yielding an ideal counterfactual.

Example of a time series design: Edwards and Beck (2002) used a powerful time series design to assess the effect of animal-assisted therapy (aquariums) on the nutritional intake of individuals with Alzheimer disease. Weight (one of the outcomes) was measured on the first of each month for 3 months before the intervention and for 4 months after it in a sample of residents in specialized units in three facilities. The researchers found that, over this 7-month period, weight declined in the 3 months

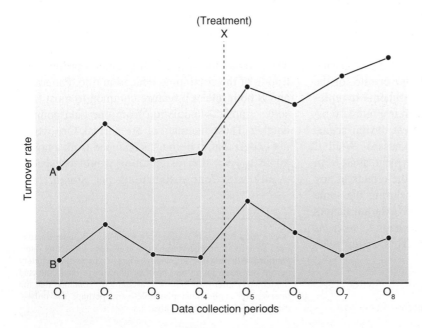

FIGURE 10.8 Two possible time series outcome patterns.

(Treatment)
X

Turnover rate

A

B

$O_1 \quad O_2 \quad O_3 \quad O_4 \quad O_5 \quad O_6 \quad O_7 \quad O_8$

Data collection periods

$$O_1 \qquad O_2 \qquad O_3 \qquad O_4 \qquad X \qquad O_5 \qquad O_6 \qquad O_7 \qquad O_8$$

$$O_1 \qquad O_2 \qquad O_3 \qquad O_4 \qquad \qquad O_5 \qquad O_6 \qquad O_7 \qquad O_8$$

FIGURE 10.9 Time series nonequivalent control group design (quasi-experimental).

$$O_1 \qquad O_2 \qquad X \qquad O_3 \qquad O_4 \qquad X \qquad O_5 \qquad O_6 \qquad X \qquad O_7 \qquad O_8$$

FIGURE 10.10 Time series with multiple institutions of treatment (quasi-experimental).

before the intervention and then increased significantly in the month the aquariums were introduced, and continued to increase in the following months.

A particularly powerful quasi-experimental design results when the time series and nonequivalent control group designs are combined, as diagrammed in Figure 10.9. In the example just described, a time series nonequivalent control group design would involve collecting data over an extended period from both the hospital introducing the continuing education mandate and another hospital not imposing the mandate. This use of information from another hospital with similar characteristics would make any inferences regarding the effects of the mandate more convincing because trends influenced by external factors would presumably be observed in both groups.

Numerous variations on the simple time series design are possible and are being used by nurse researchers. For example, additional evidence regarding the effects of a treatment can be achieved by instituting the treatment at several different points in time, strengthening the treatment over time, or instituting the treatment at one point in time and then withdrawing the treatment at a later point, sometimes with reinstitution of treatment. These three designs are diagrammed in Figures 10.10 through 10.12. Clinical nurse researchers are often in a good position to use such time series designs because measures of patient functioning are usually routinely made at multiple points over an extended period.

Example of a time series design with withdrawal and reinstitution: Hicks-Moore (2005) studied the effect of relaxing music at mealtime on agitated behaviors of nursing home residents with dementia. Music was introduced in week 2, removed in week 3, and then reinstituted in week 4. The pattern of agitated behaviors was consistent with the hypothesis that relaxing music would have a calming effect.

A particular application of a time series approach sometimes used in clinical studies is called **single-subject experiments** (sometimes referred to as *N-of-1 studies*). Single-subject studies use time series designs to gather information about an intervention based on the responses of a single patient (or a small number of patients) under controlled conditions. In the literature on single-subject methods, the most basic design involves a baseline phase of data gathering (A) and an intervention phase (B), yielding what is referred to as an AB design (the design diagrammed in Fig. 10.7). If the treatment were withdrawn, it would be an ABA design; and if a withdrawn treatment were reinstituted (as diagrammed in Fig. 10.12), it would be an ABAB design. Portney and Watkins (2000) offer valuable guidance about single-subject studies in clinical settings.

Example of a single-subject design: Landolt and colleagues (2002) used a single-subject experiment (with multiple patients) to test whether cartoon movie viewing is effective in decreasing burned children's pain behavior.

Other Quasi-Experimental Designs

Several other quasi-experimental designs are available as alternatives to an RCT. One such design, the **regression discontinuity design**, will not be elaborated here because it has rarely been used in nursing

$$O_1 \quad O_2 \quad X \quad O_3 \quad O_4 \quad X+1 \quad O_5 \quad O_6 \quad X+2 \quad O_7 \quad O_8$$

FIGURE 10.11 Time series with intensified treatment (quasi-experimental).

studies. This design, which involves *systematic* assignment of subjects to groups based on cut-off scores on a preintervention measure (e.g., giving the intervention to the most severely ill patients), is considered attractive from an ethical standpoint and merits consideration. Its features have been described in the nursing literature by Atwood and Taylor (1991).

Earlier in this chapter, we described a randomization procedure called partially randomized patient preference, or PRPP. This design has clear advantages in terms of persuading potential subjects to participate in a study because those with a strong preference get to choose their treatment condition. Those without a strong preference are randomized, but those *with* a preference are given the condition they prefer and are followed up as part of the study. The two randomized groups are part of the true experiment, but the two groups who get their preference are part of a quasi-experiment. This type of design can yield valuable information about the kind of people who prefer one condition over another, but the evidence of the effectiveness of the treatment is weak because the people who elected a certain treatment likely differ from those who elected the alternative—and these preintervention differences, rather than the alternative treatments, could account for any observed differences in outcomes at the end of the study.

Example of a PRPP design: Coward (2002) used a PRPP design in a pilot study of a support group intervention for women with breast cancer. She found that the majority of women did *not* want to be randomized, but rather had a strong preference for either being in or not being in the support group. Her article describes the challenges she faced.

Another type of quasi-experimental approach—often embedded within a true experiment—is a dose-response design, in which the outcomes of those receiving different doses of a treatment—not as a result of randomization—are compared. For example, in complex and lengthy interventions, some people attend more sessions or get more intensive treatment than others. The rationale for a quasi-experimental dose-response analysis is that if a larger dose corresponds to better outcomes, this provides supporting evidence for inferring that the treatment caused the outcome. The difficulty, however, is that people tend to get different doses of the treatment because of differences in motivation, physical function, or other characteristics that could be driving the differences in outcome—and not the different doses themselves. When a quasi-experimental dose-response analysis is conducted *within* an experiment, the dose-response evidence may well be able to enhance causal inferences.

Example of a dose-response analysis within a true experiment: Lai and Good (2005) randomly assigned community dwelling elders who had difficulty sleeping to either a control group or an intervention group that involved listening to 45-minute sedative music tapes at bedtime. Those in the intervention group experienced significantly better sleep quality (longer duration, less sleep disturbance) than those in the control group. Moreover, over the 3-week study period, sleep improved weekly, which suggested a cumulative dose effect.

Experimental and Comparison Conditions

Researchers using a quasi-experimental approach, like those adopting an experimental design, should strive to develop strong interventions that provide an opportunity for a fair test, and must develop protocols documenting what the interventions entail.

$$O_1 \quad O_2 \quad X \quad O_3 \quad O_4 \quad (-X) \quad O_5 \quad O_6 \quad X \quad O_7 \quad O_8$$

FIGURE 10.12 Time series with withdrawn and reinstituted treatment (quasi-experimental).

Researchers need to be especially careful in understanding and documenting the counterfactual in quasi-experiments. In the case of nonequivalent control group designs, this means understanding the conditions to which the comparison group is exposed. In our example of using a hospital with traditional nursing systems as a comparison for the new primary nursing system, the nature of that traditional system should be fully understood. In time series designs, the counterfactual is the condition existing before implementing the intervention. Masking should be used, to the extent possible—indeed, this is often more feasible in a quasi-experiment than in an RCT.

Strengths and Limitations of Quasi-Experiments

A major strength of quasi-experiments is that they are practical. In the real world, it may be difficult, if not impossible, to conduct true experiments. Nursing research usually occurs in real-life settings, where it may be difficult to deliver an innovative treatment randomly to some people but not to others. Quasi-experimental designs introduce some research control when full experimental rigor is not possible.

Another advantage of quasi-experiments is that, in our current era of health care consumerism, patients are not always willing to relinquish control over their treatment condition. Indeed, there is some evidence that people are increasingly unwilling to volunteer to be randomized in clinical trials (Gross & Fogg, 2001). Quasi-experimental designs, because they do not involve random assignment, are likely to be acceptable to a broader group of people. This, in turn, has implications for the generalizability of the results—but the problem is that the results are usually less conclusive.

Thus, researchers using quasi-experimental designs need to be acquainted with their weaknesses, and need to take steps to counteract those weaknesses or at least take them into account in interpreting results. When a quasi-experimental design is used, there may be several **rival hypotheses** competing with the experimental manipulation

as explanations for the results. (This is discussed further in Chapter 11.) Take as an example the case in which we administer a certain diet to a group of frail nursing home residents to assess whether this treatment results in a weight gain. If we use no comparison group or if we use a nonequivalent control group and then observe a weight gain, we must ask the questions: Is it *plausible* that some other factor caused or influenced the gain? Is it *plausible* that pretreatment differences between the experimental and comparison groups resulted in differential gain? Is it *plausible* that the elders on average gained weight simply because the most frail died or were transferred to a hospital? If the answer is "yes" to any of these questions, then the inferences that can be made about the causal effect of the intervention are weakened. The plausibility of any one threat cannot, of course, be answered unequivocally. It is usually a situation in which judgment must be exercised. Because the conclusions from quasi-experiments ultimately depend in part on human judgment, rather than on more objective criteria, cause-and-effect inferences are less convincing.

NONEXPERIMENTAL RESEARCH

Many research questions—including ones seeking to establish cause-and-effect relationships—cannot be addressed with an experimental or quasi-experimental design. For example, at the beginning of this chapter, we posed this prognosis question: Do birth weights under 1500 grams *cause* developmental delays in children? Clearly, we cannot manipulate birth weight, the independent variable. Babies are born with weights that are neither random nor subject to research control. One way to answer this question is to compare two groups of infants—babies with birth weights above and below 1500 grams at birth—in terms of their subsequent development. When researchers do not intervene by manipulating the independent variable, the study is **nonexperimental**, or, in the medical literature, **observational**.

Most nursing studies are nonexperimental, in large part because a vast number of human characteristics (e.g., birthweight, body temperature, ethnicity) inherently cannot be experimentally manipulated. Also, many variables that could *technically* be manipulated cannot be manipulated ethically. For example, if we were studying the effect of prenatal care on infant mortality, it would be unethical to provide such care to one group of pregnant women while deliberately depriving a randomly assigned second group. We would need to locate a naturally occurring group of pregnant women who had not received prenatal care. Their birth outcomes could then be compared with those of women who had received appropriate care. The problem, however, is that the two groups of women are likely to differ in terms of many other characteristics, such as age, education, and health, any of which individually or in combination could affect infant mortality, independent of prenatal care. This is precisely why experimental designs are so strong in demonstrating cause-and-effect relationships.

Another issue is that nonexperimental research is usually needed before an experimental study can be planned. Strong experimental interventions are developed on the basis of sound nonexperimental research documenting the scope of a problem and describing critical relationships between relevant variables. Thus, whereas some nonexperimental research is designed to explore causal relationships when experimental work is not possible, some studies have primarily a descriptive intent.

Correlational Research

When researchers study the effect of a potential *cause* that they cannot manipulate, they use designs that examine relationships between variables—often called **correlational designs**. A **correlation** is an interrelationship or association between two variables, that is, a tendency for variation in one variable to be related to variation in another. For example, in human adults, height and weight are correlated because there is a tendency for taller people to weigh more than shorter people.

As we mentioned early in this chapter, one of the criteria for causality is that an empirical relationship between variables must be demonstrated. It is, however, risky to infer causal relationships in correlational research, not only because of the researchers' lack of control over the independent variable, but also because of the absence of an exemplary counterfactual. In experiments, investigators make a prediction that deliberate variation of X, the independent variable, will result in a change to Y, the dependent variable. For example, they might predict that if a new medication is administered, patient improvement will result. Experimenters have direct control over the X; the experimental treatment can be administered to some and withheld from others, and the two groups can be equalized with respect to everything except the independent variable through randomization.

In correlational research, on the other hand, investigators do not control the independent variable, which often has already occurred. Although correlational studies are inherently weaker than experimental studies in elucidating cause-and-effect relationships, different designs offer different degrees of supportive evidence.

Retrospective Designs

Studies with a **retrospective design** are ones in which a phenomenon existing in the present is linked to phenomena that occurred in the past, before the study was initiated. The researcher is interested in a present "outcome" and attempts to determine antecedent factors that caused it. Most of the early studies of the link between cigarette smoking and lung cancer were retrospective. In such **case-control studies**, the researcher began with a group of people who had lung cancer (*cases*) and another group who did not (*controls*). The researcher then looks for differences between the two groups in antecedent behaviors or conditions—in our example, smoking. Thus, the signature of a retrospective study is that the researcher begins with the dependent variable and then examines whether it is correlated with one or more antecedent independent variables. Retrospective studies are often cross-sectional, with data on both the dependent and independent variables collected once.

In designing a case-control study, researchers try to identify controls without the disease or condition who are as similar as possible to the cases with regard to key extraneous variables (e.g., age, gender). Researchers sometimes use matching or other techniques to control for extraneous variables. To the degree that researchers can demonstrate comparability between cases and controls with regard to confounding traits, inferences regarding the presumed cause of the disease are enhanced. The difficulty, however, is that the two groups are almost never totally comparable with respect to all potential factors influencing the dependent variable.

Example of a case-control design:
Menihan, Phipps, and Weitzen (2006) used a case-control design to compare infants who died of sudden infant death syndrome (the cases) with controls who did not. The two groups were matched by date of birth. The researchers examined a number of antecedent factors, including birth weight, maternal characteristics, fetal heart rate variability, and sleep–wake cycles before birth.

Not all retrospective studies can be characterized as using a case-control design. Sometimes researchers use a retrospective approach to identify risk factors for different *amounts* of a problem or condition. That is, the outcome is not "caseness" but rather the *degree* of some condition. For example, a retrospective design might be used to identify factors that could be used to predict the length of time new mothers breastfed their infants. Essentially, such a design is intended to understand factors that *cause* women to make different breastfeeding decisions.

Example of a retrospective design: Hwang, Ryan, and Zerwic (2006) conducted a retrospective study to identify factors that predicted the amount of time delayed in seeking treatment for acute myocardial infarction symptoms. The independent (predictor) variables examined included patients' age, ambiguity of symptoms, and living arrangements (alone versus not alone).

Prospective Nonexperimental Designs

A nonexperimental study with a **prospective design** (called a **cohort design** by medical researchers) starts with a presumed cause and then goes forward in time to the presumed effect. For example, we might want to test the hypothesis that the incidence of rubella during pregnancy (the independent variable) is related to infant abnormalities (the dependent variable). To test this hypothesis prospectively, we would begin with a sample of pregnant women, including some who contracted rubella during their pregnancy and others who did not. The subsequent occurrence of congenital anomalies would be assessed for all subjects, and we would examine whether women with rubella were more likely than other women to bear malformed infants.

Prospective studies are more costly than retrospective studies. For one thing, a substantial follow-up period may be necessary before the dependent variable manifests itself, as is the case in prospective studies of cigarette smoking and lung cancer. Also, prospective designs may require large samples if the dependent variable of interest is rare, as in the example of malformations associated with maternal rubella. Another issue is that in a good prospective study, researchers take steps to confirm that all subjects are free from the effect (e.g., the disease) at the time the independent variable is measured, and this may in some cases be difficult or expensive to do. For example, in prospective smoking/lung cancer studies, lung cancer may be present initially but not yet diagnosed.

Despite these issues, prospective studies are considerably stronger than retrospective studies. In particular, any ambiguity about whether the presumed cause occurred before the effect is resolved in prospective research if the researcher has confirmed the initial absence of the effect. In addition, samples are more likely to be representative, and investigators may be in a position to impose controls to rule out competing explanations for the results.

Some prospective studies are exploratory. That is, the researcher measures a wide range of possible "causes" at one point in time, and then examines an outcome of interest at a later point (e.g., length of stay in hospital). Such studies are usually stronger than retrospective studies if it can be determined that the outcome was not present initially because time sequences are clear. However, they are not as powerful as prospective studies that involve specific *a priori* hypotheses and the comparison of cohorts known to differ on a presumed cause. Researchers doing exploratory retrospective or prospective studies are sometimes accused of going on "fishing expeditions" that can lead to erroneous conclusions because of spurious or idiosyncratic relationships in a particular sample of subjects.

Example of a prospective nonexperimental study: El-Masri, Hammad, and Fox-Wasylyshyn (2005) conducted a prospective cohort study to examine the power of surrogate markers of injury severity (e.g., number of blood units transfused, use of chest tubes) to predict nosocomial bloodstream infections in critically ill trauma patients.

Natural Experiments

Researchers are sometimes able to study the outcomes of a "**natural experiment**" in which a group exposed to natural or other phenomena that have important health consequences are compared with a nonexposed group. Such natural experiments are nonexperimental because the researcher does not intervene, but they are called "natural *experiments*" when people are affected essentially at random. For example, the psychological well-being of people living in a community struck with a natural disaster (e.g., a volcanic eruption) could be compared with the well-being of people living in a similar but unaffected community to determine the toll exacted by the disaster (the independent variable). Note that the independent variable does not need to be a "natural" phenomenon. It could, for example, be a fire or winning a big lottery. Moreover, the groups being compared do not need to be different people; if pre-event measures had been obtained, before–after comparisons might be profitable.

Example of a natural experiment: Liehr and colleagues (2004) were in the midst of collecting data from healthy students over a 3-day period (September 10–12, 2001) when the events of September 11 unfolded. The researchers seized the opportunity to examine what people go through in the midst of stressful upheaval. Data from both before and after the tragedy were available for the students' blood pressure, heart rate, natural language use, and television viewing.

Path Analytic Studies

Researchers interested in testing theories of causation based on nonexperimental data are increasingly using a technique known as **path analysis** (or similar techniques). Using sophisticated statistical procedures, researchers test a hypothesized causal chain among a set of independent variables, mediating variables, and a dependent variable. Path analytic procedures, which are described more fully in Chapter 23, allow researchers to test whether nonexperimental data conform sufficiently to the underlying model to justify causal inferences.

Example of a path analytic study: Lee and Laffrey (2006) used path analysis to test a hypothesized theoretical explanation of physical activity in older adults with borderline hypertension. Their analyses tested hypothesized causal pathways between background characteristics, cognitive appraisal, motivation, and physical activity.

Descriptive Research

The second broad class of nonexperimental studies is **descriptive research**. The purpose of descriptive studies is to observe, describe, and document aspects of a situation as it naturally occurs and sometimes to serve as a starting point for hypothesis generation or theory development.

Descriptive Correlational Studies

Although researchers often focus on understanding the causes of behaviors, conditions, and situations, sometimes they are better able to simply describe relationships than to comprehend causal pathways.

Many research problems are cast in noncausal terms. We ask, for example, whether men are less likely than women to bond with their newborn infants, not whether a particular configuration of sex chromosomes *caused* differences in parental attachment. Unlike other types of correlational research—such as the cigarette smoking and lung cancer investigations—the aim of **descriptive correlational research** is to describe relationships among variables rather than to infer cause-and-effect relationships.

Example of a descriptive correlational study: Phillips and colleagues (2006) conducted a descriptive correlational study to examine the relationships among spiritual well-being, sleep quality, and health status in HIV-infected men and women.

Univariate Descriptive Studies

Some descriptive studies are undertaken to describe the frequency of occurrence of a behavior or condition rather than to study relationships. **Univariate descriptive studies** are not necessarily focused on only one variable. For example, a researcher might be interested in women's experiences during menopause. The study might describe the frequency of various symptoms, the average age at menopause, and the percentage of women using medications to alleviate symptoms. There are multiple variables in this study, but the primary purpose is to describe the status of each and not to relate them to one another.

Two types of descriptive study from the field of epidemiology are especially worth noting. **Prevalence studies** are done to determine the prevalence rate of some condition (e.g., a disease or a behavior, such as smoking) at a particular point in time. Prevalence studies rely on cross-sectional designs in which data are obtained from the population at risk for the condition. The researcher takes a "snapshot" of the population at risk to determine the extent to which the condition of interest is present. The formula for a **prevalence rate** (PR) is:

$$\frac{\text{Number of cases with the condition}}{\text{Number in the population at risk}} \times K$$
$$\text{of being a case}$$

K is the number of people for whom we want to have the rate established (e.g., per 100 or per 1000 population). When data are obtained from a sample (as would usually be the case), the denominator is the size of the sample, and the numerator is the number of cases with the condition, as identified in the study. If we sampled 500 adults aged 21 years and older living in a community, administered a measure of depression, and found that 80 people met the criteria for clinical depression, then the estimated prevalence rate of clinical depression would be 16 per 100 adults in that community.

Example of a prevalence study: Rhee and colleagues (2005) used cross-sectional data from a national study of adolescent health to determine the prevalence of 10 recurrent physical symptoms of adolescents. Headaches had the highest prevalence rate (27%, i.e., 27 per 100), followed by fatigue (21%) and stomach aches (18%).

Incidence studies are used to measure the frequency of developing *new* cases. Longitudinal designs are needed to determine incidence because the researcher must first establish who is at risk for becoming a new case—that is, who is free of the condition at the outset. The formula for an **incidence rate** (IR) is as follows:

$$\frac{\text{Number of new cases with the condition}}{\text{Number in the population at risk of being}} \times K$$
$$\text{a case (free of the condition at the outset)}$$

If we continued with our previous example, suppose in October 2006 we found that 80 in a sample of 500 people were clinically depressed (PR = 16 per 100). To determine the 1-year incidence rate, we would reassess the sample in October 2007. Suppose that, of the 420 previously deemed *not* to be clinically depressed in 2001, 21 were now found to meet the criteria for depression. In this case, the estimated 1-year incidence rate would be 5 per 100 ($[21 \div 420] \times 100 = 5$).

Prevalence and incidence rates can be calculated for subgroups of the population (e.g., for men versus women). When this is done, it is possible to calculate another important descriptive index. **Relative risk** is an estimated risk for "caseness" in one group compared with another. Relative risk is computed by dividing the rate for one group by the rate for another. Suppose we found that the 1-year incidence rate for depression was 6 per 100 women and 4 per 100 men. Women's relative risk for developing depression over the 1-year period would be 1.5; that is, women would be estimated to be 1.5 times more likely to develop depression than men. Relative risk is an important index in determining the contribution of risk factors to a disease or condition (e.g., by comparing the relative risk for lung cancer for smokers versus nonsmokers).

Example of an incidence and prevalence study: Chan and co-researchers (2005) collected cross-sectional data to determine the prevalence rate of pressure ulcers in a hospital in Singapore (18.1%). Longitudinal data were also collected to establish the incidence rate within a 28-day period among those who were ulcer free initially (8.1%).

⊘ **TIP:** The quality of correlational studies that test hypothesized causal relationship is heavily dependent on design decisions—that is, how researchers design their studies to rule out competing causal explanations for the outcomes. Methods of enhancing the rigor of quantitative studies are described in the next chapter. The quality of descriptive studies, by contrast, is more heavily dependent on having a good (representative) sample (see Chapter 13) and high-quality measuring instruments (see Chapter 17).

Strengths and Limitations of Correlational Research

The quality of a study is not necessarily related to its approach; there are many excellent nonexperimental studies as well as flawed experiments. Nevertheless, nonexperimental correlational studies have several drawbacks.

Limitations of Correlational Research

As already noted, the major disadvantage of nonexperimental studies is that, relative to experimental and quasi-experimental research, they are weak in their ability to reveal causal relationships. Correlational studies are susceptible to faulty interpretations. This situation arises because the researcher works with preexisting groups that were not formed at random, but rather through **self-selection** (which is also known as *selection bias*). A researcher doing a correlational study, unlike an experimental study, cannot assume that the groups being compared are similar before the occurrence of the independent variable— the hypothesized cause. Thus, preexisting differences may be a plausible alternative explanation for any group differences on the outcome variable.

The difficulty of interpreting correlational findings stems from the fact that, in the real world, behaviors, states, attitudes, and characteristics are interrelated (correlated) in complex ways. An example may help to clarify the problems of interpreting results from correlational studies. Suppose we conducted a cross-sectional study that examined the relationship between level of depression in cancer patients and their social support (i.e., assistance and emotional sustenance through a social network). We hypothesize that social support (the independent variable) affects levels of depression (the dependent variable). Suppose we find that the patients without social support are significantly more depressed than the patients with adequate social support. We could interpret this finding to mean that patients' emotional states are influenced by the adequacy of their social supports. This relationship is diagrammed in Figure 10.13A. There are, however, alternative explanations. Perhaps there is a third variable that influences *both* social

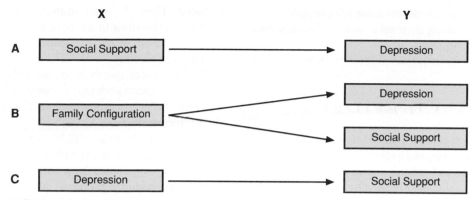

FIGURE 10.13 Alternative explanations for relationship between depression and social support in cancer patients.

support and depression, such as the patients' marital status. It may be that having a spouse is a powerful influence on how depressed cancer patients feel *and* on the quality of their social support. This set of relationships is diagramed in Figure 10.13*B*. A third possibility may be reversed causality, as shown in Figure 10.13*C*. Depressed cancer patients may find it more difficult to elicit needed social support from others than patients who are more cheerful or amiable. In this interpretation, the person's depression causes the amount of received social support, and not the other way around. Thus, interpretations of most correlational results should be considered tentative, particularly if the research has no theoretical basis.

Strengths of Correlational Research
Earlier, we discussed constraints that limit the possibility of applying experimental designs to some research problems. Correlational research will continue to play a crucial role in nursing research precisely because many interesting problems are not amenable to experimentation.

Despite our emphasis on causal relationships, it has already been noted that some kinds of research, such as descriptive research, do not focus on understanding causal networks. Furthermore, if the study is testing a causal hypothesis that has been deduced from an established theory, causal inferences may

be possible, especially if strong observational designs (e.g., a prospective design) are used.

Correlational research is often an efficient means of collecting a large amount of data about a problem. For example, it would be possible to collect extensive information about the health histories and eating habits of a large number of individuals. Researchers could then examine which health problems were associated with which diets, and could thus discover a large number of interrelationships in a relatively short amount of time. By contrast, an experimenter looks at only a few variables at a time. One experiment might manipulate foods high in cholesterol, whereas another might manipulate protein, for example.

Finally, correlational research is often strong in realism and therefore has an intrinsic appeal for solving practical problems. Unlike many experimental studies, correlational research is seldom criticized for its artificiality.

⟳ **TIP:** It is usually advantageous to design a study with as many relevant comparisons as possible. Nonequivalent control group after-only designs are weak in part because the comparative information they yield is limited. In nonexperimental studies, multiple comparison groups can be effective in dealing with self-selection, especially if the comparison groups are chosen to address competing biases. For example, in case-control studies of patients with lung cancer, one comparison group could comprise people with a respiratory disease other than lung cancer and a second could comprise those with no respiratory disorder.

DESIGNS AND RESEARCH EVIDENCE

Evidence for nursing practice depends on descriptive, correlational, and experimental research. There is often a logical progression to knowledge expansion that begins with rich description, including description from qualitative research. Descriptive studies can be invaluable in documenting the prevalence, nature, and intensity of health-related conditions and behaviors, and are critical in the development of effective interventions. Moreover, in-depth qualitative research sometimes suggests a causal link that could be the focus of more tightly controlled quantitative research. For example, Colón-Emeric and a team of researchers (2006) did case studies in two nursing homes and looked at site differences in communication patterns among the medical and nursing staff in relation to differences in information flow and innovation. Their findings suggested that a "chain of command" type of communication style may limit health care providers' ability to provide high-quality, innovative care. The study suggests a causal hypothesis that merits greater scrutiny with a larger number of nursing homes under more controlled conditions—and also suggests possibilities for interventions. Thus, although qualitative studies are low on the evidence hierarchy for supporting causal inferences (see Fig. 2.1), they may nevertheless serve as an important impetus.

Correlational studies are often undertaken in the next phase of developing an evidence base for a causal connection. Retrospective case-control studies may pave the way for more rigorous (but more expensive) prospective studies. As the evidence base builds, conceptual models may be developed and tested using path analytic designs and other theory-testing strategies. These studies can provide hints about how to structure an intervention, who can most profit from it, and when it can best be

instituted. Thus, the next important phase is to develop interventions to improve health outcomes, and to test them using experimental and quasi-experimental designs.

Not all research questions are amenable to intervention and experimentation, as noted earlier. Many important research questions will never be answered using information from Level I (meta-analyses of RCTs) or Level II studies (RCTs) on the evidence hierarchy. An important example is the question of whether smoking causes lung cancer. Despite the inability to randomize people to smoking and non-smoking groups, few people doubt that there is a causal relationship. Thinking about the criteria for causality discussed at the beginning of this chapter, there is ample evidence that an empirical relationship between smoking cigarettes and developing lung cancer exists and, through prospective studies, that smoking precedes lung cancer. The large number of studies conducted has allowed researchers to control for, and thus rule out, other possible "causes" of lung cancer. There has been a great deal of consistency and coherence in the findings. And, the criterion of biologic plausibility has been met through basic physiologic research.

Thus, it is perhaps best to think of alternative evidence hierarchies. For questions about the effects of a therapy of intervention, experimental designs are the "gold standard," and meta-analyses of multiple RCTs are at the pinnacle of the hierarchy. Advice to use an experimental design whenever possible is supported by studies that have shown that evidence from RCTs and observational studies often do not yield the same results. Often the relationship between "causes" and "effects" appear to be stronger in nonexperimental studies than in studies in which competing explanations are ruled out through randomization to different treatment conditions.

Nevertheless, for questions about prognosis or about etiology and harm, strong prospective (cohort) studies are usually the best design available for examining causal relationships. Path analytic studies with longitudinal data and a strong theoretical basis can also be powerful. Systematic reviews of multiple prospective studies, together with support from theories or biophysiologic studies, represent the strongest evidence for these types of question.

CRITIQUING GUIDELINES FOR STUDY DESIGN

The research design used in a quantitative study strongly influences the quality of evidence the study yields and therefore should be carefully scrutinized. Decisions about the design of a study have more of an impact on study quality than perhaps any other methodologic decision when the researcher is studying questions about causal influences.

Actual designs and some controlling techniques (randomization, masking) were described in this chapter, and the next chapter explains in greater detail specific strategies for enhancing research control. The guidelines in Box 10.1 are the first of two sets of questions to help you in the critique of quantitative research designs. ✴

RESEARCH EXAMPLES

Nurse researchers are conducting more intervention studies than ever before, and this trend is unlikely to abate in the near future. However, nonexperimental research has a rightful place in the repertoire of research designs for nurse researchers. In this section, we present detailed descriptions of an experimental, quasi-experimental, and nonexperimental study.

Research Example of an Experimental Study

Study: "Efficacy of a smoking-cessation intervention for elective-surgical patients" (Ratner et al., 2004)
Statement of Purpose: The purpose of the study was to determine the effectiveness of a smoking-cessation intervention for presurgical patients.
Treatment Groups: The intervention consisted of three components: (1) a presurgical counseling session that recommended smoking cessation before surgery and provided nicotine replacement gum; (2) an in-hospital postoperative counseling session within 24 hours of surgery that reinforced smoking cessation messages; and (3) telephone counseling support (9 calls over a 4-month period). Subjects in a control group received standard presurgical care.
Method: A sample of 237 smokers scheduled for elective surgery were randomly assigned to the experimental or control group. Data were collected from all subjects before random assignment and then at three follow-up points: within 24 hours of surgery, and 6 and 12 months after surgery. Smoking status was measured by self-report and through biochemical measures (CO readings of expired air while in the hospital and urinary cotinine assays returned through the mail at the two follow-up points). In addition, the researchers gathered self-reported information about smoking cessation self-efficacy, anxiety, depression, and background information such as smoking history. Nurses administered the baseline data collection instruments in a preadmission clinic before random assignment, which involved giving each subject a sealed envelope that contained a computer-generated, randomly determined group allocation. Assistants who gathered follow-up information by telephone were blinded to group assignment and hypotheses.
Key Findings:

- The treatment and control groups did not differ significantly on any demographic or smoking-related characteristics at baseline, suggesting that randomization was successful in equalizing the groups.
- Subjects in the treatment group were more likely than those in the control group to fast before surgery and to be abstinent 6 months after surgery.
- The groups did not differ with regard to smoking abstinence 12 months after surgery.

Research Example of a Quasi-Experimental Study

Study: "A quasi-experimental trial on individualized, developmentally supportive family-centered care" (Byers et al., 2006)
Statement of Purpose: The purpose of the study was to evaluate the impact of individualized, developmentally supportive family-centered care for premature infants on a range of infant outcomes (e.g., growth, behavioral stress cues, physiologic variables) and parental satisfaction.

BOX 10.1 Guidelines for Critiquing Research Designs in Quantitative Studies

1. Does the research question imply a question about a causal relationship between the independent and dependent variables?
2. What would be the strongest design for the research question? How does this compare to the design actually used?
3. Is there an intervention or treatment? Was the intervention adequately described? Was the control of comparison condition adequately described? Was an experimental or quasi-experimental design used?
4. If the design was experimental, what specific experimental design was used? Were randomization procedures adequately explained? Does the report provide evidence that randomization was successful— that is, resulted in groups that were comparable before the intervention? If cluster randomization was used, was there an adequate number of units?
5. If the design is quasi-experimental, what specific quasi-experimental design was used? Is there adequate justification for failure to randomize subjects to treatment conditions? What evidence does the report provide that any groups being compared were equivalent before the intervention?
6. If the design was nonexperimental, was the study inherently nonexperimental? If not, is there adequate justification for failure to manipulate the independent variable? What specific nonexperimental design was used? If a retrospective design was used, is there adequate justification for failure to use a prospective design? What evidence does the report provide that any groups being compared were similar with regard to important extraneous characteristics?
7. What types of comparisons are specified in the design (e.g., before-after? between-groups?) Do these comparisons adequately illuminate the relationship between the independent and dependent variables? If there are no comparisons, or flawed comparisons, how does this affect the integrity of the study and the interpretability of the results?
8. Was the study longitudinal? Was the timing of the collection of data appropriate? Was the number of data collection points reasonable?
9. Was masking/blinding used at all? If yes, who was blinded—and was this adequate? If not, is there an adequate rationale for failure to mask? Is the intervention a type that could raise expectations that in and of themselves could alter the outcomes?

Treatment Groups: The intervention group was cared for in a developmental nursery within the neonatal intensive care unit (NICU). The intervention involved individualized developmental assessments of the infants and the creation and implementation of individualized plans of care. In this model of care, the families were incorporated early and actively into the care of their high-risk infants. There was open visitation in the intervention nursery. All staff who interacted with the infants received 5 consecutive days of training on developmentally supportive care. Infants in the control nursery, which was also in the NICU of the same hospital, received traditional standards of care. The control NICU nursery had limited visitation. **Method:** A sample of 114 premature infants born at a tertiary medical center in southeastern United States participated in the study. A nonequivalent before–after quasi-experimental design was used. The control nursery was similar to the intervention nursery in terms of size, equipment, floor plan, staffing ratios, and infant acuity levels. Some background and outcome variables were retrieved from the infant's hospital records. Physiologic variables (e.g., heart rate, respiratory rate, oxygen saturation) were obtained at baseline, during caregiver activity, and after activity by means of a monitor. Behavioral stress cues were measured multiple times using observation by development specialists. Parental satisfaction was measured using a self-report scale.

Key Findings:

• The intervention and comparison group infants did not differ significantly at baseline in terms of a wide range of risk factors, including Apgar scores, gestational age, birth weight, congenital anomalies, gender, ethnicity, and maternal age.

- There were no differences between the groups in terms of days to developmental milestones, length of hospital stay, or direct cost per case. There were also no group differences in parental satisfaction.
- Stress cues were lower in the developmentally supportive care group. Infants in the intervention group had 8% less sedative/narcotics and 15% lower vasopressors costs than those in the comparison group.

Research Example of a Correlational Study

Study: "Health services use and growth patterns among older siblings of infants with prenatal drug exposure" (Bertsch, Mullins, & Chaffin, 2006)

Statement of Purpose: The purpose of the study was to examine whether the older siblings of infants with prenatal drug exposure experience adverse developmental outcomes. Like their drug-exposed infant siblings, these children tend to be raised in high-risk environments. Therefore, regardless of their own prenatal exposure to drugs, they were hypothesized to be at developmental risk.

Method: To shed light on the health care use patterns and other health-related outcomes of siblings of drug-exposed infants, their histories were compared with matched subjects who did not have a drug-exposed infant sibling. The researchers used a retrospective matched case patient/comparison subject chart review method. There were 93 case patients and 93 comparison patients who were matched first on age and gender and then on race and/or insurance status (public, private, or no coverage) to the extent possible. Hospital clinic charts were reviewed and variables such as the following were retrieved and coded: number of primary care and emergency department visits, immunizations past due, number of serious injuries, number of broken appointments, number of referrals made to child welfare, foster care placement, and height and weight percentiles.

Key Findings:

- The two groups of infants were found to be comparable in terms all four matching variables. They were also similar in terms of number of siblings and having a father living in their households.
- The case patients were found to have significantly fewer health care contacts, more deficient immunizations, and more reports of suspected maltreatment.

- The two groups did not differ in birth weight, but the case patients had lower weight gain trajectories based on growth curve modeling.

SUMMARY POINTS

- Many quantitative nursing studies aim to elucidate *cause-and-effect relationships*, and the challenge of research design is to facilitate inferences about causality.
- Various criteria have been proposed for establishing causality, the most tricky of which is to rule out the possibility that an observed relationship between the presumed cause (the independent variable) and the effect (dependent variable) does not reflect the influence of a third (extraneous) variable.
- In an idealized counterfactual model, a **counterfactual** is what would have happened to the same people simultaneously exposed *and* not exposed to the causal factor. The *effect* represents the difference between the two. Good research design entails finding a good approximation to the idealized counterfactual.
- The social science literature and medical literature use different design terms, and nurse researchers should be familiar with both.
- **Experiments** (or **randomized controlled trials, RCTs**) involve **manipulation** (the researcher manipulates the independent variable by introducing a **treatment** or **intervention**); control (including the use of a **control group** that is not given the intervention and represents the comparative counterfactual); and **randomization** or **random assignment** (with subjects allocated to experimental and control groups at random to make the groups comparable at the outset).
- The full nature of the intervention is delineated in formal protocols. Usually, everyone in the experimental group gets the same intervention, but a growing number of studies develop **patient-centered interventions (PCIs)** that are

tailored to meet individual needs or characteristics.

- Researchers can expose the control group to various conditions, including no treatment; an alternative treatment; a **placebo** or pseudointervention; standard treatment; different doses of the treatment; and a wait-list (*delayed treatment*) condition.

- Random assignment is done by methods that give every subject an equal chance of being included in any group, such as by flipping a coin or using a **table of random numbers**. Randomization is the most reliable method for equating groups on all possible characteristics that could affect study outcomes. Randomization should involve **allocation concealment** that prevents foreknowledge of upcoming assignments.

- The standard process is to randomize *individuals* to conditions after informed consent and the collection of **baseline data**, but there are variations. **Cluster randomization** involves randomly assigning larger units (e.g., hospitals, wards) to treatment conditions. **Partially randomized patient preference (PRPP) designs** involve randomizing only patients without a strong preference for condition. **Randomized consent (or Zelen) designs** randomize before informed consent.

- An **after-only** (or **posttest-only**) **design** involves collecting data only once—after the introduction of the treatment. In a **before–after** (or **pretest–posttest**) **design**, data are collected both before and after the experimental manipulation, thereby permitting an analysis of change.

- **Factorial designs**, in which two or more variables are manipulated simultaneously, allow researchers to test both **main effects** (effects from the experimentally manipulated variables) and **interaction effects** (effects resulting from combining the treatments).

- In a **randomized block design**, subjects are first divided into subgroups on a *blocking* (or *stratifying*) variable that cannot be experimentally manipulated (e.g., gender) and are *then* randomly assigned to treatment conditions separately.

- In a **crossover design**, subjects are exposed to more than one experimental condition, administered in a randomized order, and thus serve as their own controls.

- Experimental designs are considered by many to be the gold standard because they come closer than any other design in meeting the criteria for inferring causal relationships.

- Quasi-experimental designs (**controlled trials without randomization**) involve an intervention but lack randomization. Strong quasi-experimental designs include mechanisms to facilitate causal inferences.

- The **nonequivalent control group before–after design** involves the use of a **comparison group** that was not created through random assignment and the collection of pretreatment data that permit an assessment of initial group equivalence. Comparability of groups can sometimes be enhanced through *matching* on individual characteristics or by **propensity matching** on a **propensity score** for each subject.

- In a **time series design**, there is no comparison group; information on the dependent variable is collected over a period of time before and after the treatment. Time series designs are often used in **single-subject experiments**.

- There are other quasi-experimental designs, including the ethics-friendly **regression discontinuity design**, quasi-experimental **dose-response** analyses, and the quasi-experimental (nonrandomized) arms of a PRPP randomization design (i.e., groups with strong preferences).

- In evaluating the results of quasi-experiments, it is important to ask whether it is plausible that factors other than the intervention caused or affected the outcomes (i.e., whether there are **rival hypotheses** for explaining the results).

- **Nonexperimental** (or **observational**) research includes **descriptive research**—studies that summarize the status of phenomena—and **correlational studies** that examine relationships among variables but involve no manipulation of the independent variable.

- Nonexperimental research is undertaken because many variables, such as age and gender, are not amenable to randomization; also, some variables are technically manipulable but cannot ethically be manipulated.
- There are various designs for correlational studies, including **retrospective (case-control) designs** (which begin with the outcome and look back in time for antecedent causes of "caseness" by comparing cases that have a disease or condition with controls who do not); **prospective (cohort) designs** (longitudinal studies that begin with a presumed cause and look forward in time for its effect); **natural experiments** (comparisons in which one group is affected by a seemingly random event, such as a disaster, and another group is not); and **path analyses** (which test causal models developed on the basis of theory).
- Descriptive studies include both **descriptive correlational research** (which describes how phenomena are interrelated without inferring causality) and **univariate descriptive studies** (which examine the occurrence, frequency, or average value of variables without examining interrelationships).
- Descriptive studies include **prevalence studies** that document the prevalence rate of some condition at a particular point in time, and incidence studies that document the frequency of *new* cases, over a given time period. When the **incidence rates** for two groups are determined, it is possible to compute the **relative risk** of "caseness" for the two.
- The primary weakness of correlational studies is that they can harbor biases owing to **self-selection** into groups being compared.

STUDY ACTIVITIES

Chapter 10 of the *Resource Manual to Accompany Nursing Research: Generating and Assessing Evidence for Nursing Practice, 8th edition,* offers various exercises and study suggestions for reinforcing the concepts presented in this chapter. In addition, the following study questions can be addressed:

1. Assume that you have 10 individuals—Z, Y, X, W, V, U, T, S, R, and Q—who are going to participate in an experiment you are conducting. Using a table of random numbers, assign five individuals to group 1 and five to group 2.
2. A nurse researcher is interested in studying the success of several different approaches to feeding patients with dysphagia. Can the researcher use a correlational design to examine this problem? Why or why not? Could an experimental or quasi-experimental approach be used? How?
3. Insofar as possible, use the questions in Box 10.1 to critique the three research examples described at the end of the chapter.
4. Would you describe the study by Bertsch et al. (2006), summarized at the end of the chapter, as a case-control study or as a prospective study? Think carefully about what the independent and dependent variables are before answering.

STUDIES CITED IN CHAPTER 10

Methodologic or theoretical references cited in this chapter can be found in a separate section at the end of the book.

Anderson, L. A., Gross, J. B. (2004). Aromatherapy with peppermint, isopropyl alcohol, or placebo is equally effective in relieving postoperative nausea. *Journal of Perianesthesia Nursing, 19*(1), 29–35.

Axelin, A., Salantera, S., & Lehtonen, L. (2006). Facilitated tucking by parents in pain management of preterm infants: A randomized crossover trial. *Early Human Development, 82*(4), 241–247.

Bertsch, C., Mullins, S., & Chaffin, M. (2006). Health services use and growth patterns among older siblings of infants with prenatal drug exposure. *Applied Nursing Research, 19*(1), 10–15.

Byers, J., Lowman, L., Francis, J., Kaigle, L., Lutz, N., Waddell, T., & Diaz, A. (2006). A quasi-experimental trial on individualized, developmentally supportive family-centered care. *Journal of Obstetric, Gynecologic, & Neonatal Nursing, 35*(1), 105–115.

Chan, E. , Tan, S., Lee, C., & Lee, J. (2005). Prevalence, incidence, and predictors of pressure ulcers in a tertiary hospital in Singapore. *Journal of Wound Care, 14*(8), 386–388.

Colón-Emeric, C., Ammarell, N, Bailey, D., Corazzini, K., Lekan-Rutledge, D., Piven, M., Utley-Smith, Q., & Anderson, R. (2006). Patterns of medical and nursing staff communication in nursing homes: Implication and insights from complexity science. *Qualitative Health Research, 16*(2), 173–188.

Coward, D. (2002). Partial randomization design in a support group intervention study. *Western Journal of Nursing Research, 24*(4), 406–421.

Dilorio, C., Resnicow, K., McCarty, F., De, A., Dudley, W., Wang, D., & Denzmore, P. (2006). Keepin' it R.E.A.L.! Results of a mother-adolescent HIV prevention program. *Nursing Research, 55*(1), 43–51.

Edwards, N., & Beck, A. (2002). Animal-assisted therapy and nutrition in Alzheimer's disease. *Western Journal of Nursing Research, 24,* 697–712.

El-Masri, M., Hammad, T., & Fox-Wasylyshyn, S. (2005). Predicting nosocomial bloodstream infections using surrogate markers of injury severity. *Nursing Research, 54*(4), 273–279.

Gates, D., Fitzwater, E., & Succop, P. (2005). Reducing assaults against nursing home caregivers. *Nursing Research, 54*(2), 119–127.

Giesler, R., Given, B., Given, C., Rawl, S., Monahan, P., Burns, D., Azzouz, F., Reuille, K., Weinrich, S., Koch, M., & Champion, V. (2005). Improving the quality of life of patients with prostate carcinoma: A randomized trial testing the efficacy of a nurse-driven intervention. *Cancer, 104*(4), 752–762.

Hicks-Moore, S. (2005). Relaxing music at mealtime in nursing homes: Effects on agitated patients with dementia. *Journal of Gerontological Nursing, 31*(12), 26–32.

Hwang, S., Ryan, C., & Zerwic, J. (2006). The influence of age on acute myocardial infarction symptoms and patient delay in seeking treatment. *Progress in Cardiovascular Nursing, 21*(1), 20–27

Keller, C., Robinson, B., & Pickens, L. (2004). Comparison of two walking frequencies in African American postmenopausal women. *ABNF Journal, 15*(1), 3–9.

Lai, H., Chen, C., Peng, T., Chang, F., Hsieh, M., Huang, H., & Chang, S. (2006). Randomized controlled trial of music during kangaroo care on maternal state anxiety and preterm infants' responses. *International Journal of Nursing Studies, 43*(2), 139–146.

Lai, H., & Good, M. (2005). Music improves sleep quality in older adults. *Journal of Advanced Nursing, 49*(3), 234–244.

Landolt, M., Marti, D., Widner, J., & Meuli, M. (2002). Does cartoon movie distraction decrease burned children's pain behavior? *Journal of Burn Care & Rehabilitation, 23,* 61–65.

Lauver, D., Settersten, L., Kane, J., & Henriques, J. (2003). Tailored messages, external barriers, and women's utilization of professional breast cancer screening over time. *Cancer, 97*(11), 2724–2735.

Lee, Y., & Laffrey, S. (2006). Predictors of physical activity in older adults with borderline hypertension. *Nursing Research, 55*(2), 110–120.

Liehr, P., Mehl, M., Summers, L., & Pennebaker, J. (2004). Connecting with others in the midst of stressful upheaval on September 11, 2001. *Applied Nursing Research, 17*(1), 2–9.

McDonald, D. D., Wiczorek, M., & Walker, C. (2004). Factors affecting learning during health education sessions. *Clinical Nursing Research, 13,* 156–167.

McNulty, I., Katz, E., & Kim, K. Y. (2005). Thrombocytopenia following heparin flush. *Progress in Cardiovascular Nursing, 20*(4), 143–147.

Menihan, C. A., Phipps, M., & Weitzen, S. (2006). Fetal heart rate patterns and sudden infant death syndrome. *Journal of Obstetric, Gynecologic, & Neonatal Nursing, 35*(1), 116–122.

Metzger, B. L., Jarosz, P. A., & Noureddine, S. (2000). The effect of high-fat diet and exercise on the expression of genetic obesity. *Western Journal of Nursing Research, 22,* 736–748.

Movaffaghi, Z., Hasanpoor, M., Farsi, M., Hooshmand, P., & Abrishami, F. (2006). Effects of therapeutic touch on blood hemoglobin and hematocrit level. *Journal of Holistic Nursing, 24*(1), 41–48.

Nikoletti, S., Hyde, S., Shaw, T., Myers, H., & Kristjanson, L. J. (2005). Comparison of plain ice and flavoured ice for preventing oral mucositis associated with the use of 5 fluorouracil. *Journal of Clinical Nursing, 14*(6), 750–753.

Phillips, K. D., Mosck, K. S., Bopp, C. M., Dudgeon, W. A., & Hand, G. A. (2006). Spiritual well-being, sleep disturbance, and mental and physical health status in HIV-infected individuals. *Issues in Mental Health Nursing, 27*(2), 125–139.

Ratner, P., Johnson, J., Richardson, C., Bottorff, J., Moffat, B., Mackay, M., Fofonoff, D., Kingsbury, K.,

Miller, C., & Budz, B. (2004). Efficacy of a smoking-cessation intervention for elective-surgical patients. *Research in Nursing & Health, 27,* 148–161.

Rhee, H., Miles, M. S., Halpern, C. T., & Holditch-Davis, D. (2005). Prevalence of recurrent physical symptoms in U. S. adolescents. *Pediatric Nursing, 31*(4), 314–319.

Ross, C. J., Davis, T. M., & MacDonald, G. F. (2005). Cognitive-behavioral treatment combined with asthma education for adults with asthma and coexisting panic disorder. *Clinical Nursing Research,* 14(2), 131–157.

Scott, S., Raymond, P., Thompson, W., & Galt, D. (2005). Efficacy and tolerance of sodium phosphates oral solution after diet liberalization. *Gastroenterology Nursing, 28*(2), 133–139.

Shin, K. R., Kwak, S. E., Lee, J. B., & Yi, H. R. (2006). The effectiveness of hand acupuncture and moxibustion in decreasing pain and "coldness" in Korean women who had had hysterectomy. *Applied Nursing Research, 19*(1), 22–30.

Steiner, A., Walsh, B., Pickering, R., Wiles, R., Ward, J., Brooking, J., & Southampton NLU Evaluation Team. (2001). Therapeutic nursing or unblocking beds? A randomised controlled trial of a post-acute intermediate care unit. *British Medical Journal, 322*(7284), 453–460.

11

Enhancing Rigor in Quantitative Research

VALIDITY AND INFERENCE

This chapter describes strategies that can be used to strengthen quantitative research designs, including ways to enhance rigor by minimizing biases and controlling extraneous variables. Most of these strategies represent opportunities to strengthen the inferences that can be made about cause-and-effect relationships.

Validity and Validity Threats

In designing a study, a constructive approach is to think in advance of all the possible factors that could undermine the **validity** of inferences. Shadish, Cook, and Campbell (2002), in their influential book, define validity in the context of research design as "the approximate truth of an inference" (p. 34). For example, inferences that an *effect* results from a hypothesized *cause* are valid to the extent that researchers can marshal supporting evidence. Validity is always a matter of degree, not an absolute.

Validity is a property of an inference, not of a research design, but design elements profoundly affect the inferences that can be made. **Threats to validity** are reasons that an inference could be wrong. When researchers can anticipate potential

threats to validity and then introduce design features to eliminate or minimize these threats, the validity of the inference is strengthened, and thus evidence from the study is much more persuasive. We identify a number of important validity threats to encourage you to think about ways to minimize them during the design phase of a study and to evaluate them in interpreting study results.

Types of Validity

Shadish and colleagues (2002) proposed a typology of validity that identifies four different aspects of a good research design, and also catalogued dozens of threats to validity. This chapter describes the typology and briefly summarizes major threats, but we urge researchers—especially if they wish to make causal inferences in the absence of an experimental design—to consult this seminal work for further guidance on strengthening study validity.

The first type of validity, statistical conclusion validity, is more easily grasped by those who have understanding of fundamental statistical principles (see Chapter 22), but we offer a simplified explanation here. In brief, **statistical conclusion validity** concerns the validity of inferences that there truly is an empirical relationship, or correlation, between the presumed cause and the effect. The researcher's job is to provide the strongest possible evidence that the relationship is *real* and that the intervention (if any) was given a truly fair test.

Internal validity concerns the validity of inferences that, given the existence of an empirical relationship, it is the independent variable, rather than other factors, that caused the outcome. Here the researcher's job is to develop strategies to rule out the plausibility that something other than the presumed cause can account for the observed relationship.

Construct validity involves the validity of inferences "from the observed persons, settings, and cause and effect operations included in the study to the constructs that these instances might represent" (Shadish et al., 2002, p. 38). As described in Chapter 6, one aspect of construct validity concerns the degree to which an intervention is a good representation of the underlying construct that was theorized as having the potential to cause beneficial outcomes. Another concerns whether the measures of the dependent variable are good operationalizations of the constructs for which they are intended.

The fourth type is **external validity**, which is the validity that inferences about observed relationships will hold over variations in persons, setting, time, or measures of the outcomes. External validity, then, concerns the generalizability of causal inferences, and this is a critical concern for research that aims to yield evidence for evidence-based nursing practice.

These four types of validity and their associated threats are discussed in this chapter. Many of the validity threats concern inadequate control over confounding variables, and so we briefly review methods of controlling variation associated with the characteristics of study participants.

Controlling Intrinsic Source of Extraneous Variability

Participant characteristics almost always need to be controlled for quantitative findings to be interpretable. This section describes six ways of controlling confounding subject characteristics to rule out rival explanations for cause-and-effect relationships.

Randomization

Randomization is the most effective method of controlling individual confounding variables. The primary function of randomization is to secure comparable groups—that is, to equalize groups with respect to extraneous variables. A distinct advantage of random assignment, compared with other control methods, is that it controls *all* possible sources of extraneous variation, *without any conscious decision on the researcher's part about which variables need to be controlled.*

Crossover

Randomization in the context of a crossover design is an especially powerful method of ensuring equivalence between groups being compared—the subjects serve as their own controls. Such a design is not appropriate for all studies, however, because of the problem of carry-over effects. When subjects are exposed to two different conditions, they may be influenced in the second condition by their experience in the first. Because treatments are not applied simultaneously, the best approach is to use randomized ordering. When there are only two conditions, the researcher simply designates that half the subjects, at random, will receive treatment A first and that the other half will receive treatment B first. Note that, in addition to their great potential for control over confounding subject traits, crossover designs offer another advantage: fewer subjects are needed. Fifty subjects exposed to two treatments in random order yield 100 pieces of data (50×2); 50 subjects randomly assigned to two different groups yield only 50 pieces of data (25×2).

Homogeneity

When randomization and crossover are not feasible, alternative methods of controlling extraneous characteristics should be used. One such method is to use only subjects who are homogeneous with respect to both use variables—that is, the confounding variables are not allowed to vary. Suppose we were testing the effectiveness of a physical training program on the cardiovascular functioning of elders. Our quasi-experimental design involves elders from two different nursing homes, with elders in one of them receiving the physical training program. If gender were an important confounding variable (and if the two nursing homes had different proportions of men and women), we could control gender by using only men (or only women) as subjects.

Using a homogeneous sample is easy as a mechanism of controlling extraneous variables, but the price for this ease is that research findings can be generalized only to the type of subjects who participated in the study. If the physical training program were found to have beneficial effects on the cardiovascular status of a sample of women 65 to 75 years of age, its usefulness for improving the cardiovascular status of men in their 80s would require a separate study. Indeed, one noteworthy criticism of this approach is that researchers sometimes exclude subjects who are extremely ill or incapacitated, which means that the findings cannot be generalized to the very people who perhaps are most in need of interventions. Another limitation of homogeneity is that it can in some cases lower statistical conclusion validity, an issue we discuss in a later section.

> **Example of control through homogeneity:**
> Oka and Sanders (2005) studied the effect of exercise on body composition and nutritional intake in patients with heart failure. Several variables were controlled through homogeneity, including gender (only men were included), age (no one was older than 76 years), and illness severity (only those with stable class II to III heart failure were included).

◗ **TIP:** The principle of homogeneity is often used to control (hold constant) external factors as well as intrinsic participant factors. For example, it may be important to collect outcome data at the same time of the day for all participants if time could affect the outcome (e.g., fatigue). As another example, it is often desirable to maintain **constancy of conditions** in terms of locale of data collection—for example, interviewing some respondents in their own homes, but others in their places of work or in the researcher's office. In each setting, participants assume different roles (e.g., spouse, parent, employee, client), and responses to questions may be influenced to some degree by those roles.

Blocking/Stratification

Another approach to controlling extraneous variables is to include them in the research design through blocking or stratification, as discussed in the previous chapter. To pursue our example of the physical training program, if gender were the confounding variable, we could build it into the study in a randomized block design in which elderly men and women would be randomly assigned separately to treatment groups. This approach can enhance the likelihood of detecting differences between our experimental and control groups because we can eliminate the effect of the blocking variable (gender) on the dependent variable. In addition, if the blocking variable is of interest substantively, this approach gives researchers the opportunity to study differences in groups created by the blocking variable (e.g., men versus women). Stratification is most appropriate in experiments, but it is used commonly in quasi-experimental and correlational studies as well.

Matching

Matching (also known as **pair matching**) involves using knowledge of subject characteristics to create comparable groups. If matching were used in our physical training example, and age and gender were the confounding variables, we would match each subject in the physical training group with one in the comparison group with respect to age and gender. As noted in the previous chapter, there are reasons why matching is problematic. First, to match effectively, researchers must know in advance what the relevant confounding variables are. Second, after two or three variables, it often becomes impossible to pair match adequately, unless propensity score matching is used—but this method requires technical sophistication. With more than three variables, matching becomes cumbersome, if not impossible. Yet there are usually far more than three extraneous variables that could affect researchers' dependent variables. For these reasons, matching as the primary technique for controlling confounding variables should be used only when other, more powerful procedures are not feasible, as might be the case in some correlational studies (e.g., case-control designs).

Sometimes, as an alternative to pair matching, in which subjects are matched on a one-to-one basis for each matching variable, researchers use a **balanced design** with regard to key confounding variables. In such situations, researchers attempt only to ensure that the groups being compared have proportional representation with regard to extraneous variables. For example, if gender and age were the two extraneous variables of concern in our example, we would strive to ensure that the same percentage of men and women were in the two groups, and that the average age was comparable. Such an approach is less cumbersome than pair matching, but it has similar limitations. Nevertheless, both pair matching and balancing are preferable to failing to control subject characteristics at all.

Example of control through matching:
Talashek, Alba, and Patel (2006) compared inner-city teenagers who were either pregnant or never pregnant to examine factors that might predict pregnancy. Homogeneity controlled participants' area of residence (living in an inner city), and matching was used to control the teenagers' age and ethnicity.

Statistical Control

A sixth method of controlling confounding variables is through statistical analysis rather than through research design. Some of you may be unfamiliar with even basic statistical procedures, and so a detailed description of powerful **statistical control** mechanisms will not be attempted. If you have a background in statistics, you should consult Chapter 23 or a textbook on advanced statistics. Because the notion of statistical control may mystify some of you, however, we explain underlying principles with a simple illustration of a procedure called **analysis of covariance**.

In our physical training example, suppose we used a nonequivalent control group design with residents from two similar nursing homes, and we used resting heart rate as an outcome measure. There undoubtedly would be individual differences in heart rate within the overall sample—that is, it would vary from one person to the next. The research question is, Can some of the individual differences be attributed to a person's participation in the physical training program? We know that differences in resting heart rate are also related to other, extraneous characteristics, such as subjects' age. In Figure 11.1, the large circles

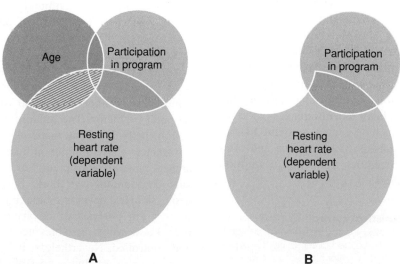

A   **B**

FIGURE 11.1 Schematic diagram illustrating the principle of analysis of covariance.

represent the total extent of individual differences for resting heart rate. A certain amount of variability can be explained by the subjects' age, which is shown as the small circle on the left in Figure 11.1**A**. Another part of the variability can perhaps be explained by subjects' participation or nonparticipation in the program, as represented as the small circle on the right. The fact that the two small circles (age and program participation) overlap indicates that there is a relationship between those two variables. In other words, subjects in the physical training group are, on average, either older or younger than those in the comparison group, and thus age should be controlled. Otherwise, it will be impossible to determine whether postintervention differences in resting heart rate should be attributed to differences in age or program participation.

Analysis of covariance controls by statistically removing the effect of extraneous variables on the dependent variable. In the illustration, the portion of heart rate variability attributable to age (the hatched area of the large circle in **A**) is removed through analysis of covariance. Figure 11.1**B** illustrates that the final analysis examines the effect of program participation on heart rate *after removing the effect of age*. By controlling heart rate variability resulting from age, we get a more accurate estimate of the effect of the training program on heart rate. Note that even after removing variability due to age, there is still individual variation not associated with the program treatment—the bottom half of the large circle in **B**. This means that the study can probably be further enhanced by controlling additional confounding variables that might account for heart rate differences in the two nursing homes, such as gender, smoking history, and so forth. Analysis of covariance and other sophisticated procedures can control multiple extraneous variables.

Example of statistical control: Phuphaibul and colleagues (2005) used a quasi-experimental design to evaluate an intervention aimed at improving the coping skills and mental health of junior high school students.

Thirteen schools were in either a control group condition, a nonintensive treatment condition, or an intensive treatment condition. Student scores on several psychosocial instruments were used as the outcome measures, and the three groups of more than 1500 students were compared after first statistically controlling baseline measures of the dependent variables.

➲ **TIP:** The confounding subject characteristics that need to be controlled vary from one study to another, but we can offer some guidance. The best variable is the dependent variable itself, measured before the independent variable occurs. In our example, controlling preprogram measures of cardiovascular functioning through analysis of covariance would be especially powerful because this would remove the effect of individual variation stemming from many other extraneous factors. Major demographic variables (e.g., age, race/ethnicity, gender, education) and health status indicators are usually good candidates to measure and control. Confounding variables that need to be controlled should be identified through a literature review.

Evaluation of Control Methods

Table 11.1 summarizes the benefits and drawbacks of the six control mechanisms. Random assignment of subjects to groups is the most effective method of managing confounding variables—that is, of approximating the ideal but unattainable counterfactual discussed in Chapter 10—because it tends to cancel out individual differences on all possible extraneous variables. Crossover designs, although an extremely useful supplement to randomization, cannot be applied to most nursing research problems. The remaining alternatives—homogeneity, blocking, matching, and analysis of covariance—have a common disadvantage: Researchers must know or predict in advance the relevant confounding variables. To select homogeneous samples, develop a blocking design, match, or perform analysis of covariance, researchers must know which variables need to be measured and controlled. Nevertheless, it is clear that randomization is not always possible. In correlational

TABLE 11.1 Methods of Control Over Participant Characteristics

METHOD	BENEFITS	LIMITATIONS
Randomization	• Controls all preintervention extraneous variables • Does not require advance knowledge of which variables to control	• Ethical and practical constraints on variables that can be manipulated • Possible artificiality of conditions
Repeated measures	• If done with randomization, strongest possible approach	• Cannot be used if there are possible carry-over effects from one condition to the next
Homogeneity	• Easy to achieve in all types of research • Could enhance interpretability of relationships	• Limits the generalizability of the results • Requires knowledge of which variables to control • Range restriction could lower statistical conclusion validity
Blocking	• Enhances the ability to detect and interpret relationships • Offers opportunity to examine blocking variable as an independent variable	• Usually restricted to a few blocking variables • Requires knowledge of which variables to control
Matching	• Enhances ability to detect and interpret relationships • May be easy if there is a large "pool" of potential available controls	• Usually restricted to a few matching variables (except when propensity matching is used) • Requires knowledge of which variables to match • May be difficult to find comparison group matches, especially if there are more than two matching variables
Statistical control	• Enhances ability to detect and interpret relationships • Relatively economical means of controlling several confounding variables	• Requires knowledge of which variables to control, and requires measurement of those variables • Requires statistical sophistication

and quasi-experimental studies, the control options available to researchers include homogeneity, blocking, matching, and analysis of covariance. The use of any of these procedures is preferable to the absence of any attempt to control intrinsic extraneous variables.

STATISTICAL CONCLUSION VALIDITY

As noted in Chapter 10, the first criterion for establishing causality is demonstrating that there is, in fact, an empirical relationship between the independent and dependent variable. Statistical methods are used to make inferences about whether such a relationship exists. Design decisions can influence whether statistical tests will actually detect true relationships, and so researchers need to make decisions that protect against reaching false statistical conclusions. Researchers need to give thought to statistical conclusion validity considerations even when they have not hypothesized causal linkages—the issue is whether relationships that exist in reality can be detected in a study. Shadish and colleagues (2002) discussed nine separate threats to statistical conclusion validity (their Table 2.2). Although we cannot discuss all aspects of statistical conclusion validity, we describe three especially important threats.

Low Statistical Power

Statistical power refers to the ability to detect true relationships among variables. Adequate statistical power can be achieved in various ways, the most straightforward of which is to use a sufficiently large sample. When small samples are used, statistical power tends to be low, and the analyses may fail to show that the independent and dependent variables are related—*even when they are*. Power and sample size are discussed in Chapters 13 and 22.

Another aspect of a powerful design concerns the construction or definition of the independent variable. Both statistically and substantively, results are clearer when differences between groups or conditions being compared are large. Researchers should aim to maximize group differences on the dependent variables by maximizing differences on the independent variable. In other words, the results are likely to be more clearcut if the groups are as different as possible. Conn and colleagues (2001) offer excellent suggestions for strengthening the power and effectiveness of nursing interventions. Advice about strengthening group differences is more easily followed in experimental than in nonexperimental research. In experiments, investigators can devise treatment

conditions that are distinct and as strong as time, money, ethics, and practicality permit. Even in nonexperimental research, however, there are frequently opportunities to operationalize independent variables in such a way that power to detect differences is enhanced.

Another aspect of statistical power concerns maximizing **precision**, which is achieved through accurate (reliable) measuring tools, controls over extraneous variables, and powerful statistical methods. Precision can best be understood through a specific example. Suppose we were studying the effect of admission into a nursing home on depression by comparing elders who were or were not admitted. Depression varies from one elderly person to another for various reasons. In the present study, we are interested in isolating—as precisely as possible—the portion of variation in depression attributable to nursing home admission. Mechanisms of research control that reduce variability attributable to confounding factors can be built into the research design, thereby enhancing precision.

In a quantitative study, the following ratio expresses what we wish to assess in this example:

$$\frac{\text{Variablity in depession}}{\text{Variability in depression due to other factors}}$$
$$\text{due to nursing home admission}$$
$$\text{(e.g. age, pain, medical condition)}$$

This ratio, although greatly simplified here, captures the essence of many statistical tests. We want to make variability in the numerator (the upper half) as large as possible relative to variability in the denominator (the lower half), to evaluate precisely the relationship between nursing home admission and levels of depression. The smaller the variability in depression due to confounding variables (e.g., age, pain), the easier it will be to detect differences in depression between elders who were or were not admitted to a nursing home. Designs that enable researchers to reduce variability caused by extraneous variables can increase statistical conclusion validity. As a purely hypothetical illustration, we will attach some numeric values* to the ratio as follows:

$$\frac{\text{Variability due to nursing home admission}}{\text{Variability due to all confounding variables}} = \frac{10}{4}$$

If we can make the bottom number smaller, say by changing it from 4 to 2, then we will have a more precise estimate of the effect of nursing home admission on depression, relative to other influences. Control mechanisms such as those described earlier help to reduce variability caused by confounding variables, and so should be considered as design options in planning a study. We illustrate this by continuing our example, singling out age as a key confounding variable. The total variability in levels of depression can be conceptualized as having the following components:

Total variability in depression = Variability due to nursing home admission + Variability due to age + Variability due to other confounding variables

This equation can be taken to mean that part of the reason why some elders are depressed and others are not is that some were admitted to a nursing home and others were not and that some were older and some were younger; in addition, other factors, such as level of pain and medical condition also had an effect on depression.

One way to increase the precision in this study would be to control age, thereby removing the variability in depression that results from age differences. We could do this, for example, by restricting the age of the sample to elders younger than 80, thereby reducing the variability in depression due to age. As a result, the effect of nursing home admission on depression becomes greater, relative to the remaining extraneous variability. Thus, this design decision (homogeneity) enabled us to get a more precise estimate of the effect of nursing home

admission on level of depression (although of course, this limits the generalizability of the findings). Research designs differ considerably in the sensitivity with which effects under study can be detected with statistical tools. Lipsey (1990) has prepared an excellent guide to assist researchers in enhancing the sensitivity of research designs.

Restriction of Range

Although the control of extraneous variation through homogeneity is an easy method to use and can help to clarify the relationship between key research variables, it can be a risky route to take. Not only does this approach limit the generalizability of study findings, it can in some circumstances threaten statistical conclusion validity. When the use of homogeneity restricts the range of values on the outcome variable, relationships between the outcome and the independent variable will be *attenuated*, and may therefore lead to an erroneous inference that the variables are unrelated.

In the example just used, we suggested the possibility of limiting the sample of nursing home residents to elders younger than 80 to reduce variability in the denominator. Our aim was to enhance the amount of variability in depression scores attributable to nursing home admission, relative to depression variability due to other factors. What if, however, few elders under 80 were depressed? With limited variability, relationships cannot be detected—the values in both the numerator and denominator are deflated. For example, if everyone had a depression score of 50, depression scores would be totally unrelated to age, pain levels, nursing home admission, and so on. Thus, in designing a study, it is important to consider whether there will be sufficient variability to support the statistical analyses envisioned. The issue of *floor effects* and *ceiling effects*, which involve range restrictions at the lower and upper end of a measure, respectively, are discussed later in this book.

➲ **TIP :** In designing a study, try to anticipate negative (nonsignificant) findings and consider whether design adjustments might affect the results. For example, suppose our study hypothesis is that environmental factors such as light and noise

---

*At this point, you should not be concerned with how these numbers can be obtained. The procedure is explained in Chapter 22.

affect the incidence of acute confusion among the hospitalized elderly. With a preliminary design in mind, try to imagine findings that *fail* to support the hypothesis. Then ask yourself what could be done to decrease the possibility of obtaining negative results, under the assumption that negative results do not reflect the truth. Could power be increased by making differences in environmental conditions sharper? Could precision be increased by controlling additional extraneous variables? Could bias be eliminated by better training of research personnel?

Unreliable Implementation of a Treatment

The strength of an intervention (and hence statistical power) can be undermined if the intervention is not as powerful in reality as it is "on paper." **Intervention fidelity** (or **treatment fidelity**) concerns the extent to which the implementation of an intervention is faithful to its plan. There is growing interest in intervention fidelity in the nursing literature and considerable advice on how to achieve it (e.g., Bellg et al., 2004; McGuire et al., 2000; Santacroce et al., 2004; Whitmer et al., 2005).

An intervention can be weakened by a number of factors, many of which researchers can influence. One issue concerns the extent to which the intervention is similar from one subject to the next. In most intervention studies, researchers strive for constancy of conditions in implementing the treatment because lack of standardization adds extraneous variation and can diminish the full force of the intervention. Even in tailored, patient-centered interventions, there are typically protocols, even though different protocols are used with different people. Using the notions just described, when standard protocols are not used or not followed, variability due to the intervention (i.e., in the numerator) can be suppressed, and variability due to extraneous factors (i.e., in the denominator) can be inflated, possibly leading to the erroneous conclusion that the intervention was ineffective. This suggests the need for a certain degree of standardization, the development of procedures manuals, thorough training of personnel, and vigilant monitoring (e.g., through observations of the deliv-

ery of the intervention) to ensure that the intervention is being implemented as planned—and to ensure that control group members have not gained access to the intervention.

Determining that the intervention was delivered as intended may need to be supplemented with efforts to ensure that the intervention was *received* as intended. This may involve a **manipulation check** to assess whether the treatment was in place, was understood, or was perceived in an intended manner. For example, if we were testing the effect of soothing versus jarring music on anxiety, we might want to determine whether subjects themselves perceived the music as soothing and jarring. Another aspect of treatment fidelity for interventions designed to promote behavioral changes concerns the concept of *enactment* (Bellg et al., 2004). Enactment refers to participants' performance of treatment-related skills, behaviors, and cognitive strategies in relevant, real-life settings.

Example of attention to treatment fidelity: Resnick and co-researchers (2005) described at length the efforts they made to ensure treatment fidelity in implementing the Exercise Plus Program, a self-efficacy based intervention to increase exercise in older women who had had a hip fracture. A treatment fidelity plan was developed that involved careful attention to the intervention design (e.g., having a standardized intervention with clear protocols), training (e.g., providing a standardized training program with a training manual), delivery (e.g., observing intervention delivery at randomly selected sessions), receipt (completing a checklist of observed activities), and enactment (reviewing calendars maintained in home settings).

Another issue is that subjects are often exposed to different conditions than were planned because of problems with **treatment adherence**. It is not unusual, for example, for those in the experimental group to elect not to participate fully in the treatment—for example, they may stop going to treatment sessions, or they may stop paying attention. To the extent possible, researchers should design the study to enhance the integrity of the treatment conditions, taking steps in particular to encourage participation among members of the treatment group. This might mean making the intervention as enjoyable and motivational as possible, and taking steps to reduce participant burden in terms of both the intervention and data collection. Nonparticipation in an intervention is rarely random, so researchers should document which subjects got what amount of treatment so that individual differences in "dose" can be taken into account in the analysis or interpretation of results.

➲ **T I P :** Except for small-scale studies, every study should have a **procedures manual** that delineates the protocols and procedures for its implementation. The Toolkit of the accompanying *Resource Manual* provides a model table of contents for such a procedures manual. The Toolkit also includes a model checklist to monitor delivery of an intervention through direct observation of intervention sessions.

INTERNAL VALIDITY

Internal validity refers to the extent to which it is possible to make an inference that the independent variable is truly causing or influencing the dependent variable and that the relationship between the two is not the spurious effect of a confounding variable. We infer from an effect to a cause by eliminating (controlling) other potential causes. The control mechanisms reviewed earlier in this chapter are all strategies for improving internal validity. If researchers are not careful in managing extraneous variation, there may be reason to challenge the conclusion that the subjects' performance on the dependent measure was caused by the independent variable.

Threats to Internal Validity

True experiments possess a high degree of internal validity because the use of manipulation and randomization usually enables the researcher to rule out most alternative explanations for the results. Researchers who use quasi-experimental or correlational designs must contend with competing explanations of what caused the outcomes. Major competing explanations, or threats to internal validity, are examined here.

Temporal Ambiguity

As we discussed in Chapter 10, a criterion for inferring a causal relationship is that the cause must precede the effect. In randomized clinical trials (RCTs), researchers themselves create the independent variable and then observe subsequent performance on an outcome variable, so establishing temporal sequencing is never a problem. In correlational studies, however, it may be unclear whether the independent variable precedes the dependent variable, or *vice versa*.

Selection

Selection (or self-selection) encompasses biases resulting from preexisting differences between groups. When individuals are not assigned randomly to groups, there is always a possibility that the groups are nonequivalent. They may differ in subtle but important ways. If the groups are nonequivalent, differences on outcomes may result from initial differences rather than from the effect of the independent variable. For example, if we found that women with a fertility problem were more likely to be depressed than women who were mothers, it would be impossible to conclude that the two groups differed in depression *because* of differences in reproductive status; women in the two groups might have been different in terms of psychological well-being from the start. The problem of selection is reduced if researchers can collect data on subject characteristics before the occurrence of the independent variable. In our example of infertility, the best design would be to collect data on women's depression before they attempted to become pregnant, and then design the study to control this.

Selection bias is one of the most problematic and frequently encountered threats to the internal validity of studies not using an experimental design. But selection can also enter into experimental designs if many subjects elect not to receive the treatment; these subjects essentially select themselves into the control condition.

History

The threat of **history** refers to the occurrence of external events that take place concurrently with the independent variable that can affect the dependent variables. For example, suppose we were studying the effectiveness of a county-wide nurse outreach program to encourage pregnant women in rural areas to improve their health-related practices before delivery (e.g., better nutritional practices, cessation of smoking, earlier prenatal care). The program might be evaluated by comparing the average birthweight of infants born in the 12 months before the outreach program with the average birthweight of those born in the 12 months after the program was introduced, using a time series design. However, suppose that 1 month after the new program was launched, a highly publicized docudrama regarding the inadequacies of prenatal care for poor women was aired on national television. Infants' birth weight might now be affected by both the intervention and the messages in the docudrama, and it becomes impossible to disentangle the two effects.

In a true experiment, history usually is not a threat to a study's internal validity because we can often assume that external events are as likely to affect the experimental as the control group. When this is the case, group differences on the dependent variables represent effects over and above those created by external factors. There are, however, exceptions. For example, when a crossover design is used, an external event may occur during the first half (or second half) of the experiment, and so treatments would be contaminated by the effect of that event. That is, some people would receive treatment A with the event and others would receive treatment A without it, and the same would be true for treatment B.

Selection biases sometimes interact with history to compound the threat to the internal validity. For example, if the comparison group is different from the treatment group, then the characteristics of the members of the comparison group could lead them to have different intervening experiences, thereby introducing both history and selection biases into the design.

Maturation

In a research context, **maturation** refers to processes occurring within subjects during the course of the study as a result of the passage of time rather than as a result of a treatment or independent variable. Examples of such processes include physical growth, emotional maturity, fatigue, and the like. For instance, if we wanted to evaluate the effects of a special sensorimotor development program for developmentally delayed children, we would have to consider that progress does occur in these children even without special assistance. A design such as a one-group pretest–posttest design, for example, would be highly susceptible to this threat.

Maturation is a relevant consideration in many areas of nursing research. Remember that maturation here does not refer to aging or development exclusively but rather to any change that occurs as a function of time. Thus, wound healing, postoperative recovery, and many other bodily changes that can occur with little or no nursing or medical intervention must be considered as an explanation for outcomes that rivals an explanation based on the effects of the independent variable.

Mortality/Attrition

Mortality is the threat that arises from attrition in groups being compared. If different kinds of people remain in the study in one group versus another, then these differences, rather than the independent variable, could account for any observed differences on the dependent variables at the end of the study. The most severely ill patients might drop out of an experimental condition because it is too demanding, or they might drop out of the comparison group because they see no personal advantage to remaining in the study. In a prospective cohort study, there may be differential attrition between groups being compared because of death, extreme illness, or geographic relocation. Attrition bias essentially is a type of selection bias that occurs after the unfolding of the study: groups initially equivalent can lose comparability because of subject loss, and it could be that the differential composition, rather than the independent variable, is the "cause" of any group differences on the dependent variables.

The risk for attrition is especially great when the length of time between points of data collection is long. A 12-month follow-up of subjects, for example, tends to produce higher rates of attrition than a 1-month follow-up. In clinical studies, the problem of attrition may be especially acute because of patient death or disability.

If attrition is random (i.e., those dropping out of a study are similar to those remaining in it with respect to extraneous characteristics), then there would not be bias. However, attrition is rarely totally random. In general, the higher the rate of attrition, the greater the likelihood of bias. Although there is no absolute standard for acceptable attrition rates, biases are usually of concern if the rate exceeds 20%.

⟶ TIP: In longitudinal studies (e.g., cohort designs), attrition can be reduced through procedures to help relocate subjects. Attrition often occurs because researchers cannot find participants, rather than because of refusals to continue in the study. One effective strategy to help in **tracing** subjects is to obtain **contact information** from participants at each point of data collection. Contact information should include the names, addresses, and telephone numbers of two or three people with whom the subject is close (e.g., parents, close friends) — people who would be likely to know how to contact participants if they moved. A sample contact information form that can be adapted for your use is provided in the Toolkit of the accompanying *Resource Manual.*

Testing and Instrumentation

Testing refers to the effects of taking a pretest on subjects' performance on a posttest. It has been documented in several studies, particularly in those dealing with opinions and attitudes, that the mere act of collecting data from people changes them. Suppose we administered to a group of nursing students a questionnaire about their attitudes toward assisted suicide. We then acquaint them with various arguments that have been made for and against assisted suicide, outcomes of court cases, and the like. At the end of instruction, we give them the same attitude measure and observe whether their attitudes have changed. The problem

is that the first administration of the questionnaire might sensitize students, resulting in attitude changes regardless of whether instruction follows. If a comparison group is not used in the study, it becomes impossible to segregate the effects of the instruction from the effects of taking the pretest. Sensitization, or testing, problems are more likely to occur when pretest data come from self-reports (e.g., a questionnaire), especially if subjects are exposed to controversial or novel material in the pretest. For some nursing studies (e.g., those that involve biophysiologic data), testing effects are not a major concern.

Another threat related to measurements is the threat of **instrumentation**. This bias reflects changes in measuring instruments or methods of measurement between two points of data collection. For example, if we used one measure of stress at baseline and a revised measure at follow-up, any differences might reflect changes in the measuring tool rather than the effect of an independent variable. Instrumentation effects can occur even if the same measure is used. For example, if the measuring tool yields more accurate measures on the second administration (e.g., if the people collecting the data are more experienced) or less accurate measures the second time (e.g., if subjects become bored or fatigued), then these differences could bias the results.

Internal Validity and Research Design

Quasi-experimental and correlational studies are especially susceptible to threats to internal validity. Table 11.2 lists the specific designs that are *most* vulnerable to the threats just described—although it should not be assumed that the threats are irrelevant in designs not listed. Each threat represents an alternative explanation (rival hypothesis) that competes with the independent variable as a cause of the dependent variable. The aim of a strong research design is to rule out these competing explanations.

An experimental design normally rules out most rival hypotheses, but even in RCTs, researchers must

TABLE 11.2	Research Designs and Threats to Internal Validity

THREAT	DESIGNS MOST SUSCEPTIBLE TO THREATS
Temporal ambiguity	Case–control Other retrospective
Selection	Nonequivalent control group (especially, posttest-only) Case-control "Natural" experiments
History	One-group pretest–posttest Time series Prospective cohort Crossover
Maturation	One-group pretest–posttest
Mortality/ attrition	Prospective cohort Longitudinal experiments and quasi-experiments
Testing instrumentation	Pretest–posttest designs

exercise caution. For example, if there is treatment infidelity or contamination between treatments, then history might be a rival explanation for any group differences (or lack of differences). Mortality can also be a salient threat in true experiments. Because the experimenter does things differently with the experimental and control groups, subjects in the groups may drop out of the study differentially. This is particularly apt to happen if the experimental treatment is painful, inconvenient, or time-consuming, or if the control condition is boring or bothersome. When this happens, subjects remaining in the study may differ from those who left in important ways, thereby nullifying the initial equivalence of the groups.

In short, researchers should consider how best to guard against and detect all possible threats to internal validity, no matter what design is used.

Internal Validity and Data Analysis

The best strategy for enhancing internal validity is to use a strong research design that includes the use of control mechanisms and careful design features discussed in this chapter. Even when this is possible (and, certainly, when this is *not* possible), it is advisable to conduct analyses to determine the nature and extent of biases that arose. When biases are detected, the information can be used to interpret substantive results; in some cases, biases can be statistically controlled.

Researchers need to be self-critics. They need to consider fully and objectively the types of biases that could have arisen within their chosen design— and then systematically search for evidence of their existence (while hoping, of course, that no evidence can be found). To the extent that biases can be ruled out or controlled, the quality of evidence the study yields will be strengthened. A few examples should illustrate how to proceed.

Selection biases should always be examined. Typically, this involves comparing groups on pretest measures, when pretest data have been collected. For example, if we were studying depression in women who delivered a baby by cesarean birth versus those who delivered vaginally, selection bias could be assessed by comparing depression in these two groups before delivery. If there are significant predelivery differences, then any postdelivery differences would have to be interpreted with initial differences in mind (or with differences controlled). In designs in which there is no pretest measure of the dependent variable, researchers should nevertheless search for selection biases by comparing groups with respect to key background variables, such as age, gender, health status, and so on. Selection biases should be analyzed even in RCTs because there is no guarantee that randomization will yield perfectly equivalent groups.

Whenever the research design involves multiple points of data collection, researchers should analyze attrition biases. This is typically achieved through a comparison of those who did and did not complete the study with regard to baseline measures of the dependent variable or other characteristics measured at the first point of data collection.

Example of assessing attrition and selection bias: Moser and Dracup (2000) studied the effect of two alternative cardiopulmonary resuscitation (CPR) training interventions against a control condition among 219 spouses of cardiac patients recovering from an acute cardiac event. At the 1-month follow-up, 196 subjects provided outcome data, for a response rate of 89.5%. The researchers found that there were no significant differences in background characteristics (e.g., race, education) between subjects completing or not completing the study, nor between subjects in the three treatment groups.

When subjects withdraw from a study, researchers are in a dilemma about whom to "count" as being "in" a condition. A procedure that is often used is an **on-protocol analysis**, which includes members in a treatment group only if they actually received the treatment. Such an analysis is problematic, however, because the sample is no longer representative of the entire group of interest, and self-selection into a nonintervention condition nullifies the comparability of groups. This type of analysis will almost always be biased toward finding positive treatment effects. A more acceptable approach is to use a principle known as **intention to treat**, which involves an analysis that assumes that each person received the treatment to which he or she was assigned. This, however, may yield an underestimate of the effects of a treatment if many subjects did not actually get the assigned treatment. If data are analyzed both ways and the outcomes are the same, researchers can have more confidence in the results. Another alternative is to include measures of the dose of treatment received into the analysis. Of course, one difficulty with an intention to treat analysis is that it is often difficult to obtain outcome data for those subjects who have dropped out of a treatment.

Example of intention to treat analysis: Dougherty and her colleagues (2002) used an experimental design to test an intervention to manage symptoms of urinary incontinence among older rural women. They used the intention-to-treat

approach: women in the experimental group remained in that group even if they failed to comply with the study protocol; and control group members remained in the control group even if they learned a technique that was part of the intervention and practiced it on their own.

In a crossover design, history is a potential threat both because an external event could differentially affect subjects in different treatment orderings and because the different orderings are in themselves a kind of differential history. The *substantive* analysis of the data involves comparing the dependent variable under treatment A versus treatment B. The analysis of bias, by contrast, involves a comparison of subjects in the different orderings (e.g., A then B versus B then A). If there are significant differences between the two orderings, then this is evidence of an **ordering bias**.

In summary, efforts to enhance the internal validity of a study should not end once the design strategy has been put in place. Researchers should seek additional opportunities to understand (and possibly to correct) the various threats to internal validity that can arise.

CONSTRUCT VALIDITY

Research cannot be undertaken without using constructs. When researchers conduct a study with specific exemplars of treatments, outcomes, settings, and people, these are all stand-ins for general constructs. Construct validity involves inferences from the particulars of the study to the higher-order constructs that they are intended to represent. Construct validity is important because constructs are the means for linking the operations used in a study to a relevant conceptualization and to mechanisms for translating the resulting evidence into practice. If studies contain construct errors, there is a risk that the evidence will be misleading.

Enhancing Construct Validity

The first step in fostering construct validity is a careful explication of the treatment (or independent variable), outcome, setting, and person constructs of interest, and the next step is to carefully select instances that match those constructs as closely as possible. Construct validity is further cultivated when researchers assess the match between the exemplars and the constructs and the degree to which any "slippage" occurred.

Construct validity has most often been a concern to researchers in connection with the measurement of outcomes, an issue we discuss at greater length in Chapter 17. However, there is a growing interest in the careful conceptualization and development of theory-based interventions in which the treatment itself has strong construct validity (e.g., Sidani & Braden, 1998). It is just as important for the independent variable (whether it be an intervention or something not amenable to experimental manipulation) to be a strong instance of the construct of interest as it is for the measurement of the dependent variable to have strong correspondence to the outcome construct. In nonexperimental research, researchers do not create and manipulate the hypothesized cause, so ensuring construct validity of the independent variable is often more difficult.

Shadish and colleagues (2002) broadened the concept of construct validity to cover persons and settings as well as outcomes and treatments. For example, some nursing interventions specifically target groups that are characterized as "disadvantaged," but there is not always agreement on how this term is defined and operationalized. Researchers select specific people to represent the construct of a disadvantaged group about which inferences will be made, and so it is important that the specific people are good exemplars of the underlying construct. The construct "disadvantaged" must be carefully delineated before a sample is selected. Similarly, if a researcher is interested in such settings as "immigrant neighborhoods" or "school-based clinics" or "nursing homes," these are constructs that require careful definition and description—and the selection of exemplars that match that setting construct. Qualitative description is often a powerful means of demonstrating the construct validity of settings.

Threats to Construct Validity

Threats to construct validity concern reasons that inferences from a particular study exemplar to an abstract construct could be erroneous. Such a threat could occur if the operationalization of the construct fails to incorporate all the relevant characteristics of the underlying construct, or it could occur if it includes extraneous content—both of which are instances of a mismatch. Shadish and colleagues (2002) identified 14 threats to construct validity (their Table 3.1) and several additional threats specific to case-control designs (their Table 4.3). Among the most noteworthy threats are the following:

1. *Reactivity to the study situation.* As discussed in Chapter 10, subjects may behave in a particular manner largely because they are aware of their participation in a study (i.e., the Hawthorne or placebo effect). When participant responses reflect, in part, their perceptions about participation in an intervention study, those perceptions become part of the treatment construct that is under study. There are several ways to reduce this problem, including masking or blinding, using outcome measures less susceptible to reactivity (e.g., information from hospital records), and using preintervention strategies to satisfy participants' desire to look competent or please the researcher.

Example of a possible Hawthorne effect:
Nes and Posso (2005) tested the efficacy of low-intensity laser therapy for reducing pain in patients with chemotherapy-induced oral mucositis. Over the course of the 5-day treatment, there was a significant decrease in the daily average pain levels before and after each treatment. The design did not include a control group, and so the researchers speculated that the results could partially reflect a Hawthorne (or placebo) effect.

2. *Researcher expectancies.* A similar threat stems from the researcher's influence on participant responses through subtle (or not-so-subtle) communication about desired out-

comes. When this happens, the researcher's expectations become part of the treatment (or nonmanipulated independent variable) construct that is being tested. Masking is a strategy to reduce this threat, but another strategy is to use observations during the course of the study to detect behavioral signals of expectations and correct them.

3. *Novelty effects.* When a treatment is new, subjects and research agents alike might alter their behavior in various ways. People may be either enthusiastic or skeptical about new methods of doing things. Results may reflect reactions to the novelty rather than to the intrinsic nature of an intervention, and so the intervention construct is clouded by novelty content.

4. *Compensatory effects.* In intervention studies, *compensatory equalization* can occur if health care staff or family members try to compensate for the control group members' failure to receive a perceived beneficial treatment. The compensatory goods or services must then be part of the construct description of the treatment conditions. *Compensatory rivalry* is a related threat arising from the control group members' desire to demonstrate that they can do as well as those who are receiving a special treatment.

5. *Treatment diffusion or contamination.* Sometimes alternative treatment conditions can get blurred, which can impede good construct descriptions of the independent variable. This may occur when participants in a control group condition receive services similar to those available in the treatment condition. More often, however, blurring occurs when those in a treatment condition essentially put themselves into the control group by dropping out of the intervention or not fully participating in it. This threat can also occur in nonexperimental studies. For example, in case-control comparisons of smokers and nonsmokers, care must be taken during screening to ensure that study participants are, in fact, appropriately categorized (e.g., some people may consider themselves non-

smokers even though they regularly smoke, but on weekends only).

Construct validity requires careful attention to what we *call* things (i.e., construct labels) so that appropriate construct inferences can be made. Enhancing construct validity in a study requires careful thought before a study is undertaken, in terms of a well-considered explication of constructs, and also requires poststudy scrutiny to assess the degree to which a match between operations and constructs was achieved.

EXTERNAL VALIDITY

External validity concerns inferences about the extent to which relationships observed in a study hold true over variations in people, conditions, and settings, as well as over variations in treatments and outcomes. External validity has emerged as a very major concern in an EBP world in which there is an interest in generalizing evidence from tightly controlled research settings to real-world clinical practice settings.

As Shadish and colleagues (2002) have noted, external validity questions may take on several different forms. For example, we may wish to ask whether relationships observed with a study sample can be generalized to a larger population—for example, whether results from a smoking cessation program found effective with pregnant teenagers in Boston can be generalized to pregnant teenagers in the United States. Many EBP questions, however, are about going from a broad study group to a *particular* client—for example, whether the pelvic muscle exercises found to be effective in alleviating urinary incontinence in one study are an effective strategy for Mary Smith. Other external validity questions are about generalizing to types of people, settings, situations, or treatments unlike those in the research. For example, can findings about a pain reduction treatment in a study of Australian women be generalized to women in the United States? Or, would a 6-week intervention to promote dietary changes in patients with diabetes be equally effective if the content were condensed into a 3-week program? Sometimes new studies are needed to answer questions about external validity, but sometimes external validity can be enhanced by decisions that the researcher makes in designing a study.

Enhancements to External Validity

One aspect of external validity concerns the *representativeness* of the exemplars used in the study. For example, if the sample is selected to be representative of the population to which the researcher wishes to generalize the results, then the findings can more readily be applied to a broader group (see Chapter 13 for sampling designs). Similarly, if the settings in which the study occurs are representative of the clinical settings in which the findings might be applied, then inferences about causes and effects in those other settings can be strengthened.

An important concept relevant to external validity is that of *replication*. Multi-site studies are powerful because more confidence in the generalizability of the results can be attained if those results have been replicated in several sites—particularly if those sites are different on dimensions considered important (e.g., size, nursing skill mix, and so on). Studies involving a heterogeneous sample of study participants can test whether study results are replicated for various subgroups of the sample—for example, whether relationships hold or intervention benefits accrue for men *and* women, or older *and* younger patients. Systematic reviews represent a crucial aid to external validity precisely because they focus on replications across time, space, people, and settings to explore whether relationships hold true.

Another issue concerns attempts to use or create study situations as similar as possible to real-world circumstances. The real world is a "messy" place from a research point of view: constancy of conditions may be desired to achieve standardization, but external validity can be imperiled if the study conditions are too artificial. For example, if nurses require 10 days of extra training to implement a promising intervention, we might ask how realistic it would be for administrators to devote resources to such training.

Threats to External Validity

In the previous chapter we discussed *interaction effects* that can occur in a factorial design when two treatments are simultaneously manipulated. The interaction question is whether the effects of treatment A hold (are comparable) for all levels of treatment B. Conceptually, questions regarding external validity are similar to this interaction question. Threats to external validity concern ways in which relationships might interact with or be moderated by variations in people, settings, time, and conditions. Shadish and colleagues (2002) described several threats to external validity, such as the following two:

1. *Interaction between relationships and people.* An effect observed with certain types of people might not be observed with other types of people. A common complaint about some RCTs is that many people are excluded not because they would not benefit from the treatment, but rather because of extraneous characteristics (e.g., cognitively impaired patients, non-English speakers). During the 1980s, the widely held perception that clinical trials were disproportionately conducted with white males led to changes in funding policies to ensure that treatment by gender and ethnicity subgroup interactions were explored.

2. *Interaction between causal effects and treatment variation.* An innovative treatment might be effective because it is paired with other elements, and sometimes those elements are intangible—for example, an enthusiastic and dedicated project director. The same "treatment" could never be totally replicated, and thus different results could be obtained in subsequent tests.

Shadish and colleagues (2002) noted that moderators of relationships are the norm, not the exception. With interventions, for example, it is normal for a treatment to "work better" for some people than for others. Thus, in thinking about external validity, the primary issue is whether there is constancy of a relationship (or constancy of causation), and not whether the *magnitude* of the effect is constant.

TRADEOFFS AND PRIORITIES IN STUDY VALIDITY

Quantitative researchers strive to design studies that are strong with respect to all four types of study validity. Sometimes, efforts to increase one type of study validity will also benefit another type. In some instances, however, the requirements for ensuring one type of validity interfere with the possibility of achieving others.

Let us take an example. Suppose we were undertaking an RCT study and went to great lengths to ensure intervention fidelity. Our efforts might include strong training of intervention agents, careful monitoring of delivery and receipt of the intervention, manipulation checks, and steps to maximize participants' adherence to treatment conditions (e.g., monetary incentives). Such efforts to strengthen intervention fidelity would have positive effects on statistical conclusion validity because the treatment was made as powerful as possible. Internal validity would be enhanced if attrition biases were minimized as a result of high levels of adherence. Intervention fidelity would also improve the construct validity of the treatment because the content delivered and received would better match the underlying construct. But what about external validity? All of the actions undertaken to ensure that the intervention is strong, construct-valid, and administered according to plan are not consistent with the realities of clinical settings. People are not normally paid to adhere to treatments, nurses are not monitored and corrected to ensure that they are following a script, training in the use of new protocols is usually brief, and so on.

This example illustrates that researchers need to give careful thought to how design decisions may affect various aspects of study validity. Of particular concern are the tradeoffs between internal and external validity.

Internal Validity and External Validity

There is considerable tension between the goals of achieving internal validity and external validity. Many of the control mechanisms that are designed to rule out competing explanations for hypothesized cause-and-effect relationships make it difficult to infer that the relationship holds true in uncontrolled real-life settings.

Internal validity was asserted to be the "*sine qua non*" of experimental research in an early influential treatise on research design (Campbell & Stanley, 1963, p. 5). The rationale, essentially, was this: If there is insufficient evidence that an intervention really caused a desired effect, why worry about generalizing the results? This high priority given to internal validity, however, is somewhat at odds with the current emphasis on evidence-based practice. The question that some are now posing is this: If study results can't be generalized and used in real-world clinical settings, who *cares* if the study has strong internal validity? Clearly, both internal and external validity are important to building an evidence base for nursing practice.

There are several "solutions" to the conflict between internal and external validity. The first (and perhaps most prevalent) approach is to emphasize one and sacrifice the other. Following a long tradition of field experimentation based on Campbell and Stanley's advice, it is often external validity that is sacrificed.

A second approach that is common in medical trials is to use a phased series of studies. In the earlier phase, there are tight controls, strict intervention protocols, and stringent criteria for including subjects in the RCT. Such studies are referred to as **efficacy studies**. Once the intervention has been deemed to be effective under tightly controlled conditions in which internal validity was the priority, it is tested with larger samples in multiple sites under less restrictive conditions, in what is referred to as **effectiveness studies** that emphasize external validity.

A third approach is to compromise. There has been recent interest in promoting designs that aim to achieve a balance between internal and external validity in a single intervention study. Such **practical (or pragmatic) clinical trials** (Glasgow, Lichtenstein, & Marcus, 2003; Glasgow et al., 2005; Tunis, Stryer, & Clancy, 2003), which will be described more fully in Chapter 12, attempt to maximize external validity with the smallest possible negative effect on internal validity.

Efforts to improve the generalizability of health care research evidence have given rise to a framework for designing and evaluating intervention research called the **RE-AIM framework** (e.g., Glasgow, 2006). The framework involves a scrutiny of five aspects of a study: its **R**each, **E**fficacy, **A**doption, **I**mplementation, and **M**aintenance. *Reach* means reaching the intended population of potential beneficiaries, which concerns the extent to which study participants have characteristics that reflect that population. *Efficacy* concerns the impact of the intervention on critical outcomes. *Adoption* concerns the number, proportion, and representativeness of settings and staff who are willing to implement the

intervention. *Implementation* concerns the consistency of delivering the intervention as intended, and also the cost of the intervention. The last component, *maintenance*, involves a consideration of the extent to which, at the individual level, outcomes are maintained over time and, at the institutional level, the extent to which the intervention becomes part of routine practices and policies. Table 11.3 summarizes some of the key planning questions for each of these five components. Detailed information about this exciting new framework and advice on how to enhance and assess the five components is available at *http://www.re-aim.org.*

⊃ TIP: The Toolkit with the accompanying *Resource Manual* includes a table listing a number of strategies that can be used to enhance the external validity of a study. The table identifies the potential consequence of each strategy for other types of study validity.

TABLE 11.3 Key Planning Questions Within the RE-AIM Framework

RE-AIM COMPONENT	PLANNING QUESTIONS
Reach	• How can I reach those who need the intervention? • How can I design the intervention and the research so as to persuade those who need it to try it?
Efficacy	• How can I plan the intervention to maximize its efficacy? • How can I design the research to maximize the potential to detect it?
Adoption	• How can I best select study sites to represent environments where the intervention might be implemented? • How can I develop organizational support for the delivery of my intervention?
Implementation	• What can I do to enhance the likelihood that the intervention is delivered properly? • How can I best assess and document the extent to which intervention fidelity occurred?
Maintenance	• How can I design the intervention so as to encourage long-term maintenance of needed behaviors? • What can I do to enhance the likelihood that the intervention is maintained and delivered over the long term?

BOX 11.1 Guidelines for Critiquing Design Elements and Study Validity in Quantitative Studies

1. Did the operationalization of the independent variable (e.g., the intervention and the counterfactual) create strong contrasts that enhanced statistical power? Was precision enhanced by controlling confounding variables? If hypotheses were not supported (e.g., a hypothesized relationship was not found), is it possible that statistical conclusion validity was compromised?
2. In intervention studies, is there evidence that attention was paid to intervention fidelity? For example, were staff adequately trained? Was the implementation of the intervention monitored? Was attention paid to both the delivery and receipt of the intervention?
3. What evidence does the report provide that selection biases were eliminated or minimized? What steps were taken to control confounding subject characteristics that could affect the comparability of groups being compared? Were these steps adequate?
4. To what extent did the study design rule out the plausibility of other threats to internal validity, such as history, attrition, and so on? What are your overall conclusions about the internal validity of the study?
5. Were there any major threats to the construct validity of the study? In intervention studies, was there a good match between the underlying conceptualization of the intervention and its operationalization? Was the intervention "pure," or was it confounded with extraneous content, such as researcher expectations? Was the setting or site a good exemplar of the type of setting envisioned in the conceptualization?
6. Was the context of the study sufficiently described to enhance its external validity? Were the setting or subjects representative of the types to which results were designed to be generalized? Were there efforts to understand whether observed relationships "held" for key subgroups?
7. Overall, did the researcher appropriately balance validity concerns? Was attention paid to certain types of threats (e.g., internal validity) at the expense of others (e.g., external validity)?

Prioritization and Design Decisions

It is, unfortunately, not possible to design a study so as to avoid all possible threats to study validity. By understanding the various threats, however, researchers can come to conclusions about the kinds of tradeoffs they are willing to make to achieve their study goals. Some threats are more worrisome than others in terms of both the likelihood of occurrence and consequences to the inferences researchers want to make. And some threats are more costly to avoid than others. Resources available for a study must be allocated so that there is a correspondence between expenditures and the importance of different types of validity. For example, with a fixed budget, researchers need to decide whether it is better to increase the size of the sample and hence power (statistical conclusion validity), or to use the money on efforts to reduce attrition from the study (internal validity).

The point here is that researchers should make conscious decisions about how to structure a study to address validity concerns. Every design decision has both a "payoff" and a cost in terms of study integrity. Being cognizant of the effects that design decisions have on the quality of research evidence is a responsibility that nurse researchers should attend to so that their evidence can have the largest possible impact on clinical practice.

TIP: A useful strategy is to create a matrix that lists various design decisions in rows of the first column (e.g., randomization to conditions), and then use the next four columns to identify the potential impact of those decisions on the four types of study validity. (In some cells, there may be no entry if there are no consequences of a design element for a given type of validity.) A sixth column could be added for estimates of the design element's financial implications, if any. The

Toolkit of the accompanying *Resource Manual* includes a model matrix as a Word document for you to use and adapt.

CRITIQUING GUIDELINES FOR STUDY VALIDITY

As noted in the previous chapter, research design decisions have a large impact on the quality of evidence that a quantitative study yields, especially if causal inferences about relationships are of concern. In critiquing a research report to evaluate its potential to contribute to nursing practice, it is crucial to make judgments about the extent to which threats to validity were minimized—or, at least, assessed and taken into consideration during the interpretation of the results.

The guidelines in Box 11.1 ⊗ focus on validity-related issues to further help you in the critique of quantitative research designs. Together with the critiquing guidelines in the previous chapter, they are likely to be the core of a strong critical evaluation of the evidence that quantitative studies yield. From an EBP perspective, it is important to remember that drawing inferences about causal relationships relies not only on how high up on the evidence hierarchy a study is (see Figure 2.1), but also, for any given level of the hierarchy, on how successful the researcher was in managing study validity and balancing competing validity demands.

RESEARCH EXAMPLE

We conclude this chapter with an example of a study that demonstrated careful attention to many aspects of study validity.

Study: "Effects of three groin compression methods on patient discomfort, distress, and vascular complications following a percutaneous coronary procedure" (Chlan, Sabo, & Savik, 2005)

Statement of Purpose: The purpose of the study was to determine which alternative groin compression methods (which are used to achieve femoral artery hemostasis during femoral sheath removal after a percutaneous coro-

nary intervention) caused less patient discomfort and distress and resulted in fewer vascular complications.

Treatment Groups: Three groin compression methods were compared: (1) the pneumatic device Femostop; (2) the C-clamp compression device; and (3) manual pressure at the groin puncture site.

Method: A sample of 306 patients undergoing percutaneous coronary procedures at an urban tertiary care hospital in the Midwestern United States were randomly assigned to one of the three compression methods. A random numbers table was used to allocate patients to conditions using the sealed envelope method. Patients rated their level of discomfort and distress before, during, and after arterial compression. The groin area was assessed for any vascular complications before sheath removal, after compression was released, and 12 and 24 hours after sheath removal.

Additional Study Validity Efforts: The researchers estimated how large a sample would be needed to achieve the power needed for statistical conclusion validity using a procedure called power analysis (see Chapter 13). Patients were excluded from the study on several grounds (e.g., if they were hemodynamically unstable, had a known groin pathology, had documented mental incompetence, could not read and write English). The researchers developed study protocols for the three compression methods, and trained 30 study nurses in their use. The nurses were required to demonstrate the required skills during training, and one of the investigators undertook spot checks for correctness of technique while the study was underway. The report suggests that masking was not used (e.g., the nurses who administered the compression gathered study data), but there was also no *a priori* hypothesis about methods. The researchers used measures of discomfort and distress that had previously been found to have construct validity. A comparison of patients in the three study groups indicated that the three groups were similar in terms of most baseline characteristics (e.g., body surface area, blood pressure, gender, medical complications, time spent in the cardiovascular lab). Time to hemostasis was found to be significantly different in the three groups, and this was controlled statistically. There was no attrition from the study.

Key Findings:

- There were no significant differences among the three groups in terms of discomfort, distress, or incidence of a vascular complication.
- The findings suggest an interaction: C-clamp contributed to less oozing when hemostasis time was less than 30 minutes, but Femostop was superior when time to hemostasis was more than 30 minutes.

○○○○○○○○○○○○○○○○○○○○○

SUMMARY POINTS

- Study validity concerns the extent to which appropriate inferences can be made. **Threats to validity** are reasons that an inference could be wrong. A key function of quantitative research design is to rule out validity threats by exercising various types of control.

- Control over extraneous subject characteristics is important to managing many validity threats. The ideal control method is random assignment to treatment conditions, which effectively controls for all possible confounding variables—especially within the context of a crossover design.

- When randomization is not possible, other control methods must be used. These include homogeneity (the use of a homogeneous sample of subjects to eliminate variability on extraneous characteristics); blocking or stratifying, as in the case of a randomized block design; **pair matching** subjects on key confounding variables to make groups more comparable (or **balanced design** of groups to achieve comparability); and **statistical control** to remove the effect of a confounding variable statistically (e.g., through **analysis of covariance**).

- Homogeneity, blocking, matching, and statistical control share two disadvantages: Researchers must know in advance which extraneous variables to control, and they are rarely able to control all of them.

- Four types of validity that affect the rigor of a quantitative study include statistical conclusion validity, internal validity, construct validity, and external validity.

- **Statistical conclusion validity** concerns the validity of inferences that there truly is an empirical relationship or correlation between variables (most often, the presumed cause and the effect).

- Threats to statistical conclusion validity include low **statistical power** (the ability to detect true relationships among variables); low **precision**

(the exactness of the relationships revealed after controlling extraneous variables); and factors that undermine a strong operationalization of the independent variable (e.g., a treatment), such as problems with implementation.

- **Intervention** (or **treatment**) **fidelity** concerns the extent to which the implementation of a treatment is faithful to its plan. Intervention fidelity is enhanced through efforts to standardize the treatment through protocols, to carefully train intervention agents, to monitor and measure the delivery and receipt of the intervention, to undertake appropriate **manipulation checks**, and to take steps to promote **treatment adherence** and avoid contamination of treatments.

- **Internal validity** concerns inferences that the outcomes of interest were caused by the independent variable, rather than by other factors extraneous to the research. Threats to internal validity include temporal ambiguity (lack of clarity about whether the presumed cause occurred before the outcome); **selection** (preexisting group differences); **history** (the occurrence of events external to an independent variable that could affect outcomes); **maturation** (changes resulting from the passage of time); **mortality** (effects attributable to subject attrition); **testing** (effects of a pretest on outcomes); and **instrumentation** (changes in the way data are gathered over time).

- **Internal validity** can be enhanced through judicious design decisions, but can also be addressed analytically (e.g., through an analysis of selection or attrition biases). When subjects withdraw from a study, an **intention to treat analysis** (analyzing outcomes for all people in their original treatment conditions) is preferred to an **on-protocol analysis** (analyzing outcomes only for those who received the condition to which they were assigned) for avoiding faulty inferences about treatment effects.

- **Construct validity** concerns inferences from the particular exemplars of a study (e.g., the specific treatments, outcomes, people, and settings) to the higher-order constructs that they are intended to represent. The first step in fostering construct validity is a careful explication of those constructs.

- Threats to construct validity can occur if the operationalization of a construct fails to incorporate all of the relevant characteristics of the construct, or if it includes extraneous content. Examples of such threats include subject reactivity, researcher expectancies, novelty effects, compensatory effects, and treatment diffusion.
- **External validity** concerns inferences about the extent to which study results can be generalized—that is, about whether relationships observed in a study hold true over variations in people, conditions, settings, outcome measures, and operationalizations of the independent variable. External validity can be enhanced through the use of representative people, settings, and so on, and through replication.
- Researchers need to prioritize and recognize tradeoffs among the various types of validity, which sometimes compete with each other. Tensions between internal and external validity are especially prominent. One solution has been to begin with a study that emphasizes internal validity (**efficacy studies**) and then if a causal relationship can be inferred, to undertake **effectiveness studies** that emphasize external validity.
- The **RE-AIM framework** (*Reach, Efficacy, Adoption, Implementation,* and *Maintenance*) is a model for designing and evaluating intervention research that is strong on multiple forms of study validity.

⬤⬤⬤⬤⬤⬤⬤⬤⬤⬤⬤⬤⬤⬤⬤⬤⬤⬤⬤

STUDY ACTIVITIES

Chapter 11 of the *Resource Manual to Accompany Nursing Research: Generating and Assessing Evidence for Nursing Practice, 8th edition*, offers various exercises and study suggestions for reinforcing the concepts presented in this chapter. In addition, the following study questions can be addressed:

1. How do you suppose the use of identical twins in a study could enhance control?
2. To the extent possible, apply the questions in Box 11.1 to the study described at the end of the chapter (by Chlan et al., 2005).

⬤⬤⬤⬤⬤⬤⬤⬤⬤⬤⬤⬤⬤⬤⬤⬤⬤⬤⬤

STUDIES CITED IN CHAPTER 11

Methodologic or theoretical references cited in this chapter can be found in a separate section at the end of the book.

Chlan, L., Sabo, J., & Savik, K. (2005). Effects of three groin compression methods on patient discomfort, distress, and vascular complications following a percutaneous coronary procedure. *Nursing Research, 54*(6), 391–398.

Dougherty, M., Dwyer, J., Pendergast, J., Boyington, A., Tomlinson, B., Coward, R., Duncan, R. P., Vogel, B., & Rooks, L. (2002). A randomized trial of behavioral management for continence with older rural women. *Research in Nursing & Health, 25,* 3–13.

Moser, D. K., & Dracup, K. (2000). Impact of cardiopulmonary resuscitation training on perceived control in spouses of recovering cardiac patients. *Research in Nursing & Health, 23,* 270–278.

Nes, A. G., & Posso, M. B. (2005). Patients with moderate chemotherapy-induced mucositis: Pain therapy using low intensity lasers. *International Nursing Review, 52*(1), 68–72.

Oka, R. K., & Sanders, M. G. (2005). The impact of exercise on body composition and nutritional intake in patients with heart failure. *Progress in Cardiovascular Nursing, 20*(4), 148–154.

Phuphaibul, R., Thanooruk, R., Leucha, Y., Sirao-ngam, Y., & Kanobdee, C. (2005). The impacts of the "Immune for Life" for teens module application on the coping behaviors and mental health of early adolescents. *Journal of Pediatric Nursing, 10*(6), 461–468.

Resnick, B., Inguito, P., Orwig, D., Yahiro, J., Hawkes, W., Werner, M., Zimmerman, S., & Magaziner, J. (2005). Treatment integrity in behavior change research. *Nursing Research, 54*(2), 139–143.

Talashek, M. L., Alba, M. L., & Patel, A. (2006). Untangling health disparities of teen pregnancy. *Journal for Specialists in Pediatric Nursing, 11*(1), 14–27.

12

Undertaking Research for Specific Purposes

A ll quantitative studies can be categorized as experimental, quasi-experimental, or non-experimental in design, as discussed in Chapter 10. And, most qualitative studies lie within one of the research traditions described in Chapter 9. This chapter describes types of research that vary according to the study purpose rather than according to research design or tradition. Several of the types discussed in this chapter involve combining both qualitative and quantitative approaches, and so we begin by first discussing such mixed method research.

MIXED METHOD RESEARCH

An emerging trend, and one that we believe will gain momentum, is the planned integration of qualitative and quantitative data within single studies or coordinated clusters of studies. This section discusses the rationale for such **mixed method** studies and presents a few applications.

Rationale for Mixed Method Studies

The dichotomy between quantitative and qualitative data represents a key methodologic distinction in the social, behavioral, and health sciences. Some argue that the paradigms that underpin qualitative and quantitative research are fundamentally incompatible. Others, however, believe that many areas of inquiry can be enriched and the evidence base enhanced through the judicious triangulation of qualitative and quantitative data. The advantages of a mixed method design include the following:

- *Complementarity.* One argument for blending qualitative and quantitative approaches is that they are complementary; they represent words and numbers, the two fundamental languages of human communication. Researchers address problems with fallible methods. By using mixed methods, researchers can allow each to do what it does best, possibly avoiding the limitations of a single approach.

- *Incrementality.* Progress on a topic tends to be incremental, relying on feedback loops. Qualitative findings can generate hypotheses to be tested quantitatively, and quantitative findings sometimes need clarification through in-depth probing. It can be productive to build such a loop into the design of a study.

- *Enhanced validity.* When a hypothesis or model is supported by multiple and complementary types of data, researchers can be more confident about the validity of their results. The use of a single approach can leave the study vulnerable to at least one (and often more than one) validity problem, such as those discussed in Chapter 11. The triangulation of methods can provide opportunities for testing alternative interpretations of the data, for examining the extent to which the context helped to shape the results, and for arriving at convergence in tapping a construct.

Perhaps the strongest argument for mixed methods research, however, is that certain questions *require* a mixed methods approach. **Pragmatism**, the paradigm that is most often associated with mixed methods research, provides a basis for asserting the "dictatorship of the research question" (Tashakkori & Teddlie, 2003, p. 21). Pragmatist researchers consider that it is the research question that should drive the inquiry, and that the question is more important than the methods used. They reject a forced choice between the traditional postpositivists' and naturalists' modes of inquiry.

Applications of Mixed Method Research

Mixed method research can be used to address various research goals. We illustrate a few applications here, and others will be discussed later in this chapter.

Instrumentation

Researchers sometimes collect qualitative data for the development and validation of formal, quantitative instruments used in research or clinical applications. The questions for a formal instrument are sometimes derived from clinical experience, theory, or prior research. When a construct is new, however, these mechanisms may be inadequate to capture its full complexity and dimensionality. A researcher's knowledge base, no matter how rich, is subjective and limited, and thus nurse researchers sometimes gather qualitative data as the basis for generating questions for quantitative instruments that are subsequently subjected to rigorous testing, as described in Chapter 18. Gilgun (2004) provides some guidance on how qualitative methods can be used in the development of clinical assessment tools.

Example of instrumentation: Beck and Gable (2000) developed the Postpartum Depression Screening Scale (PDSS), an instrument that screens new mothers for the mood disorder that can develop after delivering a baby. Scale items were based on in-depth interviews of mothers suffering from postpartum depression in a grounded theory study and two phenomenological studies. Here is an example of how items on the PDSS were developed from mothers' quotes. The quote "I was extremely obsessive with my thoughts. They would never stop. I could not control them" was developed into the item: I could not control the thoughts that kept coming into my mind (Beck & Gable, 2001).

Hypothesis Generation and Testing

In-depth qualitative studies are often fertile with insights about constructs or relationships among them. These insights then can be tested and confirmed with larger samples in quantitative studies. This most often happens in the context of discrete investigations. One problem, however, is that it usually takes years to do a study and publish the results, which means that considerable time may elapse between the qualitative insights and the formal quantitative testing of hypotheses based on those insights. A research team interested in a phenomenon might wish to collaborate in a project that has hypothesis generation and testing as an explicit goal.

Example of hypothesis generation: McClement and colleagues (2004) used qualitative and quantitative methods to develop a comprehensive understanding of the concept of *dignity* in terminally ill patients. Analysis of data from in-depth interviews with 50 palliative cancer patients resulted in a model of dignity and the generation of hypotheses about factors influencing patients' perceptions of dignity. The quantitative data were used to examine how disease-specific variables were related to dignity.

Explication

Qualitative data are sometimes used to explicate the *meaning* of quantitative descriptions or relationships. Quantitative methods can demonstrate that variables are systematically related but may fail to provide insights about *why* they are related. Such explications help to clarify important concepts and to corroborate the findings from the statistical analysis; they also help to illuminate the analysis and give guidance to the interpretation of results. Qualitative materials can be used to explicate specific statistical findings and to provide more global and dynamic views of the phenomena under study, sometimes in the form of illustrative case studies.

Example of explicating description with qualitative data: Polit, London, and Martinez (2001) conducted a mixed method study of poor urban families and, in the quantitative component, found that food insecurity and hunger were experienced by more than 50% of the families. Data from the ethnographic component was used to explicate how food insecurity was actually experienced and managed. Here is one example: *"It was hard, especially when you got kids at home saying, 'I'm hungry.'... I was doing very odd jobs that most people would not dare to do. I was making deliveries on pizza in bad neighborhoods where most people wouldn't go. I mean, I literally took my life in my own hands"* (p. 58).

Example of explicating relationships with qualitative data: Benzies, Harrison, and Magill-Evans (2004a, 2004b) collected both qualitative and quantitative data about child behavior problems. The longitudinal study of preterm and full-term infants, with follow-up when the children were age 7, included quantitative measures that allowed the researchers to examine factors predictive of the behavior problems—including parental stress during infancy. The qualitative data, based on an intensive study of four families, allowed the researchers to more fully understand the interaction of parental stress and stressful life circumstances on the one hand and children's problem behaviors on the other.

Theory Building, Testing, and Refinement

A particularly ambitious application of mixed method research is in the area of theory construction. A theory gains acceptance as it escapes disconfirmation, and the use of multiple methods provides great opportunity for potential disconfirmation of a theory. If the theory can survive these assaults, it can provide a stronger context for the organization of clinical and intellectual work.

Example of theory building: Morgan and Stewart (2002) conducted a mixed method evaluation of a dementia special care unit in a midwestern Canadian city that involved a quasi-experimental component and a grounded theory component. The study led to a better understanding of how the nursing home environment affects residents with dementia, which in turn helped to advance theory development in person–environment interaction.

Intervention Development

Qualitative research is beginning to play an increasingly important role in the development of promising nursing interventions and in efforts to test their efficacy and effectiveness. For example, Van Meijel and colleagues (2004) have proposed a model for developing evidence-based nursing interventions that relies heavily on qualitative research—with particular emphasis on understanding the diversity and complexity of clients' needs and preferences. Morse (2006a) has written a particularly useful discussion about qualitatively derived clinical interventions. There is also a growing recognition that the development of effective interventions must be based on some understanding of why people might not adhere to intervention protocols, or of the barriers they face in participating in a treatment. Intervention research is increasingly likely to be mixed method research.

Example of developmental research: Fonteyn and Bauer-Wu (2005) used qualitative methods to improve and refine a complementary therapy intervention (mindfulness meditation) for patients undergoing stem cell or autologous bone marrow transplantation. They conducted in-depth interviews with 19 patients to ascertain what participants liked and disliked, and to examine suggestions for improving the intervention.

Mixed Method Designs and Strategies

The growth in interest in mixed methods research in recent years has given rise to numerous typologies of mixed methods designs. Green and Caracelli (1997) clustered designs into two broad categories that they labeled *component designs* and *integrated designs*.

In studies with a **component design**, the qualitative and quantitative aspects are implemented as discrete components of the overall inquiry, and remain distinct during data collection and analysis. Combining the qualitative and quantitative components occurs during the interpretation and reporting phases of the project. The study by Polit and colleagues (2001), described earlier, illustrates a component design. Quantitative data were collected longitudinally from nearly 4000 women in four major cities in the United States. Longitudinal ethnographic data were collected from a small number of women in the same cities, by different researchers.

In mixed method studies with an **integrated design**, there is greater integration of the method types at all phases of the project, from the development of research questions, through data collection and analysis, to the interpretation of the results. The blending of data occurs in ways that integrate the elements from the different paradigms and offers the possibility of yielding more insightful understandings of the phenomenon under study. The previously described mixed method research by McClement and colleagues (e.g., 2004) focusing on *dignity* in dying patients exemplifies an integrated design.

Sandelowski (2000b) offered an alternative typology of mixed method designs. She used a notation system developed by Morse (1991a) that has been adopted by several mixed methods methodologists (see various writings in the excellent handbook by Tashakkori and Teddlie, 2003). The scheme focuses on two key design dimensions for a mixed methods study: (1) which approach (qualitative or quantitative) has priority, and (2) how the approaches are sequenced in a study. In this notation system, priority is designated by upper case and lower case letters: *QUAL* and *quan* designate a mixed methods study in which the dominant approach is qualitative, whereas *QUAN* and *qual* designate the reverse. If neither approach is dominant (i.e., both are equal), the notation stipulates *QUAL* and *QUAN*. Sequencing is indicated by the symbols + or →. For example, with sequential data collection, the arrow is used: *QUAN* → *qual* represents the notation for a primarily quantitative mixed method study in which qualitative data collection occurs after quantitative data collection. When both types of data collection occur concurrently, the plus sign is used (e.g., *QUAL* + *quan*). Morse's scheme makes clear that mixed method studies involve important design decisions about how to order data collection. In some cases there are important advantages to timing the approaches so that the second phase builds on knowledge gained in the first.

Using this notation, Sandelowski (2000b) developed a useful matrix that indicates the kinds of objectives that can be addressed with alternative design configurations. For example, in her Template Design #1, the qualitative approach is the dominant one and quantitative data are viewed as an adjunct. The quantitative data, which are collected concurrently with or after the qualitative data, are used to provide measured description, validation, and formal generalizations. Template Design #4, by contrast, involves qualitative data occurring before (and as an adjunct to) the quantitative portion of the study. Such a design is used when the aim is to generate questions for a quantitative instrument, or to generate hypotheses to be tested formally.

Strategies for collecting and analyzing data in mixed methods studies are continually evolving, and considerable guidance about how to productively triangulate qualitative and quantitative methods is now available—although exciting methodologic challenges remain (e.g., Brewer & Hunter, 2006; Creswell, 2003; Happ et al., 2006; Tashakkori & Teddlie, 2003). Moffatt and colleagues (2006) have written an interesting paper that offers suggestions about how to deal with (and capitalize on) situations in which the mixed method findings conflict.

Although mixed method approaches can be used in a variety of contexts, they are becoming increasingly valuable in research involving interventions, which we discuss next.

RESEARCH THAT INVOLVES INTERVENTIONS

Interventions are developed and tested in many practice and policy-related disciplines, and evidence from intervention research is increasingly being used to guide decisions in a variety of real-world applications. Different disciplines have developed their own methods and terminology in connection with evidence-based practice efforts. Nurse researchers, who have been doctorally trained in several different disciplines, have used a rich assortment of approaches. There is overlap among these approaches, but to acquaint you with relevant terms, we discuss each separately. Clinical trials are associated with medical research; evaluation research is undertaken in the fields of education, social work, and public policy; and nurses are developing their own tradition of intervention research.

Clinical Trials

Clinical trials are studies designed to assess clinical interventions. Methods associated with clinical trials were developed primarily in the context of medical research, but the vocabulary is being used by many nurse researchers.

Phases of a Full Clinical Trial

In medical and pharmaceutical research, clinical trials often adhere to a well-planned sequence of activities. Clinical trials undertaken to test a new drug or an innovative therapy often are designed in a series of four phases, as described by the U.S. National Institutes of Health, as follows:

- *Phase I* of the trial occurs after the initial development of the drug or therapy, and is designed primarily to establish safety and tolerance and to determine optimal dose or strength of the therapy. This phase typically involves small-scale studies using simple designs (e.g., before–after design without a control group). The focus is not on efficacy, but on developing the best possible (and safest) treatment.
- *Phase II* of the trial involves seeking preliminary evidence of the effectiveness of the treatment as it has been designed in Phase I. During this phase, researchers ascertain the feasibility of launching a more rigorous test, seek evidence

that the treatment holds promise, look for signs of possible side effects, and identify refinements to improve the intervention. This phase is sometimes considered a pilot test of the treatment, and may be designed either as a small-scale experiment or as a quasi-experiment.

Example of an early-phase clinical trial: Olson, Hanson, and Michaud (2003) conducted a phase II trial that compared pain levels, quality of life, and analgesic use with a sample of 24 Canadian cancer patients who received either standard opioid pain management plus Reiki or standard pain opioid management plus rest.

- *Phase III* is a full experimental test of the treatment—a randomized clinical trial (RCT) involving random assignment to an experimental or control group (or to orderings of treatment conditions) under tightly controlled conditions. The objective of this phase is to develop evidence about the treatment's *efficacy*—that is, whether the innovation is more efficacious than the standard treatment (or an alternative counterfactual). Adverse effects are also monitored. When the term *clinical trial* is used in the nursing literature, it most often is referring to a Phase III trial. Phase III RCTs often involve the use of a large and heterogeneous sample of subjects, sometimes selected from multiple, geographically dispersed sites to ensure that findings are not unique to a single setting, and to increase the sample size and hence the power of the statistical tests. Multisite clinical trials are challenging administratively, requiring strong oversight and good systems of communication, staff supervision, and data management.

Example of a multi-site Phase III RCT: A nurse-managed intervention called the Women's Initiative for Nonsmoking (WINS), developed on the basis of a well-tested smoking cessation intervention, was tailored specifically to meet the needs of women (Martin, Froelicher, & Miller, 2000). Ten hospitals in the San Francisco area participated in the trial. In each hospital, 50% of the subjects were assigned to the 3-month experimental condition or to a "usual care" group. Follow-up data are being collected at 6, 12, 24, and 30 months after baseline. Findings from this large clinical trial have begun to appear in the literature (e.g., Mahrer-Imhof et al., 2002; Froelicher et al., 2004).

- *Phase IV* of clinical trials involves studies of the *effectiveness* of an intervention in the general population. As noted in Chapter 11, the emphasis in these effectiveness studies is on the external validity of an intervention that has shown promise of efficacy under controlled (but often artificial) conditions. Phase IV efforts often examine the cost-effectiveness and clinical utility of the new treatment. In pharmaceutical research, Phase IV trials typically focus on post-approval safety surveillance and on long-term consequences over a larger population and timescale than was possible during earlier phases.

◗ TIP: Some clinical trials are designed to test whether a new intervention is as good as an established one. These are sometimes called *equivalence trials, noninferiority trials,* or trials with *positive controls.* Such trials face certain challenges, as described by Friedman, Furberg, and DeMets (1998), especially with regard to statistical conclusion validity.

Sequential Clinical Trials

Traditional Phase III clinical trials have important drawbacks in certain situations. In particular, it may take many months to recruit and randomize a sufficiently large sample; this is especially problematic if the population being treated is relatively small (e.g., people with a rare disease). Relatedly, in a standard clinical trial, it may take years to draw conclusions about the intervention's efficacy (i.e., until all data have been collected and analyzed). An alternative is the **sequential clinical trial** in which experimental data are continuously analyzed as they become available. Results accumulate over time, so that the experiment can be stopped as soon as the evidence is strong enough to support a conclusion about the intervention's efficacy.

The design for this approach involves a series of "mini-experiments." The first patient is randomly assigned (e.g., by a coin toss) to either the experimental (E) or control (C) condition. The next patient is automatically assigned to the alternative condition, creating a series of randomized paired comparisons. Most sequential trials use measures indicating preference for either the E or C condition. *Preference,* defined on the basis of clinically meaningful outcomes, is measured dichotomously (e.g., improved/did not improve). Using such preference measures, each pair of subjects is compared, yielding three possibilities: E is preferred; C is preferred; or the two are tied; ties are usually thrown out. All remaining paired comparisons are plotted on graphs for which there are preestablished boundaries with decision rules.

An example of such a graph is presented in Figure 12.1. The horizontal axis in the middle of this graph indicates the number of randomized pairs (here, 30 pairs or 60 subjects). The vertical axis indicates which way the "preference" comparison turned out. When the preference for a given pair favors E, the plotted line goes up; when it favors C, the plotted line goes down. The red butterfly-shaped lines designate decision boundaries. In this example, the first comparison resulted in a preference for the new intervention, and so the graph plots a line from the origin to one unit up. The next comparison favored the control condition, and so the plot goes down for pair number two. This procedure continues until the plot crosses one of the boundaries, which designate three **stopping rules**. When the upper boundary (U) is crossed, we would conclude that the experimental treatment is more effective. When the lower boundary (L) is crossed, the conclusion is that the control condition is more effective. Finally, when the middle boundary (M) is crossed, the decision is reached that the two treatments are equally effective. In this example, we tested 18 nontied pairs and were then able to conclude that the E condition was significantly superior to the C condition.

Sequential trials have considerable appeal for clinical studies because decisions typically can be

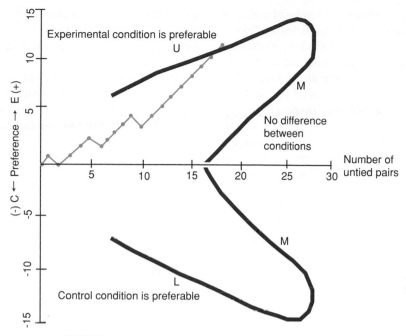

FIGURE 12.1 Example of a sequential clinical trial graph.

reached much earlier than with traditional designs. However, these trials are not always appropriate (e.g., when three conditions are being compared), or they are ambiguous if there are many ties. They may also be complicated if there are multiple outcomes for which preference has to be plotted separately. Portney and Watkins (2000) provide more information about sequential trials.

Practical Clinical Trials

The recent emphasis on evidence-based practice has underscored the importance of research evidence that can be used in real-world clinical situations. One of the problems with traditional Phase III RCTs is that, in an effort to enhance internal validity and the ability to infer causal pathways, the designs are so tightly controlled that their relevance to real-life applications comes into question. Concern about this situation has led to a call for **practical** (or **pragmatic**) **clinical trials**. Tunis, Stryer, & Clancy (2003), in an often-cited paper, defined practical clinical trials (PCTs) as "trials for which the hypotheses and study design are for-

mulated based on information needed to make a decision" (p. 1626).

PCTs address practical questions about the benefits and risks of an intervention—as well as its costs—as they would unfold in routine clinical practice. PCTs are thus sensitive to the issues under scrutiny in effectiveness (Phase IV) studies, but there is an increasing interest in developing strategies to bridge the gap between efficacy and effectiveness studies and to address issues of utility and practicality earlier in the evaluation of promising interventions. As Godwin and colleagues (2003) have noted, attempts to achieve methodologic purity in efficacy studies can result in clinically meaningless results, but efforts to achieve full generalizability should not sacrifice internal validity and yield unreliable evidence either—"achieving a creative tension between the two is crucial" (p. 28).

Suggestions about how to do this are emerging, and new strategies are likely to be developed in the years ahead. Tunis and co-authors (2003) made these recommendations for PCTs: enrollment of diverse study populations with fewer exclusions of high-risk patients; recruitment of study participants from a variety of practice settings; having a longer period of follow-up; inclusion of economic outcomes; and comparisons of clinically viable alternatives. Glasgow and colleagues (2005) expanded on the Tunis and co-researchers paper and proposed several research design options, including cluster randomization and delayed treatment designs. Carroll and Rounsaville (2003) discussed some options for **hybrid designs** that link efficacy and effectiveness research. Their suggestions combine features of traditional RCTs (e.g., random assignment, assessments of intervention fidelity) with elements of effectiveness research (e.g., assessments of the intervention's cost-effectiveness and of patient satisfaction, few restrictions on eligibility for the study).

Example of a PCT: Burton and Gibbon (2005) conducted a study that they described as a pragmatic clinical trial. They used an RCT design that randomly assigned patients with a diagnosis of stroke to either usual care or to special outreach services of education and support after hospital discharge. The intervention was tested in two hospitals in England.

➲ **TIP:** Godwin and colleagues (2003) prepared a useful table that contrasts features of an "explanatory trial" (i.e., a traditional Phase III RCT) and a pragmatic trial. The table can be accessed at *http://www.biomedcentral.com/content/supplementary/1471-2288-3-28-S1.doc.* This and other websites with material relevant to this chapter are included on a file on the accompanying CD-ROM so that you can "click" on them directly.

Evaluation Research

Evaluation research is an applied form of research whose methodologies have evolved within such fields as education and public policy. Evaluation research focuses on developing useful information about a program, practice, procedure, or policy—information that is needed by decision makers about whether to adopt, modify, or abandon a practice or program. Often (but not always), the evaluation is of a new intervention.

The term *evaluation research* is most often used when researchers are trying to determine the effectiveness of a rather complex program, rather than when they are evaluating a specific entity (e.g., alternative sterilizing solutions). Evaluation researchers tend to evaluate a program, practice, or intervention that is embedded in a political or organizational context. Evaluations often try to answer broader questions than simply whether an intervention is more effective than care as usual—for example, they often seek ways to improve the program (as in Phase II of a clinical trial) or to learn how the program actually "works" in practice.

Because of the complexity of evaluations and the programs on which they typically focus, many evaluations are mixed method studies using a component design. When a program is multidimensional, involving several distinct features or elements, there are often **black box** questions—that is, what is it about the program that is driving any observed effects? Such questions arise even when the outcomes are consistent with hypotheses.

Evaluation research plays an important role nationally. Evaluations are often the cornerstone of an area of research known as **policy research**. Nurses have become increasingly aware of the potential contribution their research can make to the formulation of national and local health policies and thus are undertaking evaluations that have implications for policies that affect the allocation of funds for health services (Wood, 2000).

In doing an evaluation, researchers often confront problems that are organizational, interpersonal, or political. Evaluation research can be threatening. Even when the focus of an evaluation is on a nontangible entity, such as a program, it is *people* who are implementing it. People tend to think that they, or their work, are being evaluated and may feel that their jobs or reputation are at stake. Thus, evaluation researchers need to have more than methodologic skills—they need to be diplomats, adept in interpersonal relations with people.

Evaluations are undertaken to answer a variety of questions about a program or policy. Some questions involve the use of an experimental (or quasi-experimental) design, but others do not. In evaluations of large-scale interventions (sometimes called **demonstrations** if they are implemented on a trial basis), evaluators may well undertake all the evaluation activities discussed here.

Process or Implementation Analysis

A **process** or **implementation analysis** is undertaken when there is a need for descriptive information about the process by which a program gets implemented and how it actually functions. A process analysis is typically designed to address such questions as the following: Does the program operate the way its designers intended (e.g., intervention fidelity)? What are the strongest and weakest aspects of the program? What exactly *is* the treatment, and how does it differ (if at all) from traditional practices? What were the barriers to implementing the program successfully? How do staff and clients feel about the intervention?

A process analysis may be undertaken with the aim of improving a new or ongoing program; in such a situation, it might be referred to as a **formative evaluation**. In other situations, the purpose of the process analysis is primarily to describe a program carefully so that it can be replicated by others—or so that people can better understand why the program was or was not effective in meeting its objectives. In either case, a process analysis involves an in-depth examination of the operation of a program, often involving a mixed method approach.

Example of a process analysis: Groner and colleagues (2005) conducted a process evaluation to assess the feasibility and acceptability of using home-health nurses to deliver a multi-component smoking relapse prevention program to new mothers. The researchers monitored how many women actually enrolled, whether the nurses were able to implement all five intervention components, and whether the intervention was acceptable to the women.

Outcome Analysis

Evaluations often focus on whether a program or policy is meeting its objectives. Evaluations that assess the worth of a program are sometimes referred to as **summative evaluations**, in contrast to formative evaluations. The intent of such evaluations is to help people decide whether the program should be discarded, replaced, continued, or replicated.

Many evaluation researchers distinguish between an outcome analysis and an impact analysis. An **outcome analysis** tends to be descriptive and does not use a rigorous experimental design. Such an analysis simply documents the extent to which the goals of the program are attained, that is, the extent to which positive outcomes occur. For example, a program may be designed to encourage women in a poor rural community to obtain prenatal care. An outcome analysis would document outcomes without rigorous comparisons. For example, the researchers might document the percentage of pregnant women in the community who had obtained prenatal care, the average month in which prenatal care was begun, and so on, and perhaps compare this information to existing preintervention community data.

Example of an outcome analysis: Valente and Nemec (2006) studied the outcomes of efforts to increase the rates of routine screening for depression and alcohol use disorders in primary care and home-based care. The intervention (a 1-hour educational program) was associated with an increase in screening rates from 50% to 80% up to 100%.

Impact Analysis

An **impact analysis** attempts to identify the **net impacts** of a program, that is, the impacts that can be attributed exclusively to the program over and above the effects of the counterfactual (e.g., standard treatment). Impact analyses use an experimental or strong quasi-experimental design because the aim of such evaluations is to attribute a causal influence to the special program. In the example cited earlier, let us suppose that the program to encourage prenatal care involved having nurses make home visits to women in the rural community to explain the benefits of early care during pregnancy. If the visits could be made to pregnant women randomly assigned to the intervention, the labor and delivery outcomes of the group of women receiving the home visits and of those not receiving them could be compared to determine the net impacts of the intervention, that is, the percentage *increase* in receipt of prenatal care among the experimental group relative to the control group. Many nursing evaluations are impact analyses, although they are not necessarily labeled as such.

Example of an impact analysis: Middleton and co-researchers (2005) studied the short-term impact of a nurse-led program of coordinated care after discharge for patients undergoing carotid endarterectomy. Patients were randomized to either the intervention—telephone liaison with the patient at 2, 6, and 12 weeks after discharge—or to the usual care control group. The intervention was found to have beneficial effects on several outcomes.

Cost Analysis

New programs or policies are often expensive to implement, but existing programs also may be expensive to operate. In our current situation of spiraling health care costs, program evaluations increasingly include a **cost analysis** (or **economic analysis**) to determine whether the benefits of the program outweigh the monetary costs. Administrators and public policy officials make decisions about resource allocations for health services not only on the basis of whether something "works" but also on the basis of whether it is economically viable. Cost analyses are typically done in connection with impact analyses and Phase III clinical trials, that is, when researchers establish persuasive evidence regarding program efficacy.

As described by Chang and Henry (1999), there are several different types of cost analyses, the two most common of which in nursing research are the following:

- **Cost/benefit analysis**, in which monetary estimates are established for both costs and benefits. One difficulty with such an analysis is that it is sometimes difficult to quantify benefits of health services in monetary terms. There is also

controversy about methods of assigning dollar amounts to the value of human life.

- **Cost-effectiveness analysis**, which is used to compare health outcomes and resource costs of alternative interventions. Costs are measured in monetary terms, but outcome effectiveness is not. The point of such analyses is to estimate what it costs to produce impacts on outcomes that cannot easily be valued in dollars. This approach avoids the pitfalls of assigning dollar values to such outcomes as quality of life. However, without information on monetary benefits, such research faces more challenges in persuading decision makers to make changes.

Example of a cost-effectiveness analysis: Stevens and colleagues (2006) compared the incremental costs associated with the provision of home-based versus hospital-based support for breastfeeding for infants during the first week of life. Mother–infant dyads were stratified by gestational age and randomized to standard hospital care or to standard care plus home support from certified nurse lactation consultants. Costs to the family and to the health care system were measured; societal costs were defined as the sum of the two. The results suggested that the costs of the two were comparable.

Cost-utility analyses, although uncommon when Chang and Henry discussed economic analyses in 1999, are now appearing in the nursing literature. This approach is preferred when morbidity and mortality are significant outcomes of interest, or when quality of life is a major concern. An index called the *quality-adjusted life year* (QALY) is frequently an important outcome indicator in cost-utility analyses.

Example of a cost-utility analysis: Raftery and colleagues (2005) undertook a cost-utility analysis of nurse-led secondary prevention clinics for coronary heart disease in connection with a randomized trial of more than 1300 patients in Scotland. The primary outcomes were costs of the clinics and the overall health service, cost per life year, and cost per quality-adjusted life year gained, all expressed as incremental gain in the special clinic group compared with the control group.

Researchers doing cost analyses need to document what it costs to operate both the new intervention and its alternative. For complex programs, economic analyses may need to show costs for individual program components. In doing cost/benefit analyses, researchers need to think carefully about an array of possible short-term costs (e.g., clients' days of work missed within 6 months after the intervention) and long-term costs (e.g., lost years of productive work life). Often the cost/benefit analyst examines economic gains and losses from several different accounting perspectives— for example, for the target group; the hospital or facility implementing the program; third-party payers; employers; taxpayers; and society as a whole (i.e., the target group and taxpayers combined). Distinguishing these different perspectives is crucial if a particular program effect is a loss for one group (e.g., taxpayers) but a gain for another (e.g., the target group).

Nurse researchers increasingly will be called on to become involved in such cost analyses. Drummond and colleagues (1997) have written an internationally acclaimed textbook on economic evaluations in health care. Duren-Winfield and her colleagues (2000) offer an excellent description of the methods used in a cost-effectiveness analysis of an exercise intervention for patients with chronic obstructive pulmonary disease, and Findorff and co-authors (2005) describe how time studies are used to calculate program costs of personnel.

Nursing Intervention Research

Both clinical trials and evaluations involve *interventions*. However, the term *intervention research* is increasingly being used by nurse researchers to describe a research approach distinguished not so much by a particular research methodology as by a distinctive *process* of planning, developing, implementing, testing, and disseminating interventions (e.g., Sidani & Braden, 1998; Whittemore & Grey, 2002). Naylor (2003) defines **nursing intervention research** as "studies either questioning existing care practices or testing innovations in care that are shaped by nursing's values and goals, guided by a

strong theoretical basis, informed by recent advances in science, and designed to improve the quality of care and health of individuals, families, communities, and society" (p. 382).

Proponents of the process are critical of the rather simplistic and atheoretical approach that is often used to design and evaluate nursing interventions. The recommended process for intervention research involves an in-depth understanding of the problem and the people for whom the intervention is being developed; careful, collaborative planning with a diverse team; and the development of an intervention theory to guide the inquiry. These recommendations suggest a systematic and progressive sequence that requires a long investment of time to "get it right," and that places developmental work at a premium.

Similar to clinical trials, nursing intervention research ideally involves several phases: (1) basic developmental research; (2) pilot research; (3) efficacy research; and (4) effectiveness research. Whittemore and Grey (2002) have proposed a fifth phase involving widespread implementation and efforts to document effects on public health. Previous chapters have provided guidance regarding designs for the pilot and full testing of an intervention, and so in this chapter, we put more emphasis on Phase I activities.

During the development phase, researchers address a number of issues relating to both the design of the intervention and strategies to test it. Table 12.1 summarizes the key issues, activities, and products or outcomes of the development phase. Conceptualization is a major focus during Phase I, and this is supported through collaborative discussions, consultations with experts, critical literature reviews, and—often—in-depth research to describe and understand the problem. As the table suggests, the development of the intervention should be *evidence based,* integrating new knowledge from descriptive research with best-practice evidence from the literature and with clinical expertise.

The construct validity of the intervention is enhanced through efforts to develop an **intervention theory** that clearly articulates what must be done to achieve desired outcomes. The theory

TABLE 12.1	Key Issues, Activities, and Products of Phase I Developmental Work for Nursing Interventions	
KEY ISSUES	**MAJOR ACTIVITIES**	**PRODUCTS AND OUTCOMES**
• Conceptualization of the problem • Conceptualization of solutions and strategies • Articulation of the evidence base for an intervention • Identification of potential pitfalls • Cultivation of interpersonal relationships	• Concept and theory development • Critical synthesis of the relevant literature • Exploratory and descriptive research • Brainstorming with colleagues and team building • Consultation with experts • Identifying key stakeholders and building partnerships with them	• Delineation of an intervention theory • Preliminary development of the content, intensity, dose, and timing of the intervention • Strategies to overcome pitfalls in implementing and testing the intervention • A design for a pilot study • A plan for sponsorship of the pilot study

indicates, based on the best available knowledge, the nature of the clinical intervention and factors that would mediate the effects of clinical procedures on expected outcomes. The intervention design, which flows from the intervention theory, specifies not only what the clinical inputs would be but also such aspects as duration and intensity of the intervention. A conceptual map, as discussed in Chapter 6, is often a useful visual tool for articulating the intervention theory and can serve as a "road map" for designing and testing the intervention. Sidani and Braden (1998) offer guidance about the components of an intervention theory.

Another part of the development work is interpersonal in nature and involves cultivation of relationships. This should occur both at the team level (e.g., putting together an enthusiastic and committed project team with diverse clinical, research, and dissemination skills) and with a variety of *stakeholders*—people who have a stake in the intervention. During the developmental phase, key stakeholders should be identified and "brought on board" to the extent possible, which may involve participatory research. Examples of stakeholders include potential beneficiaries of the intervention, members of their families, advocates for the target population, community leaders, agents of the intervention, health care administrators, and third-party payers.

The importance of getting input from key stakeholders cannot be overemphasized. It is naïve to think that an intervention theory can readily be translated into a workable and effective intervention and trial. Many of the common pitfalls of intervention research involve lack of cooperation, support, or trust among key stakeholders. The pitfalls can in some cases be avoided through developmental research designed to better understand the stakeholders' perspective. In addition to seeking information about the stakeholders' needs and concerns through in-depth research, it is wise to form an advisory group of key stakeholders and to develop channels of communication with stakeholder groups—for example, by having a project-specific website.

➔ TIP: Several strategies for designing evidence-based interventions are presented in the Toolkit of the accompanying *Resource Manual*. The Toolkit also presents a list of the most common pitfalls in intervention research. If you are developing a proposal for an intervention project, it is wise to "look savvy" about these potential pitfalls.

The second phase of nursing intervention research is a pilot test of the intervention that was developed in the initial phase, typically using simple quasi-experimental designs. The central activities during the pilot test are to secure preliminary evidence of the intervention's benefits, to refine the intervention theory and the intervention, to finalize intervention protocols for the next phase, and to assess the feasibility of a rigorous test. Part of the feasibility assessment should involve an analysis of factors that affected implementation during the pilot—factors such as recruitment, retention, and adherence problems. Qualitative research can play an especially important role in gaining insight into the feasibility of a larger-scale RCT.

The third phase, as in a classic clinical trial, is to undertake a full experimental test of the intervention. In planning a Phase III trial, care needs to be devoted to a wide array of methodologic issues that could impinge on the validity and reliability of the results, including design, sampling, data collection, and data analysis issues. The final phase focuses on effectiveness and the utility of the intervention in real-world clinical settings. The RE-AIM framework, discussed in the previous chapter, might provide some useful concepts for the design of Phase IV research. Practical clinical trials that use hybrid designs are likely to play an increasingly important role in nursing intervention research.

This model of intervention research is, at this point, more of an ideal than an actuality. For example, there are relatively few effectiveness studies in nursing research. A few research teams have begun to implement portions of the model, and efforts are likely to expand. Undertaking such a long-term, ambitious research agenda is, however, expensive, and funding for such projects will remain a challenge.

➲ **TIP:** A common problem in intervention research is inadequate development, that is, weak Phase I efforts. Avoid the common misconception that new knowledge is the product of only Phase III or Phase IV research.

Example of nursing intervention research: Duffy, Hoskins, and Dudley-Brown (2005) described the developmental work that was undertaken in designing a caring-based nursing intervention for older adults with advanced heart failure discharged from acute care. A team of nurse researchers with complementary skills and backgrounds systematically developed the intervention. The intervention was based on pilot work, findings from recent research, clinical practice guidelines, and a modification of a theoretical framework that Duffy and Hoskins had developed in earlier research. The intervention is being tested using an experimental design.

RESEARCH THAT DOES NOT INVOLVE INTERVENTIONS

The studies described in the previous section often have a nonexperimental *component*, but because they involve an intervention, they almost always involve an experimental or quasi-experimental design as well. In this section, we look at types of research that do not involve interventions and thus rely on nonexperimental designs.

Outcomes Research

Outcomes research is designed to document the effectiveness of health care services and also plays an important role in policy research. Outcomes research overlaps to some degree with evaluation research, but evaluation research more typically focuses on an appraisal of a specific (and often local) program or policy, whereas outcomes research represents a more global assessment of nursing and health care services. The impetus for outcomes research comes from the quality assessment and quality assurance functions that grew out of the professional standards review organizations in the 1970s. Outcomes research represents a response to the increasing demand from policy makers, insurers, and the public to justify care practices and systems in terms of both improved patient outcomes and costs. The focus of outcomes research in the 1980s was predominantly on patient health status and costs associated with medical care, but there is a growing interest in studying broader patient outcomes in relation to nursing care.

Although many nursing studies examine patient outcomes, specific efforts to appraise and document the quality of nursing care—as distinct from the care provided by the overall health care system—are not numerous. A major obstacle is attribution—that is, linking patient outcomes to specific nursing actions or interventions, distinct from the actions of other members of the health care team. It is also difficult in some cases to determine a causal connection between outcomes and health care interventions because factors outside the health care system (e.g., patient characteristics) affect outcomes in complex ways.

Outcomes research has used a variety of traditional designs, sampling strategies, and data collection and analysis approaches (primarily quantitative ones) but is also developing a rich array of methods that are not within the traditional research framework. The complex and multidisciplinary nature of outcomes research suggests that this evolving area will offer opportunities for methodologic creativity in the years ahead.

Models of Health Care Quality

In appraising quality in health care and nursing services, various factors need to be considered. Donabedian (1987), whose pioneering efforts created a framework for outcomes research, emphasized three factors: structure, process, and outcomes. The *structure* of care refers to broad organizational and administrative features. Structure can be appraised in terms of such attributes as size, location, range of services, type of facilities, technology, organization structure, and organizational climate. Nursing skill mix and nursing autonomy in decision making are two structural variables that have been found to be related to patient outcomes. *Processes* involve aspects of clinical management, decision making, and clinical interventions. *Outcomes* refer to the specific clinical end results of patient care. Mitchell, Ferketich, and Jennings (1998) noted that "the emphasis on evaluating quality of care has shifted from structures (having the right things) to processes

(doing the right things) to outcomes (having the right things happen)" (p. 43).

There have been several suggested modifications to Donabedian's framework for appraising health care quality, the most noteworthy of which is the Quality Health Outcomes Model developed by the American Academy of Nursing (Mitchell et al., 1998). This model is less linear and more dynamic than Donabedian's original framework, and takes client and system characteristics into account. This model does not link interventions and processes directly to outcomes, but rather the effects of interventions are seen as mediated by client and system characteristics. Mitchell and Lang (2004) report that this model, and others like it, are increasingly forming the conceptual framework for studies that evaluate quality of care.

Outcomes research usually concentrates on various linkages within such models, rather than on testing the overall model. Some studies have examined the effect of health care structures on various health care processes and outcomes, for example. Efforts have also begun on developing ways to accurately measure aspects of organizational structures and practice environments from a nursing perspective (Aiken & Patrician, 2000; Cummings, Hayduk, & Estabrooks, 2006). Most outcomes research in nursing, however, has focused on the process–patient outcomes nexus, often using large-scale data sets.

Example of research on structure: Seago, Williamson, and Atwood (2006) examined the relationship between nurse skill mix and patient outcomes over a 4-year period in three medical-surgical nursing units. The outcomes included two new failure-to-rescue (FTR) rates—FTR from medication errors and FTR from decubitus ulcers.

Nursing Processes and Interventions

To demonstrate nurses' effects on health outcomes, researchers need to carefully describe and document (quantitatively and qualitatively) nurses' clinical actions and behaviors. Examples of nursing process variables include macrolevel and microlevel nursing actions such as nurses' problem-solving skills, clinical decision making, clinical competence, nurses' autonomy and intensity, clinical leadership, and specific activities or interventions (e.g., communication, touch, clinical actions).

The work that nurses do is increasingly being documented in terms of established classification systems and taxonomies. Indeed, in the United States, the standard use of electronic health records to record all health care events, including the submission of the records to national data banks, is imminent. A number of research-based classification systems of nursing interventions are being developed, refined, and tested. Among the most prominent are the Nursing Diagnoses Taxonomy of the North American Nursing Diagnosis Association (NANDA, 2005) and the Nursing Intervention Classification (NIC) developed at the University of Iowa (Dochterman & Bulecheck, 2004). We expect that many studies in the future will link processes from these or other classification systems to health outcomes.

> **Example of classification system research:** Lunney and colleagues (2004) conducted a pilot study to assess the effects of using computer-based terms from NANDA and NIC on nurses' power to help children and to improve their outcomes. Public health nurses who used software with NANDA and NIC to record health visits were compared with those who used the same software without the classification terms.

Patient Risk Adjustment

Variations in patient outcomes depend not only on the care patients receive but also on differences in patient conditions and comorbidities. Adverse outcomes can occur no matter what nursing intervention is used. Thus, in evaluating the effects of nursing interventions on outcomes, there needs to be some way of controlling or taking into account patients' risks for poor outcomes, or the mix of risks in a caseload.

Risk adjustments have been used in a number of nursing outcomes studies. These studies typically involve the use of global measures of patient risks or patient acuity, such as the Acute Physiology and Chronic Health Evaluation (APACHE II or III) system (Knaus et al., 1985, 1991).

Outcomes

Measuring outcomes and linking them to nursing actions is critical in developing an evidence-based practice and in launching high-quality improvement efforts. Outcomes of relevance to nursing can be defined in terms of physical or physiologic function (e.g., heart rate, blood pressure, complications), psychological function (e.g., comfort, life quality, satisfaction), or social function (e.g., relations with family members). Outcomes of interest to nurses may be either short-term and temporary (e.g., postoperative body temperature) or more long-term and permanent (e.g., return to regular employment). Furthermore, outcomes may be defined in terms of the end results to individual patients receiving care, or to broader units such as a community or our entire society, and this would include cost factors.

Just as there have been efforts to develop classifications of nursing interventions, work has progressed on developing outcome classification systems. Of particular note is the Nursing-Sensitive Outcomes Classification (NOC), which has been developed by nurses at the University of Iowa College of Nursing to complement the NIC (Moorhead, Johnson, & Maas, 2004).

> **Example of outcomes research:** Using Donabedian's model as a framework, Kee and co-researchers (2005) described patient outcomes (patient adverse events, patient satisfaction with nursing care, functional status, symptom management) and explored the contributions of nursing structure and nursing processes to those outcomes in two U.S. Army military centers. Patient acuity (using the APACHE II measure) was taken into account.

Survey Research

A **survey** is designed to obtain information about the prevalence, distribution, and interrelations of variables within a population. The decennial census of the U.S. population is one example of a survey. Political opinion polls, such as those conducted by Gallup or Harris, are other examples. When surveys use samples of individuals, as they usually do, they may be referred to as **sample surveys** (as opposed to a **census**, which covers the entire population). Surveys obtain information from a sample of people by means of **self-report**—that is, study participants respond to a series of questions posed by investigators. Surveys, which yield quantitative data primarily, may be cross-sectional or longitudinal (e.g., panel studies).

The greatest advantage of survey research is its flexibility and broadness of scope. It can be applied to many populations, it can focus on a wide range of topics, and its information can be used for many purposes. The information obtained in most surveys, however, tends to be relatively superficial: surveys rarely probe deeply into such complexities as contradictions of human behavior and feelings. Survey research is better suited to extensive rather than intensive analysis. Although surveys can be conducted within the context of large-scale experiments, surveys are usually done as nonexperimental studies.

The content of a survey is limited only by the extent to which respondents are able and willing to report on the topic. Any information that can reliably be obtained by direct questioning can be gathered in a survey, although surveys include mostly questions that require brief responses (e.g., yes/no, always/sometimes/never). Often, surveys focus on what people do or how they feel: what they eat, how they care for their health, and so forth. In some instances, the emphasis is on what people plan to do—how they plan to vote, for example.

Survey data can be collected in a number of ways, but the most respected method is through **personal interviews** (or *face-to-face interviews*), in which interviewers meet in person with respondents to ask them questions. Personal interviews are often costly because they tend to involve extensive preparation (e.g., interviewer training) and a lot of personnel time. Nevertheless, personal interviews are regarded as the best method of collecting survey data because of the quality of information they yield. A further advantage of personal interviews is that the refusal rate tends to be low.

Example of a survey with personal interviews: McFarlane and colleagues (2005) conducted a personal interview survey of more than 7000 women in primary health care clinics in Texas.

Their objective was to estimate racial/ethnic differences in annual prevalence and severity of intimate partner abuse.

Telephone interviews are a less costly method of gathering survey data. When the interviewer is unknown, however, respondents may be uncooperative on the phone. Telephoning can be a convenient method of collecting information if the interview is short, specific, and not too personal, or if researchers have had prior personal contact with respondents. Telephone interviews may be difficult for certain groups of respondents, including low-income people (who do not always have a telephone) and the elderly (who may have hearing problems).

Because of the expense of collecting in-person data, survey researchers sometimes adopt what is referred to as a **mixed mode strategy**. In this approach, an interviewer first attempts to interview a sample member by telephone. If initial attempts fail (either because of a refusal or no telephone), an interviewer then attempts a personal interview or goes to the respondent's home with a cellular telephone and personally asks the person to complete the interview by phone.

Questionnaires differ from interviews in that they are self-administered. (They are sometimes referred to as **SAQs**, that is, *self-administered questionnaires*.) Respondents read the questions on a written form and give their answers in writing. Because respondents differ in their reading levels and in their ability to communicate in writing, questionnaires are *not* merely a printed form of an interview schedule. Care must be taken in a questionnaire to word questions clearly and simply. Self-administered questionnaires are economical but are not appropriate for surveying certain populations (e.g., the elderly, children). In survey research, questionnaires are often distributed through the mail, but they may also be distributed in other ways, such as over the Internet.

Example of a mailed survey: Beckstrand, Callister, and Kirchhoff (2006) mailed a survey to 1409 members of the American Association of Critical-Care Nurses to collect suggestions for improving end-of-life care in intensive care units.

Large-scale surveys are increasingly relying on new technologies to assist in data collection. Most major telephone surveys now use **computer-assisted telephone interviewing (CATI)**, and growing numbers of in-person surveys use **computer-assisted personal interviewing (CAPI)** with laptop computers. Both procedures involve developing computer programs that present interviewers with the questions to be asked on the computer screen; the interviewers then enter coded responses directly onto a computer file. CATI and CAPI surveys greatly facilitate data collection and improve data quality because there is less opportunity for interviewer error. However, considerable resources are required to substitute a computer program for paper-and-pencil forms.

Example of CATI: Lauder, Mummery, and Sharkey (2006) conducted a survey to examine the relationships between loneliness on the one hand and age, religiosity, and social capital on the other. A sample of more than 1200 people in the United Kingdom were interviewed using CATI technology.

Audio-CASI (computer-assisted self-interview) technology is the state-of-the-art approach for giving respondents more privacy than is possible in an interview (e.g., to collect information about drug use), and is especially useful for populations with literacy problems. With audio-CASI, respondents sit at a computer and listen to questions over headphones. Respondents enter their responses (usually simple codes like 1 or 2) directly onto the keyboard, without the interviewer having to see the responses. This method is discussed by Jones (2003).

There are many excellent resources for learning more about survey research, including the books by Fowler (2001) and Dillman (2000).

Secondary Analysis

Secondary analysis involves the use of data gathered in a previous study to test new hypotheses or explore new relationships. In a typical study, researchers collect far more data than are actually analyzed. Secondary analysis of existing data is efficient and economical because data collection is typically the most time-consuming and expensive part of a research project. Nurse researchers have used a secondary analysis approach with both large national data sets and smaller, more localized sets, and also are doing secondary analyses with qualitative data. Outcomes research frequently involves secondary analyses of clinical data sets.

Quantitative Secondary Analysis

A number of avenues are available for making use of an existing set of quantitative data. For example, variables and relationships among variables that were previously unanalyzed can be examined (e.g., a dependent variable in the original study could become the independent variable in the secondary analysis). In other cases, a secondary analysis focuses on a particular subgroup of the full original sample (e.g., survey data about health habits from a national sample could be analyzed to study smoking among urban teenagers).

Researchers interested in performing secondary analyses must undertake several preparatory activities. In particular, researchers need to identify, locate, and gain access to appropriate databases. They then need to do a thorough assessment of the identified data sets in terms of their appropriateness for the research question, adequacy of data quality, and technical usability of the data. (Some of these activities may be readily accomplished if the data set is being made available from a faculty member or colleague.)

A number of groups, such as university institutes and federal agencies, have made efforts to make survey data available to researchers for secondary analysis. The policies regulating public use of data vary from one organization to another, but it is not unusual for a researcher to obtain a data set at roughly the cost of duplicating data files and documentation. Thus, in some cases in which data collection originally cost hundreds of thousands of dollars, the data set can be purchased for less than 1% of the initial costs. Some universities and research institutes in universities maintain libraries of data sets from large national surveys. Large-scale data sets on health topics are available in the United States from the surveys sponsored by the

National Center for Health Statistics. For example, the National Health Interview Survey, the Health Promotion and Disease Prevention Survey, and the National Comorbidity Survey regularly gather health-related information from thousands of people all over the United States.

The use of available data from large surveys makes it possible to bypass time-consuming and costly steps in the research process, but there are some noteworthy disadvantages in working with existing data. In particular, if researchers do not play a role in collecting the data, the chances are fairly high that the data set will be deficient in one or more ways, such as in the sample used, the variables measured, and so forth. Researchers may continuously face "if only" problems: if only they had asked questions on a certain topic or had measured a particular variable differently. Additional issues to consider in doing a secondary analysis of quantitative data sets are described by Clarke and Cossette (2000) and Magee and colleagues (2006).

Example of a quantitative secondary analysis: Gleason (2006) studied racial disparities in testicular cancer using data on nearly 8000 men from a National Cancer Institute database. Gleason studied whether there were racial/ethnic differences in the relationship between men's age and their stage of testicular cancer.

TIP: There are several organizations, such as the Association of Public Data Users, that can be helpful in identifying large-scale data sets for secondary analysis. Several useful websites for locating data sets are provided on the accompanying CD-ROM.

Qualitative Secondary Analysis
Qualitative researchers, like quantitative researchers, typically collect far more data than are analyzed originally. Secondary analyses of qualitative data provide opportunities to exploit rich data sets—although there are some impediments. The first is difficulty in identifying a suitable database. The availability of large quantitative data sets, especially from government-sponsored surveys, is widely publicized, but there are few repositories of qualitative data sets. Identifying a suitable data set usually means doing a lot of investigation. Probably the most typical method is to approach researchers whose qualitative data appear to be of interest, based on reports they have written. Not all qualitative researchers, however, are willing to share their data because they themselves may intend to do further analyses.

Another issue is that data from quantitative studies are easy to maintain in computer files, and there are standard protocols for documenting what is in the data set. Qualitative data are more voluminous, and there are few established conventions for maintaining, documenting, and encoding the data in computer files. This situation is beginning to change, however, as researchers have come to recognize the value of facilitating use of rich qualitative data sets for varied purposes by multiple users (Manderson, Kehaler, & Woelz-Stirling, 2001).

Thorne (1994) has identified several types of qualitative secondary analysis. In one type, which Thorne called *analytic expansion*, researchers use their own data to answer new questions as the theory base increases or as they pursue questions at a higher level of analysis. A second type, *retrospective interpretation*, involves using an original database to examine new questions that were not thoroughly assessed in the original study. Sometimes a secondary analysis involves *cross-validation*, an effort to confirm new results beyond the ability of the original analyses. Thorne warned of potential hazards in secondary analysis of qualitative studies, such as the possibility of exaggerating the effects of the original researcher's biases, and ethical questions regarding the use of the original data sets. Another challenge concerns evaluating the quality of the data set from the primary study. Hinds and colleagues (1997) developed an assessment tool for just such a purpose. This assessment tool addresses such criteria as determining the fit of secondary research questions, completeness of the data set, and training of the primary team.

Example of a qualitative secondary analysis: Thorne and colleagues (2004) analyzed previously collected qualitative data from a larger study that explored patterns in health care communication across several chronic diseases. The new study involved an analysis of persons with multiple sclerosis and their perceptions of helpful and unhelpful communication in their health care.

Other Nonintervention Research

Nurse researchers have pursued several other types of research, most of which can use either quantitative or qualitative approaches, or a mixed method strategy.

Needs Assessments

As the name implies, a **needs assessment** is a study in which researchers collect data to estimate the needs of a group, community, or organization. The aim of such a study is to determine whether there is a need for special services or interventions, or if a program is meeting the needs of those who are supposed to benefit from it. Because resources are seldom limitless, information that can help in establishing priorities can be valuable.

There are various methods of doing needs assessments, and these methods are not mutually exclusive. The **key informant approach** collects information about a group's needs from people who are in a key position to know those needs. The key informants could be community leaders, prominent health care workers, or other knowledgeable individuals. Interviews are usually used to collect the data and are often in-depth, unstructured interviews that yield qualitative rather than quantitative data.

Needs assessments often use a **survey approach**, which involves collecting data from a sample of the group whose needs are being assessed. In a survey, questioning would not be restricted to people who have special expertise. A representative sample from the group or community would be asked about their needs. Another alternative is to use an **indicators approach**, which relies on facts and statistics available in existing reports or records. The indicators approach is cost-effective because the data are available but need organization and interpretation.

Needs assessments almost always involve the development of recommendations. Researchers conducting a needs assessment usually offer judgments about priorities based on their results (taking costs and feasibility into consideration), and may also offer advice about the means by which the most highly prioritized needs can be addressed.

Example of a needs assessment: Wollin, Yates, and Kristjanson (2006) used a key informant approach to identify the supportive needs of individuals with multiple sclerosis (MS) and their families. In-depth interviews were carried out with patients living with MS, their family members, and health care professionals.

Delphi Surveys

Delphi surveys were developed as a tool for short-term forecasting. The technique involves a panel of experts who are asked to complete several rounds of questionnaires focusing on their judgments about a topic of interest. Multiple iterations are used to achieve consensus, without the necessity of face-to-face discussion. Responses to each round of questionnaires are analyzed, summarized, and returned to the experts with a new questionnaire. The experts can then reformulate their opinions with the panel's viewpoint in mind. The process is usually repeated at least three times until a general consensus is obtained.

The Delphi technique is an efficient means of combining the expertise of a geographically dispersed group. The experts are spared the necessity of attending a formal meeting, thus saving time and expense. Another advantage is that a persuasive or prestigious expert cannot have an undue influence on the opinions of others, as could happen in a face-to-face situation. All panel members are on an equal footing. Anonymity probably encourages greater candor than might be expressed in a formal meeting.

The Delphi technique is, however, time-consuming for researchers. Experts must be solicited, questionnaires prepared and mailed, responses analyzed, results summarized, new questionnaires prepared, and so forth. The cooperation of the panel members may wane in later rounds of mailings, and so attrition bias is a potential problem. Another concern is how to define consensus (i.e., how many participants have to agree before researchers conclude that consensus has been achieved). Recommendations range from a liberal 51% to a more cautious 70%. On the whole, the Delphi technique represents a useful methodologic tool for problem solving, planning, and forecasting. Kennedy (2004) and Keeney and colleagues (2006) offer some suggestions on using this technique.

Example of a Delphi study: Tolson and co-researchers (2005) used a Delphi approach with 33 panel members to identify the most important current policies relating to the provision of high-quality nursing care in long-term care environments in Scotland. The second phase of the study involved a mail survey of more than 2000 nurses to explore nurses' awareness of, access to, and use of the policies identified in the first phase.

Replication Studies

Replication studies are direct attempts to determine whether findings obtained in an original piece of research can be duplicated in another independent study. A strong evidence-based practice requires replications. Evidence can accumulate through a series of "close-enough-to-compare" studies, but deliberate replications offer special advantages in both establishing the credibility of research findings and extending their generalizability. There are, however, relatively few *published* replication studies in the nursing literature, perhaps reflecting a bias for original research on the part of researchers, editors, and research sponsors.

There have been several attempts to classify replication strategies (Beck, 1994). One strategy is known as **identical replication** (or *literal* replication), which is an exact duplication of the original methods (e.g., sampling, measurement, analysis). Such exact duplication is rare, except in the case of a subsequent study by the original researcher. More common is **virtual replication** (or *operational* repli-

cation), which involves attempts to approximate the methods used in the reference study as closely as possible, but precise duplication is not sought. A third strategy is **systematic extension replication** (or *constructive* replication), in which methods are not duplicated, but there are deliberate attempts to test the implications of the original research. Many nursing studies that build on earlier research could be described as extension replications, but they usually are not so labeled and are not necessarily conceptualized as systematic extensions.

Beck (1994) noted that reports on replication studies should provide details about what was replicated, and how the replication was similar to or different from the original. Researchers should thoroughly critique the original research being replicated, especially if modifications were made on the basis of any shortcoming. Beck also recommended *benchmarking*—comparing the results of the original and replicated studies. The comparison should be accompanied by conclusions about both the internal and external validity of the study findings.

Many nurse researchers have called for more deliberate replication studies (e.g., Fahs et al., 2003). The push for evidence-based practice may strengthen their legitimacy as important scientific endeavors. Replications are appropriate for both intervention and observational studies, and for quantitative and qualitative research.

Example of a quantitative replication study: Hanneman and Gusick (2005) replicated an earlier study that examined oral care and positioning of patients as interventions to decrease the risk for aspiration pneumonia in hospitalized patients. In both the original study and the replication, nurses reported more frequent oral care than is documented in unit flow sheets. The replication extended the original research by including data from bedside observations of nursing actions.

Methodologic Research

Methodologic research studies are investigations of the ways of obtaining and organizing data and conducting rigorous research. Methodologic studies address the development, validation, and evaluation of research tools or methods. The growing demands for sound and reliable outcome measures and for sophisticated procedures for obtaining and analyzing data have led to an increased interest in methodologic research by nurse researchers.

Most methodologic studies are nonexperimental, often focusing on instrument development and testing. Suppose, for example, we developed and evaluated a new instrument to accurately measure patients' satisfaction with nursing care. In such a study, we would not examine levels of patient satisfaction or how satisfaction correlates with patient characteristics. Our goals are to develop a high-quality instrument that can be used by others, and to determine our success in accomplishing this. Instrument development research is becoming increasingly important, and it often involves complex and sophisticated research designs and analyses, some of which we describe in Chapter 18.

Occasionally researchers use an experimental design to test competing methodologic strategies. Suppose we wanted to test whether sending holiday and birthday cards to study participants reduced rates of attrition in longitudinal studies. Participants could be randomly assigned to a card or no-card condition. The dependent variable in this case is rates of attrition from the study.

Example of a quantitative methodologic study: Ulrich and colleagues (2005) used an RCT design to test alternative incentives to participate in a survey among nonphysician health care professionals (nurse practitioners and physician assistants). Prospective survey respondents were randomly assigned to one of three groups: no incentive, a $5 prepaid incentive in the initial mailing, or a chance to win a cash prize upon return of the survey via a lottery. The cash incentive yielded the highest response rates.

In qualitative research, methodologic issues often arise within the context of a substantive study, rather than having a study originate as a purely methodologic endeavor. In such instances, however, the researcher typically performs separate analyses designed to highlight a methodologic issue and to generate strategies for solving a methodologic problem.

Example of a qualitative methodologic study: Miranda (2004) was involved in a study in which prospective study participants were asked about their willingness to be randomly assigned to alternative interventions to address their insomnia. Most study participants were unwilling to be randomized, and Miranda analyzed the qualitative data regarding the underlying reasons for their treatment allocation preferences. The study offers useful information for the conduct of RCTs in this area.

Methodologic research may appear less compelling than substantive clinical research, but it is virtually impossible to conduct rigorous and useful research on a substantive topic with inadequate research methods.

CRITIQUING STUDIES DESCRIBED IN THIS CHAPTER

It is difficult to provide guidance on critiquing the types of studies described in this chapter because they are so varied and because many of the fundamental methodologic issues that require a critique concern the overall design. Guidelines for critiquing design-related issues were presented in the previous chapters.

You should, however, consider whether researchers took appropriate advantage of the possibilities of a mixed method design. Collecting both qualitative and quantitative data is not always necessary or practical, but in critiquing studies, you can consider whether the study would have been strengthened by triangulating different types of data. In studies in which mixed methods were used, you should carefully consider whether the inclusion of both types of data was justified and whether the researcher really made use of both types of data to enhance knowledge on the research topic. Table 12.2 provides some examples of possibilities for mixed method studies.

Box 12.1 ✹ offers a few specific questions for critiquing the types of studies included in this chapter. Separate guidelines for critiquing economic evaluations, which are more technically complex, are offered in the Toolkit of the accompanying *Resource Manual*.

TABLE 12.2 Examples of Integration Possibilities

TYPE	EXAMPLE OF QUESTION FOR QUANTITATIVE COMPONENT	EXAMPLE OF QUESTION FOR QUALITATIVE COMPONENT
Clinical trial	Are boomerang pillows more effective than straight pillows in improving the respiratory capacity of hospitalized patients?	Why did some patients complain about the boomerang pillows? How did the pillows feel?
Evaluation	How effective and cost-effective is a nurse-managed special care unit compared with traditional intensive care units?	How accepting were other health care workers of the special unit, and what problems of implementation ensued?
Outcomes research	What effect do alternative levels of nursing intensity have on the functional ability of elderly residents in long-term care facilities?	How do elderly long-term care residents interact with nurses in environments with different nursing intensity?
Needs assessment	What percentage of Haitian immigrants have unmet health care needs, and what are the highest-priority needs?	What are the barriers that prevent Haitian immigrants from getting needed health services?
Survey	How prevalent is asthma among inner-city children, and how is it treated?	How is asthma experienced by inner-city children and their parents?
Methodologic research	How accurate is a new measure of loneliness for hospitalized psychiatric patients?	Does the new measure adequately capture the dimensions and manifestations of loneliness of psychiatric patients?
Ethnography	What percentage of women in rural Appalachia seek and obtain prenatal care, and what are their birth outcomes?	How do women in rural Appalachia view their pregnancies and how do they prepare for childbirth?
Case study	How have the demographic characteristics of the caseload of St. Jude's Homeless Shelter changed over a 10-year period?	How are social, health, and psychological services integrated in St. Jude's Homeless Shelter?

RESEARCH EXAMPLES OF VARIOUS TYPES OF STUDIES

Examples of each type of research presented in this chapter have already been mentioned. Two studies are described in greater detail in this section.

Research Example of Mixed Method Nursing Intervention Research

Studies: Studies supporting the development and testing of an intervention for women with type 2 diabetes (Whittemore, Chase, et al., 2001, 2002; Whittemore, Melkus, & Grey, 2005; Whittemore, Melkus, et al., 2004)

Statement of Purpose: Prior research has found that it is often difficult for people to make the lifestyle changes

BOX 12.1 Some Guidelines for Critiquing Studies Described in Chapter 12

1. Does the study purpose match the study design? Was the best possible design (or research tradition) used to address the study purpose?
2. Is the study exclusively qualitative or exclusively quantitative? If so, could the study have been strengthened by incorporating both approaches?
3. If the study used a mixed methods design, how did the inclusion of both approaches contribute to enhanced theoretical insights or enhanced validity? In what other ways (if any) did the inclusion of both types of data strengthen the study and further the aims of the research?
4. If the study used a mixed method design, would the design be described as a component design or an integrated design? Was this approach appropriate? Comment on the timing of collecting the various types of data.
5. If the study was a clinical trial or intervention study, was adequate attention paid to developing an appropriate intervention? Was there a well-conceived intervention theory that guided the endeavor? Was the intervention adequately pilot tested?
6. If the study was a clinical trial, evaluation, or intervention study, was there an effort to understand how the intervention was implemented (i.e., a process-type analysis)? Were the financial costs and benefits assessed? If not, should they have been?
7. If the study was an evaluation or needs assessment (or a practical clinical trial), to what extent do the study results serve the practical information needs of key decision makers or intended users?
8. If the study was a survey, was the most appropriate method used to collect the data (i.e., in-person interviews, telephone interviews, mail or Internet questionnaires)?
9. If the study was a secondary analysis, to what extent was the chosen data set appropriate for addressing the research questions? What were the limitations of the data set, and were these limitations acknowledged and taken into account in interpreting the results?

needed for the self-management of diabetes. The overall purpose of this research was to develop an intervention theory and a multi-component nursing intervention to facilitate lifestyle change among women with type 2 diabetes. Phase I and II work has been completed in preparation for a full testing of the intervention in a Phase III RCT.

Phase I: As part of the Phase I effort, Whittemore and colleagues undertook activities to fully explore and understand the problem, and to develop and refine a framework. Phase I included an extensive literature review, concept development, and mixed method research. Based on the literature and guided by a modified version of the Adaptation to Chronic Illness Model, a preliminary intervention was developed that involved four 45-minute sessions over an 8-week period. Nine women, who were selected to be demographically and medically diverse, participated in the Phase I research. A rich array of data was gathered to better understand the experience of the participants. For example, all of the

nurse coaching sessions were audiotaped and transcribed, yielding 32 hours of qualitative data. Each participant also completed an in-depth interview about her experiences with her illness and with lifestyle changes needed to manage it. Quantitative data on indicators of psychological and physiologic adaptation were gathered before and after the intervention. The qualitative findings suggested that the process of integrating lifestyle change as a result of the illness was complex and involved numerous challenges. The findings helped to refine a theory of *integration* and to develop intervention protocols for the next phase. The aggregate quantitative outcomes suggested that a decrease in fasting blood glucose and an increase in health-promoting behaviors were achieved.

Phase II: The next phase was a more rigorous pilot study of the intervention. The purposes of this phase were to establish the intervention protocol, determine the timing of follow-up sessions and outcome measures, and seek preliminary evidence of the efficacy of the intervention. Based on Phase I findings, the pilot intervention involved more nurse coaching sessions over a longer period of time (six nurse coaching sessions over a 6-month period, with phone calls between some sessions). The pilot study involved randomly assigning 53 women to one of two groups—the nurse coaching intervention plus standard diabetes care, or standard care without the special intervention. In addition to experimental analyses comparing the two groups, the researchers undertook some nonexperimental, cross-sectional analyses with baseline data to explore factors affecting metabolic control and dietary self-management.

Key Phase II Findings:

- Attendance at nurse coaching sessions among those in the treatment group was high (96%).
- Women in the treatment group had several significantly better outcomes than those in the control group—for example, better diet self-management, less diabetes-related distress, better integration, and more satisfaction with care; differences in body mass index were encouraging but not statistically significant.
- In the pilot study sample, the most consistent predictors of metabolic control and dietary self-management were the women's support and self-confidence, suggesting that these should be targeted in interventions.

Research Example of a Survey, Secondary Analysis, and Methodologic Research

Studies: "Research design and subject characteristics predicting nonparticipation in a panel survey of older families with cancer (Neumark et al., 2001); "Predictors of use of complementary and alternative therapies among patients with cancer" (Fouladbakhsh et al., 2005)

The Survey: During the mid- to late-1990s, Drs. Barbara and Charles Given conducted a longitudinal survey with more than 1000 older patients who were newly diagnosed with lung, colon, breast, or prostate cancer. The panel study, called the Family Care Study, involved four rounds of telephone interviews as well as self-administered questionnaires with study participants, who were recruited over a 3-year period in multiple hospitals and cancer treatment centers in two states. The purpose of the original research was to examine the physical, emotional, and financial outcomes for patients and family members over the first year following cancer diagnosis. Key findings were presented in a report to the funding agency, NINR, and in numerous journal articles (e.g., Given et al., 2000).

Methodologic Research: The survey data set has been used in several secondary analyses, including one that focused on methodologic issues. Neumark and colleagues (2001) sought to identify factors that could account for loss of subjects in the earliest phases of sample accrual. They compared three groups: eligible patients who declined to participate (nonconsenters), patients who originally consented to participate but then later declined (early drop-outs), and subjects who actually took part in the study (participants). The researchers examined two broad types of factors that might help to explain nonparticipation in the study: subject characteristics and research design characteristics. The aim was to obtain information that would benefit others in designing studies and recruiting subjects. They found, for example, that the most powerful design factor was whether a family caregiver was approached to participate. Patients were more likely to give consent and less likely to drop out early when caregivers were also approached.

Substantive Secondary Analysis: Fouladbakhsh and colleagues (2005) used data from two similar panel studies of patients newly diagnosed with cancer, including data from the Family Care Study. Their secondary analyses focused on responses from the first two waves of data collection, relying exclusively on information from the self-administered questionnaires. The purpose of their study was to identify factors that predicted the use of complementary and alternative medicine (CAM) therapies in patients with cancer 3 months after diagnosis. The findings suggested that a substantial minority of people used CAM while undergoing conventional cancer treatment. Significant predictors of CAM included gender, marital status, cancer stage, and number of severe symptoms experienced.

SUMMARY POINTS

- Studies vary according to purpose as well as design or research tradition. For many purposes, mixed method studies are advantageous. **Mixed method** research involves the triangulation of qualitative and quantitative data in a single project.
- Mixed method studies are used for many purposes, including the development and testing of high-quality instruments, the generation and

testing of hypotheses, theory building, and intervention development.

- In mixed method studies with a **component design**, the qualitative and quantitative aspects of the study are implemented as discrete components, and are distinct during data collection and data analysis. The second broad category is **integrated designs**, in which there is greater integration of methods throughout the research process.

- **Clinical trials**, which are studies designed to assess the effectiveness of clinical interventions, often involve a series of phases. *Phase I* is designed to finalize the features of the intervention. *Phase II* involves seeking preliminary evidence of efficacy and opportunities for refinements. *Phase III* is a full experimental test of treatment *efficacy*. In *Phase IV*, the researcher focuses primarily on generalized *effectiveness* and evidence about costs and benefits.

- In a **sequential clinical trial**, experimental data from paired "mini-experiments" are continuously analyzed. Most sequential trials use measures of *preference* for either the experimental or control condition for each pair of observations. Preferences are plotted on special graphs until the plot crosses one of the boundaries, which designate **stopping rules** for the experiment.

- **Practical** (or **pragmatic) clinical trials** are studies designed to provide information to clinical decision makers. They sometimes involve **hybrid designs** that aim to reduce the gap between efficacy and effectiveness studies—that is, between internal and external validity.

- **Evaluation research** assesses the effectiveness of a program, policy, or procedure to assist decision makers in choosing a course of action. Evaluations can answer a variety of questions. **Process** or **implementation analyses** describe the process by which a program gets implemented and how it functions in practice. **Outcome analyses** *describe* the status of some condition after the introduction of an intervention.

Impact analyses test whether an intervention caused any **net impacts** relative to the counterfactual. **Cost analyses** seek to determine whether the monetary costs of a program are outweighed by benefits and include both **cost/benefit analyses** and **cost-effectiveness analyses**.

- **Nursing intervention research** is a term sometimes used to refer to a distinctive *process* of planning, developing, implementing, testing, and disseminating interventions. A key feature of this process is the development of an **intervention theory** from which the design and evaluation of an intervention flow. Intervention research proceeds in several phases, and an especially important phase is early developmental work (Phase I) that frequently involves mixed method research.

- **Outcomes research** is undertaken to document the quality and effectiveness of health care and nursing services. A model of health care quality encompasses several broad concepts, including *structure* (factors such as accessibility, range of services, facilities, and organizational climate); *process* (nursing interventions and actions); client risk factors (e.g., severity of illness and case mix of the caseload); and *outcomes* (the specific end results of patient care in terms of patient functioning).

- Survey research examines people's characteristics, behaviors, and intentions by asking them to answer questions. The preferred survey method is through **personal interviews**, in which interviewers meet respondents face-to-face and question them. **Telephone interviews** are less costly, but are inadvisable if the interview is long or if the questions are sensitive. **Questionnaires** are self-administered (i.e., questions are read by respondents, who then give written responses).

- **Secondary analysis** refers to studies in which researchers analyze previously collected data—either quantitative or qualitative. Secondary analyses are economical, but it is sometimes difficult to identify an appropriate existing data set.

- **Needs assessments** are studies to document the needs of a group or community. The three main needs assessment approaches are the **key informant**, **survey**, and **indicators approaches**.

- The **Delphi survey** is a method of problem solving in which several rounds of questionnaires are mailed to a panel of experts. Feedback from previous questionnaires is provided with each new questionnaire so that the experts can converge on a consensus in subsequent rounds.

- **Replication studies** include **identical replications** (exact duplication of methods of an earlier study in a new study); **virtual replication** (close approximation but not exact duplication of methods); and **systematic extension replication** (deliberate attempts to test the implications of the original research).

- In **methodologic research**, the investigator is concerned with the development, validation, and assessment of methodologic tools or strategies.

STUDY ACTIVITIES

Chapter 12 of the *Resource Manual to Accompany Nursing Research: Generating and Assessing Evidence for Nursing Practice*, *8th edition*, offers various exercises and study suggestions for reinforcing concepts presented in this chapter. In addition, the following study questions can be addressed:

1. Suppose you were interested in doing a survey of nurses' attitudes toward caring for AIDS patients. Would you use a personal interview, telephone interview, or questionnaire to collect your data? Defend your decision.

2. How would you design the Phase III research in the Whittemore intervention study used as a research example at the end of the chapter?

3. In the research example of the methodologic research by Neumark and colleagues (2001), what were the dependent and independent variables? How might other researchers benefit from this research?

STUDIES CITED IN CHAPTER 12

Methodologic or theoretical references cited in this chapter can be found in a separate section at the end of the book.

Aiken, L. H., & Patrician, P. A. (2000). Measuring organizational traits of hospitals: The Revised Nursing Work Index. *Nursing Research, 49*, 146–153.

Beck, C. T., & Gable, R. K. (2000). Postpartum Depression Screening Scale: Development and psychometric testing. *Nursing Research, 49*, 272–282.

Beck, C. T., & Gable, R. K. (2001). Ensuring content validity: An illustration of the process. *Journal of Nursing Measurement, 9*, 201–215.

Beckstrand, R., Callister, L., & Kirchhoff, K. (2006). Providing a "good death": Critical care nurses' suggestions for improving end-of-life care. *American Journal of Critical Care, 15*(1), 38–45.

Benzies, K. M., Harrison, M. J., & Magill-Evans, J. (2004a). Parenting and childhood behavior problems: Mothers' and fathers' voices. *Issues in Mental Health Nursing, 25*, 9–24.

Benzies, K. M., Harrison, M. J., & Magill-Evans, J. (2004b). Parenting stress, marital quality, and child behavior problems at age 7 years. *Public Health Nursing, 21*, 111–121.

Burton, C., & Gibbon, B. (2005). Expanding the role of the stroke nurse: A pragmatic clinical trial. *Journal of Advanced Nursing, 52*(6), 640–650.

Cummings, G., Hayduk, L., & Estabrooks, C. (2006). Is the Nursing Work Index measuring up? *Nursing Research, 55*(2), 92–93.

Duffy, J., Hoskins, L. M., & Dudley-Brown, S. (2005). Development and testing of a caring-based intervention for older adults with heart failure. *Journal of Cardiovascular Nursing, 20*(5), 325–333.

Fonteyn, M., & Bauer-Wu, S. (2005). Using qualitative evaluation in a feasibility study to improve and refine a complementary therapy intervention prior to subsequent research. *Complementary Therapies in Clinical Practice, 11*(4), 247–252.

Fouladbakhsh, J. M., Stommel, M., Given, B., & Given, C. (2005). Predictors of use of complementary and alternative therapies among patients with cancer. *Oncology Nursing Forum, 32*(6), 1115–1122.

Froelicher, E. S., Miller, N. H., Christopherson, D. J., Martin, K., Parker, K., Amonetti, M., Lin, Z., Sohn, M., Benowitz, N., Taylor, C. B., & Bacchetti, P. (2004). High rates of sustained smoking cessation in women hospitalized with cardiovascular disease: The women's initiative for nonsmoking (WINS). *Circulation, 109*, 587–593.

Given, C., Given, B., Azzouz, F., Stommel, M., & Kozachik, S. (2000). Comparison of changes in physical functioning of elderly patients with new diagnoses of cancer. *Medical Care, 38*(5), 482–493.

Gleason, A. M. (2006). Racial disparities in testicular cancer. *Journal of Transcultural Nursing, 17*(1), 58–64.

Groner, J., French, G., Ahijevych, K., & Wewers, M. (2005). Process evaluation of a nurse-delivered smoking relapse prevention program for new mothers. *Journal of Community Health Nursing, 22*(3), 157–167.

Hanneman, S., & Gusick, G. (2005). Frequency of oral care and positioning of patients in critical care: A replication study. *American Journal of Critical Care, 14*(5), 378–386.

Kee, C., Foley, B., Dudley, W., Jennings, B., Minick, P., & Harvey, S. (2005). Nursing structure, processes, and patient outcomes in army medical centers. *Western Journal of Nursing Research, 27*(8), 1040–1058.

Lauder, W., Mummery, K., & Sharkey, S. (2006). Social capital, age and religiosity in people who are lonely. *Journal of Clinical Nursing, 15*(3), 334–340.

Lunney, M., Parker, L., Fiore, L., Cavendish, R., & Pulcini, J. (2004). Feasibility of studying the effects of using NANDA, NIC, and NOC on nurses' power and children's outcomes. *Computers, Informatics, Nursing, 22*(6), 316–322.

Mahrer-Imhof, R., Froelicher, E. S., Li, W. W., Parker, K. M., & Benowitz, N. (2002). Women's Initiative for Nonsmoking (WINS) V: Under-use of nicotine replacement therapy. *Heart & Lung, 31*, 368–373.

Martin, K., Froelicher, E. S., & Miller, N. H. (2000). Women's Initiative for Nonsmoking (WINS) I: The intervention. *Heart & Lung, 29*, 438–445.

McClement, S. E., Chochinov, H. M., Hack, T., Kristjanson, L. J., & Harlos, M. (2004). Dignity conserving care: Application of research findings to practice. *International Journal of Palliative Nursing, 10*, 173–179.

McFarlane, J., Grofdf, J., O'Brien, J., & Watson, K. (2005). Prevalence of partner violence against 7,443 African American, white, and Hispanic women receiving care at urban public primary care clinics. *Public Health Nursing, 22*(2), 98–107.

Middleton, S., Donnelly, N., Harris, J., & Ward, J. (2005). Nursing intervention after carotid endarterectomy: A randomized trial of Coordinate Care Post-Discharge (CCPD). *Journal of Advanced Nursing, 52*(3), 250–261.

Miranda, J. (2004). An exploration of participants' treatment preferences in a partial RCT. *Canadian Journal of Nursing Research, 36*(3), 100–114.

Morgan, D, G., & Stewart, N. J. (2002). Theory building through mixed-method evaluation of a dementia special care unit. *Research in Nursing & Health, 25*, 479–488.

Neumark, D. E., Stommel, M., Given, C. W., & Given, B. A. (2001). Research design and subject characteristics predicting nonparticipation in a panel survey of older families with cancer. *Nursing Research, 50*, 363–368.

Olson, K., Hanson, J., & Michaud, M. (2003). A phase II trial of Reiki for the management of pain in advanced cancer patients. *Journal of Pain & Symptom Management, 26*, 990–997.

Polit, D. F., London, A. S., & Martinez, J. M. (2001). *The health of poor urban women*. New York: MDRC. Available at: *http://www.mdrc.org*

Raftery, J., Yao, G., Murchie, P., Campbell, N., & Ritchie, L. (2005). Cost effectiveness of nurse led secondary prevention clinics for coronary heart disease in primary care: Follow-up of a randomized controlled trial. *BMJ, 330*(7493), 707.

Seago, J. A., Williamson, A., & Atwood, C. (2006). Longitudinal analysis of nurse staffing and patient outcomes: More about failure to rescue. *Journal of Nursing Administration, 36*(1), 13–21.

Stevens, B., Guerriere, D., McKeever, P., Croxford, R., Miller K., et al. (2006). Economies of home vs. hospital breastfeeding support for newborns. *Journal of Advanced Nursing, 53*(2), 233–243.

Thorne, S., Con, A., McGuinness, L., McPerson, G., & Harris, S. (2004). Health care communication issues in multiple sclerosis: An interpretive description. *Qualitative Health Research, 14*, 5–22.

Tolson, D., Maclaren, W., Kiely, S., & Lowndes, A. (2005). Influences of policies on nursing practice in long-term care environments of older people. *Journal of Advanced Nursing, 50*(6), 661–671.

Ulrich, C., Danis, M., Koziol, D., Garrett-Mayer, E., Hubbard, R., & Grady, C. (2005). Does it pay to pay? A randomized trial of prepaid financial incentives and lottery incentives in surveys of nonphysician healthcare professionals. *Nursing Research, 54*(3), 178–183.

Valente, S., & Nemec, C. (2006). An evidence-based project to improve depression and alcohol use screening. *Journal of Nursing Care Quality, 21*(1), 93–98.

Whittemore, R., Chase, S., Mandle, C., & Roy, C. (2001). The content, integrity, and efficacy of a nurse-coaching intervention in type 2 diabetes. *Diabetes Educator, 27*, 887–898.

Whittemore, R., Chase, S., Mandle, C., & Roy, C. (2002). Lifestyle change in type 2 diabetes: A process model. *Nursing Research, 51*(1), 18–25.

Whittemore, R., Melkus, G. D., & Grey, M. (2005). Metabolic control, self-management and psychosocial adjustment in women with type 2 diabetes. *Journal of Clinical Nursing, 14,* 195–203.

Whittemore, R., Melkus, G. D., Sullivan, A., & Grey, M. (2004). A nurse-coaching intervention for women with type 2 diabetes. *Diabetes Educator, 30*(5), 795–804.

Wollin, J., Yates, P., & Kristjanson, L. (2006). Supportive and palliative care needs identified by multiple sclerosis patients and their families. *International Journal of Palliative Nursing, 12*(1), 20–26.

13

Developing a Sampling Plan

S ampling is a complex and technical topic. Yet at the same time, sampling is familiar to us all. In the course of our daily activities, we get information, make decisions, and develop predictions through sampling. A nursing student may select an elective course by sampling two or three classes on the first day of the semester. Patients may generalize about nurses' friendliness in a particular hospital based on the care they received from a sample of nurses. We all come to conclusions about phenomena based on exposure to a limited portion of those phenomena.

Researchers, too, obtain data from samples. For example, in testing the efficacy of a new asthma medication, researchers reach conclusions without administering the drug to all asthmatic patients. Researchers, however, cannot afford to draw conclusions about the effectiveness of interventions or the validity of relationships based on a sample of only three or four subjects. The consequences of making erroneous decisions are more momentous in disciplined inquiries than in private decision making.

Quantitative and qualitative researchers have different approaches to sampling. Quantitative researchers seek to select samples that will allow them to achieve statistical conclusion validity and to generalize their results. They therefore develop a **sampling plan** that specifies in advance how study participants are to be selected and how many to include. Qualitative researchers are more interested in ensuring that they can develop a rich, holistic understanding of the phenomenon of interest. They make sampling decisions during the course of data collection based on informational and theoretical needs, and typically do not develop a formal sampling plan in advance. This chapter discusses sampling issues for both quantitative and qualitative research.

BASIC SAMPLING CONCEPTS

Sampling is a critical part of the design of quantitative research. In a quantitative study, sampling has implications for all four types of study validity discussed in Chapter 11. Let us first consider some terms associated with sampling—terms that are used primarily (but not exclusively) with quantitative studies.

Populations

A **population** is the entire aggregation of cases in which a researcher is interested. For instance, if a nurse researcher were studying American nurses with doctoral degrees, the population could be defined as all U.S. citizens who are registered nurses (RNs) and who have acquired a PhD, DNSc, or other doctoral-level degree. Other possible populations might be all male patients who underwent cardiac surgery in St. Peter's Hospital during 2007, all women currently in treatment for breast cancer in Boston, or all children in Canada with cystic fibrosis. As this list illustrates, a population may be broadly defined, involving thousands of individuals, or may be narrowly specified to include only hundreds.

Populations are not restricted to human subjects. A population might consist of all the hospital records on file in a particular hospital, all the blood samples taken from clients of a health maintenance organization, or all the high schools in the United States with school-based clinics that dispense contraceptives. Whatever the basic unit, the population comprises the entire aggregate of elements in which the researcher is interested.

It is sometimes useful to make a distinction between target and accessible populations. The **accessible** or **source population** is the aggregate of cases that conform to designated criteria *and* that are accessible as subjects for a study. The **target population** is the aggregate of cases about which the researcher would like to generalize. A target population might consist of all diabetic people in the United States, but the accessible population might consist of all diabetic people who are members of a particular health plan. Researchers usually sample from an accessible population and hope to generalize to a target population.

➲ **TIP:** A key issue for the development of an evidence-based practice is information about the populations on whom research has been conducted. Many quantitative researchers fail to identify their target population, or discuss the issue of the generalizability of the results. The population of interest needs to be carefully considered in planning and reporting a study.

Eligibility Criteria

Researchers must specify criteria that define who is included in the population. Consider the population,

American nursing students. Does this population include students in all types of nursing programs? How about RNs returning to school for a bachelor's degree? Or students who took a leave of absence for a semester? Do foreign students enrolled in American nursing programs qualify? Insofar as possible, the researcher must consider the exact criteria by which it could be decided whether an individual would or would not be classified as a member of the population. The criteria that specify population characteristics are referred to as **eligibility criteria** or **inclusion criteria**. Sometimes, a population is defined in terms of characteristics that people must *not* possess (i.e., stipulating the **exclusion criteria**). For example, the population may be defined to exclude people who cannot speak English.

Specifications about the population should be driven, to the extent possible, by theoretical considerations. In thinking about ways to define the population and delineate eligibility criteria, it is important to consider whether the resulting sample is likely to be a good exemplar of the population construct in which you are interested. The construct validity of the study is enhanced when there is a good match between the eligibility criteria and the population construct.

Of course, inclusion or exclusion criteria for a study often reflect considerations other than substantive or theoretical concerns. The eligibility criteria may reflect one or more of the following:

- *Costs.* Some criteria reflect cost constraints. For example, when non–English-speaking people are excluded, this does not usually mean that the researchers are not interested in non-English speakers, but rather that they cannot afford to hire translators and multilingual data collectors.
- *Practical constraints.* Sometimes, there are other practical constraints, such as difficulty including people from rural areas, people who are hearing impaired, and so on.
- *People's ability to participate in a study.* The health condition of some people may preclude their participation. For example, people with mental impairments, who are in a coma, or who

are in an unstable medical condition may need to be excluded.

- *Design considerations.* As noted in Chapter 11, it is sometimes advantageous in terms of internal validity to define a fairly homogeneous population as a means of controlling extraneous variables.

The criteria used to define a population for a research project have implications for both the interpretation of the results and, of course, the external validity of the findings.

Example of inclusion and exclusion criteria: Sherwood and colleagues (2006) studied predictors of distress in caregivers of persons with a primary malignant brain tumor (PMBT). Caregivers were considered eligible if they were over age 21, were able to read and speak English, were providing ongoing care to someone over 21 years of age with a PMBT, and had reliable access to a telephone. Paid caregivers with no prior relationship with the care recipient were excluded.

Samples and Sampling

Sampling is the process of selecting a portion of the population to represent the entire population so that inferences about the population can be made (Fig. 13.1). A **sample** is a subset of population elements. An **element** is the most basic unit about which information is collected. In nursing research, the elements are usually humans.

Samples and sampling plans vary in quality. *The key consideration in assessing a sample in a*

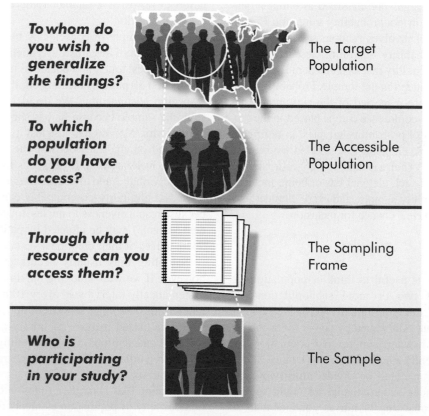

FIGURE 13.1 From the Target Population to the Study Sample.

quantitative study is its representativeness. A **representative sample** is one whose key characteristics closely approximate those of the population. If the population in a study of blood donors is 50% male and 50% female, then a representative sample would have a similar gender distribution. If the sample is not representative of the population, the external validity (and the construct validity) of the study is at risk.

Unfortunately, there is no way to make sure that a sample is representative without obtaining the information from the population. Certain sampling procedures are less likely to result in biased samples than others, but a representative sample can never be guaranteed. This may sound discouraging, but it must be remembered that researchers operate under conditions in which error is possible. Quantitative researchers strive to minimize those errors and, if possible, to estimate their magnitude.

Sampling designs are classified as either probability sampling or nonprobability sampling. **Probability sampling** involves random selection of elements. In probability sampling, researchers can specify the probability that an element of the population will be included in the sample. Probability sampling is the more respected of the two approaches because greater confidence can be placed in the representativeness of probability samples. In **nonprobability samples**, elements are selected by nonrandom methods. There is no way to estimate the probability that each element has of being included in a nonprobability sample, and every element usually does *not* have a chance for inclusion.

Strata

Sometimes, it is useful to think of populations as consisting of two or more subpopulations, or **strata**. A stratum is a mutually exclusive segment of a population, established by one or more characteristics. For instance, suppose our population was all RNs currently employed in the United States. This population could be divided into two strata based on gender. Alternatively, we could specify three strata consisting of nurses younger than 30 years of age, nurses aged 30 to 45 years, and nurses

46 years or older. Strata are often used in the sample selection process to enhance the sample's representativeness.

Sampling Bias

Researchers work with samples rather than with populations because it is more cost-effective to do so. Researchers typically have neither the time nor the resources to study all members of a population. Furthermore, it is usually possible to obtain reasonably accurate information from a sample.

Still, data from samples *can* lead to erroneous conclusions. Finding 100 people willing to participate in a study seldom poses difficulty. It is considerably more problematic to select 100 subjects who are not a biased subset of the population. **Sampling bias** refers to the systematic over-representation or under-representation of some segment of the population in terms of a characteristic relevant to the research question.

As an example of consciously biased selection, suppose we were investigating patients' responsiveness to nurses' touch and decide to use as our sample the first 50 patients meeting eligibility criteria in a specific hospital unit. We decide to omit Mr. Z from the sample because he has shown hostility to nurses. Mrs. X, who has just lost a spouse, is also excluded from the study because she is under stress. We have made conscious decisions to exclude certain individuals, and the decisions do not reflect *bona fide* eligibility criteria. This can lead to bias because responsiveness to nurses' touch (the dependent variable) may be affected by patients' feelings about nurses or their emotional state.

Sampling bias usually occurs unconsciously, however. If we were studying nursing students and systematically interviewed every 10th student who entered the nursing school library, the sample would be biased in favor of library-goers, even if we are conscientious about including every 10th student regardless of his or her appearance, gender, or other traits.

Sampling bias is partly a function of population homogeneity. If population elements were all identical with respect to key attributes, then any sample would be as good as any other. Indeed, if the population were completely homogeneous, that is, exhibited no variability at all, then a *single* element would be sufficient to draw conclusions about the population. For many physiologic attributes, it may be safe to assume reasonably high homogeneity. For example, the blood in a person's veins is relatively homogeneous and so a single blood sample is adequate. For most human attributes, however, homogeneity is the exception rather than the rule. Age, health condition, stress, attitudes—all these attributes reflect the heterogeneity of humans. When variation occurs in the population, then similar variation ideally should be reflected in a sample.

➲ **TIP:** One straightforward way to increase the generalizability of a study is to select study participants from multiple sites, such as from different hospitals, nursing homes, communities, and so on. Ideally, the different sites would be sufficiently divergent that broader representation of the population would be obtained.

NONPROBABILITY SAMPLING

Nonprobability sampling is less likely than probability sampling to produce accurate and representative samples. Despite this fact, most research samples in nursing and other disciplines are nonprobability samples. Three primary methods of nonprobability sampling in quantitative studies are convenience, quota, and purposive.

Convenience Sampling

Convenience sampling entails using the most conveniently available people as study participants. A faculty member who distributes questionnaires to nursing students in a class is using a convenience sample, or an *accidental sample*, as it is sometimes called. The nurse who conducts an observational study of women delivering twins at the local hospital is also relying on a convenience sample. The

problem with convenience sampling is that available subjects might be atypical of the population of interest with regard to critical variables.

Convenience samples do not necessarily comprise individuals known to the researchers. Stopping people at a street corner to conduct an interview is sampling by convenience. Sometimes, researchers seeking people with certain characteristics place an advertisement in a newspaper, put up signs in clinics or supermarkets, or post messages in chat rooms on the Internet. These approaches are subject to bias because people select themselves as pedestrians on certain streets or as volunteers in response to posted notices.

Snowball sampling (also called *network sampling* or *chain sampling*) is a variant of convenience sampling. With this approach, early sample members (called **seeds**) are asked to refer other people who meet the eligibility criteria. This sampling method is often used when the population is people with characteristics who might otherwise be difficult to identify (e.g., people who are afraid of hospitals). Snowballing begins with a few eligible study participants and then continues on the basis of participant referrals.

Convenience sampling is the weakest form of sampling. It is also the most commonly used sampling method in many disciplines. In heterogeneous populations, there is no other sampling approach in which the risk for sampling bias is greater.

Example of a convenience sample: Shin and Kim (2006) conducted a study to measure the thickness of subcutaneous tissue at three major injection sites among children with type 1 diabetes. They used a convenience sample of 65 children attending a diabetes camp in South Korea.

➲ **TIP:** There has been an emerging interest in developing rigorous methods of sampling *hidden populations* such as the homeless or injection drug users. Because standard probability sampling is inappropriate for such hidden populations, a technique called **respondent-driven sampling (RDS)**, a variant of snowball sampling, is being developed. RDS, unlike traditional snowballing, allows the assessment of relative inclusion probabilities based on mathematical models (Magnani et al., 2005).

TABLE 13.1	Numbers and Percentages of Students in Strata of a Population, Convenience Sample, and Quota Sample		
STRATA	**POPULATION**	**CONVENIENCE SAMPLE**	**QUOTA SAMPLE**
Male	100 (20%)	5 (5%)	20 (20%)
Female	400 (80%)	95 (95%)	80 (80%)
Total	500 (100%)	100 (100%)	100 (100%)

Quota Sampling

A **quota sample** is one in which the researcher identifies population strata and determines how many participants are needed from each stratum. By using information about population characteristics, researchers can ensure that diverse segments are represented in the sample, preferably in the proportion in which they occur in the population.

Suppose we were interested in studying nursing students' attitudes toward working with AIDS patients. The accessible population is a school of nursing with an undergraduate enrollment of 500 students; a sample of 100 students is desired. The easiest procedure would be to use a convenience sample by distributing questionnaires in classrooms. We suspect, however, that male and female students have different attitudes toward working with patients with AIDS and a convenience sample might result in too many men or women. Table 13.1 presents fictitious data showing the gender distribution for the population and for a convenience sample in the first two columns. In this example, the convenience sample over-represents women and under-represents men. We can, however, guide the selection of study participants so that the sample includes the correct number of cases from both strata. The far-right panel of Table 13.1 shows the number of men and women required for a quota sample for this example.

If we pursue this same example a bit further, you may better appreciate the dangers of a biased sample.

Suppose that one of the key questions in this study was, "Would you be willing to work on a unit that cared exclusively for AIDS patients?" The percentage of students in the population who would respond "yes" to this inquiry is shown in the first column of Table 13.2. Of course, we would not know these values; they are displayed to illustrate a point. Within the population, men are more likely than women to be willing to work on a unit with AIDS patients, yet men were seriously under-represented in the convenience sample. As a result, there is a discrepancy between the population and sample values on the outcome variable: Nearly twice as many students in the population are favorable toward working with AIDS victims (20%) than we would conclude based on results from the convenience sample (11%). The quota sample, on the other hand, does a better job of reflecting the viewpoint of the population (19%). In actual research situations, the distortions from a convenience sample may be smaller than in this example, but could be larger as well.

Quota sampling does not require sophisticated skills or a lot of effort—and it is surprising that so few researchers use this strategy. Many researchers who use a convenience sample could probably use quota sampling, and it would be advantageous to do so. Stratification should be based on one or more variables that would reflect important differences in the dependent variable under study. Such variables as gender, ethnicity, education, and medical diagnosis are often good stratifying variables.

TABLE 13.2	Students Willing to Work on AIDS Unit: Population, Convenience Sample, and Quota Sample		
	NUMBER IN POPULATION	**NUMBER IN CONVENIENCE SAMPLE**	**NUMBER IN QUOTA SAMPLE**
Willing males	28 (out of 100)	2 (out of 5)	6 (out of 20)
Willing females	72 (out of 400)	9 (out of 95)	13 (out of 80)
Total number of willing students	100 (out of 500)	11 (out of 100)	19 (out of 100)
Percentage willing	20%	11%	19%

Except for identifying the strata and the desired representation for each, quota sampling is procedurally like convenience sampling. The subjects in any subgroups constitute a convenience sample from that stratum of the population. For example, the initial sample of 100 students in Table 13.1 constituted a convenience sample from the population of 500. In the quota sample, the 20 men constitute a convenience sample of the 100 men in the population. Because of this fact, quota sampling shares many of the same weaknesses as convenience sampling. For instance, if a researcher is required by a quota sampling plan to interview 10 men between the ages of 65 and 80 years, a trip to a nursing home might be the most convenient method of obtaining those subjects. Yet this approach would fail to represent the many older men living independently in the community. Despite its problems, quota sampling represents an important improvement over convenience sampling and should be considered by quantitative researchers whose resources prevent the use of probability sampling.

Example of a quota sample: Pieper, Templin, and Ebright (2006) used quota sampling in their study of chronic venous insufficiency (CVI) in HIV-positive persons and the extent to which neuropathy increased the risk for CVI. They stratified their sample on the basis of whether or not the person had a history of injection drug use, and enrolled participants until the quotas were filled.

Purposive Sampling

Purposive sampling, or *judgmental sampling*, is based on the belief that researchers' knowledge about the population can be used to hand-pick sample members. Researchers might decide purposely to select subjects who are judged to be typical of the population or particularly knowledgeable about the issues under study. Sampling in this subjective manner, however, provides no external, objective method for assessing the typicalness of the selected subjects. Nevertheless, this method can be used to advantage in certain situations. Newly developed instruments can be effectively pretested and evaluated with a purposive sample of diverse types of people. Purposive sampling is often used when researchers want a sample of experts, as in the case of a needs assessment using the key informant approach or in Delphi surveys. Also, as discussed later in this chapter, purposive sampling is frequently used by qualitative researchers.

Example of purposive sampling: Gagnon and Grenier (2004) conducted a study to identify, validate, and rank-order quality care indicators relating to empowerment for patients with a chronic complex illness. One phase of their study involved gathering quantitative information from a purposive sample of nurses and other health care professionals selected for their expertise—at least 5 years of experience with chronic patients.

Evaluation of Nonprobability Sampling

Nonprobability samples are rarely representative of the population. When every element in the population does not have a chance of being included in the sample, it is likely that some segment of it will be systematically under-represented. And, when there is sampling bias, there is always a chance that the results could be misleading.

Why, then, are nonprobability samples used in most nursing studies? Clearly, the advantage of these sampling designs lies in their convenience and economy. Probability sampling, discussed next, requires skill and resources. There is often no option but to use a nonprobability approach. Quantitative researchers using nonprobability samples must be cautious about the inferences and conclusions drawn from the data. With care in the selection of the sample, a conservative interpretation of the results, and replication of the study with new samples, researchers find that nonprobability samples usually work reasonably well.

➲ TIP: If you use a convenience sample, you can still take steps to enhance the sample's representativeness. First, identify important extraneous variables—factors that affect variation in the dependent variable. For example, in a study of the effect of stress on health, family income would be an important extraneous variable because poor people tend to be less healthy (*and* more stressed) than more affluent ones. Then, decide how to account for this source of variation in the sampling design. One solution is to eliminate variation from extraneous variables, as discussed in Chapter 11. In the stress and health example, we might restrict the population to middle-class people. Alternatively, we could select the convenience sample from two communities known to differ socioeconomically so that our sample would reflect the experiences of both lower- and middle-class subjects. This approaches using a quota sampling method. In other words, if the population is known to be heterogeneous, you should take steps either to make it more homogeneous (thereby redefining the population) or to capture important sample variation.

PROBABILITY SAMPLING

Probability sampling involves the random selection of elements from a population. **Random sampling** involves a selection process in which each element in the population has an equal, independent chance of being selected. Probability sampling is a complex and technical topic, and books such as those by Levy and Lemeshow (1999) offer further guidance for advanced students.

➲ TIP: Random sampling should not be (although it often is) confused with random assignment, which was described in connection with experimental designs in Chapter 10. Random assignment refers to the process of allocating subjects to different treatment conditions at random. Random *assignment* has no bearing on how subjects in an experiment were selected in the first place.

Simple Random Sampling

Simple random sampling is the most basic probability sampling design. Because the more complex probability sampling designs incorporate features of simple random sampling, the procedures involved are described here in some detail.

In simple random sampling, researchers establish a **sampling frame**, the technical name for the list of the elements from which the sample will be chosen. If nursing students at the University of Connecticut were the accessible population, then a roster of those students would be the sampling frame. If the sampling unit were 500-bed or larger hospitals in Canada, then a list of all such hospitals would be the sampling frame. In practice, a population may be defined in terms of an existing sampling frame. For example, if we wanted to use a telephone directory as a sampling frame, we would have to define the population as community residents with a listed telephone number, not including cellular phones.

Once a sampling frame has been developed, elements are numbered consecutively. A table of random numbers would then be used to draw a sample of the desired size. An example of a sampling frame for a population of 50 people is presented in Table 13.3. Let us assume we want to randomly sample 20 people. As in the case of random assignment, we could find a starting place in a table of random numbers by blindly placing our finger at some point on the page. To include all numbers between 1 and 50, two-digit combinations would be read. Suppose, for the sake of the example, that we began random selection with the first number in the random number table of Table 10.2, which is 46. The person corresponding to that number,

D. Abraham, is the first subject selected to participate in the study. Number 05, H. Edelman, is the second selection, and number 23, J. Yepsen, is the third. This process would continue until the 20 subjects were chosen. The selected elements are circled in Table 13.3.

Clearly, a sample selected randomly in this fashion is not subject to researchers' biases. Although there is no guarantee that a randomly drawn sample will be representative, random selection does ensure that differences in the attributes of the sample and the population are purely a function of chance. The probability of selecting a markedly deviant sample decreases as the size of the sample increases.

Simple random sampling tends to be laborious. Developing a sampling frame, numbering all the elements, and selecting sample elements are time-consuming chores, particularly if the population is large. Imagine enumerating all the telephone subscribers listed in the New York City telephone directory! If the elements can be arranged in computer-readable form, then the computer can be programmed to select the sample automatically. In actual practice, simple random sampling is not used frequently because it is a relatively inefficient procedure. Furthermore, it is not always possible to get a listing of every element in the population, so other methods may be required.

TABLE 13.3	Sampling Frame for Simple Random Sampling Example

(1.)	N. Alexander	(26.)	C. Ball
2.	D. Brady	27.	L. Chodos
3.	D. Carroll	28.	K. DiSanto
4.	M. Dakes	29.	B. Eddy
(5.)	H. Edelman	(30.)	J. Fishon
(6.)	L. Forester	(31.)	R. Griffin
7.	J. Galt	32.	B. Hebert
8.	L. Hall	(33.)	C. Joyce
9.	R. Ivry	(34.)	S. Kane
10.	A. Janosy	35.	D. Lowe
11.	J. Kettlewell	36.	M. Montanari
12.	L. Lack	37.	B. Nicolet
(13.)	R. Mastrianni	(38.)	T. Opitz
(14.)	K. Nolte	39.	J. Portnoy
15.	N. O'Hara	40.	G. Queto
16.	T. Piekarz	41.	A. Ryan
(17.)	J. Quint	42.	S. Singleton
(18.)	M. Riggi	(43.)	L. Tower
19.	M. Solomons	44.	V. Vaccaro
20.	S. Thompson	(45.)	B. Wilmot
(21.)	C. VanWagner	(46.)	D. Abraham
22.	R. Walsh	47.	V. Brusser
(23.)	J. Yepsen	48.	O. Crampton
(24.)	M. Zimmerman	49.	R. Davis
25.	A. Arnold	(50.)	C. Eldred

Example of a simple random sample:
Boyington, Jones, & Wilson (2006) explored the presence of nursing (i.e., accessible and visible data on nurses or nursing care) on hospital websites. The sampling frame was the *U.S. News and World Report* list of the top 203 American hospitals in 2003. Fifty hospitals were selected: all 17 from the magazine's "Honor Roll" and 33 randomly selected from the remaining hospitals via an electronic number generator.

Stratified Random Sampling

In **stratified random sampling**, the population is first divided into two or more strata. As with quota sampling, the aim of stratified sampling is to enhance representativeness. Stratified sampling designs subdivide the population into homogeneous subsets from which an appropriate number of elements are selected at random.

Stratification is often based on such demographic attributes as age or gender. One difficulty is that the stratifying attributes must be known in advance and may not be readily discernible. If you were working with a telephone directory, there would be no personal information that could be used for stratification. Patient listings, student rosters, or organizational directories might contain information for meaningful stratification. Quota sampling does not have the same problem because researchers can ask prospective subjects questions that determine their eligibility for a particular stratum. In stratified sampling, however, a person's status in a stratum must be known before random selection.

The most common procedure for drawing a stratified sample is to group together elements belonging to a stratum and to select randomly the desired number of elements. To illustrate, suppose that the list in Table 13.3 consisted of 25 men (numbers 1 through 25) and 25 women (numbers 26 through 50). Using gender as the stratifying variable, we could guarantee a sample of 10 men and 10 women by randomly sampling 10 numbers from the first half of the list and 10 from the second half. As it turns out, our simple random sampling did result in 10 elements being chosen from each half of the list, but this was purely by chance. It would not have been unusual to draw, say, 8 names from one half and 12 from the other. Stratified sampling can guarantee the appropriate representation of different segments of the population.

Stratifying variables usually divide the population into unequal subpopulations. For example, if the person's race were used to stratify the population of U.S. citizens, the subpopulation of white people would be larger than that of nonwhite people. The researcher might select subjects in proportion to the size of the stratum in the population, using **proportionate stratified sampling**. If the population was students in a nursing school that had 10% African-American, 10% Hispanic, 10% Asian, and 70% white students, then a proportionate stratified sample of 100 students, with racial/ethnic background as the stratifying variable, would consist of 10, 10, 10, and 70 students from the respective strata.

When researchers are interested in understanding differences among strata, proportionate sampling may result in insufficient numbers for making comparisons. In the previous example, the researcher would not be justified in drawing conclusions about the characteristics of Hispanic nursing students based on only 10 cases. For this reason, researchers often adopt a **disproportionate sampling design** when comparisons are sought between strata of greatly unequal size. In the example, the sampling proportions might be altered to select 20 African-American, 20 Hispanic, 20 Asian, and 40 white students. This design would ensure a more adequate representation of the three racial/ethnic minorities. When disproportionate sampling is used, however, it is necessary to make an adjustment to the data to arrive at the best estimate of *overall* population values. This adjustment process, known as **weighting**, is a simple mathematic computation described in textbooks on sampling.

Stratified random sampling enables researchers to sharpen the precision and representativeness of the final sample. When it is desirable to obtain reliable information about subpopulations whose memberships are relatively small, stratification provides a means of including a sufficient number of cases in the sample by oversampling for that stratum. Stratified sampling, however, may be impossible if information on the critical variables is unavailable. Furthermore, a stratified sample requires even more labor and effort than simple random sampling because the sample must be drawn from multiple enumerated listings.

Example of stratified random sampling: Stewart and colleagues (2005) studied nursing practice issues in rural and remote areas of Canada using a mailed survey. Questionnaires were sent to a stratified random sample of rural nurses throughout Canada, using province as the stratifying variable.

Cluster Sampling

For many populations, it is impossible to get a listing of all elements. For example, the population of full-time nursing students in the United States would be difficult to list and enumerate for the purpose of drawing a simple or stratified random sample. Large-scale surveys—especially ones involving personal interviews—almost never use simple or stratified random sampling; they usually rely on cluster sampling.

In **cluster sampling**, there is a successive random sampling of units. The first unit is large groupings, or clusters. In drawing a sample of nursing students, we might first draw a random sample of nursing schools and then draw a sample of students from the selected schools. The usual procedure for selecting samples from a general population is to sample successively such administrative units as states, census tracts, and then households. Because of the successive stages in cluster sampling, this approach is often called **multistage sampling**. The resulting design can be described in terms of the number of stages (e.g., three-stage cluster sampling).

The clusters can be selected either by simple or stratified methods. For instance, in selecting clusters of nursing schools, it may be advisable to stratify on program type. The final selection from within a cluster may also be performed by simple or stratified random sampling.

For a specified number of cases, cluster sampling tends to be less accurate than simple or stratified random sampling. Despite this disadvantage, cluster sampling is more economical and practical than other types of probability sampling, particularly when the population is large and widely dispersed.

> **Example of cluster/multistage sampling:**
> Thato and colleagues (2003) studied predictors of condom use among adolescent Thai vocational students. In the first stage, the researchers randomly selected 8 private vocational schools in Bangkok, and then randomly selected students from the schools. A total of 425 students aged 18 to 22 were sampled.

Systematic Sampling

Systematic sampling involves the selection of every kth case from a list, such as every 10th person on a patient list or every 100th person in a directory of American Nurses Association members. Systematic sampling is sometimes used to sample every kth person entering a bookstore, or passing down the street, or leaving a hospital, and so forth. In such situations, unless the population is narrowly defined as all those people entering, passing by, or leaving, the sampling is essentially a sample of convenience.

Systematic sampling can, however, be applied so that an essentially random sample is drawn. If we had a list (sampling frame), the following procedure could be adopted. The desired sample size is established at some number (n). The size of the population must be known or estimated (N). By dividing N by n, the sampling interval width (k) is established. The **sampling interval** is the standard distance between elements chosen for the sample. For instance, if we were seeking a sample of 200 from a population of 40,000, then our sampling interval would be as follows:

$$k = \frac{40,000}{200} = 200$$

In other words, every 200th element on the list would be sampled. The first element should be selected randomly, using a table of random numbers. Let us say that we randomly selected number 73 from a table. The people corresponding to numbers 73, 273, 473, and so forth would be sampled. Alternatively, we could randomly select a number from 1 to the number of elements listed on a page, and then randomly select every kth unit on all pages (e.g., number 38 on every page).

Systematic sampling conducted in this manner yields essentially the same results as simple random sampling, but involves far less work. Problems would arise if the list were arranged in such a way that a certain type of element is listed at intervals coinciding with the sampling interval. For instance, if every 10th nurse listed in a nursing personnel roster were a head nurse and the sampling interval was 10, then head nurses would either always or never be included in the sample. Problems of this type are rare, fortunately. In most cases, systematic sampling is preferable to simple random sampling because the same results are obtained in a more efficient manner. Systematic sampling can also be applied to lists that have been stratified.

Example of a systematic sample: Ruchala and her colleagues (2003) surveyed a national sample of obstetric units in the United States to determine the types of intravenous fluids used to dilute oxytocin for labor induction. They mailed questionnaires to a systematic random sample of nurse managers in 700 obstetric units with 50 or more births per year as listed by the American Hospital Association.

Evaluation of Probability Sampling

Probability sampling is the only viable method of obtaining representative samples. If all the elements in the population have an equal probability of being selected, then the resulting sample is likely to do a good job of representing the population. A further advantage is that probability sampling allows researchers to estimate the magnitude of sampling error. **Sampling error** refers to differences between population values (such as the average age of the population) and sample values (such as the average age of the sample). It is a rare sample that is perfectly representative of a population; probability sampling permits estimates of the degree of error. Advanced textbooks on sampling elaborate on procedures for making such estimates.

The great drawbacks of probability sampling are its inconvenience and complexity. It is usually beyond the scope of most researchers to sample using a probability design, unless the population is narrowly defined—and if it *is* narrowly defined, probability sampling may seem like "overkill." Probability sampling is the preferred and most respected method of obtaining sample elements, but it is often impractical.

➲ **TIP:** The quality of the sampling plan is of particular importance in survey research because the purpose of surveys is to obtain descriptive information about the prevalence or average values for a population. All national surveys, such as the National Health Interview Survey in the United States, use probability samples (usually cluster samples). Probability samples are rarely used in experimental and quasi-experimental studies, in part because the main focus of such inquiries is on between-group differences rather than absolute values for a population.

SAMPLE SIZE IN QUANTITATIVE STUDIES

Quantitative researchers need to pay careful attention to the number of participants needed to achieve statistical conclusion validity. A procedure known as **power analysis** (Cohen, 1988) can be used to estimate sample size needs, but some statistical knowledge is needed before this procedure can be explained. In this section, we offer guidelines to beginning researchers; advanced students can read about power analysis in Chapter 22 or consult a sampling or statistics textbook.

Sample Size Basics

There are no simple formulas that can tell you how large a sample is needed in a given quantitative study, but we can offer a simple piece of advice: You should use the largest sample possible. The larger the sample, the more representative of the population it is likely to be. Every time researchers calculate a percentage or an average based on sample data, they are estimating a population value. Smaller samples tend to produce less accurate estimates than larger ones. In other words, the larger the sample, the smaller the sampling error.

Let us illustrate this with an example of monthly aspirin consumption in a nursing home (Table 13.4). The population consists of 15 residents whose aspirin consumption averages 16 aspirins per month, as shown in the top row of the table.

TABLE 13.4	Comparison of Population and Sample Values and Averages: Nursing Home Aspirin Consumption Example		
NUMBER OF PEOPLE IN GROUP	**GROUP**	**INDIVIDUAL DATA VALUES (NUMBER OF ASPIRINS CONSUMED, PRIOR MONTH)**	**AVERAGE**
15	Population	2, 4, 6, 8, 10, 12, 14, 16, 18, 20, 22, 24, 26, 28, 30	16.0
2	Sample 1A	6, 14	10.0
2	Sample 1B	20, 28	24.0
3	Sample 2A	16, 18, 8	14.0
3	Sample 2B	20, 14, 26	20.0
5	Sample 3A	26, 14, 18, 2, 28	17.6
5	Sample 3B	30, 2, 26, 10, 4	14.4
10	Sample 4A	22, 16, 24, 20, 2, 8, 14, 28, 20, 4	15.8
10	Sample 4B	12, 18, 8, 10, 16, 6, 28, 14, 30, 22	16.4

Eight simple random samples—two each with sample sizes of 2, 3, 5, and 10—have been drawn. Each sample average represents an estimate of the population average (i.e., 16). Under ordinary circumstances, of course, the population value would be unknown, and we would draw only one sample. With a sample size of two, our estimate might have been wrong by as many as 8 aspirins (sample 1B, average of 24), which is a 50% error. As the sample size increases, the averages get closer to the true population value, *and* the differences in the estimates between samples A and B get smaller as well. As the sample size increases, the probability of getting a markedly deviant sample diminishes. Large samples provide an opportunity to counterbalance atypical values. Unless a power analysis can be done, the safest procedure is to obtain data from as large a sample as is practically feasible.

Large samples are no assurance of accuracy, however. When nonprobability sampling methods are used, even a large sample can harbor extensive bias. The famous example illustrating this point is the 1936 American presidential poll conducted by the magazine *Literary Digest*, which predicted that Alfred M. Landon would defeat Franklin D. Roosevelt by a landslide. About 2.5 million individuals participated in this poll—a substantial sample. Biases resulted from the fact that the sample was drawn from telephone directories and automobile registrations during a depression year when only the well-to-do (who preferred Landon) had a car or telephone. Thus, a large sample cannot correct for a faulty sampling design. Nevertheless, a large nonprobability sample is preferable to a small one.

Because practical constraints such as time, subject availability, and resources often limit sample size, many nursing studies are based on relatively small samples. Indeed, the sampling plan is often one of the weakest aspects of quantitative nursing studies (this is also true of quantitative research in other disciplines). Most nursing studies use samples of convenience, and many are based on samples that are too small to provide an adequate test of the research hypotheses. Most quantitative studies are based on samples of fewer than 200 participants, and a great many studies have fewer than 100 subjects (e.g., Polit & Sherman, 1990). Power analysis is not used by many nurse researchers, and

TABLE 13.5	Three Populations of Different Homogeneity			
GROUP	**INDIVIDUAL DATA VALUES**	**LOWEST VALUE**	**HIGHEST VALUE**	**AVERAGE**
Population A	100 110 105 95 90 110 105 95 90 100	90	110	100.0
Population B	110 120 105 85 80 120 115 85 80 100	80	120	100.0
Population C	100 130 125 75 70 130 125 75 70 100	70	130	100.0
Sample A	110 90 95	90	110	98.3
Sample B	120 80 85	80	120	95.0
Sample C	125 70 75	70	125	90.0

research reports often offer no justification for the size of the study sample. When samples are too small, quantitative researchers run the risk of gathering data that will not support their hypotheses, even when their hypotheses are correct, thereby undermining statistical conclusion validity.

Factors Affecting Sample Size Requirements in Quantitative Research

Sample size requirements are affected by various factors, some of which we discuss in this section.

Homogeneity of the Population

If there is reason to believe that the population is relatively homogeneous, a small sample may be adequate. Let us demonstrate that this is so. The top half of Table 13.5 presents hypothetical values for three different populations, with only 10 people in each population. These values could reflect, for example, scores on an anxiety scale. In all three populations, the average score is 100. In population A, however, the individuals have similar anxiety scores, ranging from a low of 90 to a high of 110. In population B, the scores are more variable, and in population C, the scores are more variable still, ranging from 70 to 130.

The second half of Table 13.5 presents three sample values from the three populations. In the most homogeneous population (A), the average anxiety score for the sample is 98.3—close to the population average of 100. As the population becomes more varied, the average sample values less accurately reflect population values; there is greater sampling error when the population is heterogeneous. By increasing the sample size, the risk for sampling error would be reduced. For example, if sample C consisted of five values rather than three (say, all the even-numbered population values), then the sample average would be closer to the population average (i.e., 102 rather than 90).

For clinical studies that deal with biophysiologic processes in which variation is limited, a small sample may adequately represent the population. For most nursing studies, however, it is safer to assume a fair degree of heterogeneity, unless there is evidence from prior research to the contrary.

Effect Size

Power analysis builds on the concept of an **effect size**, which expresses the strength of relationships among research variables. If there is reason to expect that the independent and dependent variables will be strongly related, then a relatively small sample should be adequate to demonstrate the relationship statistically. For example, if we were testing a powerful new drug to treat AIDS, it might be possible to demonstrate its effectiveness with a small sample. Typically, however, interventions have modest effects, and variables are usually only moderately correlated with one another. When there is no *a priori* reason for believing that relationships will be strong (i.e., when the effect size is expected to be modest), then small samples are risky.

Cooperation and Attrition

In most studies, not everyone invited to participate in a study agrees to do so. Therefore, in developing sampling plans, it is good to begin with a realistic, evidence-based estimate of the percentage of people likely to cooperate. Thus, if your targeted sample size is 200 but you expect refusals by 50% of those invited, you would have to recruit 400 or so eligible participants.

In studies with multiple points of data collection, the number of subjects usually declines over time. This is most likely to occur if the time lag between data collection points is great, if the population is mobile or hard to locate, or if the population is at risk for death or disability. If the researcher has an ongoing relationship with participants (as might be true in clinical studies), then attrition might be low—but it is rarely nonexistent. Therefore, in estimating sample size needs, researchers should factor in anticipated loss of subjects over time.

Attrition problems are not restricted to longitudinal studies. People who initially agree to cooperate in a study may be subsequently unable or unwilling to participate for various reasons, such as death, deteriorating health, early discharge, discontinued need for an intervention, or simply a change of heart. Researchers should expect a certain amount of subject loss and recruit accordingly.

Subgroup Analyses

Researchers are sometimes interested in testing hypotheses not only for an entire population but also for subgroups. For example, we might be interested in determining whether a structured exercise program is effective in improving infants' motor skills. After testing the general hypothesis with a sample of infants, we might wish to test whether the intervention is more effective for certain infants (e.g., low-birth-weight versus normal-birth-weight infants). When a sample is divided to test for **subgroup effects**, the sample must be large enough to support these divisions of the sample.

Sensitivity of the Measures

Instruments vary in their ability to measure key concepts precisely. Biophysiologic measures are usually very sensitive—they measure phenomena accurately and can make fine discriminations in values. Psychosocial measures often contain some error and lack precision. When measuring tools are imprecise and susceptible to errors, larger samples are needed to test hypotheses adequately.

IMPLEMENTING A SAMPLING PLAN IN QUANTITATIVE STUDIES

Once decisions are made about the sampling design and sample size, the plan must be implemented. This section provides some practical information about implementing a sampling plan.

Steps in Sampling in Quantitative Studies

The steps to be undertaken in drawing a sample vary somewhat from one sampling design to the next, but a general outline of procedures can be described.

1. *Identify the population.* It is good to begin with a clear idea about the target population to which you would ideally like to be able to generalize your results. Unless you have extensive resources, you are unlikely to have access to the entire target population, and so you will also need to identify the portion of the target population that is accessible to you. Researchers sometimes *begin* by identifying an accessible population, and then decide how best to define the target population.

2. *Specify the eligibility criteria.* The criteria for eligibility in the sample should then be spelled out. The criteria should be as specific as possible

with respect to characteristics that might exclude potential subjects (e.g., extremes of poor health, inability to read English). The criteria might lead you to redefine your target population.

3. *Specify the sampling plan.* Once the accessible population has been identified, you must decide (a) the method of drawing the sample and (b) how large it will be. Sample size specifications should consider the aspects of the study discussed in the previous section. If you can perform a power analysis to determine the desired number of subjects, it is highly recommended that you do so. Similarly, if probability sampling is an option for selecting a sample, that option should be exercised. If you are not in a position to do either, we recommend using as large a sample as possible and taking steps to build representativeness into the design (e.g., by using quota sampling).

4. *Recruit the sample.* Once the sampling design has been specified, the next step is to recruit prospective study participants according to the plan (after any needed institutional permissions have been obtained) and ask for their cooperation. Issues relating to subject recruitment are discussed next.

Sample Recruitment

Recruiting subjects to participate in a study involves two major tasks: identifying eligible candidates and persuading them to participate. Researchers may need to spend time early in the project deciding the best sources for recruiting potential participants. Researchers must ask such questions as, Where do people matching my population construct live or obtain care in large numbers? Will I have direct access to subjects, or will I need administrative approval? Will there be sufficiently large numbers in one location, or will multiple sites be necessary? During the recruitment phase, it may be necessary to develop a **screening instrument**, which is a brief interview or form that allows researchers to deter-. mine whether a prospective subject meets all eligibility criteria for the study.

The next task involves actually gaining the cooperation of people who have been deemed eligible for the study. It is critical to have an effective recruitment strategy. Many people, given the right circumstances, will agree to cooperate, but—especially in intervention research—some are hesitant. Researchers should ask themselves, What will make this research experience enjoyable, worthwhile, convenient, pleasant, and nonthreatening for subjects? Factors over which researchers have control that can influence the rate of cooperation include the following:

- *Recruitment method.* Face-to-face recruitment is usually more effective than solicitation by a telephone call or a letter.
- *Courtesy.* Successful recruitment depends on using recruiters who are pleasant, courteous, nonthreatening, and enthusiastic about the study. Cooperation sometimes is enhanced if characteristics of recruiters are similar to those of prospective subjects—particularly with regard to gender, race, and ethnicity.
- *Persistence.* Although high-pressure tactics are never acceptable, persistence may sometimes be needed. When prospective subjects are first approached, their initial reaction may be to decline participation, because they might be taken off guard. If a person hesitates or gives an equivocal answer at the first attempt, recruiters should ask if they could come back at a later time.
- *Incentives.* Gifts and monetary incentives have been found to increase participation.
- *Research benefits.* The benefits of participating to the individual and to society should be carefully explained, without exaggeration or misleading information.
- *Sharing results.* Sometimes it is useful to provide people with tangible evidence of their contribution to the study by offering to send them a brief summary of the study results.
- *Convenience.* Every effort should be made to collect data at a time and location that is convenient for participants. In some cases, this may mean making arrangements for transportation or for the care of young children.

- *Endorsements.* It may be valuable to have the study endorsed or acknowledged by a person or organization that has prospective subjects' confidence, and to communicate this to them. Endorsements might come from the institution serving as the research setting, from a funding agency, or from a respected community group or person, such as a church leader. Press releases in advance of recruitment are sometimes advantageous.
- *Assurances.* Prospective subjects should be told who will see the data, what use will be made of the data, and how confidentiality will be maintained.

➲ TIP: Subject recruitment often proceeds at a slower pace than researchers anticipate. Once you have determined your sample size needs, it is a good idea to develop contingency plans for recruiting more subjects, should the initial plan prove overly optimistic. For example, a contingency plan might involve relaxing the eligibility criteria, identifying another institution through which participants could be recruited, offering incentives to make participation more attractive, or lengthening the recruitment period. When such plans are developed at the outset, it reduces the likelihood that you will have to settle for a less-than-desirable sample size.

Generalizing From Samples

Ideally, the sample is representative of the accessible population, and the accessible population is representative of the target population. By using an appropriate sampling plan, researchers can be reasonably confident that the first part of this ideal has been realized. The second part of the ideal entails greater risk. Are diabetic patients in Atlanta representative of diabetic patients in the United States? Researchers must exercise judgment in assessing the degree of similarity.

The best advice is to be realistic and conservative, and to ask challenging questions: Is it reasonable to assume that the accessible population is representative of the target population? In what ways might they differ? How would such differences affect the conclusions? If differences are great, it

would be prudent to specify a more restricted target population to which the findings could be meaningfully generalized.

Inferences about the generalizability of findings can be enhanced by comparing sample characteristics with population characteristics, when this is possible. Published information about the characteristics of many groups of interest to nurses may be available to help provide a context for evaluating sampling bias. For example, if you were studying low-income children in Chicago, you could obtain information on the Internet about salient characteristics (e.g., race/ethnicity, age distribution) of low-income American children from the U.S. Bureau of the Census. Population characteristics could then be compared with sample characteristics, and differences taken into account in interpreting the findings. Sousa, Zauszniewski, & Musil (2004) provide some suggestions for drawing conclusions about whether a convenience sample is representative of the population.

Example of comparison of characteristics:
Griffin, Polit, and Byrne (2007) conducted a survey of more than 300 pediatric nurses, whose names had been randomly selected from a list of 9000 nurses who subscribed to pediatric nursing journals. Demographic characteristics of the sample (e.g., gender, race/ethnicity, educational background) were compared with characteristics of nurses who participated in a government survey with a nationally representative sample.

SAMPLING IN QUALITATIVE RESEARCH

Qualitative studies almost always use small, nonrandom samples. This does not mean that qualitative researchers are unconcerned with the quality of their samples, but rather that they use different considerations in selecting study participants.

The Logic of Qualitative Sampling

Quantitative research is concerned with measuring attributes and relationships in a population, and therefore a representative sample is needed to ensure that the measurements accurately reflect and can be generalized to the population. The aim of most qualitative studies is to discover *meaning* and to uncover multiple realities, and so generalizability is not a guiding consideration.

Qualitative researchers begin with the following types of sampling question in mind: Who would be an information-rich data source for my study? Whom should I talk to, or what should I observe, to maximize my understanding of the phenomenon? A critical first step in qualitative sampling is selecting settings with high potential for information richness. As the study progresses, new sampling questions emerge, such as the following: Who can I talk to or observe that would confirm my understandings? Challenge or modify my understandings? Enrich my understandings? Thus, as with the overall design in qualitative studies, sampling design is an emergent one that capitalizes on early learning to guide subsequent direction.

Another point worth mentioning is that individuals are not always considered the *unit of analysis* in qualitative studies. For example, Glaser and Strauss (1967) have noted that "incidents" or experiences are often the basis for analysis. An information-rich informant can therefore contribute dozens of incidents, and so even a small number of informants can generate a large sample for analysis.

> **Example of a sample of incidents in a qualitative study:** Thulesius, Håkansson, and Petersson (2003) conducted a grounded theory study of basic processes in end-of-life cancer care in Sweden. They interviewed 64 participants (nurses, physicians, patients, and relatives) over an 8-year period. Their interviews generated more than 1000 incidents, which were used to identify *balancing* as the main social process.

➲ **TIP:** Like quantitative researchers, qualitative researchers often identify eligibility criteria for their studies. Even though they do not articulate an explicit population to whom results are intended to be generalized, qualitative researchers do establish the kinds of people who are eligible to participate in their research.

Types of Qualitative Sampling

Qualitative researchers usually eschew probability samples. A random sample is not the best method of selecting people who will make good informants, that is, people who are knowledgeable, articulate, reflective, and willing to talk at length with researchers. Various nonprobability sampling designs have been used by qualitative researchers.

Convenience Sampling

Qualitative researchers often begin with a convenience sample, which is sometimes referred to in qualitative studies as a *volunteer sample*. Volunteer samples are especially likely to be used when researchers need to have potential participants come forward and identify themselves. For example, if we wanted to study the experiences of people with frequent nightmares, we might have difficulty readily identifying potential participants. In such a situation, we might recruit sample members by placing a notice on a bulletin board, in a newspaper, or on the Internet, requesting people with frequent nightmares to contact us. In this situation, we would be less interested in obtaining a representative sample of people with nightmares than in obtaining a diverse group representing various experiences with nightmares.

Sampling by convenience may be easy and efficient, but it is not in general a preferred sampling approach, even in qualitative studies. The key in qualitative studies is to extract the greatest possible information from the few cases in the sample, and a convenience sample may not provide the most information-rich sources. However, a convenience sample may be an economical and easy way to begin the sampling process, relying on other methods as data are collected.

> **Example of a convenience sample:** Bentley and colleagues (2005) explored the experience of heart failure patients in following a low-sodium diet, to explore factors affecting nonadherence. In-depth interviews were conducted with a convenience sample of 20 patients.

Snowball Sampling

Qualitative researchers also use snowball sampling, asking early informants to make referrals to other study participants. Snowball sampling has distinct advantages over convenience sampling. The first advantage is that it may be more cost-efficient and practical. Researchers may spend less time screening people to determine whether they are appropriate for the study, for example. Furthermore, with an introduction from the referring person, researchers may have an easier time establishing a trusting relationship with new participants. Finally, researchers can more readily specify the characteristics that they want new participants to have. For example, in the study of people with nightmares, we could ask early respondents if they knew anyone else who had the same problem *and* who was articulate. We could also ask for referrals to people who would add other dimensions to the sample, such as people who vary in age, race, socioeconomic status, and so on.

A weakness of this approach is that the eventual sample might be restricted to a rather small network of acquaintances. Moreover, the quality of the referrals may be affected by whether the referring sample member trusted the researcher and truly wanted to cooperate.

⊃ **TIP:** Researchers should be careful about protecting the rights of the individuals whom early participants refer. It is wise to suggest that early informants first check with the potential referrals to make sure they are interested in participating before their names are shared with the researcher. This is especially true if the research involves a sensitive topic (e.g., drug use, suicide attempts).

Example of a snowball sample: Berggren, Bergstrom, and Edberg (2006) explored the experience of female genital mutilation among women from Somalia, Eritrea, and Sudan and their encounters with the maternal health care system in Sweden. Snowball sampling was used to recruit the women into the study. The sample consisted of 22 women—11 from Somalia, 6 from Eritrea, and 5 from Sudan.

Purposive Sampling

Qualitative sampling may begin with volunteer informants and may be supplemented with new participants through snowballing, but many qualitative studies eventually evolve to a purposive (or *purposeful*) sampling strategy—that is, selecting cases that will most benefit the study.

In purposive sampling, several strategies have been identified (Patton, 2002), only some of which are mentioned here. Note that researchers themselves do not necessarily refer to their sampling plans with Patton's labels; his classification shows the kind of diverse strategies qualitative researchers have adopted to meet the conceptual and substantive needs of their research:

- **Maximum variation sampling** involves purposefully selecting cases with a wide range of variation on dimensions of interest. By selecting participants with diverse views and perspectives, researchers invite challenges to emerging conceptualizations. Maximum variation sampling might involve ensuring that people with diverse backgrounds are represented in the sample (ensuring that there are men and women, poor and affluent people, and so on). It might also involve deliberate attempts to include people with different viewpoints about the phenomenon under study. For example, researchers might use snowballing to ask early participants for referrals to people who hold different points of view.
- **Homogeneous sampling** deliberately reduces variation and permits a more focused inquiry. Researchers may use this approach if they wish to understand a particular group of people especially well. Homogeneous sampling is often used to select people for group interviews.
- **Extreme (deviant) case sampling** provides opportunities for learning from the most unusual and extreme informants (e.g., outstanding successes and notable failures). The assumption underlying this approach is that extreme cases are rich in information because they are special in some way. In some cases, more can be learned by intensively studying extreme cases, but extreme cases can also distort understanding of a phenomenon.
- **Intensity sampling** is similar to extreme case sampling, but with less emphasis on the extremes.

Intensity samples involve information-rich cases that manifest the phenomenon of interest intensely, but not as extreme or potentially distorting manifestations. Thus, the goal in intensity sampling is to select rich cases that offer strong examples of the phenomenon.

• **Typical case sampling** involves the selection of participants who illustrate or highlight what is typical or average. The resulting information can be used to create a qualitative profile illustrating typical manifestations of the phenomenon being studied.

• **Critical case sampling** involves selecting important cases regarding the phenomenon of interest. With this approach, researchers look for the particularly good story that illuminates critical aspects of the phenomenon.

• **Criterion sampling** involves studying cases that meet a predetermined criterion of importance. Criterion sampling is sometimes used in mixed method studies in which data from the quantitative component are used to select cases meeting certain criteria for in-depth study. Sandelowski (2000b) offers a number of helpful suggestions for combining sampling strategies in mixed method research.

• **Theory-based sampling** involves the selection of people or incidents on the basis of their potential representation of important theoretical constructs. Theory-based sampling is a focused approach that is usually based on an *a priori* theory that is being examined qualitatively.

• **Sampling confirming and disconfirming cases** is often used toward the end of data collection. As researchers note trends and patterns in the data, emerging conceptualizations need to be checked. **Confirming cases** are additional cases that fit researchers' conceptualizations and offer enhanced credibility. **Disconfirming cases** are examples that do not fit and serve to challenge researchers' interpretations. These "negative" cases may offer new insights about how the original conceptualization needs to be revised or expanded.

It is important to note that almost all these sampling strategies require that researchers have some knowledge about the setting in which the study is taking place. For example, to choose extreme cases, typical cases, or critical cases, researchers must have information about the range of variation of the phenomenon and how it manifests itself. Early participants may be helpful in implementing these sampling strategies.

Quantitative researchers design their sampling plans so as to avoid sampling bias, but Morse (2003) has argued that "biasphobia" can undermine good qualitative research. With respect to sampling, she noted that the goal should be to actively and purposefully pursue the *best,* rather than the average, case. Her advice was to start with excellent examples of the phenomenon being studied, and then—once the phenomenon is better understood and there is a sense of what to look for—to examine "weaker instances and average occurrences" of the phenomenon.

⮕ TIP: Some qualitative researchers appear to call their sample *purposive* simply because they "purposely" selected people who experienced the phenomenon of interest. However, exposure to the phenomenon is an eligibility criterion—the population of interest comprises people with that exposure. If the researcher then recruits *any* person with the desired experience, the sample is selected by convenience, not purposively. Purposive sampling implies an intent to carefully choose *particular* exemplars or *types* of people who can best enhance the researcher's understanding of the phenomenon.

Theoretical Sampling

The method of sampling used in grounded theory is called **theoretical sampling**. Glaser (1978, p. 36) defined this sampling as "the process of data collection for generating theory whereby the analyst jointly collects, codes, and analyzes his data and decides what data to collect next and where to find them, in order to develop his theory as it emerges." The process of theoretical sampling is guided by the developing grounded theory. Theoretical sampling is not envisioned as a single, unidirectional line. This complex sampling technique requires researchers to be involved with multiple lines and directions as they go back and forth between data and categories as the theory emerges.

Glaser stressed that theoretical sampling is not the same as purposive sampling. Theoretical sampling's purpose is to discover categories and their properties and to offer interrelationships that occur in the substantive theory. "The basic question in theoretical sampling is, What groups or subgroups does one turn to next in data collection?" (Glaser, 1978, p. 36). These groups are not chosen before the research begins but only as they are needed for their theoretical relevance for developing further emerging categories.

Example of a theoretical sampling: Beck (2002) used theoretical sampling in her grounded theory study of mothering twins during the first year of life. A specific example of theoretical sampling concerned what the mothers kept referring to as the "blur period"—the first few months of caring for the twins. Initially, Beck interviewed mothers whose twins were about 1 year of age. Her rationale was that these mothers would be able to reflect back over the entire first year of mothering the multiples. When these mothers referred to the "blur period," Beck asked them to describe this period more fully. The mothers said they could not provide many details about this period because "it was such a blur!" Beck then chose to interview mothers whose twins were 3 months of age or younger, to ensure that mothers were still immersed in the "blur period" and would be able to provide rich detail about what this phase of mothering twins was like.

TIP: No matter what type of qualitative sampling you use, you should keep a journal or notebook to jot down ideas and reminders regarding the sampling process (e.g., who you should interview next). Memos to yourself will help you remember valuable ideas about your sample.

Sample Size in Qualitative Research

There are no rules for sample size in qualitative research. Sample size is largely a function of the purpose of the inquiry, the quality of the informants, and the type of sampling strategy used. For example, a larger sample is likely to be needed with maximum variation sampling than with typical case sampling.

In qualitative studies, sample size should be determined based on informational needs. Hence, a guiding principle in sampling is **data saturation**—that is, sampling to the point at which no new information is obtained and redundancy is achieved. Morse (2000) has noted that the number of participants needed to reach saturation depends on a number of factors. For example, the broader the scope of the research question, the more participants will likely be needed. Data quality can also affect sample size. If participants are good informants who are able to reflect on their experiences and communicate effectively, saturation can be achieved with a relatively small sample. Also, if longitudinal data are collected, fewer participants may be needed because each will provide a greater amount of information.

TIP: Sample size estimation can create practical dilemmas if you are seeking approval or funding for a project. Patton (2002) recommends that, in a proposal, researchers should specify *minimum* samples that would reasonably be adequate for understanding the phenomenon. Additional cases can then be added, as necessary, to achieve saturation.

Sampling in the Three Main Qualitative Traditions

There are similarities among the various qualitative traditions with regard to sampling: samples are usually small, probability sampling is not used, and final sampling decisions usually take place in the field during data collection. However, there are some differences as well.

Sampling in Ethnography
Ethnographers may begin by initially adopting a "big net" approach—that is, mingling with and having conversations with as many members of the culture under study as possible. Although they may

converse with many people (usually 25 to 50), they often rely heavily on a smaller number of *key informants*, who are highly knowledgeable about the culture and who develop special, ongoing relationships with the researcher. These key informants are often the researcher's main link to the "inside."

Key informants are chosen purposively, guided by the ethnographer's informed judgments. Developing a pool of potential key informants often depends on ethnographers' prior knowledge to construct a relevant framework. For example, an ethnographer might make decisions about different types of key informants to seek out based on roles (e.g., physicians, nurse practitioners) or on some other substantively meaningful distinction. Once a pool of potential key informants is developed, key considerations for final selection are their level of knowledge about the culture and how willing they are to collaborate with the ethnographer in revealing and interpreting the culture.

Sampling in ethnography typically involves more than selecting informants because observation and other means of data collection play a big role in helping researchers understand a culture. Ethnographers have to decide not only *whom* to sample, but *what* to sample as well. For example, ethnographers have to make decisions about observing *events* and *activities*, about examining *records* and *artifacts*, and about exploring *places* that provide clues about the culture. Key informants can play an important role in helping ethnographers decide what to sample.

Example of an ethnographic sample:
Sobralske (2006) conducted an ethnographic study exploring health care–seeking beliefs and behaviors of Mexican-American men living in Washington State. The researchers participated in activities within the Mexican-American community, and then recruited participants through community organizations, religious groups, schools, and personal contacts. The sample consisted of 8 key informants who varied in terms of acculturation, occupation, educational levels, and interests. The sample also included 28 secondary research participants, who were men and women with insight into health care–seeking beliefs and actions of Mexican-American men. The secondary participants helped to validate the findings from the key informants.

Sampling in Phenomenological Studies

Phenomenologists tend to rely on very small samples of participants—typically 10 or fewer. There is one guiding principle in selecting the sample for a phenomenological study: all participants must have experienced the phenomenon and must be able to articulate what it is like to have lived that experience. It might thus be said that phenomenologists use a criterion sampling method, the criterion being experience with the phenomenon under study. Although phenomenological researchers seek participants who have had the targeted experiences, they also want to explore diversity of individual experiences. Thus, as described by Porter (1999), they may specifically look for people with demographic or other differences who have shared a common experience.

Example of a sample in a phenomenological study: Nelms (2005) studied the experience of mothering among HIV-infected women. A sample of 16 women were selected to reflect a diversity of ethnicity, age, number and ages of children, and health status.

Sampling in Grounded Theory Studies

Grounded theory research is typically done with samples of about 20 to 30 people, using theoretical sampling. The goal in a grounded theory study is to select informants who can best contribute to the evolving theory. Sampling, data collection, data analysis, and theory construction occur concurrently, and so study participants are selected serially and contingently (i.e., contingent on the emerging conceptualization). Sampling might evolve as follows:

1. The researcher begins with a general notion of where and with whom to start. The first few cases may be solicited purposively, by convenience, or through snowballing.
2. In the early part of the study, a strategy such as maximum variation sampling might be used, to gain insights into the range and complexity of the phenomenon under study.
3. The sample is adjusted in an ongoing fashion. Emerging conceptualizations help to inform the sampling process.

4. Sampling continues until saturation is achieved.
5. Final sampling often includes a search for confirming and disconfirming cases to test, refine, and strengthen the theory.

Example of sampling in a grounded theory study: Meeker (2004) did a grounded theory study of end-of-life decision making among family surrogates. The sample consisted of 20 persons who had functioned as a family surrogate decision maker during the terminal phase of a family members' cancer illness. Meeker used theoretical sampling "to provide data needed to describe the categories thoroughly" (p. 208). For example, early participants reported that other family members had been supportive, and so Meeker sought participants who had experienced conflict.

CRITIQUING SAMPLING PLANS

In coming to conclusions about the quality of evidence that a study yields, the sampling plan—particularly for a quantitative study—merits special scrutiny. If the sample is seriously biased or too small, the findings may be misleading or just plain wrong.

In critiquing a description of a sampling plan, you should consider two issues. The first is whether the researcher has adequately described the sampling strategy. Ideally, research reports should include a description of the following:

- The type of sampling approach used (e.g., convenience, snowball, purposive, simple random)
- The population under study and the eligibility criteria for sample selection in quantitative studies; the nature of the setting and study group in qualitative ones (qualitative studies may also articulate eligibility criteria)
- The number of participants in the study and a rationale for the sample size
- A description of the main characteristics of participants (e.g., age, gender, medical condition, and so forth) and, in a quantitative study, of the population

- In quantitative studies, the number and characteristics of potential subjects who declined to participate in the study

If the description of the sample is inadequate, you may not be in a position to deal with the second and principal issue, which is whether the researcher made good sampling decisions. Moreover, if the description is incomplete, it will be difficult to draw conclusions about whether the evidence can be applied in your clinical practice.

Critiquing Quantitative Sampling Plans

The sampling plan in a quantitative study should be scrutinized with respect to its effects on the study's validity and the internal, external, construct, and statistical conclusion validity. If a sample is small, statistical conclusion validity will likely be undermined. If the eligibility criteria are restrictive, this could benefit internal validity—but possibly to the detriment of construct and external validity.

We have stressed that a key criterion for assessing the adequacy of a sampling plan in quantitative research is whether the sample is representative of the population. You will never be able to know for sure, of course, but if the sampling strategy is weak or if the sample size is small, there is reason to suspect some bias. When researchers have adopted a sampling plan in which the risk for bias is high, they should take steps to estimate the direction and degree of this bias so that readers can draw some informed conclusions.

Even with a rigorous sampling plan, the sample may contain some bias if not all people invited to participate in a study agree to do so. If certain segments of the population refuse to participate, then a biased sample can result, even when probability sampling is used. The research report ideally should provide information about **response rates** (i.e., the number of people participating in a study relative to the number of people sampled) and about possible **nonresponse bias**—differences between participants and those who declined to participate (also sometimes referred to as *response bias*). In a longitudinal study, attrition bias should be reported.

BOX 13.1 Guidelines for Critiquing Quantitative Sampling Designs

1. Is the population under study identified and described? Are eligibility criteria specified? Are the sample selection procedures clearly delineated?
2. Do the sample and population specifications support an inference of construct validity with regard to the population construct?
3. What type of sampling plan was used? Would an alternative sampling plan have been preferable? Was the sampling plan one that could be expected to yield a representative sample?
4. How were subjects recruited into the sample? Does the method suggest potential biases?
5. Did some factor other than the sampling plan (e.g., a low response rate) affect the representativeness of the sample?
6. Are possible sample biases or weaknesses identified?
7. Are key characteristics of the sample described (e.g., mean age, percentage female)?
8. Is the sample size sufficiently large to support statistical conclusion validity? Was the sample size justified on the basis of a power analysis or other rationale?
9. Does the sample support inferences about external validity? To whom can the study results reasonably be generalized?

In developing the sampling plan, quantitative researchers make decisions about the specification of the population as well as the selection of the sample. If the target population is defined broadly, researchers may have missed opportunities to control extraneous variables, and the gap between the accessible and the target population may be too great. One of your jobs as reviewer is to come to conclusions about the reasonableness of generalizing the findings from the researcher's sample to the accessible population and from the accessible population to a broader target population. If the sampling plan is seriously flawed, it may be risky to generalize the findings at all without replicating the study with another sample.

Box 13.1 presents some guiding questions for critiquing the sampling plan of a quantitative research report.

Critiquing Qualitative Sampling Plans

In a qualitative study, the sampling plan can be evaluated in terms of its adequacy and appropriateness (Morse, 1991b). *Adequacy* refers to the sufficiency and quality of the data the sample yielded. An adequate sample provides data without any "thin"

spots. When the researcher has truly obtained saturation with a sample, informational adequacy has been achieved, and the resulting description or theory is richly textured and complete.

Appropriateness concerns the methods used to select a sample. An appropriate sample is one resulting from the identification and use of study participants who can best supply information according to the conceptual requirements of the study. Researchers must use a strategy that will yield the fullest possible understanding of the phenomenon of interest. A sampling approach that excludes negative cases or that fails to include participants with unusual experiences may not meet the information needs of the study.

Another important issue to consider concerns the potential for transferability of the findings. The degree of transferability of study findings is a direct function of the similarity between the sample of the original study and the people at another site to which the findings might be applied. **Fittingness** is the degree of congruence between these two groups. Thus, in critiquing a report, you should see whether the researcher provided an adequately thick description of the sample and the context in which the study was carried out so that someone

BOX 13.2 Guidelines for Critiquing Qualitative Sampling Designs

1. Is the setting or context adequately described? Is the setting appropriate for the research question?
2. Are the sample selection procedures clearly delineated? What type of sampling strategy was used?
3. Were the eligibility criteria for the study specified? How were participants recruited into the study? Did the recruitment strategy yield information-rich participants?
4. Given the information needs of the study—and, if applicable, its qualitative tradition—was the sampling approach appropriate? Are dimensions of the phenomenon under study adequately represented?
5. Is the sample size adequate and appropriate for the qualitative tradition of the study? Did the researcher indicate that saturation had been achieved? Do the findings suggest a richly textured and comprehensive set of data without any apparent "holes" or thin areas?
6. Are key characteristics of the sample described (e.g., age, gender)? Is a rich description of participants and context provided, allowing for an assessment of the transferability of the findings?

interested in transferring the findings could make an informed decision.

Further guidance to critiquing sampling in a qualitative study is presented in Box 13.2.

RESEARCH EXAMPLES

In the following sections, we describe in some detail the sampling plans of two nursing studies, one quantitative and the other qualitative.

Research Example From a Quantitative Study

Study: "Level of RN educational preparation: Its impact on collaboration and the relationship between collaboration and professional identity" (Miller, 2004)

Purpose: Miller's study had two purposes: (1) to determine whether educational preparation affects nurses' perceptions of their interprofessional collaboration; and (2) to explore the relationship between such collaboration and nurses' professional identity.

Design: The researcher conducted a cross-sectional mailed survey that assessed professional identity and four dimensions of collaboration (mutual safeguarding of concerns, power/control, clarity of patient care goals, and practice spheres).

Sampling Plan: Miller drew a stratified random sample of nurses from the membership of a nursing association in a province of Canada. Using information available in the

listing, she first removed association members who were deemed unlikely to interact with professionals from other disciplines in matters related to patient care (e.g., nursing education administrators, those not in the labor market). The resulting sampling frame was then stratified by highest level of nursing preparation: those with a diploma or baccalaureate degree were in one stratum, and those with a master's or doctoral degree were in another. Before randomly selecting names, Miller determined how many nurses should be included in the sample by performing a power analysis. The power analysis assumed a modest effect size and took into account the likelihood that many people would not complete a mailed survey. The sample size for each stratum was set at 400. Of the 800 surveys mailed, 379 (47%) usable questionnaires were received: 174 from the diploma/baccalaureate degree stratum and 205 from the master's/doctoral degree stratum.

Key Findings:

- For the first three of the four dimensions of collaboration, both groups reported reasonably effective collaboration with other health professionals.
- Higher level of education was positively related to interprofessional collaboration.
- The relationship between collaboration and professional identity scores tended to be modest and mostly nonsignificant.

Research Example From a Qualitative Study

Study: "Deciding whether to continue, share, or relinquish caregiving: Caregiver views" (Caron & Bowers, 2003)

Research Purpose: The researchers conducted a study of informal caregiving in an effort to develop a substantive caregiving theory to explain the complex decision making involved in providing care to older family members.

Method: Caron and Bowers used Glaser and Strauss's grounded theory method with the goal of generating a substantive theory of caregiving decisions from their data. They conceptualized caregiving as a complex social process that lent itself well to a grounded theory approach.

Sampling Plan: The researchers generated a sample of 16 family caregivers. They first recruited 5 caregivers from a social service program, the Wisconsin Partnership Program (WPP). As the analysis progressed, sample selection was guided by factors emerging in the theory. These factors included presence or absence of cognitive impairment (Alzheimer disease or early dementia) in the care recipient, living arrangement (same or separate households), and use or nonuse of external social services in support of the caregiving. Their sample of 6 male and 10 female caregivers included 10 who were caring for relatives with cognitive impairment and 7 who were living with the family member. Four of the 16 caregivers did not have supplemental assistance from outside service providers. Although initial sample members were recruited with the WPP, the researchers recruited the remainder of their sample outside the WPP to ensure that they would be able to learn about caregiving in the absence of outside help. The remaining participants were recruited through an Alzheimer disease association and by word of mouth.

Key Findings:

- The analysis revealed various purposes of caregiving for an older adult. These purposes were found to influence whether—and how—caregivers continued to provide care or decided to share or relinquish caregiving to health care professionals.
- The two main purposes of caregiving were an interrelational purpose (in which caregivers protected and maintained the caregiver–care recipient relationship) and a pragmatic purpose (providing physical comfort and appropriate care).

SUMMARY POINTS

- **Sampling** is the process of selecting a portion of the **population**, which is an entire aggregate of cases. An **element** is the basic unit of a population about which information is collected—usually humans in nursing research.
- **Eligibility criteria** (or **inclusion criteria**) are used to establish population characteristics. Care must be taken to specify eligibility criteria so as to maximize the construct validity of the population construct.
- Researchers usually sample from an **accessible population**, but should identify the **target population** to which they would like to generalize their results.
- A key consideration in assessing a sample in a quantitative study is its *representativeness*—the extent to which the sample is similar to the population and avoids bias. **Sampling bias** refers to the systematic over-representation or under-representation of some segment of the population.
- The principal types of **nonprobability sampling** (wherein elements are selected by non-random methods) are convenience, quota, and purposive sampling. Nonprobability sampling designs are convenient and economical; a major disadvantage is their potential for bias.
- **Convenience sampling** (or *accidental sampling*) uses the most readily available or most convenient group of people for the sample. **Snowball sampling** is a type of convenience sampling in which referrals for potential participants are made by those already in the sample.
- **Quota sampling** divides the population into homogeneous **strata** (subpopulations) to ensure representation of the subgroups in the sample; within each stratum, subjects are sampled by convenience.
- In **purposive** (or *judgmental*) **sampling**, participants are hand-picked to be included in the sample based on the researcher's knowledge about the population.
- **Probability sampling** designs, which involve the random selection of elements from the population, yield more representative samples than nonprobability designs and permit estimates of the magnitude of **sampling error**.
- **Simple random sampling** involves the random selection of elements from a **sampling frame** that enumerates all the elements; **stratified**

random sampling divides the population into homogeneous subgroups from which elements are selected at random.

- **Cluster sampling** (or **multistage sampling**) involves the successive selection of random samples from larger to smaller units by either simple random or stratified random methods.
- **Systematic sampling** is the selection of every *k*th case from a list. By dividing the population size by the desired sample size, the researcher establishes the **sampling interval**, which is the standard distance between the selected elements.
- In quantitative studies, researchers should use a **power analysis** to estimate sample size needs. Large samples are preferable to small ones because larger samples enhance statistical conclusion validity and tend to be more representative, but even large samples do not *guarantee* representativeness.
- Qualitative researchers use the conceptual demands of the study to select articulate and reflective informants with certain types of experience in an emergent way, capitalizing on early learning to guide subsequent sampling decisions.
- Qualitative researchers most often use **purposive sampling** to guide them in selecting data sources that maximize information richness. Various purposive sampling strategies have been used by qualitative researchers.
- One purposive strategy is **maximum variation sampling**, which entails purposely selecting cases with a wide range of variation. Another important strategy is **sampling confirming and disconfirming cases**, that is, selecting cases that enrich and challenge the researchers' conceptualizations.
- Other types of purposive sampling include **homogeneous sampling** (deliberately reducing variation); **extreme case sampling** (selecting the most unusual or extreme cases); **intensity sampling** (selecting cases that are intense but not extreme); **typical case sampling** (selecting cases that illustrate what is typical); **critical case sampling** (selecting cases that are espe-

cially important or illustrative); **criterion sampling** (studying cases that meet a predetermined criterion of importance); and **theory-based sampling** (selecting cases on the basis of their representation of important constructs).
- Samples in qualitative studies are typically small and based on information needs. A guiding principle is **data saturation**, which involves sampling to the point at which no new information is obtained and redundancy is achieved.
- Ethnographers make numerous sampling decisions, including not only *whom* to sample but also *what* to sample (e.g., activities, events, documents, artifacts); decision making is often aided by their **key informants**, who serve as guides and interpreters of the culture.
- Phenomenologists typically work with a small sample of people (10 or fewer) who meet the criterion of having lived the experience under study.
- Grounded theory researchers typically use **theoretical sampling**, in which sampling decisions are guided in an ongoing fashion by the emerging theory. Samples of about 20 to 30 people are typical in grounded theory studies.
- Criteria for evaluating qualitative sampling are informational adequacy and appropriateness.

STUDY ACTIVITIES

Chapter 13 of the *Resource Manual to Accompany Nursing Research: Generating and Assessing Evidence for Nursing Practice, 8th edition*, offers various exercises and study suggestions for reinforcing concepts presented in this chapter. In addition, the following study questions can be addressed:

1. Answer relevant questions from Box 13.1 with regard to the study by Miller (2004), described at the end of the chapter. Also consider the following additional questions: (a) Was the sampling likely to be proportionate or disproportionate? (b) Why did Miller stratify the sample—and was the decision well advised? Did she use an appropriate stratifying variable?

(c) What are some of the likely sources of sampling bias in the final sample of 379 participants?

2. Answer relevant questions from Box 13.2 with regard to the study by Caron and Bowers (2003), described at the end of the chapter. Also consider the following additional questions: (a) What do you think the eligibility criteria for the study were? (b) Do you think it was a strength or weakness of the sampling plan to use three different approaches to recruit participants (i.e., WPP, Alzheimer disease association, word of mouth)? Why?

STUDIES CITED IN CHAPTER 13

Methodologic or theoretical references cited in this chapter can be found in a separate section at the end of the book.

Beck, C. T. (2002). Releasing the pause button: Mothering twins during the first year of life. *Qualitative Health Research, 12,* 593–608.

Bentley, N., DeJong, M., Moser, D., & Peden, A. (2005). Factors related to nonadherence to low sodium diet recommendations in heart failure patients. *European Journal of Cardiovascular Nursing, 4*(4), 331–336.

Berggren, V., Bergstrom, S., & Edberg, A. K. (2006). Being different and vulnerable: Experiences of immigrant African women who had been circumcised and sought maternity care in Sweden. *Journal of Transcultural Nursing, 17*(1), 50–57.

Boyington, A., Jones, C., & Wilson, D. (2006). Buried alive: The presence of nursing on hospital web sites. *Nursing Research, 55*(2), 103–109.

Caron, C. D., & Bowers, B. J. (2003). Deciding whether to continue, share, or relinquish caregiving: Caregiver views. *Qualitative Health Research, 13,* 1252–1271.

Gagnon, J., & Grenier, R. (2004). [Evaluation and validation of quality care indicators relative to empowerment in complex chronic disease.] *Recherche en Soins Infirmiers,* No. 76, 50–67.

Griffin, R., Polit, D., & Byrne, M. (2007). Nurse characteristics and inferences about children's pain. Manuscript submitted for publication.

Meeker, M. A. (2004). Family surrogate decision making at the end of life: Seeing them through with care and respect. *Qualitative Health Research, 14,* 204–225.

Miller, J. L. (2004). Level of RN educational preparation: Its impact on collaboration and the relationship between collaboration and professional identity. *Canadian Journal of Nursing Research, 36,* 132–147.

Nelms, T. (2005). Burden: The phenomenon of mothering with HIV. *Journal of the Association of Nurses in AIDS Care, 16*(4), 3–13.

Pieper, B., Templin, T., & Ebright, J. (2006). Chronic venous insufficiency in HIV-positive persons with and without a history of injection drug use. *Advances in Skin & Wound Care, 19*(1), 37–42.

Ruchala, P. L., Metheny, N., Essenpreis, H., & Borcherding, K. (2003). Current practice in oxytocin dilution and fluid administration for induction of labor. *Journal of Obstetric, Gynecologic, & Neonatal Nursing, 31,* 545–550.

Sherwood, P., Given, B., Given, C., Schiffman, R., Murman, D., Lovely, M., von Eye, A., Rogers, L., & Remer, S. (2006). Predictors of distress in caregivers of persons with a primary malignant tumor. *Research in Nursing & Health, 29,* 105–120.

Shin, H., & Kim, M. (2006). Subcutaneous tissue thickness in children with type 1 diabetes. *Journal of Advanced Nursing, 54*(1), 29–34.

Sobralske, M. C. (2006). Health care seeking among Mexican American men. *Journal of Transcultural Nursing, 17,* 129–138.

Stewart, N., D'Arcy, C., Pitblado, J., Morgan, D., Forbes, D., Remus, G. et al. (2005). A profile of registered nurses in rural and remote Canada. *Canadian Journal of Nursing Research, 37*(1), 122–145.

Thato, S., Charron-Prochownik, D., Dorn, L. D., Albrecht, S. A., & Stone, C. A. (2003). Predictors of condom use among adolescent Thai vocational students. *Journal of Nursing Scholarship, 35,* 157–163.

Thulesius, H., Håkansson, A., & Petersson, K. (2003). Balancing: A basic process in end-of-life care. *Qualitative Health Research, 13,* 1353–1377.

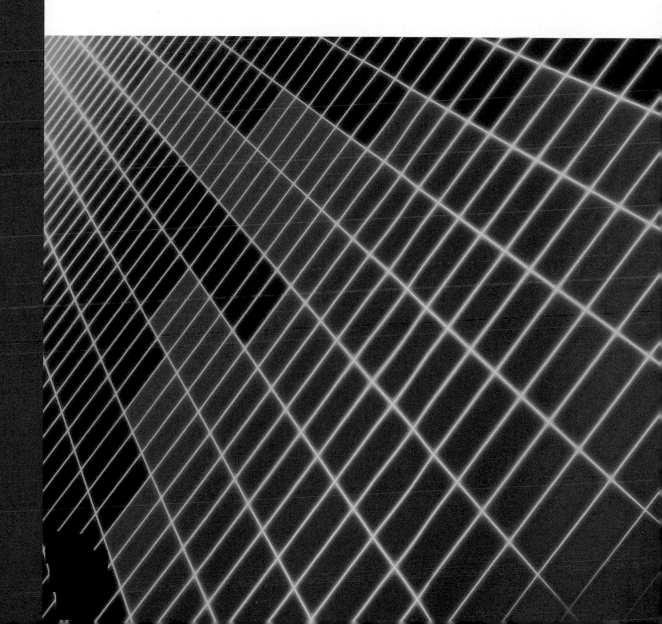

PART 4

COLLECTING RESEARCH DATA

14

Designing and Implementing a Data Collection Plan

The phenomena in which researchers are interested must ultimately be captured and translated into data that can be analyzed. Without high-quality data collection methods, the accuracy and robustness of the conclusions are subject to challenge. In quantitative studies, the tasks of defining research variables and selecting or developing appropriate methods for collecting data are among the most challenging in the research process. This chapter provides an overview of various methods of data collection for qualitative and quantitative studies, and discusses the development of a **data collection plan**.

In developing such a plan, researchers need to give thought to the kind of evidence they want to provide to their colleagues in practice settings. Some concepts—and certain measures of those concepts—are especially well-suited to the development of an evidence-based nursing practice. For example, Ingersol (2005) has identified a number of evidence-based, nurse-sensitive outcome indicators that should be given consideration in designing studies, especially for studies that test the effects of nursing interventions. Examples include achievement of appropriate self-care, health-related quality of life, functional status, risk-reduction behaviors, compliance, and health-promoting behaviors. These indicators cover the full range of data collection possibilities in nursing research in terms of type of approach, degree of structure, and the ease with which the concepts can be operationalized.

> ➡ **TIP:** The famous GIGO principle is pertinent with respect to data collection—that is, garbage in, garbage out. Poor-quality data inevitably undermine the usefulness of the study's evidence. This chapter discusses several steps researchers can take to enhance data quality, which is of utmost importance to both qualitative and quantitative researchers. More detailed discussions of data quality issues are presented in Chapter 17 (quantitative studies) and Chapter 20 (qualitative studies).

OVERVIEW OF DATA COLLECTION AND DATA SOURCES

As in the case of research designs and sampling plans, researchers must often choose from an array of alternative data collection methods and approaches. We provide an overview of approaches in this section.

Existing Data Versus Original Data

One of the first decisions that investigators make with regard to research data concerns whether to use existing data or to collect data generated specifically for the study. Most researchers develop original data, but they often can take advantage of existing information. Secondary analyses and meta-analyses, for example, rely on data that have been gathered by others. Historical research also relies on available data. As noted in Chapter 9, data for historical research are usually in the form of written historical documents: periodicals, diaries, letters, newspapers, minutes of meetings, medical documents, reports, and so forth.

Existing **records** are an important data source for nurse researchers. A wealth of data gathered for nonresearch purposes can be fruitfully exploited to answer research questions. Hospital records, patient charts, physicians' order sheets, care plan statements, and the like all constitute rich data sources to which nurse researchers may have access.

Research data obtained from records and documents are advantageous for several reasons. The most salient advantage is that they are economical; the collection of original data is often time-consuming and costly. Preexisting records also permit an examination of trends over time, if the information is collected repeatedly. Problems stemming from people's awareness of and reaction to study participation are usually completely absent when researchers obtain data from records. Furthermore, investigators do not have to rely on participants' cooperation.

On the other hand, when researchers are not responsible for collecting and recording data, they may be unaware of the records' limitations and biases. Two major sources of bias in records are **selective deposit** and **selective survival**. If the available records are not the entire set of all possible such records, researchers must address the question of how representative existing records are. Many record keepers *intend* to maintain an entire universe of records but may fail to adhere to this ideal. Lapses from the ideal may be the result of systematic biases, and careful researchers should attempt to learn just what those biases may be. (Eder and colleagues [2005] have suggested some strategies for enhancing the reliability of data extracted from medical records.)

Other difficulties also may be relevant. Sometimes records have to be verified for their authenticity,

authorship, or accuracy, a task that may be difficult if the records are old. Researchers using records must be prepared to deal with forms and file systems they do not understand. Codes and symbols that had meaning to the record keeper may have to be translated to be usable. In using records to study trends, researchers should be alert to possible changes in record-keeping procedures. For example, does a dramatic increase or decrease in the incidence of sudden infant death syndrome reflect changes in the causes or cures of this problem, or does it reflect a change in diagnosis or record keeping?

Another problem confronting researchers is the increasing difficulty of gaining access to institutional records. As mentioned in Chapter 7, federal legislation in the United States (HIPAA) has created some obstacles to accessing existing records for research purposes. Thus, although existing records may be plentiful, inexpensive, and accessible, they should not be used without paying attention to potential problems. Moreover, it is often difficult to find existing data that are ideally suited to answering a research question.

➲ **TIP:** The difference between using records and doing secondary analyses is that researchers doing a secondary analysis typically have a ready-to-analyze data set, whereas researchers using records have to assemble the data set, and considerable coding and data manipulation usually are necessary.

Example of a study using records: Adams, Horn, and Bader (2006) studied Hispanic access to hospice services in a predominantly Hispanic community in Texas. Their data were derived from a retrospective chart review of 500 patients who died in four hospices.

Major Types of Data Collection Methods

If existing data are not available for the research question, researchers must collect new data. In developing their data collection plans, researchers make many important decisions, including the decision about the basic types of data to gather. Three approaches have been used most frequently by nurse researchers: self-reports, observation, and biophysiologic measures. This section presents an overview of these methods, and subsequent chapters provide additional guidance.

Researchers' decisions about research design usually are independent of decisions about data collection methods. Researchers using an experimental design can rely on self-report data—as can a researcher doing an ethnography, for example. The research *question* may dictate which specific method of data collection to use, but researchers often have great latitude in designing a data collection plan.

Self-Reports

A good deal of information can be gathered by questioning people, a method known as **self-report**. If, for example, we were interested in learning about patients' perceptions of hospital care or about their preoperative fears, we would likely gather data by asking them relevant questions. The unique ability of humans to communicate verbally on a sophisticated level makes direct questioning a particularly important part of nurse researchers' data collection repertoire. The vast majority of nursing studies involve data collected by self-report.

The self-report method is strong in directness and versatility. If we want to know what people think, feel, or believe, the most efficient means of gathering information is to ask them about it. Perhaps the strongest argument that can be made for the self-report method is that it frequently yields information that would be difficult, if not impossible, to gather by any other means. Behaviors can be observed, but only if participants engage in them publicly. For example, it is usually impossible for researchers to observe such behaviors as child abuse or contraceptive practices. Furthermore, observers can observe only those behaviors occurring at the time of the study. Through self-reports, researchers can gather retrospective data about activities and events occurring in the past or information about behaviors in which people plan to engage in the future. Information about feelings, values, or opinions can sometimes be inferred through observation, but behaviors and feelings do not always correspond exactly. People's actions do not always indicate their state of mind. Self-report methods can be used to capture psychological characteristics through direct communication with participants.

Despite these advantages, verbal report methods have some weaknesses. The most serious issue concerns the validity and accuracy of self-reports: How can we be sure that respondents feel or act the way they say they do? How can we trust the information that respondents provide, particularly if the true answers would reveal embarrassing or socially unacceptable behavior? Investigators often have no alternative but to assume that their respondents have been frank. Yet we all have a tendency to want to present ourselves in the best light, and this may conflict with the truth. Researchers who gather self-report data should recognize the limitations of this method and should be prepared to take these shortcomings into consideration when interpreting the results.

Example of a study using self-reports: Ahl, Nystrom, and Jansson (2006) studied patients' experiences related to their decision to call an ambulance. The data came from in-depth interviews with 20 respondents.

Self-report methods normally depend on respondents' willingness to share personal information, but **projective techniques** are sometimes used to obtain data about people's way of thinking indirectly. Projective techniques present participants with a stimulus of low structure, permitting them to "read in" and then describe their own interpretations. The Rorschach test is one example of a projective technique. Other projective methods encourage self-expression through the construction of some product (e.g., drawings). The assumption is that people express their needs, motives, and emotions by working with or manipulating materials. Projective methods are used infrequently by nurse researchers, the major exception being studies using expressive methods to explore sensitive topics with children.

Example of a study using projective methods: Chaiyawat and Jezewski (2006) conducted a grounded theory study of *fear* among school-age children in Thailand. In-depth data about the children's perspectives on fear were obtained through interviews and through an analysis of their drawings.

Observation

For certain research problems, an alternative to self-reports is **observation** of people's behavior or characteristics. Information required by nurse researchers as evidence of nursing effectiveness or as clues to improving nursing practices often can be obtained through observation. Suppose, for instance, that we were interested in studying mental patients' methods of defending their personal territory, or children's reactions to the removal of a leg cast. Such phenomena are amenable to observation.

Observation can be done directly through the human senses or with the aid of technical apparatus, such as video equipment. Observational methods are quite versatile and can be used to gather a variety of information, including information about the following:

- Characteristics and conditions of individuals (e.g., the sleep–wake state of patients)
- Verbal communication (e.g., information exchange during medication administration)
- Nonverbal communication (e.g., facial expressions)
- Activities and behavior (e.g., geriatric patients' self-grooming activities)
- Skill attainment and performance (e.g., diabetic patients' skill in testing their urine for sugar and acetone)
- Environmental conditions (e.g., architectural barriers in the homes of disabled people)

Observation in natural health care environments is particularly well suited to nursing research. Nurses are in an advantageous position to observe, relatively unobtrusively, the behaviors and actions of patients, their families, and hospital staff. Moreover, nurses may, by training, be especially sensitive observers. Many nursing problems are better suited to an observational approach than to self-report techniques. Whenever people cannot be expected to describe adequately their own behaviors, observational methods may be needed. This may be the case when people are unaware of their own behavior (e.g., manifesting preoperative symptoms of anxiety), when people are embarrassed to report their activities (e.g., displays of aggression or hostility), when behaviors are emotionally laden (e.g., grieving behavior among widows), or when people are not capable of articulating their actions (e.g., young children or the mentally ill). Observation is intrinsically appealing in its ability to capture a record of behaviors and events. Furthermore, with an observational approach, humans—the observers—are used as measuring instruments and provide a uniquely sensitive and intelligent tool.

Shortcomings of observation include possible ethical difficulties and distorted behavior on the part of study participants when they are aware of being observed—a problem referred to as **reactivity**. Reactivity can be eliminated if the observations are made without people's knowledge, through some type of concealment. In some settings, concealed observations can be accomplished through the use of one-way mirrors. These strategies, however, make it difficult to obtain truly informed consent.

Another problem is **observer biases**. A number of factors interfere with objective observations, including the following:

- Emotions, prejudices, attitudes, and values of observers may result in faulty inference.
- Personal interest and commitment may color what is seen in the direction of what observers want to see.
- Anticipation of what is to be observed may affect what *is* observed.
- Hasty decisions before adequate information is collected may result in erroneous classifications or conclusions.

Observational biases probably cannot be eliminated completely, but they can be minimized through careful training.

Example of a study using observation:
Philpin (2006) observed nursing behavior in an intensive therapy unit over a 12-month period, focusing on end-of-shift information transmission among the nurses.

⮞ **TIP:** Most studies that gather observational data are done in natural settings so that people's usual behavior or characteristics can be observed. Sometimes, however, researchers create specially structured research settings (called *directed settings*) to provoke behaviors that are rare in naturalistic settings, making it inexpedient to wait for them to happen. For example, several studies have examined the behavior of bystanders in crises. Because crises are unpredictable and infrequent, investigators have staged emergencies to observe helping behavior (or lack of it) among onlookers.

Biophysiologic Measures

The trend in nursing research has been toward increased clinical investigations, resulting in a greater use of quantitative **biophysiologic measures**. Physiologic and physical variables typically require specialized technical instruments and equipment for their measurement. Because such equipment is generally available in health care settings, the costs of these measures to nurse researchers may be small or nonexistent.

A major strength of biophysiologic measures is their objectivity. Nurse A and nurse B, reading from the same spirometer output, are likely to record the same tidal volume measurements. Furthermore, barring the possibility of equipment malfunctioning, two different spirometers are likely to produce identical tidal volume readouts. Another advantage of physiologic measurements is the relative precision and sensitivity they normally offer. By *relative*, we are implicitly comparing physiologic instruments with measures of psychological phenomena, such as self-report measures of anxiety or pain. Biophysiologic measures usually yield data of exceptionally high quality.

Example of a study using biophysiologic measures: Chan and co-researchers (2006) used a randomized clinical trial (RCT) design to examine the effects of music on physiologic outcomes among patients undergoing a C-clamp procedure after percutaneous coronary interventions. Their outcomes included heart rate, respiratory rate, and oxygen saturation.

Dimensions of Data Collection Approaches

Regardless of what specific approach is used, data collection methods vary along four important dimensions: structure, quantifiability, researcher obtrusiveness, and objectivity.

Structure

Research data for quantitative studies are collected according to a structured plan that indicates what information is to be gathered and how to gather it. For example, most self-administered questionnaires are highly structured: They include a fixed set of questions to be answered in a specified sequence and with predesignated response options (e.g., agree or disagree). Structured methods give participants limited opportunities to qualify their answers or to explain the underlying meaning of their responses. Most qualitative studies, however, rely almost exclusively on unstructured or loosely structured methods of data collection.

There are advantages and disadvantages to both approaches. Structured methods often take considerable effort to develop and refine, but they yield data that are relatively easy to analyze. Structured methods are seldom appropriate for an in-depth examination of a phenomenon, however. Consider the following two methods of asking people about their levels of stress:

Structured: During the past week, would you say you felt stressed:

1. rarely or none of the time,
2. some or a little of the time,
3. occasionally or a moderate amount of the time, or
4. most or all of the time?

Unstructured: How stressed or anxious have you been this past week? Tell me about the kinds of tensions and stresses you have been experiencing.

Structured questioning would allow researchers to compute what percentage of respondents felt stressed most of the time, but would provide no information about the intensity, cause, or circumstances of the stress. The unstructured question allows for deeper and more thoughtful responses, but may pose difficulties for people who are not good at expressing themselves. Moreover, the unstructured question yields data that are considerably more difficult to analyze.

When data are collected in a highly structured fashion, the researcher must develop (or borrow) a data collection **instrument**, which is the formal written document used to collect and record information, such as a questionnaire. When unstructured methods are used, there is typically no formal instrument, although there may be a list of the types of information needed.

Quantifiability

Data that will be analyzed statistically must be quantified. For statistical analysis, all variables must be quantitatively measured—even though the variables are abstract and intangible phenomena that represent *qualities* of humans, such as hope, pain, and body image. Data that are to be analyzed qualitatively are typically collected in narrative form.

Structured data collection approaches usually yield data that are easily quantified. It may be possible (and it is sometimes useful), however, to quantify unstructured information as well. For example, responses to the unstructured question concerning stress could be categorized after the fact according to the four levels of stress indicated in the structured question. Whether it is *wise* to do so depends on the research problem, the researcher's philosophic orientation, and the nature of the responses. This is an issue to which we return in the next section.

Researcher Obtrusiveness

Data collection methods differ in the degree to which people are aware of their status as participants. If people are cognizant of their role in a study, their behavior and responses may not be "normal," and distortions can undermine the value of the research. When data are collected unobtrusively, however, ethical problems may emerge, as discussed in Chapter 7.

Study participants are most likely to distort their behavior and their responses to questions under certain circumstances. Researcher obtrusiveness is likely to be most problematic when (1) a program is being evaluated and participants have a vested interest in the evaluation outcome; (2) participants are engaged in socially unacceptable or atypical behavior; (3) participants have not complied with medical and nursing instructions; and (4) participants are the type of people who have a strong need to "look good." When researcher obtrusiveness is unavoidable under these circumstances, researchers should make an effort to put participants at ease, to stress the importance of candor and naturalistic behavior, and to train research personnel to convey a neutral and nonjudgmental demeanor.

Objectivity

Objectivity refers to the degree to which two independent researchers can arrive at similar "scores" or make similar observations regarding the concepts of interest, that is, make judgments regarding participants' attributes or behavior that are not biased by personal feelings or beliefs. Some data collection approaches require more subjective judgment than others, and some research problems require a higher degree of objectivity than others.

Researchers whose paradigmatic orientation lies in positivism usually strive for a reasonable amount of objectivity. However, in research based on the naturalistic paradigm, the subjective judgment of investigators is considered an asset because subjectivity is viewed as essential for understanding human experiences.

CONVERTING QUANTITATIVE AND QUALITATIVE DATA

Qualitative data are sometimes converted into numeric codes that can be analyzed quantitatively. It is also possible to treat data collected in a quantitative study qualitatively. In thinking about data collection, researchers might wish to consider whether either of these options would enhance their study, particularly if they are doing mixed method research.

Using Quantitative Data Qualitatively

Most data that are analyzed quantitatively actually begin as qualitative data. If we ask respondents if they have been severely depressed, moderately depressed, somewhat depressed, or not at all depressed in the previous week, they answer in words, not numbers. The words are transformed, through the process of coding, into quantitative categories. Then the numbers are analyzed statistically to determine, for example, what percentage of respondents were severely depressed in the prior week, or whether people diagnosed with cancer are more likely than others to be depressed.

However, it is possible to go back to the data and "read" them qualitatively, a process that Sandelowski (2000b) calls **qualitizing** data. For example, an entire survey interview can be read to get a glimpse of the life circumstances, problems, and experiences of an individual respondent. In such a situation, researchers can create a mini case study designed to "give life" to the patterns emerging in the quantitative analysis, to extract more information from the data, and to aid in interpreting them.

As an example, Polit, Widom, and Edin (2001) studied single mothers who were receiving public cash assistance but who were subject to new requirements that compelled them to seek employment. Based on data from 90-minute survey interviews with several thousand women, the researchers discovered that health problems of the women and their children were important barriers to sustained employment. The researchers identified a survey respondent who typified the experiences of those who had employment problems, and prepared this profile:

Example of qualitizing survey data: Miranda, a 26-year-old Mexican-American woman from Los Angeles, had had a fairly steady work record until 4 months before we spoke with her, when she had left her job as a bank cashier because her son (age 4) had serious health problems. She also had a 2-year-old daughter, and her husband, from whom she was separated, no longer lived nearby to help with child care. The bank job had paid her $210 a week before taxes, without health insurance, sick pay, or paid vacation. At the bank job, she had worked 36 hours a week, working daily from early afternoon until 8 p.m. Although at the time of the interview she was getting cash welfare assistance, food stamps, and SSI (disability) benefits on behalf of her son, her relatively high rent and utility costs (more than $700 per month) without housing assistance made it difficult for her to make ends meet, and she reported that she sometimes couldn't afford to feed her children balanced meals (Polit, Widom, & Edin, 2001, p. 2).

The aggregate survey data in this study were used *quantitatively* to describe such things as the percentage of women who left work because of health problems. The data were used *qualitatively* (as in the preceding example) to translate statistical findings into what it was like in the lives of actual respondents.

When this type of undertaking is done, researchers must be clear about what it is they wish to portray. Often, as in the example just cited, the intent is to illustrate a typical case. In such a situation, researchers look for an individual case whose quantitative values are near the average for the entire sample. However, researchers might also want to illustrate ways in which the averages fail to capture important aspects of a problem, in which case atypical (and often extreme) cases are identified to show the limitations of looking just at averages in the quantitative analysis.

Using Qualitative Data Quantitatively

A somewhat more controversial issue is the use of numbers in qualitative studies. Some qualitative researchers believe that **quantitizing** qualitative data is inappropriate. Sandelowski (2001), however, has argued that some amount of quantitizing is almost inevitable. She noted that every time qualitative researchers use terms such as *a few, some, many*, or *most*, they are implicitly conveying quantitative information about the frequency of occurrence of a theme or pattern. In addition to being inevitable, quantification of qualitative data can in some cases offer distinct benefits. Sandelowski has described how this strategy can be used to achieve several important goals:

1. *Generating meaning from qualitative data.* If qualitative data are displayed in a quantitative fashion (e.g., by displaying frequencies of certain phenomena), patterns sometimes emerge with greater clarity than they might have had the researchers simply relied on their impressions. Tabular displays can also reveal unsuspected patterns that can help in the development of hypotheses to be further tested qualitatively. Sandelowski provides an excellent example in which this procedure enabled her to see her data in a new way, and to better understand the characteristics of her sample. Whenever qualitative data are categorized, researchers are creating data that can be analyzed quantitatively (e.g., to examine the relationship between two phenomena).

2. *Documenting and confirming conclusions.* The use of numbers can assure readers that researchers' assertions are valid. If researchers can document the extent to which the emerging patterns were observed (and not observed), readers will have confidence that the data are fully accounted for. Sandelowski notes that quantitizing in this fashion can address some of the major pitfalls of qualitative analysis, which include (1) giving too much weight to dramatic or vivid accounts; (2) giving too little weight to disconfirming cases; and (3) smoothing out variation, to clean up some of the "messiness" of human experience. Thus, the use of numbers can sometimes help to confirm impressions. A procedure known as *quasi-statistics* (see Chapter 19) is used in some qualitative studies for this purpose.

3. *Re-presenting data and lives.* Qualitative researchers are especially likely to use numbers to describe important features of their samples. Thus, qualitative reports may contain tables that show characteristics of the sample as a whole (e.g., the average age, or percentage male and female), or characteristics of each individual participant.

Sandelowski also offers good advice on avoiding the misuse of numbers (e.g., overcounting, or counting that is misleading).

Example of quantitizing qualitative data:
Li and Arber (2006), who explored what strategies nurses use to construct dying patients' moral identities in three different palliative care settings, presented two tables in which their qualitative data had been categorized and counted. For example, one table presented a word count of adjectives the nurses used to describe troubled patients. The most commonly used word, "difficult," was used 58 times, followed by "anxious" (28), "bad" (25), and "confused" (25).

DEVELOPING A DATA COLLECTION PLAN IN QUANTITATIVE STUDIES

Data collection plans for quantitative studies should ideally yield accurate, valid, and meaningful data that are maximally effective in answering research questions. These are rigorous requirements, typically requiring considerable time and effort to achieve. This section discusses steps that are often undertaken in the development of a data collection plan in quantitative studies. Figure 14.1 provides an overview of the procedures used in developing such a plan.

TIP: Although the flow chart in Figure 14.1 suggests a fairly linear process, the development of a data collection plan is often an iterative one. Be prepared to backtrack and make adjustments, recognizing that the ultimate goal is not to get to the bottom of the list of steps but rather to ensure that the process yields conceptually relevant data of the highest possible quality.

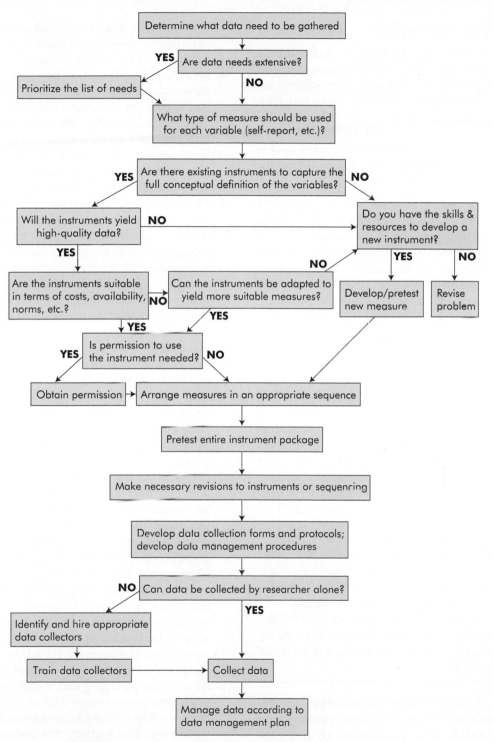

FIGURE 14.1 Developing a data collection plan for quantitative studies.

Identifying Data Needs

Researchers must usually begin by identifying the types of data needed to complete the study successfully. Typically, researchers gather information about more than just the main study variables. Advance planning may help to avoid "if only" disappointments at the analysis stage.

In a quantitative study, researchers may need to identify data requirements for accomplishing the following:

1. *Testing the hypotheses or addressing the research questions.* Researchers must include one or more measures of all the independent and dependent variables. Multiple measures of some variables may be required if a variable is complex and multifaceted or if there is an interest in obtaining corroboration through triangulation.

2. *Describing sample characteristics.* Information should be gathered about major demographic and health characteristics of the sample. We advise gathering data about participants' age, gender, race or ethnicity, educational background, marital status, and income level. This information is critical in interpreting results and understanding the population to whom the findings can be generalized. If the sample includes participants with a health problem, data on the nature of that problem also should be gathered (e.g., severity of health problem, types of treatment obtained, length of stay in hospital).

TIP: Because the need to collect information about sample characteristics is nearly universal, we have included a sample demographic form in the Toolkit of the accompanying *Resource Manual.* The demographic questionnaire can be adapted and expanded, as needed. We have also included annotated guidelines for asking a few key demographic questions for varying circumstances and desired levels of precision.

---

3. *Controlling extraneous variables.* As discussed in Chapter 11, various approaches can be used to control extraneous variables, and many of them require the measurement of those variables. For example, when analysis of covariance is used, each variable that is statistically controlled must be measured.

4. *Analyzing potential biases.* Data that can help the researcher to identify potential biases usually should be collected. For example, researchers should gather information that would help to identify selection biases in a nonequivalent control group design. Researchers should give some thought to potential biases and then determine how they could be assessed.

5. *Understanding subgroup effects.* It is often desirable to answer the research questions not only for the entire sample but also for key subgroups of participants. For example, we may wish to know if a special intervention for indigent pregnant women is equally effective for primiparas and multiparas. In such a situation, we would need to collect information about the participants' childbearing history so that we could divide the sample and analyze for separate subgroup effects.

6. *Interpreting results.* Researchers should try to anticipate alternative results, and then determine what types of data would best help in interpreting them. For example, if we hypothesized that the presence of school-based clinics in high schools would lower the incidence of sexually transmitted diseases among students but found that the incidence remained constant after the clinic was established, what type of information would we want to help us interpret this result (e.g., information about the students' frequency of intercourse, number of partners, use of condoms, and so on)?

7. *Checking the manipulation.* When researchers manipulate the independent variable in intervention studies, it is sometimes useful to determine whether the manipulation actually occurred. Such a manipulation check can help in interpreting negative results. As an example, if a researcher were studying the impact of a new hospital policy on the morale of the nursing staff, it might be important to determine the nurses' level of awareness of the new policy; if the results indicate no change in staff morale, this could reflect lack of awareness of the policy rather than indifference to it.

8. *Obtaining administrative information.* It is almost always necessary to gather administrative information to help in project management. Administrative information might include participant identification numbers, dates of actual data collection, where data collection occurred, reasons that a potential subject did not participate in the study, and contact information if the study is longitudinal.

⮕ **TIP:** Although this list is especially appropriate in quantitative studies, several of the types of data listed would also be gathered in qualitative studies (e.g., characteristics of the sample, administrative information).

The list of possible data needs may seem daunting, but many categories overlap. For example, participant characteristics (for sample description) are often key extraneous variables, or useful in creating subgroups. If time or resource constraints make it impossible to collect the full range of variables, then researchers should prioritize data needs and be aware of how the absence of certain variables could affect the study's integrity.

It is often useful, in identifying and prioritizing data needs, to develop a matrix with key pieces of information so that decisions can be made in a systematic way. A matrix can also help to identify "holes" (types of data that are missing) and redundancies. Figure 14.2 presents a hypothetical (and partial) example of such a matrix for an intervention study that tests the effects of humor on stress and immune function in hospitalized patients with cancer. Other columns could be added to this matrix— for example, if there are time constraints or worries about burdening participants, an additional column might contain estimates of the amount of time needed to collect the information. (This matrix is included in the Toolkit of the accompanying *Resource Manual* for you to use and adapt). ✷ The important point is that researchers should understand their data needs and take steps to ensure the fullest possible coverage within the constraints of time, resources, and respondent burden issues.

⮕ **TIP:** In developing instruments, it may be necessary to evaluate tradeoffs between data quality and data quantity. If compromises have to be made, it is usually preferable to forego quantity. For example, it is better to have an excellent measure of the dependent variable without supplementary measures for interpreting outcomes than to have mediocre measures of all desired variables. When data quality for key variables is poor, the results cannot be trusted, so additional information cannot possibly help to clarify the findings.

Selecting Types of Measures

After data needs have been identified, the next step is to select a data collection method for each variable. It is common, and often advantageous, to combine self-reports, observations, or physiologic measures in a single study. Researchers also combine measures that vary in terms of the four basic dimensions. In reviewing data needs, researchers should determine how best to capture each variable in terms of its conceptual or theoretical definition.

Research considerations are not the only factors that drive decisions about methods to use in collecting data. The decisions must also be guided by ethical considerations (e.g., whether covert data collection is warranted), cost constraints, the availability of appropriate staff to help with data collection, and other considerations discussed in the next section. Data collection is often the costliest and most time-consuming portion of a study. Because of this, researchers often have to make a number of compromises about the type or amount of data collected.

Selecting and Developing Instruments

Once preliminary decisions have been made regarding the basic data collection methods to be used, researchers should determine whether there are instruments available for measuring study constructs, as will often be the case. We provide some guidance on locating instruments in Chapter 16.

Potential data collection instruments should then be assessed to determine their appropriateness. The

VARIABLE	PURPOSE*	METHOD	INSTRUMENT	DATA QUALITY INFORMATION**
Use of humor	A (IV)	Creation of groups through random assignment	—	
Use of humor	F (IV)	Self-administered scale	Rating of staff humor—developed for study	
Stress	A (DV)	Self-administered scale	Symptoms of Stress Inventory	Test–retest reliability: 0.82, high concurrent validity (Jones)
Stress	A, B (DV)	Self-administered scale	Visual Analog Scale—stress	Test–retest reliability: 0.78; good construct validity (Lee)
Stress	A, B (DV)	Autonomic nervous system response	Heart rate, blood pressure, skin conductance	
Immune function	A (DV)	NK cell activity	Chromium-51 release cytotoxicity assay	
Immune function	A, B (DV)	Lymphocyte proliferation	Mononuclear cell cultures	
Depression	A (DV)	Self-administered scale	Center for Epidemiologic Studies Depression Scale	Alpha = 0.89, good construct and criterion-related validity (Smith)
Type of cancer, treatment, prognosis	C, D, E, H	Records	Hospital chart	
Demographic information	C, D, E, H	Records	Age, gender, marital status (admission form)	
Address, phone number	G	Records	Admission form	
Staff reactions to intervention	I	Self-administered questionnaire	Open-ended questions	

Purpose Codes: (IV = independent variable; DV = dependent variable)
A. To address research questions or test hypotheses (key variables)
B. To triangulate/corroborate
C. To describe sample characteristics
D. To control extraneous variation
E. To analyze potential biases
F. To perform a manipulation check
G. To secure administrative/contact information
H. To understand subgroup differences
I. To help interpret results

* Information in this column is fictitious, entered here for illustrative purposes.

FIGURE 14.2 ⊗ Example of a partial data matrix for an intervention study on the use of humor with hospitalized patients with cancer.

primary consideration is whether the instrument is conceptually relevant: Does the instrument capture your conceptual definition of the variable? The next factor to consider is whether the instrument will yield data of sufficiently high quality. Approaches to evaluating data quality are discussed in Chapter 17. Additional criteria that may affect researchers' decisions in selecting an instrument are as follows:

1. *Resources*. Resource constraints sometimes prevent the use of the highest-quality measures. There may be some direct costs associated with the measure (e.g., some psychological tests must be purchased), but the biggest data collection cost involves compensation to data collectors if you cannot do it single-handedly—that is, if you have to hire interviewers or observers. In such a situation, the instrument's administration time may determine whether it is a viable option. Also, if the data collection procedures are burdensome, it may be necessary to pay a subject stipend. Data collection costs should be carefully considered, especially if the use of expensive methods means that you will be forced to cut costs elsewhere (e.g., using a smaller sample).

2. *Availability and familiarity*. In selecting measures, you may need to consider how readily available or accessible various instruments are, especially biophysiologic ones. Similarly, data collection strategies with which you have had experience are in general preferable to new measures because administration is usually smoother and more efficient in such cases.

3. *Norms and comparability*. You may find it desirable to select a measure for which there are relevant norms. **Norms** indicate the "normal" values and distribution of values on the measure for a specified population. Many standardized tests and scales (e.g., the SF-36 Health Survey from the Medical Outcomes Study) have national norms. Norms are useful because they offer, in essence, a built-in comparison group. For similar reasons, you may find it advantageous to adopt an instrument because it was used in other similar studies and

therefore provides a supplementary context for interpreting your findings. When a study is an intentional replication, it is often essential to use the same instruments as in the original study, even if higher-quality measures are available.

4. *Population appropriateness*. The measure must be chosen with the characteristics of the target population in mind. Characteristics of special importance include participants' age, their literacy levels, and their cultural or ethnic backgrounds. If there is concern about participants' reading skills, it may be necessary to calculate the readability of a prospective instrument. If participants include members of minority groups, you should strive to find instruments that are culturally appropriate. If non–English-speaking participants are included in the sample, then the selection of a measure may be based, in part, on the availability of a translated version of the measure.

5. *Administration issues*. Some instruments have special requirements that need to be considered. For example, obtaining information about the developmental status of children sometimes requires the skills of a professional psychologist. Another administration issue is that some instruments require or assume stringent conditions with regard to the time of administration, privacy of the setting, and so on. In such a case, requirements for obtaining valid measures must match attributes of the research setting.

6. *Reputation*. Instruments designed to measure the same construct often differ in the reputation they enjoy among specialists working in a field, even if they are comparable with regard to documented quality. Therefore, it may be useful to seek the advice of knowledgeable people, preferably ones with personal, direct experience using the instruments.

Based on such considerations, you may conclude that existing instruments are not suitable for all research variables. In such a situation, you will be faced with either adapting an existing instrument to make it more appropriate, or developing a new one. Creating a new instrument should be considered a last resort, especially for novice researchers, because it is difficult to develop accurate and valid measuring tools. However, there are situations in which there may not be an acceptable alternative. Chapter 18 provides guidance on developing self-report instruments, but it sometimes may make more sense to modify the research question so that existing instruments can be used.

If you are fortunate in identifying a suitable instrument, your next step likely will be to obtain written permission from the author (or the publisher, if it is a commercially distributed instrument) to use or adapt it. In general, copyrighted materials always require permission. Instruments that have been developed under a government grant are usually in the public domain, and so do not require permission because they have been supported with taxpayers' dollars. When in doubt, however, it is best to obtain permission. By contacting the author of an instrument to obtain permission, you can also request more information about the instrument and its quality than was available in a published report. (A sample letter requesting permission to use an instrument is available in the Toolkit). ✸

Pretesting the Data Collection Package

Researchers who develop a new instrument in methodologic studies almost invariably subject it to rigorous **pretesting** so that it can be evaluated and refined. However, even when the data collection plan involves existing instruments, it is wise to conduct a small pretest.

One purpose of a pretest is to determine how much time it takes to administer the entire instrument package and whether participants find it burdensome. Typically, researchers use multiple instruments, and it may be difficult to estimate how long it will take to administer the complete set. Such estimates may be required for informed consent purposes or for developing a project budget. If the pretest instruments require more time than is acceptable, it may be necessary to eliminate certain variables or instruments, guided by the prioritization list established earlier.

Pretests can serve many other purposes, including the following:

- Identifying parts of the instrument package that are difficult for pretest subjects to read or understand or that may have been misinterpreted by them
- Identifying any instruments or questions that participants find objectionable or offensive
- Determining whether the sequencing of questions or instruments is sensible
- Determining needs for training data collection staff
- Determining whether the measures yield data with sufficient variability

The last purpose requires explanation. For most research questions, the instruments ideally discriminate among participants with different levels of an attribute. If we are asking, for example, whether women experience greater depression than men when they learn of a cancer diagnosis, we need an instrument capable of distinguishing between people with higher and lower levels of depression. If an instrument yields data with limited variability, then it will be impossible to detect a difference in depression between men and women—even when such a difference actually exists. Thus, researchers should look at pretest variation on key research variables. If, to pursue the example, the entire pretest sample looks very depressed (or not at all depressed), it may be necessary to modify the instruments.

Example of pretesting: Nyamathi and colleagues (2005) studied the predictors of perceived health status in a sample of 415 homeless adults with tuberculosis. The study involved collecting an extensive array of data through self-reports. All the instruments had been previously tested with homeless people, and many were pretested in group settings to determine clarity and sensitivity to the population.

Developing Data Collection Forms and Procedures

After the instrument package has been finalized, researchers face a number of administrative tasks. First, appropriate forms must be developed. In some studies, many forms are required: screening forms to determine eligibility, informed consent forms, records of attempted contacts with participants, forms for recording the actual data, contact information sheets, and administrative logs for recording the receipt of data. It is prudent to design forms that are attractively formatted, legible, and inviting to use, especially if they are to be used by subjects themselves. Care should also be taken to design forms to ensure confidentiality. For example, identifying information (e.g., names, addresses) is often recorded on a page that can be detached and kept separate from other data.

⊃ TIP: Whenever possible, try to avoid reinventing the wheel. It is inefficient and unnecessary to start from scratch — not only in developing instruments but also in creating forms, training materials, and so on. Ask seasoned researchers if they have materials you could borrow or adapt.

In most quantitative studies, researchers also develop **data collection protocols** that spell out the procedures to be used in data collection. These protocols describe such things as the following:

* Conditions that must be met for collecting the data (e.g., Can others be present at the time of data collection? Where must data collection occur?)
* Specific procedures for collecting the data, including requirements for sequencing instruments and recording information
* Information to provide participants who ask routine questions about the study (i.e., answers to FAQs). Examples include the following: How will the information from this study be used? How did you get my name, and why are you asking me? How long will this take? Who will have access to this information? Can I see the study results? Whom can I contact if I have a complaint about the process? Will I be paid or reimbursed for expenses?
* Procedures to follow in the event that a participant becomes distraught or disoriented, or for any other reason cannot complete the data collection

Procedures and forms are usually required for managing collected data, especially if data are being gathered from multiple sites or over an extended period. For example, in an observational study, a data management form might record, for each case, the date the observation was scheduled to take place, the date it actually took place, the date the observation form was received back in some central location, and the date the data were coded and entered onto a computer file.

Researchers also need to make decisions about how to actually gather, record, and manage their data. Technological advances continue to offer new options for handling data. As noted in Chapter 12, survey researchers are increasingly using sophisticated computer programs to facilitate collecting, recording and encoding self-report data (e.g., CATI, CAPI). The Internet is being used to gather data from geographically dispersed populations, and handheld computers or personal digital assistants (PDAs) are beginning to play a role. Courtney and Craven (2005) and Guadagno and colleagues (2004) offer some suggestions about new technology and data collection.

⊃ TIP: Document everything you do as you develop and implement your data collection plan, and save your documentation. You may need the information later when you write your research report, request funding for a follow-up study, or help other researchers.

IMPLEMENTING A DATA COLLECTION PLAN IN A QUANTITATIVE STUDY

Data quality in a quantitative study is affected by both the data collection plan and how the plan is implemented.

Selecting Research Personnel

An important decision concerns who will actually collect the research data. In small studies, the researchers in charge often collect the data themselves. In larger studies, however, this may not be feasible. When data are collected by others, it is important to select appropriate people. In general, they should be neutral agents through whom data passes—that is, their characteristics or behavior should not affect the substance of the data. Some considerations that should be kept in mind when selecting research personnel are as follows:

- *Experience.* Research staff ideally have had prior experience collecting data. For example, for a self-report study, it is advantageous to use people with interviewing experience. If it is necessary to use those without experience, look for people who can readily acquire the necessary skills (e.g., an interviewer should have good verbal and social skills).

- *Congruity with sample characteristics.* To the extent possible, data collectors should match study participants with respect to such characteristics as racial or cultural background and gender. In some studies, this is an absolute requirement (e.g., hiring a person who speaks the language of an immigrant sample). The greater the sensitivity of the questions, the greater the desirability of matching characteristics. For example, in a study of the sexual behavior of pregnant African-American teenagers, the interviewers would ideally be African-American women.

- *Unremarkable appearance.* Extremes of appearance should be avoided because participants may react to extremes and alter their behavior or responses accordingly. For example, data collectors should in general not be very old or very young. They should not dress extremely casually (e.g., in shorts and tee shirts), nor very formally (e.g., with elaborate jewelry). While on the job, data collectors should never wear anything that conveys their political, social, or religious views (e.g., political buttons, jewelry with peace symbols).

- *Personality.* Data collectors should be pleasant (but not effusive), sociable (but not overly talkative or overbearing), and nonjudgmental (but not apathetic or unfeeling about partici-

pants' lives). The goal is to have nonthreatening staff who can encourage candor and put participants at ease without interjecting their own values.

- *Availability.* Data collectors should ideally be available for the entire data collection period to avoid having to recruit and train new staff. If the study is longitudinal, it is advantageous to hire people who could potentially be available for subsequent rounds of data collection.

In some situations, researchers cannot select research personnel. For example, the data collectors may be staff nurses employed at a hospital or graduate students in a school of nursing. Training of the data collection staff is particularly important in such situations.

> **Example of care in selecting research personnel:** Gary and Yarandi (2004) studied depression among southern rural African-American women. The research staff, who both recruited and interviewed study participants, were nurses who were members of the local affiliate of the National Black Nurses Association and who were trained by the lead researchers.

Training Data Collectors

Depending on the prior experience of data collectors, training will need to cover both general procedures (e.g., how to conduct a research interview) and ones specific to the study (e.g., how to administer a particular set of questions or make certain observations). Training can often be accomplished in a single day, but in complex projects, it may require more time. The lead researcher is usually the best person to conduct the training and to develop training materials.

The data collection protocols, discussed in the previous section, usually are a good foundation for a **training manual**. The manual normally includes background materials (e.g., the study aims), general instructions, specific instructions, and copies of all the data collection and administrative forms. Table 14.1 presents an example of a table of contents for a training manual in a quantitative

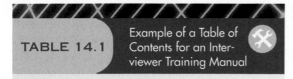

TABLE 14.1 Example of a Table of Contents for an Interviewer Training Manual

interview study. This table of contents is included in the Toolkit of the accompanying *Resource Manual*. Models for some of the sections in this table of contents (Sections II.C, III.C, and III.D) are also available in the Toolkit for your use and adaptation.

The agenda for the training should cover the content of the training manual, elaborating on any portion that is especially difficult or complex. The training usually includes demonstrations of fictitious data collection sessions, performed either live or on videotape. Finally, the training usually involves having the trainees do trial runs of data collection (*mock interviews*) in front of the trainers to demonstrate their understanding of the instructions. Thompson, Pickler, and Reyna (2005) provide some additional tips relating to the training of research personnel and the clinical coordination of research.

Example of data collector training: In a survey that provided the data for the report by Polit, London, and Martinez (2001), about 100 interviewers were trained in four research sites to interview nearly 4000 welfare mothers. Each training session lasted 3 days, including a half day of training on the use of CAPI. At the end of the training, several trainees were not kept on as interviewers because they were not skillful in mastering their assignments.

DATA COLLECTION ISSUES IN QUALITATIVE STUDIES

In qualitative studies, data collection usually is more fluid than in quantitative research, and decisions about what to collect evolve in the field. For example, as the researcher begins to gather and digest information, it may become apparent that it would be fruitful to pursue a line of questioning that had not originally been anticipated. However, even while allowing for and profiting from this flexibility, qualitative researchers make a number of up-front decisions about data collection. Moreover, qualitative researchers need to be prepared for problematic situations that can arise in the field. The best prearranged plans for data collection sometimes fall through. Creativity for workable solutions and new strategies is often needed.

Example of need for flexibility in a qualitative study: Irwin and Johnson (2005) conducted a study that involved interviews with 6-year-old children about their health. The researchers discussed how they had to be creative and had to individualize the interview experience with the child participants—for example, in developing strategies to build rapport with them. They used several forms of play (drawing, role-playing) to enhance their level of comfort but learned that if the form of play did not match the needs of the child, barriers to rapport building were created. Irwin and Johnson also noted the need to be flexible and to "think outside the box" when it came to selecting a setting for the interview.

Types of Data for Qualitative Studies

Qualitative researchers typically go into the field knowing the most likely sources of data, while not ruling out other possible data sources that might come to light as data collection progresses. The primary method of collecting qualitative data is through self-report, that is, by interviewing study participants. Observation is often a part of many qualitative studies as well. Physiologic data are rarely collected in a naturalistic inquiry, except perhaps to describe participants' characteristics or to ascertain eligibility for the sample.

Table 14.2 compares the types of data used by researchers in the three main qualitative traditions, as well as other aspects of the data collection process for each tradition. Ethnographers almost always collect a wide array of data, with observation and interviews being the most important methods. Ethnographers also gather or examine products of the culture under study, such as documents, records, artifacts, photographs, and so on. Phenomenologists and grounded theory researchers rely primarily on in-depth interviews with individual participants, although observation also plays an important role in some grounded theory studies.

The adopted approach also has implications for how the researcher as "self" is used (Lipson, 1991). Researchers conducting phenomenological studies use themselves to collect rich description of human experiences and to develop relationships in which intensive interviews are conducted with a small number of people. Grounded theorists use themselves not only to collect data but also to process the data and generate categories for the emerging theory. Ethnographers use themselves as observers who collect data not only through informal interviews but also through active participation in field settings.

In qualitative studies, there are usually relatively few forms and protocols developed before going into the field. However, a form might be needed for gathering demographic and administrative information. Also, a preliminary list of questions to be asked or observations to be made during the initial data collection is often useful.

Field Issues in Qualitative Studies

The collection of qualitative data in the field often gives rise to several important issues, which are particularly salient in ethnographies. Ethnographic researchers, in addition to the matters discussed in this section, must deal with such issues as gaining entrée, negotiating for space and privacy for interviewing and recording data, deciding on an appropriate role (i.e., the extent to which they will actually participate in the culture's activities), and taking care not to exit from the field prematurely. Ethnographers also need to be able to cope with culture shock and should have a high tolerance for uncertainty and ambiguity (Agar, 1980).

Gaining Trust

Researchers who do qualitative research must, to an even greater extent than quantitative researchers, gain and maintain a high level of trust with participants. Researchers need to develop strategies in the field to establish credibility among those being studied. This may in some cases be a delicate balancing act because researchers must try as much as possible to "be like" the people being studied while at the same time keeping a certain distance. "Being like" participants means that researchers should be sensitive to such issues as styles of dress, modes of speech,

TABLE 14.2	Comparison of Data Collection Issues in Three Qualitative Traditions		
ISSUE	**ETHNOGRAPHY**	**PHENOMENOLOGY**	**GROUNDED THEORY**
Types of data	Primarily observation and interviews, plus artifacts, documents, photographs, genealogies, maps, social network diagrams	Primarily in-depth interviews, sometimes diaries, other written materials	Primarily individual interviews, sometimes group interviews, observation, participant journals, documents
Unit of data collection	Cultural systems	Individuals	Individuals
Data collection points	Mainly longitudinal	Mainly cross-sectional	Cross-sectional or longitudinal
Length of time for data collection	Typically long, many months or years	Typically moderate	Typically moderate
Data recording	Field notes, logs, interview notes/ recordings	Interview notes/recordings	Interview notes/record- ings, memoing, observational notes
Salient field issues	Gaining entrée, reactivity, determining a role, learning how to participate, encouraging candor and other interview logistics, loss of objectivity, premature exit, reflexivity	Bracketing one's views, building rapport, encouraging candor, listening while preparing what to ask next, keeping "on track," handling emotionality	Building rapport, encouraging candor, listening while preparing what to ask next, keeping "on track," handling emotionality

customs, and schedules. In ethnographic research, it is important not to take sides on any controversial issue and not to appear too strongly affiliated with a particular subgroup of the culture—especially with leaders or prominent members of the culture. It is not usually possible to gain the trust of the group if researchers appear close to those in power.

The Pace of Data Collection

In qualitative studies, data collection is often a powerful and exhausting experience, especially if the phenomenon being studied concerns an illness experience or other stressful life event (e.g.,

domestic violence). Moreover, collecting high-quality qualitative data requires intense concentration and energy. Regardless of the type of data being collected, the process can be an emotional strain for which researchers need to be prepared. One way to deal with this is to collect data at a pace that minimizes the emotional impact. For example, in an interview study, it may be prudent to limit interviewing to no more than one a day, and to engage in emotionally releasing activities (e.g., exercising) between interviews. It may also be helpful to debrief about any feelings of distress with a co-researcher, colleague, or advisor.

Emotional Involvement With Participants

Qualitative researchers need to guard against getting too emotionally involved with participants, a pitfall that has been referred to as "**going native**." Researchers who get too close to participants run several risks, including compromising their ability to collect objectively the most meaningful and trustworthy data, and becoming overwhelmed with participants' suffering. It is important, of course, to be supportive and to listen carefully to people's concerns and difficulties, but it usually is not advisable to intervene and try to solve participants' problems, or to share personal problems with them. If participants need help, it is better to give advice about where they can get it than to give it directly.

Reflexivity

As noted in Chapter 8, reflexivity is an important concept in qualitative data collection. Reflexivity refers to researchers' awareness of themselves as part of the data they are collecting. Researchers need to be conscious of the part they play in their own study, and reflect on their own behavior and how it can affect the data they obtain.

Example of reflexivity: Hutchinson, Marsiglio, and Cohan (2002), who were studying young men's developing procreative identity, described their reflexive analysis of the challenges of conducting in-depth interviews with young men. The researchers pondered, for example, how language they used as researchers could affect the kind of data they got from participants. They discovered in their analysis the importance of "turning points" in the young men's experiences, but reflexively demanded: "Under what interview conditions, if any, is it useful to use the words *turning point* if participants had not yet introduced it themselves?" (p. 52).

➲ **TIP:** In qualitative studies, data are often collected by a single researcher working alone, in which case issues such as the selection and training of data collection personnel are not relevant. Nevertheless, self-training and self-preparation are important. When a team of researchers works together on a study, as appears to be happening more frequently than in the past, considerable attention needs to be paid to team issues related to fieldwork — and to group decision making and planning in general (Hall et al., 2005).

Recording and Storing Qualitative Data

In addition to thinking about the types of data to be gathered, qualitative researchers need to plan ahead for how data will be recorded and stored. Interview data, common to all qualitative traditions, can be recorded in two ways: by taking detailed notes of what participants say, or by audio recording (or video recording) what they say. To ensure that interview data are the actual verbatim responses of study participants, it is strongly recommended that qualitative interviews be recorded and subsequently transcribed, rather than relying on interviewer notes. Notes tend to be incomplete, and may be biased by the interviewer's memory or personal views. Moreover, note taking can distract researchers, whose main job is to listen intently and direct the flow of questioning based on what has already been said.

Environmental distractions are a common pitfall in recording interviews. A quiet setting with as little noise as possible is ideal, but this is not always possible for clinical nurse researchers. The second author of this book (Beck) has conducted many challenging interviews. As an example, a mother of three children was interviewed in her living room about her experience with postpartum depression. A time had been prearranged to conduct the interview while her two toddlers were napping. When Beck arrived, the mother apologized: her toddlers had napped earlier than usual, so they would be up during the visit. Beck placed the tape recorder as high up on the couch as possible to keep it out of the reach of the toddlers who kept trying to get it during most of the interview. The television was on to occupy the toddlers, and the 6-week-old baby was especially fussy that day, crying through most of the interview. The noise level in the background of the tape made accurate transcription difficult.

When observations are made, detailed observational notes must be maintained, unless it is possible to videotape. Observational notes should be made shortly after an observational session and are often entered onto a computer file. Whatever method is used to record observations, researchers need to go into the field with the equipment or supplies needed to record their data, and to be sure that the equipment is functioning properly.

➲ **TIP :** It is wise to use good-quality equipment to ensure proper audio and video recording. For example, for recording interviews, make sure that the microphone is adequately sensitive for the acoustics of the environment, or use lapel microphones for both respondents and interviewers.

Grounded theory researchers write analytic memos to themselves. These memos can vary in length from a sentence to multiple pages. These memos document researchers' ideas about how the theory is developing (e.g., how some themes are interrelated).

If assistants are used to collect the data, qualitative researchers need to be as concerned as quantitative researchers about hiring appropriate staff, and training them to collect high-quality data. In particular, the data collectors must be trained to elicit rich and vivid descriptions. Qualitative interviewers need to be good listeners; they need to hear all that is being said, rather than trying to anticipate what is coming next. A good data collector must have both self-awareness and an awareness of the participant (e.g., by paying attention to nonverbal behavior). Qualitative data collectors must be able to create an atmosphere that safely allows for the sharing of experiences and feelings. Respect and authentic caring for participants are critical.

Storage of data while in the field can be problematic because researchers may not have a safe or secure storage space. When this is the case, they often devise a way to keep the data physically with them at all times until it can be secured (e.g., in a fanny pack). Of course, all data tapes or forms should be carefully labeled with an identification number, the date the data were collected, and (if relevant) the name or identification number of the data collector.

With regard to final storage of qualitative data, an important issue to consider is how the analysis will be done—manually, or with the assistance of computers. Increasingly, qualitative researchers are using computer programs to facilitate the organization of vast amounts of narrative information, and this has implications for how the data should be stored. Researchers should ideally be familiar with the computer program to be used before deciding on how to store their data.

➲ **TIP :** It is a wise strategy to have backup copies of your data. Backing up files is imperative (and easy) for data stored on computers, but if computers are not being used, photocopies of written or transcribed materials should be maintained in a separate location. If you expect a delay between taping and transcribing an interview, you should also consider making backup copies of the tapes, which can sometimes get erased through static electricity.

CRITIQUING DATA COLLECTION PLANS

The goal of a data collection plan is to produce data that are of exceptional quality. Every decision a researcher makes about the data collection methods and procedures is likely to affect data quality—and hence the quality of the overall study. These decisions should be critiqued in drawing conclusions about the study's capacity to answer the research questions or test study hypotheses.

The chapters that follow discuss specific data collection strategies (Chapters 15 and 16), the development of new instruments (Chapter 18), and methods of enhancing and assessing data quality (Chapters 17 and 20). Each of these chapters offers assistance in critiquing aspects of data collection in a research project. The critiquing guidelines in this chapter, presented in Box 14.1, focus on global decisions about the design and implementation of a data collection plan. ✪ Unfortunately, data collection procedures are often not described in detail in research reports owing to space constraints in journals.

RESEARCH EXAMPLES

In this section, we provide details about the data collection plan for a quantitative and a qualitative study, which were described with greater care than is typical.

BOX 14.1 Guidelines for Critiquing Data Collection Plans

1. Did the researcher make the right decision about collecting new data versus using existing data for the study?
2. Did the researcher make good data collection decisions with regard to structure, quantification, researcher obtrusiveness, and objectivity?
3. Were the right methods used to collect the data (self-report, etc.)? Was triangulation of methods used appropriately—i.e., were multiple methods sensibly used?
4. Was the right amount of data collected? Were data collected to address the varied needs of the study? Were *too many* data collected in terms of burdening study participants—and, if so, how might this have affected data quality?
5. Did the researcher select good instruments, in terms of congruence with underlying constructs, data quality, reputation, efficiency, and so on? Were new instruments developed unnecessarily?
6. Was the set of data collection instruments adequately pretested?
7. Did the report provide adequate information about data collectors and data collection procedures?
8. Who collected the data? Were data collectors judiciously chosen? Did they have traits that undermined the collection of unbiased, high-quality data, or did their traits enhance data quality?
9. Was the training of data collectors described? Was the training adequate? Were steps taken to improve data collectors' ability to elicit or produce high-quality data, or to monitor their performance?
10. Where and under what circumstances were data gathered? Was the setting for data collection appropriate?
11. Were other people present during data collection? Could the presence of others have resulted in any biases?
12. In a qualitative study, was adequate attention paid to the challenges of doing fieldwork? Were data recorded and stored in an appropriate fashion?

Research Example of Data Collection in a Quantitative Study

Study: "Parental caregiving and developmental outcomes of infants of mothers with HIV" (Holditch-Davis et al., 2001)

Purpose: The purpose of the research was to describe the development of infants of mothers with HIV. The study also explored the longitudinal effects of child characteristics, parental and family characteristics, and parenting quality on children's developmental outcomes.

Design: This nonexperimental study was a longitudinal follow-up study of 81 infants born to women with HIV. Data were first collected when the infants were about 2 to 5 months of age, and then at 6, 12, 18, and 24 months.

Data Collection Plan: The data collection plan was complex, involving structured self-report measures, developmental tests, and in-home observations. Existing data from medical records were also used. The researchers

took care to develop an efficient data collection plan; for example, demographic and medical data were obtained through medical records rather than by asking the mothers. The research team selected high-quality self-report measures with solid reputations; they also evaluated data quality within their own research sample, and found evidence of acceptably good quality. Procedures for gathering observational measures were described in some detail. For example, at 12, 18, and 24 months, observers spent 1 hour observing mother–infant interactions, recording negative interactions, positive interactions, and so on. Well-trained observers were used to collect data: Before making real observations, observers had to achieve a high level of agreement in their categorization of behaviors with one of the investigators. A full 3 to 6 months of practice was required to achieve acceptable performance standards. The dependent variables were measures of the infants' mental and motor development. One test was a respected scale of language development,

the Preschool Language Scale. This test was administered by research assistants who had been trained by a doctorally prepared speech pathologist. Another measure was the Bayley Scales of Infant Development, considered the premier measure of its type. Because this scale must be professionally administered, clinical psychologists who had no knowledge of the infants' performance on other tests administered it. The report carefully documented the attention the researchers paid to ensuring the highest possible quality data. The study data were used to examine substantive questions, control extraneous variables, test for bias, and describe the research sample.
Findings:

- Quality of caregiving (especially positive attention) had a positive effect on all developmental outcomes, even when background variables were statistically controlled.
- Infants with changes in their primary caregiver had lower developmental scores than infants remaining with consistent caregivers.

Research Example of Data Collection in a Qualitative Study

Study: "Black non-Hispanic mothers' perceptions about the promotion of infant-feeding methods by nurses and physicians" (Cricco-Lizza, 2006); "The milk of human kindness: Environmental and human interactions in a WIC clinic that influence infant-feeding decisions of Black women" (Cricco-Lizza, 2005)
Purpose: The overall purpose of this study was to explore the context of Black women's infant feeding decisions within an urban Women, Infants, and Children (WIC) clinic.
Design: Cricco-Lizza undertook an ethnographic study that involved 18 months of fieldwork in a New York metropolitan area WIC clinic.
Data Collection Plan: The main forms of data collection for this study were unstructured self-reports (interviews and informal conversations) and participant observation. With regard to the observational data, Cricco-Lizza observed the WIC clinic operations, focusing in particular on the interactions of 130 Black mothers with their babies, significant others, other WIC mothers, and WIC staff. Observations occurred in the waiting room and in group nutrition education classes. Observation sessions—63 in total—were each about 2 hours long and took place two or three times per week at varying times and days. While observing the mothers in the clinic waiting room, the

researcher also initiated informal discussions with some of them about their infant-feeding beliefs and motherhood experiences. Data obtained through observation were recorded as field notes. After completing an observation session, the researcher immediately constructed an outline of salient events that was later expanded to included specific, detailed information about behaviors, conversations, and the setting. The field notes were typed up shortly after each session. From the group of 130 women who were observed, Cricco-Lizza purposively selected 11 primiparous key informants who were willing to be interviewed several times through their pregnancy and the postpartum period. Six women used formula feeding and five women breastfed. In-depth interviews (which were tape recorded and then transcribed) were conducted during pregnancy, during the early postpartum period, and again 1 month later. The interviews, which followed a formal protocol, captured a range of information about the childbirth experience and infant feeding beliefs and practices. Formal interviews were supplemented by informal interviews in face-to-face meetings and telephone conversations with the key informants. The informal meetings occurred in the women's homes, hospitals, malls, the WIC clinic, and fast-food restaurants. A total of 147 telephone conversations occurred, and the calls provided rich information about important events that happened unexpectedly in the women's lives. Notes from the conversations were recorded immediately. The researcher had between 11 and 32 "data points" (formal and informal interviews) for each key informant. Throughout data collection, the researcher made no recommendations about infant feeding methods. All data were collected by the researcher herself, and she personally verified the accuracy of each transcribed interview, line by line. Thousands of pages of transcribed interviews and field notes were amassed during the study, and various steps were used to ensure the trustworthiness of the data.
Findings:

- The WIC clinic environment set a positive tone for the delivery of service, and the mothers saw the clinic as an important source of support.
- WIC influenced the women's infant feeding decisions. Despite the fact that WIC provided free formula that facilitated bottle-feeding, personalized breastfeeding promotion by trusted WIC staff resulted in breastfeeding decisions by many women.
- However, informants reported limited breastfeeding education and support from nurses and physicians during the childbearing period.

SUMMARY POINTS

- Some researchers use existing data in their studies—for example, those doing historical research, meta-analyses, secondary analyses, or an analysis of **records**. Existing records and documents are an economical source of research data, but two major potential biases in records are **selective deposit** and **selective survival**.

- Data collection methods vary along four dimensions: structure, quantifiability, researcher obtrusiveness, and objectivity.

- It is sometimes useful for quantitative researchers to **qualitize** their data to provide a richer understanding of phenomena or test their interpretations; and qualitative researchers can sometimes profit from **quantitizing** their data to generate new meaning or to document and confirm their conclusions.

- Most nursing research studies involve the use of **self-reports**, that is, data obtained by directly questioning people about the phenomena of interest. Self-reports are strong with respect to their directness and versatility; the major drawback is the potential for respondents' deliberate or unconscious misrepresentations.

- **Projective techniques** are data collection methods that rely on people's projection of psychological traits in response to vaguely structured stimuli. Expressive projective methods take the form of play, drawing, or role playing.

- Observational methods involve obtaining data through the direct observation of phenomena. A wide variety of human activity and traits are amenable to observation, but observation is subject to various **observer biases** and to distorted behavior by study participants (**reactivity**).

- **Biophysiologic measures** tend to yield high-quality data that are objective and valid, and often cost-efficient for nurse researchers.

- Quantitative researchers typically develop a detailed **data collection plan** before they actually begin to collect their data. For highly structured data, researchers often use formal data collection **instruments**.

- An early step in developing a data collection plan is the identification and prioritization of all data needs. In addition to addressing research questions, data may be needed to describe the sample, control extraneous variables, analyze biases, understand subgroup effects, interpret results, perform manipulation checks, and obtain administrative information.

- After data needs have been identified, existing measures of the variables should be sought for use or adaptation. The construction of new instruments requires considerable time and skill and should be undertaken only as a last resort.

- The selection of existing instruments should be based on such considerations as conceptual suitability, expected data quality, cost, population appropriateness, and reputation.

- Even when existing instruments are used, the instrument package should be **pretested** to determine its length, clarity, and overall adequacy.

- When researchers cannot collect the data without assistance, they should carefully select data collection staff and formally train them.

- Qualitative studies typically adopt data collection plans that are flexible and that evolve as the study progresses.

- Self-reports are the most frequently used type of data collection method in qualitative studies, followed by observation. Ethnographies are especially likely to combine these two data sources with others such as the products of the culture (e.g., photographs, documents, artifacts).

- Qualitative researchers are confronted with a number of special fieldwork issues. These include gaining participants' trust, pacing data collection to avoid being overwhelmed by the intensity of data, avoiding emotional involvement with participants ("**going native**"), and maintaining reflexivity (awareness of the part they play in the study and possible effects on their data).

- Qualitative researchers need to plan in advance for how their data will be recorded and stored. If technical equipment is used (e.g., audio recorders, video recorders), care must be taken to select high-quality equipment that functions properly in the field.

● ●

STUDY SUGGESTIONS

Chapter 14 of the *Resource Manual to Accompany Nursing Research: Generating and Assessing Evidence for Nursing Practice, 8th edition*, offers various exercises and study suggestions for reinforcing concepts presented in this chapter. In addition, the following study questions can be addressed:

1. Read a recent research report in a nursing journal, paying especially close attention to the data collection plan. What information about procedures that may affect data quality is missing from the report? How, if at all, does this absence affect your acceptance of the researchers' conclusions?

2. Apply the questions in Box 14.1, to the extent possible, to the research examples at the end of the chapter.

● ●

STUDIES CITED IN CHAPTER 14

Methodologic or theoretical references cited in this chapter can be found in a separate section at the end of the book.

Adams, C., Horn, K., & Bader, J. (2006). Hispanic access to hospice services in a predominantly Hispanic community. *American Journal of Hospice and Palliative Care, 23*(1), 9–16.

Ahl, C., Nystrom, M., & Jansson, L. (2006). Making up one's mind: Patients' experiences of calling an ambulance. *Accident & Emergency Nursing, 14*(1), 11–19.

Chaiyawat, W., & Jezewski, M. (2006). Thai school-age children's perception of fear. *Journal of Transcultural Nursing, 17*(1), 74–81.

Chan, M., Wong, O., Chan, H., Fong, M., Lai, S., Lo, C., Ho, S., Ng, S., & Leung, S. (2006). Effects of music on patients undergoing a C-clamp procedure after percutaneous coronary interventions. *Journal of Advanced Nursing, 53*(6), 669–679.

Cricco-Lizza, R. (2005). The milk of human kindness: Environmental and human interactions in a WIC clinic that influence infant-feeding decisions of Black women. *Qualitative Health Research, 15*(4), 525–538.

Cricco-Lizza, R. (2006). Black non-Hispanic mothers' perceptions about the promotion of infant-feeding methods by nurses and physicians. *Journal of Obstetric, Gynecologic, & Neonatal Nursing, 35*(2), 173–180.

Gary, F. A., & Yarandi, H. N. (2004). Depression among southern rural African American women. *Nursing Research, 53*(4), 251–259.

Holditch-Davis, D., Miles, M. S., Burchinal, M., O'Donnell, K., McKinney, R., & Lim, W. (2001). Parental caregiving and developmental outcomes of infants of mothers with HIV. *Nursing Research, 50*, 5–14.

Hutchinson, S., Marsiglio, W., & Cohan, M. (2002). Interviewing young men about sex and procreation: Methodological issues. *Qualitative Health Research, 12*, 42–60.

Li, S., & Arber, A. (2006). The construction of troubled and credible patients: A study of emotion talk in palliative care settings. *Qualitative Health Research, 16*(1), 27–46.

Nyamathi, A., Berg, J., Jones, T., & Leake, B. (2005). Predictors of perceived health status of tuberculosis-infected homeless. *Western Journal of Nursing Research, 27*(7), 896–910.

Philpin, S. (2006). "Handing over": Transmission of information between nurses in an intensive therapy unit. *Nursing in Critical Care, 11*(2), 86–93.

Polit, D. F., London, A. S., & Martinez, J. M. (2001). *The health of poor urban women*. New York: MDRC. (Available at *http://www.mdrc.org*)

Polit, D. F., Widom, R., & Edin, K. (2001). *Is work enough: Experiences of current and former welfare mothers who work*. New York: MDRC. (Available at *http://www.mdrc.org*)

15

Collecting Unstructured Data

This chapter and the next one describe some specific strategies for collecting research data. As noted in the previous chapter, the degree of structure used in data collection represents a key dimension along which data collection approaches vary. In this chapter, we describe methods of gathering unstructured or semistructured data that are used most typically in qualitative studies. Chapter 16 discusses structured methods used in quantitative research.

QUALITATIVE SELF-REPORT TECHNIQUES

Unstructured or loosely structured self-report methods provide narrative data for qualitative analysis. Qualitative researchers usually do not have a specific set of questions that must be asked in a particular order and worded in a given way. Instead, they start with some general questions or topics and allow respondents to tell their stories in a conversational fashion. Most (but not all) narrative self-report data are collected through interviews rather than by questionnaire.

Unstructured interviews encourage respondents to define the important dimensions of a phenomenon and to elaborate on what is relevant to them, rather than being guided by investigators' *a priori* notions of relevance. Researchers in virtually all qualitative traditions gather unstructured or loosely structured self-report data.

Types of Qualitative Self-Reports

Researchers use various approaches in collecting qualitative self-report data. The main methods are described here.

Unstructured Interviews

Researchers who do not have a preconceived view of the content or flow of information to be gathered may conduct completely **unstructured interviews**. Unstructured interviews are conversational and interactive, and are the mode of choice when researchers do not have a clear idea of what it is they do not know. Researchers using unstructured interviews do not begin with a series of prepared questions because they do not yet know what to ask or even where to begin. In conducting unstructured interviews, researchers let participants tell their stories, with little interruption. Phenomenological, grounded theory, and ethnographic studies usually rely heavily on unstructured interviews.

Researchers using a completely unstructured approach often begin by informally asking a broad question (sometimes called a **grand tour question**) relating to the research topic, such as, "What happened when you first learned you had AIDS?"

Subsequent questions are more focused and are guided by responses to the broad question. Some respondents may request direction after the initial broad question is posed, perhaps asking, "Where should I begin?" Respondents should be encouraged to begin wherever they wish.

Van Manen (1990) provided suggestions for guiding a phenomenological interview in a manner likely to produce rich descriptions of the experience under study:

- "Describe the experience from the inside, as it were; almost like a state of mind: the feelings, the mood, the emotions, etc.
- Focus on a particular example or incident of the object of experience: describe specific events, an adventure, a happening, a particular experience.
- Try to focus on an example of the experience that stands out for its vividness, or as it was the first time.
- Attend to how the body feels, how things smell(ed), how they sound(ed), etc." (pp. 64–65).

Kahn (2000), discussing unstructured interviews in hermeneutic phenomenological studies, recommended interviews that resemble conversations. If the experience under study is an ongoing one, Kahn suggested obtaining as much detail as possible about the participant's daily life. For example, a question that can be used is, "Pick a normal day for you and tell me what happened" (p. 62). If the experience being studied is primarily in the past, then Kahn advocated a retrospective approach. The interviewer begins with a general question such as, "What does this experience mean to you?" (p. 63), and then probes for more detail until the experience is thoroughly described.

Example of unstructured interviews in a phenomenological study: DeSanto-Madeya (2006) conducted a phenomenological study to explore the meaning of living with a spinal cord injury 5 to 10 years after the injury. Unstructured interviews were conducted in the spinal cord–injured person's home. The interviews were initiated with the following statement: "Please describe your experiences, including circumstances, situations, thoughts, and feelings that you think reflect your experiences of living with a spinal cord injury." Interviews lasted between 1 and 2 hours each.

In grounded theory, the interviewing technique changes as the theory is developed. At the outset, interviews are similar to open-ended conversations using unstructured interviews. Glaser and Strauss (1967) suggested researchers initially should just sit back and listen to participants' stories. Later, as the theory emerges, researchers ask more direct questions related to categories in the grounded theory. The more direct questions can be answered rather quickly, and so the interviews tend to get shorter as the grounded theory develops.

Ethnographic interviews are also unstructured. Spradley (1979) describes three types of question used to guide interviews: descriptive, structural, and contrast (Spradley, 1979). *Descriptive questions* ask participants to describe their experiences in their own language, and are the backbone of ethnographic interviews. *Structural questions* are more focused and help to develop the range of terms in a category or domain. Last are *contrast questions*, which are asked to distinguish differences in the meaning of terms and symbols.

Example of ethnographic interviewing: Bannister (1999) conducted an ethnographic study of midlife women's experience of their changing bodies using Spradley's method. An example of a descriptive question was, "I wonder if you could tell me about your experience of your changing body?" (p. 524). An example of a structural question was, "Corinne, you said, 'I see myself getting older.' Are there other phrases you might use to describe this?" (p. 524). Last, an example of a contrast question was, "Mary, how would you describe the difference between your comments, 'How others view me' and 'How I view myself?'" (p. 524).

Completely unstructured methods most typically are used in face-to-face interview situations in naturalistic settings. It is, however, possible to use the Internet for collecting unstructured data, and this is particularly advantageous for "interviewing" respondents who are geographically distant. Mann and Stewart (2001) offer advice about Internet interviewing.

Example of unstructured Internet interviewing: Beck (2004) conducted a phenomenological study through the Internet on posttraumatic stress disorder (PTSD) due to childbirth. A recruitment notice was posted on the website of Trauma and Birth Stress, a charitable trust in New Zealand that provided support for women who have experienced birth trauma. Women who were interested e-mailed Beck, who sent directions for the study to prospective participants by e-mail attachment. Each mother was asked to respond to the following statement: Please describe in as much detail as you wish to share your experience of PTSD after childbirth." Women sent Beck their stories by e-mail attachment. (This study appears in its entirety in Appendix D of the accompanying *Resource Manual*).

➲ **TIP:** An advantage of Internet interviewing is that participants' narratives are already typed, thus avoiding the major expense of transcribing taped interviews. In an Internet environment, however, researchers need to devote their time and effort into crafting individual e-mail responses to make sure all participants feel valued and understand that their narratives made a contribution to the study.

Semistructured Interviews

Researchers sometimes want to be sure that a specific set of topics is covered in their qualitative interviews. They know what they want to ask, but cannot predict what the answers will be. Their role in the process is somewhat structured, whereas the participants' is not. In such **focused** or **semistructured interviews**, researchers prepare in advance a written **topic guide**, which is a list of areas or questions to be covered with each participant. The interviewer's function is to encourage participants to talk freely about all the topics on the list, and to tell stories in their own words. This technique ensures that researchers will obtain all the information required, and gives people the freedom to respond in their own words, provide as much detail as they wish, and offer illustrations and explanations.

In preparing the list of questions, care needs to be taken to order questions in a logical sequence, perhaps chronologically, or perhaps from the general to the specific. (However, interviewers need to be attentive because sometimes respondents spontaneously give information about questions that are later on the list.) The list of questions might include suggestions for follow-up questions or **probes** designed to elicit more detailed information. Examples of such probes include, "What happened next?" and "When that happened, how did you feel?" Care should be taken not to include questions that require one- or two-word responses, such as "yes" or "no." The goal is to ask questions that give respondents an opportunity to provide rich, detailed information about the phenomenon under study.

In deciding whether to use a semistructured or unstructured interview, it is important to consider not only the research tradition, but also the state of knowledge on a topic. Gibson (1998) used both approaches in a study of the experiences and expectations of patients discharged from an acute psychiatric hospital. Gibson found that unstructured interviews resulted in greater depth and detail than semistructured interviews, and that respondents preferred unstructured interviews.

Example of a semistructured interview: Clarke and colleagues (2006) studied gender differences in how cancer patients perceive the social support they receive from health care staff in the United Kingdom. Semistructured interviews were conducted with 16 patients undergoing cancer treatment. An example of a question they asked is, "Are there ways staff could do more to support patients like yourself?" and a suggested follow-up probe was, "In what ways could staff have supported you better?" (p. 68).

Focus Group Interviews

Focus group interviews are becoming increasingly popular in the study of health problems. In a focus group interview, a group of four or more people is assembled for a discussion. The interviewer (often called a **moderator**) guides the discussion according to a written set of questions or topics to be covered, as in a semistructured interview. Focus group sessions are carefully planned discussions that take advantage of group dynamics for accessing rich information in an efficient manner.

Typically, the people selected for a group are a fairly homogeneous group, to promote a comfortable group dynamic. People usually feel more at ease expressing their views when they share a similar background with other group members. Thus, if the overall sample is diverse, it is usually best to organize focus groups for people with similar characteristics (e.g., in terms of race/ethnicity, age, gender, or experience).

Several writers have suggested that the optimal group size for focus groups is 6 to 12 people, but Côté-Arsenault and Morrison-Beedy (1999) advocate smaller groups of about 5 participants when the topic is emotionally charged or sensitive. Groups of four or fewer may not generate sufficient interaction, however, particularly because not everyone is equally comfortable in expressing their views.

◐ TIP : In recruiting group members, it is usually wise to recruit one or two more people than is considered optimal, because of the risk of no-shows. Monetary incentives can help reduce this risk. It is also important to call the recruits the night before the session to remind them of the appointment and confirm attendance.

The setting for the focus group sessions should be selected carefully and, ideally, should be a neutral one. Churches, hospitals, or other settings that are strongly identified with particular values or expected behaviors may not be suitable, depending on the topic. The location should be one that is comfortable, not intimidating, accessible, and easy to find. It should also be acoustically amenable to audiotaping.

Moderators play a critical role in the success of focus group interviews. An important job of moderators is to solicit input from all group members, and not let a few vocal people dominate the discussion. It is sometimes useful to have more than one moderator, so that particular cues can be followed up by more than one listener. Researchers other than the moderator should be present, to take detailed notes about each session.

A major advantage of a group format is that it is efficient—researchers obtain the viewpoints of many individuals in a short time. Moreover, focus groups capitalize on the fact that members react to what is being said by others, thereby potentially leading to richer or deeper expressions of opinion. Also, focus group interviews are usually stimulating to respondents. One disadvantage is that some people are uncomfortable about expressing their views in front of a group. Another concern is that the dynamics of the session may foster a group culture that could inhibit individual expression as "group think" takes hold. Studies of focus groups have shown, however, that they are similar to individual interviews in terms of number or quality of ideas generated (Kidd & Parshall, 2000). Some critics have worried, however, about whether data from focus groups are as "natural" as data obtained from individual interviews (Morgan, 2001).

Key to an effective focus group is the researcher's *questioning route*, that is, the series of questions used to guide the interview. Krueger and Casey (2000) provide helpful guidelines for developing a good questioning route. A typical 2-hour focus group session should include about 12 questions. A good strategy is for the sequence of questions to move from general to specific.

Focus groups have been used by researchers in many qualitative research traditions, and can play a particularly important role in feminist, critical theory, and participatory action research. Nurse researchers have offered excellent guidance on studies with focus groups (e.g., Côté-Arsenault & Morrison-Beedy, 2005; Morrison-Beedy, Côté-Arsenault, & Feinstein, 2001), and several books on how to do focus group research are available (e.g., Bader & Rossi, 2002; Kreuger & Casey, 2000). The Toolkit of the accompanying *Resource Manual* also has additional resources on focus groups, and several websites relating to focus group methods are suggested on the accompanying student CD-ROM. ✪ ◉

Joint Interviews

Nurse researchers are sometimes interested in phenomena that involve interpersonal relationships, or that require understanding the perspective of more than one person. For example, the phenomenon might be the grief that mothers *and* fathers experience on losing a child, or the experiences of AIDS patients *and* their caretakers. In such cases, it can be productive to conduct **joint interviews** in which two or more parties are simultaneously questioned, using either an unstructured or semistructured format. Unlike focus group interviews, which typically involve group members who do not know each other, joint or dyadic interviews are done with people who are intimately related.

Joint interviews usually supplement rather than replace individual interviews because there are things that cannot readily be discussed in front of the other party (e.g., criticisms of the other person's behavior). However, joint interviews can be especially helpful when researchers want to *observe* the dynamics between two key actors. Morris (2001) provides some useful guidelines and raises important issues in the conduct of joint interviews.

Life Histories

Life histories are narrative self-disclosures about individual life experiences. Ethnographers frequently use individual life histories to learn about cultural patterns. A famous example of this is Oscar Lewis' life history of poor families in Mexico, which gave rise to the controversial concept of *culture* of poverty.

With a life history approach, researchers ask respondents to provide, often in chronologic sequence, a narration of their ideas and experiences, either orally or in writing. Life histories may take months, or even years, to record, with researchers providing only gentle guidance in the telling of the story. Narrated life histories are often backed up by intensive observation of the person, interviews with friends or family members, or a scrutiny of letters, photographs, or other materials.

Leininger (1985) noted that comparative life histories are especially valuable for the study of the patterns and meanings of health and health care, especially among elderly people. Her highly regarded essay provides a protocol for obtaining a life health care history.

Oral Histories

Researchers use the technique known as **oral history** to gather personal recollections of events and their perceived causes and consequences. Oral histories, unlike life histories, typically focus on describing important themes rather than individuals. Oral histories are a method for connecting individual experiences with broader social and cultural contexts.

Oral histories are an important method for historical researchers when the topic under study is the not-too-distant past, and people who experienced the event can still be asked about those experiences. Oral histories are also a tool used by feminist researchers and other researchers with an ideological perspective because oral histories are a way to reach groups that have been ignored or oppressed.

Depending on the focus of the oral history, researchers can conduct interviews with a number of persons or concentrate on multiple interviews with one individual. Researchers usually use unstructured interviews to collect oral history data.

Example of oral histories: LeVasseur (2003) analyzed the oral histories of 18 combat nurses who served in the Vietnam War. The following themes emerged: disruption and disorientation, loss of idealism, moral conflict, responsibility and powerlessness, professional peak, and becoming real.

Critical Incidents

The **critical incidents technique** is a method of gathering information about people's behaviors by examining specific incidents relating to the behavior under investigation (Flanagan, 1954). The technique, as the name suggests, focuses on a factual incident, which may be defined as an observable and integral episode of human behavior. The word *critical* means that the incident must have had a discernible impact on some outcome; it must make either a positive or negative contribution to the accomplishment of some activity of interest. For example, if we were interested in understanding the use of humor in clinical practice, we might ask a sample of nurses the following questions: "Think of the last time you used humor in your interactions with a hospital patient. What led up to the situation? Exactly what did you do? How did the patient react? Why did you feel it would be all right to use a humorous approach? What happened next?"

The technique differs from other self-report approaches in that it focuses on something specific about which respondents can be expected to testify as expert witnesses. Usually, data on 100 or more critical incidents are collected, but this typically involves interviews with a much smaller number of people because each participant can often describe multiple incidents. The critical incident technique has been used in both individual and focus group interviews.

Example of a critical incident study: Bormann and colleagues (2006) studied the outcomes of a stress management program. The 5-week program taught a "mind–body–spiritual" technique of silently repeating a mantra—a word or phrase with spiritual meaning. Three months later, critical incident interviews with 55 participants yielded 147 incidents involving applications of the technique.

Diaries and Journals

Personal **diaries** have long been used as a source of data in historical research. It is also possible to generate new data for a nonhistorical study by asking study participants to maintain a diary or journal over a specified period. Diaries can be useful in providing an intimate and detailed description of a person's everyday life.

The diaries may be completely unstructured; for example, individuals who have undergone organ transplantation could be asked simply to spend 10 to 15 minutes a day jotting down their thoughts and feelings. Frequently, however, subjects are requested to make entries into a diary regarding some specific aspect of their experience, sometimes in a semistructured format (e.g., about their eating or sleeping patterns). Nurse researchers have used health diaries to collect information about how people prevent illness, maintain health, experience morbidity, and treat health problems.

Although diaries are a useful means of learning about ongoing experiences, one limitation is that they can be used only by people with adequate literacy skills, although there are examples of studies in which diary entries were audiotaped rather than written out. Diaries also depend on a high level of participant cooperation.

Example of diaries: Jacelon and Imperio (2005) described how they used diaries to explore the strategies that older adults use to manage their chronic health problems. Study participants were asked to maintain a diary over a 2-week period for at least 15 minutes a day. They were given a list of questions to help them focus their thoughts on aspects of the concept of personal integrity. Participants were given three options for maintaining the diary—written, audiotaped, and telephone conversation.

The Think-Aloud Method

The **think-aloud method** is a technique for collecting data about cognitive processes, such as thinking, problem solving, and decision making. This method involves having people use audio-recording devices to talk about decisions as they are being made or while problems are being solved, over an extended period (e.g., throughout a shift). The method produces an inventory of decisions as they occur in a naturalistic context, and allows researchers to examine sequences of decisions or thoughts, as well as the context in which they occur (Fonteyn, Kuipers, & Grober, 1993). Think-aloud procedures have been used in a number of studies of clinical nurses' decision making and reasoning processes.

The think-aloud method has been used in both naturalistic and simulated settings. Although simulated settings offer the opportunity of controlling the context of the thought process (e.g., presenting people with a common problem to be solved), naturalistic settings offer the best opportunity for understanding clinical processes.

Think-aloud sessions are sometimes followed up with personal interviews or focus group interviews in which the tape may be played (or excerpts from the transcript quoted). Participants are then questioned about aspects of their reasoning and decision making.

Example of the think-aloud method: Simmons and colleagues (2003) used the think-aloud method to explore the clinical reasoning strategies of experienced nurses as they considered assessment findings of patients.

Photo Elicitation Interviews

Photo elicitation involves an interview stimulated and guided by photographic images. This procedure, most often used in ethnographies, has been described as a method that can break down barriers between researchers and study participants, and promote a more collaborative discussion (Harper, 1994). The photographs typically are ones that researchers or associates have made of the participants' world, through which researchers can gain insights into a new culture. Participants may need to be continually reassured that their taken-for-granted explanations of the photos are providing new and useful information.

Photo elicitation can also be used with photos that participants have in their homes, although in such case researchers have less time to frame useful questions, and no opportunity to select the photos that will be the stimulus for discussion. Researchers have also used the technique of asking participants to take photographs themselves and then interpret them.

Example of photo elicitation: Turner (2005) explored the meaning and experience of *hope* in young people living in Australia. The researcher gave participants disposable cameras and asked them to take pictures that, in their view, showed hope. Then Turner conducted in-depth interviews with the youth, with questions prompted, in part, by the photographs.

Self-Report Narratives on the Internet

In addition to the possibility of gathering narrative data on the Internet through structured or semi-structured "interview" methods, a potentially rich data source for qualitative researchers involves narrative self-reports available directly on the Internet. For example, researchers can enter into long conversations with other users in a chat room. Also, data that can be analyzed qualitatively are simply "out there," as when a researcher enters a chat room or goes to a bulletin board and analyzes the content of the existing, unsolicited messages.

Using the Internet to access narrative data has obvious advantages. This approach is economical and allows researchers to obtain information from geographically dispersed and perhaps remote Internet users (Fitzpatrick & Montgomery, 2004). However, a number of ethical concerns have been raised, and authenticity and other methodologic challenges need to be considered (Kralik et al., 2006; Moloney et al., 2003; Robinson, 2001).

Example of Internet data use: Klemm and Wheeler (2005) evaluated messages posted over a 2-month period on an online cancer caregiver listserve. They found that supportive and hopeful statements prevailed.

Gathering Qualitative Self-Report Data

The purpose of gathering narrative self-report data is to enable researchers to construct reality in a way that is consistent with the constructions of the people being studied. This goal requires researchers to take steps to overcome communication barriers and to enhance the flow of meaning. Asking good questions and eliciting good narrative data are far more difficult than they appear. This section offers some suggestions about gathering qualitative self-report data through in-depth interviews. Further suggestions are offered by Fontana and Frey (2003), Rubin and Rubin (2005), and Gubrium and Holstein (2001).

Preparing for the Interview

Although qualitative interviews are conversational, this does not mean that they are entered into casually. The conversations are purposeful ones that require advance thought and preparation. For example, careful thought should be given to the wording of questions. To the extent possible, the wording should make sense to respondents and reflect their world view.

An important issue is that researchers and respondents should have a common vocabulary. If the researcher is studying a different culture or a subgroup that uses distinctive terms or slang, efforts should be made before data collection begins to understand those terms and their nuances.

Researchers usually prepare for the interview by developing, mentally or in writing, the broad questions to be asked (or at least the initial questions, in unstructured interviews). Sometimes it is useful to do a practice interview with a stand-in respondent. If there are questions that are especially sensitive, it is a good idea to ask such questions late in the interview when rapport has been established.

➲ **TIP:** Memorize central questions if you have written them out, so that you will be able to maintain eye contact with participants.

It is also important to decide in advance how to present oneself—as a researcher, as a nurse, as an ordinary person as much like participants as possible, as a humble "learner," and so on. One advantage of assuming the nurse role is that people often trust nurses. On the other hand, people may be overly deferent if nurses are perceived as better educated or more knowledgeable than they are themselves. Moreover, participants may use the interview as an opportunity to ask numerous health questions, or to solicit opinions about particular health practitioners.

Another part of the preparation involves decisions about places where the interviews can be conducted. Warren (2001) advocates letting participants choose the setting. It is, however, important to think about possibilities to suggest to them. In-home interviews are often preferred because interviewers then have the opportunity to observe the participants' world, and to take observational notes. When in-home interviews are not desired by participants (e.g., if they are worried that the interview would be overheard by household members and prefer more privacy), it is wise to have alternative suggestions, such as in an office, in a coffee shop, and so on. The important thing is to select places that offer some privacy, that protect insofar as possible against interruptions, and that are adequate for recording the interview. Of course, in some cases, the setting will be dictated by circumstances, as when interviews take place while participants are hospitalized.

For interviews done in the field, researchers must anticipate the equipment and supplies that will be needed. Preparing a checklist of all such items is helpful. The checklist typically would include audiotaping equipment, batteries, tapes, consent and demographic forms, notepads, and pens. Other possibilities include laptop computers, incentive payments, cookies or donuts to help break the ice, and distracting toys or picture books if it is likely that children will be home. It may be necessary to bring proper identification to assure participants of the legitimacy of the visit. And, if the topic under study is likely to elicit emotional narratives, tissues should be readily at hand.

⮕ **T I P :** Use high-quality tapes for audiotaping interviews. Make sure that the size of the tape corresponds to the size used in the transcription equipment.

Conducting the Interview

Qualitative interviews are typically long—sometimes lasting up to several hours. Researchers often find that the respondents' construction of their experience only begins to emerge after lengthy, in-depth dialogues. Interviewers must prepare respondents for the interview by putting them at ease. Part of this process involves sharing pertinent information about the study (e.g., about protection of confidentiality), and another part is using the first few minutes for pleasantries and ice-breaking exchanges of conversation before actual questioning begins. Up-front "small talk" can help to overcome stage fright, which can occur for both interviewers and respondents. Participants may be particularly nervous when the interviews are being tape-recorded, which is the preferred method of recording information. They typically forget about the tape recorder after the interview is underway, so the first few minutes should be used to help both parties "settle in."

⮕ **T I P :** If possible, place the actual tape-recording equipment on the floor or somewhere out of sight.

Study participants will not share much information with interviewers if they do not trust them. Close rapport with respondents provides access to richer information and to personal, intimate details of their stories. Interviewer personality plays a role in developing rapport: Good interviewers are usually congenial, friendly people who have the capacity to see the situation from the respondent's perspective.

Nonverbal communication can be critical in conveying concern and interest. Facial expressions, postures, nods, and so on, help to set the tone for the interview. Gaglio, Nelson, and King (2006) offered some insights concerning the development of rapport in primary care settings.

The most critical interviewing skill for in-depth interviews is being a good listener. It is especially important not to interrupt respondents, to "lead" them, to offer advice or opinions, to counsel them, or to share personal experiences. The interviewer's job is to listen intently to the respondents' stories, a task that is often exhausting. Only by attending carefully to what respondents are saying can in-depth interviewers develop appropriate follow-up questions. Even when a topic guide is used, interviewers must not let the flow of dialogue be bound by those questions. In semistructured interviews, many questions that appear on a topic guide are answered spontaneously over the course of the interview, usually out of sequence.

⮕ **T I P :** In-depth interviewers must be comfortable with pauses and silences, and should let participants set the pace. Interviewers can encourage respondents with nonspecific prompts, such as "Mmhm."

In-depth interviewers need to be prepared for strong emotions, such as anger, fear, or grief, to surface. Narrative disclosures can "bring it all back" for respondents, which can be a cathartic or therapeutic experience if interviewers create an atmosphere of concern and caring—but it can also be stressful.

Interviewers may need to manage a number of potential crises during the interviews. One that happens at least once in most qualitative studies is the failed or improper recording of the interview. Thus, even when interviews are tape-recorded, notes should be taken during or immediately after the interview to ensure the highest possible reliability of data and to prevent a total information loss. Interruptions (usually the telephone) and other distractions are another common problem. If respondents are willing, telephones can be controlled by unplugging them or taking the receiver off the hook. Interruptions by personal intrusions of friends or family members may be more difficult to manage. In some cases, the interview may need to be terminated and rescheduled—for example, when a woman is discussing domestic violence and the perpetrator enters and stays in the room.

Interviewers should strive for a positive closure to the interview. The last questions in in-depth interviews should usually be along these lines: "Is there anything else you would like to tell me?" or "Are there any other questions that you think I should have asked you?" Such probes can often elicit a wealth of important information. In closing, interviewers normally ask respondents whether they would mind being contacted again, in the event that additional questions come to mind after reflecting on the information, or in case interpretations of the information need to be verified.

➲ **TIP:** It is usually unwise to schedule back-to-back interviews. It is important not to rush or cut short the first interview to be on time for the next one, and you may sometimes be too emotionally drained to do a second interview in one day. It is also important to have an opportunity to write out notes, impressions, and analytic ideas, and it is best to do this when an interview is fresh in your mind.

Postinterview Procedures

Tape-recorded interviews should be listened to and checked for audibility and completeness soon after the interview is over. If there have been problems with the recording, the interview should be reconstructed in as much detail as possible. Listening to the interview may also suggest possible follow-up questions that could be asked if respondents are recontacted. Morse and Field (1995) recommend that interviewers listen to the tapes objectively and critique their own interviewing style, so that improvements can be made in subsequent interviews.

Steps also need to be taken to ensure that the transcription of interviews is done with rigor. It is

prudent to hire experienced transcribers, to check the quality of initial transcriptions, and to give the transcribers feedback. Transcribers can sometimes unwittingly change the meaning of data by misspelling words, by omitting words, or by not adequately entering information about pauses, laughter, crying, or volume of the respondents' speech (e.g., shouting).

➲ **TIP:** If transcribers need to be hired, transcriptions can be the most expensive part of a study. It generally takes about 3 hours of transcription time for every hour of interviewing. New, improved voice recognition computer software is available to help with transcribing interviews.

Evaluation of Unstructured Self-Report Approaches

In-depth interviews are an extremely flexible approach to gathering data and, in many research contexts, offer distinct advantages. In clinical situations, for example, it is often appropriate to let people talk freely about their problems and concerns, allowing them to take much of the initiative in directing the flow of information. Unstructured self-reports may allow investigators to ascertain what the basic issues or problems are, how sensitive or controversial the topic is, how easy it is to secure respondents' cooperation in discussing the issues, how individuals conceptualize and talk about the problems, and what range of opinions or behaviors exist relevant to the topic. In-depth interviews may also help elucidate the underlying meaning of a pattern or relationship repeatedly observed in more structured research.

On the other hand, qualitative methods are extremely time-consuming and demanding of researchers' skills in gathering, analyzing, and interpreting the resulting data. Also, samples tend to be small because of the quantity of information produced, so it may be difficult to know whether findings are idiosyncratic.

UNSTRUCTURED OBSERVATIONAL METHODS: PARTICIPANT OBSERVATION

Qualitative researchers sometimes collect unstructured or loosely structured observational data, often as an important supplement to self-report data. The aim of their research is to understand the behaviors and experiences of people as they actually occur in naturalistic settings. Qualitative researchers seek to observe people and their environments with a minimum of structure and interference.

Unstructured observational data are most often gathered in field settings through a process known as **participant observation**. Participant observers participate in the functioning of the social group under investigation and strive to observe, ask questions, and record information within the contexts, structures, and symbols that are relevant to group members. Bogdan (1972) defined participant observation as ". . . research characterized by a prolonged period of intense social interaction between the researcher and the subjects, in the milieu of the latter, during which time data . . . are unobtrusively and systematically collected" (p. 3).

Example of participant observation: Shin, Cho, & Kim (2005) undertook an ethnographic study to learn about the meaning of death to elderly women of a Korean clan. In addition to interviews with 14 key informants and other secondary informants, the researchers undertook participant observation of the daily lives of clan members, and of the rituals of death and ancestor worship.

Not all qualitative observational research is *participant* observation (i.e., with observations occurring from *within* the group under study). Some unstructured observations involve watching and recording unfolding behaviors without the observers interacting with participants in activities. If a key research objective, however, is to learn how group interactions and activities give meaning to human behaviors and experiences, then participant observation is an appropriate method.

The members of any group or culture are influenced by assumptions they take for granted, and observers can, through active participation as members, gain access to these assumptions. Participant observation is used by grounded theory researchers, ethnographers, and researchers with ideological perspectives.

Example of unstructured nonparticipant observation: El-Nemer, Downe, and Small (2006) used unstructured observational methods to explore the care given to 21 Egyptian women during their labor and delivery. Women were observed in the labor and delivery room, with observations comprising a total of 180 hours.

The Participant Observer Role in Participant Observation

The role that observers play in the groups under study is important because the observers' social position determines what they are likely to see. That is, the behaviors that are likely to be available for observation depend on observers' position in a network of relations.

Leininger and McFarland (2006) describe a participant observer's role as evolving through a four-phase sequence:

1. Primarily observation and active listening
2. Primarily observation with limited participation
3. Primarily participation with continued observation
4. Primary reflection and reconfirmation of findings with informants

In the initial phase, researchers observe and listen to those under study to obtain a broad view of the situation. This phase allows both observers and the observed to "size up" each other, to become acquainted, and to become more comfortable interacting. This first phase is sometimes referred to as "learning the ropes." In the next phase, observation is enhanced by a modest degree of participation. By participating in the group's activities, researchers can study not only people's behaviors, but also people's reactions to them. In phase 3, researchers strive to become more active participants, learning by the actual experience of doing rather than just by watching and listening. In phase 4, researchers reflect on the total process of what transpired and how people interacted with and reacted to them.

Junker (1960) described a somewhat different continuum that does not assume an evolving process: complete participant, participant as observer, observer as participant, and complete observer. Complete participants conceal their identity as researchers, entering the group ostensibly as regular members. For example, a nurse researcher might accept a job as a clinical nurse with the express intent of studying, in a concealed fashion, some aspect of the clinical environment. At the other extreme, complete observers do not attempt participation in the group's activities, but rather make observations as outsiders. At both extremes, observers may have difficulty asking probing questions—albeit for different reasons. Complete participants may arouse suspicion if they make inquiries not congruent with a total participant role, and complete observers may not have personal access to, or the trust of, those being observed. Most observational fieldwork lies in between these two extremes and may shift over time.

Example of participant observer roles:
Woodgate (2005) studied adolescents' experiences with cancer through in-depth interviews and unstructured observations. Adolescents were observed in inpatient and outpatient units over the 2-year period of fieldwork. Woodgate described her approach as "moderate participant observation" (p. 10), in which she made an effort to maintain an unobtrusive balance between participation and observation.

➲ **TIP:** Being a fully participating member of a group does not *necessarily* offer the best perspective for studying a phenomenon—just as being an actor in a play does not offer the most advantageous view of the performance.

Getting Started

Observers must overcome at least two initial hurdles: gaining entrée into the social group or culture under study, and establishing rapport and developing trust within the social group. Without gaining entrée, the study cannot proceed; but without the group's trust, researchers could be restricted to what Leininger (1985) referred to as "front stage" knowledge, that is, information distorted by the group's protective facades. The observer's goal is to "get back stage"— to learn about the realities of the group's experiences and behaviors. This section discusses some practical and interpersonal aspects of getting started in the field.

Gaining an Overview

Before fieldwork begins, or in the very earliest stage of fieldwork, it is usually useful to gather some written or pictorial descriptive information that provides an overview of the setting. In an institutional setting, for example, it is helpful to obtain a floor plan, an organizational chart, an annual report, and so on. Then, a preliminary personal tour of the setting should be undertaken to gain familiarity with its ambiance and to note major activities, social groupings, transactions, and events.

In community studies, ethnographers sometimes conduct what is referred to as a **windshield survey** (or *windshield tour*), which involves an intensive exploration (sometimes in an automobile, and hence the name) to "map" important features of the community under study. Such community mapping can include documenting community resources (e.g., churches, businesses, public transportation, community centers), community liabilities (e.g., vacant lots, empty stores, public housing units), and social and environmental characteristics (e.g., condition of streets and buildings, traffic patterns, types of signs, children playing in public places).

Example of a windshield survey: In the mixed method study of the health and well-being of low-income families in four U.S. cities (Polit, London, & Martinez, 2001), the ethnographic component involved windshield surveys in 12 neighborhoods (3 per city). The protocol for this windshield survey is included in the Toolkit section of the accompanying *Resource Manual.* ✪

Establishing Rapport

After gaining entrée into the research setting and obtaining permissions and suggestions from gate-keepers, the next step is to enter the field. In some cases, it may be possible just to "blend in" or ease into a social group, but often researchers walk into a "head-turning" situation in which there is considerable curiosity because they stand out as strangers. Participant observers often find that, for their own comfort level and also for that of participants, it is best to have a brief, simple explanation about their presence. Except in rare cases, deception is neither necessary nor recommended, but vagueness has many advantages. People rarely want to know *exactly* what researchers are studying, they simply want an introduction and enough information to satisfy their curiosity and erase any suspicions they may have about the researchers' ulterior motives.

After initial introductions with members of the group, it is usually best to keep a fairly low profile. At the beginning, researchers are not yet familiar with the customs, language, and norms of the group, and it is critical to learn these things. Politeness and friendliness are, of course, essential, but effusive socializing is not appropriate at the early stages of fieldwork.

➲ **TIP:** At this point, your job is to listen intently and learn what it is going to take to fit into the group, that is, what you need to do to become accepted as a member. To the extent possible, you should downplay any expertise you might have because you do not want to distance yourself from participants. Your overall goal is to gain people's trust and to move relationships to a deeper level.

As rapport is developed and trust is established, researchers can begin to play a more active participatory role and to collect observational data in earnest.

Gathering Unstructured Observational Data

Participant observers typically place few restrictions on the nature of the data collected, in keeping with the goal of minimizing observer-imposed meanings and structure. Nevertheless, participant observers often have a broad plan for the types of information to be gathered. Among the aspects likely to be considered relevant are the following:

1. *The physical setting.* What are the main features of the physical setting? What is the context within which human behavior unfolds? What types of behaviors and characteristics are promoted (or constrained) by the physical environment? How does the environment contribute to what is happening?

2. *The participants.* What are the characteristics of the people being observed? How many people are there? What are their roles? Who is given free access to the setting—who "belongs"? What brings these people together?

3. *Activities and interactions.* What is going on—what are people doing and saying, and how are they behaving? Is there a discernible progression of activities? How do people interact with one another? What methods do they use to communicate, and how frequently do they do so? What is the tone of their communications? What type of emotions do they show during their interactions? How are participants interconnected to one another or to activities underway?

4. *Frequency and duration.* When did the activity or event begin, and when is it scheduled to end? How much time has elapsed? Is the activity a recurring one, and if so, how regularly does it recur? How typical of such activities is the one that is under observation?

5. *Precipitating factors.* Why is the event or interaction happening? What contributes to how the event or interaction unfolds?

6. *Organization.* How is the event or interaction organized? How are relationships structured? What norms or rules are in operation?

7. *Intangible factors.* What did *not* happen (especially if it ought to have happened)? Are participants saying one thing verbally but communicating other messages nonverbally? What types of things were disruptive to the activity or situation?

Clearly, this is far more information than can be absorbed in a single session (and not all categories may be relevant to the research question). However, this framework provides a starting point for thinking about observational possibilities while in the field. (This list of features amenable to in-depth observation is included in the Toolkit as a Word document so that it can be adapted to fit the needs of specific studies.) ⊗

➡ **TIP:** When we enter a social setting in our everyday lives, we unconsciously process many of the questions on this list. Usually, however, we do not consciously *attend* to our observations and impressions in any systematic way, and are not careful about making note of the details that contribute to our impressions. This is precisely what participant observers must learn to do.

Spradley (1980) distinguished three levels of observation that typically occur during fieldwork. The first level is **descriptive observation**, which tends to be broad and is used to help observers figure out what is going on. During these descriptive observations, researchers make every attempt to observe as much as possible. Later in the inquiry, observers do **focused observations** on more carefully selected events and interactions. Based on the research aims and on what has been learned from the descriptive observations, participant observers begin to focus more sharply on key aspects of the setting. From these focused observations, they may develop a system for organizing observations, such as a taxonomy or category system. Finally, **selective observations** are the most highly focused, and are undertaken to facilitate comparisons between categories or activities. Spradley describes these levels as analogous to a funnel, with an increasingly narrow and more systematic focus.

While in the field, participant observers have to make decisions about how to sample observations and to select observational locations. **Single positioning** means staying in a single location for a period to observe behaviors and transactions in that location. **Multiple positioning** involves moving around the site to observe behaviors from different locations. **Mobile positioning** involves following a person throughout a given activity or period. It is usually useful to use a combination of positioning approaches in selecting observational locations.

Because participant observers cannot spend a lifetime in one site and because they cannot be in more than one place at a time, observation is almost always supplemented with information obtained in unstructured interviews or conversations. For example, informants may be asked to describe what went on in a meeting that the observer was unable to attend, or to describe events that occurred before the observer entered the field. In such a case, the informant functions as the observer's observer.

Recording Observations

Participant observers may find it tempting to put more emphasis on the *participation* and *observation* parts of their research than on the recording of those activities. Without systematic daily recording of the observational data, however, the project will flounder. Observational information cannot be trusted to memory; it must be diligently recorded as soon after the observations as possible.

Types of Observational Records

The most common forms of record keeping in participant observation are logs and field notes, but photographs and videotapes may also be used. A **log** (or **field diary**) is a daily record of events and conversations in the field. A log is a historical listing of how researchers have spent their time and can be used for planning purposes, for keeping track of expenses, and for reviewing what work has already been completed. Box 15.1 presents an example of a log entry from Beck's (2002) study of mothers of multiples.

Field notes are much broader, more analytic, and more interpretive than a simple listing of occurrences. Field notes represent the participant observer's efforts to record information and also to synthesize and understand the data. The next sections discuss the content of field notes and the process of writing them.

BOX 15.1 Example of a Log Entry

Log entry for Mothers of Multiples Support Group Meeting (Beck, 2002)
July 15, 1999 10–11:30 AM
This is my fourth meeting that I have attended. Nine mothers came this morning with their twins. One other woman attended. She was pregnant with twins. She came to the support group for advice from the other mothers regarding such issues as what type of stroller to buy, etc. All the moms sat on the floor with their infants placed on blankets on the floor next to them. Toddlers and older children played together off to the side with a box of toys. I sat next to a mom new to the group with her twin 4-month-old girls. I helped her hold and feed one of the twins. On my other side was a mom who had signed up at the last meeting to participate in my study. I hadn't called her yet to set up an appointment. She asked how my research was going. We then set up an appointment for next Thursday at 10 AM at her home for me to interview her. The new mother that I sat next to also was eager to participate in the study. In fact she said we could do the interview right after the meeting ends today but I couldn't, due to another meeting. We scheduled an interview appointment for next Thursday at 1 PM. I also set up a third appointment for an interview for next week with I.K. for Monday at 1 PM. She had participated in an earlier study of mine. She came right over to me this morning at the support group meeting.

⮕ **TIP:** Field notes are important in many types of studies, not just in studies involving participant observation. For example, field notes are critical in process evaluations and in inquiries relating to intervention fidelity.

The Content of Field Notes

Participant observers' field notes contain a narrative account of what is happening in the field; they serve as the data for analysis. Most "field" notes are not written while observers are literally in the field but rather are written after an observational session in the field has been completed.

Field notes are usually lengthy and time-consuming to prepare. Observers need to discipline themselves to provide a wealth of detail, the meaning and importance of which may not emerge for weeks. Descriptions of what has transpired must include enough contextual information about time, place, and actors to portray the situation fully. *Thick description* is the goal for participation observers' field notes.

⮕ **TIP:** Especially in the early stages of fieldwork, a general rule of thumb is this: When in doubt, write it down.

Field notes are both descriptive and reflective. **Descriptive notes** (or **observational notes**) are objective descriptions of observed events and conversations; information about actions, dialogue, and context are recorded as completely and objectively as possible. Sometimes descriptive notes are recorded on loosely structured forms analogous to topic guides to ensure that key information is captured. ✳

Reflective notes, which document the researcher's personal experiences, reflections, and progress while in the field, can serve a number of different purposes:

• **Methodologic notes** are reflections about the strategies and methods used in the observations. Sometimes participant observers do things that do not "work," and methodologic notes document their thoughts about new strategies or thoughts about why a strategy that was used was especially effective. Methodologic notes also can provide instructions or reminders about how subsequent observations will be made.

• **Theoretical notes** (or **analytical notes**) document researchers' thoughts about how to make sense of what is going on. These notes are the

---

BOX 15.2 Example of Field Notes: Mothering Multiples Grounded Theory Study

Observational Notes: O.L. attended the mothers of multiples support group again this month but she looked worn out today. She wasn't as bubbly as she had been at the March meeting. She explained why she wasn't doing as well this month. She and her husband had just found out that their house has lead-based paint in it. Both twins do have increased lead levels. She and her husband are in the process of buying a new home.

Theoretical Notes: So far all the mothers have stressed the need for routine in order to survive the first year of caring for twins. Mothers, however, have varying definitions of routine. I.R. had the firmest routine with her twins. B.L. is more flexible with her routine, i.e., the twins are always fed at the same time but aren't put down for naps or bed at night at the same time. Whenever one of the twins wants to go to sleep is fine with her. B.L. does have a daily routine in regards to housework. For example, when the twins are down in the morning for a nap, she makes their bottles up for the day (14 bottles total).

Methodologic Notes: The first sign-up sheet I passed around at the Mothers of Multiples Support Group for women to sign up to participate in interviews for my grounded theory study only consisted of two columns: one for the mother's name and one for her telephone number. I need to revise this sign-up sheet to include extra columns for the age of the multiples, the town where the mother lives, and older siblings and their ages. My plan is to start interviewing mothers with multiples around 1 year of age so that the moms can reflect back over the process of mothering their infants for the first 12 months of their lives.

Right now I have no idea of the ages of the infants of the mothers who signed up to be interviewed. I will need to call the nurse in charge of this support group to find out the ages.

Personal Notes: Today was an especially challenging interview. The mom had picked the early afternoon for me to come to her home to interview her because that is the time her 2-year-old son would be napping. When I arrived at her house her 2-year-old ran up to me and said hi. The mom explained that he had taken an earlier nap that day and that he would be up during the interview. So in the living room with us during our interview were her two twin daughters (3 months old) swinging in the swings and her 2-year-old son. One of the twins was quite cranky for the first half hour of the interview. During the interview the 2-year-old sat on my lap and looked at the two books I had brought as a little present. If I didn't keep him occupied with the books, he would keep trying to reach for the microphone of the tape recorder.

From Beck, C.T. (2002). Releasing the pause button: Mothering twins during the first year of life. *Qualitative Health Research, 12,* 593–608.

---

researchers' efforts to attach meaning to observations while in the field, and serve as a starting point for subsequent analysis.

• **Personal notes** are comments about researchers' own feelings while in the field. Almost inevitably, field experiences give rise to personal emotions and challenge researchers' assumptions. It is essential to reflect on such feelings because there is no other way to determine whether the feelings are influencing what is being observed or what is being done in the participant role. Personal notes can also contain reflections relating to ethical dilemmas.

Box 15.2 presents examples of various types of field notes from Beck's (2002) study of mothering multiples.

Reflective notes are typically not integrated into the descriptive notes, but are kept separately as parallel notes; they may be maintained in a journal or series of self-memos. Strauss and Corbin (1990) argue that these reflective memos or journals help researchers to achieve analytic distance from the actual data, and therefore play a critical role in the project's success.

➲ **T I P :** Personal notes should begin even before entering the field. By writing down your feelings, assumptions, and expectations, you will have a baseline against which to compare feelings and experiences that emerge in the field.

The Process of Writing Field Notes

The success of participant observation depends on the quality of the field notes. This section describes some techniques for enhancing their quality.

A fundamental issue concerns the timing of field note preparation: Field notes should be written as soon as possible after an observation is made. The longer the interval between an observation and field note preparation, the greater the risk of forgetting or distorting the data. If the delay is long, intricate details will be lost; moreover, memory of what was observed may be biased by things that happen subsequently.

➲ **T I P :** Be sure not to talk to anyone about your observation before you have had a chance to write up the observational notes. Such discussions could color what you record.

Participant observers cannot usually write their field notes while they are in the field observing, in part because this would distract them from their job of being keen observers, and also because it would undermine their role as ordinary group participants. Researchers must develop the skill of making detailed mental notes that can later be committed to a permanent record. In addition, observers usually try to jot down unobtrusively a phrase or sentence that will later serve as a reminder of an event, conversation, or impression. Many experienced field workers use the tactic of frequent trips to the bathroom to record these **jottings**, either in a small notebook, into a recording device, or onto a PDA. With the widespread use of cell phones, researchers can also excuse themselves to make a call, and

"phone in" their jottings to an answering machine. Observers use the jottings and mental recordings to develop more extensive field notes.

➲ **T I P :** It is important to schedule enough time for properly recording field notes after an observation. An hour of observation can take 3 or 4 hours to record, so advance planning is essential. Try to find a quiet place for recording field notes, preferably a location where you can work undisturbed for several hours. Because most researchers now record field notes onto computers, the place will ideally be able to accommodate computer equipment.

Observational field notes need to be as complete and detailed as possible. This means that hundreds of pages of field notes typically will be created, and so systems need to be developed for recording and managing them. For example, each entry should have the date and time the observation was made, the location, and the name of the observer (if several are working together as a team). It is useful to give observational sessions a name that will trigger a memory (e.g., "Emotional Outburst by a Patient With Ovarian Cancer").

Thought also needs to be given to how to record participants' dialogue. The goal is to record conversations as accurately as possible, but it is not always possible to maintain verbatim records because tape-recordings are seldom made if researchers are trying to maintain a stance as regular participants. Procedures need to be developed to distinguish different levels of accuracy in recording dialogue (e.g., by using quotation marks and italics for true verbatim recordings, and a different designation for paraphrasing).

Observation, participation, and record keeping are exhausting, labor-intensive activities. It is important to establish the proper pace of these activities to ensure the highest possible quality notes for analysis.

Evaluation of Participant Observation

Participant observation can provide a deeper and richer understanding of human behaviors and social situations than is possible with more structured procedures. Participant observation is particularly valuable for its ability to "get inside" a particular situation and lead to a more complete understanding of its complexities. Furthermore, this approach is inherently flexible and therefore gives observers the freedom to reconceptualize problems after becoming more familiar with the situation. Participant observation is the preferred method for answering questions about intangible phenomena that are difficult for insiders to explain or articulate because these phenomena are taken for granted (e.g., group norms, cultural patterns, approaches to problem solving).

Like all research methods, however, there are potential problems with participant observation. The risks for observer bias and observer influence are prominent difficulties. Observers may lose objectivity in viewing and recording actual observations; they may also inappropriately sample events and situations to be observed. Once researchers begin to participate in a group's activities, the possibility of emotional involvement becomes a salient concern. Researchers in their member role may fail to attend to scientifically relevant aspects of the situation or may develop a myopic view on issues of importance to the group. Participant observation may thus be an unsuitable approach when the risk for identification is strong. Another important issue concerns the ethical dilemmas that often emerge in participant observation studies. Finally, participant observation depends more on the observational and interpersonal skills of the observer than do highly structured techniques—skills that may be difficult to cultivate.

On the whole, participant observation and other unstructured observational methods are extremely profitable for in-depth research in which researchers wish to develop a comprehensive conceptualization of phenomena within a social setting or culture.

CRITIQUING THE COLLECTION OF UNSTRUCTURED DATA

It is usually not easy to critique the decisions that a researcher has made in collecting qualitative data because details about those decisions are sel-

dom spelled out in research reports. In particular, there is often scant information about participant observation. It is not uncommon for a report to simply say that the researcher undertook participant observation, without descriptions of how much time was spent in the field, what exactly was observed, how observations were recorded, or what level of participation was involved. In fact, we strongly suspect that many projects described as having used a participant observation approach were unstructured observations with little or no actual participation. Thus, one aspect of a critique is likely to involve an appraisal of how much information the research report provided about the data collection methods used. Even though space constraints in journals make it impossible for researchers to fully elaborate their methods, researchers do have a responsibility to communicate basic information about their approach so that readers can better assess the quality of evidence that the study yields. Examples of questions asked and types of observations made are important.

As we will discuss more fully in Chapter 20, triangulation of methods provides important opportunities for qualitative researchers to enhance the quality of their data. Thus, an important issue to consider in evaluating unstructured data is whether the types and amount of data collected are sufficiently rich to support an in depth, holistic understanding of the phenomena under study.

Box 15.3 provides some guidelines for critiquing the collection of unstructured data. The guidelines are available in the Toolkit for your use and adaptation. ✪

●◗◗◗◗◗◗◗◗◗◗◗◗◗◗◗◗◗◗◗●

RESEARCH EXAMPLE

This section provides an example of a qualitative study that collected unstructured self-report and observational data.

Study: "Surfacing the life phases of a mental health support group" (Mohr, 2004)

Statement of Purpose: The purpose of this study was to explore how mental health advocacy and support groups

Box 15.3 Guidelines for Critiquing Unstructured Data Collection Methods

1. Was the collection of unstructured data appropriate to the study aims?
2. Given the research question and the characteristics of study participants, did the researcher use the best method of capturing study phenomena (i.e., self-reports, observation)? Should supplementary data collection methods have been used to enrich the data available for analysis?
3. If self-report methods were used, did the researcher make good decisions about the specific method used to solicit information (e.g., focus group interviews, critical incident interviews, and so on)? Was the modality of obtaining the data appropriate (e.g., in-person interviews, Internet questioning)?
4. If a topic guide was used, did the report present examples of specific questions? Were the questions appropriate and comprehensive? Did the wording minimize the risk for biases? Did the wording encourage full and rich responses?
5. Were interviews tape-recorded and transcribed? Were steps taken to ensure the accuracy of transcriptions? If interviews were not tape-recorded, what steps were taken to ensure the accuracy of the data?
6. Were self-report data gathered in a manner that promoted high-quality responses (e.g., in terms of privacy, efforts to put respondents at ease)? Who collected the data, and were they adequately prepared for the task?
7. If observational methods were used, did the report adequately describe what the observations entailed? What did the researcher actually observe, in what types of setting did the observations occur, and how often and over how long a period were observations made? Were decisions about positioning described? Were risks for observational bias addressed?
8. What role did the researcher assume in terms of being an observer and a participant? Was this role appropriate?
9. How were observational data recorded? Did the recording method maximize data quality?

start and develop, and what challenges threaten their long-term survival.

Design: Mohr's ethnographic study focused on a family support program that was associated with a system of care for children with emotional and behavioral disabilities. Mohr explained to the entire support group membership that the purpose of an ethnography is to study and describe a culture through physical association with people in their natural settings. She also explained that, as a researcher, she could have varying levels of involvement. The group agreed to have Mohr function as a participating observer, rather than simply as an observer. Her family history (she had psychiatrically ill relatives) enhanced her acceptance and credibility with group members.

Data Collection: Between 1999 and 2001, Mohr attended 25 regular support group sessions and recorded field notes describing the meetings: who attended, where they sat, who came late or early, who presented, who asked questions, and who made comments. In each observation session, Mohr paid careful attention to the structure and content of group activities and to its processes. Then, in 2001, Mohr conducted focused interviews with five group leaders and seven other members of the group. The interviews were designed to help Mohr understand the informants' views on the support group's culture, the processes of formation and maintenance, and the role of the group in the informants' lives. The interviews were audiotaped and professionally transcribed, and tapes were compared against the transcripts for completion and accuracy. In all, the data from the 2½-year study consisted of 703 pages of field notes, personal reflections, interview transcripts, and documents generated by the support group.

Reflexivity: In her report, Mohr shared some of her thoughts about the data collection process, and acknowledged that the role of participant observer was challenging. Here is an example: "It was not a straightforward matter to collect data and to participate in a group and be legitimately involved from an affective perspective yet attentive to the collection of data. My roles as a family member, clinician, and researcher were ones that required considerable juggling, self-reflection, and clarification during and after each meeting" (p. 64).

Key Findings:

- The data revealed a dynamic pattern of group evolution that included several distinct sequential phases.
- The phases through which the support group evolved included exploring, shaping and shaking, structuring, turbulence, and maintenance.
- Mohr noted that the group dynamics and the group's responses to challenges have implications for strategies to enhance the likelihood of survival of such groups.

SUMMARY POINTS

- Unstructured and loosely structured self-reports, which provide respondents and interviewers latitude in formulating questions and answers, yield rich narrative data for qualitative analysis.
- Methods of collecting qualitative self-report data include the following: (1) **unstructured interviews**, which are conversational discussions on the topic of interest; (2) **semistructured** (or **focused**) **interviews**, in which interviewers are guided by a **topic guide** of questions to be asked; (3) **focus group interviews**, which involve discussions with small, homogeneous groups about topics covered in a topic guide; (4) **joint interviews**, which involve simultaneously talking with members of a dyad (e.g., two spouses); (5) **life histories**, which encourage respondents to narrate, in chronological sequence, their life experiences; (6) **oral histories**, which are used to gather personal recollections of events and their perceived causes and consequences; (7) **critical incidents technique**, which involves probes about the circumstances surrounding a behavior or incident that is critical to an outcome of interest; (8) **diaries** and journals, in which respondents are asked to maintain daily records about some aspects of

their lives; (9) the **think-aloud method**, which involves having people use audio-recording devices to talk about decisions as they are making them; (10) **photo elicitation**, which is stimulated and guided by photographic images; and (11) solicited or unsolicited narrative communications on the Internet.

- In preparing for in-depth interviews, researchers learn about the language and customs of participants, formulate broad questions, make decisions about how to present themselves, develop ideas about interview settings, and take stock of equipment needs.
- Conducting good in-depth interviews requires considerable interviewer skill in putting people at ease, developing trust, listening intently, and managing possible crises in the field.
- In-depth self-report methods tend to yield data of considerable richness and are useful in gaining an understanding about little-researched phenomena, but they are time-consuming and yield a large volume of data that are challenging to analyze.
- Qualitative researchers sometimes collect unstructured observational data, often through **participant observation**. Participant observers obtain information about the dynamics of social groups or cultures within members' own frame of reference.
- In the initial phase of participant observation studies, researchers are primarily observers getting a preliminary understanding of the site. As time passes, researchers become more active participants.
- Observations tend to become more focused over time, ranging from **descriptive observation** (broad observations) to **focused observation** of more carefully selected events or interactions, and then to **selective observations** designed to facilitate comparisons.
- Participant observers usually select events to be observed through a combination of **single positioning** (observing from a fixed location), **multiple positioning** (moving around the site to observe in different locations), and **mobile positioning** (following a person around a site).

- **Logs** of daily events and **field notes** are the major methods of recording unstructured observational data. Field notes are both descriptive and reflective.
- **Descriptive notes** (sometimes called **observational notes**) are detailed, objective accounts of what transpired in an observational session. Observers strive for detailed, thick description.
- **Reflective notes** include **methodologic notes** that document observers' thoughts about their strategies; **theoretical notes** (or **analytic notes**) that represent ongoing efforts to make sense of the data; and **personal notes** that document observers' feelings and experiences.

STUDY ACTIVITIES

Chapter 15 of the *Resource Manual to Accompany Nursing Research: Generating and Assessing Evidence for Nursing Practice, 8th edition*, offers various exercises and study suggestions for reinforcing concepts presented in this chapter. In addition, the following study questions can be addressed:

1. Identify which qualitative self-report methods might be appropriate for the following research problems, and provide a rationale:
   a. What are the coping strategies of parents who have lost a child through sudden infant death syndrome?
   b. How do nurses in emergency departments make decisions about their activities?
   c. What are the health beliefs and practices of Haitian immigrants in the United States?
   d. What is it like to experience having a family member undergo open heart surgery?
2. Suppose you were interested in observing fathers' behavior in the delivery room during the birth of their first child. Identify the observer-observed relationship that you would recommend adopting for such a study, and defend your recommendation. What are the

possible drawbacks of your approach, and how might you deal with them?
3. Apply relevant questions in Box 15.3 to the research example at the end of the chapter (Mohr, 2004), referring to the full journal article as necessary.

STUDIES CITED IN CHAPTER 15

Methodologic or theoretical references cited in this chapter can be found in a separate section at the end of the book.

Bannister, E. M. (1999). Women's midlife experience of their changing bodies. *Qualitative Health Research, 9*, 520–537.

Beck, C. T. (2002). Releasing the pause button: Mothering twins during the first year of life. *Qualitative Health Research, 12*, 593–608.

Beck, C. T. (2004). Post-traumatic stress disorder due to childbirth: The aftermath. *Nursing Research, 53*(4), 216–223.

Bormann, J., Oman, D., Kemppainen, J., Becker, S., Gershwin, M., & Kelly, A. (2006). Mantrum repetition for stress management in veterans and employees: A critical incident study. *Journal of Advanced Nursing, 53*(5), 502–512.

Clarke, S., Booth, L., Velikova, G., & Hewison, J. (2006). Social support: Gender differences in cancer patients in the United Kingdom. *Cancer Nursing, 29*(1), 66–72.

DeSanto-Madeya, S. (2006). The meaning of living with spinal cord injury 5 to 10 years after the injury. *Western Journal of Nursing Research, 28*(3), 265–289.

El-Nemer, A., Downe, S., & Small, N. (2006). "She would help me from the heart:" An ethnography of Egyptian women in labor. *Social Science and Medicine, 62*(1), 81–92.

Hassouneh-Phillips, D. (2005). Understanding abuse of women with physical disabilities. *Advances in Nursing Science, 28*(1), 70–80.

Jacelon, C. S., & Imperio, K. (2005). Participant diaries as a source of data in research with older adults. *Qualitative Health Research, 15*(7), 991–997.

Kalischuk, R. G., & Davies, B. (2001). A theory of healing in the aftermath of youth suicide. *Journal of Holistic Nursing, 19*, 163–186.

Klemm, P. & Wheeler, E. (2005). Cancer caregivers online: Hope, emotional roller coaster, and physical/emotional/psychological responses. *Computers, Informatics, Nursing, 23*(1), 38–45.

LeVasseur, J. J. (2003). The proving grounds: Combat nursing in Vietnam. *Nursing Outlook, 51,* 31–36.

McDevitt, J., Snyder, M., Miller, A., & Wilbur, J. (2006). Perceptions of barriers and benefits to physical activity among outpatients in psychiatric rehabilitation. *Journal of Nursing Scholarship, 38*(1), 50–55.

Mohr, W. K. (2004). Surfacing the life phases of a mental health support group. *Qualitative Health Report, 14,* 61–77.

Polit, D. F., London, A. S., & Martinez, J. M. (2001). *The health of poor urban women.* New York: MDRC.

Shin, K. R., Cho, M. C., & Kim, J. S. (2005). The meaning of death as experienced by elderly women of a Korean clan. *Qualitative Health Research, 15*(1), 5–18.

Simmons, B., Lanuza, D., Fonteyn, M., Hicks, F., & Holm, K. (2003). Clinical reasoning in experienced nurses. *Western Journal of Nursing Research, 25,* 701–719.

Turner, DeS. (2005). Hope seen through the eyes of 10 Australian young people. *Journal of Advanced Nursing, 52*(5), 508–515.

Woodgate, R. (2005). A different way of being: Adolescents' experiences with cancer. *Cancer Nursing, 28*(1), 8–15.

16

Collecting Structured Data

S tructured data collection involves having a fixed, rather than flexible, approach to gathering information. Both the people collecting the data and the people providing the information are constrained during the collection of structured data. Constraints are imposed so that there is consistency in what is asked and how answers are reported, in an effort to enhance objectivity and reduce biases. The most widely used data collection method by nurse researchers is structured self-reports.

STRUCTURED SELF-REPORT INSTRUMENTS

Researchers collecting structured self-report data use a formal, written instrument. The instrument is an **interview schedule** when the questions are asked orally in either face-to-face or telephone interviews. It is called a **questionnaire** or an SAQ (self-administered questionnaire) when respondents complete the instrument themselves, usually on a paper-and-pencil instrument (PAPI) but sometimes directly onto a computer. Sometimes researchers embed an SAQ into an interview schedule, with interviewers asking some questions orally but respondents answering others in writing. This section discusses the development and administration of structured self-report instruments.

Types of Structured Questions

Structured instruments consist of a set of questions (sometimes called **items**), in which the wording of both the questions and, in most cases, response alternatives is predetermined. When structured interviews or questionnaires are used, subjects are asked to respond to the same questions, in the same order, and with the same set of response options. In developing structured instruments, much effort is usually devoted to the content, form, and wording of questions.

Open and Closed Questions

Structured instruments vary in *degree* of structure through different combinations of open-ended and closed-ended questions. **Open-ended questions** allow respondents to respond in their own words, in narrative fashion. The question, "What was the biggest problem you faced after your surgery?" is an example of an open-ended question (such as would be used in qualitative studies). In questionnaires, respondents are asked to give a written reply to open-ended items, and therefore, adequate space must be provided to permit a full response. Interviewers are expected to quote responses verbatim or as closely as possible, as would be the case in qualitative interviews that are not tape-recorded.

Closed-ended (or **fixed-alternative**) **questions** offer respondents response options, from which they must choose the one that most closely matches the appropriate answer. The alternatives may range from the simple "yes" or "no" variety (e.g., "Have you smoked a cigarette within the past 24 hours?") to complex expressions of opinion or behavior.

Both open- and closed-ended questions have certain strengths and weaknesses. Good closed-ended items are often difficult to construct but easy to administer and, especially, to analyze. With closed-ended questions, researchers need only tabulate the number of responses to each alternative to gain some understanding of what the sample as a whole thinks about an issue. The analysis of open-ended items, on the other hand, is more difficult and time-consuming. The usual procedure is to develop categories and assign open-ended responses to them. That is, researchers essentially transform open-ended responses to fixed categories in a *post hoc* fashion so that tabulations can be made.

Closed-ended items are more efficient than open-ended questions because respondents can complete more closed- than open-ended questions in a given amount of time. In questionnaires, participants may be less willing to compose written responses than to check off or circle appropriate alternatives. Closed-ended items are also preferred with respondents who are unable to express themselves well verbally. Furthermore, some questions are less objectionable in closed form than in open form. Take the following example:

1. What was your family's total annual income last year?
2. In what range was your family's total annual income last year?
   - ❏ 1. Under $25,000,
   - ❏ 2. $25,000 to $49,999,
   - ❏ 3. $50,000 to $74,999,
   - ❏ 4. $75,000 to $99,999, or
   - ❏ 5. $100,000 or more

The second question gives respondents a greater measure of privacy than the blunter open-ended question, and there is less demand for precision.

These advantages of closed-ended questions are offset by some shortcomings. The major drawback is the possibility that researchers may have neglected or overlooked potentially important responses. The omission of possible alternatives can lead to inadequate understanding of the issues or to outright bias if respondents choose an alternative that misrepresents their position. When the area of research is relatively new, open-ended questions are often better than closed-ended ones for avoiding bias.

Another objection to closed-ended items is that they can be superficial. Open-ended questions allow for a richer and fuller perspective on the topic of interest, if respondents are verbally expressive and cooperative. Some of this richness may be lost when researchers tabulate answers by developing a system of classification, but excerpts taken directly from the open-ended responses can be valuable in imparting the flavor of the replies in a report.

Finally, some respondents may object to being forced into choosing from response options that do not reflect their opinions precisely. Open-ended questions give freedom to respondents and, therefore, offer the possibility of spontaneity and elaboration.

Decisions about the mix of open- and closed-ended questions in a structured instrument are based on a number of considerations, such as the sensitivity of the questions, the verbal ability of respondents, the amount of time available, and the amount of prior research on the topic. Combinations of both types are recommended to offset the strengths and weaknesses of each. Questionnaires typically use closed-ended questions predominantly, to minimize respondents' writing burden. Interview schedules, on the other hand, tend to be more variable in their mixture of these two question types.

Specific Types of Closed-Ended Questions

The analytic advantages of closed-ended questions are compelling for certain research questions. Various types of closed-ended questions, many of which are illustrated in Table 16.1, are discussed here. These various question types can be intermixed within a structured instrument.

- **Dichotomous questions** require respondents to make a choice between two response alternatives,

| TABLE 16.1 | Examples of Closed-Ended Questions |

QUESTION TYPE	EXAMPLE
1. Dichotomous question	Have you ever been hospitalized? 1. Yes 2. No
2. Multiple-choice question	How important is it to you to avoid a pregnancy at this time? 1. Extremely important 2. Very important 3. Somewhat important 4. Not important
3. Cafeteria question	People have different opinions about the use of estrogen replacement therapy for women at menopause. Which of the following statements best represents your point of view? 1. Estrogen replacement is dangerous and should be banned. 2. Estrogen replacement has undesirable risks that suggest the need for caution in its use. 3. I am undecided about my views on estrogen replacement. 4. Estrogen replacement has many beneficial effects that merit its use. 5. Estrogen replacement is a wonder treatment that should be administered to most menopausal women.
4. Rank-order question	People value different things in life. Below is a list of things that many people value. Please indicate their order of importance to you by placing a "1" beside the most important, "2" beside the second-most important, and so on. ____ Career achievement/work ____ Family relationships ____ Friendships, social interactions ____ Health ____ Money ____ Religion
5. Forced-choice question	Which statement most closely represents your point of view? 1. What happens to me is my own doing. 2. Sometimes I feel I don't have enough control over my life.
6. Rating question	On a scale from 0 to 10, where 0 means "extremely dissatisfied" and 10 means "extremely satisfied," how satisfied were you with the nursing care you received during your hospitalization? 0　1　2　3　4　5　6　7　8　9　10 Extremely dissatisfied　　　　　　　　Extremely satisfied

such as yes/no or male/female. Dichotomous questions are considered most appropriate for gathering factual information.

- **Multiple-choice questions** offer more than two response alternatives. Dichotomous items sometimes are considered too restrictive by respondents, who may resent being forced to see an issue as either "yes" or "no." Graded alternatives are preferable for opinion or attitude questions because they give researchers more information (intensity as well as direction of opinion) and because they give respondents a chance to express a range of views. Multiple-choice questions most commonly offer three to seven alternatives.

- **Cafeteria questions** are a special type of multiple-choice question that asks respondents to select a response that most closely corresponds to their view. Response options are usually full expressions of a position on the topic.

- **Rank-order questions** ask respondents to rank target concepts along a continuum, such as most to least important. Respondents are asked to assign a 1 to the concept that is most important, a 2 to the concept that is second in importance, and so on. Rank-order questions can be useful but need to be handled carefully because respondents sometimes misunderstand them. Rank-order questions should involve 10 or fewer rankings.

- **Forced-choice questions** require respondents to choose between two statements that represent polar positions or characteristics. Several personality tests use a forced-choice format.

- **Rating questions** ask respondents to evaluate something along an ordered dimension. Rating questions are typically **bipolar**, with end points specifying opposite extremes on a continuum. The end points and sometimes intermediary points along the scale are verbally labeled. The number of gradations or points along the scale can vary but often is an odd number, such as 7, 9, or 11, to allow for a neutral midpoint. (In the example in Table 16.1, the rating question has 11 points, numbered 0 to 10.)

- **Checklists** include several questions with the same response format. A checklist is a two-dimensional arrangement in which a series of questions is listed along one dimension (usually vertically) and response alternatives are listed along the other. Checklists (sometimes called **matrix questions**) are relatively efficient and easy to understand, but because they are difficult to read orally, they are used more frequently in SAQs than in interviews. Figure 16.1 presents an example of a checklist.

- **Visual analogue scales (VAS)** are used to measure subjective experiences, such as pain, fatigue, nausea, and dyspnea. The VAS is a straight horizontal or vertical line, the end anchors of which are labeled as the extreme limits of the sensation or feeling being measured. Subjects are asked to

The next question is about things that may have happened to you personally. Please indicate how recently, if ever, these things happened to you:

	Yes, within past 12 months	Yes, 2–3 years ago	Yes, more than 3 years ago	No, never
a. Has someone ever yelled at you all the time or put you down on purpose?	1	2	3	4
b. Has someone ever tried to control your every move?	1	2	3	4
c. Has someone ever threatened you with physical harm?	1	2	3	4
d. Has someone ever hit, slapped, kicked, or physically harmed you?	1	2	3	4

FIGURE 16.1 Example of a checklist.

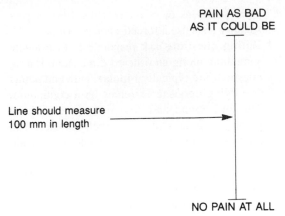

FIGURE 16.2 ✪ Example of a visual analogue scale.

mark a point on the line corresponding to the amount of sensation experienced. Traditionally, the VAS line is 100 mm in length, which facilitates the derivation of a score from 0 to 100 through simple measurement of the distance from one end of the scale to the subject's mark on the line. An example of a VAS is presented in Figure 16.2. ✪

In certain situations, researchers collect information about activities and dates, and in such situations, it is useful to use an **event history calendar** (Martyn & Belli, 2002). Such calendars are matrixes that plot time on one dimension (usually the horizontal dimension) and the events or activities of interest on the other. The person recording the data (either the study participant or an interviewer) draws lines to indicate the stop and start dates of the specified events or behaviors. Event history calendars are especially useful in collecting information about the occurrence and sequencing of events retrospectively. Data quality about past occurrences is enhanced because the calendar helps participants relate the timing of some events to the timing of others. An example of an event history calendar is included in the Toolkit section of the accompanying *Resource Manual.* ✪

In some cases an alternative to collecting event history information retrospectively is to ask participants to maintain information in a structured **diary** form on an ongoing basis over a specified time period. This is the approach often used to collect quantitative information about sleeping, eating, or exercising behavior.

> **Example of a structured diary:** Glesson-Kreig (2006) assessed the effect of keeping daily diaries on physical activity levels and self-efficacy for physical activity in persons with type 2 diabetes. Diabetic adults were randomly assigned to either the intervention group, which maintained daily diaries of activity for 6 weeks, or the control group. Each day, participants recorded type of activity (e.g., walking, swimming), duration of activity in minutes, and activity intensity (slow, moderate, or brisk) on forms the researchers provided.

Composite Scales and Other Structured Self-Reports

Several special types of structured self-reports are used by nurse researchers and are discussed in this section. The most important are composite social-psychological scales that are often incorporated into a questionnaire or interview package. A **scale** provides a numeric score to place respondents on a continuum with respect to an attribute being measured, like a scale for measuring people's weight. Scales are used to discriminate quantitatively among people with different attitudes, fears, perceptions, and needs. Scales are created by combining several closed-ended items (such as those described in the previous section) into a single composite score. Many sophisticated scaling techniques have been developed, only two of which are discussed in this book.* We also briefly discuss other self-report methods, including cognitive and neurologic tests, vignettes, and Q sorts.

Likert Scales

The most widely used scaling technique is the **Likert scale**, named after the psychologist Rensis

---

* One early type of psychosocial scale was the **Thurstone scale**, named after the psychologist L. L. Thurstone. Thurstone's approach to scaling is elaborate and time-consuming and has fallen into relative disuse. Another scaling method, developed by Louis Guttman in the 1940s, is known as the **Guttman** or **cumulative scales**. Advanced scaling procedures include **ratio scaling**, **magnitude estimation scaling**, **multidimensional scaling**, and **multiple scalogram analysis**. Textbooks on psychological scaling and psychometric procedures should be consulted for more information about these scaling strategies.

Likert. A Likert scale consists of several declarative items that express a viewpoint on a topic. Respondents typically are asked to indicate the degree to which they agree or disagree with the opinion expressed by the statement.

Table 16.2 presents an illustrative six-item Likert-type scale for measuring young adults' attitudes toward condom use. Likert scales often include 10 or more statements; the example in Table 16.2 is shown only to

illustrate key features. After respondents complete a Likert scale, their responses are scored. Typically, agreement with positively worded items and disagreement with negatively worded items are assigned higher scores. (See Chapter 18, however, for a discussion of problems with including both positive and negative items on a scale.) The first item in Table 16.2 is positively worded; agreement indicates a favorable attitude toward condom use. Thus, a higher score

		RESPONSES†					SCORE	
DIRECTION OF SCORING*	**ITEM**	**SA**	**A**	**?**	**D**	**SD**	**Person 1 (✓)**	**Person 2 (✗)**
+	1. Using a condom shows you care about your partner.		✓			✗	4	1
−	2. My partner would be angry if I talked about using condoms.			✗		✓	5	3
−	3. I wouldn't enjoy sex as much if my partner and I used condoms.		✗		✓		4	2
+	4. Condoms are a good protection against AIDS and other sexually transmitted diseases.			✓	✗		3	2
+	5. My partner would respect me if I insisted on using condoms.	✓				✗	5	1
−	6. I would be too embarrassed to ask my partner about using a condom.		✗			✓	5	2
	Total score						26	11

TABLE 16.2 — Example of a Likert Scale to Measure Attitudes Toward Condoms

*Researchers would not indicate the direction of scoring on a Likert scale administered to subjects. The scoring direction is indicated in this table for illustrative purposes only.

†SA, strongly agree; A, agree; ?, uncertain; D, disagree; SD, strongly disagree.

would be assigned to those agreeing with this item than to those disagreeing with it. With five response alternatives, a score of 5 would be given to those strongly agreeing, 4 to those agreeing, and so forth. The responses of two hypothetical respondents are shown by a check or an X, and their scores for each item are shown in far right columns. Person 1, who agreed with the first item, has a score of 4, whereas person 2, who strongly disagreed, has a score of 1. The second item is negatively worded, and so scoring is reversed—a 1 is assigned to those who strongly agree, and so forth. This reversal is needed so that a high score consistently reflects positive attitudes toward condoms. A person's total score is determined by adding together individual item scores. Such scales are often called **summated rating scales** because of this feature. The total scores of the two respondents to items in Table 16.2 are shown at the bottom of the table. The scores reflect a considerably more positive attitude toward condoms on the part of person 1 than person 2.

The summation feature of such scales makes it possible to make fine discriminations among people with different points of view. A single question allows people to be put into only five categories. A six-item scale, such as the one in Table 16.2, permits finer gradation—from a minimum possible score of $6 (6 \times 1)$ to a maximum possible score of $30 (6 \times 5)$.

Although traditional Likert scales were used to measure attitudes, summated rating scales can be used to measure a wide array of attributes. In such cases, the bipolar scale would not be agree/disagree but might be always true/never true, extremely likely/extremely unlikely, and so on.

Constructing a good Likert-type scale requires considerable skill and work. Chapter 18 of this book describes the steps involved in developing and testing such scales.

> **Example of a summated rating scale:** Lehoux and colleagues (2006) constructed Likert scales to measure the attitudes and perceptions of hospital-based nurses to high-tech home care interventions (e.g., peritoneal dialysis, parenteral nutrition).

Semantic Differential Scales

Another technique for measuring psychosocial traits is the **semantic differential (SD)**. With the SD, respondents are asked to rate a concept (e.g., low-carbohydrate diet, low-fat diet, high-protein diet) on a series of bipolar adjectives, such as effective/ineffective, good/bad, or strong/weak. Respondents place a check at the appropriate point on 7-point rating scales extending from one extreme of the dimension to the other. Figure 16.3 shows an example of the format for an SD for rating the concept *nurse practitioners*.

Semantic differentials are flexible and easy to construct. The concept being rated can be virtually anything—a person, situation, abstract idea, controversial issue, and so forth. The concept can be

NURSE PRACTITIONERS

competent	7*	6	5	4	3	2	1	incompetent
worthless	1	2	3	4	5	6	7	valuable
important								unimportant
pleasant								unpleasant
bad								good
cold								warm
responsible								irresponsible
successful								unsuccessful

*The score values would not be printed on the form administered to actual subjects. The numbers are presented here solely for the purpose of illustrating how semantic differentials are scored.

FIGURE 16.3 Example of a semantic differential.

presented as a word, as a phrase, or even as visual material (e.g., photos, drawings). Typically, several concepts are included on an SD so that comparisons can be made across concepts (e.g., male nurse, female nurse, male physician, female physician).

Researchers also have leeway in selecting the bipolar scales, but two considerations should guide the selection. First, the adjective pairs should be appropriate for the concepts being used and for the information being sought. The addition of the adjective pair tall/short in Figure 16.3 would add little understanding of how people react to nurse practitioners.

The second consideration in selecting adjective pairs is the extent to which the adjectives measure the same dimension of the concept. Research with SD scales suggests that adjective pairs tend to cluster along three independent dimensions: evaluation, potency, and activity. The most important group of adjectives are evaluative ones, such as effective/ineffective, valuable/worthless, good/bad, and so forth. Potency adjectives include strong/weak and large/ small, and examples of activity adjectives are active/passive and fast/slow. These three dimensions need to be considered separately because people's *evaluative* ratings of a concept are independent of their *activity* or *potency* ratings. For example, two people who associate high levels of activity with the concept "nurse practitioners" might have divergent views on the evaluation dimension. Researchers must decide whether to represent all three dimensions or whether only one or two are needed. Each dimension must be scored separately.

Scoring of SD responses is essentially the same as for Likert scales. Scores from 1 to 7 are assigned to each bipolar scale response, with higher scores usually associated with the positively worded adjective. Responses are then summed across the bipolar scales to yield a total score.

Example of a study using an SD: Rempusheski and O'Hara (2005) developed a semantic differential scale called the Grandparent Perceptions of Family Scale (GPFS). The GPFS involves having respondents rate stimuli (e.g., "How I view my grandchild") with regard to 22 bipolar adjective pairs. Three adjective pairs were in the action subscale (e.g., active/ passive), 11 were in the evaluative subscale (e.g., happy/sad), and 8 were in the potency subscale (e.g., emotionally strong/emotionally weak).

➲ TIP: Most nurse researchers use existing scales rather than developing their own. Box 16.1 provides citations for locating existing scales, and some helpful websites are included on the accompanying student CD-ROM. Additionally, both the nursing and nonnursing literature should be consulted for references to scale-development studies. Finally, a good place to look for existing instruments is in the Health and Psychosocial Instruments (HaPI) database, which can be accessed through OVID. Note that many scales and test instruments must be purchased from the publisher, or require the author's permission to use them.

Cognitive and Neuropsychological Tests

Nurse researchers sometimes are interested in assessing the cognitive skills of study participants. There are several different types of **cognitive tests**. For example, *intelligence tests* are attempts to evaluate a person's global ability to perceive relationships and solve problems, and *aptitude tests* are designed to measure a person's potential for achievement. Of the many such tests available, some have been developed for individual (one-on-one) administration, whereas others have been developed for group use. Individual tests, such as the Stanford-Binet IQ test, must be administered by a person who has received training as a tester. Group tests of ability (e.g., the Scholastic Assessment Test), can be administered with little training. Nurse researchers have been particularly likely to use ability tests in studies of high-risk groups, such as low-birth-weight children.

Example of a study using cognitive tests: Herman (2004) administered subtests of the Wechsler Adult Intelligence Scale, as well as other cognitive tests, to schizophrenic inpatients to assess whether there were differences between patients who were and patients who were not dually diagnosed with substance abuse disorders.

Some cognitive tests are specially designed to assess neuropsychological functioning among those with potential cognitive impairments, such as the Mini-Mental State Examination (MMSE). These tests capture varying types of competence, such as the ability to concentrate and the ability to remember.

BOX 16.1 References for Self-Report and Observational Scales/ Psychological Measures

Aiken, L. R., & Aiken, L. A. (1996). *Rating scales and checklists: Evaluating behavior, personality, and attitudes.* New York: John Wiley & Sons.

Anastasi, A., & Urbina, S. (1997). *Psychological testing* (7th ed.). Englewood Cliffs, NJ: Prentice-Hall.

Fischer, J., & Corcoran, K. (2000). *Measures for clinical practice* (3rd ed.). New York: The Free Press.

Frank-Stromberg, M., & Olsen, S. J. (Eds.). (2003). *Instruments for clinical health-care research* (3rd ed.). Sudbury, MA: Jones and Bartlett.

Kerig, P., & Lindahl, K. (2000). *Family observational coding systems: Resources for systematic research.* Mahwah, NJ: Lawrence Erlbaum.

McDowell, I., & Newell, C. (1996). *Measuring health: A guide to rating scales and questionnaires* (2nd ed.). New York: Oxford University Press.

Murphy, L. L., Plake, B. S., Impara, J. C., & Spies, R. (Eds.). (2002). *Tests in print VI.* Lincoln, NE: The Buros Institute.

Robinson, J. P., Shaver, P. R., & Wrightsman, L. S. (Eds.). (1991). *Measures of personality and social psychological attitudes* (3rd ed.). New York: Academic Press.

Spies, P., Plake, B., & Murphy, L. (Eds.). (2003). *The 16th mental measurements yearbook.* Lincoln, NE: The Buros Institute.

Strickland, O. L., & Dilorio, C., Eds. (2003). *Measurement of nursing outcomes* (2nd ed.). New York: Springer.

Waltz, C. F., Dilorio, C., Strickland, O. L., & Jenkins, L. (2003). *Measurement of nursing outcomes: Vol. I. Client outcomes and quality of care* (2nd ed.). New York: Springer.

Nurses have used such tests extensively in studies of elderly patients and patients with Alzheimer disease. Good sources for learning more about ability tests are the books by Anastasi and Urbina (1997) and Spies and colleagues (2003) (See Box 16.1).

Example of a study measuring neuropsychological function: Insel and Cole (2005) tested the effectiveness of an intervention to improve older adults' remembering to take medications for chronic illness. Study participants were tested for cognitive functioning using the MMSE, and the association between MMSE scores and medication adherence was examined.

Q Sorts

In a **Q sort,** participants are presented with a set of cards on which words or phrases are written. Participants are asked to sort the cards along a specified bipolar dimension, such as most important/ least important. Typically, there are between 50 and 100 cards to be sorted into 9 or 11 piles, with the number of cards to be placed in each pile predetermined by the researcher (e.g., 2 cards in piles 1 and 9, 4 cards in piles 2 and 8). It is difficult to achieve stable and reliable results with fewer than 50 cards, but the task becomes tedious and difficult with more than 100.

The sorting instructions and objects to be sorted in a Q sort can vary. For example, attitudes can be studied by writing attitudinal statements on the cards and asking participants to sort them on a continuum from "totally disagree" to "totally agree." Or, patients could be asked to rate nursing behaviors on a continuum from least helpful to most helpful.

Q sorts are versatile and can be applied to a wide variety of problems. Requiring people to place a predetermined number of cards in each pile can reduce biases that are common in Likert scales. On the other hand, it is difficult and time-consuming to administer Q sorts to a large sample of people. Some critics argue that the forced distribution of cards according to researchers' specifications is artificial and excludes information about how participants would ordinarily distribute their responses. Another issue is that Q sorts cannot be incorporated into mailed or Internet questionnaires or administered in telephone interviews, but they can be included in studies involving face-to-face interactions with respondents.

Example of a Q sort: Chang and colleagues (2005) used a Q sort to explore cancer patients' views about caring behaviors. Statements describing 50 caring behaviors were placed on the cards, and participants were asked to place the cards in piles on a 7-point "most important" to "least important" continuum. Cards were to be distributed with 1 card in piles 1 and 7, 4 cards in piles 2 and 6, 10 cards in piles 3 and 5, and the remaining 20 cards in pile 4.

Vignettes

Another self-report approach involves the use of **vignettes**, which are brief descriptions of events or situations to which respondents are asked to react. The descriptions, which can either be fictitious or based on fact, are structured to elicit information about respondents' perceptions, opinions, or knowledge about some phenomenon. The vignettes are usually written narrative descriptions, but researchers have also used videotaped vignettes. The questions posed to respondents after the vignettes may be either open ended (e.g., How would you describe this patients' level of confusion?) or closed ended (e.g., Rate how confused you think this patient is on the 7-point scale below). Usually 3 to 5 vignettes are included in an instrument.

Sometimes the underlying purpose of vignette studies is not revealed to participants, especially if the technique is used as an indirect measure of attitudes, prejudices, and stereotypes using embedded descriptors, as in the following example.

Example of vignettes: Griffin, Polit, and Byrne (in press) distributed vignette packets describing three hospitalized children to a national sample of 342 pediatric nurses to determine whether the nurses' pain management decisions were affected by characteristics of the children. All three vignettes described children in pain: one described either a boy or a girl, another described a white or African-American child, and the third described a physically attractive or unattractive child. Nurses answered questions about the pain treatments they would administer without being aware that the child characteristics had been experimentally manipulated.

Vignettes are an economical means of eliciting information about how people might behave in situations that would be difficult to observe in daily life. Also, vignettes often represent an interesting task for subjects. Finally, vignettes can be incorporated into questionnaires distributed by mail or over the Internet, and are therefore an inexpensive data collection strategy. The principal problem with vignettes concerns the validity of responses. If respondents describe how they would react in a situation portrayed in the vignette, how accurate is that description of their actual behavior? Thus, although the use of vignettes can be profitable, potential biases should be taken into account in interpreting results.

TIP: Some of the methods described in this chapter might be appealing because they are unusual and may therefore seem like a creative approach to collecting data. However, the prime considerations in selecting a data collection method should always be the conceptual congruence between the constructs of interest and the method, and the quality of data that the method yields.

Questionnaires Versus Interviews

In developing their data collection plans, researchers need to decide whether to collect data through interviews or questionnaires. Each method has advantages and disadvantages.

Advantages of Questionnaires

Self-administered questionnaires, which can be distributed in person, by mail, or over the Internet, offer some advantages. The strengths of questionnaires include the following:

- *Cost.* Questionnaires, relative to interviews, are much less costly and require less time and energy to administer. Distributing questionnaires to groups (e.g., to residents of a nursing home) is clearly an inexpensive and expedient approach. And, with a fixed amount of funds or time, a larger and more geographically diverse sample can be obtained with mailed or Internet questionnaires than with interviews.

• *Anonymity*. Unlike interviews, questionnaires offer the possibility of complete anonymity. A guarantee of anonymity can be crucial in obtaining candid responses, particularly if the questions are personal or sensitive. Anonymous questionnaires often result in a higher proportion of socially unacceptable responses (i.e., responses that place respondents in an unfavorable light) than interviews.

• *Interviewer bias*. The absence of an interviewer ensures that there will be no interviewer bias. Interviewers ideally are neutral agents through whom questions and answers are passed. Studies have shown, however, that this ideal is difficult to achieve. Respondents and interviewers interact as humans, and this interaction can affect responses.

Internet surveys are especially economical, and can in some cases yield a data set directly amenable to analysis, without having to have staff entering data (the same is also true for CAPI and CATI interviews). Internet surveys also provide opportunities for interactively providing participants with customized feedback, and for prompts that can minimize missing responses.

Advantages of Interviews

The strengths of interviews outweigh those of questionnaires. It is true that interviews are costly, prevent anonymity, and bear the risk of interviewer bias. Nevertheless, interviews are considered superior to questionnaires for most research purposes because of the following advantages:

• *Response rates*. Response rates tend to be high in face-to-face interviews. People are more reluctant to refuse to talk to an interviewer who directly solicits their cooperation than to discard or ignore a questionnaire. A well-designed and properly conducted interview study normally achieves response rates in the vicinity of 80% to 90%, whereas mailed and Internet questionnaires typically achieve response rates of 50% or lower. Because nonresponse is not random, low response rates can introduce serious biases. (However, if questionnaires are personally distributed to people in a particular setting—e.g., maternity patients about to be discharged from the hospital—reasonably good response rates can be achieved.)

• *Audience*. Many people simply cannot fill out a questionnaire. Examples include young children and blind, elderly, illiterate, or uneducated individuals. Interviews, on the other hand, are feasible with most people. For Internet questionnaires, a particularly important drawback is that not everyone has access to computers or uses them regularly.

• *Clarity*. Interviews offer some protection against ambiguous or confusing questions. Interviewers can determine whether questions have been misunderstood and can clarify matters. In questionnaires, misinterpreted questions can go undetected by researchers, and thus responses may be misleading.

• *Depth of questioning*. The information obtained from questionnaires tends to be more superficial than interview data, largely because questionnaires typically contain mostly closed-ended items. Open-ended questions are avoided in questionnaires because most people dislike having to compose and write out a reply. Much of the richness and complexity of respondents' experiences are lost if closed-ended items are used exclusively. Furthermore, interviewers can enhance the quality of self-report data through probing.

• *Missing information*. Respondents are less likely to give "don't know" responses or to leave a question unanswered in an interview than on questionnaires.

• *Order of questions*. In an interview, researchers have control over question ordering. Questionnaire respondents are at liberty to skip around from one section of the instrument to another. Sometimes a different ordering of questions from the one originally intended could bias responses.

• *Sample control.* Interviews permit greater control over the sample. Interviewers know whether the people being interviewed are the intended respondents. People who receive questionnaires, by contrast, can pass the instrument on to a friend, relative, and so forth, and this can change the sample composition. Internet surveys are especially vulnerable to the risk that people not targeted by researchers will respond, unless there are password protections.

• *Supplementary data.* Finally, face-to-face interviews can result in additional data through observation. Interviewers are in a position to observe or judge the respondents' level of understanding, degree of cooperativeness, social class, lifestyle, and so forth. Such information can be useful in interpreting responses.

Many advantages of face-to-face interviews also apply to telephone interviews. Long or detailed interviews or ones with sensitive questions usually are not well suited for telephone administration, but for relatively brief instruments, telephone interviews are more economical than personal interviews and tend to yield a higher response rate than mailed or Internet questionnaires.

Designing Structured Self-Report Instruments

Assembling a high-quality structured self-report instrument is a challenging and time-consuming task. To design useful, accurate instruments, researchers must carefully analyze the research requirements and attend to minute details. The steps for developing structured self-report instruments follow closely the ones we outlined in Chapter 14, but a few additional considerations should be mentioned.

Once data needs have been identified, related constructs should be clustered into separate **modules** or areas of questioning. For example, an interview schedule may consist of a module on demographic information, another on health symptoms, a third on stressful life events, and a fourth on health-promoting activities.

Some thought needs to be given to sequencing modules, and questions within modules, to arrive at an order that is psychologically meaningful and encourages candor and cooperation. The schedule should begin with questions that are interesting, motivating, and not too sensitive. The instrument also needs to be arranged to minimize bias. The possibility that earlier questions might influence responses to subsequent questions should be kept in mind. Whenever both general and specific questions about a topic are included, general questions should be placed first to avoid "coaching."

Every instrument should be prefaced by introductory comments about the nature and purpose of the study. In interviews, introductory information would be conveyed to respondents by the interviewer, who would typically follow a script. In questionnaires, the introduction usually takes the form of an accompanying **cover letter**. The introduction should be carefully constructed because it represents the first point of contact with potential respondents. An example of a cover letter for a mailed questionnaire is presented in Figure 16.4. (This cover letter is included in a Word file in the Toolkit in the accompanying *Resource Manual* for you to use and adapt.)

When a first draft of the instrument is in reasonably good order, it should be reviewed by experts in questionnaire construction, by substantive content area specialists, and by someone capable of detecting technical problems, such as spelling mistakes, grammatical errors, and so forth. When these various people have provided feedback, a revised version of the instrument can be pretested. The pretest should be administered to a small sample of individuals (usually 10 to 20) who are similar to actual participants.

In the remainder of this section, we offer some specific suggestions for designing high-quality self-report instruments. Additional guidance is offered in books by Fowler (1995) and Bradburn, Sudman, and Wansink (2004).

Tips for Wording Questions

Although we all are accustomed to asking questions, the proper phrasing of questions for a study is

Dear Community Resident:

We are conducting a study to examine how men who are approaching retirement age (55 to 65 years old) feel about various issues relating to their health care. This study, which is sponsored by the National Institutes of Health, will enable health care providers to better meet the needs of men in your age group. Would you please assist us in this study by completing the enclosed questionnaire? Your opinions and experiences are very important to us and are needed to give an accurate picture of the health-related needs of men in the Capital District.

Your name was selected at random from a list of residents in your community. The questionnaire is completely anonymous, so you are not asked to put your name on it or identify yourself in any way. We hope, therefore, that you will feel comfortable giving your honest opinions. If you prefer not to answer any particular question, feel free to leave it blank. Please *do* answer questions if you can, though. If you have any comments or concerns about any questions, just write your comments in the margin of the questionnaire or feel free to contact me by e-mail (dfp1@yahoo.com) or by phone (518-587-3994).

A postage-paid return envelope is enclosed for your convenience. Please take a few minutes to complete and return the questionnaire to us—it should only take about 15 to 20 minutes of your time. **In appreciation for your cooperation, you will be entered into a raffle to win a $250 American Express gift certificate.** Simply return the self-addressed, stamped postcard separately from the questionnaire. To be included in the raffle, your questionnaire must be returned to us by July 10. The raffle winner will be notified by July 17.

Your participation in the study is completely voluntary. By returning your study booklet, you will be granting your consent to participate in the study. Thank you in advance for your assistance.

FIGURE 16.4 ✸ Example of a cover letter for a mailed questionnaire.

a challenging task. In wording their questions, researchers should keep four important considerations in mind.

1. *Clarity*. Questions should be worded clearly and unambiguously. This is usually easier said than done. Respondents do not necessarily understand what information is needed and do not always have the same mind-set as the researchers.
2. *Ability of respondents to give information.* Researchers need to consider whether respon-dents can be expected to understand the question or are qualified to provide meaningful information.
3. *Bias*. Questions should be worded in a manner that will minimize the risk for response biases.
4. *Sensitivity*. Researchers should strive to be courteous, considerate, and sensitive to the needs and rights of respondents, especially when asking questions of a private nature.

Here are some specific suggestions with regard to these four considerations (additional guidance on wording items for composite scales is provided in Chapter 18):

- Clarify in your own mind the information you are seeking. The question, "When do you usually eat your evening meal?" might elicit such responses as "around 6 PM," or "when my son gets home from soccer practice," or "when I feel like cooking." The question itself contains no words that are difficult, but the question is unclear because the researcher's intent is not apparent.

- Avoid technical terms (e.g., parity) if more common terms (e.g., number of children) are equally appropriate. Use words that are simple enough for the *least* educated respondents in your sample. Don't assume that even nurses have extensive knowledge of all aspects of nursing and medical terminology.

- Do not assume that respondents will be aware of, or informed about, issues or questions in which you are interested. Furthermore, avoid giving the impression that they *ought* to be informed. Questions on complex or specialized issues sometimes can be worded in such a way that respondents will be comfortable admitting ignorance (e.g., "Many people have not had a chance to learn much about factors that increase the risk for asthma. Do you happen to know of any contributing factors?"). Another approach is to preface a question by a short statement of explanation about terminology or issues.

- Avoid leading questions that suggest a particular kind of answer. A question such as, "Do you agree that nurse-midwives play an indispensable role in the health team?" is not neutral.

- State a range of alternatives within the question itself when possible. For instance, the question, "Do you prefer to get up early in the morning on weekends?" is more suggestive of the "right" answer than "Do you prefer to get up early in the morning or to sleep late on weekends?"

- For questions that deal with controversial opinions or socially unacceptable behavior (e.g., excessive drinking, noncompliance with medical instructions), closed-ended questions may be preferred. It is easier to check off having engaged in socially disapproved actions than to verbalize those actions in response to open-ended questions. Moreover, when controversial behaviors are presented as options, respondents are more likely to believe that their behavior is not unique, and admission of such behavior becomes less difficult.

- Impersonal wording of questions is sometimes useful in minimizing embarrassment and encouraging honesty. To illustrate this point, compare these two statements with which respondents might be asked to agree or disagree: (1) "I am personally dissatisfied with the nursing care I received during my hospitalization," (2) "The quality of nursing care in this hospital is unsatisfactory." A respondent might feel more comfortable admitting dissatisfaction with nursing care in the less personally worded second question.

Tips for Preparing Response Alternatives

If closed-ended questions are used, researchers also need to develop response alternatives. Below are some suggestions for preparing them.

- Response options should cover all significant alternatives. If respondents are forced to choose a response from options provided by researchers, they should feel reasonably comfortable with the available options. As a precaution, researchers often have as one response option a phrase such as "Other—please specify."

- Alternatives should be mutually exclusive. The following categories for a question on a person's age are *not* mutually exclusive: 30 years or younger, 30–40 years, 40–50 years, or 50 years or older. People who are exactly 30, 40, or 50 would qualify for two categories.

- There should be an underlying rationale for ordering alternatives. Options often can be placed in order of decreasing or increasing favorability, agreement, or intensity. When options have no "natural" order, alphabetic ordering of the alternatives can avoid leading respondents to a particular response (e.g., see the rank order question, number 4, in Table 16.1).

- Response alternatives should not be too lengthy. One sentence or phrase for each alternative should almost always be sufficient to express a concept. Response alternatives should be about equal in length.

Tips for Formatting an Instrument

The appearance and layout of an instrument may seem a matter of minor administrative importance. However, a poorly designed format can have substantive consequences if respondents (or interviewers) become confused, miss questions, or answer questions they should have omitted. The format is especially important in questionnaires because respondents cannot typically seek assistance. The following suggestions may be helpful in laying out an instrument:

- Try not to compress too many questions into too small a space. An extra page of questions is better than a form that appears cluttered and confusing and that provides inadequate space for responses to open-ended questions.
- Set off the response options from the question or stem itself. Response alternative are usually aligned vertically (see Table 16.1). In questionnaires, respondents can be asked either to circle their answer or to place a check in the appropriate box.
- Give special care to formatting **filter questions**, which are designed to route respondents through different sets of questions depending on their responses. In interview schedules, the typical procedure is to use **skip patterns** that instruct interviewers to skip to a specific question (e.g., SKIP TO Q10). In SAQs, skip instructions may be confusing. It is usually better to put questions appropriate to a subset of respondents apart from the main series of questions, as illustrated in Box 16.2, part B. An important advantage of CAPI, CATI, audio-CASI, and some Internet surveys is that skip patterns are built into the computer program, leaving no room for human error.
- Avoid forcing all respondents to go through inapplicable questions in an SAQ. That is, ques-

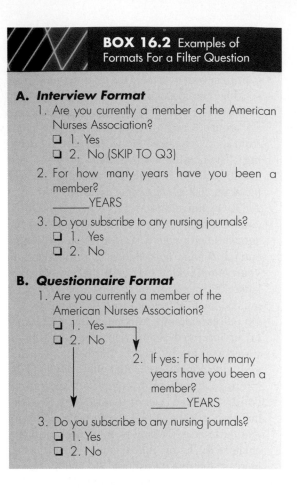

BOX 16.2 Examples of Formats For a Filter Question

A. _Interview Format_

1. Are you currently a member of the American Nurses Association?
   - ❑ 1. Yes
   - ❑ 2. No (SKIP TO Q3)

2. For how many years have you been a member?
   _____YEARS

3. Do you subscribe to any nursing journals?
   - ❑ 1. Yes
   - ❑ 2. No

B. _Questionnaire Format_

1. Are you currently a member of the American Nurses Association?
   - ❑ 1. Yes
   - ❑ 2. No

     2. If yes: For how many years have you been a member?
     _____YEARS

3. Do you subscribe to any nursing journals?
   - ❑ 1. Yes
   - ❑ 2. No

tion 2 in Box 16.2, part B could have been worded as follows: "If you are a member of the American Nurses Association, for how long have you been a member?" Nonmembers may not be sure how to handle this question and may be annoyed at having to read through irrelevant material.

Administering Structured Self-Report Instruments

Administering interview schedules and questionnaires requires different skills and involves different considerations. In this section, we examine issues in the administration of structured instruments, and ways of handling difficulties.

Collecting Interview Data

The quality of interview data relies heavily on interviewer proficiency. Interviewers for large survey organizations receive extensive general training in addition to specific training for individual studies. Although we cannot in this introductory book cover all the principles of good interviewing, we can identify some major issues. Additional guidance can be found in the book by Fowler and Mangione (1990).

A primary task of interviewers is to put respondents at ease so that they will feel comfortable in expressing opinions honestly. Respondents' personal reactions to interviewers can affect their willingness to participate. Interviewers, therefore, should always be punctual (if an appointment has been made), courteous, and friendly. Interviewers should strive to appear unbiased and to create a permissive atmosphere that encourages candor. All opinions of respondents should be accepted as natural; interviewers should not express surprise, disapproval, or even approval.

When a structured interview schedule is being used, interviewers should follow question wording precisely. Similarly, interviewers should not offer spontaneous explanations of what questions mean. Repetitions of the questions are usually adequate to dispel misunderstandings, particularly if the instrument has been properly pretested. Interviewers should not read questions mechanically. A natural, conversational tone is essential in building rapport with respondents, and this tone is impossible to achieve if interviewers are not thoroughly familiar with the questions.

When closed-ended questions have lengthy or complicated response alternatives, or when a series of questions has the same response alternatives, interviewers should hand subjects a **show card** that lists response options. People cannot be expected to remember detailed unfamiliar material and may choose the last alternative if they cannot recall earlier ones. (An example of a show card is included in the Toolkit for this chapter in the accompanying *Resource Manual*). ✪

Answers to closed-ended items are recorded by checking or circling the appropriate alternative, but responses to open-ended questions must be re-corded in full. Interviewers should not paraphrase or summarize respondents' replies.

Obtaining complete, relevant responses to open-ended questions is not always an easy matter. Respondents may reply to seemingly straightforward questions with irrelevant remarks or partial answers. Some may say, "I don't know" to avoid giving their opinions on sensitive topics, or to stall while they think over the question. In such cases, the interviewers' job is to *probe*. The purpose of a probe is to elicit more useful information than respondents volunteered during their initial reply. A probe can take many forms: Sometimes it involves a repetition of the original question, and sometimes it is a long pause intended to communicate to respondents that they should continue. Frequently, it is necessary to encourage a more complete response by a nondirective supplementary question, such as, "How is that?" Interviewers must be careful to use only *neutral* probes that do not influence the content of a response. Box 16.3 gives some examples of neutral, nondirective probes used by professional interviewers to get more complete responses to questions. The ability to probe well is perhaps the greatest test of an interviewer's skill. To know when to probe and how to select the best probes, interviewers must comprehend fully the purpose of each question and the type of information being sought. (The Toolkit for Chapter 14 of the accompanying *Resource Manual* has

BOX 16.3 Examples of Neutral, Nondirective Probes

- Is there anything else?
- Go on.
- Are there any other reasons?
- How do you mean?
- Could you please tell me more about that?
- Would you tell me what you have in mind?
- There are no right or wrong answers; I'd just like to get your thinking.
- Could you please explain that?
- Could you please give me an example?

supplementary material relating to interviewer training that might be useful.) ✹

Guidelines for telephone interviews are essentially the same as those for face-to-face interviews, but additional effort usually is required to build rapport over the telephone. In both cases, interviewers should strive to make the interview a pleasant and satisfying experience in which respondents are made to understand that the information they are providing is important.

Collecting Questionnaire Data Through In-Person Distribution

Questionnaires can be distributed in various ways, including personal distribution, through the mail, and over the Internet. The most convenient procedure is to distribute questionnaires to a group of people who complete the instrument together at the same time. This approach has the obvious advantages of maximizing the number of completed questionnaires and allowing researchers to clarify any possible misunderstandings. Group administrations are often possible in educational settings and in some clinical situations.

Personal presentation of questionnaires to individual respondents is another alternative. Personal contact with respondents has a positive effect on response rates for SAQs. Furthermore, researchers can help explain or clarify particular items or the study purpose. Personal involvement may be relatively time-consuming and expensive if questionnaires have to be delivered and picked up at respondents' homes. The distribution of questionnaires in clinical settings, on the other hand, is often inexpensive and efficient and is likely to yield a high rate of completed questionnaires.

Example of personal distribution of questionnaires: Gray (2006) studied pregnant women's self-appraisal of risks to themselves and their babies. Questionnaires were distributed to a sample of women who were medically categorized as high risk in a large level-three maternity service. Of the 214 expectant women invited to participate in the study, 176 completed questionnaires (82% response rate), either during their hospital stay or during a regularly scheduled clinic appointment.

Collecting Questionnaire Data Through the Mail

For surveys of a broad population, questionnaires are often mailed to respondents. This approach is cost-effective for reaching geographically dispersed respondents, but it tends to yield low response rates. When only a subsample of respondents return their questionnaires, it may be unreasonable to assume that those who responded were typical of the overall sample. That is, researchers are faced with the possibility that people who did not complete a questionnaire would have answered questions differently from those who did return it.

If the response rate is high, the risk for nonresponse bias may be negligible. A response rate greater than 65% is probably sufficient for most purposes, but lower response rates are the norm. Researchers should attempt to discover how representative respondents are, relative to the selected sample, in terms of basic demographic characteristics, such as age, gender, and race/ethnicity. This comparison may lead researchers to conclude that respondents and nonrespondents are sufficiently similar. When demographic differences are found, investigators can make inferences about the direction of biases.

Response rates can be affected by the manner in which the questionnaires are designed and mailed. The physical appearance of the questionnaire can influence its appeal, so some thought should be given to the layout, quality and color of paper, method of reproduction, and typographic quality of the instrument. The standard procedure for distributing mailed questionnaires is to include a stamped, addressed return envelope. Failure to enclose a return envelope can have an adverse effect on response rates.

➲ **TIP:** People are more likely to complete a mailed questionnaire if they are encouraged to do so by someone whose name (or position) they recognize. If possible, include a letter of endorsement from someone visible (e.g., a hospital or government official), or write the cover letter on the stationery of a well-respected organization.

The use of **follow-up reminders** is effective in achieving higher response rates for mailed (and Internet) questionnaires. This procedure involves additional mailings urging nonrespondents to complete and return their forms. Follow-up reminders are typically sent about 10 to 14 days after the initial mailing. Sometimes reminders simply involve a letter or postcard of encouragement to nonrespondents. It is preferable, however, to enclose a second copy of the questionnaire with the reminder letter because many nonrespondents will have misplaced the original or thrown it away. Telephone follow-ups can be even more successful, but are costly and time-consuming. With anonymous questionnaires, researchers may be unable to distinguish between respondents and nonrespondents for the purpose of sending follow-up letters. In such a situation, the simplest procedure is to send out a follow-up reminder to the entire sample, thanking those who have already answered and asking others to cooperate. Dillman (2000) offers excellent advice for achieving acceptable response rates in mailed and Internet surveys. ✪

Example of mailed questionnaires: Mantler and colleagues (2006) surveyed a sample of Canadian nurses to examine their reactions to sign-on bonuses and recruitment incentives for employment. Questionnaire packets were mailed to the home addresses of 2000 RNs with a postage-paid return envelope. A total of 833 completed questionnaires were returned, for a response rate of 41%.

Collecting Questionnaire Data Through the Internet

The Internet is an economical medium for distributing questionnaires. Surveys using the Internet appear to be an especially promising approach for accessing groups of people interested in very specific topic domains. Using the Internet to distribute questionnaires requires appropriate equipment and some technical skills, but there are a growing number of aids for doing such surveys.

Surveys can be administered through the Internet in several ways. One method is to design a questionnaire in a word processing program (e.g.,

Microsoft Word, WordPerfect), as would usually be the case for mailed questionnaires. The file containing the questionnaire is then attached to e-mail messages and distributed to a list of potential respondents. Respondents can complete the questionnaire and return it as an e-mail attachment, or they can print it and return it by mail or fax. This method may be problematic if respondents have trouble opening attachments or if they use a different word processing program. Surveys sent by e-mail messages also run the risk of not getting delivered to the intended party, either because e-mail addresses have changed or because the e-mail messages are blocked by Internet security filters. Blocks are especially common for messages with attachments (Baernholdt & Clarke, 2006).

Example of an e-mailed survey: Yetter-Read (2004) used an e-mail listserve to recruit participants, administer a survey, and send electronic gift certificates in a study of psychological responses to being a carrier of the gene for phenylketonuria. The return rate for the survey was 51%.

Internet surveys can also be administered as a **web-based survey**. This approach requires researchers to have their own website on which the survey form is placed. Respondents typically access the website by a hypertext link (i.e., by clicking on the hypertext, which sends the user to the website). For example, respondents may be invited to participate in the survey through an e-mail message that includes the hyperlink to the survey, or they may be invited to participate when they enter a website related in content to the survey (e.g., the website of a cancer support organization). There are also mechanisms for having the survey website included on search engines. However, it is important to weigh the tradeoffs between having a broad population and receiving survey data from inappropriate respondents.

Web-based forms are designed for online response, and may in some cases be programmed to include interactive features. By having dynamic features, respondents can receive as well as give information—a feature that increases people's motivation to participate. For example, respondents can be given information about their own responses (e.g., how they scored on a scale) or about responses of other participants. A major advantage of web-based forms is that the entered data are directly amenable to analysis. They are, however, more expensive than e-mail surveys.

Example of a web-based survey: Knue, Doellman, and Jacobs (2006) conducted a web-based survey to obtain information from intravenous therapy nurses about their use of peripherally inserted central catheters in children. Respondents were solicited by e-mails that were sent four different times to members of a venous listserve. The e-mails communicated information about the study purpose, the criteria for survey submission, and the link to the web-based survey. (Information about response rates was not provided in the report.)

There will undoubtedly be a growth of Internet surveys in the years ahead. They tend to be economical and can reach a broad audience. However, samples are almost never representative (unless the population is narrowly defined), and response rates in e-mailed surveys tend to be low—often even lower than mailed questionnaires. Several reference books are available to help researchers who wish to launch an Internet survey. For example, the books by Best and Krueger (2004), Dillman (2000), and Fitzpatrick and Montgomery (2004) provide useful information. There are also commercial vendors that can help with programming requirements. Some links to such vendors are included on the accompanying student CD-ROM. Weber and colleagues (2005) offer useful information about web-based data collection and management.

Evaluation of Structured Self-Reports

Structured self-reports represent a powerful mechanism for obtaining data, and are the most widely used method of data collection by nurse researchers. They are versatile, are capable of soliciting information about a wide range of topics, and yield information that can be readily analyzed using well-established statistical procedures. Questions can be constructed with care and worded in a manner that encourages candor. In an unstructured interview, respondents answer different questions, and there is no way to know whether the manner in which the questions were worded actually affected responses. On the other hand, the questions tend to be much more superficial than questions in unstructured interviews because most structured questions are closed ended.

Structured self-reports are susceptible to the risk for various **response biases**—many of which are also possible in unstructured self-reports. Respondents may provide biased responses reflecting their reaction to the behavior, perceived expectations, or appearance of the interviewers, for example. Perhaps the most pervasive problem is people's tendency to present a favorable image of themselves. **Social desirability response bias** refers to the tendency of some individuals to misrepresent their responses consistently by giving answers that are congruent with prevailing social values or professional expectations. This problem is often difficult to combat. Subtle, indirect, and delicately worded questioning sometimes can help to alleviate this response bias. The creation of a permissive atmosphere and provisions for respondent anonymity also encourage frankness. In an interview situation, interviewer training is essential.

Some response biases are most commonly observed in composite scales. These biases are sometimes referred to as **response set biases**. Scale scores are seldom entirely pure and accurate measures of the critical variable. A number of irrelevant factors are also being measured at the same time. Because response set factors can bias responses to a considerable degree, investigators who construct scales must attempt to eliminate or minimize them.

Extreme response sets are a bias reflecting consistent selection of extreme alternatives (e.g., "strongly agree"). These extreme responses distort the findings because they do not necessarily signify the most intense feelings about the phenomenon under study, but rather a characteristic of the respondent. There is little a researcher can do to counteract this bias, but there are procedures for detecting it.

Some people have been found to agree with statements regardless of content. Such people are called **yea-sayers**, and the bias is known as the

acquiescence response set. A less common problem is the opposite tendency for other individuals, called **nay-sayers**, to disagree with statements independently of question content.

It is important for researchers using self-reports to give the issue of response biases some thought. If an instrument or scale is being developed for general use by others, evidence should be gathered to demonstrate that the scale is sufficiently free from response biases to measure the critical variable. In structured self-report studies, it is imperative to gather evidence that the data obtained are accurate and valid—issues we discuss in the next chapter.

STRUCTURED OBSERVATION

Structured observation involves the collection of observational data using formal instruments and protocols that dictate what to observe, how long to observe it, and how to record the needed information. Unlike participant observation, structured observation typically is not intended to capture a broad slice of ordinary life, but rather to document specific behaviors, actions, and events. Observers using structured observation are still required to make some inferences and exercise judgment, but they are restrained with regard to the kinds of phenomena that will be watched and recorded. The creativity of structured observation lies not in the observation itself but rather in the formulation of a system for accurately categorizing, recording, and encoding the observations. Because structured techniques depend on plans developed before the actual observation, they are not appropriate when researchers have limited knowledge about the phenomena under investigation.

➲ **TIP:** Researchers often use structured observations in lieu of self-reports in situations in which study participants cannot be asked questions—or cannot be expected to provide reliable answers. Many structured observational instruments are designed to capture the behaviors of infants and children, or older people whose communication skills are impaired.

In selecting behaviors, conversation, or attributes to be observed, researchers must decide what constitutes a *unit*. There are two basic approaches, which actually are end points of a continuum. The **molar approach** entails observing large units of behavior and treating them as a whole. For example, psychiatric nurse researchers might study patient mood swings. An entire constellation of verbal and nonverbal behaviors might be construed as signaling aggressive behaviors, for example. At the other extreme, the **molecular approach** uses small, highly specific behaviors or verbal segments as observational units. Each action, gesture, or phrase is treated as a separate entity. The choice of approaches depends mostly on the nature of the research problem. The molar approach is more susceptible to observer errors because of greater ambiguity in what is being observed. On the other hand, in reducing observations to concrete, specific elements, investigators may fail to understand how small elements work in concert in a behavior pattern.

Methods of Recording Structured Observations

Researchers recording structured observations typically use either a checklist or a rating scale. Both types of record-keeping instruments specify in advance the behaviors or events to be observed and are designed to produce numeric information.

➲ **TIP:** Compared with the abundance of books designed to provide guidance in developing self-report instruments, there are relatively few resources for researchers who want to design their own observational instruments, except if the focus of the observation is on interpersonal interactions (e.g., Bakeman & Gottman, 1997; Kerig & Lindahl, 2000).

Category Systems and Checklists

The most common approach for organizing structured observations involves constructing a category system to classify observed phenomena. A **category system** represents an attempt to designate in a systematic fashion the qualitative behaviors and events transpiring in the observational setting.

Some category systems are constructed so that *all* observed behaviors within a specified domain (e.g., utterances) can be classified into one and only one category. In such an exhaustive system, the categories are mutually exclusive.

Example of exhaustive categories: Holditch-Davis and colleagues (2004) made longitudinal observations of the behavior patterns and sleep–wake states of preterm infants at high risk for developmental problems. The infants' muscle tone, motor activity, respiration, and eye movements were used to classify their sleep–wake states into one of five mutually exclusive categories: quiet waking, active waking, sleep–wake transition, active sleep, and quiet sleep.

When observers use an exhaustive system—that is, when all behaviors of a certain type, such as verbal interaction, are observed and recorded—researchers must be careful to define categories so that observers know when one behavior ends and a new one begins. Another essential feature is that referent behaviors should be mutually exclusive. If overlapping categories are not eliminated, observers will have difficulty deciding how to classify a particular observation. The underlying assumption in the use of such a category system is that behaviors, events, or attributes that are allocated to a particular category are equivalent to every other behavior, event, or attribute in that same category.

A contrasting technique is to develop a system in which only particular types of behavior (which may or may not be manifested) are categorized. For example, if we were studying autistic children's aggressive behavior, we might develop such categories as "strikes another child," or "kicks or hits walls or floor." In such a category system, many behaviors—all the ones that are nonaggressive—would not be classified. Nonexhaustive systems are adequate for many purposes, but one risk is that resulting data might be difficult to interpret. Problems may arise if a large number of behaviors are not categorized or if long segments of the observation sessions do not involve the target behaviors. In such situations, investigators may have trouble placing categorized behavior into an interpretable context, unless there is a method to capture the amount of time in which the target behaviors occurred, relative to the total time under observation.

Example of nonexhaustive categories: Harrison, Roane, and Weaver (2004) developed a system to categorize infant behavioral signs of distress (startle, yawn, grimace, clenched fist, tremor, and hiccups). Behaviors unrelated to distress were not categorized. The actual measure used in the analysis was the percentage of observational intervals in which distress cues occurred out of all observational intervals.

A critical requirement for a good category system is the careful and explicit definition of behaviors and characteristics to be observed. Each category must be explained in detail so that observers have relatively clearcut criteria for determining the occurrence of a specified phenomenon. Virtually all category systems require observers to make some inferences, to a greater or lesser degree.

Example of low observer inference: Walker and colleagues (2003) made observations of maternal behavior in rats following repeated pain to their pups. Mother rats were observed after their pups were separated from them and then reunited after receiving a painful procedure. Various maternal behaviors were coded. One was *nesting*, defined as "the time when the mother was over her pups in the crouching position and more than 3 pups were attached to the nipples" (p. 255).

In this system, assuming that observers were properly trained, relatively little inference would be required to allocate the mother rat's behavior to the proper category. Other category systems, however, require more inference.

Example of moderate observer inference: Drummond and colleagues (2005) studied the effect of a family problem-solving intervention on cooperative parenting communication, which was measured with an observational instrument that required moderate inference. For example, parents were videotaped playing with their child, and parental initiations, responses, nonengaged behaviors, and praise were categorized. Examples of parental responses that needed to be coded were "repeating," "expansion," "seeking clarification," and "negative feedback."

In such category systems, even when categories are defined in detail, a moderately heavy inferential burden is placed on observers. The decision concerning how much observer inference is appropriate depends on a number of factors, including the research purposes and the observers' skills. Beginning researchers are advised to construct or use category systems that require low to moderate inference.

Category systems are the basis for constructing a **checklist**, which is the instrument observers use to record observed phenomena. The checklist is usually formatted with the list of behaviors or events from the category system on the left and space for tallying the frequency or duration of occurrence of behaviors on the right. With nonexhaustive category systems, categories of behaviors that may or may not be manifested by participants are listed on the checklist. The observer's tasks are to watch for instances of these behaviors and to record their occurrence.

With exhaustive checklists, the observers' task is to place all behaviors in only one category for each element. By **element**, we refer to either a unit of behavior, such as a sentence in a conversation, or a time interval. To illustrate, suppose we were studying the problem-solving behavior of a group of public health workers discussing a new intervention for the homeless. Our category system involves eight categories: (1) seeks information, (2) gives information, (3) describes problem, (4) offers suggestion, (5) opposes suggestion, (6) supports suggestion, (7) summarizes, and (8) miscellaneous. Observers would be required to classify every group member's contribution—using, for example, each sentence as the element—in terms of one of these eight categories.

Another approach with exhaustive systems is to categorize relevant behaviors at regular time intervals. For example, in a category system for infants' motor activities, the researcher might use 15-second time intervals as the element; observers would categorize infant movements within 15-second periods.

Rating Scales

The major alternative to a checklist for recording structured observations is a **rating scale** that requires observers to rate a phenomenon along a descriptive continuum that is typically bipolar. The ratings are quantified for subsequent statistical analysis.

Observers may be required to rate behaviors or events at specified intervals throughout the observational period (e.g., every 10 minutes). Alternatively, observers may rate entire events or transactions after observations are completed. Postobservation ratings require observers to integrate a number of activities and to judge which point on a scale most closely fits their interpretation of the overall situation. For example, suppose we were observing children's behavior during a scratch test for allergies. After each session, observers might be asked to rate the children's overall anxiety during the procedure on a graphic rating scale such as the following:

Rate how calm or nervous the child was during the procedure:

1	2	3	4	5	6	7
Extremely calm			Neither calm nor nervous			Extremely nervous

---

⮕ **T I P :** Global observational rating scales are sometimes included at the end of structured interviews. For example, in a study of the health problems of nearly 4000 welfare mothers, interviewers were asked to observe and rate the safety of the home environment with regard to potential health hazards to the children on a 5-point scale, from completely safe to extremely unsafe (Polit, London, & Martinez, 2001).

Rating scales can also be used as an extension of checklists, in which observers not only record the occurrence of a behavior but also rate some qualitative aspect of it, such as its magnitude or intensity. A particularly good example is Weiss's (1992) Tactile Interaction Index (TII) for observing patterns of interpersonal touch. The TII comprises four dimensions: location (part of body touched, such as arm, abdomen); action (the specific gesture or movement used, such as grabbing, hitting, patting); duration (temporal length of the touch); and intensity. Observers using the index must both classify the nature and duration of the touch *and* rate intensity on a 4-point scale: light, moderate, strong, or deep. When rating scales are coupled with a category scheme in this fashion, considerable information about a phenomenon can be obtained, but it places an immense burden on observers, particularly if there is extensive activity.

> **Example of observational ratings:** The NEECHAM Confusion Scale is an observational measure designed to detect the presence and severity of acute confusion. Two of its three subscales (Processing and Behavior) involve behavioral dimensions along which an observed elder is rated. For example, one rating in the Processing subscale concerns alertness/responsiveness, and the ratings are from 0 (responsiveness depressed) to 4 (full attentiveness). The NEECHAM has been used extensively for both clinical and research purposes. For example, Miller and colleagues (2004) used NEECHAM scores as outcome measures in an assessment of the Elder Care Supportive Interventions Protocol.

➲ TIP: It is usually useful to spend a period of time with study participants before the actual observations and recording of data. Having a warm-up period helps to relax people (especially if audio or video equipment is being used) and can be helpful to observers (e.g., if participants have a linguistic style to which observers must adjust, such as a strong regional accent).

Constructing Versus Borrowing Structured Observational Instruments

The development and testing of new observational instruments typically require months of effort. Researchers may have no alternative but to design new observational instruments if existing ones are inappropriate. As with self-report instruments, however, we encourage researchers to explore the literature fully for available observational instruments, even if they must be adapted. The use of an existing system not only saves considerable work but also facilitates comparisons among studies.

A few source books describe available observational instruments for certain research applications (e.g., Frank-Stromberg & Olsen, 2003), but the best source for such instruments is recent research literature on the study topic. For example, if you wanted to conduct an observational study of infant pain, a good place to begin would be recent research on this or similar topics to obtain information on how infant pain was operationalized.

Sampling for Structured Observations

Researchers must decide how, when, and for how long structured observational instruments will be used. Observations are usually done for a specific amount of time, and the amount of time is standardized across study participants.

Observational sampling is sometimes needed to obtain representative examples of behaviors without having to observe for prolonged periods. Note that observational sampling concerns the selection of *behaviors* (or conversational segments) to be observed, not the selection of study participants.

One method is **time sampling**, which involves the selection of time periods during which observations will occur. The time frames may be systematically selected (e.g., every 60 seconds at 5-minute intervals), selected at random, or selected by a quota system. As an example, suppose we were studying mothers' interactions with their handicapped children in a playground setting. During a 1-hour observation period, we sample moments to observe, rather than observing the entire session. Let us say that observations are made in 3-minute intervals. If we used a systematic sampling approach, we would observe for 3 minutes, then cease observing for a prespecified period, say 3 minutes. With this scheme, a total of ten 3-minute observations would be made. A second approach is to sample randomly 3-minute periods from the total of 20 such periods in an hour; a third is to use all 20 periods. The decision with regard to the length and number of periods for creating a suitable sample must be made in accordance with research aims. In establishing time units, a key consideration is determining a psychologically meaningful time frame. A good deal of pretesting and experimentation with different sampling plans may be necessary.

> **Example of time sampling:** Billinghurst, Morgan, and Arthur (2003) studied the frequency of rhythm disturbance events among patients on remote cardiac telemetry and examined how many of the events were detected by telemetry nurses. Observational data were collected in a coronary respiratory care unit over a 9-day period. Two-hour blocks of time were randomly selected within 8-hour time periods.

Event sampling is a second system for obtaining observations. This approach uses integral behavioral sets or events for observation. Event sampling requires that the investigator either have some knowledge about the occurrence of events, or be in a position to await (or arrange) their occurrence. Examples of integral events suitable for event sampling include shift changes of nurses in a hospital, cast removals of pediatric patients, and cardiac arrests in the emergency department. This approach is preferable to time sampling when the events of interest are infrequent and are at risk of being missed if time sampling is used. Event sampling also has the advantage that situations are observed in their entirety rather than being fragmented into segments, and so may be preferred for making molar observations. Still, when behaviors and events are frequent—especially for molecular observations—time sampling has the virtue of enhancing the representativeness of observed behaviors.

Example of event sampling: White-Traut and colleagues (2005) analyzed observational data from videotapes of the prefeeding behavior of healthy premature infants. Infants were videotaped immediately before the first three oral feedings. The coding of infant behaviors focused on feeding readiness cues and behavioral state (e.g., crying, alert, sleeping).

Mechanical Aids in Observations

The health care field has a rich array of observational equipment that can reveal conditions or attributes that are ordinarily imperceptible. Nasal specula, stethoscopes, bronchoscopes, radiographic and imaging equipment, ultrasound technology, and a myriad of other medical instruments make it possible to gather observational information about people's health status and functioning for both clinical and research purposes.

In addition to equipment for enhancing physiologic observations, mechanical devices are available for recording behaviors and events, making analysis or categorization at a later time possible. When the behavior of interest is primarily auditory, recordings can be obtained and used as a per-

manent record, and technological advances have vastly improved the quality, sensitivity, and unobtrusiveness of recording equipment. Other technological instruments to aid auditory observation have been developed, such as laser devices that are capable of recording sounds by being directed on a window to a room, and voice tremor detectors that are sensitive to stress. Auditory recordings can also be subjected to computerized speech software analysis to obtain objective quantitative measures of certain features of the recordings (e.g., volume, pitch).

When visual records are desired, videotapes can be used. In addition to being permanent, videotapes can capture complex behaviors that might elude notice by on-the-spot observers. Visual records are also more capable than the naked eye of capturing fine units of behavior, such as micro-momentary facial expressions. Videotapes offer the possibility of checking the accuracy of coders or the recording skills of participant observers and so are useful as a training aid. Finally, it is often easier to conceal a camera than a human observer. Video records also have a number of drawbacks, some of which are fairly technical, such as lighting requirements, lens limitations, and so forth. Other problems result from the fact that the camera angle adopted could present a lopsided view of an event or situation. Also, some participants may be more self-conscious in front of a video camera than they would otherwise be. Still, for many applications, permanent visual records offer unparalleled opportunities to expand the range and scope of observational studies.

Also of interest is the growing technology for assisting with the encoding and recording of observations made directly by on-the-spot observers. For example, there is equipment that permits observers to enter observational data directly into a computer as the observation occurs, and in some cases, the equipment can record physiologic data concurrently.

Example of the use of equipment: Samselle and colleagues (2005) analyzed data from 20 videotapes of women giving birth to examine the relationship between care provider communications and maternal pushing behavior. Observers categorized the mothers' pushing effort as *spontaneous* or *directed*, following a set of explicit classification criteria; timed the length of each maternal bearing down; and calculated total pushing time.

Example of observations by nonresearch personnel: McGuiness, Ryan, & Robinson (2005) studied the risks of children adopted from the former Soviet Union, and the protective influences of the adoptive families. A key outcome variable concerned the children's competence, which was assessed by asking parents to complete the Child Behavior Checklist.

Structured Observations by Nonresearch Observers

The research discussed thus far involves observations made and recorded by researchers or observer assistants. Sometimes, however, researchers ask others not connected with the research team to provide structured observational data, based on their observations of the characteristics, activities, and behaviors of others. This method has much in common (in terms of format and scoring) with self-report scales; the primary difference is that the person completing the scale is asked to describe the attributes and behaviors of *another* person, based on their observations of that person. For example, a mother might be asked to describe the behavior problems of her preschool child, or staff nurses might be asked to evaluate the functional capacity of nursing home residents.

Obtaining observational data from nonresearchers has practical advantages: It is economical compared with using trained observers. For example, observers might have to watch children for hours or days to describe the nature and intensity of behavior problems, whereas parents or teachers could do this readily. Some behaviors might never lend themselves to outsider observation because of reactivity, occurrence in private situations, or infrequency (e.g., sleepwalking).

On the other hand, such methods may have the same problems as self-report scales (e.g., response-set bias) in addition to observer bias. Observer bias may in some cases be extreme, such as often happens when parents are asked to provide information about their children. Nonresearch observers are typically not trained, and interobserver agreement usually cannot be determined. Thus, this approach has some problems but will inevitably continue to be used because, in many cases, there are no alternatives.

Evaluation of Structured Observation

Structured observation is an important method of data collection, particularly for systematically recording aspects of people's behaviors when they are not capable of describing them through self-reports. Observational methods are particularly valuable for gathering information about infants and children, and about older people who are confused, agitated, or unable to communicate.

Observations, like self-reports, are vulnerable to biases. One source of bias comes from those being observed. As with self-reports, study participants may distort their behaviors in the direction of "looking good." They may also behave atypically because of their awareness of being observed, or their shyness in front of strangers or in front of a camera.

Biases can also reflect human perceptual errors and inadequacies, which are a continuous threat to data quality. Observation and interpretation are demanding tasks, requiring attention, sensation, perception, and conception. To accomplish these activities in a completely objective fashion is challenging and perhaps impossible. Biases are especially likely to operate when a high degree of observer inference is required.

Several types of observational bias are especially common. One bias is the **enhancement of contrast effect**, in which observers distort observations in the direction of dividing content into clearcut entities. The converse effect—a bias toward **central tendency**—occurs when extreme events are distorted toward a middle ground. With **assimilatory biases**, observers distort observations in the direction of identity with previous inputs. This bias would have the effect of miscategorizing information in the direction of regularity and orderliness. Assimilation to the observer's expectations and attitudes also occurs.

Rating scales and other evaluative observations are also susceptible to bias. The **halo effect** is the tendency of observers to be influenced by one characteristic in judging other, unrelated characteristics. For example, if we formed a positive general impression of a person, we would probably be likely to rate that person as intelligent, loyal, and dependable simply because these traits are positively valued. Rating scales may reflect observers' personality. The **error of leniency** is the tendency for observers to rate everything positively, and the **error of severity** is the contrasting tendency to rate too harshly.

The careful construction and pretesting of checklists and rating scales, and the proper training and preparation of observers, are techniques that can play an important role in minimizing or estimating biases. If people are to become good instruments for collecting observational data, then they must be trained to observe in such a way that accuracy is maximized and biases are minimized. Even when the principal investigator is the primary observer, self-training and dry runs are essential. The setting during the trial period should resemble as closely as possible the settings that will be the focus of actual observations.

Ideally, training should include practice sessions during which the comparability of the observers' recordings is assessed. That is, two or more independent observers should watch a trial event or situation, and observational coding should then be compared. Procedures for establishing the **interrater reliability** of structured observational instruments are described in the next chapter.

➡ **T I P :** Observations should be made in a neutral and nonjudgmental manner. People being observed are more likely to mask their emotions or behave atypically if they think they are being critically appraised. Even positive cues (such as nodding approval) should be withheld because approval may induce repetition of a behavior that might not otherwise have occurred. (Positive cues may be impossible to withhold in participant observation studies, which makes it all the more important for observers to be reflective and to keep personal notes.)

BIOPHYSIOLOGIC MEASURES

The trend in nursing research has been toward increased use of measures to assess the physiologic status of study participants, and to evaluate clinical outcomes. The National Institute for Nursing Research has, in fact, emphasized the need for more physiologically based nursing research. Many clinically relevant variables do not, of course, require biophysiologic instrumentation for their measurement. Data on physiologic activity or dysfunction can often be gathered through direct observation (e.g., cyanosis, edema, wound status), and other biophysiologic data can be gathered by asking people directly (e.g., ratings of pain). This section focuses on biophysiologic phenomena that are measured through specialized technical equipment.

Settings in which nurses work are typically filled with a wide variety of technical instruments for measuring physiologic functions. It is beyond the scope of this book to describe the many kinds of biophysiologic measures available to nurse researchers. Our goals are to present an overview of biophysiologic measures, to illustrate their use in research, and to note considerations in decisions to use them.

Purposes of Collecting Biophysiologic Data

Clinical nursing studies involve biophysiologic instruments both for creating independent variables (e.g., an intervention using biofeedback equipment) and for measuring dependent variables. For the most part, our discussion focuses on the use of biophysiologic measures as dependent (outcome) variables. Most nursing studies in which biophysiologic measures have been used fall into one of six classes:

1. *Studies of basic biophysiologic processes that have relevance for nursing care.* These studies involve normal, healthy participants or an animal species. For example, Graves, Ramsay, & McCarthy (2006) examined the effects of indomethacin and NS398—a nonspecific and specific COX inhibitor, respectively—on

muscle mass in mice bearing two types of tumor-induced skeletal muscle wasting.

2. *Descriptions of the physiologic outcomes of nursing and health care.* These studies do not focus on specific interventions, but rather are designed to document standard procedures or to learn how standard procedures affect patients' physiologic outcomes. For example, LaMar and Dowling (2006) examined the incidence of infection (from blood cultures, urine cultures, stool cultures, and so on) for cobedded preterm twins.

3. *Evaluations of a specific nursing intervention.* These evaluation studies differ from those in the second category in that they involve the testing of a new intervention, usually in comparison with standard methods of care or with alternative interventions. Typically, these studies involve a hypothesis stating that the innovation will result in improved biophysiologic outcomes among patients. As an example, Liehr and colleagues (2006) tested the effectiveness of adding story-centered care (carefully attending to the patient's narratives) to standard care in lowering the blood pressure of people with stage 1 hypertension.

4. *Product assessments.* Some studies are designed to evaluate products to enhance patient health or comfort, rather than to evaluate nursing actions. For example, Chertok, Schneider, and Blackburn (2006) compared physiologic outcomes (maternal prolactin and cortisol levels) of breastfeeding with and without ultrathin nipple shields.

5. *Studies to evaluate the measurement and recording of biophysiologic information gathered by nurses.* The accurate measurement of biophysiologic phenomena is crucial, and therefore a growing number of studies focus on improving clinical measurements. For instance, Chin-Peuckert and colleagues (2004) hypothesized that warm infusion solution should be used for urodynamic evaluations of children. The outcome measures included maximum cystometric bladder capacity, maximum flow rate, and pressure at maximum flow.

6. *Studies of the correlates of physiologic functioning in patients with health problems.* Researchers study possible antecedents and consequences of biophysiologic indicators to gain insight into potential treatments or modes of care. Nurse researchers have also studied biophysiologic outcomes in relation to social or psychological characteristics. In some cases, the studies are prospective and are designed to identify antecedents to physiologic problems. In other cases, the researcher is trying to describe concurrently the psychological status of people with different physiologic conditions. As an example, Meynell and Barosso (2005) studied the relationship between fatigue intensity and measures derived from bioimpedance analysis (e.g., body cell mass, fat-free mass) in HIV-positive people.

Types of Biophysiologic Measures

Physiologic measurements can be classified in one of two major categories. *In vivo* **measurements** are those performed directly in or on living organisms. Examples include measures of oxygen saturation, blood pressure, and body temperature. An *in vitro* **measurement**, by contrast, is performed outside the organism's body, as in the case of measuring serum potassium concentration in the blood.

In vivo measures often involve the use of highly complex instrumentation systems. An **instrumentation system** is the apparatus and equipment used to measure one or more attributes of a subject and the presentation of that measurement data in a manner that humans can interpret. Organism–instrument systems involve up to six major components: (1) a stimulus; (2) a subject; (3) sensing equipment (e.g., transducers); (4) signal-conditioning equipment (to reduce interference signals); (5) display equipment; and (6) recording, data processing, and transmission equipment. Not all instrumentation systems involve all six components. Some systems, such as an electronic thermometer, are simple, but others are extremely complex. For example, some electronic monitors yield simultaneous measures of such physiologic variables as cardiac responsiveness, respiratory rate and rhythm, core temperature, and muscular activity.

In vivo instruments have been developed to measure all bodily functions, and technological improvements continue to advance our ability to measure biophysiologic phenomena more accurately, more conveniently, and more rapidly than ever before. The uses to which such instruments have been put by nurse researchers are richly diverse and impressive.

Example of a study with *in vivo* measures:
Kim and colleagues (2006) studied cardiopulmonary responses to a moderate-intensity aerobic exercise intervention in women newly diagnosed with breast cancer. Outcome measures included heart rate, systolic blood pressure, and oxygen consumption (e.g., $\dot{V}O_2$ peak).

With *in vitro* measures, data are gathered by extracting physiologic material from subjects and submitting it for laboratory analysis. Nurse researchers may or may not be involved in the extraction of the material; however, the analysis is normally done by specialized laboratory technicians. Usually, each laboratory establishes a range of normal values for each measurement, and this information is critical for interpreting the results.

Several classes of laboratory analysis have been used in studies by nurse researchers, including chemical measurements (e.g., measures of hormone levels or potassium levels); microbiologic measures (e.g., bacterial counts); and cytologic *or* histologic measures (e.g., tissue biopsies). It is impossible, of course, to catalog the thousands of laboratory tests available. Laboratory analyses of blood and urine samples are the most frequently used *in vitro* measures in nursing investigations.

Example of a study with *in vitro* measures:
Miketova and colleagues (2005) studied oxidative stress as a possible mechanism of chemotherapy-induced central nervous system injury in children with acute lymphoblastic leukemia. Unoxidized and oxidized components of phosphatidylcholine were measured in cerebral spinal fluid samples.

Selecting a Biophysiologic Measure

For nurses unfamiliar with the hundreds of biophysiologic measures available in institutional settings, the selection of appropriate research measures may pose a challenge. There are, unfortunately, no comprehensive handbooks to guide interested researchers to the measures, instruments, and interpretations that may be required in collecting physiologic data. Probably the best approach is to consult knowledgeable colleagues or experts at a local institution. It also may be possible to obtain useful information on biophysiologic measures from research articles on a problem similar to your own, a review article on the central phenomenon under investigation, manufacturers' catalogs, and exhibits of manufacturers at professional conferences.

Obviously, the most basic issue to address in selecting a physiologic measure is whether it will yield good information about the research variable. In some cases, researchers need to consider whether the variable should be measured by observation or self-report instead of (or in addition to) using biophysiologic equipment. For example, stress could be measured by asking people questions (e.g., using the State–Trait Anxiety Inventory); by observing their behavior during exposure to stressful stimuli; or by measuring heart rate, blood pressure, or levels of adrenocorticotropic hormone in urine samples.

Several other considerations should be kept in mind in selecting a biophysiologic measure. Some key questions include the following:

- Is the equipment or laboratory analysis you need readily available to you? If not, can it be borrowed, rented, or purchased?
- If equipment must be purchased, is it affordable? Can funding be acquired to cover the purchase (or rental) price?
- Can you operate the required equipment and interpret its results, or do you need training? Are there resources available to help you with operation and interpretation?
- Will you have difficulty obtaining permission to use the equipment from an Institutional Review Board or other institutional authority?

• Does the measure need to be direct (e.g., a direct measure of blood pressure by way of an arterial line), or is an indirect measure (e.g., blood pressure measurement by way of a sphygmomanometer) sufficient?

• Is continuous monitoring necessary (e.g., electrocardiogram readings), or is a point-in-time measure adequate?

• Do your activities during data collection permit you to record data simultaneously, or do you need an instrument system with recording equipment (or a research assistant)?

• Is a mechanical stimulus needed to get meaningful measurements? Does available equipment include the required stimulus?

• Is a single measure of the dependent variable sufficient, or are multiple measures preferable? If multiple measures are better, what burden does this place on you and on participants?

• Are your measures likely to be influenced by reactivity (i.e., subjects' awareness of their subject status)? If so, can alternative or supplementary nonreactive measures be identified, or can the extent of reactivity bias be assessed?

• Can your research variable be measured using a noninvasive procedure, or is an invasive procedure required?

• Is the measure you plan to use sufficiently accurate and sensitive to variation?

• Are you thoroughly familiar with rules and safety precautions, such as grounding procedures, especially when using electrical equipment?

Evaluation of Biophysiologic Measures

Biophysiologic measures offer the following advantages to nurse researchers:

• Biophysiologic measures are accurate and precise compared with psychological measures (e.g., self-report measures of anxiety).

• Biophysiologic measures are objective. Two nurses reading from the same thermistor thermometer are likely to record the same temperature measurements, and two different thermistor thermometers are likely to produce identical readouts. Patients cannot easily distort measurements of biophysiologic functioning deliberately.

• Biophysiologic instrumentation provides valid measures of the targeted variables: thermometers can be depended on to measure temperature and not blood volume, and so forth. For nonbiophysiologic measures, the question of whether an instrument is really measuring the target concept is an ongoing concern.

• Because equipment for obtaining biophysiologic measurements is available in hospital settings, the cost of collecting biophysiologic data may be low or nonexistent.

Biophysiologic measures also have a few disadvantages:

• The measuring tool may affect the variables it is attempting to measure. The presence of a sensing device, such as a transducer, located in a blood vessel partially blocks that vessel and, hence, alters the pressure–flow characteristics being measured.

• There are normally interferences that create artifacts in biophysiologic measures. For example, noise generated in a measuring instrument interferes with the signal being produced.

• Energy must often be applied to the organism when taking the biophysiologic measurements; extreme caution must continually be exercised to avoid the risk for damaging cells by high-energy concentrations.

• The difficulty in choosing biophysiologic measures for nursing studies lies not in their shortage, nor in their questionable utility, nor in their inferiority to other methods. Indeed, they are plentiful, often highly reliable and valid, and extremely useful in clinical nursing studies. However, care must be exercised in selecting appropriate instruments or laboratory analyses with regard to practical, ethical, medical, and technical considerations.

BOX 16.4 Guidelines for Critiquing Structured Data Collection Methods

1. Was the collection of structured data appropriate to the study aims?
2. Given the research question and the characteristics of study participants, did the researcher use the best method of capturing study phenomena (i.e., self-reports, observation, biophysiologic measures)? Should supplementary data collection methods have been used to enrich the data available for analysis?
3. If self-report methods were used, did the researcher make good decisions about the specific method used to solicit self-report information (e.g., mix of open- and closed-ended questions, use of composite scales)?
4. Was the instrument package adequately described in terms of reading level of the questions, length of time to complete it, number of modules included, and so on?
5. Was the mode of obtaining the self-report data appropriate (e.g., in-person interviews, mailed SAQs, Internet questioning)?
6. Were self-report data gathered in a manner that promoted high-quality and unbiased responses (e.g., in terms of privacy, efforts to put respondents at ease)? Who collected the data, and were they adequately trained for the task?
7. If observational methods were used, did the report adequately describe what specific constructs were observed? What was the unit of observation—was the approach molar or molecular?
8. Was a category system or rating system used to organize and record observations? Was the category system exhaustive? How much inference was required of the observers? Were decisions about exhaustiveness and degree of observer inference appropriate?
9. What methods were used to sample observational units? Was the sampling approach a good one, and did it likely yield a representative sample of behavior?
10. To what degree were observer biases controlled or minimized? Who collected the observational data, and were they appropriately trained?
11. Were biophysiologic measures used in the study, and was this appropriate? Were appropriate methods used to measure the variables of interest? Did the researcher appear to have the skills necessary for proper interpretation of biophysiologic measures?

CRITIQUING STRUCTURED METHODS OF DATA COLLECTION

It is usually easier to critique a researcher's data collection decisions for structured than for unstructured methods. A researcher can more readily report, for example, that the State–Trait Anxiety Inventory was used to measure anxiety than to provide detailed and transparent information about how the experience of anxiety was captured in a qualitative study. Nevertheless, the amount of detail provided even in quantitative reports is rarely extensive because of space constraints in journals.

A full critique of data collection plans is rarely feasible.

Box 16.4 ⊗ provides some guidelines for critiquing the collection of structured data. The guidelines are available in the Toolkit for your use and adaptation. Further guidance on drawing conclusions about data quality in studies using structured methods is provided in Chapter 17.

RESEARCH EXAMPLES

Two examples that illustrate a variety of structured data collection approaches follow.

Research Example of Structured Observation

Study: "Improving outcomes of nursing home interactions" (Williams, 2006)

Statement of Purpose: The purpose of this study was to evaluate the effectiveness of an intervention designed to improve resident–staff communication in three nursing homes.

Design: The educational intervention involved three 1-hour sessions within a 2-week period in each facility, using an established program. A single group before–after design was used to assess whether the intervention improved nursing home staff's communication skills and helped to reduce *elderspeak*—a patronizing communication style. Data were collected at baseline, and then again within 1 week of completing the intervention and 2 months later.

Data Collection: Digital minidisk audio recorders were used to record communication between staff and residents. At all three points of data collection, staff participants were recorded for 2 hours while caring for residents. Williams remained on the unit during the observation sessions, but did not interrupt staff in their usual routines during the 2-hour recording sessions. The first 5 minutes of each 2-hour session were deleted to allow time for participant adjustment. Then the first five conversations of each staff member with different residents were selected for coding and analysis. Only interactions lasting at least 1 minute were included. A total of 526 staff–resident conversations were transcribed. The transcripts were then coded for four psycholinguistic measures of elderspeak, using a system previously established by other researchers. The four measures (e.g., use of diminutives, mean length of utterances) were coded by trained assistants who were blinded to when the recordings were made (i.e., before or after the intervention). Additionally, a rating scale was used to rate the emotional tone of the conversations. The ratings involved 5-point Likert-type scales (with ratings ranging from *not at all* to *very*) that measure three dimensions: care, respect, and control. For example, the *control* subscale includes the descriptors dominating, controlling, directive, and bossy. A subset of 138 conversations, randomly selected to represent all three data collection periods, were rated by raters who were not the same people as the ones who coded the conversations for elderspeak.

Key Findings:

- Psycholinguistic features of elderspeak were significantly reduced after the intervention. In particular, the use of diminutives declined significantly.

- Postintervention conversations were more respectful, less controlling, and more caring than baseline conversations.

Research Example of Structured Self-Reports and Biophysiologic Measures

Study: "Randomized controlled trial on lifestyle modification in hypertensive patients" (Cakir & Pinar, 2006)

Statement of Purpose: The purpose of this study was to test the effects of a comprehensive lifestyle modification intervention on blood pressure and other cardiovascular risk factors in hypertensive patients living in Istanbul, Turkey.

Design: A sample of 70 hypertensive patients were randomly assigned to a comprehensive lifestyle intervention group or to a control group. Participants in the intervention group participated in classes over a 3-month period at an outpatient hypertension clinic. Control group members were provided routine outpatient services. Data were collected at baseline and then 6 months later.

Data Collection: The primary outcome measure was systolic blood pressure (SBP). Additional outcomes included diastolic blood pressure, fasting lipids, obesity parameters, alcohol consumption, smoking, and stress management. Blood pressure measurements were done in an education room that was quiet and free from temperature extremes. Participants were seated in a chair with back supports and instructed to place their feet flat on the floor. They were also instructed to remove constricting clothing and to refrain from talking. Three blood pressure measurements were taken in a standardized manner at 2-minute intervals, and the average of the three was used in the data analysis. Fasting blood samples were obtained by venous puncture, and lipid measures (TC, HDL-C, LDL-C) were obtained. Body mass index (BMI) was calculated as weight (kg) divided by the square of height (m^2). Waist circumference was measured on the metric scale. Behavioral changes were measured by administering the Health Promoting Lifestyle Profile (HPLP) scale. The HPLP is a 48-item self-report scale that captures frequency of engaging in activities aimed at increasing health and well-being. Responses are scaled from 1 (*never*) to 4 (*routine*), with higher scores reflecting more frequent practice of health behaviors. The scale includes six subscales: self-realization, health responsibility, exercise, nutrition, interpersonal support, and stress management. Finally, incidences of alcohol consumption and smoking were obtained from a questionnaire and patient diaries.

Key Findings:
- At the end of 6 months, blood pressure, body weight, BMI, waist circumference, and fasting lipids (except HDL-C) significantly declined in the intervention group but not in the control group.
- There were also significant improvements in self-reported lifestyle behaviors as captured in the HPLP among those in the treatment group.

SUMMARY POINTS

- Structured methods of data collection involve placing constraints on both those collecting the data and those providing it.
- Structured self-report *instruments* (which include **interview schedules** or **question-naires**) may include open- or closed-ended questions. **Open-ended questions** permit respondents to reply in narrative fashion, whereas **closed-ended** (or **fixed-alternative**) **questions** offer response options from which respondents must choose.
- Types of closed-ended questions include (1) **dichotomous questions**, which require a choice between two options (e.g., yes/no); (2) **multiple-choice questions**, which offer a range of alternatives; (3) **cafeteria questions**, in which respondents are asked to select a statement best representing their view; (4) **rank-order questions**, in which respondents are asked to rank a list of alternatives along a continuum; (5) **forced-choice questions**, which require respondents to choose between two competing positions; (6) **rating questions**, which ask respondents to make judgments along an ordered, bipolar dimension; (7) **checklists** or **matrix questions**, in which several questions requiring the same response format are listed; and (8) **visual analogue scales** (VAS), which are continua used to measure subjective experiences such as pain. **Event history calendars** and diaries are used to capture information about the occurrence of events.

- Composite psychosocial **scales** are multiple-item self-report tools for measuring the degree to which individuals possess or are characterized by target traits or attributes.
- **Likert scales** comprise a series of statements worded favorably or unfavorably toward a phenomenon. Respondents indicate degree of agreement or disagreement with each statement; a total score is computed by the summing item scores, each of which is scored for the intensity and direction of favorability expressed. Likert scales are also called **summated rating scales**.
- **Semantic differentials** (SDs) consist of a series of bipolar rating scales on which respondents indicate their reaction toward some phenomenon; scales can measure an evaluative (e.g., good/bad), activity (e.g., active/passive), or potency (e.g., strong/weak) dimension.
- Various aspects of cognitive functioning can be measured by **cognitive tests**, including intelligence, aptitude, or neuropsychological functioning.
- **Q sorts**, in which people sort a set of card statements into piles according to specified criteria, can be used to measure attitudes, personality, and other psychological traits.
- **Vignettes** are brief descriptions of an event or situation to which respondents are asked to react. They are used to assess respondents' hypothetical behaviors, opinions, and perceptions.
- Questionnaires are less costly and time-consuming than interviews, offer the possibility of anonymity, and run no risk of interviewer bias; however, interviews tend to yield higher response rates, to be suitable for a wider variety of people, and to yield richer data than questionnaires.
- Data quality in interviews depends heavily on interviewers' interpersonal skills. Interviewers must put respondents at ease and build rapport with them, and need to be skillful at *probing* for additional information when respondents give incomplete or irrelevant responses.
- Group administration is the most convenient and economical way to distribute questionnaires.

Another approach is to mail them, but this method is plagued with the risk for low response rates, which can result in a biased sample. Questionnaires can also be distributed through the Internet, either by an e-mail attachment or as a **web-based survey** that participants access through a hypertext link and respond to directly. Internet surveys rarely yield representative samples because response rates are low and not everyone has access to computers.

- A number of techniques, such as the use of **follow-up reminders** and good **cover letters**, are designed to increase response rates.

- Structured self-reports are a valuable research tool but are vulnerable to the risk for reporting biases, which are often called **response set biases**. Such biases stem the tendency of some people to respond to questions in characteristic ways, independently of content.

- The **social desirability response bias** stems from a person's desire to appear in a favorable light. The **extreme response set** results when a person characteristically endorses extreme response alternatives. Another response bias is known as **acquiescence response set**, which is a **yea-sayer**'s tendency to agree with statements regardless of their content. A converse problem arises when people (**nay-sayers**) disagree with most statements.

- Structured observational methods impose constraints on observers to enhance the accuracy and objectivity of the observations and to obtain an adequate representation of the phenomena of interest.

- Researchers focus on different *units of observation*. The **molar approach** entails observations of large segments of behaviors as integral units; the **molecular approach** treats small, specific actions as separate entities.

- **Checklists** are tools for recording the occurrence or frequency of predesignated behaviors, events, or characteristics. Checklists are based on **category systems** for encoding observed phenomena into discrete categories. Some checklists categorize exhaustively all behaviors of a particular type (e.g., body movements) in an ongoing fashion, whereas others record particular behaviors while ignoring others.

- With **rating scales**, another record-keeping device for structured observations, observers are required to rate phenomena along a dimension that is typically bipolar (e.g., passive/aggressive); ratings are made either at specific intervals (e.g., every 15 minutes) or after observations are completed.

- Some structured observations use sampling to select behaviors or events to be observed. **Time sampling** involves the specification of the duration and frequency of both observational periods and intersession intervals. **Event sampling** selects integral behaviors or events of a special type for observation.

- Technological advances have greatly augmented researchers' capacity to collect, record, and preserve observational data. Such devices as audiotape recorders and videotape cameras permit behaviors and events to be described or categorized after their occurrence.

- Observational methods are an excellent method of operationalizing some constructs, but are subject to various biases. The greater the degree of observer inference, the more likely that perceptual errors and distortions will occur. The most prevalent observer biases include the **enhancement of contrast effect**, **central tendency bias**, the **halo effect**, **assimilatory biases**, **errors of leniency**, and **errors of severity**.

- For certain research problems, alternatives to self-report and observation—especially biophysiologic measures—may be appropriate data collection techniques. Biophysiologic measures can be classified as either *in vivo* **measurements** (those performed within or on living organisms, like blood pressure measurement) or *in vitro* **measurements** (those performed outside the organism's body, such as blood tests).

- Biophysiologic measures have the advantage of being objective, accurate, and precise, but care must be taken in using such measures with regard to practical, technical, and ethical considerations.

STUDY ACTIVITIES

Chapter 16 of the *Resource Manual to Accompany Nursing Research: Generating and Assessing Evidence for Nursing Practice, 8th edition*, offers various exercises and study suggestions for reinforcing concepts presented in this chapter. In addition, the following study questions can be addressed:

1. Voluntary nonemployment of nurses contributes to nursing shortages. Suppose you were planning to conduct a statewide study of the plans and intentions of nonemployed registered nurses in your state. Would you ask mostly open-ended or closed-ended questions? Would you adopt an interview or questionnaire approach? If a questionnaire, how would you distribute it?

2. Suppose that the study of nonemployed nurses were done by a mailed questionnaire. Draft a cover letter to accompany it.

3. A nurse researcher is planning to study temper tantrums displayed by hospitalized children. Would you recommend using a time sampling approach? Why or why not?

4. Use the critiquing guidelines in Box 16.4 to critique the data collection of the two studies used as research examples at the end of this chapter.

STUDIES CITED IN CHAPTER 16

Methodologic or theoretical references cited in this chapter can be found in a separate section at the end of the book.

Billinghurst, F., Morgan, B., & Arthur, H. M. (2003). Patient and nurse-related implications of remote cardiac telemetry. *Clinical Nursing Research, 12,* 356–370.

Cakir, H., & Pinar, R. (2006). Randomized trial on lifestyle modification in hypertensive patients. *Western Journal of Nursing Research, 28*(2), 190–209.

Chang, Y., Lin, Y., Chang, H., & Lin, C. (2005). Cancer patients and staff ratings of caring behaviors. *Cancer Nursing, 28*(5), 331–229.

Chertok, I., Schneider, J., & Blackburn, S. (2006). A pilot study of maternal and term infant outcomes associated with ultrathin nipple shield use. *Journal of Obstetric, Gynecologic, & Neonatal Nursing, 35*(2), 265–272.

Chin-Peuckert, L., Rennick, J. E., Jednak, R., Capolicchio, J., & Salle, J. L. (2004). Should warm infusion solution be used for urodynamic studies in children? A prospective randomized study. *Journal of Urology, 172,* 1657–1661.

Drummond, J., Fleming, D., McDonald, L., & Kysela, G. M. (2005). Randomized controlled trial of a family problem-solving intervention. *Clinical Nursing Research, 14,* 57–80.

Glesson-Kreig, J. M. (2006). Self-monitoring of physical activity: Effects of self-efficacy and behavior in people with type 2 diabetes. *Diabetes Educator, 32,* 69–77.

Graves, E., Ramsay, E., & McCarthy, D. (2006). Inhibitors of COX activity preserve muscle mass in mice bearing the Lewis lung carcinoma, but not the B16 melanoma. *Research in Nursing & Health, 29*(2), 87–97.

Gray, B. A. (2006). Hospitalization history and differences in self-rated pregnancy risk. *Western Journal of Nursing Research, 28*(2), 216–229.

Griffin, R., Polit, D., & Byrne, M. (in press). Stereotyping and nurses' recommendations for treating pain in hospitalized children. *Research in Nursing & Health, 30.*

Harrison, L., Roane, C., & Weaver, M. (2004). The relationship between physiological and behavioral measures of stress in preterm infants. *Journal of Obstetric, Gynecologic, & Neonatal Nursing, 33*(2), 236–245.

Herman, M. (2004). Neurocognitive functioning and quality of life among dually diagnosed and non-substance abusing schizophrenia inpatients. *International Journal of Mental Health Nursing, 13*(4), 282–291.

Holditch-Davis, D., Scher, M., Schwartz, R., & Hudson-Barr, D. (2004). Sleeping and waking state development in preterm infants. *Early Human Development, 80*(1), 43–64.

Insel, K. C., & Cole, L. (2005). Individualizing memory strategies to improve medication adherence. *Applied Nursing Research, 18*(4), 199–204.

Kim, C., Kang, D., Smith, B., & Landers, K. (2006). Cardiopulmonary responses and adherence to exercise in women newly diagnosed with breast cancer undergoing adjuvant therapy. *Cancer Nursing, 29*(2), 156–165.

Knue, M., Doellman, D., & Jacobs, B. (2006), Peripherally inserted central catheters in children: A survey of practice patterns. *Journal of Infusion Nursing, 29*(1), 28–34.

LaMar, K., & Dowling, D. A. (2006). Incidence of infection for preterm twins cared for in cobedding in the neonatal intensive care unit. *Journal of Obstetric, Gynecologic, & Neonatal Nursing, 35*(2), 193–198.

Lehoux, P., Richard, L., Pineault, R., & Saint-Arnaud, J. (2006). Delivery of high-tech home care by hospital-based nursing units in Quebec. *Canadian Journal of Nursing Leadership, 19*(1), 44–55.

Liehr, P., Meininger, J., Vogler, R., Chan, W., Frazier, L., Smalling, S., & Fuentes, F. (2006). Adding story-centered care to standard care lifestyle intervention for people with stage 1 hypertension. *Applied Nursing Research, 19*(1), 16–21.

Mantler, J., Armstrong-Stassen, M., Horsbaugh, M., & Cameron, S. (2006). Reactions of hospital staff nurses to recruitment incentives. *Western Journal of Nursing Research, 28*(1), 70–84.

McGuinness, T., Ryan, R., & Robinson, C. (2005). Protective influences of families for children adopted from the former Soviet Union. *Journal of Nursing Scholarship, 37*(3), 216–221.

Meynell, J., & Barroso, J. (2005). Bioimpedance analysis and HIV-related fatigue. *Journal of the Association of Nurses in AIDS Care, 16*(2), 13–22.

Miketova, P., Kaemingk, K., Hockenberry, M., Pasvogel, A., Hutter, J., Krull, K., & Moore, I. (2005). Oxidative changes in cerebral spinal fluid phosphatidylcholine during treatment for acute lymphoblastic leukemia. *Biological Research for Nursing, 6*(3), 187–195.

Miller, J., Campbell, J., Moore, K., & Schofield, A. (2004). Elder care supportive intervention protocol: Reducing discomfort in confused, hospitalized older adults. *Journal of Gerontological Nursing, 30*(8), 10–18.

Polit, D. F., London, A. S., & Martinez, J. M. (2001). *The health of poor urban women.* New York: MDRC.

Rempusheski, V. F., & O'Hara, C. (2005). Psychometric properties of the Grandparent Perceptions of Family Scale (GPFS). *Nursing Research, 54*(6), 419–427.

Samselle, C., Miller, J., Leucha, Y., Fischer, K., & Rosten, L. (2005). Provider support of spontaneous pushing during second stage labor. *Journal of Obstetric, Gynecologic, & Neonatal Nursing, 34*(6), 695–702.

Walker, C. D., Kudreikis, K., Sherrard, A., & Johnston, C. C. (2003). Repeated neonatal pain influences maternal behavior, but not stress responsiveness in rat offspring. *Developmental Brain Research, 140,* 253–261.

Weiss, S. J. (1992). Measurement of the sensory qualities in tactile interaction. *Nursing Research, 41,* 82–86.

White-Traut, R., Berbaum, M., Lessen, B., McFarlin, B., & Cardenas, L. (2005). Feeding readiness in preterm infants. *MCN: The American Journal of Maternal/Child Nursing, 30*(1), 52–59.

Williams. K. N., (2006). Improving outcomes of nursing home interactions. *Research in Nursing & Health, 29*(2), 121–133.

Yetter-Read, C. (2004). Conducting a client-focused survey using e-mail. *Computers, Informatics, Nursing, 22*(2), 83–89.

17

Assessing Measurement Quality in Quantitative Studies

A n ideal data collection procedure is one that captures a construct in a way that is relevant, accurate, truthful, and sensitive. For most concepts of interest to nurse researchers, there are few data collection procedures that match this ideal. Biophysiologic methods have a higher chance of success in attaining these goals than self-report or observational methods, but no method is flawless. In this chapter, we discuss criteria for evaluating the quality of data obtained with structured instruments. We begin by discussing principles of measurement. Our discussion is, for the most part, based on **classical measurement theory (CMT)**, which has predominated views with regard to the measurement of affective measures (i.e., psychosocial constructs such as social support or depression). An alternative measurement theory (item response theory, or IRT) is gaining in popularity, especially for the measurement of cognitive constructs (e.g., achievement or ability). We discuss IRT briefly in Chapter 18.

MEASUREMENT

Quantitative studies derive data through the measurement of variables. **Measurement** involves the assignment of numbers to represent the amount of an attribute present in an object or person, using a specified set of rules. As this definition implies, quantification and measurement go hand in hand. A famous quote by early American psychologist L. L. Thurstone states a fundamental position: "Whatever exists, exists in some amount and can be measured." Attributes are not constant: They vary from day to day, from situation to situation, or from one person to another. This variability is presumed to be capable of a numeric expression that signifies *how much* of an attribute is present. The purpose of assigning numbers is to differentiate between people or objects that possess varying degrees of the critical attribute.

Rules and Measurement

Measurement involves assigning numbers to objects according to rules, rather than haphazardly. Rules for measuring temperature, weight, blood pressure, and other physical attributes are familiar to us. Rules for measuring many variables for nursing research studies, however, have to be invented. Whether the data are collected by observation, self-report, or some other method, researchers must specify criteria for assigning the numeric values to the characteristic of interest.

As an example, suppose we were studying attitudes toward distributing condoms in school clinics

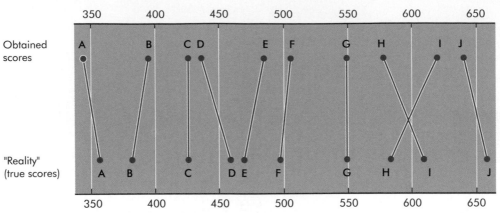

FIGURE 17.1 Relationship between obtained and true scores for a hypothetical set of test scores.

and asked parents to express their extent of agreement with the following statement:

Teenagers should have access to contraceptives in school clinics.
- ❏ Strongly disagree
- ❏ Disagree
- ❏ Slightly disagree
- ❏ Neither agree nor disagree
- ❏ Slightly agree
- ❏ Agree
- ❏ Strongly agree

Responses to this question can be quantified by developing a system for assigning numbers to them. Note that *any* rule would satisfy the definition of measurement. We could assign the value of 30 to "strongly agree," 27 to "agree," 20 to "slightly agree," and so on, but there is no justification for doing so. In measuring attributes, researchers strive to use good, meaningful rules. Without any *a priori* information about the "distance" between the options, the most practical approach is to assign a 7 to "strongly agree" and a 1 to "strongly disagree." This rule would quantitatively differentiate, in increments of one point, among people with seven different opinions about the statement. With a new instrument, researchers seldom know in advance if their rules are the best possible. New measurement rules reflect researchers' hypotheses about how attributes function and vary. The adequacy of the hypotheses—that is, the worth of the instruments—needs to be assessed empirically.

Researchers endeavor to link numeric values to reality. To state this goal more technically, measurement procedures should be isomorphic to reality. The term *isomorphism* signifies equivalence or similarity between two phenomena. An instrument cannot be useful unless the measures resulting from it correspond with the real world.

To illustrate the concept of isomorphism, suppose a standardized test was administered to 10 students, who obtained the following scores: 345, 395, 430, 435, 490, 505, 550, 570, 620, and 640. These values are shown at the top of Figure 17.1. Now suppose that in reality the true scores of these students on a hypothetically perfect test were as follows: 360, 375, 430, 465, 470, 500, 550, 610, 590, and 670, as shown at the bottom of Figure 17.1. This figure shows that, although not perfect, the test came fairly close to representing true scores; only two people (H and I) were improperly ordered. This example illustrates a measure whose isomorphism with reality is high, but improvable.

Researchers almost always work with fallible measures. Instruments that measure psychological phenomena are less likely to correspond to reality than physical measures, but few instruments are error free.

Advantages of Measurement

What exactly does measurement accomplish? Consider how handicapped health care professionals would be in the absence of measurement. What would happen, for example, if there were no measures of body temperature or blood pressure? Subjective evaluations of clinical outcomes would have to be used. A principal strength of measurement is that it removes subjectivity and guesswork. Because measurement is based on explicit rules, resulting information tends to be objective, that is, it can be independently verified. Two people measuring the weight of a person using the same scale would likely get identical results. Not all measures are completely objective, but most incorporate mechanisms for minimizing subjectivity.

Measurement also makes it possible to obtain reasonably precise information. Instead of describing Nathan as "rather tall," we can depict him as being 6 feet, 3 inches tall. If we chose, we could obtain even greater precision. With precise measures, researchers can more readily differentiate among people with different degrees of an attribute.

Finally, measurement is a language of communication. Numbers are less vague than words and therefore can communicate information more accurately. If a researcher reported that the average oral temperature of a sample of patients was "somewhat high," different readers might develop different conceptions about the sample's physiologic state. However, if the researcher reported an average temperature of 99.6°F, there would be no ambiguity.

Errors of Measurement

Both the procedures involved in applying measurements and the objects being measured are susceptible to influences that can alter the resulting data. Some influences can be controlled to a certain degree, and attempts should always be made to do so, but such efforts are rarely completely successful.

Instruments that are not perfectly accurate yield measurements containing some error. Within classical measurement theory, any **observed** (or **obtained**) **score** can be decomposed conceptually into two parts—an error component and a true component. This can be written symbolically as follows:

Obtained score = true score ± error

or

$$X_O = X_T \pm X_E$$

The first term in the equation is an observed score—for example, a systolic blood pressure reading or a score on an anxiety scale. X_T is the value that would be obtained with an infallible measure. The **true score** is hypothetical—it can never be known because measures are *not* infallible. The final term in the equation is the **error of measurement**. The difference between true and obtained scores is the result of factors that distort the measurement.

Decomposing obtained scores in this fashion highlights an important point. When researchers measure an attribute, they are also *measuring attributes* that are not of interest. The true score component is what they hope to isolate; the error component is a composite of other factors that are also being measured, contrary to their wishes. This concept can be illustrated with an exaggerated example. Suppose a researcher measured the weight of 10 people on a spring scale. As subjects step on the scale, the researcher places a hand on their shoulders and applies some pressure. The resulting measures (the X_Os) will be biased upward because the scores reflect both actual weight (X_T) and the researcher's pressure (X_E). Errors of measurement are problematic because their value is unknown and also because they often are variable. In this example, the amount of pressure applied likely would vary from one subject to the next. In other words, the proportion of true score component in an obtained score varies from one person to the next.

Many factors contribute to errors of measurement. Some errors are random or variable, whereas others are systematic, which represent *bias*. The most common influences on measurement error are the following:

1. *Situational contaminants.* Scores can be affected by the conditions under which they are produced. A participant's awareness of an observer's presence (reactivity) is one source

of bias. The anonymity of the response situation, the friendliness of researchers, or the location of the data gathering can affect participants' responses. Other environmental factors, such as temperature, lighting, and time of day, can represent sources of measurement error.

2. *Transitory personal factors*. A person's score can be influenced by such temporary personal states as fatigue, hunger, anxiety, or mood. In some cases, such factors directly affect the measurement, as when anxiety affects a pulse rate measurement. In other cases, personal factors can alter scores by influencing people's motivation to cooperate, act naturally, or do their best.

3. *Response-set biases*. Relatively enduring characteristics of respondents can interfere with accurate measures. Response sets such as social desirability, acquiescence, and extreme responses are potential problems in self-report measures, particularly in psychological scales (see Chapter 16).

4. *Administration variations*. Alterations in the methods of collecting data from one person to the next can result in score variations unrelated to variations in the target attribute. If observers alter their coding categories, if interviewers improvise question wording, if test administrators change the test instructions, or if some physiologic measures are taken before a feeding and others are taken after a feeding, then measurement errors can potentially occur.

5. *Instrument clarity*. If the directions for obtaining measures are poorly understood, then scores may be affected by misunderstanding. For example, questions in a self-report instrument may be interpreted differently by different respondents, leading to a distorted measure of the variable. Observers may miscategorize observations if the classification scheme is unclear.

6. *Item sampling*. Errors can be introduced as a result of the sampling of items used in the measure. For example, a nursing student's score on a 100-item test of nursing knowledge will be influenced somewhat by *which* 100 questions are included. A person might get 95 questions correct on one test but only 92 right on another similar test.

7. *Instrument format*. Technical characteristics of an instrument can influence measurements. Open-ended questions may yield different information than closed-ended ones. Oral responses to a question may be at odds with written responses to the same question. The ordering of questions in an instrument may also influence responses.

The Toolkit for Chapter 17 of the *Resource Manual* includes a list of suggestions for enhancing data quality and minimizing measurement error in quantitative studies. ✪

RELIABILITY OF MEASURING INSTRUMENTS

The reliability of a quantitative instrument is a major criterion for assessing its quality and adequacy. An instrument's **reliability** is the consistency with which it measures the target attribute. If a scale weighed a person at 120 pounds one minute and 150 pounds the next, we would consider it unreliable. The less variation an instrument produces in repeated measurements, the higher its reliability. Thus, reliability can be equated with a measure's stability, consistency, or dependability.

Reliability also concerns a measure's accuracy. An instrument is reliable to the extent that its measures reflect true scores—that is, to the extent that measurement errors are absent from obtained scores. A reliable measure maximizes the true score component and minimizes the error component.

These two ways of explaining reliability (consistency and accuracy) are not so different as they might appear. Errors of measurement that impinge on an instrument's accuracy also affect its consistency. The example of the scale with variable weight readings illustrates this point. Suppose that the true weight of a person is 125 pounds, but that two independent measurements yielded 120 and 150 pounds. In terms of the equation presented in the previous section, we could express the measurements as follows:

$$120 = 125 - 5$$
$$150 = 125 + 25$$

The errors of measurement for the two trials (-5 and $+25$, respectively) resulted in scores that are inconsistent *and* inaccurate.

The reliability of an instrument can be assessed in various ways, and the appropriate method depends on the nature of the instrument and on the aspect of reliability of greatest concern. Three key aspects are stability, internal consistency, and equivalence.

Stability

The **stability** of an instrument is the extent to which similar results are obtained on two separate occasions. The reliability estimate focuses on the instrument's susceptibility to extraneous influences over time, such as participant fatigue.

Assessments of an instrument's stability involve procedures that evaluate **test–retest reliability**. Researchers administer the same measure to a sample twice and then compare the scores. The comparison is performed objectively by computing a **reliability coefficient**, which is an index of the magnitude of the test's reliability.

To explain reliability coefficients, we must briefly discuss a statistic called the **correlation coefficient**. We have pointed out repeatedly that researchers strive to detect and explain relationships among phenomena. For example, is there a relationship between patients' gastric acidity levels and level of stress experienced? The correlation coefficient is a tool for quantitatively describing the magnitude and direction of a relationship between two variables. The computation of this index does not concern us here. It is more important to understand how to read a correlation coefficient.

Two variables that are obviously related are people's height and weight. Tall people tend to be heavier than short people. We would say that there was a **perfect relationship** if the tallest person in a population were the heaviest, the second tallest person

were the second heaviest, and so forth. Correlation coefficients summarize how perfect relationships are. The possible values for a correlation coefficient range from -1.00 through $.00$ to $+1.00$. If height and weight were perfectly correlated, the correlation coefficient expressing this relationship would be 1.00. Because the relationship exists but is not perfect, the correlation coefficient is typically in the vicinity of .50 or .60. The relationship between height and weight can be described as a **positive relationship** because increases in height tend to be associated with increases in weight.

When two variables are totally unrelated, the correlation coefficient equals zero. One might expect that women's dress sizes are unrelated to their intelligence. Large women are as likely to perform well on I.Q. tests as small women. The correlation coefficient summarizing such a relationship would presumably be in the vicinity of .00.

Correlation coefficients running from .00 to -1.00 express **inverse** or **negative relationships**. When two variables are inversely related, increases in one variable are associated with *decreases* in the second variable. Suppose that there is an inverse relationship between people's age and the amount of sleep they get. This means that, on average, the older the person, the fewer the hours of sleep. If the relationship were perfect (e.g., if the oldest person in a population got the least sleep, and so on), the correlation coefficient would be -1.00. In actuality, the relationship between age and sleep is probably modest—in the vicinity of $-.15$ or $-.20$. A correlation coefficient of this magnitude describes a weak relationship wherein older people *tend* to sleep fewer hours and younger people tend to sleep more, but nevertheless some younger people sleep few hours, and some older people sleep a lot.

Now we can discuss the use of correlation coefficients to compute reliability estimates. With test–retest reliability, an instrument is administered twice to the same people. Suppose we wanted to assess the stability of a self-esteem scale. Self-esteem is a fairly stable attribute that does not fluctuate much from day to day, so we would expect a reliable measure of it to yield consistent scores on two occasions. To check the instrument's stability,

| TABLE 17.1 | Fictitious Data for Test-Retest Reliability of Self-Esteem Scale | |

SUBJECT NUMBER	TIME 1	TIME 2
1	55	57
2	49	46
3	78	74
4	37	35
5	44	46
6	50	56
7	58	55
8	62	66
9	48	50
10	67	63 $r = .95$

we administer the scale 2 weeks apart to 10 people. Fictitious data for this example are presented in Table 17.1. It can be seen that, in general, differences in scores on the two testings are not large. The reliability coefficient for test–retest estimates is the correlation coefficient between the two sets of scores. In this example, the computed reliability coefficient is .95, which is high.

The value of the reliability coefficient theoretically can range between −1.00 and +1.00, like other correlation coefficients. A negative coefficient would have been obtained in our example if those with high self-esteem scores at time 1 had low scores at time 2, and *vice versa*. In practice, reliability coefficients normally range between .00 and 1.00. The higher the coefficient, the more stable the measure. Reliability coefficients above .80 usually are considered good. In some situations, a higher coefficient may be required, or a lower one may be acceptable.

The test–retest method is a relatively easy approach to estimating reliability, and can be used with self-report, observational, and physiologic measures. The test–retest approach has certain disadvantages, however. One issue is that many traits *do* change over time, independently of the measure's stability. Attitudes, behaviors, knowledge, physical

condition, and so forth can be modified by experiences between testings. Test–retest procedures confound changes from measurement error and those from true changes in the attribute being measured. Still, there are many relatively enduring attributes for which a test–retest approach is suitable.

Stability estimates suffer from other problems, however. One possibility is that people's responses (or observers' coding) on the second administration will be influenced by their memory of initial responses, regardless of the actual values the second day. Such memory interference results in spuriously high reliability coefficients. Another difficulty is that people may actually change *as a result of* the first administration. Finally, people may not be as careful using the same instrument a second time. If they find the process boring on the second occasion, then responses could be haphazard, resulting in a spuriously low estimate of stability.

On the whole, reliability coefficients tend to be higher for short-term retests than for long-term retests (i.e., those greater than 1 or 2 months), because of actual changes in the attribute being measured. Stability indexes are most appropriate for relatively enduring characteristics such as personality, abilities, or certain physical attributes such as adult height.

Even though most test–retest efforts involve the calculation of a standard correlation coefficient, as just described, other methods are sometimes used. For example, Yen and Lo (2002) describe how an *intraclass correlation* approach offers advantages because of the ability of this index to detect systematic error.

Example of test–retest reliability: Welch and colleagues (2006) developed the Beliefs About Dietary Compliance Scale to measure perceived benefits and barriers to limiting dietary sodium. The 1-week test–retest reliability was .68 for the "Benefits" subscale and .86 for the "Barriers" subscale.

Internal Consistency

Scales and tests that involve summing item scores are almost always evaluated for their internal consistency. Scales designed to measure an attribute ideally are composed of items that measure that attribute and nothing else. On a scale to measure nurses' empathy, it would be inappropriate to include an item that measures diagnostic competence. An instrument may be said to be **internally consistent** or *homogeneous* to the extent that its items measure the same trait.

Internal consistency reliability is the most widely used reliability approach among nurse researchers. Its popularity reflects the fact that it is economical (it requires only one test administration) and is the best means of assessing an especially important source of measurement error in psychosocial instruments, the sampling of items.

◐ **T I P :** Many scales contain multiple subscales or subtests, each of which tap distinct, but related, concepts (e.g., a measure of independent functioning might include subscales for motor activities, communication, and socializing). The internal consistency of *each* subscale is typically assessed and, if subscale scores are summed for an overall score, the scale's internal consistency is also assessed.

The most widely used method for evaluating internal consistency is **coefficient alpha** (or **Cronbach's alpha**). Coefficient alpha can be interpreted like other reliability coefficients described here; the normal range of values is between .00 and +1.00, and higher values reflect a higher internal consistency. It is beyond the scope of this text to explain this method in detail, but more information is available in textbooks on psychometrics (e.g., Nunnally & Bernstein, 1994; Waltz, Strickland, & Lenz, 2005). Most statistical software can be used to calculate alpha. The research example at the end of Chapter 18 presents some output for a reliability analysis.

In summary, coefficient alpha is usually used as an index of internal consistency to estimate the extent to which different subparts of an instrument (i.e., items) are reliably measuring the critical attribute. Cronbach's alpha does not, however, evaluate fluctuations over time as a source of unreliability.

Example of internal consistency reliability:
Wu, Larrabee, and Putman (2006) conducted a psychometric study involving a shortened version of the Caring Behavior Inventory. The 24-item short form had high internal consistency ($\alpha = .96$), with alphas for the four subscales ranging from .83 to .98.

Equivalence

Equivalence, in the context of reliability assessment, primarily concerns the degree to which two or more independent observers or coders agree about the scoring on an instrument. If there is a high level of agreement, then the assumption is that measurement errors have been minimized. Nurse researchers are especially likely to use this approach with observational measures, although it can be used in other applications—for example, for evaluating the consistency of coding open-ended questions or the accuracy of extracting data from records onto a form.

The reliability of ratings and classifications can be enhanced by careful training and the specification of clearly defined, nonoverlapping categories. Even when such care is taken, researchers should assess the reliability of observational instruments and coding systems. In this case, "instrument" includes both the category or rating system *and* the observers or coders making the measurements.

Interrater (or *interobserver*) **reliability** can be assessed using a variety of approaches, which can be categorized as consensus, consistency, and measurement approaches (Stemler, 2004). Many of the indexes of interrater reliability used by nurse researchers are of the consensus type, which are based on the assumption that the goal is to have observers share a common interpretation of the construct under observation, and to reach consensus (exact agreement). Consensus measures of interrater reliability for observational coding involve having two or more trained observers watching an event simultaneously, and independently recording data according to the instrument's instructions. The data can then be used to compute an index of agreement between observers. (For coders, information would be independently coded into categories and then intercoder agreement would be assessed.) When ratings are dichotomous, one procedure is to calculate the proportion of agreements, using the following equation:

$$\frac{\text{Number of agreement}}{\text{Number of agreement} + \text{disagreements}}$$

This simple formula unfortunately tends to overestimate agreements because it fails to account for agreement by chance. If a behavior being observed were coded for absence versus presence, the observers would agree 50% of the time by chance alone. The most widely used statistic in this situation is Cohen's **kappa** (Cohen, 1960), which adjusts for chance agreements. **Multirater kappa** (Fleiss, 1971) can be used when more than two raters are independently rating the same thing. Different standards have been proposed for acceptable levels of kappa, but there is some agreement that a value of .60 is minimally acceptable, and that values of .75 and higher are excellent. Numerous other measures of interrater agreement have been developed for situations in which there are two or more raters and two or more rating categories (see, for example, Lindell & Brandt, 1999).

For certain types of data (e.g., ratings on a multipoint scale), correlation techniques are suitable, and these typically capture consistency rather than consensus. For example, a correlation coefficient can be computed to demonstrate the strength of the relationship between one rater's scores and another's. An index known as the **intraclass correlation coefficient** can also be used to assess interrater reliability (Shrout & Fleiss, 1979).

> **Example of interrater reliability:** Immers, Schuurmans, and van de Bijl (2005) assessed interrater reliability for measuring *confusion* using the observational NEECHAM scale. A total of 39 ratings by ICU nurses were compared with ratings by one of the researchers. The computed value of Cohen's kappa was .60.

Interpretation of Reliability Coefficients

Reliability coefficients are important indicators of an instrument's quality. Unreliable measures reduce statistical power and hence affect statistical conclusion validity. If data fail to support a hypothesis, one possibility is that the instruments were unreliable—not necessarily that the expected relationships do not exist. Knowledge about an instrument's reliability thus is critical in interpreting research results, especially if research hypotheses are not supported.

For group-level comparisons, coefficients in the vicinity of .70 may be adequate (especially at the subscale level), but coefficients of .80 or greater are highly desirable. By group-level comparisons, we mean that researchers compare scores of groups, such as male versus female or experimental versus control subjects. If measures are used for making decisions about individuals, then reliability coefficients ideally should be .90 or better. For instance, if a test score was used as a criterion for admission to a graduate nursing program, then the accuracy of the test would be of critical importance to both individual applicants and the school of nursing.

Reliability coefficients have a special interpretation that should be briefly explained without elaborating on technical details. This interpretation relates to the earlier discussion of decomposing observed scores into error components and true components. Suppose we administered a scale that measures hope to 50 cancer patients. It would be expected that the scores would vary from one person to another—that is, some people would be more hopeful than others. Some variability in scores is true variability, reflecting real individual differences in hopefulness; some variability, however, is error. Thus,

$$V_O = V_T + V_E$$

where V_O = observed total variability in scores
V_T = true variability
V_E = variability owing to errors

A reliability coefficient is directly associated with this equation. *Reliability is the proportion of true variability to the total obtained variability,* or

$$r = \frac{V_T}{V_O}$$

If, for example, the reliability coefficient were .85, then 85% of the variability in obtained scores would represent true individual differences, and 15% of the variability would reflect extraneous fluctuations. Looked at in this way, it should be clearer why instruments with reliability lower than .70 are risky to use.

Factors Affecting Reliability

Various things affect an instrument's reliability, and these factors are useful to keep in mind in developing an instrument or selecting one for use. First, the reliability of composite self-report and observational scales is partly a function of their length (i.e., number of items). To improve reliability, more items tapping the same concept should be added. Items that have no discriminating power (i.e., that elicit similar responses from everyone) should, however, be removed. Item analysis procedures for guiding decisions about item retention, modification, or deletion are outlined in Chapter 18.

With observational scales, reliability can usually be improved by greater precision in defining categories, or greater clarity in explaining the underlying dimension for rating scales. The most effective means of enhancing reliability in observational studies, however, is thorough training of observers.

The reliability of an instrument is related in part to the heterogeneity of the sample with which it is used. The more homogeneous the sample (i.e., the more similar their scores), the lower the reliability coefficient will be. This is because instruments are designed to measure differences among those being measured. If the sample is homogeneous, then it is more difficult for the instrument to discriminate reliably among those who possess varying degrees of the attribute being measured. For example, a depression scale will be less reliable when administered to a homeless sample than when it is used with a general population.

Choosing an instrument previously demonstrated to be reliable is no guarantee of its high quality in a new study. An instrument's reliability is not a fixed entity. *The reliability of an instrument is a property not of the instrument but rather of the instrument when administered to a certain sample under certain conditions.* A scale that reliably

measures dependence in hospitalized adults may be unreliable with nursing homes residents. This means that in selecting an instrument, it is important to know the characteristics of the group with whom it was developed. If the group is similar to the population for a new study, then the reliability estimate provided by the scale developer is probably a reasonably good index of the instrument's accuracy in the new study.

➲ TIP: You should not be satisfied with an instrument that will *probably* be reliable in your study. The recommended procedure is to compute new estimates of reliability whenever research data are collected. For physiologic measures that are relatively impervious to fluctuations from personal or situational factors, this procedure may be unnecessary. However, observational tools, self-report measures, and tests of knowledge—all of which are susceptible to measurement errors—should be subjected to a reliability check as a routine step in the research process.

Finally, reliability estimates vary according to the procedures used to obtain them. A scale's test–retest reliability is rarely the same value as its internal consistency reliability. In selecting an instrument, researchers need to determine which aspect of reliability (stability, internal consistency, or equivalence) is most relevant.

Example of different reliability estimates: Gulick (2003) adapted the Postpartum Support Questionnaire (PSQ) for use with mothers with multiple sclerosis. She evaluated the adapted scale using both test–retest and internal consistency approaches. As an example of her findings, the coefficient alphas for the Emotional Support subscale were .90 and .91 at 1 and 3 months postpartum, respectively. The subscale's test–retest reliability over this 2-month period was .68.

VALIDITY

The second important criterion for evaluating a quantitative instrument is its validity. **Validity** is the degree to which an instrument measures what it is supposed to measure. When researchers develop an instrument to measure hopelessness, how can they be sure that resulting scores validly reflect this construct and not something else, like depression?

Reliability and validity are not independent qualities of an instrument. *A measuring device that is unreliable cannot possibly be valid.* An instrument cannot validly measure an attribute if it is inconsistent and inaccurate. An unreliable instrument contains too much error to be a valid indicator of the target variable. An instrument can, however, be reliable without being valid. Suppose we had the idea to assess patients' anxiety by measuring the circumference of their wrists. We could obtain highly accurate, consistent, and precise measurements of wrist circumferences, but such measures would not be valid indicators of anxiety. Thus, the high reliability of an instrument provides no evidence of its validity; low reliability of a measure *is* evidence of low validity.

Like reliability, validity has different aspects and assessment approaches. Unlike reliability, however, an instrument's validity is difficult to establish. There are no equations that can easily be applied to the scores of a hopelessness scale to estimate how good a job the scale is doing in measuring the critical variable. Validation efforts should be viewed as evidence-gathering enterprises, in which the goal is to assemble sufficient evidence from which validity can be inferred. Thus, the more evidence gathered, using various methods to assess validity, the stronger the inference.

➲ **TIP:** Instrument developers usually gather evidence of the validity and reliability of their instruments in a thorough **psychometric assessment** before making the instruments available for general use. If you use an existing instrument, choose one with demonstrated high reliability and validity. If you select an instrument for which there is no published psychometric information, try contacting the instrument developer and ask about its psychometric properties.

Face Validity

Face validity refers to whether the instrument *looks* as though it is measuring the appropriate construct. Although face validity should not be considered strong evidence for an instrument's validity, it is helpful for a measure to have face validity if other types of validity have also been demonstrated. For example, it might be easier to persuade people to participate in a study if the instruments being used have face validity.

Example of face validity: McDowell and colleagues (2005) adapted the 20-item Diabetes Management Self-Efficacy Scale for use with Australian populations. Face validity was established through consultation with diabetes educators and people with type 2 diabetes.

Content Validity

Content validity concerns the degree to which an instrument has an appropriate sample of items for the construct being measured and adequately covers the construct domain. Content validity is relevant for both affective measures (i.e., measures relating to feelings, emotions, and psychological traits) and cognitive measures.

For cognitive measures, the content validity question is, How representative are the questions on this test of the universe of questions on this topic? For example, suppose we were testing students' knowledge about major nursing theories. The test would not be content valid if it omitted questions about, for example, Orem's self-care theory.

Content validity is also relevant in the development of affective measures, as we discuss at some length in the next chapter. Researchers designing a new instrument should begin with a thorough conceptualization of the construct so that the instrument can capture the full content domain. Such a conceptualization might come from a variety of sources, including rich first-hand knowledge, an exhaustive literature review, consultation with experts, or findings from a qualitative inquiry.

Example of using qualitative data to enhance content validity: McSweeney and colleagues (2004) developed the McSweeney Acute and Prodromal Myocardial Infarction Symptom Survey, an instrument specifically designed to detect early symptoms of MI in women. The list of symptoms for the instrument was derived from two in-depth studies, the first with 20 women who had experienced an MI, and the second involving two interviews with 40 additional women shortly after an MI experience.

An instrument's content validity is necessarily based on judgment. There are no completely objective methods of ensuring the adequate content coverage of an instrument. However, it is becoming increasingly common to use a panel of substantive experts to evaluate and document the content validity of new instruments.

There are various approaches to assessing content validity using an expert panel, but nurse researchers have been in the forefront of developing an approach that involves the calculation of a **content validity index (CVI).** The experts are asked to evaluate individual items on the new measure as well as the overall instrument. Two key issues in such an evaluation are whether individual items are relevant and appropriate in terms of the construct, and whether the items adequately measure all dimensions of the construct.

At the item level, a common procedure is to have experts rate items on a 4-point scale of relevance. Although there are several variations of labeling the 4 ordinal points, the scale that seems to be used most often (e.g., Davis, 1992) is as follows: 1 = not relevant, 2 = somewhat relevant, 3 = quite relevant, 4 = highly relevant. Then, for each item, the item CVI (I-CVI) is computed as the number of raters giving a rating of either 3 or 4, divided by the number of experts—that is, the proportion in agreement about relevance. For example, an item rated as "quite" or "highly" relevant by 4 out of 5 judges would have an I-CVI of .80, which is considered an acceptable value.

There have been two approaches to calculating scale-level CVIs (S-CVIs), and unfortunately instrument development papers almost never indicate which approach was used (Polit & Beck, 2006). One approach is to calculate the percentage of items on the scale for which *all* judges agreed on content validity. In other words, if a 10-item scale had 6 items for which the I-CVIs were 1.00, then

the S-CVI would be .60. We call this method the S-CVI/UA (universal agreement) approach. Because disagreements (as well as agreements) can occur by chance, and because disagreements could reflect expert bias or misunderstandings, we find this approach too stringent.

A second approach is to compute the S-CVI by averaging the I-CVIs. We recommend this averaging approach, which we refer to as S-CVI/Ave, and also suggest a value of .90 as the standard for establishing excellent content validity (Polit & Beck, 2006). Validation of a scale should be done with a minimum of three experts, but a larger group is preferable. Further guidance is offered in Chapter 18.

> **Example of using a content validity index:**
> Lindgren (2005) described the development and testing of the Health Practices in Pregnancy Questionnaire. The content validity of this 18 item scale was rated by three nurse experts. The S-CVI, using the averaging approach, was calculated to be .83.

Criterion-Related Validity

Establishing **criterion-related validity** involves determining the relationship between an instrument and an external criterion. The instrument is said to be valid if its scores correlate highly with scores on the criterion. For example, if a measure of attitudes toward premarital sex correlates highly with subsequent loss of virginity in a sample of teenagers, then the attitude scale would have good validity. For criterion-related validity, the key issue is whether the instrument is a useful predictor of other behaviors, experiences, or conditions.

One requirement of this approach is the availability of a reliable and valid criterion with which measures on the instrument can be compared. This is, unfortunately, seldom easy. If we were developing an instrument to measure the nursing effectiveness of nursing students, we might use supervisory ratings as our criterion—but can we be sure that these ratings are valid and reliable? The ratings might themselves need validation. Criterion-related validity is most appropriate when there is a concrete, reliable criterion. For example, a scale to

TABLE 17.2	Fictitious Data for Criterion-Related Validity Example

SUBJECT	SCORE ON PROFESSIONALISM SCALE	NUMBER OF PUBLICATIONS
1	25	2
2	30	4
3	17	0
4	20	1
5	22	0
6	27	2
7	29	5
8	19	1
9	28	3
10	15	1

$r = .83$

measure smokers' motivation to quit smoking has a clearcut, objective criterion (subsequent smoking).

Once a criterion is selected, criterion validity can be assessed easily. A correlation coefficient is computed between scores on the instrument and the criterion. The magnitude of the coefficient (the validity coefficient) is a direct estimate of how valid the instrument is, according to this validation method. To illustrate, suppose we developed a scale to measure nurses' professionalism. We administer the instrument to a sample of nurses and also ask the nurses to indicate how many articles they have published. The publications variable was chosen as one of many potential objective criteria of professionalism. Fictitious data are presented in Table 17.2. The correlation coefficient of .83 indicates that the professionalism scale correlates fairly well with the number of published articles. Whether the scale is really measuring professionalism is a different issue—an issue that is the concern of construct validation discussed in the next section.

A distinction is sometimes made between two types of criterion-related validity. **Predictive validity** refers to the adequacy of an instrument in differentiating between people's performance on some future criterion. When a school of nursing correlates incoming students' high school grades with subsequent grade-point averages, the predictive validity of the high school grades for nursing school performance is being evaluated.

Example of predictive validity: Perraud and co-researchers (2006) developed a scale—the Depression Coping Self-Efficacy Scale—to measure depressed individuals' confidence in their ability to follow treatment recommendations. Scale scores at discharge from a psychiatric hospital were found to be predictive of rehospitalization 6 to 8 weeks later.

Concurrent validity refers to an instrument's ability to distinguish individuals who differ on a present criterion. For example, a psychological test to differentiate between those patients in a mental institution who can and cannot be released could be correlated with current behavioral ratings of health care personnel. The difference between predictive and concurrent validity, then, is the difference in the timing of obtaining measurements on a criterion.

Example of concurrent validity: Warms and Belza (2004) assessed the concurrent validity of using "actigraphy" as an approach to measuring physical activity for wheelchair users with spinal cord injury. Activity counts by actigraphy were correlated with the patients' self-reported activity intensity.

Validation by means of the criterion-related approach is most often used in applied or practically oriented research. Criterion-related validity is helpful in assisting decision makers by giving them some assurance that their decisions will be effective, fair, and, in short, valid.

Construct Validity

As discussed in Chapter 11, **construct validity** is a key criterion for assessing the quality of a study, and construct validity has most often been addressed in terms of measurement issues. As noted earlier, construct validity concerns inferences from the particulars of the study (in this case, the measures used to operationalize variables) to the higher-order constructs of interest. The key construct validity questions with regard to measurement are: What is this instrument really measuring? Does it adequately measure the abstract concept of interest? Unfortunately, the more abstract the concept, the more difficult it is to establish construct validity; at the same time, the more abstract the concept, the less suitable it is to rely on criterion-related validity. Actually, it is really not just a question of suitability: What objective criterion is there for such concepts as empathy, role conflict, or separation anxiety? Despite the difficulty of construct validation, it is an activity vital to the development of a strong evidence base. The constructs in which nurse researchers are interested must be validly measured.

Validating an instrument in terms of construct validity is a challenging task. Construct validation is essentially a hypothesis-testing endeavor, typically linked to a theoretical perspective regarding the construct. In validating a measure of death anxiety, we would be less concerned with its relationship to a criterion than with its correspondence to a cogent conceptualization of death anxiety. Construct validation can be approached in several ways, but it always involves logical analysis and hypothesis tests. Constructs are explicated in terms of other abstract concepts; researchers develop hypotheses about the manner in which the target construct will function in relation to other constructs.

There are a number of ways to gather evidence about the construct validity of a scale, most of

which are discussed in this section. It should also be noted, however, that if the instrument developer has taken strong steps to enhance the content validity of the instrument, construct validity will also be strengthened.

Known Groups

One construct validation approach is the **known-groups technique**. In this procedure, the instrument is administered to groups hypothesized to differ on the critical attribute because of some known characteristic. For instance, in validating a measure of fear of the labor experience, we could contrast the scores of primiparas and multiparas. We would expect that women who had never given birth would be more anxious than women who had done so, and so we might question the instrument's validity if such differences did not emerge. We would not necessarily expect large differences; some primiparas would feel little anxiety, and some multiparas would express some fears. On the whole, however, we would anticipate differences in average group scores.

> **Example of the known-groups technique:**
> Weiss, Ryan, and Lokken (2006) adapted the Perceived Readiness for Discharge After Birth Scale (PRDBS). They examined the construct validity of the scale using the known-groups approach, comparing several groups of mothers hypothesized to differ in their perceived readiness for discharge—for example, breastfeeding versus bottle-feeding mothers, primiparas versus multiparas, and those with and without clinical variances during postpartum hospitalization.

Hypothesized Relationships

A similar method of construct validation involves testing hypothesized relationships, often on the basis of theory. This is really a variant of the known-groups approach, which involves hypotheses about the relationship between the measure of the construct and a variable representing group membership. A researcher might reason as follows:

* According to theory, construct X is positively related to construct Y.
* Instrument A is a measure of construct X; instrument B is a measure of construct Y.

- Scores on A and B are correlated positively, as predicted.
- Therefore, it is inferred that A and B are valid measures of X and Y.

This logical analysis is fallible and does not constitute proof of construct validity, but yields important evidence. Construct validation is essentially an evidence-building enterprise.

Example of testing relationships: Knauth and Skowron (2004) did a psychometric evaluation of the Differentiation of Self Inventory (DSI) for adolescents. The DSI, a scale developed to measure a major concept in Bowen family theory, was hypothesized based on this theory to be associated with both chronic anxiety and symptoms of psychological distress. The hypotheses were supported in a test with 363 high school students.

Convergent and Discriminant Validity

An important construct validation tool is a procedure known as the **multitrait–multimethod matrix method** (**MTMM**) (Campbell & Fiske, 1959). This procedure involves the concepts of convergence and discriminability. **Convergence** is evidence that different methods of measuring a construct yield similar results. Different measurement approaches should converge on the construct. **Discriminability** is the ability to differentiate the construct from other similar constructs. Campbell and Fiske argued that evidence of both convergence and discriminability should be brought to bear in the construct validity question.

To help explain the MTMM approach, fictitious data from a study to validate a "need for autonomy" measure are presented in Table 17.3. In using this approach, researchers must measure the critical concept by two or more methods. Suppose we measured need for autonomy in nursing home residents by (1) giving a sample of residents a self-report summated rating scale (the measure we are attempting to validate); (2) asking nurses to rate residents after observing them in a task designed to elicit autonomy or dependence; and (3) having residents react to a pictorial (projective) stimulus depicting an autonomy-relevant situation.

A second requirement of the full MTMM is to measure a differentiating construct, using the same measuring methods. In the current example, suppose we wanted to differentiate "need for autonomy" from "need for affiliation." The discriminant concept must be similar to the focal concept, as in our example: We would expect that people with high need for autonomy would tend to be relatively low on need for affiliation. The point of including both concepts in a single validation study is to gather evidence that the two concepts are distinct, rather than two different labels for the same underlying attribute.

| TABLE 17.3 | Example of a Multitrait–Multimethod Matrix |

METHOD	TRAITS	SELF-REPORT (1)		OBSERVATION (2)		PROJECTIVE (3)	
		AUT$_1$	AFF$_1$	AUT$_2$	AFF$_2$	AUT$_3$	AFF$_3$
Self-report (1)	AUT$_1$	(.88)					
	AFF$_1$	−.38	(.86)				
Observation (2)	AUT$_2$	.60	−.19	(.79)			
	AFF$_2$	−.21	.58	−.39	(.80)		
Projective (3)	AUT$_3$	.51	−.18	.55	−.12	(.74)	
	AFF$_3$	−.14	.49	−.17	.54	−.32	(.72)

AUT, need for autonomy trait; AFF, need for affiliation trait.

The numbers in Table 17.3 represent the correlation coefficients between scores on six different measures (two traits × three methods). For instance, the coefficient of −.38 at the intersection of AUT_1–AFF_1 expresses the relationship between self-report scores on the need for autonomy and need for affiliation measures. Recall that a minus sign before the correlation coefficient signifies an inverse relationship. In this case, the −.38 tells us that there was a slight tendency for people scoring high on the need for autonomy scale to score low on the need for affiliation scale. (The numbers in parentheses along the diagonal of this matrix are the reliability coefficients.)

Various aspects of the MTMM matrix have a bearing on construct validity. The most direct evidence (**convergent validity**) comes from the correlations between two different methods measuring the same trait. In the case of AUT_1–AUT_2, the coefficient is .60, which is reasonably high. Convergent validity should be large enough to encourage further scrutiny of the matrix. Second, the convergent validity entries should be higher, in absolute magnitude,* than correlations between measures that have neither method nor trait in common. That is, AUT_1–AUT_2 (.60) should be greater than AUT_2–AFF_1 (−.21) or AUT_1–AFF_2 (−.19), as it is in fact. This requirement is a minimum one that, if it fails, should cause researchers to have serious doubts about the measures. Third, convergent validity coefficients should be greater than coefficients between measures of different traits by a single method. Once again, the matrix in Table 17.3 fulfills this criterion: AUT_1–AUT_2 (.60) and AUT_2–AUT_3 (.55) are higher in absolute value than AUT_1–AFF_1 (−.38), AUT_2–AFF_2 (−.39), and AUT_3–AFF_3 (−.32). The last two requirements provide evidence for **discriminant validity**.

The evidence is seldom as clearcut as in this contrived example. Indeed, a common problem with the MTMM is interpreting the pattern of coefficients. Another issue is that there are no clearcut criteria for determining whether MTMM requirements have been met—that is, there are no objective means of assessing the magnitude of similarities and differences within the matrix. The MTMM is nevertheless a valuable tool for exploring construct validity. Researchers sometimes decide to use MTMM concepts even when the full model is not feasible, as in focusing only on convergent validity. Executing any part of the model is better than no effort at construct validation. 🌐

Example of convergent and discriminant validity: Radwin and colleagues (2005) developed and tested four scales to measure desired health outcomes that would reflect high-quality cancer nursing care (Fortitude Scale, Trust in Nurses Scale, Cancer Patient Optimism Scale, and Authentic Self Representation Scale). Using specialized software, the Multitrait/Multi-Item Analysis Program, their analysis provided preliminary evidence of the scales' convergent and discriminant validity.

Factor Analysis

Another approach to construct validation uses a statistical procedure known as factor analysis. Although factor analysis, which is discussed in Chapter 18, is computationally complex, it is conceptually rather simple. **Factor analysis** is a method for identifying clusters of related variables—that is, dimensions underlying a central construct. Each dimension, called a **factor**, represents a relatively unitary attribute. The procedure is used to identify and group together different items measuring an underlying attribute. In effect, factor analysis constitutes another means of testing hypotheses about the interrelationships among variables, and for looking at the convergent and discriminant validity of a large set of items. Indeed, a procedure known as **confirmatory factor analysis** is sometimes used as a method for analyzing MTMM data (Ferketich, Figueredo, & Knapp, 1991; Lowe & Ryan-Wenger, 1992).

Example of factor analysis in construct validation: Shellman (2006) developed the Eldercare Cultural Self-Efficacy Scale, which was designed to assess nursing students' confidence in caring for ethnically diverse elders. Responses to the scale items by a sample of 248 nursing students were factor analyzed, which revealed four dimensions (e.g., Assessing for Lifestyle and Social Patterns, Determining Cultural Beliefs).

---

*The **absolute magnitude** refers to the value without a plus or minus sign. A value of −.50 is of a higher absolute magnitude than +.40.

Interpretation of Validity

Like reliability, validity is not an all-or-nothing characteristic of an instrument. An instrument does not possess or lack validity; it is a question of degree. An instrument's validity is not proved, established, or verified but rather is supported to a greater or lesser extent by evidence.

Strictly speaking, researchers do not validate an instrument but rather an application of it. A measure of anxiety may be valid for presurgical patients on the day of an operation but may not be valid for nursing students on the day of a test. Of course, some instruments may be valid for a wide range of uses with different types of samples, but each use requires new supporting evidence. The more evidence that can be gathered that an instrument is measuring what it is supposed to be measuring, the more confidence researchers will have in its validity.

◯ TIP: When you select an instrument, you should seek evidence of the scale's psychometric soundness by examining the report of the instrument developers. However, you also should consider evidence from others who have used the scale. Each time the scale "performs" as hypothesized, this constitutes supplementary evidence for its validity. Conversely, if hypotheses involving the use of the scale are not supported, this suggests potential validity problems (although, of course, other factors may be responsible for nonsupported hypotheses, such as a small sample or a weak design).

SENSITIVITY, SPECIFICITY, AND LIKELIHOOD RATIOS

Reliability and validity are the two most important criteria for evaluating quantitative instruments. High reliability and validity of measuring tools are necessary for high-quality quantitative research.

Researchers sometimes need to consider other qualities of an instrument. In particular, sensitivity and specificity are criteria that are important in evaluating instruments designed as screening or diagnostic tools (e.g., a scale to measure risk for osteoporosis). Screening and diagnostic instruments can be self-report, observational, or biophysiologic measures.

Sensitivity is the ability of a measure to identify a "case" correctly, that is, to screen *in* or diagnose a condition correctly. A measure's sensitivity is its rate of yielding "true positives." **Specificity** is the measure's ability to identify noncases correctly, that is, to screen *out* those without the condition correctly. Specificity is an instrument's rate of yielding "true negatives." To determine an instrument's sensitivity and specificity, researchers need a reliable and valid criterion of "caseness" against which scores on the instrument can be assessed.

Calculating Sensitivity, Specificity, and Other Indicators

Suppose we wanted to evaluate whether adolescents' self-reports about their smoking were accurate, and we asked 100 teenagers aged 13 to 15 about whether they had smoked a cigarette in the previous 24 hours. The "gold standard" for nicotine consumption is cotinine levels in a body fluid, and so let us assume that we did a urinary cotinine assay. Some fictitious data are shown in Table 17.4.

Sensitivity, in this example, is calculated as the proportion of teenagers who said they smoked *and* who had high concentrations of cotinine, divided by all real smokers as indicated by the urine test. Put another way, it is the true positives divided by all positives. In this case, there was considerable underreporting of smoking, and so the sensitivity of the self-report was only .50. Specificity is the proportion of teenagers who accurately reported they did not smoke, or the true negatives divided by all negatives. In our example, specificity is .83. There was considerably less over-reporting of smoking ("faking bad") than under-reporting ("faking good"). It should be noted that sensitivity and specificity are often reported as percentages rather than proportions, simply by multiplying the proportions by 100.

Often, additional indicators are calculated with data such as shown in this table. **Predictive values** are posterior probabilities—the probability of an outcome after the results are known. A **positive**

TABLE 17.4	Fictitious Data to Illustrate Sensitivity, Specificity, and Likelihood Ratios		
	URINARY COTININE LEVEL		
SELF-REPORTED SMOKING	**Positive (Cotinine > 200 ng/mL)**	**Negative (Cotinine ≤ 200 ng/mL)**	**Total**
Yes, smoked	A (true positive) 20	B (false positive) 10	A + B 30
No, did not smoke	C (false negative) 20	D (true negative) 50	C + D 70
Total	A + C 40	B + D 60	A + B + C + D 100

Sensitivity = A/(A + C)   = .50
Specificity = D/(B + D)   = .83
Positive predictive value (PPV) = A/(A + B)   = .67
Negative predictive value (NPV) = D/(C = D)   = .71
Likelihood ratio—positive (LR+) = sensitivity/(1 − specificity)   = 2.99
Likelihood ratio—negative (LR−) = (1 − sensitivity)/specificity   = .60

predictive value (or PPV) is the proportion of people with a positive result who have the target outcome or disease. In our example, the PPV is the proportion of teens who said they smoke who actually *do* smoke, according to the cotinine test results. Two out of three of those who reported smoking had high concentrations of cotinine, and so PPV = .67. A **negative predictive value** (NPV) is the proportion of people who have a negative test result who do not have the target outcome or disease. As shown in Table 17.4, 50 out of the 70 teenagers who reported not smoking actually were nonsmokers, and so the NPV in our example is .71.

Example of sensitivity, specificity, and predictive values: Kwong and colleagues (2005) developed a modified Braden scale for use in acute care hospitals in mainland China. They compared the modified scale to the original scale and to another pressure ulcer risk scale. Sensitivity was the same for all three scales (89%), as was negative predictive value (100%), but specificity

(75%) and positive predictive value (7%) were highest for the modified Braden.

In the medical community, reporting **likelihood ratios** has come into favor because it summarizes the relationship between specificity and sensitivity in a single number. The likelihood ratio addresses the question, How much more likely are we to find that an indicator is positive among those *with* the outcome of concern compared with those for whom the indicator is negative? For a positive test result, then, the likelihood ratio (LR+) is the ratio of true-positive results to false-positive results. The formula for LR+ is sensitivity, divided by 1 minus specificity. For the data in Table 17.4, LR+ is 2.99: we are about three times as likely to find that a self-report of smoking occurs for a true smoker than it does for a nonsmoker. For a negative test result, the likelihood ratio (LR−) is the ratio of false-negative results to true-negative results. For the data in Table 17.4, the LR− is .60. In our example, we are about half as likely to find that a self-report of nonsmoking is false than we are to find that it reflects a true nonsmoker. When a test is high on both sensitivity and specificity (which is not especially true in our example), the likelihood ratio is high, and discrimination is good.

Example of likelihood ratios: Holland and co-researchers (2006) developed and validated a screening instrument to determine early in a hospital stay the adult patients who would need specialized discharge planning services. For the sample of nearly 1000 patients used to develop the instrument, the sensitivity was 79%, and the specificity was 76%. The LR+ was 3.29, and the LR− was 0.27.

Receiver Operator Characteristic (ROC) Curves

All the indicators that we calculated for the data in Table 17.4 are contingent upon the critical value that we established for cotinine concentration. Sensitivity and specificity would be quite different if we had used 100 ng/mL as indicative of smoking status, rather than 200 ng/mL. There is almost invariably a tradeoff between the sensitivity and specificity of a measure. When sensitivity is increased to include more true positives, the number of true negatives declines. Therefore, a critical task in developing new diagnostic or screening measures is to develop the appropriate **cutoff point**, that is, the score used to distinguish cases and noncases.

To determine the best cutoff point, researchers often are guided by a **receiver operating characteristic curve (ROC curve)** (Fletcher, Fletcher, & Wagner, 2005). To construct an ROC curve, the sensitivity of an instrument (i.e., the rate of correctly identifying a case *vis-à-vis* a well-established criterion) is plotted against the false-positive rate (i.e., the rate of incorrectly diagnosing someone as a case, which is the inverse of its specificity) over a range of different scores. The score (cutoff point) that yields the best balance between sensitivity and specificity can then be determined. The optimum cutoff is at or near the shoulder of the ROC curve.

ROC curves can best be explained with an illustration. Figure 17.2 presents an ROC curve from a study in which a goal was to establish cutoff points for scores on the Braden-Q scale for predicting pressure ulcer risk in children (Curley et al., 2003). In this figure, sensitivity and 1 minus specificity are plotted for each possible score of the Braden Q scale. The upper left corner represents sensitivity at its highest possible value (1.0) and false positives at

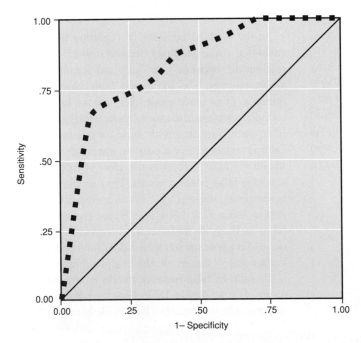

FIGURE 17.2 Receiver operating characteristic (ROC) curve for Braden Q Scale. (From Curley, M. A. Q., Razmus, I. S., Roberts, K. E., & Wypij, D. [2003] Predicting Pressure Ulcer Risk in Pediatric Patients: The Braden Q Scale. *Nursing Research, 52*[1], 27.)

its lowest possible value (.00). Screening instruments that do an excellent job of discriminating have points that crowd close to the upper left corner, which indicates that as sensitivity increases, there is relatively little loss in specificity. ROC curves that are closer to a diagonal, from lower left to upper right, are indicative of an instrument with poor discriminatory power.

The overall utility of an instrument can be calculated as the proportion of the area under the ROC curve, an index referred to as **area under the curve**, or **AUC**. The larger the area, the more accurate the instrument. The AUC for the data portrayed in Figure 17.2 is .83. The cutoff score in this example was established at 16. At this cutoff value, the sensitivity was .88, and the specificity was .58. The researchers used these preliminary analyses to improve on the Braden Q scale and achieved even better results.

In selecting an appropriate cutoff point, the final decision is likely to be driven by clinical or economic factors and not just statistical ones. The financial and emotional costs of misclassifying people may be greater for false positives than false negatives, or *vice versa*.

OTHER CRITERIA FOR ASSESSING QUANTITATIVE MEASURES

Although we have already discussed the major criteria that are used to evaluate the quality of measuring instruments, we briefly mention a few others.

Efficiency

Instruments of comparable reliability and validity may differ in their efficiency. A depression scale that requires 5 minutes of people's time is efficient compared with a depression scale that requires 20 minutes to complete. In most studies, efficient instruments are desirable because they reduce the burden on participants (and may thus enhance data quality).

One aspect of efficiency is the number of items on the instrument. Long instruments tend to be more reliable than shorter ones. There is, however, a point of diminishing returns. As an example, consider a 40-item scale to measure social support that has an internal consistency reliability of .94. We can use a formula, known as the **Spearman-Brown formula**, to estimate how reliable the scale would be with fewer items. As an example, if we wanted to shorten the scale to 30 items, the formula would result in an estimated reliability of .92.* Thus, a 25% reduction in the instrument's length resulted in a negligible decrease in reliability, from .94 to .92. Most researchers likely would sacrifice a modest amount of reliability in exchange for reducing subjects' response burden and data collection costs.

Efficiency is more characteristic of certain types of data collection procedures than others. In self-reports, closed-ended questions are more efficient than open-ended ones, for example. A researcher may decide that other advantages (such as depth of information) offset a certain degree of inefficiency. Other things being equal, however, it is desirable to select as efficient an instrument as possible.

Other Criteria

A few remaining qualities that sometimes are considered in assessing a quantitative instrument can be noted. Most of the following six criteria are actually aspects of the reliability and validity issues:

1. *Comprehensibility.* Subjects and researchers should be able to comprehend the behaviors required to secure accurate and valid measures.
2. *Precision.* An instrument should discriminate between people with different amounts of an attribute as precisely as possible.

---

*The equation (and the worked-out example) for this situation is as follows:

$$r^1 = \frac{kr}{1 + [(k - 1)r]} = \frac{.75(.94)}{1 + [(-.25)(.94)]} = .92$$

where k = the factor by which the instrument is being decreased, in this case, $k = 30 \div 40 = .75$; r = reliability for the full scale, here, .94; and r^1 = reliability estimate for the shorter scale.

3. *Speededness*. For most instruments, researchers should allow adequate time to obtain complete measurements without rushing the measuring process.
4. *Range*. The instrument should be capable of achieving a meaningful measure from the smallest expected value of the variable to the largest.
5. *Linearity*. A researcher normally strives to construct measures that are equally accurate and sensitive over the entire range of values.
6. *Reactivity*. The instrument should, insofar as possible, avoid affecting the attribute being measured.

DATA QUALITY WITH SINGLE INDICATORS

The discussion in this chapter has primarily focused on methods of evaluating data quality for multi-item self-report and observational scales, which are the methods most widely used by nurse researchers to measure key constructs. Textbooks on research methods or measurement rarely say much about reliability or validity for single questions (e.g., "What is your date of birth?") or single-item scales, such as visual analogue scales.

The truth of the matter is that it is not easy to evaluate data quality in such situations. This is of great concern in large national surveys, such as the National Longitudinal Study of Adolescent Health. Population estimates of, say, the average number of times adolescents have been hospitalized, or the percentage who have ever used marijuana, are based on reports in response to individual (non-scaled) questions, and so the accuracy of the responses is vital. Accuracy should also be of concern to nurse researchers, of course. We touch briefly here on data quality assessment for single indicators, but note that data quality concerns in such situations mostly involve efforts to minimize error rather than attempts to evaluate it.

The two basic strategies for estimating measurement error in such situations are a test–retest approach, and external verification. In the former, the same questions that are of interest for assessment purposes are asked on two separate occasions.

When this happens for the express purpose of assessing consistency (in what is called a *response variance reinterview* by survey researchers), the second administration typically involves a subsample of respondents and an abbreviated instrument with key questions. Survey researchers compute various statistical indexes (e.g., an *index of inconsistency*) to help them understand and interpret response differences—that is, measurement error—in the two administrations (Subcommittee on Measuring and Reporting the Quality of Survey Data, 2001). Although few nurse researchers would have the resources to undertake such an enterprise, there may be opportunities to use the underlying principle for critical pieces of information. For example, in a self-report instrument, it might be possible to ask the same question twice (e.g., early and later), or to ask the question in slightly different ways in the same questionnaire. Also, if a study is longitudinal, factual information (e.g., date of birth) could be gathered twice to assess any discrepancies.

The second approach is to verify information provided in the primary data gathering method against an external source—a form of criterion-related validation. For example, information from a question about birth date could be checked against birth records. Responses to questions about health status, diagnosis, or health care could be checked against medical records. Measurement errors are then estimated based on a comparison of the two types of information. Of course, it should not necessarily be assumed that records are free of error, but they may be less prone to certain types of bias. Other forms of external verification may be available, should this be considered desirable. In particular, **proxy reports** (obtaining information from another source, such as a family member) might be an option. Patrician (2004) offers some additional guidance regarding the use of single-item scales.

Reliability and validity might also be a concern with regard to biophysiologic measures, although such measures tend to yield data of high quality, compared with psychosocial measures. However, researchers using biophysiologic measures should also give data quality some thought rather than assuming it will be error free. Instruments may not be properly calibrated, the person doing the tests may not be following laboratory protocols, and laboratory procedures can vary from one lab to the next. Measurement errors can also occur because of patient circumstances, such as insufficient sleep. Moreover, if physiologic measures are taken from charts, the possibility of error needs to be considered. DeKeyser and Pugh (1990) offer guidance with regard to measurement errors arising from physiologic measures.

CRITIQUING DATA QUALITY IN QUANTITATIVE STUDIES

If data are seriously flawed, the study cannot contribute useful evidence. Therefore, in drawing conclusions about a study, it is important to consider whether researchers have taken appropriate steps to collect data that accurately reflect reality. Research consumers have the right—indeed, the obligation—to ask, Can I trust the data? Do the data accurately and validly reflect the construct under study?

Information about data quality should be provided in every quantitative research report because it is not possible to come to conclusions about the quality of evidence of the study without such information. Reliability estimates are usually reported because they are easy to communicate. Ideally—especially for composite scales—the report should provide reliability coefficients based on data from the study itself, not just from previous research. Interrater or interobserver reliability is especially crucial for coming to conclusions about data quality in observational studies. The values of the reliability coefficients should, of course, be sufficiently high to support confidence in the findings. It is especially important to scrutinize reliability information in studies with nonsignificant findings because the unreliability of measures can undermine statistical conclusion validity.

Validity is more difficult to document in a report than reliability. At a minimum, researchers should defend their choice of existing measures based on

validity information from the developers, and they should cite the relevant publication. If a study used a screening or diagnostic measure, information should also be provided about its sensitivity and specificity.

Box 17.1 provides some guidelines for critiquing aspects of data quality of quantitative measures. The guidelines are available in the Toolkit of the accompanying *Resource Manual* for your use and adaptation. ⊗

RESEARCH EXAMPLE

In this section, we describe a study that used both self-report and biophysiologic measures. We focus on the researchers' documentation of data quality in their study.

Study: "Subjective fatigue, influencing variables, and consequences in chronic obstructive pulmonary disease" (Kapella et al., 2006)

Statement of Purpose: The purpose of this study was to test a hypothesized theoretical explanation of functional performance in patients with chronic obstructive pulmonary disease. The analyses tested hypothesized causal pathways between anxious and depressed mood states, airflow obstruction, and sleep quality and functional performance.

Design: Data were collected from 130 patients with chronic obstructive pulmonary disease (COPD) using a cross-sectional design. Biophysiologic data were gathered either in a hospital setting or in participants' homes. Self-report data were gathered primarily through questionnaires. Participants were asked to complete the instrument packet in the morning and to return it by mail within 1 week.

Instruments and Data Quality: Kapella and her co-researchers administered a wide number of self-report scales, only some of which will be discussed here. The researchers took care to describe their instruments with exemplary detail, and to discuss data quality issues. Fatigue, one of the key variables in this study, was assessed using three instruments, one of which was the Numerical Rating Scales (NRSs). NRSs were used to measure the frequency, intensity, and distress of the feeling of fatigue. Possible scores range from 3 to 15. The report summarized prior efforts to document the validity of the scale for people with COPD. The researchers also provided new evidence to support the convergent and discriminant validity of the NRSs.

BOX 17.1 Guidelines for Critiquing Data Quality in Quantitative Studies

1. Is there congruence between the research variables as conceptualized (i.e., as discussed in the introduction of the report) and as operationalized (i.e., as described in the method section)?
2. If operational definitions (or scoring procedures) are specified, do they clearly indicate the rules of measurement? Do the rules seem sensible? Were data collected in such a way that measurement errors were minimized?
3. Does the report offer evidence of the reliability of measures? Does the evidence come from the research sample itself, or is it based on other studies? If the latter, is it reasonable to conclude that data quality would be similar for the research sample as for the reliability sample (e.g., are sample characteristics similar)?
4. If reliability is reported, which estimation method was used? Was this method appropriate? Should an alternative or additional method of reliability appraisal have been used? Is the reliability sufficiently high?
5. Does the report offer evidence of the validity of the measures? Does the evidence come from the research sample itself, or is it based on other studies? If the latter, is it reasonable to believe that data quality would be similar for the research sample as for the validity sample (e.g., are the sample characteristics similar)?
6. If validity information is reported, which validity approach was used? Was this method appropriate? Does the validity of the instrument appear to be adequate?
7. If there is no reliability or validity information, what conclusion can you reach about the quality of the data in the study?
8. If a diagnostic or screening tool was used, is information provided about its sensitivity and specificity, and were these qualities adequate?
9. Were the research hypotheses supported? If not, might data quality play a role in the failure to confirm the hypotheses?

For example, the scores correlated significantly (convergent validity) with study participants' scores on the Global Fatigue Severity Scale of the Fatigue Assessment Instrument (FAI). The computed value of Cronbach's alpha for the NRSs was .89. The reliability coefficients for the four subscales of the FAI were also good, ranging from .78 to .92. Self-report scales were also used to measure dyspnea, functional performance, sleep quality, and anxious and depressed mood. For example, the measure of functional performance was the Functional Performance Inventory (FPI), a 65-item instrument that had previously been found to be valid and reliable with people with COPD. Cronbach's alpha for the FPI in the present study was .92. Finally, spirometry was performed on participants according to standardized methods and yielded a measure of airflow obstruction (FEV_1) that was used as an indicator of disease severity. The report described the procedure and norms used to calculate the percentage of predicted normal values.
Key Findings:

- There was a strong relationship between dyspnea and fatigue.
- Dyspnea, depressed mood, and sleep quality were moderately successful in predicting levels of fatigue.

- Fatigue, dyspnea, and airflow obstruction helped to predict functional performance.

SUMMARY POINTS

- **Measurement** involves the assignment of numbers to objects to represent the amount of an attribute, using a specified set of rules. Researchers strive to develop or use measurements whose rules are *isomorphic* with reality.
- Few quantitative measuring instruments are infallible. Sources of measurement error include situational contaminants, response-set biases, and transitory personal factors, such as fatigue.
- **Obtained scores** from an instrument consist of a **true score** component (the value that would be obtained for a hypothetical perfect measure of the attribute) and an error component, or **error of measurement**, that represents measurement inaccuracies.

- **Reliability**, one of two primary criteria for assessing a quantitative instrument, is the degree of consistency or accuracy with which an instrument measures an attribute. The higher the reliability of an instrument, the lower the amount of error in obtained scores.
- There are different methods for assessing an instrument's reliability and for computing a **reliability coefficient**. A reliability coefficient typically is based on the computation of a **correlation coefficient** that indicates the magnitude and direction of a relationship between two variables.
- Correlation coefficients can range from –1.00 (a perfect **negative relationship**) through zero to +1.00 (a perfect **positive relationship**). Reliability coefficients usually range from .00 to 1.00, with higher values reflecting greater reliability.
- The **stability** aspect of reliability, which concerns the extent to which an instrument yields the same results on repeated administrations, is evaluated by **test–retest reliability** procedures.
- **Internal consistency reliability**, which refers to the extent to which all the instrument's items are measuring the same attribute, is usually assessed using **Cronbach's alpha** method.
- When the reliability assessment focuses on **equivalence** between observers in rating or coding behaviors, estimates of **interrater** (or *interobserver*) **reliability** are obtained. When a consensus measure capturing interrater agreement within a small number of categories is desired, the **kappa** statistic is often used; for consistency of ratings, the **intraclass correlation coefficient** is often appropriate.
- Reliability coefficients reflect the proportion of true variability in a set of scores to the total obtained variability.
- **Validity** is the degree to which an instrument measures what it is supposed to be measuring.
- **Face validity** refers to whether the instrument appears, on the face of it, to be measuring the appropriate construct.
- **Content validity** is concerned with the sampling adequacy of the content being measured.

- Expert ratings on the relevance of items can be used to compute **content validity index (CVI)** information. Item-level CVIs (I-CVIs) represent the percentage of experts rating each item as relevant, and scale-level CVIs using the averaging calculation method (S-CVI/Ave) are the average of all I-CVI values.
- **Criterion-related validity** (which includes both **predictive validity** and **concurrent validity**) focuses on the correlation between the instrument and an outside criterion.
- **Construct validity,** an instrument's adequacy in measuring the focal construct, is primarily a hypothesis-testing endeavor. One construct validation method is the **known-groups technique**, which contrasts scores of groups hypothesized to differ on the attribute; another is **factor analysis**, a statistical procedure for identifying unitary clusters of items or measures.
- Another construct validity approach is the **multitrait–multimethod matrix technique**, which is based on the concepts of convergence and discriminability. **Convergence** refers to evidence that different methods of measuring the same attribute yield similar results. **Discriminability** refers to the ability to differentiate the construct being measured from other, similar concepts.
- A **psychometric assessment** of a new instrument is usually undertaken to gather evidence about validity, reliability, and other quality criteria.
- Sensitivity and specificity are important criteria for screening and diagnostic instruments. **Sensitivity** is the instrument's ability to identify a case correctly (i.e., its rate of yielding true positives). **Specificity** is the instrument's ability to identify noncases correctly (i.e., its rate of yielding true negatives). Other related indexes include the measure's **positive predictive value** (PPV), **negative predictive value** (NPV), and **likelihood ratios**.
- Sensitivity is sometimes plotted against specificity in a **receiver operating characteristic curve** (**ROC curve**) to determine the optimum **cutoff point** for caseness.

STUDY ACTIVITIES

Chapter 17 of the accompanying *Resource Manual for Nursing Research: Generating and Assessing Evidence for Nursing Practice, 8th edition*, offers various exercises and study suggestions for reinforcing the concepts presented in this chapter. In addition, the following study questions can be addressed:

1. Explain in your own words the meaning of the following correlation coefficients:
   a. The relationship between intelligence and grade-point average was found to be .72.
   b. The correlation coefficient between age and gregariousness was −.20.
   c. It was revealed that patients' compliance with nursing instructions was related to their length of stay in the hospital ($r = -.50$).
2. An instructor has developed an instrument to measure knowledge of research terminology. Would you say that more reliable measurements would be yielded before or after a year of instruction on research methodology, using the exact same test, or would there be no difference? Why?
3. Use the critiquing guidelines in Box 17.1 to evaluate data quality in the study by Kapella and colleagues (2006), referring to the original study if possible.

STUDIES CITED IN CHAPTER 17

Methodologic or theoretical references cited in this chapter can be found in a separate section at the end of the book.

Curley, M. A. Q., Razmus, I. S., Roberts, K. E., & Wypij, D. (2003). Predicting pressure ulcer risk in pediatric patients. *Nursing Research, 52,* 22–33.

Gulick, E. E. (2003). Adaptation of the Postpartum Support Questionnaire for mothers with multiple sclerosis. *Research in Nursing and Health, 26,* 30–39.

Holland, D., Harris, M., Leibson, C., Pankrantz, V., & Krichbaum, K. (2006). Development and validation of a screen for specialized discharge planning services. *Nursing Research, 55*(1), 62–71.

Immers, H., Schuurmans, M., & van de Bijl, J. (2005). Recognition of delirium in ICU patients: A diagnostic study of the NEECHAM confusion scale in ICU patients. *BMC Nursing, 4,* 7–13.

Kapella, M., Larson, J., Patel, M., Covey, M., & Berry, J. (2006). Subjective fatigue, influencing variables, and consequences in chronic obstructive pulmonary disease. *Nursing Research, 55*(1), 10–17.

Knauth, D. G., & Skowron, E. A. (2004). Psychometric evaluation of the Differentiation of Self Inventory for adolescents. *Nursing Research, 53,* 163–171.

Kwong, E., Pang, S., Wong, T., Ho, J., Shano-ling, X., & Li-jun, T. (2005). Predicting pressure ulcer risk with the modified Braden, Braden, and Norton scales in acute care hospitals in Mainland China. *Applied Nursing Research, 18*(2), 122–128.

Lindgren, K. (2005). Testing the Health Practices in Pregnancy Questionnaire—II. *Journal of Obstetric, Gynecologic, & Neonatal Nursing, 34,* 465–472.

McDowell, J., Courtney, M., Edwards, H., & Shortridge-Baggett, L. (2005). Validation of the Australian/English version of the Diabetes Management Self-Efficacy Scale. *International Journal of Nursing Practice, 11,* 177–184.

McSweeney, J. C., O'Sullivan, P., Cody, M., & Crane, P. B. (2004). Development of the McSweeney Acute and Prodromal Myocardial Infarction Symptom Survey. *Journal of Cardiovascular Nursing, 19,* 58–67.

Perraud, S., Fogg, L., Kopytko, E., & Gross, D. (2006). Predictive validity of the Depression Coping Self-Efficacy Scale (DCSES). *Research in Nursing & Health, 29*(2), 147–160.

Radwin, L., Washko, M., Suchy, K., & Tyman, K. (2005). Development and pilot testing of four health outcome scales. *Oncology Nursing Forum, 32*(1), 92–96.

Shellman, J. (2006). Development and psychometric evaluation of the Eldercare Cultural Self-Efficacy Scale. *International Journal of Nursing Education Scholarship, 3,* 10–20.

Warms, C. A., & Belza, B. L. (2004). Actigraphy as a measure of physical activity for wheelchair users with spinal cord injury. *Nursing Research, 53,* 136–143.

Weiss, M., Ryan, P., & Lokken, L. (2006). Validity and reliability of the Perceived Readiness for Discharge After Birth Scale. *Journal of Obstetric, Gynecologic, & Neonatal Nursing, 35*(1), 34–45.

Welch, J., Bennett, S., Delp, R., & Agarwal, R. (2006). Benefits of and barriers to dietary sodium adherence. *Western Journal of Nursing Research, 28*(2), 162–180.

Wu, Y., Larrabee, J., & Putman, H. (2006). Caring Behaviors Inventory: A reduction of the 42-item instrument. *Nursing Research, 55*(1), 18–25.

18

Developing and Testing Self-Report Scales

S ome researchers find that, despite diligent efforts, they are unable to identify an appropriate instrument to operationalize a construct of interest. This may occur when the construct is new, but more often it is due to shortcomings of existing instruments. Because this situation occurs fairly regularly, this chapter is designed to provide an overview of the steps involved in the development of high-quality self-report scales.

The scope of this chapter is fairly narrow, although it covers the vast majority of measures that nurse researchers construct and use. First, as the title of the chapter suggests, we focus on structured *self-report* measures rather than observational ones (although many of the same steps would apply for observational scales). Second, we describe methods of developing *multi-item* scales (i.e., not one-item visual analogue scales). Third, we exclude scale types that are infrequently used in nursing, such as semantic differential scales or Guttman scales. Fourth, we concentrate primarily on scales rooted in classical measurement theory rather than on scales based on item response theory. We will be using examples of scales to measure the *affective domain* (e.g., measures of attitudes, psychological traits, emotions, and so on) rather than scales to measure the *cognitive domain* (e.g., achievement, performance, knowledge), but many of the principles apply to both domains.

⯈ TIP: The development of high-quality scales is a lengthy and labor-intensive process, and it is also one that requires a fair amount of statistical sophistication. We urge you to think carefully about embarking on a scale-development endeavor, and to consider involving a psychometric consultant if you proceed.

BEGINNING STEPS: CONCEPTUALIZATION AND ITEM GENERATION

Conceptualizing the Construct

The importance of a sound and thorough conceptualization of the construct to be measured cannot be overemphasized. You will not be able to quantify an attribute adequately unless you thoroughly understand the **latent variable** (the underlying construct) you wish to capture. In measurement theory, the latent variable, which is not directly observable, is the *cause* of the scores on the measure. That is, the strength of the latent variable is presumed to trigger a certain numeric value on the scale. You cannot develop items to produce the right score value, and you cannot expect good content and construct validity in your scale, if you are not clear about the construct, its dimensions, and its nuances.

The first step in scale development, then, is to become an *expert* on the construct. This means becoming knowledgeable about any relevant theory, about research relating to the construct, and about any existing (albeit imperfect) instruments. Scale developers almost always begin with a thorough review of the relevant literature, on which they can base conceptual definitions of their constructs.

Most complex constructs have a number of different facets or dimensions, and it is important to identify and understand each one. In part, this is a content validity consideration: for the overall scale to be content valid, there must be items representing all facets of the construct. Identifying dimensions also has methodologic implications. All scales—or subscales of a broader scale—need to be unidimensional and internally homogeneous, and so an adequate number of items (operational definitions) of each dimension need to be developed.

During the early conceptualization stage, you will also need to think about (and be clear about) related constructs that need to be differentiated from the construct of interest. If you are measuring, say, self-esteem, you have to be sure you can differentiate it from similar but distinct constructs, such as self-confidence. So, in thinking about the dimensions of the target construct, you should be sure that they are truly aspects of the construct and not a different construct altogether.

Before you can begin to develop a scale, you will also need to have an explicit conceptualization of the population for whom the scale is intended. For example, an anxiety scale for a general population may not be suitable if your interest is in measuring childbearing anxiety in pregnant women. There are arguments for developing patient-specific scales, particularly with respect to the relevancy of items. On the other hand, developing a highly focused scale with low "bandwidth," while possibly enhancing "fidelity" (Cronbach, 1990), reduces the scale's generalizability and researchers' ability to make comparisons across populations. The point is that in developing a scale, you should have a clear view of how and with whom the scale will be used.

Understanding the population for whom the scale is intended is critical for developing good items, even beyond the obvious implications for item content. Without a good grasp of the population, it will be difficult to consider such issues as reading levels and cultural appropriateness in wording the items.

For instruments that are being developed for wide-scale use, it is generally recommended that an expert panel be established to review domain specifications, in an early effort to ensure the content validity of the scale (AERA, APA, & NCME Joint Committee, 1985). An iterative, Delphi survey–type approach with opportunities for refinement by the expert panel is often useful (Berk, 1990).

Deciding on the Type of Scale

Before items can be generated, you will need to decide on the type of scale you wish to create because item characteristics vary by scale type. There is a wide variety of scaling options, but we have narrowed our focus to the most widely used scale types because this is a research methods textbook and not a book on measurement or psychometrics. For those interested in such scaling approaches as semantic differentials, Guttman scaling, Thurstone scaling, multidimensional scaling, econometric methods, ipsative (forced-choice) scaling, or other approaches, we refer you to other references (e.g., Gable & Wolfe, 1993; Nunnally & Bernstein, 1994; Streiner & Norman, 2003; Waltz, Strickland, & Lenz, 2005).

In this chapter we concentrate on the development of multi-item summated rating scales, which is also the focus of several other books on scale development that can be consulted for greater elaboration (DeVellis, 2003; Streiner & Norman, 2003). Two broad categories of scales fall into this category: traditional Likert scales and latent trait scales.

Traditional Likert scales, discussed in Chapter 16, are based in classical measurement theory (CMT). Items on Likert scales, it may be recalled, are declarative statements followed by a bipolar response scale that often reflects an agree/disagree continuum. In CMT, the scale developer selects items that are presumed to be roughly comparable indicators of the underlying construct, and the items gain strength in approximating a hypothetical true score through their aggregation. Traditional Likert scales, then, rely on items that are deliberately redundant, in the hope that multiple indicators of the construct will converge on the true score and balance out and reduce the error term.

Item response theory (IRT), an alternative to CMT, has been widely used in the development of cognitive tests, but its use in developing and evaluating affective measures is growing. IRT methods differentiate error much more finely than CMT methods, particularly with respect to characteristics of the items in a scale. The goal of IRT is to allow researchers to determine the characteristics of items independent of who completes them. **Latent trait scales** are developed using an IRT framework, and although it is beyond the scope of this book to elaborate upon the complex statistical procedures involved in testing latent trait scales, we can provide a few brief comments and references for those who wish further guidance.

Latent trait scales can use formats like the ones used in CMT, and so a Likert-type format is fine—in fact, a person completing a Likert scale would likely not know whether it had been developed within the CMT or IRT framework. But a person *developing* a Likert-type scale should decide in advance which measurement approach is being used because the items used in the scale would be different. Whereas the items on a CMT Likert scale are designed to be similar to each other to tap the underlying construct in a comparable manner, items on a latent trait (IRT) Likert scale are carefully chosen and refined to tap different degrees of the attribute being measured.

As an example, suppose we were developing a scale to measure risk-taking behavior in adolescents. In a CMT scale, the items might include statements about risk taking of similar intensity, with which respondents would agree or disagree. The aggregate of responses would array respondents along a continuum indicating varying propensity to take risks. In an IRT scale, the items themselves would be chosen to reflect different levels of

risk taking (e.g., smoking cigarettes, using drugs, driving a car at 100 miles an hour without a seat belt). Each of these items could be described as having a different *difficulty*. It is "easier" to agree with or admit to lower-risk items than higher-risk items. Item difficulty is one of the main parameters (there are others) that can be analyzed in IRT scale development. When item difficulty is the only parameter being considered in an IRT analysis, researchers often say that are using a **Rasch model**.

IRT is a more sophisticated approach than CMT for assessing the strengths and weaknesses of individual items, but it is more complex and uses software that is not as readily available—at least, as of the time of this writing. DeVellis (2003) believes that CMT scaling approaches will continue to prevail for affective measures, but suggests that IRT scaling is especially appropriate when the scale involves items that are inherently hierarchical. Those interested in latent trait scales and IRT should consult Hambleton, Swaminathan, and Rogers (1991) or Embretson and Reise (2000).

Example of an IRT-based scale: Doorenbos and colleagues (2005) used IRT to construct a multi-item scale of symptoms in women with breast cancer.

Developing an Item Pool: Getting Started

The next step is to develop a pool of possible items for the scale. Items—which collectively constitute the operational definition of the construct—need to be carefully crafted to reflect the latent variable they are designed to measure. This is often easier to do as a team effort because different people articulate a similar idea in diverse ways. But regardless of whether you are doing this alone or as part of a team effort, you may be asking, Where do items for a scale come from? Here are some possible sources:

1. *Existing instruments.* In some cases, it might be possible to adapt an existing instrument rather than starting from scratch. Although adaptations often require adding and deleting items, they also may involve rewording items— for example, to make them more culturally

appropriate, or to use simpler language for a population with low reading skills. If you adapt items, you should get permission from the author of the original scale because published scales are copyright protected.

2. *The literature.* Ideas for item content often come from a thorough understanding of the literature. Because at this point you would already be an "expert" on the construct, this should be an obvious source for possible items.

3. *Concept analysis.* A related source of ideas for items is a concept analysis—which you may already have undertaken as a preliminary step in the scale development process. Walker and Avant (2004) offer concept analysis strategies that could be used to develop items for a scale.

4. *In-depth qualitative research.* As mentioned in Chapter 12, in-depth inquiry relating to the key construct is a particularly rich source for scale items. Undertaking qualitative research, such as a phenomenological study, can help you to better understand the dimensions of a phenomenon, and can also give you the actual words to use for items. Tilden, Nelson, and May (1990), Beck and Gable (2001b), and Gilgun (2004) offer some guidance on the use of qualitative research as a mechanism for enhancing the content validity of a new scale.

5. *Focus groups.* Focus groups may also be an efficient means of determining how people express their ideas relating to the construct. If you are unable to undertake a focus group or other in-depth study before generating your items, be sure to pay particular attention to the verbatim quotes in qualitative reports relating to your construct.

6. *Clinical observations.* Patients in clinical settings may be an excellent source of items. Ideas for items may come from direct observation of patients' behaviors in relevant situations, or from listening to their comments and conversations with others.

Examples of Sources of Items: Abdallah and colleagues (2005) developed items for their scale to measure nurse practitioner activities through in-depth interviews, participant observation, and a focus group. McGilton (2003) used a concept analysis approach in developing her scales on supportive leadership for charge nurses and unit managers. Smith, Thurkettle, and de la Cruz (2004) derived items for their scale to measure nurses' use of intuition through a literature review and informal interviews with nursing students.

DeVellis (2003) urges scale developers to get started writing scale items without a lot of editing and critical review in the early stages. Perhaps a good way to begin if you are struggling is to develop a simple statement with the key construct mentioned in it. For example, if the construct is test anxiety, you might start with, "I get anxious when I take a test." This could be followed by similar statement worded differently (e.g., "Taking tests makes me nervous").

Making Decisions About Item Features

Either before you begin to generate items, or as you are doing it, you will need to make decisions about such issues as the number of items to develop, the number and form of the response options, whether to include both positively and negatively worded items, and how to deal with time.

Number of Items

In the CMT framework, a **domain sampling model** is frequently assumed, which involves the random sampling of a homogeneous set of items from a hypothetical universe of items relating to the construct. Of course, sampling from a *universe* of all possible items does not happen in reality for affective measures, but it is a principle worth keeping in mind in developing items. The idea is to generate a fairly exhaustive set of item possibilities, given the theoretical demands of the construct. For a traditional Likert scale, redundancy (except for trivial word substitutions) is a good thing—the goal is to measure the construct of interest with a set of items that capture the central theme in slightly different ways so that irrelevant idiosyncracies of individual items will cancel each other out.

Although there is no magic number for how many items should be developed, our advice is to generate a very large pool of items. As you proceed through the scale development process, many items will be discarded. Moreover, longer scales tend to be more reliable, so starting with a large number of items helps to ensure that you will eventually have a final scale with good internal consistency. DeVellis (2003) recommends starting with 3 to 4 times as many items as you will have in your final scale (e.g., 30 to 40 items for a 10-item scale), but at a minimum there should be 50% more (e.g., 15 items for a 10-item scale).

Response Options

Scale items involve both a stem (usually a declarative statement), and a set of response options. Traditional Likert scales often involve response options on a continuum of agreement, as previously noted, but other continua are also possible, such as frequency (never/always), importance (very important/unimportant), quality (excellent/very poor), and likelihood (definitely/definitely not).

How many response options should be given to respondents? There is no simple answer, but you should keep in mind the goal of a scale is to array people on a continuum, and so variability is essential. Variability can be enhanced by including a lot of items, by offering numerous response options, or both. However, there is not much merit in creating the illusion of precision when it does not exist. With a 0 to 100 range of scores, for example, the difference between a 96 and a 98 might not be meaningful.

Most Likert scales are created with 5 or 7 options, with verbal descriptors attached to each option and—often—with numbers placed under the descriptors to facilitate coding and to further help respondents find an appropriate place on the underlying continuum. An odd number of items provides respondents with an opportunity to be neutral or ambivalent (i.e., to choose a midpoint), and so some scale developers prefer an even number (e.g., 4 or 6) to force even mild leanings and avoid equivocation. However, inasmuch as some respondents may actually *be* neutral or ambivalent, a midpoint

options allows them to express it. The midpoint can be labeled with such phrases as "neither agree nor disagree," "undecided," "agree and disagree equally," or simply "?".

⮕ **T I P :** Here are some frequently used words for response options, with the midpoint term not listed:

- Strongly disagree, disagree, agree, strongly agree
- Disagree strongly, disagree moderately, disagree slightly, agree slightly, agree moderately, agree strongly
- Never, rarely (or seldom), occasionally (or sometimes), frequently (or usually), always
- Very important, important, moderately important, of little importance, unimportant
- Definitely not, probably not, possibly, probably, very probably, definitely

---

Positive and Negative Stems

A generation ago, on the advice of leading psychometricians, scale developers deliberately sought to include both positively and negatively worded statements in their scales, and to reverse-score the negative items. An example might be two items such as these on a scale of depression: "I frequently feel blue," and "I am happy most of the time." The objective was to include items that would minimize the possibility of an acquiescence response set—the tendency to agree with statements regardless of their content.

There is now sufficient evidence to suggest that it is not prudent to include both types of items on a scale. Some respondents appear to be confused by reversing polarities. Answering negative item stems appears to be an especially difficult cognitive task for younger respondents. Some research suggests that acquiescence can be minimized by putting the most positive response options (e.g., strongly agree) at the end of the list rather than at the beginning.

Item Intensity

In a traditional Likert scale, the intensity of the statements (stems) should be fairly similar, and fairly strongly worded. If items are so mildly stated that almost anyone would agree with them, the scale will not be able to discriminate between people with different amounts of the underlying latent variable. For example, an item such as "Good health is important" would generate almost universal agreement. On the other hand, statements should not be so extremely worded as to result in almost universal rejection. For example, "Nurses who do not have a B.S. degree should be shot," is obviously a poor measure of people's attitudes toward nursing credentials.

For a latent trait scale, scale developers would seek a range of item intensities. Even on such an IRT-based scale, however, there is no point in including items with which almost everyone would either agree or disagree.

Item Time Frames

Some items make an explicit reference to a time frame (e.g., "In the past few days I have had trouble falling asleep), but others do not (e.g., "I have trouble falling asleep"). Sometimes instructions to a scale can designate a temporal frame of reference (e.g., "In answering the following questions, please indicate how you have felt in the past week"). And yet other scales ask respondents to respond in terms of a time frame: "In the past week, I have had trouble falling asleep: Every day, 5–6 days . . . Never."

A time frame should not emerge as a consequence of item development. You should decide in advance, based on your conceptual understanding of the construct and the needs for which the scale is being constructed, how to deal with time.

> **Example of handling time in a scale:** The Postpartum Depression Screening Scale asks respondents to indicate their emotional state in the past 2 weeks—for example, over the past 2 weeks I: " . . . felt so all alone" or ". . .cried a lot for no reason" (Beck & Gable, 2000, 2001a). This 2-week timeframe was chosen because it parallels the duration of symptoms required for a diagnosis of major depressive episode according to the *DSM-IV* criteria.

Wording the Items

Items should be worded in such a manner that every respondent is answering the same question. A number of resources are available to guide you in wording good items (e.g., Fowler, 1995; Streiner & Norman, 2003). Some suggestions on question wording are provided in Chapter 16, and here we provide just a few additional tips to wording clear, comprehensible items that tap the core construct and minimize response error:

1. *Clarity.* Scale developers should obviously strive for item clarity and avoid ambiguities. Words should be carefully chosen with the educational background and reading level of the population for whom the scale is intended in mind. In most cases, this will mean developing a scale at the 6th- to 7th-grade reading level. But even beyond reading level, you should do your best to select words that everyone will understand, and to have everyone reach the same conclusion about what the words mean.

2. *Jargon.* Jargon should generally be avoided. Be especially cautious about using terms that might be well-known in health care circles (e.g., lesion) but not familiar to the average person.

3. *Length.* Avoid long sentences or phrases. Simple sentences are the easiest to comprehend. In particular, eliminate unnecessary words. For example, "It is fair to say that in the scheme of things I do not get enough sleep," could more simply be worded, "I usually do not get enough sleep." There is some evidence that item length and validity coefficients are inversely related (Holden, Fekken, & Jackson, 1985).

4. *Double negatives.* It is often preferable to word things in an affirmative way ("I am usually happy" than in a negative way ("I am not usually sad"), but double negatives should always be avoided ("I am *not* usually *un*happy").

5. *Double-barreled items.* Avoid putting two or more ideas in a single item. For example, "I am afraid of insects and snakes" is a bad item because a person who is afraid of insects but not snakes (or *vice versa*) would not know how to respond.

Some additional issues are important for scale developers who know or anticipate that the scale will be translated into other languages, as we discuss in a subsequent section.

> **Examples of well-worded items:** Here are two items from the purposeful action Medication-Taking Questionnaire for hypertensive patients (Johnson & Rogers, 2006): "I would rather treat my blood pressure without pills" and "I am OK if I do not take my blood pressure pills." Respondents indicate agreement or disagreement with items on a 7-point scale. (The report appears in its entirety in Appendix I of the accompanying *Resource Manual*).

PRELIMINARY EVALUATION OF ITEMS

Internal Review

Once a sufficiently large pool of items has been generated, it is time for critical appraisal. Review should begin with thoughtful inspection by the scale developers, with care devoted to such issues as whether individual items capture the construct, are grammatical, and are well worded. The initial review should also consider whether the items taken together adequately embrace the full nuances of the construct—that is, whether additional items need to be generated to enhance the scale's content validity.

It is also imperative to assess the scale's **readability** (unless the scale is intended for a population with known high literacy, such as people with advanced degrees). There are a lot of different approaches for assessing the reading level of written documents, but unfortunately many of these methods are either time-consuming or require several hundreds of words of text, and thus are not suited to evaluating scale items (Streiner & Norman, 2003).

Many word processing programs provide some information about readability. In Microsoft Word, for example, you could type your items on a list and then get readability statistics for the items as a whole or for individual items using the Spelling and Grammar option on the Tools menu. For example, take the following two sets of items for tapping fatigue:

Set A	Set B
I am frequently exhausted.	I am often tired.
I invariably get insufficient sleep.	I don't get enough sleep.

The Word software tells us that the items in set A have a *Flesch-Kincaid grade level* of 12.0 and a *Flesch reading ease score* of 4.8. (The reading ease score rates text on a 100-point scale, with higher values associated with greater ease, using a formula that considers average sentence length and the average number of syllables.) Set B, by contrast, has a grade level of 1.8 and a reading ease score of 89.4. Streiner and Norman (2003) recommend that word processing–based readability information be interpreted cautiously, but it is clear from the foregoing analysis that the second set of items would be far superior to the first set for a population that includes respondents with limited education. A general principle is to avoid long sentences and words with four or more syllables.

> **Example of assessing readability:** Janssen, Dennis, and Reime (2006) developed a scale to measure satisfaction with intrapartum and postpartum hospital care, the Care in Obstetrics: A Measure for Testing Satisfaction (COMFORTS) Scale. The final Flesch reading level of the scale was grade 6.

Input From the Target Population

Even before the scale items are actually administered to respondents from the population of interest for the purpose of psychometric analysis, it is often productive to get some preliminary feedback from a small number of people. One approach is to pretest the items with a sample of about 10 to 20 people drawn from the target population. These respondents can be asked some simple questions (e.g., Are there statements that confused you? Did you understand the meaning of each question? Were the directions for completing the form clear?). *Cognitive questioning* is an excellent technique for discovering how others process the words and ideas presented to them in structured questions. ⊗ Streiner and Norman (2003, pp. 65–66) describe several other techniques that can be used to detect ambiguities and language problems in a pretest.

◆ TIP: When questioning pretest respondents about the clarity or meaning of the items, avoid using the word "item," which is research jargon (i.e., do not say, "Are there *items* that confused you?").

Additionally, it is a good idea to peruse the pretest answers to see if response patterns suggest the need for item revisions or deletions. For example, items with virtually no variability (e.g., everyone agrees or disagrees) should be revised or omitted because they cannot contribute to the scale's ability to discriminate among people with varying degrees of the underlying construct. Streiner and Norman (2003) warn that if the pretest fails to suggest any changes, this probably indicates a flaw in the pretest rather than problem-free items.

As an alternative or supplement to pretests, focus groups can also be used at this stage in scale development. Two or three groups can be convened to discuss whether, from the participants' perspective, the items are understandable, linguistically and culturally appropriate, inoffensive, and relevant to the construct.

External Review by Experts

External review of the revised items by a panel of experts is all but essential to establish the scale's content validity. It is advisable to undertake two rounds of review, if feasible—the first to refine or weed out faulty items or to add new items to cover the domain adequately, and the second to formally assess the content validity of the items and scale. We discuss some procedures in such a two-step strategy, although the two steps are sometimes combined.

Selecting and Recruiting the Experts
The panel of experts needs to include people with strong credentials with regard to the construct being measured. Criteria such as the following can be used in identifying substantive experts: documented clinical experience, published papers on the topic in refereed journals, presentations at national professional meetings, or an ongoing program of research on the topic. The experts should be knowledgeable about the key construct *and* the target population. Also, if the construct has close links to a theory (e.g., Orem's self-care theory), then experts on the theory should also be included. In the first round of review, it is also desirable to include experts on scale construction.

In the initial phase of a two-part review, we advise a good mix of experts, so a panel with 8 to 12 members is likely to be necessary. It is also prudent to include a mix of experts in terms of roles (e.g., clinicians, faculty, researchers) as well as relevant disciplines. For example, for a scale designed to measure fear of dying in the elderly, the experts might include nurses, gerontologists, and psychiatrists. If the scale is intended for broad use, it might also be advantageous to recruit experts from various areas of the country, because of possible regional variations in language. The second panel for formally assessing the content validity of a more refined set of items should consist of three to five experts in the content area.

Example of an expert panel: Wynd and Schaefer (2002) invited 12 experts to review the Osteoporosis Risk Assessment Tool (ORAT). Experts were sought if they had clinical and research knowledge about osteoporosis risk in adults, based on their credentials and record of research. The experts included physicians, nurses with advanced clinical practice, and nurse researchers, selected for widespread geographic representation.

Grant and Davis (1997) offer advice on information to include in a cover letter soliciting the cooperation of potential experts. The panel of experts is typically sent (usually via mail or e-mail) a packet of materials, including background information relating to the construct and target population, reviewer instructions, and a questionnaire soliciting the expert's opinion. A critical component of the packet is a careful explanation of the conceptual underpinnings of the construct, including an explication of the various dimensions encompassed by the construct to be captured in subscales. The panel may also be given a brief overview of the literature, as well as a bibliography. ✱ The Toolkit of the *Resource Manual* includes a sample cover letter and other material relating to expert review (as Word documents that can be adapted).

Preliminary Expert Review: Content Validation of Items

The job of the experts is to evaluate both individual items and the overall scale (and any subscales), using guidelines established by the scale developer. The first panel of experts is usually invited to rate each item along several dimensions, and so the task is complex. Among the dimensions often used are the following: clarity of wording; relevance of the item to the underlying construct or a specific dimension of the construct; and appropriateness of the item for the target population (e.g., developmental or cultural appropriateness). Experts could

either be asked to make judgments dichotomously (e.g., unclear/clear) or along a continuum. Relevance, for example, is often rated as follows: 1 = not relevant, 2 = somewhat relevant, 3 = quite relevant, 4 = highly relevant. Figure 18.1 ✱ shows a possible format for a content validation assessment of relevance.

The questionnaire usually asks for elaboration (qualitative information) for items judged to be unclear, not relevant, or not appropriate, such as how the item might be worded more clearly, or why the item is deemed to be not relevant. Another dimension that could be included for each item in a first-phase evaluation concerns an overall recommendation—for example: retain the item exactly as worded; make major revisions to the item; make minor revisions to the item; and drop the item entirely.

For scales encompassing multiple aspects of a construct that require subscales, an alternative procedure for evaluating item relevance is to ask the

---

The scale items shown below have been developed to measure one dimension of the construct of safe sexual behaviors among adolescents, namely **assertiveness.** Please read each item and score it for its relevance in representing this concept.

Assertiveness is defined as the use of verbal and interpersonal skills to negotiate protection during sexual activities.

Item	**Relevance Rating**			
	Not Relevant	Somewhat Relevant	Quite Relevant	Highly Relevant
1. I ask my partner about his/her sexual history before having intercourse.	1	2	3	4
2. I don't have sex without asking the person if he/she has been tested for HIV/AIDS.	1	2	3	4
3. When I am having sex with someone for the first time, I insist that we use a condom.	1	2	3	4
4. I don't let my partner talk me into having sex without knowing something about how risky it would be.	1	2	3	4

Please comment on any of these items, including possible revisions or substitutions, or your thoughts about why an item is not relevant to the concept of assertiveness. Please suggest any additional items you feel would improve the measurement of assertiveness relating to adolescents' safe sexual behaviors.

FIGURE 18.1 Example of a content validity form.

experts to match each item with a specific dimension of the construct (e.g., to which of the four dimensions does item 2 belong?). Gable and Wolfe (1993) offer guidelines and formats for undertaking such a task.

In addition to evaluating each item, the initial panel of experts should be asked to consider whether the items taken as a whole adequately cover the construct domain. The items on a scale constitute the operational definition of the construct, so it is important to assess whether the operational definition taps each dimension adequately. Specific guidance on items or subdomains that should be added should be solicited from the experts. For scales constructed within an IRT framework, the experts should also be asked whether they perceive the items as a whole to span a continuum of difficulty (i.e., whether the underlying hierarchy is adequately captured).

If there is agreement among the experts, the next step is straightforward: their opinion is used to guide decisions about retaining, revising, deleting, or adding items. When there is disagreement, however, it may require further investigation. Perhaps the experts did not understand the task, perhaps some have a tendency to give high (or low) ratings, perhaps the conceptual definitions were ambiguous, and so on. In other words, you may need to evaluate the experts and your own instructions as well as the items and the scale.

The typical formula for evaluating agreement among experts on individual items is the number agreeing, divided by the number of experts. When the dimension being rated is relevance, the standard method for computing a content validity index *at the item level* (I-CVI) is the number giving a rating of either 3 or 4 on the 4-point relevance scale, divided by the number of raters. For example, if five experts rated an item as 3 and one rated the item as 2, the I-CVI would be .83. Because of the risk for chance agreement when ratings are dichotomous—relevant versus not relevant—we recommend that I-CVIs should be .78 or higher (Polit, Beck, & Owen, in press). This means that there must be 100% agreement of relevance among

raters when there are four or fewer content experts. When there are five to eight experts, one rating of "not relevant" can be tolerated, and when there are nine or more experts, even more can disagree on relevance.

Items with lower than desired I-CVIs need careful scrutiny. It may be necessary to recontact the experts to better understand genuine differences of opinion or to strive for greater consensus. If there are legitimate disagreements among the experts on individual items (or if there is strong agreement about lack of relevance), the items should be revised or dropped.

Content Validation of the Scale

In the second round of content validation, a smaller group of experts (perhaps three to five) can be used to evaluate the relevance of the revised set of items and to compute the scale content validity (S-CVI). Lynn (1986) suggests that the raters can be drawn from the same pool of experts as in the first phase, but they can also be a new group. We recommend using a subset of experts from the first panel because then information from the first round can be used to select the most qualified judges. With information from round 1, for example, you can perhaps identify experts who did not understand the task, who had a tendency to give high (or low) ratings, who were not as familiar with the construct as you thought, or who otherwise seemed biased. In other words, data from the first round can be analyzed with a view toward evaluating the performance of the experts, not just the items. This analysis might also require in-depth discussion with some of the experts to fully understand the reason for any incongruent or anomalous ratings.

With respect to the analysis of the experts from their quantitative ratings, here are some suggestions. First, it may be imprudent to select experts who rated every item as "highly relevant" (or "not relevant"). Second, it would not be wise to invite back an expert who gave high ratings to items that were judged by most others to not be relevant, or *vice versa*. Third, the proportion of items judged relevant should be computed for all judges. For example, if the first expert rated 8 out of 10 items as relevant, the proportion for that judge would be .80. The patterns of proportions across experts can be examined for "outliers." If the average proportion across raters is, for example, .80, you might want to have a discussion with experts whose average proportion was either very low (e.g., .50) or very high (e.g., 1.0) to determine whether they understood the task. Or, you might simply avoid inviting this expert back for the second round. Qualitative feedback from an expert in round 1 in the form of useful comments about the items might indicate both content capability and a strong commitment to the project. Finally, items known not to be relevant can be included in the first round to identify judges who rate irrelevant items as relevant and thus may not really be experts after all.

Once the panel is selected and ratings of relevance are obtained for the revised set of items, the S-CVI can be computed. There is, unfortunately, more than one way to compute an S-CVI, and computation methods are almost never reported in scale development papers (Polit & Beck, 2006). As discussed in Chapter 17, we recommend the approach that averages across I-CVIs (S-CVI/Ave). On a 10-item scale, for example, if the I-CVIs for 5 items were .80 and the I-CVIs for the remaining 5 items were 1.00, then the S-CVI/Ave would be .90. We recommend an S-CVI/Ave of .90 or higher.

In summary, we recommend that for a scale to be judged as having excellent content validity, it would be composed of items that had I-CVIs of .78 or higher and an S-CVI (using the averaging approach) of .90 or higher. This requires strong items, outstanding experts, and clear instructions to the experts regarding the underlying constructs and the rating task.

⟶ TIP: When you describe your content validation efforts in a report, be specific about your criteria for accepting items (i.e., the cut-off value for your I-CVIs) and the scale (the S-CVI). You will also need to specify what method you used to compute the S-CVI. Finally, your report should indicate the range of obtained values for the I-CVIs.

ADMINISTRATION TO A DEVELOPMENT SAMPLE

At this point, you will have whittled down and refined your item pool based on your own and others' careful scrutiny. The next step in scale development is to undertake a quantitative assessment of the items, which requires that they be administered to a fairly large development sample. As with content validation, this may involve a two-part process, with preliminary assessment occurring in the first phase and subsequent efforts to establish construct validity and fully establish psychometric adequacy of the final scale in the second.

Testing a new instrument is a full study in and of itself, and care must be taken to design the study so that it will yield useful evidence regarding the worth of the scale. If you have reached this point, you already have done a literature review, developed a strong conceptual basis for your study, and developed the instrument. Now you need to develop a sampling plan and a data collection strategy.

Developing a Sampling Plan

The development sample should be drawn from the population for whom the scale has been devised. An ideal development sample is representative of the population and large enough to support complex analyses. If it is not possible to administer the pool of items to a random sample from the target population (as is typical), it is nevertheless worthwhile to recruit a sample from multiple, geographically distant sites to enhance representativeness and to guard against the risk for geographic variation in interpreting scale items. Other strategies to enhance representativeness should be sought, as well—for example, making sure that the sample includes older and younger respondents, men and women, people with varying educational and ethnic backgrounds, and so on, if these characteristics are relevant. One other note is that if you do not plan on a follow-up study to confirm the psychometric properties of the final scale, you should consider taking steps to ensure that the sample includes the right kind of people for a "known-groups" analysis.

How large is a "large" sample? There is neither consensus among experts nor hard-and-fast rules, unfortunately. Some suggest that 300 is an adequate number to support a factor analysis (e.g., Nunnally & Bernstein, 1994), whereas others offer guidance in terms of a ratio of items to respondents. Recommendations range from 3 or 4 people per item to 40 or 50 per item (Knapp & Brown, 1995). Ten respondents per item is the number that seems to be most often recommended. That means that if you have 20 items, your sample should probably be at least 200. The main issue with regard to sample size is that covariation among the items might not be stable if there are too few observations.

Developing a Data Collection Plan

Decisions have to be made concerning how to administer the instrument (e.g., by mailed or distributed questionnaires, over the Internet), and what to include in the instrument. In deciding on a mode of administration, you should choose an approach that best approximates how the scale typically would be administered after it is finalized. There is no sense collecting development data in an oral interview if the scale usually would be administered in writing, or *vice versa*. Thought should also be given to administration setting. For example, if the scale is designed as a screening tool for hospitalized patients, then hospitals should be the setting for collecting the development data.

The essential things to include on the instrument are the items themselves and basic demographic information. Thought should also be given to including other measures on the instrument, however—especially if you do not anticipate a second study for the purposes of establishing the scale's validity. In such a situation, it would be important to include validation measures in the initial study.

One type of validation measure concerns constructs similar to, but distinct from, the construct being captured by the new scale to evaluate discriminant validity. Measures of other constructs hypothesized to be related to the target construct

should also be considered. If the data confirm a relationship predicted by theory or prior research, this would lend evidence to the new scale's validity. Finally, it may be useful to include measures to assess response biases, especially social desirability. Inferences about items that are influenced by this bias can be made by examining the items' correlations with a measure of social desirability. (More complex approaches to evaluating and addressing the effects of social desirability and "faking bad" biases are discussed in Streiner and Norman, Chapter 6.) Brief 10-item (Strahan & Gerbasi, 1972) and 13-item (Reynolds, 1982) social desirability scales have been developed.

➲ TIP: In deciding on what other measures to include in the study, it is important to remember that respondents' motivation to cooperate may decline as the instrument package gets longer.

Preparing for Data Collection

As in all data collection efforts, care should be taken to make the instrument attractive, professional looking, and easy to read and understand. The use of color or graphics may enhance response rates. Colleagues, friends, or family members should be asked to evaluate the appearance of the instrument before it is reproduced.

Instructions for completing the instrument should be clear. There should be no ambiguity about what is expected of respondents, and guidance in understanding the end anchor points of response options should be provided if points along the continuum are not explicitly labeled. The instructions should encourage candor. Sometimes social desirability can be minimized through statements that indicate there are no right or wrong answers. Of course, anonymity also reduces social desirability bias, and is recommended—unless there is a desire to administer the scale a second time for the purposes of estimating test–retest reliability. Pett, Lackey, and Sullivan (2003) offer useful suggestions for laying out an instrument and for developing instructions to respondents.

One other consideration is how to sequence the items in the instrument. At issue is something that is referred to as a *proximity effect*, the tendency to be influenced in responding to an item by the response given to the previous item. This effect would tend to artificially inflate estimates of internal consistency. One approach to deal with this is the random ordering of items. An alternative, for scales designed to measure several related dimensions, is to systematically alternate items that are expected to be scored into different subscales.

Example of item ordering: Beck and Gable's (2000) Postpartum Depression Screening Scale (PDSS) consists of seven subscales. Items on the PDSS are ordered so that one item from each of the seven subscales is presented before going on to the next series. Items on the "Suicidal Thoughts" subscale are always last in the series because of the emotion-laden content of these items.

ANALYSIS OF SCALE DEVELOPMENT DATA

The analysis of data from multi-item scales is a topic on which entire books have been written. We provide only an overview here, together with suggestions for further reading. We assume that readers of this section have basic familiarity with statistics. Those who need a refresher should consult Chapters 21 through 23.

Basic Item Analysis

The performance of each item on the preliminary scale needs to be evaluated empirically. Within classical measurement theory, what is desired is an item that has a high correlation with the true score of the underlying construct. We cannot assess this directly, but if each item is a measure of that latent variable, then the items should correlate with one another.

The best way to assess degree of **inter-item correlation** is to inspect the correlation matrix of all the items. If there are items with substantial negative inter-item correlations, some should perhaps be reverse-scored, using the computer to create a new variable (e.g., NEWITEM = 8 – OLDITEM, for 7-point scales). However, negative correlations, unless intentional, are likely to reflect problems with some of the items. And if negative correlations persist after reverse scoring (unless there is a separate subscale for negative items), the troubling items should probably be deleted. For items on the same subscale, inter-item correlations between .30 and .70 are often recommended (e.g., Ferketich, 1991), with correlations lower than .30 suggesting little congruence with the underlying construct and ones higher than .70 suggesting over-redundancy. Knapp and Brown (1995), however, suggest that several of these item analysis guidelines have no firm empirical basis and that cut-off values may be scale specific. Indeed, in the case of item inter-item correlation, a great deal depends on the number of items in the scale. An average inter-item correlation of .57 is needed to achieve a coefficient alpha of .80 on a 3-item scale, but an average of only .29 is needed for a 10-item scale (DeVellis, 2003).

A next step is to compute preliminary total scale scores (or subscale scores if appropriate) and then to calculate the correlation between individual items and the total scores on the scales they are intended to represent. If item scores do not correlate well with scale scores, it is probably measuring something else and will lower the reliability of the scale. There are two types of **item–scale correlations**, one in which the total score includes the item under consideration (*uncorrected*), and another in which the individual item is removed from the calculation of the total scale score. The latter (*corrected*) approach is preferable because the inclusion of the item on the scale inflates the correlation coefficients, and the inflation factor increases as the number of items on the scale decreases. The standard advice is to eliminate items whose correlation with the total scale is less than .30, but values as high as .50 have been recommended by some. Whether one accepts these criteria or not, higher item–total correlations are more desirable than lower ones.

DeVellis (2003) also advocates looking at basic descriptive information for each item, as a double check. Items should clearly have good variability—without it, they will not correlate with the total scale and will not fare well in a reliability or factor analysis. Means for the items that are close to the center of the range of possible scores are also desirable (e.g., a mean near 4 on a 7-point scale). Items with means near one extreme or the other tend not to discriminate well among respondents.

Other item analysis techniques have been developed, many in connection with measures of cognitive abilities. Some scale developers compute item *p* levels or *difficulty levels,* which are indicators of how "difficult" each item is. For example, if 60 people agreed with an item and 40 disagreed with it, it could be said that the *p* level for the item was .60 because 60% found it "easy" to agree. Items in the middle range of difficulty are most desirable. Another index that is too complex to explain here is the *discrimination index*, which examines the discriminative ability of each item. As mentioned earlier, item response theory has given rise to a number of excellent diagnostic tools for examining the performance of individual items. These and other item analysis techniques are described elsewhere (e.g., Gable & Wolfe, 1993; Nunnally & Bernstein, 1994; Waltz et al., 2005)

Example of item analysis: Heo and co-researchers (2005) undertook several item analytic procedures with data from a sample of 638 patients in their evaluation of the Minnesota Living With Heart Failure Questionnaire. They computed item–total correlations, inter-item correlations, item *p* levels, and a discrimination index. As a result of these and other analyses, they recommended that 5 items be deleted.

Exploratory Factor Analysis

A set of items is not necessarily a scale—the items form a scale only if they have a common underlying construct. **Factor analysis** disentangles complex interrelationships among items and identifies items that "go together" as unified concepts. This section deals with a type of factor analysis known as **exploratory factor analysis (EFA)**, which essentially assumes no *a priori* hypotheses about dimensionality of a set of items. Another type—confirmatory factor analysis—uses more complex modeling and estimation procedures, as described later.

Suppose we developed 50 Likert-type items measuring women's attitudes toward menopause. We could form a scale by adding together scores from several individual items, but which items should be combined? Would it be reasonable to combine all 50 items? Probably not, because the 50 items are not all tapping the same thing—there are various *dimensions* to women's attitude toward menopause. One dimension may relate to aging, and another to loss of reproductive ability. Other items may involve sexuality, and yet others may concern avoidance of monthly aggravation. These multiple dimensions to women's attitudes toward menopause should be captured on separate subscales. Women's attitude on one dimension may be independent of their attitude on another. Identifying dimensions of a construct is often done during the early conceptualization phase and when the items are being evaluated by experts. Preconceptions about dimensions, however, do not always "pan out" when tested against actual responses. Factor analysis offers an objective, empirical method of clarifying the underlying dimensionality of a large set of measures. Underlying dimensions thus identified are called **factors**, which are weighted combinations of items in the analysis.

Factor Extraction

EFA involves two phases. The first phase (**factor extraction**) condenses items in the data matrix into a smaller number of factors and thus is used to define the number of underlying dimensions. The general goal is to extract clusters of highly interrelated items from a correlation matrix. There are various methods of performing the first step, each of which uses different criteria for assigning weights to items. The most widely used factor extraction method is called **principal components analysis (PCA)**, but another recommended method is called **common factor analysis**. The pros and cons of these two alternative approaches to factor extraction have been nicely summarized by Pett and colleagues (2003). Our discussion focuses on PCA, although there is overlap between the two

TABLE 18.1	Summary of Factor Extraction Results

FACTOR	EIGENVALUE	PERCENTAGE OF VARIANCE EXPLAINED	CUMULATIVE PERCENTAGE OF VARIANCE EXPLAINED
1	12.32	29.2	29.2
2	8.57	23.3	52.5
3	6.91	15.6	68.1
4	2.02	8.4	76.5
5	1.09	6.2	82.7
6	.98	5.8	88.5
7	.80	4.5	93.0
8	.62	3.1	96.1
9	.47	2.2	98.3
10	.25	1.7	100.0

methods. The two procedures usually (although not always) lead to the same conclusions about underlying dimensionality.

Factor extraction results in an *unrotated factor matrix,* which contains coefficients or *weights* for all original items on each extracted factor. Each factor that is extracted is a weighted linear combination of all the original items. For example, with three items, a factor would be item 1 (times a weight) + item 2 (times a weight) + item 3 (times a weight). In the PCA method, weights for the first factor are computed such that the average squared weight is maximized, permitting a maximum amount of variance to be extracted by the first factor. The second factor, or linear weighted combination, is formed so that the highest possible amount of variance is extracted from what *remains* after the first factor has been taken into account. The factors thus represent independent sources of variation in the data matrix.

Factoring should continue until there is no further meaningful variance left, and so a criterion must be applied to determine when to stop extraction and move on to the second phase. There are several possible criteria, a fact that makes factor analysis a semisubjective process. Several of the most commonly used criteria can be described by

illustrating information generated in a factor analysis. Table 18.1 presents fictitious values for eigenvalues, percentages of variance accounted for, and cumulative percentages of variance accounted for, for 10 factors. **Eigenvalues** are equal to the sum of the squared weights for the factor. Many researchers establish as their cut-off point for factor extraction eigenvalues greater than 1.00. In our example, the first 5 factors meet this criterion. Some believe that the eigenvalue rule is too generous, that is, extracts too many factors (e.g., DeVellis, 2003). Another cut-off benchmark, referred to as the *scree test,* is based on a principle of discontinuity: A sharp drop in the percentage of explained variance indicates the appropriate termination point. In Table 18.1, we might argue that there is considerable discontinuity between the third and fourth factors—that is, that 3 factors should be extracted. Yet another guideline concerns the amount of variance explained by the factors. Some advocate that the number of factors extracted should account for at least 60% of the total variance, and that for any factor to be meaningful, it must account for at least 5% of the variance. In our table, the first 3 factors account for 68.1% of the total variance; 6 factors contribute 5% or more to the total variance.

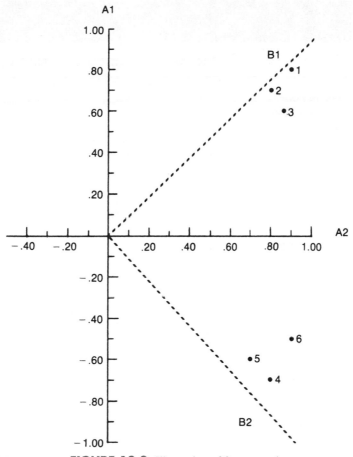

FIGURE 18.2 Illustration of factor rotation.

So, should we extract 3, 5, or 6 factors? One approach is to see whether there is any convergence among these guidelines. In our example, two of them (the scree test and total variance test) suggest 3 factors. Another approach is to determine whether any of the rules yields a number consistent with our original conceptualization about dimensionality. In our example, if we had designed the items to represent three theoretically meaningful subscales, we might consider 3 factors to be the right number because there is sufficient empirical support for that conclusion. Indeed, some have argued that restricting the factor solution to a pre-specified number of factors that is consistent with the original conceptualization can yield important

information regarding how much variance is accounted for by the factors.

Factor Rotation
The second phase of factor analysis—**factor rotation**—is performed on factors that have met the extraction criteria, to make the factors more interpretable. The concept of rotation can be best explained graphically. Figure 18.2 shows two coordinate systems, marked by axes A1 and A2 and B1 and B2. The primary axes (A1 and A2) represent factors I and II, respectively, as defined *before* rotation. The points 1 through 6 represent 6 items in this two-dimensional space. The weights associated with each item can be determined in reference to

| TABLE 18.2 | Factor Loadings: School-Age Temperament Inventory | | | |

ITEM	FACTOR 1	FACTOR 2	FACTOR 3	FACTOR 4
1. Does not complete homework[a]	.04	**.82**	−.01	.07
2. Is shy with adults he (she) doesn't know	.02	.00	**.78**	.00
3. Runs when entering or leaving	.16	.03	.00	**.79**
4. Is bashful when meeting new children	.09	.01	**.80**	−.01
5. Stays with homework until finished	.04	**.84**	.00	.06
6. Yells or snaps at others when angry	**.79**[b]	.05	.04	.12
7. Runs or jumps when going down stairs	.18	.11	.05	**.74**
8. Is moody when corrected for misbehavior	**.75**	.10	.13	.02
9. Runs to where he (she) wants to go	.09	.07	−.10	**.77**
10. Responds intensely to disapproval	**.78**	.11	.06	.12
11. Has difficulty completing assignments[a]	.08	**.78**	.01	.04
12. Seems uncomfortable at someone's house	.11	.06	**.75**	.06

[a]Item was reverse-coded before factor analysis.

[b]Bolded entries represent high loadings on a factor and are used to name and interpret the factor.

Adapted from Table 1 of McClowry, S. G., Halverson, C. F., & Sanson, A. (2003). A re-examination of the validity and reliability of the School-Age Temperament Inventory. *Nursing Research, 52*(3), 176–182.

these axes. For instance, before rotation, item 1 has a weight of .80 on factor I and .85 on factor II, and item 6 has a weight of −.45 on factor I and .90 on factor II. Unrotated axes account for a maximum amount of variance but rarely provide a structure with conceptual meaning. Interpretability is enhanced by rotating the axes so that clusters of items are distinctly associated with a factor. In the figure, B1 and B2 represent rotated factors. After rotation, items 1, 2, and 3 have large weights on factor I and small weights on factor II, and the reverse is true for items 4, 5, and 6.

Researchers choose from two classes of rotation. Figure 18.2 illustrates **orthogonal rotation**, in which factors are kept at right angles to one another. Orthogonal rotations maintain the independence of factors—that is, orthogonal factors are uncorrelated with one another. **Oblique rotations**, on the other hand, permit rotated axes to depart from a 90-degree angle. In our figure, an oblique rotation would have put axis B1 between items 2 and 3 and axis B2 between items 5 and 6. This

placement strengthens the clustering of items around an associated factor, but results in correlated factors. Some researchers argue that orthogonal rotation leads to greater theoretical clarity; others claim that it is unrealistic. Those advocating oblique rotation point out that if the concepts *are* correlated, then the analysis should reflect this fact. In developing a scale with multiple dimensions, we likely would expect the dimensions to be correlated, and so oblique rotation might well reveal more theoretically meaningful results. This can be determined empirically: if an oblique rotation is specified, information about correlation between factors is provided. If the correlations are low (e.g., less than .15 or .20), an orthogonal rotation may be preferred because it yields a simpler model.

Researchers work with a **rotated factor matrix** in interpreting the factor analysis. An example of such a matrix is displayed in Table 18.2. This matrix was adapted from a table for a factor analysis of the School-Age Temperament Inventory (SATI), and only shows information for 12 of the scale's 38 items

(McClowry, Halverson, & Sanson, 2003). The entries under each factor are the weights, called **factor loadings**. For orthogonally rotated factors, factor loadings can range from −1.00 to +1.00 and can be interpreted like correlation coefficients—they express the correlation between individual items and factors, that is, the underlying dimensions. In this example, item 1 is highly correlated with factor 2, .82. By examining factor loadings, it is possible to find which items "belong" to a factor. For example, items 6, 8, and 10 have sizable loadings on factor 1. (Loadings with an absolute value of .40 or higher often are used as cutoff values, although smaller values are acceptable if the item pool is large.) The underlying dimensionality of the data can then be interpreted. By inspecting the content of items 6, 8, and 10, we can search for a common theme that makes the items go together. The developers of the SATI called this first factor Negative Reactivity. Items 1, 5, and 11 have high loadings on factor 2, which they named Task Persistence. Factors 3 and 4 are called Approach/Withdrawal and Activity, respectively. The naming of factors is a process of identifying underlying constructs—and in most cases, this naming would have occurred during the early phases of conceptualization.

The results of the factor analysis can be used not only to identify the dimensionality of the construct but also to make decisions about item retention and deletion. If items have very low loadings on all factors, they may be good candidates for deletion (or revision, if you can detect wording problems that may have caused different respondents to infer different meaning from the item). Items that have fairly high loadings on multiple factors may also indicate the need for rewording. Items with marginal loadings (e.g., .35) but that appear to have good content validity probably should be retained for the reliability analysis.

Example of exploratory factor analysis:
Klakovich and de la Cruz (2006) developed a scale to measure interpersonal communication in nursing, the Interpersonal Communication Assessment Scale (ICAS). The 54-item scale was tested with 246 clinical faculty. Exploratory factor analysis resulted in a 3-factor solution, and the factors were labeled Advocacy, Therapeutic Use of Self, and Validation.

Reliability Analysis

After we have selected a final set of items based on the item analysis and factor analysis, a reliability analysis should be undertaken to calculate coefficient alpha. Alpha, it may be recalled, provides an estimate of the proportion of variance in the scale scores that is attributable to the true score and thus is a key indicator of the scale's quality.

Most computer programs for doing reliability analysis provide extensive information about the overall scale and individual items, including many item analysis diagnostics we described earlier. Especially important at this point in scale development is information about the value of coefficient alpha for the scale—and for a hypothetical scale in which each individual item is removed. If the overall alpha is extremely high, it may be prudent at this point to eliminate redundancy by deleting items that do not make a sizeable contribution to alpha. (Sometimes removal of an item actually *increases* alpha.) In some cases, a modest reduction in reliability is worth the benefit of lowering respondent burden. Scale developers must consider the best tradeoff between brevity and reliability.

One thing that should be kept in mind is that reliabilities tend to capitalize on chance factors in a sample of respondents, and will often be lower in a new sample. Thus, you should aim for reliabilities a bit higher in the development sample than ones you would consider minimally acceptable so that if the alphas deteriorate they will still be adequate. This is especially true if the development sample is small.

⊃ TIP: If you have the good fortune to have a very large sample, you should consider dividing the sample in half, running the factor analysis and reliability analysis with one subsample, and then re-running them with the second as a cross-validation of factor structure and scale reliabilities.

FINAL STEPS: SCALE REFINEMENT AND VALIDATION

In some scale development efforts, the bulk of the work is over at this point. For example, if you developed a scale as part of a larger substantive project because you were unable to identify a good measure of a key construct, you may be ready at this point to pursue your substantive analyses. If, however, you are developing a scale that you expect others will want to use, a few more steps remain.

Revising the Scale

The analyses undertaken in the development study often suggest the need to reword items, and may also indicate that more items need to be developed. For example, if any alpha coefficients for subscales are lower than .80 or so, consideration should be given to adding a couple of items for subsequent testing. In thinking about new items, a good strategy is to examine the items that had high factor loadings. The ones with high loadings presumably correlate most strongly with the latent variable and may offer powerful clues for new items.

There may be other reasons for adding new items. For example, if a confirmatory factor analysis is envisioned as part of a scale validation effort, it is important to have at least 4 items for each factor (subscale) because there are technical problems with dimensions having 3 or fewer items.

Finally, you should carefully examine the content of the items remaining in your scale. Sometimes alphas are inflated by items that have similar wording, so it is wise to make decisions about retaining or removing items not only on the basis of their contribution to alpha, but also on the basis of content validity considerations. It is likely to prove worthwhile to re-examine data on the I-CVIs of each item in making final decisions.

Scoring and Transforming the Scale

Scoring the scale is often easy with Likert-type items: item scores are typically just added together (with reverse-scoring of items, if appropriate) to form subscale scores, and subscale scores are added together to form total scale scores. However, scoring in this manner on the final scale should be a conscious decision.

When individual items are simply added together, the implicit assumption is that all of the items are equally important indicators of the latent variable. If there are theoretical or empirical reasons for suspecting otherwise, a system of weighting the items (so that more important items are given more weight in the total score) might be considered. For example, a scale to assess a person's risk for a disease or condition (e.g., risk for cardiovascular disease) might benefit from weighting some items (e.g., high blood pressure) more heavily than others. Weighting is sometimes accomplished empirically, for example, by using factor loadings from a PCA to weight items. Weighting is discussed more extensively in Streiner and Norman (2003), and Pett and colleagues (2003) provide detailed information about factor scores. An interesting approach to weighting is called the *scale product technique*. This method, which combines features of traditional Likert scales with a scaling method called *Thurstone scaling*, is described by Lynn and McMillen (2004).

A related consideration is whether the scores should be *transformed*. If, for example, subscales have different numbers of items, the means will almost surely vary even if the average intensity is similar across dimensions—making it difficult to make comparisons across dimensions. For this reason, some scale developers deliberately try to construct scales that have an equal number of items per subscale. Another approach is to transform scores, most typically through the use of *standard scores* or *z scores* (see Streiner & Norman, 2003).

Conducting a Validation Study

Developing evidence regarding the psychometric adequacy of a scale is an ongoing task. Scale developers ideally should take steps to gather new data about the worth of their instrument in a validation study. Those who are not able to carry out a second study should strive to undertake many of the activities described in this section with data from the original development study. Designing a validation study entails much of the same issues (and advice) as designing a development study, in terms of sample composition, sample size, data collection strategies, and so on. Thus, we focus here on activities undertaken in a validation study. Although the activities we describe primarily concern validity, it should go without saying that internal consistency reliability should be recomputed in the validation sample.

Confirmatory Factor Analysis

Confirmatory factor analysis (CFA) is playing an increasingly important role in validation studies. CFA is preferable to EFA as an approach to construct validity because CFA is a hypothesis testing approach—testing the hypothesis that the items belong to specific factors, rather than having the dimensionality of a set of items emerge empirically, as in EFA.

CFA, as the term has come to be used, is a subset of an advanced class of statistical techniques referred to as *structural equation modeling* (SEM), which we discuss in Chapter 23. One frequently used program for SEM is called LISREL (Linear Structural Relations analysis)—a name that is sometimes used synonymously with SEM and particular methods for analyzing covariance structures. (Other programs for SEM analysis include EQS and Amos.)

CFA differs from EFA in a number of respects, many of which are quite technical. One concerns the estimation procedure. As described in Chapter 23, most multivariate procedures used by nurse researchers employ *least-squares estimation*. In SEM, the most frequently used estimation procedure is **maximum likelihood estimation**. (Maximum likelihood estimators are ones that estimate the parameters most likely to have generated the observed measurements.) Least-squares procedures are based on several stringent assumptions that are generally untenable—for example, the assumption that variables are measured without error. SEM approaches can accommodate measurement error and avoid other restrictions as well.

CFA involves the testing of a **measurement model**, which stipulates the hypothesized relationships among underlying latent variables and the *manifest variables*—that is, the items. In evaluating the measurement model, CFA tests causal relationships between measured and latent variables, correlations between pairs of latent variables, and correlations among the errors associated with the measured variables. The measurement model is thus essentially a factor analytic model that seeks to confirm a hypothesized factor structure. Loadings on the factors (the *latent variables*) provide a method for evaluating relationships between observed variables (the items) and unobserved variables (the factors or dimensions of a construct).

We illustrate with a simplified example involving a scale designed to measure two aspects of fatigue: physical fatigue and mental fatigue. In our example, depicted in Figure 18.3, both types of fatigue are captured by five items each: items I1 to I5 for physical fatigue and items I6 to I10 for mental fatigue. According to the model, people's item responses are *caused by* their physical and mental fatigue (and thus the straight arrows indicating hypothesized causal paths), and are also affected by error (e_1 through e_{10}). Moreover, it is hypothesized that the error terms are correlated, as indicated by the curved lines connecting the errors. Correlated measurement errors on the items might arise as a result of the person's desire to "look good" or to acquiesce—factors that would systematically affect all item scores. The figure also shows that the two latent fatigue variables are hypothesized to be correlated.

The hypothesized measurement model then would be tested against actual data. The analysis would provide loadings of the observed variables on the latent variables, the correlation between the two latent variables, and the correlations between the error terms. The analysis would also indicate whether the overall model fit is good, based on a **goodness-of-fit statistic**. If the hypothesized model is not a good fit to the study data, the measurement model could be respecified and retested.

CFA is a highly complex topic, and we have described only its most basic characteristics. Further reading on the topic is imperative for those desiring to pursue it (e.g., Gable & Wolfe, 1993; Nunnally & Bernstein, 1994).

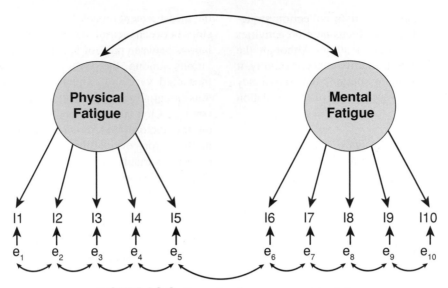

FIGURE 18.3 Example of a measurement model.

Example of confirmatory factor analysis:
Havens and Vessey (2005) undertook a psychometric assessment of the Decisional Involvement Scale, a diagnostic measure of nurse decisional involvement in patient care. Confirmatory factor analysis was undertaken with two independent samples of staff RNs (N = 849 and 650). Six subscales were confirmed with both samples.

Other Validation Activities

A validation effort would not be complete without undertaking additional activities designed to provide evidence of the scale's criterion-related or construct validity, such as the ones described in Chapter 17. As a reminder, the primary means of generating evidence for either type of validity is essentially correlational. In criterion-related validity, scores on the new scale must be correlated with some external criterion—ideally one with very strong reliability and validity itself. In construct validity, scores on the scale are correlated with various things, such as measures of constructs that would theoretically correlate with the target construct; membership in a group whose performance on the construct could be predicted (i.e., known

groups); supplementary measures of the same construct (convergent validity); and measures of a closely related but distinguishable construct (divergent validity). It is desirable to produce as much validity evidence as possible, so thought should be given to including multiple additional measures in the validation instrument, and to selecting a sample that will permit a known groups approach.

If a CFA is not possible (perhaps because of the inaccessibility of the software or lack of training in using it), it is nevertheless advisable to undertake a "confirmatory" factor analysis using the more traditional methods, such as PCA. Comparisons between the original and new factor analyses can be made with respect to factor structure, loadings, variance accounted for, eigenvalues, and so on. In the new analysis, the number of factors to be extracted and rotated can also be prespecified because this is now the working hypothesis about the underlying dimensionality of the construct. Although subjective comparisons between the two analyses are likely to prove adequate, there are also statistical methods for comparing factor solutions (Tabachnik & Fidell, 2006). For example, an index known as Cattell's *salient similarity index* can be computed to compare patterns of factor loadings.

Establishing Cut-off Points

Scales are designed to produce scores along a continuum, but there are constructs for which it is important to dichotomize the scale scores. One familiar example is classroom and licensing examinations: there must be a score (cut-off point) that distinguishes those who pass and those who fail. Diagnostic and screening scales need to provide information about whether there is "caseness" or not.

Various methods—both empirical and subjective—have been developed for establishing cut-off points on scales (Streiner & Norman, 2003). As described in Chapter 17, the method that has the most credibility is the construction of receiver operating characteristic (ROC) curves and its associated indicators. The data for undertaking such an analysis would typically come from a validation study. Scale developers who intend to develop ROC curves need to develop highly reliable criteria for dividing people into groups (e.g., those with and those without the condition being screened), and the criteria must be independent of participants' responses on the scale.

Establishing Norms

In some cases, it might be desirable to *standardize* a new scale and establish norms. This typically occurs if the expectation is that (1) the scale will be widely used, and used by people who find it important to have well-grounded comparative information to help them evaluate scores; and (2) average scale scores will vary markedly by members of well-defined subpopulations. Norms are most commonly established for key demographic characteristics, such as age and gender.

A first decision to make concerns the scope of the norms. For example, *national norms* describe scores achieved for a national sample of respondents, whereas *international norms* are derived from samples from respondents from many countries.

Localized norms are also possible, but are obviously restricted in their utility.

Sampling is the most critical aspect of a standardization effort. The sample used to establish norms should be geographically dispersed (within the desired scope) and representative of the population for whom the scale is intended. In most cases, this means using probability sampling. Usually a very large standardization sample is required so that the descriptive information for the subgroups of interest is stable. The greater the precision desired (i.e., the smaller the degree of error that can be tolerated), the larger the sample needs to be.

After the scale is administered to the standardization sample, various descriptive statistics are computed, and information that can be used as a basis for evaluating comparative performance must be developed. Norms are often expressed in terms of percentiles. For example, an adult male with a score of 72 on the scale might be at the 80th percentile, but a female with the same score might be at the 89th percentile. Excellent guidelines for norming instruments have been developed by Waltz and her colleagues (2005) and Nunnally and Bernstein (1994).

Producing the Final Instrument, a Manual, and Reports

Once all of the evidence has been gathered, scale developers can proceed to finalize their instrument. Care should be taken to design an attractive, easy-to-use, and legible form.

If you expect the scale to be used by others, you should also develop a manual for its use. The manual should include not only the items, but also the underlying conceptual rationale; the process that was used to develop, refine, and evaluate items; instructions for the use of the scale, including scoring and interpretation; information about norms and cut-off points, if relevant; and information about the scale's psychometric properties. Guidelines for preparing manuals are published in *Standards for Educational and Psychological Testing* (AERA, APA, & NCME Joint Committee, 1985).

Once the final instrument has been completed, scale developers should consider registering a copyright, even if they do not plan to publish the scale commercially. Information on this process in the United States can be found at *http://www.copyright.gov.* ✪ If the developers would like to have their scale available commercially, they would need to seek out a test publisher. A member directory of test publishers can be obtained from the Association of Test Publishers (*http://www.testpublishers.org*). ✪ Scale developers can send query letters to a number of different test publishers simultaneously to assess interest in the instrument. Along with the query letter, it is a good idea to include a copy of the scale, a prospectus for its psychometric manual, and the curriculum vita of the developer. If publishers are interested in publishing the scale, the developers must sign a contract and transfer the copyright.

> **Example of commercial publication:**
> Beck and Gable decided to pursue commercial publication of the PDSS. They sent a cover letter, prospectus, copy of the PDSS, and their curriculum vitae to 10 companies that published clinical instruments. A copy of the query letter submitted to Western Psychological Services (WPS), with whom they signed a contract, can be found in the Toolkit of the accompanying *Resource Manual*, together with a sample table of contents for an instrument manual.

Finally, scale development and validation activities should be reported in the nursing literature so that others can benefit. An editorial in the journal *Research in Nursing & Health* provides guidance regarding information to include in an instrument development paper (Froman & Schmitt, 2003).

TRANSLATING SCALES INTO OTHER LANGUAGES

Scales are increasingly being used with people who differ in language and culture. Developing culturally and linguistically equivalent scales in other languages requires nearly as much care and effort as developing an original scale. We provide a brief overview and offer suggestions for further reading on this important topic.

Centered Versus Decentered Translations

Translation is often approached in a "centered" way, in which the scale is translated into another language, with no effect on the wording of the original instrument. In such a *centered* (or asymmetric) *translation*, loyalty to the original scale items is maintained. Such translations typically occur after the fact, that is, after the original scale has been validated and used, and has been identified as a candidate for translation because it has desirable features.

By contrast, the translation process in a *decentered translation* involves the possibility of modifications to items on the original scale. Such decentered (or symmetric) translations often reflect the goal of replacing culturally exclusive language with more universally understood language. This approach is often (although not always) adopted when the developer knows in advance that the scale will be used in two languages, and so translation activities are built into the scale development process.

➔ **TIP:** When a translation is anticipated up-front, scale developers should consider doing the following when they are crafting items: (1) avoid metaphors, idioms, and colloquialisms; (2) use specific words rather than ones open to interpretation, such as "daily" rather than "frequently"; (3) avoid pronouns — repeat nouns if necessary to avoid ambiguity; (4) write in the present tense and avoid the subjunctive mode, such as "should"; and (5) use words with a Latin root if the target language is a Romance language such as Spanish or French (Hilton & Skrutkowski, 2002; Lange, 2002).

> **Example of a decentered translation:** Yeh (2002) translated the California Critical Thinking Disposition Inventory into Chinese using a decentered translation approach.

Conceptual Equivalence

The goal of a translation is to achieve equivalence between an original version of a scale and a translated version. *Equivalence*, however, is in itself a complex concept. Over a dozen different types of equivalencies have been proposed by various authors, although only a few are given consideration in a typical translation effort (Beck, Bernal, & Froman, 2003; Streiner & Norman, 2003).

A particularly important consideration early in a translation effort concerns *conceptual equivalence.* Do people in the two cultures view the central construct in the same way? As an example, consider *obesity.* A person who is obese in some mainstream Western cultures might not be considered obese elsewhere. A related question is, Does the construct even have *meaning* in the other culture? For example, does the construct of *pleasure* or *enjoyment* have meaning in devastatingly poor societies in which daily survival is a struggle? (Note that conceptual equivalence is an important issue even among subcultures that speak the same language.) Thus, one of the first tasks that must be undertaken in a translation effort is to ascertain whether the meaning of the construct as defined in the scale reflects the meaning of the construct within the "target" culture. Experts knowledgeable about the culture in question often need to be consulted in this early step.

Semantic Equivalence: Back Translations

Semantic equivalence concerns the extent to which the *meaning* of each item is the same in the target culture after translation as it was in the original. Literal translations are almost never satisfactory. The translation needs to preserve the underlying meaning of the original wording rather than the exact wording.

The most respected translation process for achieving semantic equivalence involves **back-translation** (Brislin, 1970), in which an instrument is translated from the original *source language* into a *target language*, and then translated back into the source language by translators who are unfamiliar with the original wording. The process typically involves a number of important steps.

Selecting and Preparing Translators
The first step is to select translators. At a minimum, two translators are needed, but four or more working as a team is usually desirable. For example, for translations from English to Spanish, it is important to include native Spanish speakers from various regions because of regional linguistic and cultural variations (e.g., Mexico, Puerto Rico, Central America, etc.). Translations are typically done *into* the native tongue of the translator. So, for example, for an English-to-French translation, the items would first be translated by a native French speaker and the back-translation would be translated by a native English speaker. Being bilingual is not a sufficient qualification for doing a translation: ideally, translators would have some training and experience as professionals, have first-hand familiarity with both cultures, and be capable of understanding the conceptual underpinnings of the construct.

The scale developer needs to carefully explain the construct, and the intent of each item and the scale, to the translators. Translators should also be given guidance about expectations for their performance—for example, they need to be told how much flexibility they have in doing the translation, what reading level to aim for, whether colloquialisms are discouraged, the importance of semantic equivalence, and so on.

⊃ **T I P :** It is sometimes productive to have two independent versions of the translations, a procedure that was used by Wang, Lee, and Fetzer (2006) in their translation of the High School Questionnaire: Profile of Experiences into Chinese. One translation was done by a person who taught English in Taiwan, and the second version was done by a graduate student majoring in English.

Undertaking an Iterative Process
The translation/back-translation process is often an iterative one, requiring multiple rounds of translation, review, and group discussion to arrive at consensus. It begins with the translation of items, followed by the back translation by translators blinded to the original wording. Then a comparison is made between the wording of original items and their back-translated counterparts to detect any possible alterations resulting from the translation. The theory is that if the original and back-translated versions

are identical, the translated item is equivalent in meaning.

⊃ **TIP:** It has been found that some back-translators infer the original item wording (even when the translation is poor), rather than actually translating from the target language back to the source language, so it is advisable to instruct back-translators to treat the target-language version as the original.

More often than not, the original and back-translated versions are *not* identical. If there are serious differences, it may be fruitful to have a group discussion among the translators, and then begin the process anew with a second group of translators after making changes to either the qualifications of the translators, item wording in the source language, or instructions to the translators (or some combination of these). Jones and her colleagues (2001), in their translation of an English coping scale into Tagalog (the Philippine language), used three bilingual teams.

Example of a back-translated item: Beck and colleagues (2003) provided the following example from the development of the Spanish version of the PDSS:

Original item: I was afraid that I would never be my normal self again.
Translated item: Temia no volver a ser otra vez la misma de antes.
Back-translated item: I was afraid I was not going to be the same person as before.

When the original and back-translated items are reasonably close, it is time to involve a committee to review what has transpired and to arrive at a consensus about the translated version of the scale items. The committee may be the team of translators but may also be three or more bilingual persons who have not participated in the translation process. Committee members are given complete information on each item—the original version, translated versions, and back-translated versions. They may also be given supplementary information, such as the desired reading level and the *actual* reading level of the various versions. Committee work may

require several hours of discussion before consensus is reached.

The committee may conclude that a back-translated item is a better match to the translated item than the original wording. In such a case, if a decentering approach has been used, the wording of the original item should be changed to reflect a more universally understood construction.

Testing the Translated Version

After any final editing (e.g., for grammatical or spelling corrections), the translated scale needs to be tested, in a manner analogous to testing the original scale. Pretesting with a small sample of members of the target culture is important, and cognitive questioning is especially valuable with a translated instrument.

Another important tool for further evaluating the semantic equivalence of the original and translated scale is to pretest both versions with a sample of bilingual people. Two forms of the instrument should be prepared (source language first on one, target language first on the other), with forms distributed randomly to the pretest sample. Then responses on the two forms can be compared, both at the scale level and at the item level. Jones and her colleagues (2001) found that the statistical analysis of their pretest data was very useful in identifying discrepancies in meaning between the two language versions that had previously gone undetected.

Finally, the translated scale should be submitted to a full psychometric evaluation with a large sample of respondents. These efforts not only provide evidence of the soundness of the translated scale, but also support inferences about equivalence. For example, if the internal consistency of the translated scale is substantially lower than the original, there is clearly something wrong with the translation. Confirmatory factor analysis is another strategy that is useful in facilitating conclusions about both the conceptual and semantic equivalence of the scales. Other construct validation procedures ideally would also be used with a sample from the new culture (e.g., known groups).

Example of a scale translation study: Chien and Norman (2004) undertook a translation of the Family Burden Interview Schedule (FBIS) from English into Chinese. The scale was translated, back-translated, and evaluated by 15 bilingual health professionals. The translated and original scales were then completed by 30 bilingual family caregivers. Item equivalence of the two versions, assessed with a weighted kappa statistic, was acceptable, and correlations between the scale scores were high. In a second phase, the Chinese FBIS was administered to 185 family caregivers. Internal consistency reliability was .87 for the total scale. Validation efforts (including known-groups technique, theoretically driven correlations, and factor analysis) indicated good construct validity of the translated scale.

CRITIQUING SCALE DEVELOPMENT STUDIES

Reports on scale development efforts appear regularly in many nursing journals. If you are planning to use a scale in a substantive study, you should carefully review the methods used to construct and validate the scale—and to translate it, if a translated version is under consideration. You should also determine whether the evidence regarding the psychometric adequacy of the scale is sufficiently sound to merit its use. Remember that you run the risk of undermining the statistical conclusion validity of your study (i.e., of having insufficient power for testing your hypotheses) if you use a scale with weak reliability. Box 18.1 provides guidelines for evaluating a research report on the development and validation of a scale.

RESEARCH EXAMPLE

Studies: "Postpartum Depression Screening Scale: Development and psychometric testing" (Beck & Gable, 2000); "Further validation of the Postpartum Depression Screening Scale" (Beck & Gable, 2001a); "Postpartum Depression Screening Scale: Spanish version" (Beck & Gable, 2003)

Background: Beck studied postpartum depression (PPD) in a series of qualitative studies, using both a

---

BOX 18.1 Guidelines for Critiquing Instrument Development and Validation Reports

1. Does the report offer a clear definition of the construct? Does it provide sufficient context for the study through a summary of the literature and discussion of relevant theory? Is the population for whom the scale is intended adequately described?
2. Does the report indicate how items were generated? Do the procedures seem sound?
3. Does the report provide information about content validation efforts? Is there evidence of good content validity?
4. Were appropriate efforts made to refine the scale (e.g., through pretests, item analysis)?
5. Was the development or validation sample appropriate in terms of representativeness and size?
6. Was factor analysis used to examine or validate the dimensionality of the scale? If yes, does the report offer evidence to support the factor structure and the naming of factors?
7. Were appropriate methods used to assess the scale's reliability? Were reliability estimates sufficiently high?
8. Were appropriate methods used to assess the scale's validity? Is the evidence regarding validity persuasive? What other validation methods would have strengthened the study?
9. Does the report provide information for scoring the scale and interpreting scale scores—for example, means and standard deviations, cut-off scores, norms?
10. If the study involves a translation, were appropriate procedures (e.g., back translation, a committee approach, validation efforts) used to ensure scale equivalency?

phenomenological approach (1992, 1996) and a grounded theory approach (1993). Based on her in-depth understanding of PPD, she began in the late 1990s to develop a scale that could be used to screen for PPD, the Postpartum Depression Screening Scale (PDSS).

Statement of Purpose: The methodologic studies, which Beck undertook with an expert psychometrician, were designed to develop, refine, and validate a scale to screen women for postpartum depression, and to translate the scale into Spanish (Beck & Gable, 2000, 2001a, 2001b, 2001c, 2003, 2005; Beck et al., 2003).

Scale Development: The PDSS is a Likert scale designed to tap seven dimensions, such as sleeping/eating disturbances and mental confusion. A 56-item pilot form of the PDSS was initially developed with 8 items per dimension, using a 5-point response scale. Beck's program of research on PPD and her knowledge of the literature were used for specifying the domain. Themes from Beck's qualitative research were used to develop seven dimensions, and to craft the items to operationalize those dimensions. The reading level of the final PDSS was assessed to be at the 3rd-grade level, and the Flesch reading ease score is 92.7.

Content Validity: Content validity was enhanced by using direct quotes from the qualitative studies as items on the scale (e.g., "I felt like I was losing my mind"). The pilot form was subjected to two content validation procedures, including ratings of perceived "fit" with a dimension by a panel of five content experts. Feedback from these procedures led to some item revisions.

Construct Validity: The PDSS was administered to a sample of 525 new mothers in six states (Beck & Gable, 2000). Preliminary item analyses resulted in the deletion of several items, based on item-total correlations. The PDSS was finalized as a 35-item scale with seven subscales, each with 5 items. This version of the PDSS was subjected to confirmatory factor analyses, which involved a validation of Beck's hypotheses about how individual items mapped onto underlying constructs, such as cognitive impairment. Item response theory was also used, and provided supporting evidence of the scale's construct validity. In a subsequent study, Beck and Gable (2001a) administered the PDSS and two other depression scales to 150 new mothers and tested hypotheses about how scores on the PDSS would correlate with scores on other scales. The results indicated good convergent validity.

Criterion-Related Validity: In the second study, Beck and Gable correlated scores on the PDSS with an expert clinician's diagnosis of PPD for each woman. The validity coefficient was .70, which was higher than the correlations between the diagnosis and scores on the other two depression scales, indicating its superiority as a screening instrument.

Internal Consistency Reliability: In both studies, Beck and Gable evaluated the internal consistency reliability of the PDSS and its subscales. Subscale reliability was high, ranging from .83 to .94 in the first study and from .80 to .91 in the second study. Figure 18.4 shows the reliability analysis printout for the five items on the Mental Confusion subscale from the first study. In the top panel, the first column identifies subscale items by number: I11, I18, and so on. I11, for example, is the item, "I felt like I was losing my mind." The item means and standard deviations suggest a good amount of variability on each item. The next panel presents intercorrelations among the 5 items. The correlations are fairly high, ranging from .6012 for items I25 with I53 to .8143 for items I11 with I25. In the panel near the bottom labeled "Item-total Statistics," the fourth column ("Corrected Item-Total Correlation") presents correlation coefficients for the relationship between women's score on an item and their score on the total subscale (after removing the item from the scale). I11 has a corrected item-total correlation of .7991, which is very high; all five items have excellent correlations with the total score. The sixth (final) column indicates what the internal consistency would be if an item were deleted. If I11 were removed from the subscale and only the 4 other items remained, the reliability coefficient would be .8876; in the panel below, we see that the reliability for the 5-item subscale is even higher: alpha = .9120. Deleting any of the 5 items on the subscale would reduce its internal consistency, but only by a rather small amount.

Sensitivity and Specificity: In the second validation study, ROC curves were constructed to examine the sensitivity and specificity of the PDSS at different cut-off points, using the expert diagnosis to establish true positives and true negatives for PPD. In the validation study, 46 of the 150 mothers had a diagnosis of major or minor depression. To illustrate the tradeoffs the researchers made, the ROC curve (Fig. 18.5) revealed that with a cut-off score of 95 on the PDSS to screen in PPD cases, the sensitivity would be only .41, meaning that only 41% of the women actually diagnosed with PPD would be identified. A score of 95 has a specificity of 1.00, meaning that all cases *without* an actual PPD diagnosis would be accurately screened out. At the other extreme, a cut-off score of 45 would have 1.00 sensitivity but only .28 specificity (i.e., 72% false-positive rate), an unacceptable

****** Method 2 (covariance matrix) will be used for this analysis ******

R E L I A B I L I T Y   A N A L Y S I S   -   S C A L E   (A L P H A)

1.   I11
2.   I18
3.   I25
4.   I39
5.   I53

		Mean	Std Dev	Cases
1.	I11	2.3640	1.4243	522.0
2.	I18	2.2146	1.2697	522.0
3.	I25	2.2050	1.3736	522.0
4.	I39	2.3985	1.3511	522.0
5.	I53	2.2759	1.3491	522.0

Correlation Matrix

	I11	I18	I25	I39	I53
I11	1.0000				
I18	.6540	1.0000			
I25	.8143	.6031	1.0000		
I39	.6456	.6594	.6519	1.0000	
I53	.6469	.7508	.6012	.7240	1.0000

N of Cases =   522.0

Item Means	Mean	Minimum	Maximum	Range	Max/Min	Variance
	2.2916	2.2050	2.3985	.1935	1.0877	.0076

Item Variances	Mean	Minimum	Maximum	Range	Max/Min	Vaiancer
	1.8347	1.6122	2.0285	.4163	1.2582	.0225

Item-total Statistics

	Scale Mean if Item Deleted	Scale Variance if Item Deleted	Corrected Item-Total Correlation	Squared Multiple Correlation	Alpha if Item Deleted
I11	9.0939	21.3712	.7991	.7145	.8876
I18	9.2433	23.0060	.7639	.6231	.8951
I25	9.2529	22.0972	.7696	.6912	.8937
I39	9.0594	22.2901	.7687	.6097	.8938
I53	9.1820	22.1760	.7812	.6662	.8912

R E L I A B I L I T Y   A N A L Y S I S   -   S C A L E   (A L P H A)

Reliability Coefficients   5 items

Alpha =   .9120 Standardized item alpha =   .9122

FIGURE 18.4 Reliability analysis for the Mental Confusion subscale of the Postpartum Depression Screening Scale.

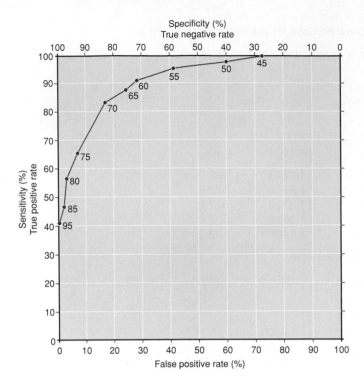

FIGURE 18.5 Receiver operating characteristic (ROC) curve for Postpartum Depression Screening Scale (PDSS): major or minor postpartum depression. Area = 0.91 (SD = 0.03). (Used with permission from Beck, C. T., & Gable, R. K. [2001]. Further validation of the Postpartum Depression Screening Scale. *Nursing Research, 50,* 161.)

rate of overdiagnosis. Based on their results, Beck and Gable recommended a cut-off score of 60, which would accurately screen in 91% of PPD cases, and would mistakenly screen in 28% of subjects who do not have PPD. Beck and Gable determined that using this cut-off point would have correctly classified 85% of their sample. In their ROC analysis, the area under the curve was excellent, .91.

Spanish Translation: Beck collaborated with translation experts to develop a Spanish version of the PDSS. Eight bilingual translators from four different backgrounds (Mexican, Puerto Rican, Cuban, and other South American) translated and back-translated the scale items. The translators met as a committee to review each others' wordings and to arrive at a consensus. The English and Spanish versions were then administered to a bilingual sample of 34 people, in random order. Scores on the two versions correlated highly (e.g., .98 on the "Sleeping/Eating Disturbances" subscale). The alpha reliability coefficient was .95 for the total Spanish scale, and ranged from .76 to .90 for the subscales. Confirmatory factor analysis yielded information that was judged to indicate an adequate fit with the hypothesized measurement model. The

cut-off point for the Spanish version was also determined to be 60.

SUMMARY POINTS

- Scale development begins with a sound conceptualization of the construct (the **latent variable**) to be measured, including its dimensionality.
- After deciding on the type of scale to construct, items must be generated; common sources for items include existing instruments, the research literature, concept analyses, in-depth studies, focus groups, and clinical observations.
- In classical measurement theory, a **domain sampling model** is often assumed, in which the basic notion is to sample a homogeneous set of items from a hypothetical universe of items.
- In generating items, a number of decisions must be made, including how many items to generate

(typically a large number initially), what to use as the continuum for the response options, how many response options there should be, whether to include positive and negative item stems in the scale, how intensely worded the items should be, and what to do about references to time.

- After items are generated, they should be inspected for clarity, length, inappropriate use of jargon, and good wording; the scale's **read-ability** should also be assessed.

- External review of the preliminary pool of items should also be undertaken, including review by members of the target population (e.g., either through a small pretest or review in a focus group).

- Content validity should be built into the scale both through careful efforts to conceptualize the construct, and through content validation procedures by a panel of experts—including the calculation of a quantitative index such as the CVI to summarize the experts' judgments of the relevance of scale items.

- Once content validity has been established at a satisfactory level, the scale must be administered to a development sample—typically 200 or more respondents who are representative of the target population.

- Data collected from the development sample are then analyzed using a number of techniques, including **item analysis** (e.g., a scrutiny of **inter-item correlations** and **item–scale correlations**), **exploratory factor analysis (EFA)**, and reliability analysis.

- EFA is used to reduce a large set of variables into a smaller set of underlying dimensions, called **factors**. Mathematically, each factor is a linear combination of variables in a data matrix.

- The first phase of factor analysis (**factor extraction**) identifies clusters of items that are strongly intercorrelated and is used to define the number of underlying dimensions in the items empirically; the most widely used factor extraction method is called **principal components analysis (PCA)**, but another important alternative is called **common factor analysis**.

- The second phase of factor analysis involves **factor rotation**, which enhances the interpretability of the factors by aligning items more distinctly with a particular factor. Rotation can be either **orthogonal** (which maintains the independence of the factors) or **oblique** (which allows intercorrelated factors). **Factor loadings** of the items on the rotated factor matrix are then used to interpret and name the factors.

- After the scale is finalized based on the preliminary analyses, a second study is often undertaken to validate the scale, using a variety of validation techniques; one widely used approach is **confirmatory factor analysis (CFA)**.

- CFA involves tests of a **measurement model**, which stipulates the hypothesized relationship between latent variables and *manifest variables*. CFA is a subset of sophisticated statistical techniques referred to as **structural equation modeling**.

- Some scales—especially ones that will be used to make assessments of diagnoses of individuals—benefit in interpretation through the establishment of cut-off points or norms.

- Well-constructed scales with good psychometric properties are increasingly likely to be translated for use in other cultures. Translations are often **centered** on the original language, but a **decentered** approach, which would allow modifications to the wording of items in the original scale, may be preferred when it is anticipated during the development phase that the scale will be used in two languages.

- Both *conceptual equivalence* and *semantic equivalence* are critical to the success of a translated effort. The "gold standard" for semantic equivalence involves **back-translation**, in which the scale is first translated from the *source language* into the *target language*, and then translated back to the source language by translators blind to the original wording. The next step typically involves a committee that convenes with the goal of arriving at a consensus translation.

- The translated version is then tested in a manner similar to the original scale. Evidence for semantic equivalence and psychometric soundness comes from pretests of both original and translated scales with a sample of bilingual people, and from comparison of reliabilities, factor structures, and other validity estimates between the two scales.

STUDY ACTIVITIES

Chapter 18 of the accompanying *Resource Manual for Nursing Research: Generating and Assessing Evidence for Nursing Practice, 8th edition*, offers various exercises and study suggestions for reinforcing the concepts presented in this chapter. In addition, the following study questions can be addressed:

1. Read a recent scale development paper and see how many of the steps discussed in this chapter were followed. Which omitted steps (if any) jeopardize the evidence about the scale's quality?
2. In Figure 18.4, if Beck and Gable had wanted a 4-item subscale rather than a 5-item subscale, which item would they have eliminated?
3. Use the critiquing guidelines in Box 18.1 to evaluate scale development procedures in the studies by Beck and Gable (2000, 2001a, 2003), referring to the original studies if possible.

STUDIES CITED IN CHAPTER 18

Methodologic or theoretical references cited in this chapter can be found in a separate section at the end of the book.

Abdallah, L., Fawcett, J., Kane, R., Dick, K., & Chen, J. (2005). Development and psychometric testing of the EverCare Nurse Practitioner Role and Activity Scale (ENPRAS). *Journal of the American Academy of Nurse Practitioners, 17,* 21–26.

Beck, C. T. (1992). The lived experience of postpartum depression: A phenomenological study. *Nursing Research, 41,* 166–170.

Beck, C. T. (1993). Teetering on the edge: A substantive theory of postpartum depression. *Nursing Research, 42,* 42–48.

Beck, C. T. (1996). Postpartum depressed mothers' experience interacting with their children. *Nursing Research, 45,* 98–104.

Beck, C. T., & Gable, R. K. (2000). Postpartum Depression Screening Scale: Development and psychometric testing. *Nursing Research, 49,* 272–282.

Beck, C. T., & Gable, R. K. (2001a). Further validation of the Postpartum Depression Screening Scale. *Nursing Research, 50,* 155–164.

Beck, C. T., & Gable, R. K. (2003). Postpartum Depression Screening Scale: Spanish version. *Nursing Research, 52,* 296–306.

Beck, C. T., & Gable, R. K. (2005). Screening performance of the Postpartum Depression Screening Scale:—Spanish version. *Journal of Transcultural Nursing, 16*(4), 331–338.

Chien, W., & Norman, I. (2004). The validity and reliability of a Chinese version of the Family Burden Interview Schedule. *Nursing Research, 53,* 314–322.

Doorenbos, A. Z., Verbitsky, N., Given, B., & Given, C. (2005). An analytic strategy for modeling multiple-item responses: A breast cancer symptom example. *Nursing Research, 54,* 229–234.

Havens, D., & Vasey, J. (2005). The staff nurse Decisional Involvement Scale. *Nursing Research, 54*(6), 376–383.

Heo, S., Moser, D. K., Riegel, B., Hall, L. A., & Christman, N. (2005). Testing the psychometric properties of the Minnesota Living with Heart Failure Questionnaire. *Nursing Research, 54,* 265–272.

Janssen, P., Dennis, C., & Reime, B. (2006). Development and psychometric testing of the Care in Obstetrics: Measure for Testing Satisfaction (COMFORTS) Scale. *Research in Nursing & Health, 29*(1), 51–60.

Johnson, M., & Rogers, S. (2006). Development of the purposeful action Medication-Taking Questionnaire. *Western Journal of Nursing Research, 28*(3), 335–351.

Klakovich, M., & de la Cruz, F. (2006). Validating the Interpersonal Communication Assessment Scale. *Journal of Professional Nursing, 22*(1), 60–67.

McClowry, S. G., Halverson, C. F., & Sanson, A. (2003). A re-examination of the validity and reliability of the School-Age Temperament Inventory. *Nursing Research, 52,* 176–182.

McGilton, K. S. (2003). Development and psychometric evaluation of supportive leadership scales. *Canadian Journal of Nursing Research, 35,* 72–86.

Smith, A. J., Thurkettle, M. A., & de la Cruz, F. A. (2004). Use of intuition by nursing students: Instrument development and testing. *Journal of Advanced Nursing, 47,* 614–622.

Wynd, C. A., & Schaefer, M. A. (2002). The Osteoporosis Risk Assessment Tool: Establishing content validity through a panel of experts. *Applied Nursing Research, 16,* 184–188.

Yeh, M. L. (2002). Assessing the reliability and validity of the Chinese version of the California Critical Thinking Disposition Inventory. *International Journal of Nursing Studies, 39*(2), 123–132.

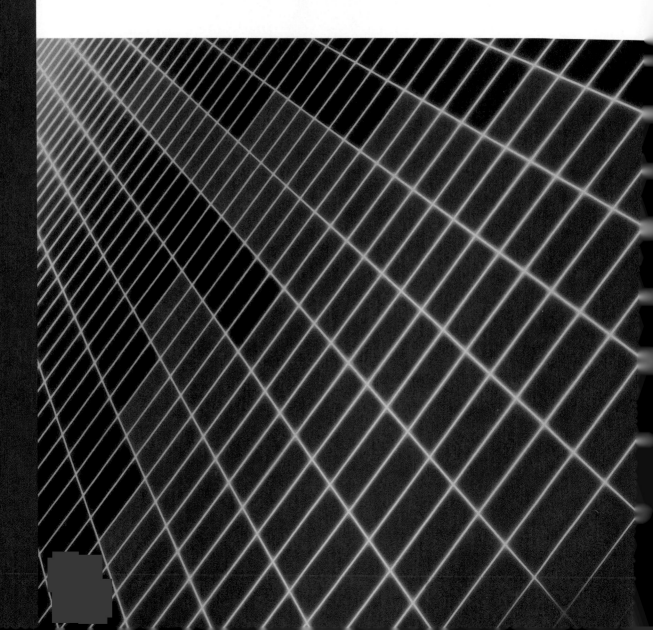

PART 5

ANALYZING AND INTERPRETING RESEARCH DATA

19

Analyzing Qualitative Data

Qualitative data take the form of loosely structured, narrative materials, such as verbatim dialogue between an interviewer and a respondent, field notes of participant observers, or diaries kept by study participants. This chapter describes methods for analyzing such qualitative data.

INTRODUCTION TO QUALITATIVE ANALYSIS

The purpose of data analysis is to organize, provide structure to, and elicit meaning from research data. In qualitative studies, data collection and data analysis usually occur simultaneously, rather than after data are collected. The search for important themes and concepts begins from the moment data collection gets underway.

Qualitative analysis is a labor-intensive activity that requires creativity, conceptual sensitivity, and sheer hard work. In this section, we discuss some general considerations relating to qualitative analysis.

Qualitative Analysis Challenges

Qualitative data analysis is a particularly challenging enterprise, for three major reasons. First, there are no universal rules for analyzing qualitative data.

The absence of standard analytic procedures makes it difficult to explain how to do such analyses, and how to present findings in a way that their validity is apparent. Some of the procedures that we describe in the next chapter are important tools for enhancing the trustworthiness of the analysis.

The second challenge of qualitative analysis is the enormous amount of work required. Qualitative analysts must organize and make sense of pages and pages of narrative materials. In a multimethod study by one of us (Polit), the qualitative data consisted of transcribed interviews with more than 100 poor women discussing life stressors and health problems. The transcriptions ranged from 30 to 50 pages, resulting in more than 3000 pages that had to be read, reread, and then organized, integrated, and interpreted.

The final challenge comes in reducing data for reporting purposes. Quantitative results can often be summarized in a few tables. Qualitative researchers, by contrast, must balance the need to be concise with the need to maintain the richness and evidentiary value of their data.

➲ **TIP:** Qualitative analyses are more difficult to *do* than quantitative ones, but qualitative findings are usually easier to understand than quantitative ones because the stories are often told in everyday language. Qualitative analyses are often harder

507

to evaluate critically than quantitative analyses, however, because readers cannot know first-hand if researchers adequately captured thematic patterns in the data.

Analysis Styles

Crabtree and Miller (1999) observed that there are nearly as many qualitative analysis strategies as there are qualitative researchers, but they identified three major analysis styles along a continuum. At one end is a style that is more standardized, and at the other is a style that is more intuitive and interpretive. The three prototypical styles are as follows:

- *Template analysis style.* In this style, researchers develop a **template** or analysis guide to which the narrative data are applied. The units for the template are typically behaviors, events, or linguistic expressions (e.g., phrases). Researchers begin with a rudimentary template before collecting data, but the template undergoes revision as more data are gathered. The analysis of the resulting data, sorted according to the template, is interpretive, not statistical. This style is most likely to be adopted by researchers whose research tradition is ethnography, ethology, discourse analysis, and ethnoscience.

- *Editing analysis style.* Researchers using an editing style act as interpreters who read through the data in search of meaningful segments and units. Once segments are identified, they develop a **category scheme** and corresponding codes that can be used to sort and organize the data. The researchers then search for the patterns and structure that connect the categories. Researchers whose research traditions are grounded theory, phenomenology, hermeneutics, and ethnomethodology use procedures that fall within the editing analysis style.

- *Immersion/crystallization style.* This style involves the analyst's total immersion in and reflection of the text materials, resulting in an intuitive crystallization of the data. This highly interpretive, subjective style is less frequently encountered in the nursing research literature than the other two styles.

Researchers seldom use terms like *template analysis style* or *editing style* in their reports. These terms are primarily *post hoc* characterizations of styles adopted by qualitative researchers. However, King (1998) has described the process of undertaking a template analysis, and his approach has been adopted by some nurse researchers undertaking descriptive qualitative studies.

Example of a template analysis: Fereday and Muir-Cochrane (2006) presented a detailed description of how they used a hybrid approach to coding their data for a study about the role of performance feedback in nursing practice. Their approach integrated inductively derived codes based on their data with coding from a preestablished, theoretically driven template.

The Qualitative Analysis Process

The analysis of qualitative data is an active and interactive process. Qualitative researchers typically scrutinize their data carefully and deliberately, often reading the data over and over in a search for meaning and deeper understanding. Insights and theories cannot emerge until researchers become completely familiar with their data. Morse and Field (1995) noted that qualitative analysis is a "process of fitting data together, of making the invisible obvious, of linking and attributing consequences to antecedents. It is a process of conjecture and verification, of correction and modification, of suggestion and defense" (p. 126).

QUALITATIVE DATA MANAGEMENT AND ORGANIZATION

Qualitative analysis is supported and facilitated by several tasks that help to organize and manage the mass of narrative data, as described next.

Transcribing Qualitative Data

Audiotaped interviews and field notes are major data sources in qualitative studies. Verbatim transcription of the tapes is a critical step in preparing for data analysis, and researchers need to ensure that transcriptions are accurate, that they validly reflect the totality of the interview experience, and that they facilitate analysis.

Transcription conventions are essential. For example, transcribers have to indicate, through symbols in the written text, who is speaking (e.g., "I" for interviewer, "P" for participant), overlaps in speaking turns, time elapsed between utterances when there are gaps, nonlinguistic utterances (e.g., sighs, sobs, laughter), emphasis of words, and so on. Silverman (1993) offers some guidance with regard to transcription conventions.

Transcription errors are almost inevitable, which means that researchers need to check the accuracy of transcribed data. Poland (1995) notes that there are three categories of error:

1. *Deliberate alterations of the data.* Transcribers may intentionally "fix" data to make the transcriptions look more like what they "should" look like. Such alterations are not done out of malice, but rather reflect a desire to be helpful. For example, transcribers may alter profanities, omit sounds such as phones ringing, or "tidy up" the text by deleting "ums" and "uhs." It is crucial to impress on transcribers the importance of verbatim accounts.

2. *Accidental alterations of the data.* Inadvertent transcription errors are more common. One pervasive problem concerns proper punctuation. The insertion or omission of commas, periods, or question marks can alter the interpretation of the text. A common error is misinterpreting words and substituting ones that change the meaning of the dialogue. For example, the actual words might be, "this was totally moot," but the transcription might read, "this was totally mute." Researchers should take steps to verify accuracy before analysis gets underway.

3. *Unavoidable alterations.* Data are unavoidably altered by the fact that transcriptions capture only a portion of an interview experience. For example, transcriptions will inevitably miss many nonverbal cues, such as body language, intonation, and so on.

> **➲ TIP:** When checking the accuracy of transcribed data, it is critical to listen to the taped interview while doing the cross-check. This is also a good time to insert in the transcription any nonverbal behavior you captured in your field notes.

Researchers should begin data analysis with the best-possible quality data, which requires careful training of transcribers, ongoing feedback, and continuous efforts to verify accuracy. MacLean, Meyer, & Estable (2004) offer suggestions for improving the accuracy of transcripts. One such suggestion is to work with a transcriptionist at the start of the project to establish guidelines for handling potential problems. For example, how will the researcher be alerted that the transcriptionist was unable to understand certain portions of the tape recording? The researcher can teach the transcriptionist his or her notation preferences for inaudible sections (e.g., cannot hear, poor tape quality, too much background noise). MacLean and colleagues (2004) urged researchers to provide transcriptionists with lists of terms and acronyms that might be unfamiliar. Transcriptionists also need to be prepared for dealing with emotionally difficult material. Transcribing emotion-laden interviews can result in inaccuracies if transcriptionists deny or "mis-hear" the words.

Lapadat (2000) offered other strategies to enhance transcription rigor. She suggested keeping a log of decision points while transcribing (e.g., What has the transcriber chosen not to transcribe?). Lapadat also suggested developing a codebook to record transcription conventions that were adopted or newly created for the project.

Developing a Category Scheme

Qualitative researchers begin their analysis by organizing their data—that is, by developing a method to classify and index their data. Researchers must be able to gain access to parts of the data, without having to repeatedly reread the data set in its entirety. This phase of data analysis is essentially reductionist—data must be converted to smaller, more manageable units that can be retrieved and reviewed.

The most widely used procedure is to develop a category scheme and then to code data according to the categories. A preliminary category system (a template) is sometimes drafted before data collection, but more typically, qualitative analysts develop categories based on a scrutiny of actual data. There are no straightforward or easy guidelines for this task. Developing a high-quality category scheme involves a careful reading of the data, with an eye to identifying underlying concepts and clusters of concepts. The nature of the categories may vary in level of detail or specificity, as well as in level of abstraction.

Researchers whose aims are primarily descriptive tend to use categories that are fairly concrete. For example, the category scheme may focus on differentiating various types of actions or events, or different phases in a chronologic unfolding of an experience. In developing a category scheme, related concepts are often grouped together to facilitate the coding process.

> **Example of a descriptive category scheme:**
> The coding scheme used by Polit, London, & Martinez (2000) to categorize data relating to food insecurity and hunger in low-income families is an example of a category system that was concrete and descriptive. For example, one major coding category was "Strategies used to avoid hunger." The subcategories used to code the interview included eight strategies, such as "Stretching food, eating smaller portions" and "Eating old or unsafe food."

Studies designed to develop a theory are more likely to involve abstract, conceptual categories. In creating conceptual categories, researchers must break the data into segments, closely examine them, and compare them to other segments for similarities and dissimilarities to determine what the meaning of those phenomena are. (This is part of the process referred to as *constant comparison* by grounded theory researchers.) The researcher asks questions such as the following about discrete events, incidents, or statements:

What is this?
What is going on?

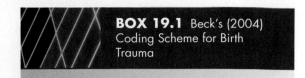

BOX 19.1 Beck's (2004) Coding Scheme for Birth Trauma

Theme 1. To care for me: Was that too much to ask?
A. Feeling abandoned and alone
B. Stripped of dignity
C. Lack of interest in a woman as a unique person
D. Lack of support and reassurance

Theme 2. To communicate with me: Why was this neglected?
A. Labor and delivery staff failed to communicate with the patients.
B. Labor and delivery staff spoke as if the woman in labor was not present.
C. Clinicians failed to communicate among themselves.

Theme 3. To provide safe care: You betrayed my trust and I felt powerless.
A. Perceived unsafe care
B. Feared for their own safety and that of their unborn infants
C. Felt powerless

Theme 4. The end justifies the means: At whose expense? At what price?
A. Traumatic deliveries were glossed over.
B. Successful outcome of the baby took center stage.
C. The mother was made to feel guilty.
D. No one wanted to listen to the mother.

What does it stand for?
What else is like this?
What is this distinct from?

Important concepts that emerge from close examination of the data are then given a label that forms the basis for a category scheme. These names are necessarily abstractions, but the labels are usually sufficiently graphic that the nature of the material to which they refer is clear—and often provocative.

> **Example of a conceptual category scheme:**
> Box 19.1 shows the category scheme developed by Beck (2004) to categorize data from her Internet

interviews on birth trauma. The coding scheme included four major thematic categories with subcodes. For example, an excerpt that described a mother's feelings of humiliation would be coded under category 1B (i.e., being stripped of her dignity).

⊃ **TIP :** A good category scheme is critical to a thoughtful analysis, and so a substantial sample of the data should be read before the scheme is drafted. To the extent possible, you should read materials that vary along key dimensions, to capture a range of content. The dimensions might be informant characteristics (e.g., men versus women) or aspects of the data collection experience (e.g., data from different sites).

Coding Qualitative Data

Once a category scheme has been developed, the data are read in their entirety and coded for correspondence to the categories—a task that is seldom easy. Researchers may have difficulty deciding on the most appropriate code, or may not fully comprehend the underlying meaning of some aspect of the data. It may take a second or third reading of the material to grasp its nuances.

Also, researchers often discover in going through the data that the initial category system was incomplete. It is common for categories to emerge that were not initially identified. When this happens, it is risky to assume that the category was absent in materials that have already been coded. A concept might not be identified as salient until it has emerged three or four times. In such a case, it would be necessary to reread all previously coded material to have a truly complete grasp of that category. Making changes midway is often painful and frustrating, but without an effective category system, it is not possible to integrate important themes adequately.

Another issue is that narrative materials usually are not linear. For example, paragraphs from transcribed interviews may contain elements relating to three or four different categories, embedded in a complex fashion.

Example of a multitopic segment: An example of a multitopic segment of an interview from Beck's (2004) phenomenological study of birth trauma is shown in Figure 19.1. The codes in the margin represent codes from the scheme presented in Box 19.1.

It is sometimes recommended that a single member of the research team code the entire data set, to ensure the highest possible coding consistency across interviews or observations. Nevertheless, at least a portion of the interviews should be coded by two or more people early in the coding process, if possible, to evaluate and enhance reliability.

⊃ **TIP :** It is wise to develop a codebook—written documentation describing the exact definition of the various categories used to code the data. Good qualitative codebooks usually include one or more actual excerpts that typify materials coded in each category. The Toolkit section of the accompanying *Resource Manual* includes an example of a codebook from Beck's work.

Manual Methods of Organizing Qualitative Data

Traditional manual methods of organizing qualitative data are becoming less common as a result of the widespread use of computer software that can perform indexing functions. Here, we briefly describe some manual methods of data management; the next section describes computer methods.

When the amount of data is small, or when a category system is simple, researchers sometimes use colored paper clips or Post-It Notes to code narrative content. For example, if we were analyzing interviews about women's thoughts about menopause, we might use blue paper clips for text relating to loss of fertility, red clips for text on menopausal side effects, yellow clips for text relating to aging, and so on. Then we could pull out all material with a certain color clip to examine one aspect of menopausal attitudes at a time.

In analyzing data from a phenomenological study, researchers sometimes use file cards, placing

At some point a fetal scalp monitor was introduced then what seemed to be very shortly after that, my own OB came in and said my baby was in fetal distress and that a c-section was probably needed given that I was only 6 cms. This floored me in every imaginable way-emotionally, physically, and mentally. I'd labored in what I thought was "well mannered" for 12 hours. NO ONE had told me they were monitoring my baby. NO ONE told me they suspected she was in distress. Then BOOM, my baby is in trouble and my almost picture-perfect labor is gone. After that point, things became blurry because I can only see them through what I describe as an emotional fog. I lost it in front of everybody which I rarely do.

2 A

2 A
As they wheeled me into the theatre, I asked again where was my husband. They said he was on his way. They wheeled me in and told me to curl my back for the epidural. There were a few nurses there and I remember them talking about me as if I wasn't there. Didn't they realize that I could hear them? The needle must have gone in 4 or 5 times. I was crying. I was scared and the epidural hurt a bloody lot. Some one please help me. I felt all alone. And I was thinking that I don't want another baby and go through this again. I recall thinking how much more pain do I have to put up with? Was my baby going to be all right? I needed reassurance but none was given.

2B

2 A

1D

Then another man took over the epidural and asked me to sit up and bend over while he put the needle in. I started to feel numb below my waist. I felt a pin prick and felt my tummy being pulled apart. It was awful as I couldn't see or feel anything.

1A

3C

1C
So my trauma was a result of that emergency caesarean. It happened so fast. Of feeling so scared and alone and having to go through it all alone with out my husband there. The nurses didn't tell me anything about what was going on. I felt powerless. I also felt the hospital staff could have given me some indication that I may have had to have an emergency caesarean instead of letting me think that I was going to have a natural labor. I also wished that the doctor herself could have come to see how I was doing afterwards. I think it would have helped me a lot if she had come and talked about how I was doing and how I felt and why I had to have an emergency c-section.

2A

2A

4B

4D
All people kept telling me after my daughter was born was how lucky I was and that I could have lost her. I know I was lucky but telling that does not help how I felt. With them telling me that, I felt guilty for feeling the way I did. I wanted some attention too. I wanted to be looked after and listened to. I tried several times to bring up how I felt but it was brushed away with the "I've been through that before and so what" response. I really felt like I was in the wrong to feel the way I did because I had a healthy baby.

4C

FIGURE 19.1 Coded excerpt from Beck's (2004) Study.

each significant statement from the interviews on a file card of its own. The file cards are then sorted into piles representing themes. Some researchers use different-colored file cards for each participant's data.

Before the advent of computer programs for managing qualitative data, a typical procedure was to develop **conceptual files**. In this approach, researchers create a physical file for each category, and insert all material relating to that category into the file. To create conceptual files, researchers must first go through all the data, writing relevant codes in the margins, as in Figure 19.1. Then they cut up a copy of the material by category area, and place the cut-out excerpt into the file for that category. All of the content on a particular topic then can be retrieved by going to the applicable file folder.

Creating such conceptual files is cumbersome and labor intensive. This is particularly true when segments of the narrative materials have multiple codes, as is true for the excerpt in Figure 19.1. For example, there would need to be three copies of the last paragraph—one for each file corresponding to the three codes used for this paragraph. Researchers must also be sensitive to the need to provide enough context that the cut-up material can be understood (e.g., including material preceding or following the directly relevant materials). Finally, researchers must usually include pertinent administrative information. For example, for interview data, each excerpt would need to include the ID number for the participant so that researchers could, if necessary, obtain additional information from the master copy.

> **Example of manual data organization:**
> Manns and Chad (2001) explored quality of life among people with a quadriplegic or paraplegic spinal cord injury. Transcribed interviews with 15 informants were read several times. Their report described how categories were developed from the data, and how they used the file folder method to organize categorized material.

Computer Programs for Managing Qualitative Data

Computer assisted qualitative data analysis software (CAQDAS) can help to remove some of the work of cutting and pasting pages of narrative material. These programs permit the entire data file to be entered onto the computer, each portion of an interview or observational record coded, and then portions of the text corresponding to specified codes retrieved and printed (or shown on a screen) for analysis. The software can also be used to examine relationships between codes. Software cannot, however, *do* the coding, and it cannot tell the researcher how to analyze the data. Researchers must continue their role as analysts and critical thinkers.

Dozens of CAQDAS have been developed. The main types of software packages that are available to handle and manage qualitative data include: text retrievers, code and retrieve, theory building, concept maps and diagrams, and data conversion/collection (Taylor, 2005; Weitzman & Miles, 1995). Below is a brief description of these types of software.

Text retrievers are programs that help researchers locate text and terms in databases and documents. *Code-and-retrieve packages* permit researchers to code text. Chunks of the text are marked and linked to a name given by the researcher to indicate that piece of the text's content. The software can then collect together all the parts of the text labeled with the same code.

More sophisticated *theory-building software*, the most frequently used type of CAQDAS, permits researchers to build relationships between concepts, develop hierarchies of codes, diagram, and create hyperlinks to create nonhierarchical networks. Examples of theory-building packages include ATLAS/TI, HyperRESEARCH, and NVivo7. NVivo7, the latest software from Qualitative Solutions and Research (QSR), combines the best of two earlier packages (NVivo2 and NUD*IST 6). NVivo7 helps researchers find patterns in their data and explore hunches, and enables them to display and analyze relationships in the data.

Software for **concept mapping** and diagramming permits researchers to construct more sophisticated diagrams than theory-building software. Concept maps are a means for organizing and representing knowledge. Concept maps include concepts (enclosed in circles or boxes) and relationships between them (indicated by connecting lines). The connecting lines are labeled with *linking words* (e.g., "necessary for," "begin with") that describe the relationship between the two concepts. Propositions—meaningful statements that indicate how two or more concepts are connected—can then be formed based on the concept maps (Novak & Canas, 2006). CmapTools, an example of concept mapping software (*http://www.ihmc.us*), was developed at the Institute for Human and Machine Cognition (IHMC) and is available without charge to educational and not-for-profit organizations.

Data conversion/collection software converts audio into text. Voice recognition software can convert spoken voice into text and is attractive because of the time and expense needed to transcribe audiotaped interviews. Voice recognition software is designed for a single user. The software must be "trained" to recognize the voice of the user, typically an oral transcriptionist. After training is completed, the user can listen to short segments of the taped interview and repeat into the computer exactly what he or she just heard. Estimates of the time required to train software for voice recognition have averaged about 10 hours (Fogg & Wightman, 2000).

Voice recognition programs are available from a number of vendors. Their performance is highly variable and depends on such factors as the capability of the computer on which the software is installed, the quality of the microphone, and the amount of background noise (Fogg & Wightman, 2000). The inability of voice recognition software to automatically punctuate is one of its disadvantages. The oral transcriptionist must specifically state the punctuation, such as "period" and "comma". Oral transcriptionists also still need to make edits to the text to correct re-dictation errors. MacLean and colleagues (2004) used voice recognition software to transcribe their interviews in their research on health promotion initiatives and discussed some problems they encountered. For instance, the voice recognition program consistently misinterpreted common homonyms like "here" and "hear" and "to," "too," and "two," resulting in inaccuracies in the transcript. Thus, the time-saving advantages of using voice recognition software may be small.

⊃ **TIP:** When first using qualitative data analysis software, choosing a software package that is best for your study can be overwhelming. It can be helpful to contact distributors of such software and ask for free demonstration disks.

Computer programs offer many advantages for managing qualitative data, but some people prefer manual methods because they allow researchers to get closer to the data. Others have raised objections to having a process that is basically cognitive turned into an activity that is mechanical and technical (e.g., Seidel, 1993). MacMillan and Koenig (2004) warned of misunderstandings and misuse of software programs in qualitative analysis. They stressed that CAQDAS needs to be reviewed within the epistemologic framework of the qualitative research method chosen for the study. Despite concerns, many researchers have switched to computerized data management. Proponents insist that it frees up their time and permits them to pay greater attention to more important conceptual issues.

CAQDAS is constantly revised and upgraded, so it is hard to stay current on this topic. The website for the CAQDAS Networking Project is particularly useful, and includes a paper on choosing a CAQDAS software package (Lewins & Silver, 2006). This and other relevant websites are listed on the CD-ROM included with this book for you to "click" on directly.

Example of using computers to manage qualitative data: Wotton, Borbasi, and Redden (2005) studied nurses' perceptions of factors influencing palliative care for patients with end-stage heart failure. Interviews with 17 nurses were audiotaped and transcribed. The NVivo software was used to manage the data and also to explore connections between themes and subthemes that emerged in the data.

➡ TIP: Articles that describe how specific qualitative data analysis software has been used are especially helpful to read before starting your own project. For example, Bringer, Johnston, and Brackenridge (2004) described in detail their use of the software program NVivo in a grounded theory study. A number of print screens from their analysis are included in the article as illustrations.

ANALYTIC PROCEDURES

Data *management* in qualitative research is reductionist in nature: It involves converting large masses of data into smaller, more manageable segments. By contrast, qualitative data *analysis* is constructionist: It involves putting segments together into meaningful conceptual patterns. Qualitative analysis is an inductive process that involves determining the pervasiveness of key ideas. Although there are various approaches to qualitative data analysis, some elements are common to several of them. We provide some general guidelines, followed by a description of procedures used by ethnographers, phenomenologists, and grounded theory researchers. We also provide information about analyzing data from focus group interviews and briefly note a strategy for analyzing triangulated qualitative and quantitative data.

A General Analytic Overview

The analysis of qualitative materials begins with a search for broad categories or themes. In their thorough review of how the term *theme* is used among qualitative researchers, DeSantis and Ugarriza (2000) offered this definition: "A **theme** is an abstract entity that brings meaning and identity to a current experience and its variant manifestations. As such, a theme captures and unifies the nature or basis of the experience into a meaningful whole" (p. 362).

Themes emerge from the data. They often develop within categories of data (i.e., within categories of the coding scheme used for indexing materials), but may also cut across them. For example, in Beck's (2004) study (see Box 19.1), one theme that emerged was the clinicians' neglect of communication, including failure to communicate with their patients in labor and delivery (code 2A) and failure to communicate amongst themselves (code 2C).

The search for themes involves not only discovering commonalities across participants but also seeking natural variation. Themes are never universal. Researchers must attend not only to what themes arise but also to how they are patterned. Does the theme apply only to certain types of people or in certain communities? In certain contexts? At certain periods? What are the conditions that precede the observed phenomenon, and what are the apparent consequences of it? In other words, the qualitative analyst must be sensitive to *relationships* within the data.

Researchers' search for themes, regularities, and patterns in the data can sometimes be facilitated by charting devices that enable them to summarize the evolution of behaviors, events, and processes. For example, for qualitative studies that focus on dynamic experiences—such as decision making—it is often useful to develop flow charts or time-lines that highlight time sequences, major decision points and events, and factors affecting the decisions.

Example of a time-line: In Beck's (2002) grounded theory study of mothering twins during the first year of life, time-lines highlighting a mother's 24-hour schedule were helpful. Figure 19.2 presents an example for a 23-year-old mother of twins who had been born premature and were in the neonatal intensive care unit for 2 months. The twins had recently been discharged from the hospital. Until the twins were 3 months old, the mother maintained the twins on the same feeding schedule as they had been on in the hospital—every 3 hours. The time-line in the figure illustrates a typical 24-hour period for this mother during the 4 weeks after hospital discharge.

The identification of key themes and categories is seldom a tidy, linear process— iteration is almost always necessary. That is, researchers derive themes from the narrative materials, go back to the materials with the themes in mind to see if the

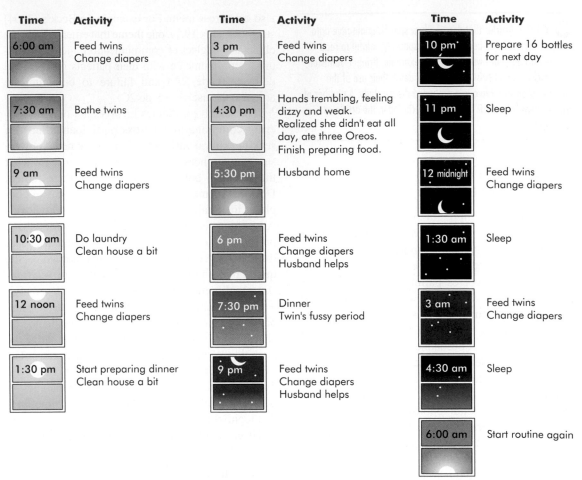

Time	Activity	Time	Activity	Time	Activity
6:00 am	Feed twins Change diapers	3 pm	Feed twins Change diapers	10 pm	Prepare 16 bottles for next day
7:30 am	Bathe twins	4:30 pm	Hands trembling, feeling dizzy and weak. Realized she didn't eat all day, ate three Oreos. Finish preparing food.	11 pm	Sleep
9 am	Feed twins Change diapers	5:30 pm	Husband home	12 midnight	Feed twins Change diapers
10:30 am	Do laundry Clean house a bit	6 pm	Feed twins Change diapers Husband helps	1:30 am	Sleep
12 noon	Feed twins Change diapers	7:30 pm	Dinner Twin's fussy period	3 am	Feed twins Change diapers
1:30 pm	Start preparing dinner Clean house a bit	9 pm	Feed twins Change diapers Husband helps	4:30 am	Sleep
				6:00 am	Start routine again

FIGURE 19.2 Example of a timeline for mothering multiples study.

materials really do fit, and then refine the themes as necessary. Sometimes apparent insights early in the process have to be abandoned.

Example of abandoning an early conceptualization: Strang and colleagues' (2006) study of the experiences of family caregivers of relatives with dementia illustrated this: "We coded data categories in stages with each stage representing a higher level of conceptual complexity . . . the interplay within the caregiver dyad reminded us of *dancing*. As the analysis progressed, the dance metaphor failed to fully represent the increasingly complex nature of the interactions between caregiver and the family member with dementia. We abandoned it completely" (p. 32).

Some qualitative researchers—especially phenomenologists—use metaphors as an analytic strategy, as the preceding example suggests. A **metaphor** is a symbolic comparison using figurative language to evoke a visual analogy. Metaphors can be a powerfully creative and expressive tool for qualitative analysts. As a literary device, metaphors can permit greater insight and understanding in qualitative data analysis, in addition to helping link parts to the whole. Thorne and Darbyshire (2005) have, however, criticized the overuse of metaphors in qualitative research. They pointed out that, although metaphoric allusions can be a powerful and memorable approach to articulating human experience, they can run the risk of "supplanting creative insight with hackneyed cliché masquerading as profundity" (p. 1111).

> **Example of a metaphor:** SmithBattle (2005) conducted a longitudinal study of mothers who gave birth as teenagers. The women were interviewed four times between 1988 (when the infants were 8 to 10 months old) and 2001 (when the mothers were about 30 years old). The researcher used the metaphor of a *narrative spine* to describe how the mothers' lives unfolded during the 12-year period. "The narrative spines of some mothers were large and supported well-developed, coherent 'chapters' on mothering, adult love, and work. For others, mothering provided a 'backbone' for a meaningful life . . ." (p. 831).

A further step involves validation. In this phase, the concern is whether the themes inferred accurately represent the perspectives of the people interviewed or observed. Several validation procedures can be used, which we will discuss in Chapter 20. If more than one researcher is working on the study, sessions in which the themes are reviewed and specific cases discussed can be highly productive. Such investigator triangulation cannot ensure thematic validity, but it can minimize idiosyncratic biases.

In validating and refining themes, some researchers introduce **quasi-statistics**—a tabulation of the frequency with which certain themes or insights are supported by the data. The frequencies cannot be interpreted in the same way as frequencies generated in survey studies because of imprecision in the enumeration of the themes, but, as Becker (1970) pointed out,

• • •

Quasi-statistics may allow the investigator to dispose of certain troublesome null hypotheses. A simple frequency count of the number of times a given phenomenon appears may make untenable the null hypothesis that the phenomenon is infrequent. A comparison of the number of such instances with the number of negative cases—instances in which some alternative phenomenon that would not be predicted by his theory appears—may make possible a stronger conclusion, especially if the theory was developed early

enough in the observational period to allow a systematic search for negative cases (p. 81).

• • •

Sandelowski (2001) believes that numbers are underutilized in qualitative research because of two myths: first, that real qualitative researchers *do not* count, and second, that qualitative researchers *cannot* count. Numbers are helpful in highlighting the complexity and work of qualitative research and in generating meaning from the data. Numbers are also useful in documenting and testing interpretations and conclusions and in describing events and experiences. Sandelowski has warned, however, of the pitfalls of overcounting.

> **Example of tabulating data:** Wilde (2003) studied the experiences of long-term users of indwelling urinary catheters. She tabulated aspects of the participants' acceptance of the catheter, and their experience of stigma and vulnerability in living with a catheter, in two "theme grids." For example, many of the 14 study participants noted that they considered the catheter to be "part of me" (64%). A majority also explicitly mentioned that one of their coping mechanisms was to hide the catheter (57%).

In the final analysis stage, researchers strive to weave the thematic pieces together into an integrated whole. The various themes need to be interrelated to provide an overall structure (such as a theory or integrated description) to the data. The integration task is a difficult one because it demands creativity and intellectual rigor if it is to be successful.

Qualitative Content Analysis

In the remainder of this section, we discuss analytic procedures used by ethnographers, phenomenologists, and grounded theory researchers. Qualitative researchers who conduct descriptive qualitative studies not based in a specific tradition may, however, simply say that they performed a content analysis. **Qualitative content analysis** is the analysis of the content of narrative data to identify prominent themes and patterns among the themes. Qualitative content analysis involves breaking down data into smaller *units*, coding and naming the units according to the content they represent, and grouping coded material based on shared concepts.

Krippendorff (2005) identified five definitions of units: physical, syntactical, categorical, propositional, and thematic distinctions. These definitions refer to the types of cognitive operations coders need to do to identify units within a text. *Physical* units are defined by time, length, or size—but not by type of information. *Syntactical* distinctions are based on grammatical divisions within the data—that is, words, sentences, paragraphs. *Categorical* distinctions define units by identifying something they have in common, that is, by membership in a category. *Propositional* distinctions divide units based on specific constructions such as a proposition or a clause. Lastly, *thematic* distinctions delineate units according to themes.

Krippendorff (2005) suggested *clustering* as a way to represent the results of content analyses. Clustering is based on similarities among units of analysis and hierarchies that conceptualize the text on different levels of abstraction. The steps of clustering can be displayed in **dendrograms**, which are treelike diagrams. Dendrograms indicate when and which units are merged. Hsieh and Shannon (2005) offered a good discussion of three different approaches to content analysis.

> **Example of a content analysis:** Beck (2005) undertook a content analysis of the benefits of women participating in Internet interviews regarding their traumatic childbirths. Her paper included an example of a dendrogram.

Analysis of Ethnographic Data

Analysis begins from the moment ethnographers set foot in the field. Ethnographers are continually looking for *patterns* in the behavior and thoughts of the participants, comparing one pattern against another, and analyzing many patterns simultaneously (Fetterman, 1989). As they analyze patterns of everyday life, ethnographers acquire a deeper understanding of the culture being studied. Maps, flow charts, and organizational charts are also useful tools that help to crystallize and illustrate the data being collected. Matrices (two-dimensional displays) can also help to highlight a comparison graphically, to cross-reference categories, and to discover emerging patterns.

Spradley's (1979) research sequence is often used for data analysis in an ethnographic study. His method is based on the premise that language is the primary means that relates cultural meaning in a culture. The task of ethnographers is to describe cultural symbols and to identify their coding rules. His sequence of 12 steps, which includes both data collection and data analysis, is as follows:

1. Locating an informant
2. Interviewing an informant
3. Making an ethnographic record
4. Asking descriptive questions
5. Analyzing ethnographic interviews
6. Making a domain analysis
7. Asking structural questions
8. Making a taxonomic analysis
9. Asking contrast questions
10. Making a componential analysis
11. Discovering cultural themes
12. Writing the ethnography

Thus, in Spradley's method, there are four levels of data analysis, the first of which is **domain analysis**. Domains, which are units of cultural knowledge, are broad categories that encompass smaller categories. There is no preestablished number of domains to be uncovered in an ethnographic study. During this first level of data analysis, ethnographers identify relational patterns among terms in the domains that are used by members of the culture. The ethnographer focuses on the cultural meaning of terms and symbols (objects and events) used in a culture, and their interrelationships.

In **taxonomic analysis**, the second level of data analysis, ethnographers decide how many domains the data analysis will encompass. Will only one or two domains be analyzed in depth, or will a number of domains be studied less intensively? After making this decision, a **taxonomy**—a system of classifying and organizing terms—is developed to illustrate the internal organization of a domain and the relationship among the subcategories of the domain.

In **componential analysis**, multiple relationships among terms in the domains are examined. The ethnographer analyzes data for similarities and differences among cultural terms in a domain. Finally, in **theme analysis**, cultural themes are uncovered. Domains are connected in cultural themes, which help to provide a holistic view of the culture being studied. The discovery of cultural meaning is the outcome.

Example using Spradley's method: Tzeng and Lipson (2004) investigated experiences of patients and family members after a suicide attempt within the cultural context of Taiwan. Data from interviews and participant observations were analyzed in an ongoing fashion. The analysis began with the coding of categories and terms, which they "associated into higher order domains" (p. 348). They also undertook a componential analysis by conducting "a back and forth process to establish different categories: searching for contrasts among these domains, grouping some together as dimensions, and combining related dimensions" (p. 348). The postsuicide stigma suffered by patients and their families was based on such cultural themes as "Suicide is bu-hsiao" (nonfilial piety).

Other approaches to ethnographic analysis have also been developed. For example, in their ethnonursing research method, Leininger and McFarland (2006) provided ethnographers with a four-phase ethnonursing data analysis guide. In the first phase, ethnographers collect, describe, and record data. The second phase involves identifying and categorizing descriptors. In phase 3, data are analyzed to discover repetitive patterns in their context. The fourth and final phase involves abstracting major themes and presenting findings.

Example using Leininger's method: DeOliveira and Hoga (2005) studied the process of seeking and undergoing surgical contraception by low-income Brazilian women. Using Leininger's ethnonursing research method, the researchers interviewed 7 key informants and 11 additional informants. The cultural theme was that "being *operada* was the realization of a great dream" (p. 5).

Phenomenological Analysis

Schools of phenomenology have developed different approaches to data analysis. Three frequently used methods for descriptive phenomenology are the methods of Colaizzi (1978), Giorgi (1985), and Van Kaam (1966), all of whom are from the Duquesne school of phenomenology, based on Husserl's philosophy. Table 19.1 presents a comparison of these three methods of analysis. The basic outcome of all three methods is the description of the meaning of an experience, often through the identification of essential themes.

Phenomenologists search for common patterns shared by particular instances. There are, however, some important differences among these three approaches. Colaizzi's method, for example, is the only one that calls for returning to study participants, Giorgi's analysis to validate results relies solely on researchers. His view is that it is inappropriate either to return to participants to validate findings or to use external judges to review the analysis. Van Kaam's method requires that intersubjective agreement be reached with other expert judges.

Example of a study using Colaizzi's method: Beck (2006) explored the experiences of mothers regarding the yearly anniversary of their traumatic childbirths. Thirty-seven women participated over the Internet in this study. Mothers sent their stories describing their experiences of their anniversaries on attachment to Beck. These stories were analyzed using Colaizzi's method for data analysis. Four themes revealed the essence of women's experiences of the anniversary of their birth trauma: (1) the prologue: an agonizing time, (2) the actual day: a celebration of a birthday or the torment of an anniversary, (3) the epilogue: a fragile state, and (4) subsequent anniversaries: for better or worse.

A second school of phenomenology is the Utrecht school. Phenomenologists using this Dutch approach combine characteristics of descriptive and interpretive phenomenology. Van Manen's (1990) method is an example of this combined approach, in which researchers try to grasp the essential meaning of the experience being studied. According to Van Manen, thematic aspects of experience can be uncovered or isolated from participants' descriptions of the experience by three methods: (1) the holistic approach, (2) the selective or highlighting approach, and (3) the detailed or line-by-line approach. In the **holistic approach**, researchers view the text as a

TABLE 19.1	Comparison of Three Phenomenological Analytic Methods	

COLAIZZI (1978)	GIORGI (1985)	VAN KAAM (1966)
1. Read all protocols to acquire a feeling for them.	1. Read the entire set of protocols to get a sense of the whole.	1. List and group preliminarily the descriptive expressions that must be agreed upon by expert judges. Final listing presents percentages of these categories in that particular sample.
2. Review each protocol and extract significant statements.	2. Discriminate units from participants' description of phenomenon being studied.	2. Reduce the concrete, vague, and overlapping expressions of the participants to more descriptive terms. (Intersubjective agreement among judges needed.)
3. Spell out the meaning of each significant statement (i.e., formulate meanings).	3. Articulate the psychological insight in each of the meaning units.	3. Eliminate elements not inherent in the phenomenon being studied or that represent blending of two related phenomena.
4. Organize the formulated meanings into clusters of themes. a. Refer these clusters back to the original protocols to validate them. b. Note discrepancies among or between the various clusters, avoiding the temptation of ignoring data or themes that do not fit.	4. Synthesize all of the transformed meaning units into a consistent statement regarding participants' experiences (referred to as the "structure of the experience"); can be expressed on a specific or general level.	4. Write a hypothetical identification and description of the phenomenon being studied.
5. Integrate results into an exhaustive description of the phenomenon under study.		5. Apply hypothetical description to randomly selected cases from the sample. If necessary, revise the hypothesized description, which must then be tested again on a new random sample.
6. Formulate an exhaustive description of the phenomenon under study in as unequivocal a statement of identification as possible.		6. Consider the hypothesized identification as a valid identification and description once preceding operations have been carried out successfully.
7. Ask participants about the findings thus far as a final validating step.		

whole and try to capture its meanings. In the **selective approach**, researchers highlight or pull out statements or phrases that seem essential to the experience under study. In the **detailed approach**, researchers analyze every sentence. Once themes have been identified, they become the objects of reflection and interpretation through follow-up interviews with participants. Through this process, essential themes are discovered.

Van Manen (2006) stressed that this phenomenological method cannot be separated from the practice of writing. Writing up the results of qualitative analysis is an active struggle to understand and recognize the lived meanings of the phenomena studied. The text written by a phenomenological researcher must lead readers to a "questioning wonder." The words chosen by the writer need to take the reader into a "wondrous landscape" as the reader is drawn into the textual meaning (Van Manen, 2002, p. 4).

Example of a study using Van Manen's method: Trybulski (2005) studied women's postabortion experiences 15 or more years after they had the procedure. Trybulski described in detail how Van Manen's approach was used to analyze data from 16 women. The thematic analysis involved using all three of Van Manen's approaches: "The holistic or sententious analysis yielded a sense of the experience as a whole. In the selective or highlighting review, multiple readings of the text uncovered essential experiential statements. Finally, the investigator read the text in a detailed fashion, considering each sentence and sentence cluster for its contribution to the understanding of the experience" (p. 565).

In addition to identifying themes from participants' descriptions, Van Manen also called for gleaning thematic descriptions from artistic sources. Van Manen urged qualitative researchers to keep in mind that literature, music, painting, and other art forms can provide a wealth of experiential information that can increase insights as the phenomenologist tries to interpret and grasp the essential meaning of the experience being studied. Experiential descriptions in literature and art help challenge and stretch phenomenologists' interpretive sensibilities.

Example of a phenomenological analysis using artistic expressions: Lauterbach (2007) investigated mothers' experiences with the death of a wished-for baby. Poetry, literature, and art helped Lauterbach's interpretation of the mothers' experiences. For instance, Herbert Mason's poem "The Memory of Death," in which he reflected on the death of his child, and Robert Frost's poem "Home Burial," in which Frost described gender differences in the experience of infant death, were used in data analysis. Memorial art in cemeteries and funeral photographs also provided insight.

A third school of phenomenology is an interpretive approach called Heideggerian hermeneutics. Central to analyzing data in a hermeneutic study is the notion of the **hermeneutic circle**. The circle signifies a methodologic process in which, to reach understanding, there is continual movement between the parts and the whole of the text being analyzed. Gadamer (1975) stressed that, to interpret a text, researchers cannot separate themselves from the meanings of the text and must strive to understand possibilities that the text can reveal. Ricoeur (1981) broadened this notion of text to include not just the written text but also any human action or situation.

Example of Gadamerian hermeneutics: Tapp (2004) studied dilemmas of family support during cardiac recovery. Her data were derived from transcripts of videotaped clinical sessions with six families. Guided by Gadamer's writings, Tapp's interpretation of the text occurred at three levels: "First, the transcripts for each session were reviewed to identify salient events, meanings, and patterns related to experiences . . . that . . . . illustrated attempts to offer or receive support. Second, all of the sessions for each family were then reviewed for thematic patterns across their unique situation. . . . Interpretive memoing traced emerging understandings of support within each family situation and within their relationships. Finally, the salient events, family concerns, and recurrent patterns were compared between and across the six family situations" (p. 566).

Diekelmann, Allen, and Tanner (1989) have proposed a seven-stage process of data analysis in hermeneutics that involves collaborative effort by a team of researchers. The goal of this process is to describe shared practices and common meanings. Diekelmann and colleagues' stages include the following

1. All the interviews or texts are read for an overall understanding.
2. Interpretive summaries of each interview are written.
3. A team of researchers analyzes selected transcribed interviews or texts.
4. Any disagreements on interpretation are resolved by going back to the text.
5. Common meanings and shared practices are identified by comparing and contrasting the text.
6. Relationships among themes emerge.
7. A draft of the themes along with exemplars from texts are presented to the team. Responses or suggestions are incorporated into the final draft.

According to Diekelmann and colleagues, the discovery in step 6 of a **constitutive pattern**—a pattern that expresses the relationships among relational themes and is present in all the interviews or texts—forms the highest level of hermeneutical analysis. A situation is constitutive when it gives actual content to a person's self-understanding or to a person's way of being in the world.

Example using Diekelmann's hermeneutical analysis: Cheung and Hocking (2004) used Diekelmann's method to explore spousal carers' experience of caring for victims of multiple sclerosis. First, the researchers read all transcripts from their interviews with 10 spousal caregivers in Australia to gain an overall understanding. Then they read and reread the transcripts in search of similar categories and themes. Next, they analyzed data for relational themes that cut across all texts. Finally, they examined the data to identify a constitutive pattern that described the ways in which participants' experiences of caring for their partner had changed their way of living and their personal meanings. The constitutive pattern that emerged from the data was called "Weaving Through a Web of Paradoxes."

Benner (1994) offered another analytic approach for hermeneutic phenomenology. Her interpretive analysis consists of three interrelated processes: the search for paradigm cases, thematic analysis, and analysis of exemplars. **Paradigm cases** are "strong instances of concerns or ways of being in the world" (Benner, 1994, p. 113). Paradigm cases are used early in the analytic process as a strategy for gaining understanding. Thematic analysis is done to compare and contrast similarities across cases. Lastly, paradigm cases and thematic analysis can be enhanced by *exemplars* that illuminate aspects of a paradigm case or theme. The presentation of paradigm cases and exemplars in research reports allows readers to play a role in consensual validation of the results by deciding whether the cases support the researchers' conclusions.

Example using Benner's hermeneutical analysis: Raingruber and Kent (2003) conducted an interpretive phenomenological study of faculty and student experiences with sensations and perceptions experienced during traumatic clinical events. The researchers interviewed students and faculty in nursing and social work. Using Benner's interpretive analysis, one paradigm case and 12 exemplars were described in support of their conclusion that nursing faculty and students experienced strong physical sensations during traumatic situations. In the paradigm case, "Trina, a social work student, described suddenly feeling like her body was 'a ripe apple ready to drop from the tree when a little boy surprised her by calling her momma'" (p. 455).

Grounded Theory Analysis

The grounded theory method emerged in the 1960s in connection with a research program—which focused on dying in hospitals—by two sociologists, Glaser and Strauss (1967). The two co-originators eventually split and developed divergent schools of thought, which have been called the "Glaserian" and "Straussian" versions of grounded theory (Walker & Myrick, 2006). The division between the two mainly concerns the manner in which the data are analyzed.

Glaser and Strauss's Grounded Theory Method

Grounded theory in both systems of analysis uses the **constant comparative** method of data analysis.

This method involves a comparison of elements present in one data source (e.g., in one interview) with those in another. The process is continued until the content of each source has been compared with the content in all sources. In this fashion, commonalities are identified.

The concept of fit is an important element in Glaserian grounded theory analysis. **Fit** is the process of identifying characteristics of one piece of data and comparing them with the characteristics of another datum to determine whether they are similar. In the analytic process, fit is used to sort and reduce data. Fit enables the researcher to determine whether data can be placed in the same category or if they can be related to one another. However, Glaser (1992) warned qualitative researchers not to force an analytic fit, noting that "if you torture data enough it will give up!" (p. 123). Forcing a fit hinders the development of a relevant theory. *Fit* is also an important issue when a grounded theory is applied in new contexts: the theory must closely "fit" the substantive area where it will be used (Glaser & Strauss, 1967).

Coding in the Glaserian grounded theory approach is used to conceptualize data into patterns. The substance of the topic under study is conceptualized through **substantive codes**, whereas **theoretical codes** provide insights into how substantive codes relate to each other. There are two types of substantive codes: open and selective. **Open coding**, used in the first stage of the constant comparative analysis, captures what is going on in the data. Open codes may be the actual words used by the participants. Through open coding, data are broken down into incidents, and their similarities and differences are examined. During open coding, researchers ask, "What category or property of a category does this incident indicate?" (Glaser, 1978, p. 57).

There are three different levels of open coding that vary in degree of abstraction. **Level I codes** (or *in vivo* codes) are derived directly from the language of the substantive area. They have vivid imagery and "grab." Table 19.2 presents five level I codes from interviews in Beck's (2002) grounded theory study on mothering twins, along with excerpts associated with those codes. (A figure showing Beck's hierarchy of codes, from level I to one of her level III codes, is presented in the Toolkit section of the accompanying *Resource Manual*).

As researchers constantly compare new level I codes with previously identified ones, they condense them into broader **level II codes**. For example, in Table 19.2, Beck's five level I codes were collapsed into the level II code, "Reaping the Blessings." **Level III codes** (or theoretical constructs) are the most abstract. These constructs "add scope beyond local meanings" (Glaser, 1978, p. 70) to the generated theory. Collapsing level II codes aids in identifying constructs.

Open coding ends when the core category is discovered, and then selective coding begins. The **core category** is a pattern of behavior that is relevant or problematic for study participants. In **selective coding** (which can also have three levels of abstraction), researchers code only those data that are related to the core variable. One kind of core variable is a **basic social process (BSP)** that evolves over time in two or more phases. All BSPs are core variables, but not all core variables have to be BSPs.

Glaser (1978) provided nine criteria to help researchers decide on a core category:

1. It must be central, meaning that it is related to many categories.
2. It must reoccur frequently in the data.
3. It takes more time to saturate than other categories.
4. It relates meaningfully and easily to other categories.
5. It has clear and grabbing implications for formal theory.
6. It has considerable carry-through.
7. It is completely variable.
8. It is a dimension of the problem.
9. It can be any kind of theoretical code.

Theoretical codes help grounded theorists to weave the broken pieces of data back together. Theoretical codes have the tremendous power "to grab," which Glaser (2005) called "theoretical

TABLE 19.2 Collapsing Level I Codes into the Level II Code of "REAPING THE BLESSINGS" (Beck, 2002)

QUOTE	LEVEL I CODE
I enjoy just watching the twins interact so much. Especially now that they are mobile. They are not walking yet but they are crawling. I will tell you they are already playing. Like one will go around the corner and kind of peek around and they play hide and seek. They crawl after each other. (3)	Enjoying Twins
With twins it's amazing. She was sick and she had a fever. He was the one acting sick. She didn't seem like she was sick at all. He was. We watched him for like 6–8 hours. We gave her the medicine and he started calming down. Like WOW! That is so weird. Cause you read about it but it's like, Oh come on! You know that doesn't really happen and it does. It's really neat to see. (15)	Amazing
These days it's really neat cause you go to the store or you go out and people are like "Oh, they are twins, how nice." And I say, "Yeah they are. Look, look at my kids." (15)	Getting Attention
I just feel blessed to have two. I just feel like I am twice as lucky as a mom who has one baby. I mean that's the best part. It's just that instead of having one baby to watch grow and change and develop and become a toddler and school-age child you have two. (11)	Feeling Blessed
It's very exciting. It's interesting and it's fun to see them and how the twin bond really is. There really is a twin bond. You read about it and you hear about it but until you experience it, you just don't understand. One time they were both crying and they were fed. They were changed and burped. There was nothing wrong. I couldn't figure out what was wrong. So I said to myself, "I am just going to put them together and close the door." I put them in my bed together and they patty-caked their hands and put their noses together and just looked at each other and went right to sleep. (15)	Twin Bonding

code capture" (p. 74). Theoretical codes provide a grounded theory with a greater explanatory power because they enhance the abstract meaning of the relationships among categories. Glaser (1978) first proposed 18 families of theoretical codes that researchers can use to conceptualize how substantive codes relate to each other (Box 19.2). Recently, Glaser (2005) opened up endless possibilities for theoretical codes that researchers can use. He provided examples of theoretical codes from biochemistry (bias random walk), from economics (amplifying causal looping), and from political science (conjectural causation). The larger the array of theoretical codes available, the less tendency a researcher will have to force on the developing theory a pet or favorite theoretical code (Glaser, 2005).

Throughout coding and analysis, grounded theory analysts document their ideas about the data, themes, and emerging conceptual scheme in **memos**. Memos preserve ideas that may initially not seem productive but may later prove valuable once further developed. Memos also encourage researchers to reflect on and describe patterns in the data, relationships between categories, and emergent conceptualizations.

BOX 19.2 Families of Theoretical Codes for Grounded Theory Analysis

1. The six C's: causes, contexts, contingencies, consequences, covariances, and conditions
2. Process: stages, phases, passages, transitions
3. Degree: intensity, range, grades, continuum
4. Dimension: elements, parts, sections
5. Type: kinds, styles, forms
6. Strategy: tactics, techniques, maneuverings
7. Interaction: mutual effects, interdependence, reciprocity
8. Identity–self: self-image, self-worth, self-concept
9. Cutting point: boundaries, critical junctures, turning points
10. Means–goal: purpose, end, products
11. Cultural: social values, beliefs
12. Consensus: agreements, uniformities, conformity
13. Mainline: socialization, recruiting, social order
14. Theoretical: density, integration, clarity, fit, relevance
15. Ordering/elaboration: structural ordering, temporal ordering, conceptual ordering
16. Unit: group, organization, collective
17. Reading: hypotheses, concepts, problems
18. Models: pictorial models of a theory

Adapted from Glaser, B. G. (1978). *Theoretical sensitivity.* Mill Valley, CA: Sociological Press.

TIP: The Toolkit of the *Resource Manual* includes an example of a memo from Beck's work. Glaser (1978) offered guidelines for preparing effective memos to generate substantive theory, including the following:

- Keep memos separate from data.
- Stop coding when an idea for a memo occurs, so as not to lose the thought.
- A memo can be brought on by literally forcing it, by beginning to write about a code.
- Memos can be modified as growth and realizations occur.
- In writing memos, do not focus on persons; instead, talk conceptually about the substantive codes as they are theoretically coded.
- When you have two ideas, write each idea up as a separate memo to prevent confusion.
- Always remain flexible with memoing approaches.

Glaser's grounded theory method is concerned with the *generation* of categories and hypotheses rather than testing them. The product of the typical grounded theory analysis is a theoretical model that endeavors to explain a pattern of behavior that is both relevant and problematic for study participants. Once the basic problem emerges, the grounded theorist goes on to discover the process these participants experience in coping with or resolving this problem.

Example of Glaser and Strauss's grounded theory analysis: Figure 19.3 presents Beck's (2002) model from a grounded theory study that conceptualized "Releasing the Pause Button" as the core category and process through which mothers of twins progressed as they attempted to resume their lives after giving birth. According to this model, the process involves four phases: Draining Power, Pausing Own Life, Striving to Reset, and Resuming Own Life. Beck used 10 coding families in her theoretical coding for the Releasing the Pause Button process. The family *cutting point* provides an illustration. Three months seemed to be the turning point for mothers, when life started to become more manageable. Here is an excerpt from an interview that Beck coded as a cutting point: "Three months came around and the twins sort of slept through the night and it made a huge, huge difference."

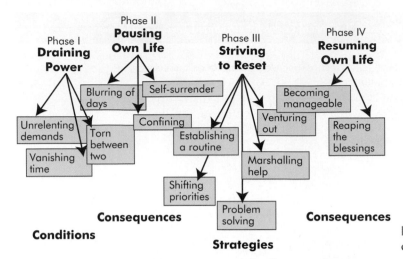

FIGURE 19.3 Beck's (2002) model of mothering twins.

Although Glaser and Straus cautioned against consulting the literature before a basic theoretical framework is stabilized, they also viewed grounded theory as an "ever modifying process" (Glaser, 1978, p. 5) that could benefit from scrutiny of other work. Glaser discussed the evolution of grounded theories through the process of **emergent fit**, to prevent individual substantive theories from being "respected little islands of knowledge" (p. 148). As Glaser pointed out, generating grounded theory does not necessarily require discovering all new categories or ignoring ones previously identified in the literature: "The task is, rather, to develop an emergent fit between the data and a pre-existent category that might work. Therefore, as in the refitting of a generated category as data emerge, so must an extant category be carefully fitted as data emerge to be sure it works. In the bargain, like the generated category, it may be modified to fit and work. In this sense the extant category was not merely borrowed but earned its way into the emerging theory" (p. 4). Through constant comparison, researchers can compare concepts emerging from the data with similar concepts from existing theory or research to determine which parts have emergent fit with the theory being generated.

Example of emergent fit: Wuest (2000) described how she grappled with reconciling emergent fit with Glaser's warning to avoid reading the literature until a grounded theory is well on its way. She used examples from her grounded theory study on negotiating with helping systems (e.g., health care, education, religion) to illustrate how emergent fit with existing research on relationships in health care was used to support her emerging theory. Constant comparison provided the checks and balances on using preexisting knowledge.

Strauss and Corbin's Approach

The Strauss and Corbin (1998) approach to grounded theory analysis differs from the original Glaser and Strauss method with regard to method, processes, and outcomes. Table 19.3 summarizes major analytic differences between these two grounded theory analysis methods.

Glaser (1978) stressed that to generate a grounded theory, the basic problem must emerge from the data—it must be discovered. The theory is, from the very start, grounded in the data, rather than starting with a preconceived problem. Strauss and Corbin, however, stated that the research itself is only one of four possible sources of a research problem. Research problems can, for example, come from the literature or a researcher's personal and professional experience.

The Strauss and Corbin method involves three types of coding: open, axial, and selective coding. In **open coding**, data are broken down into parts and compared for similarities and differences. Similar

TABLE 19.3	Comparison of Glaser's and Strauss/Corbin's Methods	
	GLASER	**STRAUSS & CORBIN**
Initial data analysis	Breaking down and conceptualizing data involves comparison of incident to incident so patterns emerge	Breaking down and conceptualizing data includes taking apart a single sentence, observation, and incident
Types of coding	Open, selective, theoretical	Open, axial, selective
Connections between categories	18 coding families	Paradigm model (conditions, contexts, action/interactional strategies, and consequences)
Outcome	Emergent theory (discovery)	Conceptual description (verification)

actions, events, and objects are grouped together as more abstract concepts, which are called categories. In open coding, the researcher focuses on generating categories and their properties and dimensions. In **axial coding**, the analyst systematically develops categories and links them with subcategories. Strauss and Corbin (1998) term this process of relating categories and their subcategories as "axial because coding occurs around the axis of a category, linking categories at the level of properties and dimensions" (p.123). What is called the *paradigm* is used to help identify linkages among categories. The basic components of the paradigm include conditions, actions/interactions, and consequences. **Selective coding** is the process by which the findings are integrated and refined. The first step in integrating the findings is to decide on the **central category** (sometimes called the *core category*), which is the main theme of the research. Recommended techniques to facilitate identifying the central category are writing the storyline, using diagrams, and reviewing and organizing memos.

The outcome of the Strauss and Corbin approach is, as Glaser (1992) termed it, a full conceptual description. The original grounded theory method (Glaser & Strauss, 1967), by contrast, generates a theory that explains how a basic social problem that emerged from the data is processed in a social setting.

Example of Strauss and Corbin's grounded theory analysis: Negarandeh and co-researchers (2006) studied the barriers and facilitators influencing the role of patient advocacy among Iranian nurses. Interview data were gathered from 24 nurses working in a university hospital in Tehran. Each interview was transcribed and analyzed before the next interview occurred, with analysis providing direction for subsequent interviews. Analysis, using the Strauss and Corbin approach, started with open coding: "Through open coding, the interview transcripts were reviewed several times and the data reduced to the codes and then the categories were formed from the codes, in a manner that similar codes were grouped into the same categories. The focus of axial coding was on specifying a category in the context in which it had appeared. This process allowed links to be made between categories and their subcategories, and then selective coding developed the main categories and their interrelations."

Analysis of Focus Group Data

Focus group interviews yield rich and complex data that pose special analytic challenges. Indeed, there is little consensus about the analysis of focus group data, despite its use by researchers in several qualitative research traditions.

Focus group interviews are especially difficult to transcribe, partly because of technical problems. For example, it is difficult to place microphones so that the voices of all group members are picked up with equal clarity, particularly because participants tend to speak at different volumes. An additional issue is the inevitability that several participants will speak at once, making it impossible for transcriptionists to discern everything being said.

A controversial issue in the analysis of focus group data is whether the unit of analysis is the group or individual participants. Some writers (e.g., Morrison-Beedy, Côté-Arsenault, & Feinstein, 2001) maintain that the group is the proper unit of analysis. Analysis of group-level data involves a scrutiny of themes, interactions, and sequences within and between groups. Others, however (e.g., Carey & Smith, 1994; Kidd & Parshall, 2000), argue that analysis should occur at both the group and the individual level. Those who insist that only group-level analysis is appropriate argue that what individuals say in focus groups cannot be treated as personal disclosures because they are inevitably influenced by the dynamics of the group. However, even in personal interviews, individual responses are shaped by social processes, and analysis of individual-level data (independent of group) is thought by some analysts to add important insights.

Carey and Smith (1994) advocated a third level of analysis—namely, the analysis of individual responses *in relation* to group context (e.g., whether a participant's view is in accord with or in contrast to majority opinion). Duggleby (2005) observed that two methods for analyzing focus group interaction data have been suggested—first, describing interactions as a means of interpreting the findings, and second, incorporating the group interaction data directly into the transcripts. She proposed a third alternative: a *congruent methodologic approach* that analyzes interaction data in the same manner as group or individual data.

For those who wish to analyze data from individual participants, it is essential to maintain information about what each person said—a task that is impossible to do if researchers are relying solely on audiotapes. Videotapes, as supplements to audiotapes, are sometimes used to identify who said what in focus group sessions. More frequently, however, researchers have several members of the research team in attendance at the sessions, whose job it is to take detailed field notes about the order of speakers and about significant nonverbal behavior, such as pounding or clenching of fists, crying, aggressive body language, and so on.

Transcription quality is especially important in focus group interviews: Emotional content as well as words must be faithfully recorded because participants are responding not only to the questions being posed but also to the experience of being in a group. Field notes, debriefing notes, and verbatim transcripts ideally must be integrated to yield a more comprehensive transcript for analysis.

Example of integrating focus group data:
Morrison-Beedy and colleagues (2001) provided several examples of integrating data across sources from their focus group research. For example, one verbatim quote was, "It was no big deal." This was supplemented with data from the field notes that the woman's eyes were cast downward as she said this, and that the words were delivered sarcastically. The complete transcript for this entry, which includes researcher interpretation in brackets, was as follows: "'It was no big deal.' (said sarcastically, with eyes looking downward). [It really was a very big deal to her, but others had not acknowledged that.]" (p. 52).

Because of group dynamics, focus group analysts must be sensitive to both the thematic content of these interviews and to how, when, and why themes are developed. Some of the issues that could be central to focus group analysis are the following:

- Does an issue raised in a focus group constitute a *theme* or merely a strongly held viewpoint of one or two members?
- Do the same issues or themes arise in more than one group?
- If there are group differences, why might this be the case—were participants different in characteristics and experiences, or did group processes affect the discussions?
- Are some issues sufficiently salient that they not only are discussed in direct response to specific questions posed by the moderator but also spontaneously emerge at multiple points in the session?
- Do group members find certain issues both interesting *and* important?

Some focus group analysts, such as Kidd and Parshall (2000), use quantitative methods as adjuncts to their qualitative analysis. Using qualitative analysis software, they conduct such analyses as assessing similarities and differences between groups, determining coding frequencies to aid pattern detection, examining codes in relation to participant characteristics, and examining how much dialogue individual members contributed. They use such methods not so that interpretation can be based on frequencies, but so that they can better understand context and identify issues that require further critical scrutiny and interpretation.

➲ **TIP:** Focus group data are sometimes analyzed according to the procedures of a formal research tradition, such as grounded theory.

Analysis of Triangulated Qualitative–Quantitative Data

Chapter 12 described the growth of mixed method research that triangulates qualitative and quantitative data within the context of a single study or coordinated sequence of studies. Typically, data from such studies are integrated after the fact. That is, quantitative data are analyzed statistically, narrative data are analyzed through qualitative methods, and then researchers interpret overall patterns in light of findings from the two study components.

There is, however, emerging interest in exploring alternative methods of analysis. One such approach is the construction of a **meta-matrix** that permits researchers to see important patterns and themes across data sources. This method, which can also be used to integrate multiple types of qualitative data (e.g., interviews and observational field notes), involves the development of a two- or three-dimensional matrix that aligns various types of data (Miles & Huberman, 1994). Typically, one dimension is for particular study participants. Then, for each participant, a chart is constructed in which data from multiple data sources are entered, so that the analyst can see at a glance such information as scores on psychosocial scales (e.g., scores on the

Center for Epidemiological Studies Depression scale), comments from open-ended dialogue with participants (e.g., verbatim narratives relating to depression), hospital record data (e.g., physiologic information), and the researchers' own reflexive comments. A third dimension can be added if there are multiple sources of data relating to multiple constructs (e.g., depression, pain). An example of a simple meta-matrix is included in the Toolkit with the accompanying *Resource Manual*. ✖

The construction of a meta-matrix allows researchers to explore whether statistical conclusions are supported by the qualitative data for individual study participants, and *vice versa*. Patterns of regularities, as well as anomalies, may be easier to see through detailed inspection of such matrices, and can allow for fuller exploration of all sources of data simultaneously.

Example of a meta-matrix: Wendler (2001) constructed a meta-matrix for her study of the impact of a therapeutic intervention, Tellington touch, on patient anxiety, pain, and physiologic status. She gathered quantitative data on such variables as blood pressure, state anxiety, pain levels, and nicotine and caffeine use. Participants also responded to open-ended questions. The clinician completed field notes on impressions, and spontaneous participant comments and participant observers provided field notes on behaviors. These multiple sources of data were analyzed quantitatively and qualitatively, and then subsequently arrayed in a meta-matrix, which yielded important insights.

INTERPRETATION OF QUALITATIVE FINDINGS

Interpretation and analysis of qualitative data occur virtually simultaneously, in an iterative process. That is, researchers interpret the data as they read and re-read them, categorize and code them, inductively develop a thematic analysis, and integrate the themes into a unified whole.

It is difficult to provide guidance about the process of interpretation in qualitative studies, but there is considerable agreement that the ability to "make meaning" from qualitative texts depends on researchers' immersion in and closeness to the data. **Incubation** is the process of *living* the data, a process in which researchers must try to understand their meanings, find their essential patterns, and draw legitimate, insightful conclusions. Another key ingredient in interpretation and "meaning making" is researchers' self-awareness and the ability to reflect on their own world view and perspectives—that is, reflexivity.

Creativity also plays an important role in uncovering meaning in the data. Chandler, in writing about the transition from *saturation* to *illumination,* wrote that, "Strategies for creativity take time and require incubation for new ideas to percolate. Insight into the incubation of data is critical to the final theoretical revelations" (Chandler, in Hunter et al., 2002, p. 396). Thus, researchers need to give themselves sufficient time to achieve the *aha* that comes with making meaning beyond the facts.

Efforts to validate the analysis are necessarily efforts to validate interpretations as well. Prudent qualitative researchers hold their interpretations up for closer scrutiny—self-scrutiny as well as review by peers and outside reviewers. Even when researchers have undertaken peer debriefings and other strategies described in the next chapter, these procedures do not constitute proof that results and interpretations are credible. For both qualitative and quantitative researchers, it is important to consider possible alternative explanations for the findings and to take into account methodologic or other limitations that could have affected study results.

Example of seeking alternative explanations: Cheek and Ballantyne (2001) studied family members' selection process for a long-term care facility for elderly patients being discharged from an acute setting. In describing their methods, they explicitly noted that "attention throughout was paid to looking for rival or competing themes or explanations" (p. 225). In their analysis, they made a conscious effort to weigh alternatives.

In drawing conclusions, qualitative researchers should consider the transferability of the findings. Although qualitative researchers rarely seek to make generalizations, they often strive to develop an understanding of how the study results can be usefully applied. The central question is: In what other types of settings and contexts could one expect the phenomena under study to be manifested in a similar fashion?

CRITIQUING QUALITATIVE ANALYSIS

Evaluating a qualitative analysis in a research report is not easy to do, even for experienced researchers. The main problem is that readers do not have access to the information they would need to determine whether researchers exercised good judgment and critical insight in coding the narrative materials, developing a thematic analysis, and integrating materials into a meaningful whole. Researchers are seldom able to include more than a handful of examples of actual data in a journal article. Moreover, the process they used to inductively abstract meaning from the data is difficult to describe and illustrate.

In a critique of qualitative analysis, a primary task usually is determining whether researchers took sufficient steps to validate inferences and conclusions. A major focus of a critique of qualitative analyses, then, is whether the researchers have adequately documented the analytic process. The report should provide information about the approach used to analyze the data. For example, a report for a grounded theory study should indicate whether the researchers used the Glaser and Strauss or the Strauss and Corbin method.

Critiquing analytic decisions is substantially less clearcut in a qualitative than in a quantitative study. For example, it would be inappropriate to critique a phenomenological analysis for following Giorgi's approach rather than Colaizzi's approach. Both are respected methods of conducting a phenomenological study—although phenomenologists themselves may have cogent reasons for preferring one approach over the other.

One aspect of a qualitative analysis that *can* be critiqued, however, is whether the researchers have

Box 19.3 Guidelines for Critiquing Qualitative Analyses

1. Given the nature of the data, was the data analysis approach appropriate for the research design?
2. Is the category scheme described? If so, does the scheme appear logical and complete? Does there seem to be unnecessary overlap or redundancy in the categories?
3. Were manual methods used to index and organize the data, or was a computer program used?
4. Does the report adequately describe the process by which the actual analysis was performed? Does the report indicate whose approach to data analysis was used (e.g., Glaser's or Strauss's, in grounded theory studies)? Was this method consistently and appropriately applied?
5. What major themes or processes emerged? If excerpts from the data are provided, do the themes appear to capture the meaning of the narratives—that is, does it appear that the researcher adequately interpreted the data and conceptualized the themes? Is the analysis parsimonious—could two or more themes be collapsed into a broader and perhaps more useful conceptualization?
6. What evidence does the report provide that the analysis is accurate and replicable? Were data displayed in a manner that allows you to verify the researcher's conclusions?
7. Was a conceptual map, model, or diagram effectively displayed to communicate important processes?
8. Was the context of the phenomenon adequately described? Does the report give you a clear picture of the social or emotional world of study participants?
9. Did the analysis yield a meaningful and insightful picture of the phenomenon under study? Is the resulting theory or description trivial or obvious?

documented that they have used one approach consistently and have been faithful to the integrity of its procedures. Thus, for example, if researchers say they are using the Glaser and Strauss approach to grounded theory analysis, they should not also include elements from the Strauss and Corbin method. An even more serious problem occurs when, as sometimes happens, the researchers "muddle" traditions. For example, researchers who describe their study as a grounded theory study should not present *themes* because grounded theory analysis does not yield themes. Furthermore, researchers who attempt to blend elements from two traditions may not have a clear grasp of the analytic precepts of either one. For example, a researcher who claims to have undertaken an ethnography using a grounded theory approach to analysis may not be well informed about the underlying goals and philosophies of these two traditions.

Some further guidelines that may be helpful in evaluating qualitative analyses are presented in Box 19.3.

RESEARCH EXAMPLES

Example of an Ethnographic Analysis

Study: "Sources of practice knowledge among nurses" (Estabrooks et al., 2005)

Statement of Purpose: The purpose of this study was to explore and identify nurses' sources of practice knowledge.

Method: This report was based on two large studies that used an ethnographic case study design to examine factors that influence nurses' use of research in their practice. The cases for the first study were five pediatric units, and those for the second were two adult patient care units, drawn from four tertiary level hospitals in Alberta and Ontario. Data included transcribed individual and focus group interviews with nurses in the hospitals, as well as field notes from participant observation. Card-sorting interviews were also conducted to uncover the structure of the knowledge sources domain. In each setting, data were collected by a research assistant (a master's prepared nurse), who spent 6 months on the unit.

Analysis: Interview transcripts and field notes were entered into the computer program called NUD*IST for subsequent coding and analysis. Data were coded using a line-by-line process. Initial codes, which were based on a reading of the first interviews, were reviewed by the research team until consensus on the coding scheme was achieved. Spradley's procedures were used to develop a taxonomy. The process was a dynamic one, involving "repeated re-categorization of initial categories, and further sorting and analysis of each large (and saturated) category" (p. 462).

Key Findings: Nurses' sources of practice knowledge were categorized into four broad groupings, and these groupings formed the structure of the taxonomy.

- The category of *social interactions* dominated the findings; these interactions are processes through which nurses communicate and exchange information between and among each other, other health care professionals, and patients.
- *Experiential knowledge*, the second category, is knowledge gained during the regular course of nursing practice.
- *Documentary sources* included written materials, including unit-based sources (e.g., patients' charts) and off-unit sources (e.g., journal articles); use of these latter sources was limited.
- *A priori knowledge* is knowledge that a nurse brings to the unit, including knowledge gained in nursing school and from prior experiences.

Example of a Phenomenological Analysis

Study: "The lived experience of pregnancy while carrying a child with a known, nonlethal congenital abnormality" (Hedrick, 2005)

Statement of Purpose: The purpose of this study was to gain an understanding of the experience of pregnancy for women carrying a child with a known, nonlethal congenital abnormality (e.g., Down syndrome, congenital heart defect).

Method: This phenomenological study involved in-depth interviews with 15 pregnant women whose child had been diagnosed with a fetal abnormality. All of the mothers were informed of their fetus's diagnosis in the second trimester. Gestational age at the time of the interview ranged from 24 to 36 weeks. Redundancy of information was observed by the 11th interview, but 4 additional interviews were completed to ensure a description of the full experience. Interviews were taped and transcribed for subsequent analysis.

Analysis: Interview data were analyzed according to the four steps described by Giorgi (1985), as outlined in Table 19.1. The first step was developing an understanding of the whole of each interview by reading and reflecting on each one. The second step involved reading each successive transcript thoroughly and breaking each down into distinct *meaning units*. Meaning units consisted of words, phrases, sentences, or passages. Meaning units were coded by the investigator, but were also coded by a second qualitative nurse researcher to ensure accuracy and completeness. The third step involved transformation of the participants' words "into the language of science associated with nursing" (p. 734). In the final step, the transformed meaning units were synthesized into an overall description of the phenomenon. This final description "contained all the transformed meaning units and gave structure to the data to accurately communicate the lived experience" (p. 734) of these women's pregnancies.

Key Findings:

- For the women in the study, the pregnancy experience was of a paradoxical nature, reflecting both positive and negative emotions and expectations.
- Three major themes emerged: (1) time is good, but it is also the enemy; (2) you grieve, but you do not grieve; and (3) my baby's not perfect, but he or she is still mine.

Example of a Grounded Theory Analysis

Study: "Moral reckoning in nursing" (Nathaniel, 2006)

Statement of Purpose: The purpose of this study was to elucidate the experiences and consequences of professional nurses' moral distress, and to formulate an explanatory theory of moral distress and its consequences.

Method: This grounded theory study involved in-depth interviews with 21 registered nurses. Informants were highly educated (most had graduate degrees) and experienced (80% had more than 10 years of experience). All had been involved in a troubling patient care situation that caused distress. The study began with a broad research question: What transpires in morally laden situations in which nurses experience distress? The initial question was narrowed and redirected as the research progressed. Because the nature of the information was considered sensitive, Nathaniel did not tape-record the interviews. She made brief, contemporaneous notes, and then detailed field notes were prepared immediately following the interviews.

Analysis: Interview data were analyzed using the classic Glaserian method. Analysis began with the first episode of data gathering. Using constant comparison, data were analyzed sentence by sentence as they were coded. Nathaniel began with open coding, which led to theoretical sampling and the generation of memos. As analysis proceeded, core social psychological processes began to emerge. This in turn furnished the foundation for subsequent selective coding and memoing around the identified core category of *moral reckoning* in nursing. As the interviews were coded and compared, moral distress—which was the original focus of the study—failed to emerge as a major category. "The core variable, moral reckoning, was identified when it emerged as the one to which all others were related" (p. 423).

Key Findings:

- Moral distress occurred in nurses who were in the midst of the moral reckoning process; moral reckoning is broader, both temporally and psychosocially, than moral distress.
- Moral reckoning was conceptualized as a three-stage process that begins with a stage of ease, which is then interrupted by a situational bind that challenges the nurse's core beliefs. This compels the nurses into the stage of resolution, in which he or she either gives up or makes a stand. The final stage is the stage of reflection.

SUMMARY POINTS

- Qualitative analysis is a challenging, labor-intensive activity, guided by few standardized rules.
- Although there are no universal strategies, three prototypical analytic styles have been identified: (1) a *template analysis style* that involves the development of an analysis guide (**template**) to sort the data; (2) an *editing analysis style* that involves an interpretation of the data on which a **category scheme** is based; and (3) an *immersion/crystallization style* that is characterized by the analyst's total immersion in and reflection of text materials.
- The first major step in analyzing qualitative data is to organize and index the materials for easy retrieval, typically by coding the content of the data according to a category scheme.
- Traditionally, researchers have organized their data by developing **conceptual files**, which are

physical files in which coded excerpts of data relevant to specific categories are placed. Now, however, computer programs (CAQDAS) are widely used to perform basic indexing functions, and to facilitate data analysis.

- The actual analysis of data begins with a search for **themes**, which involves the discovery not only of commonalities across subjects but also of natural variation and patterns in the data. Some qualitative analysts use **metaphors** or figurative comparisons to evoke a visual and symbolic analogy.
- The next analytic step usually involves a validation of the thematic analysis. Some researchers use **quasi-statistics**, which involves a tabulation of the frequency with which certain themes or relations are supported by the data.
- In a final analytic step, the analyst tries to weave the thematic strands together into an integrated picture of the phenomenon under investigation.
- Some researchers identify neither a specific approach nor a specific research tradition; those whose focus is qualitative description often say that they used **qualitative content analysis** as their analytic method.
- In ethnographies, analysis begins as the researcher enters the field. Ethnographers continually search for *patterns* in the behavior and expressions of study participants.
- One approach to analyzing ethnographic data is Spradley's method, which involves four levels of data analysis: **domain analysis** (identifying *domains*, or units of cultural knowledge); **taxonomic analysis** (selecting key domains and constructing **taxonomies** or systems of classification); **componential analysis** (comparing and contrasting terms in a domain); and a **theme analysis** (to uncover cultural themes).
- Leininger's method of ethnonursing research involves four phases: collecting and recording data; categorizing descriptors; searching for repetitive patterns; and abstracting major themes.
- There are numerous different approaches to phenomenological analysis, including the descriptive methods of Colaizzi, Giorgi, and Van Kaam, in which the goal is to find common

patterns of experiences shared by particular instances.

- In Van Manen's approach, which involves efforts to grasp the essential meaning of the experience being studied, researchers search for themes, using either a **holistic approach** (viewing text as a whole); a **selective approach** (pulling out key statements and phrases); or a **detailed approach** (analyzing every sentence).
- Central to analyzing data in a hermeneutic study is the notion of the **hermeneutic circle**, which signifies a methodologic process in which there is continual movement between the parts and the whole of the text under analysis.
- In hermeneutics, there are several choices for data analysis. Diekelmann's method calls for the discovery of a **constitutive pattern**, which expresses the relationships among themes. Benner's approach consists of three processes: searching for **paradigm cases**, thematic analysis, and analysis of *exemplars.*
- Grounded theory uses the **constant comparative** method of data analysis. **Fit** is the process of identifying characteristics of one piece of data and comparing them with those of another datum to see if they are similar.
- One approach to grounded theory is the Glaser and Strauss (Glaserian) method, in which there are two broad types of codes: **substantive codes** (in which the empirical substance of the topic is conceptualized) and **theoretical codes** (in which the relationships among the substantive codes are conceptualized).
- Substantive coding involves **open coding** to capture what is going on in the data, and then **selective coding,** in which only variables relating to a core category are coded. The **core category,** a behavior pattern that has relevance for participants, is sometimes a **basic social process (BSP)** that involves an evolutionary process of coping or adaptation.
- In the Glaser and Strauss method, open codes begin with **level I** (*in vivo*) **codes,** which are collapsed into a higher level of abstraction in **level II codes.** Level II codes are then used to formulate **level III codes,** which are theoretical constructs.

- Through constant comparison, the researcher compares concepts emerging from the data with similar concepts from existing theory or research to determine which parts have **emergent fit** with the theory being generated.
- The Strauss and Corbin method is an alternative grounded theory method whose outcome is a full conceptual description. This approach to grounded theory analysis involves three types of coding: **open coding** (in which categories are generated), **axial coding** (where categories are linked with subcategories), and **selective coding** (in which the findings are integrated and refined).
- A controversy in the analysis of focus group data is whether the unit of analysis is the group or individual participants—some analysts examine the data at both levels. A third analytic option is the analysis of group interactions.
- One approach to analyzing triangulated data from multiple sources (e.g., qualitative and quantitative data) is the construction of a **meta-matrix** that arrays such data in a table so the analyst can inspect patterns and themes across data sources.

STUDY ACTIVITIES

Chapter 19 of the *Resource Manual to Accompany Nursing Research: Generating and Assessing Evidence for Nursing Practice, 8th edition*, offers various exercises and study suggestions for reinforcing concepts presented in this chapter. In addition, the following study questions can be addressed:

1. Read a recent qualitative nursing study. If a different investigator had gone into the field to study the same problem, how likely is it that the conclusions would have been the same? How transferable are the researcher's findings? What did the researcher learn that he or she would probably not have learned with a more structured and quantified approach?

2. Apply relevant questions in Box 19.3 to one of the three research examples at the end of the chapter, referring to the full journal article as necessary.

ooooooooooooooooooooooo

STUDIES CITED IN CHAPTER 19

Methodologic or theoretical references cited in this chapter can be found in a separate section at the end of the book.

Beck, C. T. (2002). Releasing the pause button: Mothering twins during the first year of life. *Qualitative Health Research, 12,* 593–608.

Beck, C. T. (2004). Birth trauma: In the eye of the beholder. *Nursing Research, 53,* 28–35.

Beck, C. T. (2005). Benefits of participating in Internet interviews: Women helping women. *Qualitative Health Research, 15,* 411–422.

Beck, C. T. (2006). Anniversary of birth trauma: Failure to rescue. *Nursing Research, 55*(6), 381–390.

Cheek, J., & Ballantyne, A. (2001). Moving them on and in: The process of searching for and selecting an aged care facility. *Qualitative Health Research, 11,* 221–237.

Cheung, J., & Hocking, P. (2004). The experience of spousal carers of people with multiple sclerosis. *Qualitative Health Research, 14,* 153–166.

DeOliveira, E. A., & Hoga, L. A. (2005). The process of seeking and undergoing surgical contraception: An ethnographic study in a Brazilian community. *Journal of Transcultural Nursing, 16,* 5–14.

Estabrooks, C., Rutakumwa, W., O'Leary, K., Profetto-McGrath, J., Milner, M., Levers, M. J., & Scott-Findlay, S. (2005). Sources of practice knowledge among nurses. *Qualitative Health Research, 15,* 460–476.

Fereday, J., & Muir-Cochrane, E. (2006). Demonstrating rigor using thematic analysis: A hybrid approach of inductive and deductive coding and theme development. *International Journal of Qualitative Methods, 5*(1), Article 7. Retrieved January 5, 2007, from *http://www.ualberta.ca/~iiqm/buckissues/5_1/pdf/fereday.pdf*

Hedrick, J. (2005). The lived experience of pregnancy while carrying a child with known, nonlethal congenital abnormality. *Journal of Obstetric, Gynecologic, & Neonatal Nursing, 34*(6), 732–740.

Lauterbach, S. (2007). Meanings in mothers' experience with infant death. In P. L. Munhall (Ed.). *Nursing research: A qualitative perspective* (2nd ed., pp. 211–238). Sudbury, MA: Jones and Bartlett.

Manns, P. J., & Chad, K. E. (2001). Components of quality of life for persons with a quadriplegic and paraplegic spinal cord injury. *Qualitative Health Research, 11,* 795–811.

Nathaniel, A. K. (2006). Moral reckoning in nursing. *Western Journal of Nursing Research, 28*(4), 419–438.

Negarandeh, R., Oskouie, F., Ahmadi, F., Nikravesh, M., & Hallberg, I. (2006). Patient advocacy: Barriers and facilitators. *BMC Nursing, 5,* 3.

Polit, D. F., London, A., & Martinez, J. M. (2000). Food security and hunger in poor, mother-headed families in four U.S. cities. New York: MDRC.

Raingruber, B., & Kent, M. (2003). Attending to embodied responses: A way to identify practice based and human meanings associated with secondary trauma. *Qualitative Health Research, 13,* 449–468.

SmithBattle, L. (2005). Teenage mothers at age 30. *Western Journal of Nursing Research, 27*(7), 831–850.

Strang, V., Koop, P., Dupuis-Blanchard, S., Nordstrom, M., & Thompson, B. (2006). Family caregivers and transition to long-term care. *Clinical Nursing Research, 15*(1), 27–45.

Tapp, D. M. (2004). Dilemmas of family support during cardiac recovery: Nagging as a gesture of support. *Western Journal of Nursing Research, 26,* 561–580.

Trybulski, J. (2005). The long-term phenomena of women's postabortion experiences. *Western Journal of Nursing Research, 27*(5), 559–576.

Tzeng, W., & Lipson, J. G. (2004). The cultural context of suicide stigma in Taiwan. *Qualitative Health Research, 14,* 345–358.

Wendler, M. C. (2001). Triangulation using a meta-matrix. *Journal of Advanced Nursing, 35,* 521–525.

Wilde, M. H. (2003). Life with an indwelling urinary catheter: The dialectic of stigma and acceptance. *Qualitative Health Research, 13,* 1189–1204.

Wotton, K., Borbasi, S., & Redden, M. (2005). When all else has failed: Nurses' perception of factors influencing palliative care for patients with end-stage heart failure. *Journal of Cardiovascular Nursing, 20*(1), 18–25.

Wuest, J. (2000). Negotiating with helping systems: An example of grounded theory evolving through emergent fit. *Qualitative Health Research, 10,* 51–70.

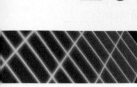

20

Enhancing Quality and Integrity in Qualitative Research

S trategies for enhancing the integrity of qualitative studies flow throughout the project. Integrity in qualitative research is an all-encompassing issue that begins as questions are formulated and continues through the preparation of a report. For this reason, we have chosen to describe these strategies after introducing basic concepts relating to the design of qualitative studies and the collection and analysis of qualitative data. For those learning to do qualitative research, we consider this a particularly important chapter.

PERSPECTIVES ON QUALITY IN QUALITATIVE RESEARCH

Qualitative researchers agree on the importance of doing high-quality research, yet few issues in qualitative inquiry have generated more controversy than efforts to define what is meant by "high quality." Although it is beyond the scope of this book to explain arguments of the debate in detail, we provide an overview that is intended to help you identify a position that is compatible with your philosophical and methodologic views.

Debates About Rigor and Validity

One of the most contentious issues in the debate about quality concerns the use of terms such as *rigor* and *validity*—terms that are shunned by some because they are associated with the positivist paradigm and are seen as inappropriate goals for research conducted in the naturalistic or critical paradigms. Those who advocate different criteria and terms for evaluating quality in qualitative research argue that the issues at stake in the various paradigms are fundamentally different in terms of philosophical underpinnings and goals, and therefore require altogether different terminology. For these critics, the concepts of rigor and validity are empirical analytic terms that does not fit into an interpretive approach that values insight and creativity (e.g., Denzin & Lincoln, 2000). As Sandelowski (1993b) put it, "We can preserve or kill the spirit of qualitative work; we can soften our notion of rigor to include the playfulness, soulfulness, imagination, and technique we associate with more artistic endeavors, or we can further harden it by the uncritical application of rules. The choice is ours: rigor or rigor mortis" (p. 8).

Others challenge opposition to the term *validity*. Whittemore, Chase, and Mandle (2001), for example, argued that validity is an appropriate term in all paradigms, noting that the dictionary definition of validity (the state or quality of being sound, just, and well-founded) lends itself equally to qualitative and quantitative research. Similarly, Morse and colleagues (2002) posited that "the broad and abstract concepts of reliability and validity can be applied to all research because the goal of finding plausible and credible outcome explanations is central to all research" (p. 3). Another, more pragmatic, argument favoring the use of "mainstream" terms such as validity and rigor is precisely that they *are* mainstream. In a world dominated by quantitative researchers whose evidence hierarchies place qualitative studies on a low rung, and whose quality criteria are used to make decisions about research funding, some feel that it is useful to use terms and criteria that are recognizable and widely accepted.

Sparkes (2001) contended that the debate over validity is not a simple dichotomy, and suggested that there are four possible perspectives on the issue. The first, which he called the *replication perspective*, is that validity is an appropriate criterion for assessing quality in both qualitative and quantitative studies, although qualitative researchers must use different procedures to achieve it. Those who adopt a *parallel perspective* maintain that a separate set of evaluative criteria needs to be developed for qualitative inquiry. This perspective resulted in the development of standards for the **trustworthiness** of qualitative research that parallel the standards of reliability and validity in quantitative research (Lincoln & Guba, 1985). The third perspective in Sparke's typology is the *diversification of meanings perspective*, which is characterized by efforts to establish new forms of validity that do not have reference points in traditional quantitative research. As but one example, Lather (1986) discussed *catalytic validity* in connection with critical and feminist research as the degree to which the research process energized study participants and altered their consciousness. The final perspective in Sparke's typology was what he called the *letting-go-of-validity perspective*, which involves a total abandonment of the concept of validity. Wolcott (1994), an ethnographer, represented this perspective in his discussion of the absurdity of validity. Yet, as Wolcott (1995) himself noted, validity can be dismissed, but the issue itself will not go away: "Qualitative researchers need to understand what the debate is about and *have* a position; they do not have to resolve the issue itself" (p. 170).

Generic Versus Specific Standards

Another issue in the controversy surrounding quality criteria for qualitative inquiry concerns whether there should be a generic set of standards, or whether specific standards are needed for different types of inquiry—for example, for ethnographers and grounded theory researchers. Rolfe (2006) has raised the possibility that each study is individual and unique, and that it may be futile to apply predetermined criteria of any kind in assessing the quality of studies—be they qualitative or quantitative.

Many writers have accepted the notion that research conducted within different qualitative traditions must attend to different concerns, and that techniques for enhancing and demonstrating research integrity vary. Watson and Girard (2004), for example, proposed that quality standards should be reflective of the research method used, and that they must be "congruent with the philosophical underpinnings supporting the research tradition endorsed" (p. 875). Reflecting this viewpoint of having criteria aligned with tradition, many writers have offered standards for specific forms of qualitative inquiry, such as grounded theory (Chiovitti & Piran, 2003); phenomenology and hermeneutics (Koch, 1994; Whitehead, 2004); ethnography (LeCompte & Goetz, 1982; Hammersley, 1992); descriptive qualitative research (Milne & Oberle, 2005); and critical research (Lather, 1986; Reason, 1981).

Some writers believe, however, that there are some quality criteria that are fairly universal within the naturalistic paradigm. In their synthesis of criteria for developing evidence of validity in qualitative studies, Whittemore and associates (2001) proposed four primary criteria that they viewed as essential to *all* qualitative inquiry.

Standards for Conduct Versus Assessment of Qualitative Research

Yet another issue concerns whose point of view is being considered in the quality standards. Morse and colleagues (2002) contended that many of the established standards are relevant for *assessment* rather than as guides to conducting high-quality qualitative research. They believe that Lincoln and Guba's criteria, which are often considered the gold standard, are best described as *post hoc* tools that reviewers can use to evaluate trustworthiness at the end of a study: "While strategies of trustworthiness may be useful in attempting to *evaluate* rigor, they do not in themselves *ensure* rigor" (p. 9).

As an example of how the viewpoint of evaluators has been given prominence, one suggested indicator of integrity is **researcher credibility**—that is, the faith that can be put in the researcher (Patton, 1999, 2002). While such an indicator might affect readers' confidence in the integrity of the inquiry, it clearly is not a *strategy* that researchers can adopt to make their study more rigorous.

Morse and colleagues (2002) and others (e.g., Tobin & Begley, 2004) have argued that there needs to be more emphasis on verification strategies for researchers to use throughout the inquiry "so that reliability and validity are actively attained, rather than proclaimed by external reviewers on the completion of the project" (p. 9). In their view, responsibility for ensuring rigor should rest with researchers rather than with external judges. They advocated a proactive stance to integrity that would involve constant self-scrutiny, investigator responsiveness, and verification efforts. Morse (2006b) noted that "good qualitative inquiry must be verified reflexively in each step of the analysis. This means that it is self-correcting" (p. 6).

From the point of view of qualitative researchers, the ongoing question must be: How can I be confident that my account is an accurate and insightful representation? From the point of view of a critical reader, the question is: How can I trust that the researcher has offered an accurate and insightful representation? The evidence and strategies needed for answering these questions overlap, but are not identical.

Terminology Proliferation and Confusion

The result of all these tensions and controversies is that there is no common vocabulary for quality criteria

in qualitative research—nor, for that matter, for the goals of high-quality qualitative research. Terms such as *goodness, integrity, truth value, rigor, trustworthiness*, and so on abound, and for each proposed descriptor, several papers refuting it as appropriate are published. As Kahn (1993) astutely observed, there is a certain inevitability to this dilemma, given qualitative researchers' focus on language.

With regard to actual criteria for quality in qualitative research, dozens (if not hundreds) of terms have been suggested. Whittemore and colleagues (2001) presented a table that summarized the validity criteria suggested by developers of 10 different frameworks for judging validity. The 10 frameworks include such terms as plausibility, relevance, credibility, consistency, fittingness, neutrality, and applicability—to name only a handful.

Establishing a consensus on what the quality criteria for qualitative inquiry should be, and what they should be named, remains elusive, and it is unlikely that a consensus will be achieved in the near future, if ever. Some feel that the ongoing debate is healthy and productive, whereas others feel that "the situation is confusing and has resulted in a deteriorating ability to actually discern rigor" (Morse et al., 2002, p. 5).

Given the lack of consensus, and the heated arguments supporting and contesting various frameworks, it is difficult to provide guidance about how qualitative researchers should proceed. We present information about *criteria* from two frameworks in the section that follows, and then describe *strategies* for diminishing threats to integrity and attaining high quality in qualitative research. We recommend that these frameworks and strategies be viewed as points of departure for explorations on how to make a qualitative study as rigorous/trustworthy/insightful/valid as possible.

FRAMEWORKS OF QUALITY CRITERIA

Although not without critics, the criteria often thought of as the gold standard for qualitative researchers are those outlined by Lincoln and

Guba (1985), and later augmented by Guba and Lincoln (1994). The second framework described here is the synthesis proposed by Whittemore and colleagues (2001).

An important point in thinking about criteria for qualitative inquiry is that attention needs to be paid to both "art" and "science," to interpretation and description. Creativity and insightfulness need to be encouraged and sustained, but not at the expense of scientific excellence. And the quest for rigor cannot sacrifice inspiration and elegant abstractions, or else the results are likely to be "perfectly healthy but dead" (Morse, 2006b, p. 6). Good qualitative work is both descriptively sound and explicit, and interpretively rich and innovative.

Lincoln and Guba's Framework

Lincoln and Guba (1985) suggested four criteria for developing the *trustworthiness* of a qualitative inquiry: credibility, dependability, confirmability, and transferability. These four criteria for trustworthiness represent parallels to the positivists' criteria of internal validity, reliability, objectivity, and external validity, respectively. This framework provided the initial platform upon which much of the current controversy on rigor emerged. In their later writings, responding to numerous criticisms and to their own evolving conceptualizations, a fifth criterion that is more distinctively within the naturalistic paradigm was added: authenticity (Guba and Lincoln, 1994).

Credibility
Credibility is viewed by Lincoln and Guba as an overriding goal of qualitative research, and is a criterion identified in several of the 10 frameworks mentioned in the Whittemore and associates (2001) review. **Credibility** refers to confidence in the truth of the data and interpretations of them. Qualitative researchers must strive to establish confidence in the truth of the findings for the particular participants and contexts in the research. Lincoln and Guba pointed out that credibility involves two aspects: first, carrying out the study in a way that enhances the believability of the find-

ings, and second, taking steps to *demonstrate* credibility to external readers.

Dependability
The second criterion in the Lincoln and Guba framework is **dependability**, which refers to the stability (reliability) of data over time and over conditions. The dependability question is: Would the findings of an inquiry be repeated if it were replicated with the same (or similar) participants in the same (or similar) context? Credibility cannot be attained in the absence of dependability, just as validity in quantitative research cannot be achieved in the absence of reliability.

Confirmability
Confirmability refers to objectivity, that is, the potential for congruence between two or more independent people about the data's accuracy, relevance, or meaning. This criterion is concerned with establishing that the data represent the information participants provided, and that the interpretations of those data are not figments of the inquirer's imagination. For this criterion to be achieved, the findings must reflect the participants' voice and the conditions of the inquiry, and not the biases, motivations, or perspectives of the researcher.

Transferability
Transferability refers essentially to the generalizability of the data, that is, the extent to which the findings can be transferred to or have applicability in other settings or groups. As Lincoln and Guba noted, the responsibility of the investigator is to provide sufficient descriptive data in the research report so that consumers can evaluate the applicability of the data to other contexts: "Thus the naturalist cannot specify the external validity of an inquiry; he or she can provide only the thick description necessary to enable someone interested in making a transfer to reach a conclusion about whether transfer can be contemplated as a possibility" (p. 316).

➲ **TIP:** You may run across the term *fittingness*, which was a term used earlier by Guba and Lincoln (1981) to refer to the degree to which research findings have meaning to others in similar situations. In later work, however, they used the term *transferability*. Similarly, in their initial discussions of quality criteria, they used the term *auditability*, a concept that was later refined and called *dependability*.

Authenticity

Authenticity refers to the extent to which the researchers fairly and faithfully show a range of different realities. Authenticity emerges in a report when it conveys the feeling tone of participants' lives as they are lived. A text has authenticity if it invites readers into a vicarious experience of the lives being described, and enables readers to develop a heightened sensitivity to the issues being depicted. When a text achieves authenticity, readers are better able to understand the lives being portrayed "in the round," with some sense of the mood, feeling, experience, language, and context of those lives.

Whittemore and Colleagues' Framework

Whittemore and colleagues (2001), in their synthesis of qualitative criteria from 10 prominent systems (including that of Lincoln and Guba), used the term *validity* as the overarching goal. In their view, there are four primary criteria that are essential to all qualitative inquiry, whereas six secondary criteria provide supplementary benchmarks of validity and are not relevant to every study. Researchers must decide, based on the goals of their research, the optimal weight that should be given to each criterion.

The primary criteria include credibility, authenticity, criticality, and integrity. The six secondary criteria include explicitness, vividness, creativity, thoroughness, congruence, and sensitivity. Thus, the terminology overlaps with that of Lincoln and Guba's framework with regard to two criteria (credibility and authenticity), whereas the other eight represent either concepts not captured in the Lincoln and Guba framework or nuanced variations. We briefly define each of these eight terms, and then offer questions relating to the attainment of these criteria (Table 20.1).

Criticality refers to the researcher's critical appraisal of every decision made throughout the research process. **Integrity** is demonstrated by ongoing self-reflection and self-scrutiny to ensure that interpretations are valid and grounded in the data. Criticality and integrity are strongly interrelated and are sometimes considered jointly (e.g., Milne & Oberle, 2005).

In terms of secondary criteria, **explicitness** (similar to auditability) is the ability to follow the researcher's decisions and interpretive efforts by means of carefully maintained records and explicitly presented results. **Vividness** involves the presentation of rich, vivid, faithful, and artful descriptions that highlight salient themes in the data. **Creativity** reflects challenges to traditional ways of thinking and is demonstrated through innovative approaches to collecting, analyzing, and interpreting data. **Thoroughness** refers to adequacy of the data as a result of sound sampling and data collection decisions (saturation), as well as to the full development of ideas. **Congruence** refers to interconnectedness between methods and question, between the current study and earlier ones, and between theory and approach; it also refers to connections between study findings and contexts outside the study situation. Finally, **sensitivity** refers to the degree to which the research was implemented in a manner that reflects respectful sensitivity to and concern for the people, groups, and communities being studied.

Table 20.1 presents these 10 criteria, together with two sets of questions. The first set is intended as a guide to researchers in their thinking about quality issues during the conduct of a study. The second set consists of questions that are relevant after a study is completed. Researchers can use these questions as a means of self-evaluation, and those who scrutinize a study can apply them to evaluate both the process and the product of qualitative inquiry. ✷ The questions in Table 20.1, formatted onto worksheets, are available in a Word document in the Toolkit of the accompanying *Resource Manual*.

STRATEGIES TO ENHANCE QUALITY IN QUALITATIVE INQUIRY

The criteria for establishing integrity in a qualitative study are complex and challenging—regardless of

CRITERIA	QUESTIONS FOR SELF-SCRUTINY DURING A STUDY	QUESTIONS FOR *POST HOC* ASSESSMENTS OF A STUDY
Primary Criteria		
Credibility	What steps can I take to ensure that participants' experiences and context are represented in a comprehensive and believable way? What verification procedures can I use?	Do the research results reflect participants' experiences and context in a believable way?
Authenticity	How can I ensure that I will adequately represent the multiple realities and voices of those being studied?	Has the researcher adequately represented the multiple realities of those being studied? Has an emic perspective been portrayed?
Criticality	What procedures can I use to support critical self-reflection and critical thinking about key decisions during the research? How can I cultivate responsiveness to the data?	Is there evidence that the inquiry involved critical appraisal of key decisions?
Integrity	Have I put in place adequate checks on the validity of my interpretations? Have I grounded my interpretations in the data?	Does the research reflect ongoing, repetitive checks on the many aspects of validity? Are the findings humbly presented?
Secondary Criteria		
Explicitness	Have I maintained adequate records documenting decisions and interpretive processes? Have I taken steps to expose my own biases or perspectives?	Have methodologic decisions been explained and justified? Have biases been identified? Is evidence presented in support of conclusions and interpretations?
Vividness	Have I faithfully used the data to provide a rich, evocative, and compelling description, without using excessive detail?	Have rich, evocative, and compelling descriptions been presented?
Creativity	Have I sufficiently stretched my imagination and creative powers to develop insightful interpretations?	Do the findings illuminate in an insightful and original way? Are new perspectives and rich imagination brought to bear on the inquiry?
Thoroughness	Have I been sufficiently thorough in ensuring sampling and data adequacy? Have I explored the full scope of the phenomenon and convincingly answered the research question?	Has sufficient attention been paid to sampling adequacy, information richness, data saturation, and contextual completeness?
Congruence	Have I taken adequate steps to ensure logical, philosophical, theoretical, and methodologic congruency? Have I ensured that readers will be able to identify congruence with other settings?	Is there congruity between the questions and methods, the methods and participants, the data and categories? Do themes fit together coherently? Is there adequate information for determining the fit with other contexts?
Sensitivity	Have my methods and questions reflected an ethical and sensitive respect for study participants and the groups, communities, and cultures to which they belong?	Has the research been undertaken in a way that is sensitive to the cultural, social, and political contexts of those being studied?

*Criteria are from Whittemore and colleagues' (2001) synthesis of qualitative validity criteria. Questions reflect the thinking of Whittemore et al., and other sources.

the names people attach to them. A variety of strategies have been proposed to address these challenges, and this section describes many of them.

Some quality enhancement strategies are linked to a specific criterion—for example, maintaining records to document methodologic decisions is a strategy that addresses the *explicitness* criterion in the Whittemore and colleagues framework. Many strategies, however, simultaneously address multiple criteria. For this reason, we have not organized strategies according to quality criteria—for example, which strategies to use to address *credibility*. Instead, we have organized strategies according to different phases of an inquiry, namely data generation, coding and analysis, and report preparation. This organization is imperfect, owing to the nonlinear and iterative nature of research activities in qualitative studies, and so we acknowledge upfront that some activities described under one aspect of a study are likely to have relevance under another.

Table 20.2 offers some guidance about how various quality enhancement strategies map onto the criteria in the Lincoln and Guba framework and the Whittemore framework.

Quality Enhancement Strategies in Generating Data

Several strategies that qualitative researchers use to enrich and strengthen their studies have been mentioned in earlier chapters and will not be elaborated here. For example, intensive listening during an interview, careful probing to obtain rich and comprehensive data, and audiotaping interviews for transcription are all strategies to enhance data quality, as are methods to gain people's trust during fieldwork (see Chapter 15). In this section, we focus on some additional strategies that are used primarily (although not exclusively) during the collection of qualitative data. Note, however, that many of these strategies represent design options that need to be considered during the planning phase of a project and cannot be postponed until fieldwork has begun.

Prolonged Engagement and Persistent Observation

An important step in establishing rigor and integrity in qualitative studies is **prolonged engagement** (Lincoln & Guba, 1985)—the investment of sufficient time collecting data to have an in-depth understanding of the culture, language, or views of the people or group under study, to test for misinformation and distortions, and to ensure saturation of important categories. Prolonged engagement is also essential for building trust and rapport with informants, which in turn makes it more likely that useful, accurate, and rich information will be obtained. Thus, in planning a qualitative study, researchers need to ensure that they have adequate time and resources to stay engaged in fieldwork for a sufficiently long period of time.

⮕ **TIP:** Thorne and Darbyshire (2005) have pointed out that *premature closure* can be a problem in qualitative research. Without a commitment to prolonged engagement, researchers sometimes make an inappropriate claim of saturation simply because they have reached a convenient stopping point.

Example of prolonged engagement: Plach, Stevens, and Keigher (2005) conducted a study of older women living with HIV or AIDS. The nine study participants were interviewed 10 times each over a 2-year period to gain an in-depth understanding of their experience with symptom management, adherence to medical regimens, and personal efforts to maintain their health.

High-quality data collection in naturalistic inquiries also involves **persistent observation**, which concerns the salience of the data being gathered and recorded. Persistent observation refers to the researchers' focus on the characteristics or aspects of a situation or a conversation that are relevant to the phenomena being studied. As Lincoln and Guba (1985) noted, "If prolonged engagement provides scope, persistent observation provides depth" (p. 304).

Example of persistent observation: Beck (2002) conducted a grounded theory study of mothering twins during the first year of life. In addition to prolonged engagement for 10 months of fieldwork, she engaged in persistent observation. After interviewing mothers in their homes, Beck often stayed and helped them with their twins, using the time for persistent observation of the mothers caretaking (e.g., details of what and how the mothers talked to their twins).

Data and Method Triangulation

As noted in an earlier chapter, triangulation refers to the use of multiple referents to draw conclusions about what constitutes truth, and has been compared with convergent validation. The aim of triangulation is to "overcome the intrinsic bias that comes from single-method, single-observer, and single-theory studies" (Denzin, 1989, p. 313). Patton (1999) also advocated triangulation, arguing that "no single method ever adequately solves the problem of rival explanation" (p. 1192). Triangulation can also help to capture a more complete and contextualized portrait of the phenomenon under study. Denzin (1989) identified four types of triangulation (data triangulation, investigator triangulation, method triangulation, and theory triangulation), and many other types have been proposed. Two types are described here because of their relevance to data collection.

Data triangulation involves the use of multiple data sources for the purpose of validating conclusions. There are three types of data triangulation: time, space, and person. **Time triangulation** involves collecting data on the same phenomenon or about the same people at different points in time. Time triangulation can involve gathering data at different times of the day, or at different times in the year. This concept is similar to test–retest reliability assessment—the point is not to study a phenomenon longitudinally to determine how it changes, but to determine the congruence of the phenomenon across time. **Space triangulation** involves collecting data on the same phenomenon in multiple sites, to test for cross-site consistency. Finally, **person** triangulation involves collecting data from different types or levels of people (e.g., individuals, groups such as families,

and collectives such as communities), with the aim of validating data through multiple perspectives on the phenomenon.

Example of data (person/space) triangulation: Piven and colleagues (2006) studied how the relationships of Minimum Data Set (MDS) coordinators with other staff in nursing homes influenced care processes. Data were gathered from MDS coordinators in two nursing homes. Many other nursing home staff in the two sites also provided data for the study, including staff from administration, nursing, social work, rehabilitative services, and dietary services.

Method triangulation involves using multiple methods of data collection about the same phenomenon. In qualitative studies, researchers often use a rich blend of unstructured data collection methods (e.g., interviews, observations, documents) to develop a comprehensive understanding of a phenomenon. Multiple data collection methods provide an opportunity to evaluate the extent to which a consistent and coherent picture of the phenomenon emerges.

Example of method triangulation: Woodgate (2006) studied sources and forms of social support available to adolescents with cancer. Multiple forms of data were gathered in this longitudinal study, including individual interviews with 15 adolescents, two focus group interviews, and participant observation, which involved observing the adolescents in the inpatient and outpatient units during various periods and during different points in time.

Comprehensive and Vivid Recording of Information

In addition to taking steps to record data from interviews accurately, researchers need to carefully and thoughtfully prepare field notes that are rich with descriptions of what transpired in the field. Even if interviews are the only source of data, researchers should record descriptions of the participants' demeanor and behaviors during the interactions, and they should thoroughly describe the interview context.

Other record-keeping activities are also important. A log of decisions needs to be maintained, and

TABLE 20.2	Quality Enhancement Strategies in Relation to Quality Criteria for Qualitative Inquiry

STRATEGY	CRITERIA: GUBA & LINCOLN[a]					CRITERIA: WHITTEMORE ET AL.[b]							
	Dep.	Conf.	Trans.	Cred.	Auth.	Crit.	Integ.	Explic.	Viv.	Creat.	Thor.	Congr.	Sens.
Throughout the Inquiry													
Reflexivity/reflective journaling				X	X		X					X	
Careful documentation, decision trail	X	X				X	X	X					
Data Generation													
Prolonged engagement				X	X						X		X
Persistent observation				X	X		X				X		X
Comprehensive field notes			X	X			X			X	X		
Theoretically driven sampling											X		
Audiotaping & verbatim transcription				X	X			X	X				
Triangulation (data, method)	X			X							X	X	
Saturation of data			X	X							X		
Member checking	X			X		X							
Data Coding/Analysis													
Transcription rigor/data cleaning				X		X							
Intercoder checks; development of a codebook		X		X		X							
Triangulation (investigator, theory, analysis)		X		X		X						X	
Stepwise replication	X	X				X							
Search for disconfirming evidence/negative case analysis				X		X	X				X		
Peer review/debriefing		X		X		X							
Inquiry audit	X	X				X	X	X				X	
Presentation of Findings													
Documentation of quality enhancement efforts		X		X			X	X			X		
Thick, vivid description			X		X			X	X			X	X
Impactful, evocative writing					X					X	X		X
Documentation of researcher credentials, background				X			X				X		
Documentation of reflexivity				X			X	X			X		

[a]The criteria from the Lincoln and Guba (1985, 1996) framework include dependability (Dep.), confirmability (Conf.), transferability (Trans.), credibility (Cred.), and authenticity (Auth.); the last two criteria are identical to two primary criteria in the Whittemore et al. (2001) framework.

[b]The criteria from the Whittemore et al. (2001) framework include, in addition to credibility and authenticity, criticality (Crit.), integrity (Integ.), explicitness (Expl.), vividness (Viv.), creativity (Creat.), thoroughness (Thor.), congruence (Congr.), and sensitivity (Sens.)

reflective journals help to enhance rigor. Thoroughness in record keeping helps readers and external reviewers to develop confidence in the data.

Researchers sometimes specifically develop an **audit trail**, that is, a systematic collection of materials and documentation that would allow an independent auditor to come to conclusions about the data. Six classes of records are useful in creating an adequate audit trail: (1) the raw data (e.g., interview transcripts); (2) data reduction and analysis products (e.g., theoretical notes, working hypotheses); (3) process notes (e.g., methodologic notes); (4) materials relating to researchers' intentions and dispositions (e.g., reflexive notes); (5) instrument development information (e.g., pilot forms); and (6) data reconstruction products (e.g., drafts of the final report).

➲ **TIP:** As Morse and colleagues (2002) have noted, diligence in maintaining information does not in and of itself ensure the validity of the inquiry. They pointed out that "audit trails may be kept as proof of the decisions made throughout the project, but they do not identify the quality of those decisions, the rationale behind those decisions, or the responsiveness and sensitivity of the investigator to data" (pp. 6–7).

Example of an audit trail: In their in-depth study of Chinese Canadians' beliefs toward organ donation, Molzahn and colleagues (2005) maintained an audit trail to document all methodologic decisions, the evolution of the findings, and the researchers' orientation to the problem.

Member Checking

Lincoln and Guba considered member checking a particularly important technique for establishing the credibility of qualitative data. In a **member check**, researchers provide feedback to study participants about emerging interpretations, and obtain participants' reactions. The argument is that if researchers' interpretations are good representations of participants' realities, participants should be given an opportunity to react to them.

Member checking with participants can be carried out in an ongoing way as data are being collected (e.g., through deliberate probing to ensure that interviewers have understood participants' meanings), and more formally after data have been fully analyzed. Member checking is sometimes done in writing. For example, researchers can ask participants to review and comment on case summaries, interpretive notes, thematic summaries, or drafts of the research report. Member checks are more typically done in face-to-face discussions with individual participants or small groups of participants.

➲ **TIP:** For focus group studies, it is usually recommended that member checking occur *in situ*. That is, moderators develop a summary of major themes or viewpoints in real time, and present that summary to focus group participants at the end of the session for their feedback. Especially rich data often emerge from participants' reactions to those summaries.

Despite the potential contribution that member checking can make to a study's credibility, several issues need to be kept in mind. One is that some participants may be unwilling to engage in this process. Some—especially if the research topic is emotionally charged—may feel they have attained closure once they have shared their concerns, feelings, and experiences. Further discussion might not be welcomed. Others may decline being involved in member checking because they are afraid it might arouse suspicions of their families. Choudhry (2001), in her study of the challenges faced by elderly women from India who had immigrated to Canada, got many refusals when she asked participants to examine transcripts of their interviews. Participants feared that a second visit to their homes might arouse suspicions among their family members and increase their sense of loss and regret.

➲ **TIP:** If member checking is used as a validation strategy, participants should be encouraged to provide critical feedback about factual errors or interpretive deficiencies. In writing about the study, it is important to be explicit about how member checking was done and what role it played as a validation strategy. Readers cannot develop much confidence in the study simply by learning that member checking was done.

Another issue is that member checks can lead to misleading conclusions of credibility if participants "share some common myth or front, or conspire to mislead or cover up" (Lincoln & Guba, p. 315). At the other extreme, some participants might fail to express disagreement with researchers' interpretations either out of politeness or in the belief that researchers are "smarter" or more knowledgeable than they themselves are. Thorne and Darbyshire (2005), in fact, caution against what they irreverently called *Adulatory Validity*, which they described as "the epistemological pat on the back for a job well done, or just possibly it might be part of a mutual stroking ritual that satisfies the agendas of both researcher and researched" (p. 1110). They noted that member checking tends to privilege interpretations that place study participants in the most charitable light.

Thorne and Darbyshire are not alone in their concerns about member checking as a validation strategy. Indeed, few strategies for enhancing data quality are as controversial as member checking. Morse (1999), for example, disputed the idea that participants have more analytic and interpretive authority than the researcher. Giorgi (1989) also argued that asking participants to evaluate the researcher's psychological interpretation of their own descriptions exceeds the role of participants. Morse and colleagues (2002), as well as Sandelowski (1993b), have worried that because study results have been synthesized, decontextualized, and abstracted from and across various participants, individual participants may not recognize their own experiences or perspectives during a member check. Even more scathingly, some critics view member checking as antithetical to the epistemology of qualitative inquiry. Smith (1993), in particular, has criticized the philosophical contradictions inherent in this strategy, arguing that it is inconsistent with inquiry that purports to reveal multiple realities and multiple ways of knowing.

⮕ **TIP:** It is important to strive for methodologic congruence with regard to member checking. For example, if Giorgi's phenomenological methods are used in an inquiry, member checking would not be undertaken, but member checking *is* called for in phenomenological studies following Colaizzi's approach.

Example of member checking: Chiovitti and Piran (2003) conducted a grounded theory study of psychiatric nurses' experiences of caring for patients in hospitals. They described how they used member checking to test their theoretical constructions against participants' meanings of phenomena. As their grounded theory was being developed, their open codes were checked and verified, through direct questioning, for their relevance to participants' meanings. "Participants were invited to refine, develop, and revise the emerging theoretical structure" (p. 431). The researchers provided an example of how two open codes were checked against participants' meaning before combining the two codes into a higher-level axial code.

Strategies Relating to Coding and Analysis

Excellent qualitative inquiry is likely to involve the simultaneous collection and analysis of data, and so several of the strategies described in the preceding section are relevant to ensuring both analytic integrity and high-quality data. Member checking, for example, can occur in an ongoing fashion as part of the data collection process, but typically also involves participants' review of preliminary analytic constructions. Also, we discussed some strategies for analytic validation in Chapter 19 (e.g., using quasi-statistics). In this section we introduce a few additional strategies that are more clearly aligned with the coding, analysis, and interpretation of qualitative data.

Investigator and Theory Triangulation

The overall purpose of triangulation is to provide a basis for convergence on the truth; triangulation offers opportunities to sort out "true" information from irrelevant or erroneous information by using multiple methods and perspectives. During analysis, several types of triangulation are pertinent. **Investigator triangulation** refers to the use of two or more researchers to make data collection, coding, and analytic decisions. The underlying premise is that through collaboration, investigators can reduce the possibility of biased decisions and idiosyncratic interpretations of the data.

Conceptually, investigator triangulation is analogous to interrater reliability in quantitative studies, and is a strategy that is often used in coding qualitative data. Some researchers take formal steps to compare two or more independent category schemes or a subset of independent coding decisions.

Example of independent coding: Mentes, Chang, and Morris (2006) studied the perspectives of nursing home staff on the problem of dehydration in skilled nursing facilities, using data from focus group interviews in three nursing homes. Here is how they described their coding: "In coding the data, two reviewers independently read the transcripts and came up with an initial checklist of codes and then compiled a master list of codes after comparing the checklists and reconciling differences in the coding. Using the master code list, the two reviewers then independently applied the code" (p. 396).

➲ **TIP:** Coding consistency, whether it be intracoder or intercoder, depends on having clearly defined categories and decision rules that are documented in a code book or coding "dictionary."

If investigators bring to the analysis task a complementary blend of skills and expertise, the analysis and interpretation can potentially benefit from divergent perspectives. Blending diverse methodologic, disciplinary, and clinical skills also can contribute to other types of triangulation.

Example of investigator triangulation: Snethen and a team of co-researchers (2006) studied family interaction and decision making relating to children's participation in pediatric clinical trials. The team was composed of specialists in the fields of cultural diversity, ethics, pediatrics, and women's health. Their approach was to have a team member take responsibility for developing a case summary of families after examining transcripts relating to the full family unit (mothers, fathers, affected children, and siblings). Data matrices were developed to assist in comparing both within and across the 14 family units. The team then met over a 2-day period to review, discuss, analyze and interpret the case summaries.

➲ **TIP:** Investigator triangulation is extremely useful in focus group studies, and immediate postsession debriefings are highly recommended. In such debriefings—which should themselves be tape-recorded—team members who were present during the session meet to discuss issues and themes that arose. They also should share their views about group dynamics, such as coercive group members, censoring of controversial opinions, individual conformity to group viewpoints, and discrepancies between verbal and nonverbal behavior.

One form of investigator triangulation is a procedure referred to as **stepwise replication**, a strategy that is most often mentioned in connection with the Lincoln and Guba criterion of dependability. This technique involves having a research team that can be divided into two groups. These groups deal with data sources separately and conduct, essentially, independent inquiries through which data can be compared. Ongoing, regular communication between the groups is essential for the success of this procedure.

Example of stepwise replication: Williams and co-researchers (2000) used stepwise replication in a study of coping with normal results from predictive gene testing for neurodegenerative disorders. Ten participants were interviewed three times. Three researchers read through transcripts of the first set of interviews and made marginal notes for coding. The three researchers compared their codes and revised them until agreement was reached. All transcripts from the remaining interviews were coded independently, and the researchers met periodically to compare codes and reach a consensus.

With **theory triangulation**, researchers use competing theories or hypotheses in the analysis and interpretation of their data. Qualitative researchers who develop alternative hypotheses while still in the field can test the validity of each because the flexible design of qualitative studies provides ongoing opportunities to direct the inquiry. Theory triangulation can help researchers to rule out rival hypotheses and to prevent premature conceptualizations.

Although Denzin's (1989) seminal work discussed four types of triangulation as a method of converging on valid understandings about a phenomenon, other types have been suggested. For example, Kimchi, Polivka, and Stephenson (1991) have described **analysis triangulation** (i.e., using two or more analytic techniques to analyze the same set of data). This approach offers another opportunity to validate the meanings inherent in a qualitative data set. Analysis triangulation can also involve using multiple units of analysis (e.g., individuals, dyads, families).

➜ T I P : Farmer and colleagues (2006) provided a useful description of the triangulation protocol they used in the Canadian Heart Health Dissemination Project that illustrates how triangulation was operationalized.

Searching for Disconfirming Evidence and Competing Explanations

A powerful verification procedure that occurs at the intersection of data collection and data analysis involves a systematic search for data that will challenge a categorization or explanation that has emerged early in the analysis. The search for disconfirming evidence occurs through purposive or theoretical sampling methods. As noted in Chapter 13, the purposive sampling of individuals who can offer conflicting accounts or points of view can greatly strengthen a comprehensive understanding of a phenomenon. Clearly, this strategy depends on concurrent data collection and data analysis: researchers cannot look for disconfirming data unless they have a sense of what they need to know. Indeed, Morse and colleagues (2002) consider the iterative interaction between data and analysis essential to verification in qualitative inquiry.

Example of searching for disconfirming evidence: Tuckett (2005) conducted a study of truth telling in high-level aged care in a nursing home. One of his sampling decisions was driven by his desire to search for disconfirming or challenging evidence. One of the RNs in the nursing home was what Tuckett considered an atypical case. The RN not only was a team leader but also was the daughter of one of the nursing home residents. Her understanding about truth telling included her roles both as an RN and as a daughter of a patient. Tuckett chose to include her in his sample because "rather than set her views aside as 'different,' she was purposefully followed-up in an interview because she gave me an insight into the consequences of this dual role/relationship and its impact on her understandings of truth telling" (p. 35).

Lincoln and Guba (1985) discussed the related activity of **negative case analysis**. This strategy (sometimes called *deviant case analysis*) is a process by which researchers revise their interpretations by including cases that appear to disconfirm earlier hypotheses. The goal of this procedure is to continuously refine a hypothesis or theory until it accounts for *all* cases.

Patton (1999) similarly encouraged a systematic exploration for rival themes and explanations during the analysis: "Failure to find strong supporting evidence for alternative ways of presenting the data or contrary explanations helps increase confidence in the original, principal explanation generated by the analyst" (p. 1191). He noted that this strategy can be addressed both inductively and logically. Inductively, the strategy involves seeking other ways of organizing the data that might lead to different conclusions and interpretations. Logically, it means conceptualizing other logical possibilities and then searching for evidence that those competing explanations can be supported by the data.

Example of a search for rival explanations: Whitehead (2004) described her efforts to search for rival explanations in a hermeneutic study to explore the lived experience of people with chronic fatigue syndrome/myalgic encephalitis: "During analysis, I engaged in a systematic search for alternative themes, divergent patterns, and rival explanations of the data. The aim was not to disprove the alternatives but to look for data that supported alternative explanations. When patterns and trends were identified, attention was given to findings that both did and did not support these, and I continued to allow individual accounts to be heard" (p. 515).

Peer Review and Debriefing

Another quality enhancement strategy involves external validation. **Peer debriefing** involves sessions with peers to review and explore various aspects of the inquiry. Peer debriefing exposes researchers to the searching questions of others who are experienced in either the methods of naturalistic inquiry, the phenomenon being studied, or both.

In a peer debriefing session, researchers might present written or oral summaries of the data that have been gathered, categories and themes that are emerging, and researchers' interpretations of the data. In some cases, taped interviews might be played. Among the questions that peer debriefers might address are the following:

- Is there evidence of researcher bias?
- Have the researchers been sufficiently reflexive?
- Do the gathered data adequately portray the phenomenon?
- If there are important omissions, what strategies might remedy this problem?
- Are there any apparent errors of fact?
- Are there possible errors of interpretation?
- Are there competing interpretations? More comprehensive or parsimonious interpretations?
- Have all important themes been identified?
- Are the themes and interpretations knit together into a cogent, useful, and creative conceptualization of the phenomenon?

Example of peer debriefing: In her study of women diagnosed with polycystic ovary syndrome, Snyder (2006) debriefed with two other researchers. At each phase of her thematic analysis, Snyder consulted with the peer reviewers until agreement was achieved. Both reviewers were doctorally prepared nurses with qualitative research experience.

Inquiry Audits

A similar, but more formal, approach is to undertake an inquiry audit, a procedure that is considered a means of enhancing the dependability and confirmability of a study. An **inquiry audit** involves a scrutiny of the data and relevant supporting documents by an external reviewer. Such an audit requires careful documentation of all aspects of the inquiry, as previously discussed. Once the audit trail materials are assembled, the inquiry auditor proceeds to audit, in a fashion analogous to a financial audit, the trustworthiness of the data and the meanings attached to them. Although the auditing task is complex, it can serve as a tool for persuading others that qualitative data are worthy of

confidence. Relatively few comprehensive inquiry audits have been reported in the literature, but some studies report partial audits or the assembling of auditable materials. Rodgers and Cowles (1993) present useful information about inquiry audits.

Example of an inquiry audit: Erwin, Meyer, and McClain (2005) provided a detailed account of how they used an audit to address issues of trustworthiness in their study of violence in the lives of high-risk urban teenagers. The audit involved a 5-phase process that unfolded over a 6-week period: engagement of the auditor, familiarization with the study, evaluation of the strengths and weaknesses of the study, articulation of the audit findings, and presentation of the audit report to the entire research team. The researchers concluded that "Positioning the audit before producing final results allows researchers to address many study limitations, uncover potential sources of bias in the thematic structure, and systematically plan subsequent steps in an emerging design" (p. 707).

Strategies Relating to Presentation

The strategies discussed thus far are steps that researchers can undertake to convince *themselves* that their study has integrity and credibility. This section describes some issues relating to convincing *others* of the high quality of the inquiry.

Disclosure of Quality Enhancement Strategies

It should go without saying that a large part of demonstrating integrity to others in a research report involves providing a good description of the quality enhancement activities that were undertaken. Yet many research reports fail to include information that would give readers confidence in the integrity of the research. Some qualitative reports do not address the subject of rigor, validity, integrity, or trustworthiness at all, whereas others pay lip service to validity concerns, simply noting, for example, that reflexive journals and audit trail were maintained. Just as clinicians seek *evidence* relating to the health care needs of clients, readers of reports need evidence that the findings are believable and true. It is important to include enough information about quality enhancement strategies used in the inquiry so that readers can draw their own conclusions about the quality of the study. The research example at the end of this chapter is exemplary with regard to the level of information provided to readers.

Thick and Contextualized Description

Thick description, as noted in previous chapters, refers to a rich, thorough, and vivid description of the research context, the people who participated in the study, and the experiences and processes observed during the inquiry. The prevailing sentiment is that if there is to be transferability of the findings, the burden rests with the investigator to provide sufficient information to permit judgments about contextual similarity. Lucid and textured descriptions, with the judicious inclusion of verbatim quotes from study participants, also contribute to other quality criteria, including the authenticity and vividness of a qualitative study.

➲ TIP : Sandelowski (2004) cautioned as follows: ". . . the phrase *thick description* likely ought not to appear in write-ups of qualitative research at all, as it is among those qualitative research words that should be seen but not written" (p. 215). Her advice, although specifically addressed to ethnographers, applies equally well to all qualitative researchers: "Ethnographers should not talk about thick description but rather demonstrate thick description in the interpretations of cultures they present as their findings" (p. 215).

Example of thick description: Some of the research context not described in the write-up of Beck's (2004) birth trauma study (but shared in oral presentations of the findings) included powerful and graphic photographs that some mothers sent her over the Internet. Mothers shared them with Beck to help bring alive their written stories. For example, one mother sent three photos of herself because she said a picture is worth a 1000 words and she wanted to vividly show the immediate impact of birth trauma on a woman. The first photo was of the mother smiling before her traumatic delivery of twins. The next two pictures were of the mother with her newborn twins while still in the delivery room. She wrote in her e-mail to the researcher, "Cheryl, focus on my eyes. There is nobody home!" Her eyes were vacant. When Beck showed these pictures (with permission of the mother) during one of her presentations at a nursing research conference, one of the attendees said, after Beck had finished her presentation, that the mother looked as if she had lost her soul during the birth of her twins.

In high-quality qualitative studies, descriptions typically need to go beyond a faithful and thorough rendering of information. Powerful description often has an evocative quality and the capacity for emotional impact. However, qualitative researchers must be careful not to misrepresent their findings by sharing only the most dramatic, poignant, or sensational stories. Thorne and Darbyshire (2005) cautioned against what they called "lachrymal validity," a criterion for evaluating research according to the extent to which the report can wring tears from its readers! At the same time, they noted that the opposite problem with some reports is that they are "bloodless." Bloodless findings are characterized by a tendency of some researchers to "play it safe in writing up the research, reporting the obvious (possibly in the most thinly 'salami-sliced' 'findings' articles), failing to apply any inductive analytic spin to the sequence, structure, or form of the findings" (p. 1109).

Researcher Credibility

As previously noted, an aspect of credibility discussed by Patton (1999, 2002) is *researcher credibility*. In qualitative studies, researchers *are* the data collecting instruments—as well as creators of the analytic process. Therefore, researcher qualifications, experience, and reflexivity are relevant in establishing confidence in the data. Patton has argued that, from the perspective of the readers, trustworthiness of the inquiry is enhanced if the report contains information about the researchers, including information about credentials. In addition, the report may need to make clear the personal connections they had to the people, topic, or community under study. For example, it is relevant for a reader of a report on the coping mechanisms of AIDS patients to know that the researcher is HIV positive. Patton (2002) recommended that researchers report "any personal and professional information that may have affected data collection, analysis and interpretation—either negatively or positively . . ." (p. 566).

Example of researcher credibility: D'Abundo and Chally (2004) conducted a grounded theory study of women battling an eating disorder. Here is what they wrote in the report about their backgrounds: "Eating disorders primarily occur in White middle-to-upper class women and girls, and both researchers were demographically similar to the research population. One researcher had a family member who had the disease. The other had struggled with atypical eating as an adolescent" (pp. 1095–1096).

Researcher credibility is also enhanced when research reports describe the researchers' efforts to be self-reflective and to take their own prejudices and perspectives into account. During her study of the experience of chronic fatigue syndrome, Whitehead (2004) maintained a reflective journal and used excerpts from it to illustrate how researcher credibility could be enhanced through this process.

DEVELOPMENT OF A QUALITY-MINDED OUTLOOK

Conducting high-quality qualitative research is not just about methods and strategies—that is, it is not just about what researchers *do*. It is also about who the researchers *are*—that is, about their outlook, their self-demands, and their ingenuity. As Morse and colleagues (2002) succinctly put it, "Research is only as good as the investigator" (p. 10). Attributes that good qualitative researchers must possess are difficult to teach, but it is nevertheless important to know what those attributes are so they can be cultivated. We express several important attributes, therefore, as *commitments* that researchers can strive to achieve.

1. **Commitment to Transparency.** Good qualitative inquiry cannot be a secretive enterprise that masks decisions, biases, and limitations from outside scrutiny. Conscientious qualitative researchers take steps to maintain the records needed to document a decision trail, and to justify the decisions. A commitment to transparency also means seeking opportunities to have decisions reviewed by others. To the extent possible, researchers should seek opportunities to demonstrate transparency in their writing, including how themes and categories were formulated from the initial participant data.

2. **Commitment to Absorption and Diligence.** Meticulousness and thoroughness are essential to high-quality research. Researchers who are not thorough run the risk of having thin, unsaturated data that undermine a full and rich description of the phenomenon of interest. The concept of *replication* within the study is crucial: there must be sufficient, and redundant, data to account for all aspects of the phenomenon (Morse et al., 2002). In good qualitative research, investigators cannot avoid the tedium of reading and re-reading their data, returning repeatedly to check whether their interpretations are true to their data. Thoroughness also implies that researchers will seek opportunities to challenge their early conceptualizations, and to find multiple sources of corroborating evidence both internally (i.e., within the study data) and externally (e.g., in the literature).

3. **Commitment to Verification.** Confidence in the data, and in the analysis and interpretation of those data, is possible only when researchers are committed to instituting verification and self-correcting procedures throughout the study. Morse and colleagues (2002) have written at length about the importance of verification, noting that verification is "the process of checking, confirming, making sure, and being certain" (p. 9). A strong commitment to verification strengthens methodologic coherence and helps to ensure that errors and missteps are corrected before they undermine the entire enterprise.

4. **Commitment to Reflexivity.** Although there is not always agreement about the *forms* that self-reflection will assume in qualitative inquiry (e.g., *bracketing* is advised by some but considered impossible by others), there is widespread agreement that researchers need to devote time and energy to carefully analyzing and documenting their presuppositions, biases, and ongoing emotions. Reflexivity involves a continual self-scrutiny of subjective responses, as well as interpersonal transactions with study participants. Developing a reflexive posture means continually asking, How might my previous experiences, my values, my background, my prejudices be shaping my analysis and interpretations?

5. Commitment to Participant-Driven Inquiry.
In good qualitative research, the inquiry is driven forward by the participants, not the researcher. Researchers must continually remain responsiveness to the flow and content of interactions with, and observations of, their informants. Participants shape the scope and breadth of questioning, and they help to guide sampling decisions. The analysis and interpretation must give voice to those who participated in the inquiry.

6. Commitment to Insightful Interpretation.
Morse (2006b) has written that *insight* is a major process in qualitative inquiry but has been neglected and overlooked as a topic of discussion—perhaps because it is not an easily acquired commodity. Morse argued that insight requires researchers to be *ready* for insight—they must have considerable knowledge about their data and be able to link them in meaningful ways to relevant literature. Patton (1999) similarly noted, quoting Pasteur, that "Chance favors the prepared mind" (p. 1191). Thus, immersion in one's own data and having good-quality data are essential. Morse also noted, however, that qualitative researchers need to give themselves "*permission* to use insight and the confidence to do it well" (p. 3). Relatedly, Morse and colleagues (2002) urged researchers to *think theoretically*, which "requires macro-micro perspectives, inching forward without making cognitive leaps, constantly checking and rechecking, and building a solid foundation" (p. 13).

CRITIQUING DATA QUALITY IN QUALITATIVE STUDIES

For qualitative research to be judged trustworthy, investigators must *earn* the trust of their readers. Many qualitative reports do not provide much information about the researchers' efforts to ensure that their research is strong with respect to the quality criteria described in this chapter, but there appears to be a promising trend toward greater transparency and forthrightness about quality issues. In a world that is very conscious about the quality of research evidence, qualitative researchers need to be proactive in doing high-quality research. They also need to share their quality enhancement strategies with readers so that readers can draw their own conclusions about the quality of the evidence and its relevance to their own practice.

Part of the difficulty that qualitative researchers face in demonstrating trustworthiness and authenticity is that page constraints in journals impose conflicting demands. It takes a precious amount of space to present quality enhancement strategies adequately and convincingly. Using space for such documentation means that there is less space for the thick description of context and the rich verbatim accounts that are also necessary in high-quality qualitative research. Qualitative research is often characterized by the need for critical compromises. It is well to keep such compromises in mind in critiquing qualitative research reports.

BOX 20.1 Guidelines for Evaluating Quality and Integrity in Qualitative Studies

1. Does the report discuss efforts to enhance or evaluate the quality of the data and the overall inquiry? If so, is the description sufficiently detailed and clear? If not, is there other information that allows you to draw inferences about the quality of the data, the analysis, and the interpretations?

2. Which specific techniques (if any) did the researcher use to enhance the quality of the inquiry? Were these strategies used judiciously and to good effect?

3. What quality enhancement strategies were *not* used? Would supplementary strategies have strengthened your confidence in the study and its evidence?

4. Given the efforts to enhance data quality, what can you conclude about the study's validity, integrity, or rigor?

Table 20.1 offered questions that are useful in considering whether researchers have attended important quality criteria. As noted earlier, not all questions are equally relevant for all types of qualitative inquiry. Reports that explicitly state which criteria guided the inquiry demonstrate sensitivity to readers' needs. Some further guidelines that may be helpful in evaluating qualitative analyses are presented in Box 20.1. ✪

RESEARCH EXAMPLE

Study: "The process of preparedness in communicating with children" (Yearwood & McClowry, 2006)

Statement of Purpose: The purpose of this study was to explore the cultural meaning of parent–child communication in inner-city families with children at risk for behavioral problems.

Method: Data for this qualitative study were collected over an 18-month period. Study participants were recruited from a larger sample of participants who took part in an intervention (called Insight) in three inner-city schools. The sample included children, parents, teachers, and facilitators from the intervention portion of the larger study. Parents, the primary informants, were mainly African-American single mothers. A total of 40 parents participated.

Quality Enhancement Strategies: Yearwood and McClowry's report provided abundant detail about the efforts they made to enhance the trustworthiness and integrity of their study. Triangulation was an important strategy. Data were collected at multiple sites (space triangulation), from different perspectives (person triangulation), and using multiple methods—personal interviews, focus group interviews, and extensive observation (method triangulation). The investigators' strategies included both prolonged engagement (18 months in the field) and persistent observation, which entailed extensive periods of observation "in all three schools, during meetings in the community with school personnel, during Insight team meetings, during walks or drives throughout the community of interest, and while reading or looking at media coverage of community events" (p. 43). The ongoing presence of the researchers in the schools enabled them to gain the trust of the study parents, "who more freely displayed their communication behaviors with their children and talked about community dynamics affecting some of their actions" (p. 45). The researchers maintained detailed field notes, in which they recorded impressions, activities, and interactions. Data collection and analysis occurred simultaneously, and the report described how the researchers made adjustments in their methodologic strategies while they were in the field. Data collection continued even after saturation was achieved to ensure that those enrolled later in the main study would have an opportunity to contribute to the qualitative component. All interviews and focus group sessions were tape-recorded and subsequently transcribed. The report indicated that "The researcher reviewed all transcriptions multiple times, checking for accuracy in an iterative process while coding openly" (p. 44). The researchers made a deliberate effort in their analyses to look at negative cases. Member checking was used by sharing early emerging patterns with participants who came into the study later, and by sharing findings with groups of parents. Finally, an independent audit was undertaken by two doctoral-level nurse researchers, one of whom was an expert in qualitative methods and the other of whom was an expert in cultural dynamics. The audit entailed a review of the raw data, theoretical notes, and a draft of the final report.

Key Findings: The findings from this study indicated that the parents used a complex communication process with their high-risk children. Factors that influenced their communications included the immediacy of safety concerns and the child's temperament. The parents' ultimate communication goal was to equip their children with tools to help them to safely navigate their school and community environments.

SUMMARY POINTS

- There are several controversies that surround the issue of *quality* in qualitative studies, one of which involves terminology. Some have argued that terms such as *rigor* and *validity* are quantitative terms not suitable as goals in qualitative inquiry, but others are equally adamant that these terms are appropriate.
- Other controversies involve what criteria to use as indicators of validity or integrity, whether there should be generic or study-specific criteria, what strategies to use to address the quality criteria, and whose perspective (researchers or external critics) should prevail.
- The framework that has been used most often in discussions about quality criteria (although it

has been subjected to much criticism) is that of Lincoln and Guba, who identified five criteria for evaluating the **trustworthiness** of data and interpretations: credibility, dependability, confirmability, transferability, and (added to their framework at a later date) authenticity.

- **Credibility**, which refers to confidence in the truth value of the findings, is sometimes said to be the qualitative equivalent of internal validity. **Dependability** refers to the stability of data over time and over conditions, and is somewhat analogous to the concept of reliability in quantitative studies. **Confirmability** refers to the objectivity or neutrality of the data. **Transferability**, the analogue of external validity, is the extent to which findings from the data can be transferred to other settings or groups. **Authenticity** refers to the extent to which researchers fairly and faithfully show a range of different realities and convey the feeling tone of lives as they are lived.

- An alternative framework, representing a synthesis of 10 qualitative validity schemes (the Whittemore and colleagues framework), proposed four primary criteria (credibility, authenticity, criticality, and integrity) and six secondary criteria (explicitness, vividness, creativity, thoroughness, congruence, and sensitivity). The primary criteria can be applied to any qualitative inquiry, but the secondary criteria can be given different weight depending on study goals.

- **Criticality** refers to the researcher's critical appraisal of every research decision. **Integrity** is demonstrated by ongoing self-scrutiny to ensure that interpretations are valid and grounded in the data.

- **Explicitness** is the ability to follow the researcher's decisions through careful documentation. **Vividness** involves rich and vivid descriptions. **Creativity** reflects challenges to traditional ways of thinking. **Thoroughness** refers to comprehensive data and the full development of ideas. **Congruence** is interconnectedness between parts of the inquiry and the whole, and between study findings and external contexts. **Sensitivity**, the sixth of the secondary criteria in the Whittemore framework, is the degree to which an inquiry reflects respect and compassion for those being studied.

- Strategies for enhancing the quality of qualitative data as they are being collected include **prolonged engagement**, which strives for adequate scope of data coverage; **persistent observation**, which is aimed at achieving adequate depth; comprehensive and vivid recording of information (including maintenance of an **audit trail** of key decisions); triangulation; and member checking.

- Triangulation is the process of using multiple referents to draw conclusions about what constitutes the truth. During data collection, key forms of triangulation include **data triangulation** (using multiple data sources to validate conclusions) and **method triangulation** (using multiple methods, such as interviews and observations, to collect data about the same phenomenon.

- **Member checks** involve asking study participants to review and react to study data and emerging categories, themes, and conceptualizations. Member checking is among the most controversial methods of addressing quality issues in qualitative inquiry.

- Strategies for enhancing quality during the coding and analysis of qualitative data include **investigator triangulation** (independent coding and analysis of at least a portion of the data by two or more researchers); **theory triangulation** (use of competing theories or hypotheses in the analysis and interpretation of data); **stepwise replication** (dividing the research team into two groups that conduct independent inquiries that can be compared and merged); searching for disconfirming evidence; searching for rival explanations and undertaking a **negative case analysis** (revising interpretations to account for cases that appear to disconfirm early conclusions); external validation through **peer debriefings** (exposing the inquiry to the searching questions of peers); and launching a formal **inquiry audit** (a formal scrutiny of the research process and audit trail documents by an independent external auditor).

- Strategies that can be used to convince readers of reports of the high quality of qualitative inquiries include disclosure of the quality enhancement strategies in which the researcher engaged; using *thick description* to vividly portray contextualized information about the study participants and the central phenomenon; and making efforts to be transparent about researcher credentials and reflexivity so that **researcher credibility** can be established.

• Doing high-quality qualitative research is not just about *method* and what the researchers *do*—it is also about who they *are.* To become an outstanding qualitative researcher, there must be a commitment to transparency, thoroughness, verification, reflexivity, participant-driven inquiry, and insightful and artful interpretation.

●◎●◎●◎●◎●◎●◎●◎●◎●◎●◎●

STUDY ACTIVITIES

Chapter 20 of the *Resource Manual to Accompany Nursing Research: Generating and Assessing Evidence for Nursing Practice, 8th edition*, offers various exercises and study suggestions for reinforcing concepts presented in this chapter. In addition, the following study questions can be addressed:

1. You have been asked to be a peer reviewer for a team of nurse researchers who are conducting a phenomenological study of the experiences of physical abuse during pregnancy. What specific questions would you ask the team during debriefing, and what documents would you want the researchers to share?

2. Apply relevant questions in Table 20.1 and Box 20.1 to the research example at the end of the chapter, referring to the full journal article as necessary.

●◎●◎●◎●◎●◎●◎●◎●◎●◎●◎●

STUDIES CITED IN CHAPTER 20

Methodologic or theoretical references cited in this chapter can be found in a separate section at the end of the book.

Beck, C. T. (2002). Releasing the pause button: Mothering twins during the first year of life. *Qualitative Health Research, 12,* 593–608.

Beck, C. T. (2004). Birth trauma: In the eye of the beholder. *Nursing Research, 53,* 28–35.

Choudhry, U. K. (2001). Uprooting and resettlement experiences of South Asian immigrant women. *Western Journal of Nursing Research, 23,* 376–393.

D'Abundo, M., & Chally, P. (2004). Struggling with recovery: Participant perspectives on battling an eating disorder. *Qualitative Health Research, 14*(8), 1094–1106.

Mentes, J., Chang, B., & Morris, J. (2006). Keeping nursing home residents hydrated. *Western Journal of Nursing Research, 28*(4), 392–406.

Molzahn, A. E., Starzomski, R., McDonald, M., & O'Loughlin, C. (2005). Chinese Canadian beliefs toward organ donation. *Qualitative Health Research, 15,* 82–98.

Piven, M., Ammarell, M., Bailey, D., Corazzini, K., Colón-Emeric, C., Lekan-Rutledge, D., Utley-Smith, Q., & Anderson. R. (2006). MDS coordinator relationships and nursing home care processes. *Western Journal of Nursing Research, 28*(3), 294–309.

Plach, S., Stevens, P., & Keigher, S. (2005). Self-care of women growing older with HIV and/or AIDS. *Western Journal of Nursing Research, 27*(5), 534–553.

Snethen, J., Broome, M., Knafl, K., Deatrick, J., & Angst, D. (2006). Family patterns of decision-making in pediatric clinical trials. *Research in Nursing & Health, 29*(3), 223–232.

Snyder, B. (2006). The lived experience of women diagnosed with polycystic ovary syndrome. *Journal of Obstetric, Gynecologic, & Neonatal Nursing, 35*(3), 385–392.

Tuckett, A. G. (2005). Part II. Rigour in qualitative research: Complexities and solutions. *Nurse Researcher, 13,* 29–42.

Williams, J. K., Schutte, D. L., Evers, C., & Holkup, P. A. (2000). Redefinition: Coping with normal results from predictive gene testing for neurodegenerative disorders. *Research in Nursing & Health, 23,* 260–269.

Woodgate, R. L. (2006). The importance of being there: Perspectives of social support by adolescents with cancer. *Journal of Pediatric Oncology Nursing, 23*(3), 122–134.

Yearwood, E. L., & McClowry, S. (2006). The process of preparedness in communicating with children. *Journal of Family Nursing, 12*(1), 38–55.

21

Describing Data Through Statistics

Without statistics, quantitative data would be a chaotic mass of numbers. Statistical procedures enable researchers to organize, interpret, and communicate numeric information.

This textbook does not emphasize the theory or mathematic basis of statistics. Even computation is underplayed because this is not a statistics textbook and, in any event, statistics are seldom calculated by hand. We focus on how to use statistics in different situations, and how to understand what they mean once they have been applied. Mathematic talent is not required to use or understand statistical analysis—only logical thinking ability is needed.

Statistics are either descriptive or inferential. **Descriptive statistics** are used to describe and synthesize data. Averages and percentages are examples of descriptive statistics. Actually, when such indexes are calculated from population data, they are called **parameters**. A descriptive index from a sample is a **statistic**. Research questions are about parameters, but researchers calculate statistics to estimate them and use **inferential statistics** to make inferences about the population. This chapter discusses descriptive statistics, and Chapter 22 focuses on inferential statistics. First, however, we discuss the concept of levels of measurement because the analyses that can be performed depend on how variables are measured.

LEVELS OF MEASUREMENT

Scientists have developed a system for categorizing measures. The four **levels of measurement** are nominal, ordinal, interval, and ratio.

Nominal Measurement

The lowest level of measurement is **nominal measurement**, which involves assigning numbers to classify characteristics into categories. Examples of variables amenable to nominal measurement include gender, blood type, and marital status.

The numbers assigned in nominal measurement have no quantitative meaning. If we code males as 1 and females as 2, the number 2 does not mean "more than" 1. The numbers are merely symbols representing different values of the gender attribute—we could reverse the code and use 1 for females, 2 for males. Indeed, we could have used alphabetical symbols, such as M and F—although we recommend numeric codes.

Nominal measurement provides no information about an attribute except equivalence and nonequivalence. If we were to "measure" the gender of Nate, Ryan, Norah, and Lauren by assigning them the codes 1, 1, 2, and 2, respectively, this means Nate and Ryan are equivalent on the gender attribute but are not equivalent to Norah and Lauren.

Nominal measures must have categories that are mutually exclusive and collectively exhaustive. For example, if we were measuring marital status, we might use the following codes: 1 = married, 2 = separated or divorced, 3 = widowed. Each subject must be classifiable into one and only one category. The requirement for collective exhaustiveness would not be met if, for example, there were subjects in the sample who had never been married.

The numbers in nominal measurement cannot be treated mathematically. It is, for example, nonsensical to calculate the average gender of a sample, but we can state frequencies of occurrence within the categories. In a sample of 50 patients, if there are 30 men and 20 women, we could say that 60% of the subjects are male and 40% are female. No further mathematic operation is meaningful with nominal data.

It may strike you as odd to think of nominal categorization as measurement. Nominal measurement does, however, involve assigning numbers to attributes according to rules. The rules are not sophisticated, but they are rules nonetheless.

Example of nominal measures: Chen and Narsavage (2006) studied factors related to hospital readmission among patients with chronic obstructive pulmonary disease (COPD) in Taiwan. Their dependent variables (readmission for a COPD diagnosis versus not at 14 and 90 days after discharge) were nominal-level variables, as were several other variables describing the sample (e.g., gender, smoking status, religion, marital status).

Ordinal Measurement

Next in the measurement hierarchy is **ordinal measurement**, which involves sorting objects based on their relative ranking on an attribute. This level of measurement goes beyond mere categorization: Attributes are *ordered* according to some criterion. Ordinal measurement captures information not only about equivalence but also about relative rank among objects.

Consider this scheme for coding a client's ability to perform activities of daily living: (1) completely dependent, (2) needs another person's assistance, (3) needs mechanical assistance, (4) completely independent. In this case, the measurement is ordinal. The numbers signify incremental ability to perform activities of daily living. Individuals assigned a value of four are equivalent to each other with regard to functional ability *and*, relative to those in the other categories, have more of that attribute.

Ordinal measurement does not, however, tell us anything about how much greater one level is than another. We do not know if being completely independent is twice as good as needing mechanical assistance. Nor do we know if the difference between needing another person's assistance and needing mechanical assistance is the same as that between needing mechanical assistance and being completely independent. Ordinal measurement tells us only the relative ranking of the attribute's levels.

As with nominal measures, mathematic operations with ordinal-level data are restricted—for example, averages are usually meaningless. Frequency counts, percentages, and several other statistical procedures to be discussed later are appropriate for analyzing ordinal-level data.

Example of ordinal measures: Shin and colleagues (2006) tested the effectiveness of a tailored intervention designed to increase exercise among Korean adults with chronic disease. The participants' stage of engaging in exercise was classified before and after the intervention on an ordinal scale: precontemplation, contemplation, and active.

Interval Measurement

Interval measurement occurs when researchers can specify the rank-ordering of objects on an attribute and can assume equivalent distance between them. The Fahrenheit temperature scale is an example: a temperature of 60°F is 10°F warmer than 50°F. A 10°F difference similarly separates

40°F and 30°F, and the two differences in temperature are equivalent. Interval measures are thus more informative than ordinal measures, but interval measures do not give information about absolute magnitude. For example, it cannot be said that 60°F is twice as hot as 30°F, or three times as hot as 20°F. The Fahrenheit scale involves an arbitrary zero point. Zero on the thermometer does not signify a total absence of heat. In interval scales, there is no real or rational zero point. Most psychological tests are based on interval scales.

Interval scales expand analytic possibilities—in particular, interval-level data can be averaged meaningfully. It is reasonable, for example, to compute an average daily temperature for hospital patients. Many widely used statistical procedures require interval measurements.

Example of interval measures: Miller and colleagues (2006) studied the effects of acculturation and other factors on depressed mood in midlife immigrant women from the former Soviet Union. Most of the variables in the analysis were measured with interval-level Likert-type scales, including the dependent variable. Depressed mood was measured by the Center for Epidemiologic Studies Depression Scale (CES-D), a 20-item scale with scores that can range from 0 to 60.

Ratio Measurement

The highest level of measurement is **ratio measurement**. Ratio scales have a rational, meaningful zero. Ratio measures provide information concerning the ordering of objects on the critical attribute, the intervals between objects, *and* the absolute magnitude of the attribute. Many physical measures provide ratio-level data. A person's weight, for example, is measured on a ratio scale because zero weight is an actual possibility. It is acceptable to say that someone who weighs 200 pounds is twice as heavy as someone who weighs 100 pounds.

Because ratio scales have an absolute zero, all arithmetic operations are permissible. One can meaningfully add, subtract, multiply, and divide numbers on a ratio scale. All the statistical procedures suitable for interval-level data are also appropriate for ratio-level data.

Example of ratio measures: Bastani and colleagues (2006) tested a relaxation intervention for anxious primigravid Iranian women, using an experimental design. Several dependent variables were pregnancy outcomes measured on a ratio scale, including the infant's birth weight and gestational age at birth.

➲ TIP: Nominal-level measures are often called categorical. Variables measured on an interval- or ratio-level scale may be referred to as continuous variables.

Comparison of the Levels

The four levels of measurement constitute a hierarchy, with ratio scales at the top and nominal measurement at the base. Moving from a higher to a lower level of measurement results in an information loss, as we demonstrate with an example of people's weight. Table 21.1 presents fictitious data for 10 subjects named in column 1. The second column shows ratio-level data, that is, actual weight in pounds. In the third column, the ratio data have been converted to interval measures by assigning a score of 0 to the lightest individual (Alaine), a score of 5 to the person 5 pounds heavier than the lightest person (Caitlin), and so forth. Note that the resulting scores are still amenable to addition and subtraction; differences in pounds are equally far apart, even though they are at different parts of the scale. The data no longer tell us, however, anything about the subjects' weights. Alaine could be a 10-pound infant or a 125-pound adult.

In the fourth column of Table 21.1, sample members were rank-ordered from the lightest (assigned the score of 1) to the heaviest (assigned the score of 10), yielding an ordinal measure. Now even more information is missing. The data provide no indication of how much heavier Alexander is than Alaine. The difference separating them could be 5 pounds or 150 pounds.

The final column presents nominal measurements in which people were classified as either

| TABLE 21.1 | Fictitious Data for Four Levels of Measurement: Subjects' Weight (pounds) |

SUBJECTS	RATIO-LEVEL	INTERVAL-LEVEL	ORDINAL-LEVEL	NOMINAL
Alexander	180	70	10	2
Alaine	110	0	1	1
Derek	165	55	8	2
Amanda	130	20	5	1
Terence	175	65	9	2
Caitlin	115	5	2	1
Danielle	125	15	4	1
James	150	40	7	1
Bob	145	35	6	1
Andrea	120	10	3	1

heavy or *light*. The criterion used to categorize people was weight greater than, or less than or equal to, 150 pounds. Within a category, there is no information as to who is heavier than whom. With this level of measurement, Alexander, Derek, and Terence are equivalent with regard to the attribute heavy/light, as defined by the classification criterion.

This example illustrates that at every successive level in the measurement hierarchy, information is lost. It also illustrates another point: With information at one level, it is possible to convert data to a lower level, but the converse is not true. If we were given only the nominal measurements, it would be impossible to reconstruct actual weights.

It is not always easy to identify a variable's level of measurement. Nominal and ratio measures usually are discernible with little difficulty, but the distinction between ordinal and interval measures is more problematic. Some methodologists argue that most psychological measures that are treated as interval measures are really only ordinal measures. Although instruments such as Likert scales produce data that are, strictly speaking, ordinal, many analysts believe that treating them as interval measures results in too few errors to warrant using less powerful statistical procedures.

➲ TIP: In operationalizing variables, it is usually best to use the highest measurement level possible. Higher levels of measurement yield more information and are amenable to more powerful analyses than lower levels (Owen & Froman, 2005). There are, however, a few exceptions, because sometimes group membership is more meaningful than continuous scores, especially for clinicians who need meaningful "cut points" for making decisions. For example, for some purposes, it may be more relevant to designate infants as being of low versus normal birth weight (nominal level) than to use actual birth weight values (ratio level).

FREQUENCY DISTRIBUTIONS

Unanalyzed quantitative data are overwhelming. It is not even possible to discern general trends until some order is imposed on the data. Consider the 60 numbers in Table 21.2. Let us assume that these numbers are the scores of 60 preoperative patients on a 6-item measure of anxiety—scores that we will consider to be on an interval scale. Visual inspection of the numbers does not help us understand patients' anxiety.

TABLE 21.2 Patients' Anxiety Scores

22	27	25	19	24	25	23	29	24	20
26	16	20	26	17	22	24	18	26	28
15	24	23	22	21	24	20	25	18	27
24	23	16	25	30	29	27	21	23	24
26	18	30	21	17	25	22	24	29	28
20	25	26	24	23	19	27	28	25	26

A set of data can be described in terms of three characteristics: the shape of the distribution of values, central tendency, and variability. Central tendency and variability are dealt with in subsequent sections.

Constructing Frequency Distributions

Frequency distributions are used to organize numeric data. A **frequency distribution** is a systematic arrangement of values from lowest to highest, together with a count of the number of times each value was obtained. The 60 fictitious anxiety scores are presented as a frequency distribution in Table 21.3. We can now see at a glance what the highest and lowest scores were, what the most common score was, where the bulk of scores clustered, and how many patients were in the sample (total sample size is typically depicted as *N* in research reports). None of this was apparent before the data were organized.

TABLE 21.3 Frequency Distribution of Patients' Anxiety Scores

SCORE (X)	TALLIES	FREQUENCY (f)	PERCENTAGE (%)
15	I	1	1.7
16	II	2	3.3
17	II	2	3.3
18	III	3	5.0
19	II	2	3.3
20	IIII	4	6.7
21	III	3	5.0
22	IIII	4	6.7
23	IIII	5	8.3
24	IIII IIII	9	15.0
25	IIII II	7	11.7
26	IIII I	6	10.0
27	IIII	4	6.7
28	III	3	5.0
29	III	3	5.0
30	II	2	3.3
		$N = 60 = \Sigma f$	$\Sigma\% = 100.0\%$

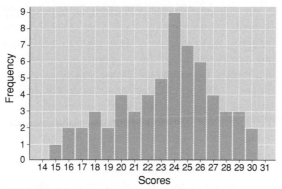

FIGURE 21.1 Histogram of patients' anxiety scores.

Frequency distributions consist of two parts: observed values (the Xs) and the frequency of cases at each value (the fs). Values are listed in numeric order in one column, and corresponding frequencies are listed in another. Table 21.3 shows the intermediary step of tallying by the method of four vertical bars and then a slash for the fifth observation. In frequency distributions, the score values must be mutually exclusive and collectively exhaustive. The sum of numbers in the frequency column must equal the sample size. In less verbal terms, $\Sigma f = N$, which means the sum of (signified by the Greek letter sigma, Σ) the frequencies (f) equals the sample size (N).

It is usually useful to display not only frequency counts but also percentages for each score value, as shown in the fourth column of Table 21.3. Just as the sum of all frequencies should equal N, the sum of all percentages should equal 100.

Sometimes researchers display frequency data in graphs, which can communicate a lot of information quickly. The most widely used graphs for displaying interval- and ratio-level data are **histograms** and **frequency polygons**, which are constructed in a similar fashion. First, score values are arrayed on a horizontal dimension, with the lowest value on the left, ascending to the highest value on the right. Frequencies or percentages are displayed vertically. A histogram is constructed by drawing bars above the score classes to the height corresponding to the frequency for that score class. Figure 21.1 shows a histogram for the anxiety score data.

Instead of vertical bars, frequency polygons use dots connected by straight lines to show frequencies. A dot corresponding to the frequency is placed above each score (Fig. 21.2). It is customary to connect the line to the base at the score below the minimum value obtained and above the maximum value obtained. In this example, however, the graph is terminated at 30 and brought down to the base at that point with a dotted line because a score of 31 was impossible.

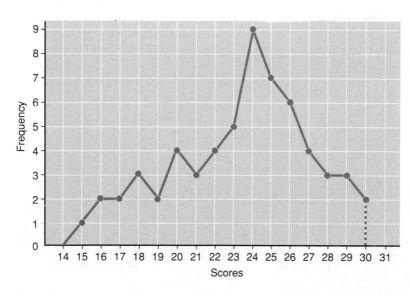

FIGURE 21.2 Frequency polygon of patients' anxiety scores.

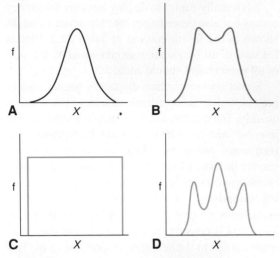

FIGURE 21.3 Examples of symmetric distributions.

Shapes of Distributions

A frequency polygon can assume many shapes. A distribution is **symmetric** if, when folded over, the two halves are superimposed on one another. Symmetric distributions thus consist of two halves that are mirror images of one another. All the distributions in Figure 21.3 are symmetric. With real data sets, distributions are rarely perfectly symmetric, but minor discrepancies are ignored in characterizing a distribution's shape.

In **asymmetric** or **skewed distributions**, the peak is off center, and one tail is longer than the other. When the longer tail points to the right, the distribution is **positively skewed,** as in Figure

21.4A. Personal income, for example, is positively skewed. Most people have low to moderate incomes, with relatively few people with high incomes in the tail. If the tail points to the left, the distribution is **negatively skewed**, as illustrated in Figure 21.4B. An example of a negatively skewed attribute is age at death. Here, most people are at the upper end of the distribution, with relatively few dying at an early age. Patients' anxiety scores (see Fig. 21.2) were negatively skewed, with high scores more common than low ones.

A second aspect of a distribution's shape is **modality**. A **unimodal distribution** has only one peak (i.e., a value with high frequency), whereas a **multimodal distribution** has two or more peaks. The most common multimodal distribution has two peaks, and is called **bimodal**. Figure 21.3A is unimodal, and multimodal distributions are illustrated in Figure 21.3B and D. Symmetry and modality are independent aspects of a distribution. Knowledge of skewness does not tell you anything about how many peaks the distribution has.

Some distributions are found so frequently that they have special names. Of particular importance is the **normal distribution** (sometimes called a *Gaussian distribution* or *bell-shaped curve*). A normal distribution is symmetric, unimodal, and not too peaked, as shown in Figure 21.3A. Many human attributes approximate a normal distribution. Examples include height and intelligence. The normal distribution plays a key role in inferential statistics.

FIGURE 21.4 Examples of skewed distributions.

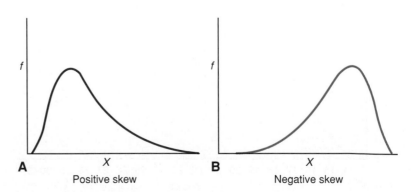

CENTRAL TENDENCY

Frequency distributions are a good way to organize data and clarify patterns. Often, however, a pattern is of less interest than an overall summary. Researchers usually ask such questions as, "What is the average oxygen consumption of myocardial infarction patients during bathing?" or "What is the average weight loss of patients with cancer?" Such questions seek a single number that best represents a distribution of values. Because an index of "typicalness" is more likely to come from the center of a distribution than from an extreme, such indexes are called measures of **central tendency**. Lay people use the term *average* to designate central tendency. Researchers avoid this ambiguous term because there are three kinds of indexes of central tendency: the mode, the median, and the mean.

The Mode

The **mode** is the most frequently occurring score value in a distribution. The mode is determined by inspecting a frequency distribution. In the following distribution, we can readily see that the mode is 53:

50 51 51 52 53 53 53 53 54 55 56

The score of 53 occurred four times, a higher frequency than for any other number. The mode of patients' anxiety scores (see Table 21.3) is 24. In multimodal distributions, there is more than one score value that has high frequencies.

Modes are a quick way to determine a "popular" score, but are rather unstable. By *unstable*, we mean that modes tend to fluctuate widely from sample to sample drawn from the same population. The mode is used primarily to describe typical values for nominal-level measures. For instance, researchers often characterize their samples by providing modal information on nominal-level demographics, as in the following example: "The typical (modal) subject was a married white woman."

The Median

The **median** is the point in a distribution above which and below which 50% of cases fall. As an example, consider the following set of values:

2 2 3 3 4 5 6 7 8 9

The value that divides the cases exactly in half is 4.5, the median for this set of numbers. The point that has 50% of the cases above and below it is halfway between 4 and 5. For the patient anxiety scores, the median is 24. An important characteristic of the median is that it does not take into account the quantitative values of scores—it is an index of average *position* in a distribution and is thus insensitive to extremes. In the above set of numbers, if the value of 9 were changed to 99, the median would remain 4.5. Because of this property, the median is often the preferred index of central tendency when a distribution is skewed. In research reports, the median may be abbreviated as **Md** or **Mdn**.

The Mean

The **mean**—often symbolized as M or $\overline{X}$—is the sum of all scores, divided by the number of scores—what people usually refer to as the *average*. The mean of the patients' anxiety scores is 23.4 (1405 ÷ 60). Let us compute the mean weight of eight subjects with the following weights: 85, 109, 120, 135, 158, 177, 181, and 195:

$$\overline{X} = \frac{85 + 109 + 120 + 135 + 158 + 177 + 181 + 195}{8} = 145$$

Unlike the median, the mean is affected by every score. If we were to exchange the 195-pound subject in this example for one weighing 275 pounds, the mean would increase from 145 to 155. A substitution of this kind would leave the median unchanged.

The mean is the most widely used measure of central tendency. Many important tests of statistical significance, described in Chapter 22, are based on the mean. When researchers work with interval-level or ratio-level measurements, the mean, rather than the median or mode, is usually the statistic reported.

Comparison of the Mode, Median, and Mean

The mean is the most stable index of central tendency. If repeated samples were drawn from a population, means would fluctuate less than modes or medians. Because of its stability, the mean is the most useful estimate of central tendency. Sometimes, however, the primary concern is to understand what is typical, in which case a median might be preferred. If we wanted to know about the economic well-being of U.S. citizens, for example, we would get a distorted impression by considering mean income, which would be inflated by the wealth of a minority. The median would better reflect how a typical person fares financially.

When a distribution of scores is symmetric and unimodal, the three indexes of central tendency coincide. In skewed distributions, the values of the mode, median, and mean differ. The mean is always pulled in the direction of the long tail, as shown in Figure 21.5. A variable's level of measurement plays a role in determining the appropriate index of central tendency to use. In general, the mode is most suitable for nominal measures, the mode or median is appropriate for ordinal measures, and the mean is appropriate for interval and ratio measures.

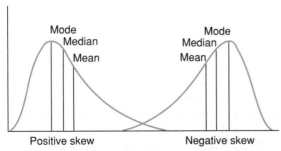

FIGURE 21.5 Relationships of central tendency indexes in skewed distributions.

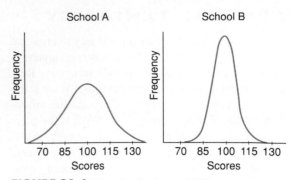

FIGURE 21.6 Two distributions of different variability.

VARIABILITY

Two distributions with identical means could differ in several respects—for example, they could have different shapes. The characteristic of concern in this section is the **variability** of distributions, that is, how spread out or dispersed the data are.

Consider the two distributions in Figure 21.6, which represent hypothetical scores for students from two schools on an IQ test. Both distributions have a mean of 100, but the score patterns are different. School A has a wide range of scores, with some below 70 and some above 130. In school B, by contrast, there are few low scores but also few high scores. School A is more **heterogeneous** (i.e., more variable) than school B, and school B is more **homogeneous** than school A.

Researchers compute an index of variability to express the extent to which scores in a distribution differ from one another. The most common indexes are the range and standard deviation. (Other indexes are described in statistics textbooks.)

The Range

The **range** is simply the highest score minus the lowest score in a distribution. In the example of patients' anxiety scores, the range is 15 (30 − 15). In the examples shown in Figure 21.6, the range for school A is about 80 (140 − 60), and the range for school B is about 50 (125 − 75).

The chief virtue of the range is its computational ease, but the range, being based on only two scores, is highly unstable. From sample to sample drawn from the same population, the range tends to fluctuate widely. Another limitation is that the range ignores variations in scores between the two extremes. In school B of Figure 21,6, suppose one student obtained a score of 60 and one other student obtained a score of 140. The range of both schools would then be 80, despite clear differences in heterogeneity. For these reasons, the range is used largely as a gross descriptive index.

Standard Deviation

With interval- or ratio-level data, the most widely used measure of variability is the standard deviation. The **standard deviation** indicates the *average amount* of deviation of values from the mean. Like the mean, the standard deviation is calculated using every score.

A variability index needs to capture the degree to which scores deviate from one another. This concept of deviation is represented in the range by the presence of a minus sign, which produces an index of deviation, or difference, between two score points. The standard deviation is similarly based on score differences. In fact, the first step in calculating a standard deviation is to compute deviation scores for each subject. A **deviation score** (symbolized as x) is the difference between an individual score and the mean; that is, $x = X - \bar{X}$. If a person weighed 150 pounds and the sample mean were 140, then the person's deviation score would be $+10$.

Because what we are looking for is an *average* deviation, you might think that a good variability index could be computed by summing deviation scores and then dividing by the number of cases. This gets us close to a good solution, but the difficulty is that the sum of a set of deviation scores is always zero. Table 21.4 presents an example of deviation scores computed for nine numbers. As shown in the second column, the sum of the x's is zero. Deviations above the mean always balance exactly deviations below the mean.

The standard deviation overcomes this problem by squaring each deviation score before summing.

TABLE 21.4 Computation of a Standard Deviation

X	$x = X - \bar{X}$	$x^2 = (X - \bar{X})^2$
4	−3	9
5	−2	4
6	−1	1
7	0	0
7	0	0
7	0	0
8	1	1
9	2	4
10	3	9
$\Sigma X = 63$	$\Sigma x = 0$	$\Sigma x^2 = 28$
$\bar{X} = 7$		

$$SD = \sqrt{\frac{28}{9}} = \sqrt{3.11} = 1.76$$

After dividing by the number of cases, the square root is taken to bring the index back to the original unit of measurement. The formula for the standard deviation* is as follows:

$$SD = \sqrt{\frac{\Sigma x^2}{N}}$$

A standard deviation has been completely worked out for the data in Table 21.4. First, a deviation score is calculated for each of the nine raw scores by subtracting the mean ($\bar{X} = 7$) from them. The third column shows that each deviation score is squared, thereby converting all values to positive numbers. The squared deviation scores are summed ($\Sigma x^2 = 28$), divided by 9 (N), and a square root taken to yield an SD of 1.76. In research reports, the standard deviation is often abbreviated as **s** or **SD**. Most researchers routinely report the means and standard deviation of key variables.

*Some statistical texts indicate that the formula for an unbiased estimate of the population SD uses $N - 1$ rather than N in the denominator. Knapp (1970) clarifies that N is appropriate when the researcher is interested in *describing* variation in sample data.

⊃ **TIP:** Occasionally, the standard deviation is simply shown in relation to the mean without a formal label. For example, the patients' anxiety scores might be shown as M = 23.4 (3.7) or M = 23.4 ± 3.7, where 23.4 is the mean and 3.7 is the standard deviation.

Sometimes one finds a reference to an index of variability called the *variance*. The **variance** is simply the value of the standard deviation before a square root has been taken. In other words, variance = SD^2. In our example, the variance is 1.76^2, or 3.11. The variance is rarely reported because it is not in the same unit of measurement as the original data, but it is an important component in inferential statistical tests that we discuss later.

A standard deviation is more difficult to interpret than other statistics, like the mean or range. In our example, we calculated an SD of 1.76. One might well ask, 1.76 *what*? What does the number mean? First, as we already know, the standard deviation is a variability index for a set of scores. If two distributions had a mean of 25.0, but one had an SD of 7.0 and the other had an SD of 3.0, we would immediately know that the second sample was more homogeneous.

Second, think of a standard deviation as an average of deviations from the mean. The mean tells us the single best value for summarizing a distribution; a standard deviation tells us how much, on average, scores deviate from that mean. A standard deviation might thus be interpreted as indicating our degree of error when we use a mean to describe the entire sample.

The standard deviation can also be used to interpret individual scores in a distribution. Suppose we had weight data from a sample whose mean weight was 125.0 pounds with SD = 10.0. The standard deviation provides a *standard* of variability. Weights greater than 1 SD away from the mean (i.e., greater than 135 or less than 115 pounds) are greater than the average variability for that distribution.

In normal and near-normal distributions, there are roughly 3 SDs above and 3 SDs below the mean. To illustrate, suppose we had normally distributed scores with a mean of 50 and an SD of 10 (Fig. 21.7). In a normal distribution, a fixed percentage of cases falls within certain distances from the mean.

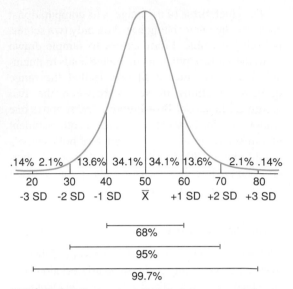

FIGURE 21.7 Standard deviations in a normal distribution.

Sixty-eight percent of cases fall within 1 SD of the mean (34% above and 34% below the mean). In our example, nearly 7 out of 10 scores fall between 40 and 60. Ninety-five percent of scores in a normal distribution fall within 2 SDs from the mean. Only a handful of cases—about 2% at each extreme—lie more than 2 SDs from the mean. In the figure, we can see that a person with a score of 70 had a higher score than about 98% of the sample.

In summary, the SD is a useful variability index for describing a distribution and interpreting individual scores. Like the mean, the standard deviation is a stable estimate of a parameter and is the preferred index of a distribution's variability.

⊃ **TIP:** Descriptive statistics (percentages, means, standard deviations, and so on) are used for various purposes, but are most often used to summarize sample characteristics, describe key research variables, and document methodologic features (e.g., response rates). They are seldom used to answer research questions—inferential statistics (see Chapter 22) are usually used for this purpose. The Toolkit of the accompanying *Resource Manual* includes some table templates for displaying descriptive information.

TABLE 21.5	Example of Descriptive Statistics: Selected Psychosocial Risks and Resources for Low-Income Women		
	N	RANGE OF ACTUAL SCORES	MEAN (SD)
Stress (Prenatal Psychosocial Profile, PPP)	130	11–54	18.3 (5.7)
Depression (Beck Depression Inventory)	128	2–59	13.6 (9.9)
Spirituality (Spiritual Perspective Scale)	130	14–60	48.0 (9.2)
Total social support (PPP scale)	129	13–132	98.8 (30.5)

Adapted from Jesse, D. E., Graham, M., & Swanson, M. (2006). Psychosocial and spiritual factors associated with smoking and substance use during pregnancy in African American and white low-income women. *Journal of Obstetric, Gynecologic, & Neonatal Nursing, 35*(1), 68–77.

Example of descriptive statistics: Table 21.5 presents descriptive statistics based on data from a study of factors associated with smoking and substance use during pregnancy among low-income women (Jesse, Graham, & Swanson, 2006). The table shows, for four psychosocial risk or resource factors, the actual range of scores, the mean score value, and the standard deviation. Based on this information, we can see that the scores were quite heterogeneous, and that the distributions were usually skewed. For example, the mean on the spirituality scale (48.0) was much higher than the midpoint between the lowest and highest values (37.0), indicating a negative skew.

BIVARIATE DESCRIPTIVE STATISTICS

So far we have focused on descriptions of single variables. The mean, mode, standard deviation, and so forth are **univariate** (one-variable) **descriptive statistics** that describe one variable at a time. Most research is about relationships between variables, and **bivariate** (two-variable) **descriptive statistics** describe such relationships. The two most commonly used methods of describing two-variable relationships are through contingency tables and correlation indexes.

Contingency Tables

A **contingency table** (or **crosstab***)* is a two-dimensional frequency distribution in which the frequencies of two variables are *crosstabulated.* Suppose we had data on patients' gender and whether they were nonsmokers, light smokers (<1 pack of cigarettes a day), or heavy smokers (≥1 pack a day). The question is whether there is a tendency for men to smoke more heavily than women, or *vice versa* (i.e., whether there is a relationship between smoking and gender). Fictitious data on these two variables are shown in a contingency table in Table 21.6. Six **cells** are created by placing one variable (gender) along one dimension and the other variable (smoking status) along the other dimension. After subjects' data are allocated to the appropriate cells, percentages are computed. The crosstab allows us to see at a glance that, in this sample, women were more likely than men to be nonsmokers (45.4% versus 27.3%) and less likely to be heavy smokers (18.2% versus 36.4%). Contingency tables usually are used with nominal data or ordinal data that have few ranks. In the present example, gender is a nominal measure, and smoking status, as defined, is an ordinal measure.

TABLE 21.6	Contingency Table for Gender and Smoking Status Relationship					
	GENDER					
	WOMEN		**MEN**		**TOTAL**	
SMOKING STATUS	*n*	%	*n*	%	*n*	%
Nonsmoker	10	45.4	6	27.3	16	36.4
Light smoker	8	36.4	8	36.4	16	36.4
Heavy smoker	4	18.2	8	36.4	12	27.3
TOTAL	22	100.0	22	100.0	44	100.0

Example of a contingency table: Table 21.7 presents a contingency table from an actual study that examined the relationship between degree of psychological distress and the use of psychotropic drugs in a sample of elders from Québec (Voyer et al., 2003). Overall, 15.3% of the sample of more than 3000 elders reported using an anxiolytic, sedative, or hypnotic (ASH) drug; 5.9% reported being in high psychological distress. About one third (33.4%) of those in high distress reported using an ASH drug, compared with only 8.9% of those in low distress.

A comparison of Tables 21.6 and 21.7 illustrates that crosstabulated data can be presented in two ways: Percentages for each cell can be computed based on either row totals or column totals. In Table 21.6, the number 10 in the first cell (non-smoking women) was divided by the *column* total (i.e., total number of women—22) to arrive at the percentage of women who were nonsmokers (45.4%). The table *could* have shown 62.5% in this cell—the percentage of nonsmokers who were women (10 ÷ 16). In Table 21.7, the number 81 in the first cell was divided by the row total of 915 (i.e., the number of elders in low distress) to yield 8.9%—the percentage of those in low distress who are ASH users. Computed the other way, the researchers would have gotten 17.6% (81 + 461)—the percentage of ASH drug users who were in low distress. Either approach is acceptable, but

the former is sometimes preferred because then the column percentages add up to 100%. Readers of reports need to determine which method was used to understand the findings.

Correlation

Relationships between two variables are usually described through **correlation** procedures. Correlation coefficients, briefly described in Chapter 17, can be computed with two variables measured on either the ordinal, interval, or ratio scale. The correlation question is: To what extent are two variables related to each other? For example, to what degree are anxiety scores and blood pressure readings related? This question can be answered graphically or by calculating an index that describes the *magnitude* and *direction* of the relationship.

Correlations between two variables can be graphed on a **scatter plot** (*scatter diagram*) using a coordinate graph with the two variables laid out at right angles. Values for one variable (X) are scaled on the horizontal axis, and values for the second variable (Y) are scaled vertically, as shown in Figure 21.8. This graph presents data for 10 subjects (a–j). For subject *a*, the values for X and Y are 2 and 1, respectively. To graph subject *a*'s position, we go two units to the right along the X axis, and one unit up on the Y axis. This procedure is

TABLE 21.7	Example of a Contingency Table: Psychological Distress and Consumption of Anxiolytic, Sedative, and Hypnotic (ASH) Drugs in the Elderly						
	CONSUMPTION OF ASH DRUGS						
	Consumption		**No Consumption**		**TOTAL**		
DEGREE OF PSYCHOLOGICAL DISTRESS	**n**	**%**	**n**	**%**	**N**	**%**	
Low	81	8.9	834	91.1	915	30.4	
Intermediate	320	16.7	1599	83.3	1919	63.7	
High	60	33.6	118	66.5	178	5.9	
Total	461	15.3	2551	84.7	3012	100.0	

Calculations and adaptations from Voyer, P., McCubbin, M., Preville, M., & Boyer, R. (2003). Factors in duration of anxiolytic, sedative, and hypnotic drug use in the elderly. *Canadian Journal of Nursing Research, 35*(4), 126–149.

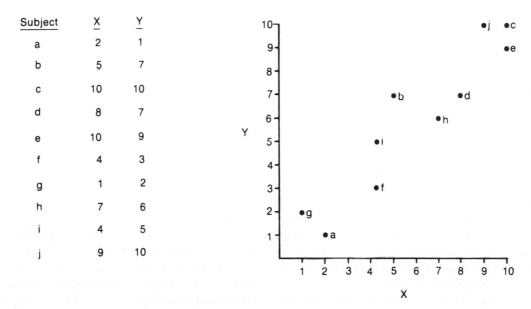

Subject	X	Y
a	2	1
b	5	7
c	10	10
d	8	7
e	10	9
f	4	3
g	1	2
h	7	6
i	4	5
j	9	10

FIGURE 21.8 Construction of a scatter plot.

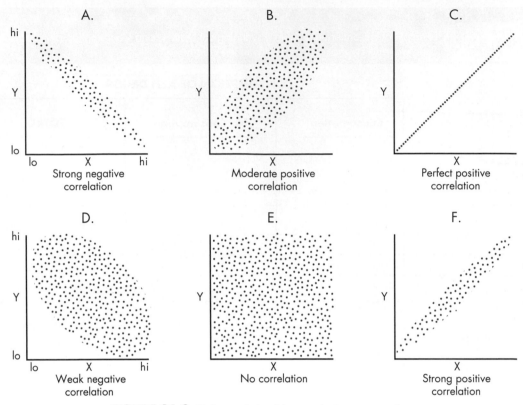

FIGURE 21.9 Various relationships graphed on scatter plots.

followed for all subjects. The letters on the plot are shown to help identify subjects, but normally only dots appear.

In a scatter plot, the direction of the slope of points indicates the direction of the correlation. As noted in Chapter 17, a positive correlation occurs when high values on one variable are associated with high values on a second variable. If the slope of points begins at the lower left corner and extends to the upper right corner, the relationship is positive. In the current example, X and Y are positively related. People with high scores on variable X tended to have high scores on variable Y, and low scorers on X tended to score low on Y.

A negative (or inverse) relationship is one in which high values on one variable are related to low values on the other. Negative relationships on a scatter plot are depicted by points that slope from the upper left corner to the lower right corner, as in Figure 21.9A and D.

When relationships are perfect, it is possible to predict perfectly the value of one variable by knowing the value of the second. For instance, if all people who were 6 feet, 2 inches tall weighed 180 pounds, and all people who were 6 feet, 1 inch tall weighed 175 pounds, and so on, then weight and height would be perfectly, positively related. In such a situation, we would only need to know a person's height to know his or her weight, or *vice versa*. On a scatter plot, a perfect relationship is represented by a sloped straight line, as in Figure 21.9C. When a relationship is not perfect, as is usually the case, one can interpret the *degree* of correlation by seeing how closely the points cluster around a straight line. The more closely packed the points are around a diagonal slope, the stronger the correlation. When the points are scattered all over the graph, the relationship is low or nonexistent. Various degrees and directions of relationships are presented in Figure 21.9.

It is more efficient to express relationships by computing a correlation coefficient, an index with values ranging from -1.00 for a perfect negative correlation, through zero for no relationship, to $+1.00$ for a perfect positive correlation. All correlations that fall between .00 and -1.00 are negative, and ones that fall between .00 and $+1.00$ are positive. The higher the absolute value of the coefficient (i.e., the value disregarding the sign), the stronger the relationship. A correlation of $-.80$, for instance, is much stronger than a correlation of $+.20$.

The most widely used correlation index is the **product–moment correlation coefficient**, also referred to as **Pearson's r**. This coefficient is computed with variables measured on either an interval or ratio scale. The correlation index usually used for ordinal-level measures is **Spearman's rho (ρ)**. The calculation of these correlation statistics is laborious and seldom performed by hand. (Computational formulas are available in statistics textbooks, such as those by Munro [2004] or Polit [1996].)

It is difficult to offer guidelines on what to interpret as strong or weak relationships because it depends on the variables in question. If we measured patients' body temperatures orally and rectally, a correlation (r) of .70 between the two measurements would be low. For most psychosocial variables (e.g., stress and severity of illness), an r of .70 is high; correlations between such variables are typically in the .20 to .40 range. Perfect correlations ($+1.00$ and -1.00) are rare.

Correlation coefficients are often reported in tables displaying a two-dimensional **correlation matrix**, in which every variable is displayed in both a row and a column and coefficients are displayed at the intersections. An example of a correlation matrix is presented at the end of this chapter.

> **TIP:** Many of the statistics discussed in this chapter *can* be used for inferential as well as descriptive purposes, as we discuss in the next chapter.

DESCRIBING RISK

The evidence-based practice (EBP) movement has made clinical decision making based on research findings an important issue. There are a number of descriptive statistical indexes that can be used to interpret findings and facilitate such decision making. These indexes reflect the growing realization that risks (and risk reduction) must be interpreted within a context. If an intervention reduces the risk for an adverse event three times over, but the initial risk is miniscule, the intervention may have too high a cost/benefit ratio to be practical. Both absolute change and relative change in risks are important in clinical decision making.

The indexes described in this section are often not reported in journals articles, but rather must be calculated by potential users of research information. We suspect that increasing numbers of researchers will be presenting such calculations in their reports in the years ahead. Further information about the use and interpretation of these indexes can be found in the books by DiCenso, Guyatt, and Ciliska (2005) and Guyatt and Rennie (2002).

The focus in this section is on describing dichotomous outcomes (e.g., alive/dead, had a fall/did not have a fall) in relation to exposure versus nonexposure to a treatment. This situation results in a 2 × 2 contingency table with four cells, as depicted in Table 21.8. Methods to capture effects for continuous outcomes are discussed in the next chapter.

Table 21.8 labels the four cells in the contingency table so that computations for the various indexes can be explained. *Cell a* is the number with an undesirable outcome (e.g., death) in an intervention group; *cell b* is the number with a desirable outcome (e.g., survival) in an intervention group; and *cells c* and *d* are the two outcome possibilities for a nontreated (control) group. We can now

| TABLE 21.8 | Indexes of Risk and Association in a 2 × 2 Table for an Intervention Study |

EXPOSURE TO AN INTERVENTION	OUTCOME		TOTAL
	Yes (Undesirable Outcome)	**No** (Desirable Outcome)	
Yes (Exposed to the intervention)	a	b	a + b
No (Not exposed to the intervention)	c	d	c + d
TOTAL	a + c	b + d	a + b + c + d

Absolute risk, exposed group (AR_E) $= a/(a + b)$

Absolute risk, non-exposed group (AR_{NE}) $= c/(c + d)$

Absolute risk reduction (ARR) $= (c/(c + d)) - (a/(a + b))$ or $AR_{NE} - AR_E$

Relative risk (RR) $= \dfrac{a/(a + b)}{c/(c + d)}$ or $\dfrac{AR_E}{AR_{NE}}$

Relative risk reduction (RRR) $= \dfrac{(c/(c + d)) - (a/(a + b))}{c/(c + d)}$ or $\dfrac{ARR}{AR_{NE}}$

Odds ratio (OR) $= \dfrac{ad}{bc}$ or $\dfrac{a/b}{c/d}$

Number needed to treat $= \dfrac{1}{(c/(c + d)) - (a/(a + b))}$ or $\dfrac{1}{ARR}$

explain the meaning and calculation of several indexes that are of particular interest to clinicians.

TIP: Note that the computations shown in Table 21.8 specifically reflect *risk* indexes that assume that the intervention exposure will be beneficial, and that information for the *undesirable* outcome (risk) will be in cells a and c. If good outcomes rather than risks were put in cells a and c, the formula would have to be modified. For example, AR_E would then be b/(a + b), and so on. Similarly, if the research question involved the association between an adverse event and a hypothesized risk factor (e.g., the risk that high cholesterol is associated with a cardiovascular accident), the group exposed to the risk factor (e.g., those with high cholesterol) should be in the *bottom* row (cells c and d) and not the top row—or, again, the formulas would need

to be adapted. As a general rule, to use the formulas shown in Table 21.8, the cell in the lower left corner (cell c) should be expected to reflect the highest frequency of undesirable outcomes.

Absolute Risk

Absolute risk can be computed for both those exposed to an intervention or risk factor, and for those not exposed. **Absolute risk** is simply the proportion of people who experienced an undesirable outcome in each group. We illustrate this and other indexes with fictitious data from a hypothetical intervention study in which 200 smokers were randomly assigned to a smoking cessation intervention or to a control group (Table 21.9). Smoking status 3 months

TABLE 21.9	Hypothetical Data for Smoking Cessation Example			
EXPOSURE TO SMOKING CESSATION INTERVENTION	**OUTCOME**			**TOTAL**
	Continued Smoking	**Stopped Smoking**		
Yes, exposed (experimental group)	50	50		100
No, not exposed (control group)	80	20		100
TOTAL	130	70		200

Absolute risk, exposed group (AR_E) $= 50/100 = .50$
Absolute risk, non-exposed group (AR_{NE}) $= 80/100 = .80$
Absolute risk reduction (ARR) $= .80 - .50 = .30$
Relative risk (RR) $- .50/.80 - .625$
Relative risk reduction (RRR) $= .30/.80 = .375$
Odds ratio (OR) $= \dfrac{(50/50)}{(80/20)} = .25$
Number needed to treat $= 1/.30 = 3.33$

after the intervention is the outcome variable. In this example, the absolute risk of continued smoking was .50 in the intervention group and .80 in the control group. The risk for an undesirable outcome for a treatment group is sometimes called the *experimental event rate (EER),* and the risk for an adverse outcome for untreated (or unexposed) people is sometimes referred to as the *baseline risk rate,* or the *control event rate (CER).* In the absence of the intervention, 20% of those in the experimental group would presumably have stopped smoking anyway, but the intervention boosted the rate to 50%.

Absolute Risk Reduction

The **absolute risk reduction (ARR)**, which is sometimes called the *risk difference* or *RD,* represents a comparison of the two risks. It is computed by subtracting the absolute risk for the treated group from the absolute risk for the untreated group. This index indicates the estimated proportion of people who

would be spared from the undesirable outcome through exposure to the intervention. In our example, the value of ARR is .30: 30% of the control group subjects would presumably have stopped smoking if they had received the intervention, over and above the 20% who stopped without the intervention.

Relative Risk

The index called **relative risk (RR)**, or the *risk ratio*, represents the estimated proportion of the original risk for an adverse outcome (in our example, continued smoking) that persists when people are exposed to the intervention. To compute an RR, the absolute risk for exposed subjects is divided by the absolute risk for nonexposed subjects. In our fictitious example, the RR is .625. This means that the risk for continued smoking after the smoking cessation intervention is estimated to be 62.5% of what it would have been in its absence.

Relative Risk Reduction

Another useful index for evaluating the effectiveness of an intervention is the **relative risk reduction (RRR)**. The RRR is the estimated proportion of baseline (untreated) risk that is reduced through exposure to the intervention. This index is computed by dividing the ARR by the absolute risk for the control group. In our example, RRR = .375. This means that the smoking cessation intervention decreased the relative risk for continued smoking by 37.5%, compared with not having had the intervention.

Odds Ratio

The **odds ratio (OR)** is the most widely reported index among those described in this section, even though it is less intuitively meaningful than an index of risk. The **odds**, in this context, is the proportion of subjects *with* the adverse outcome relative to those *without* it. In our example, the odds of continued smoking for the experimental group is 50 (the number who continued smoking) divided by 50 (the number who stopped), or 1. The odds for the control group is 80 divided by 20, or 4. The **odds ratio** is the ratio of these two odds, or .25 in our example. The estimated odds of continuing to smoke are one fourth as high among those in the intervention group as among those in the control group. Turned around, we could say that the estimated odds of continued smoking are 4 times higher among smokers who do not get the intervention as among those who do.

➔ TIP: Odds ratios can be computed when the independent variable is not dichotomous, using a statistical procedure described in Chapter 23. For example, we could estimate the odds ratio for obesity among adults in four different age groups (26 to 35, 36 to 45, 46 to 55, and 56 to 65), using one of the groups as a reference.

Number Needed to Treat

One final index of interest in the current EBP environment is the **number needed to treat (NNT)**, which represents an estimate of how many people would need to receive a treatment or intervention to prevent one undesirable outcome. The NNT is computed by dividing 1 by the value of the absolute risk reduction. In our example, ARR = .30, and so NNT is 3.33. About three smokers would need to be exposed to the intervention to avoid one person's continued smoking. The NNT is inversely related to the RRR. An intervention that is twice as effective with regard to relative risk reduction will cut the number needed to treat in half. The NNT is especially valuable for decision makers because it can be integrated with monetary information to determine whether an intervention is cost-effective.

Example of RR, OR, and NNT: Downe, Gerrett, and Renfrew (2004) conducted a clinical trial to estimate whether the rate of instrumental birth in nulliparous women using epidural analgesia is affected by the mother's position during the second stage of labor. A sample of 107 women was randomized to either the lateral position or a supported sitting position. Lateral position was associated with lower rates of instrumental birth: lateral group, 33%, versus sitting group, 52%. The RR was .64, the NNT was 5, and the OR was 2.2. The rate for episiotomies was also lower in the lateral position group, with RR = .66 and NNT = 5.

➔ TIP: Various tools are available on the Internet to facilitate the calculation of indexes described in this section, including the website for the Centre for Evidence-Based Medicine's EBM toolbox (*http://www.cebm.net/toolbox.asp*) and the University of British Columbia's Clinical Significance Calculator (*http://www.healthcare.ubc.ca/calc/clinsig.html*). These and other useful websites are available on the accompanying student CD-ROM for you to click on directly.

THE COMPUTER AND DESCRIPTIVE STATISTICS

Researchers almost invariably use a computer to calculate statistics. This section aims to familiarize you with printouts from a widely used computer program called Statistical Package for the Social Sciences (SPSS).

TABLE 21.10	Fictitious Data on Law-Income Pregnant Adolescents				
GROUP*	INFANT BIRTH WEIGHT	REPEAT PREGNANCY †	MOTHER'S AGE (YEARS)	NO. OF PRIOR PREGNANCIES	SMOKING STATUS ‡
1	107	1	17	1	1
1	101	0	14	0	0
1	119	0	21	3	0
1	128	1	20	2	0
1	89	0	15	1	1
1	99	0	19	0	1
1	111	0	19	1	0
1	117	1	18	1	1
1	102	1	17	0	0
1	120	0	20	0	0
1	76	0	13	0	1
1	116	0	18	0	1
1	100	1	16	0	0
1	115	0	18	0	0
1	113	0	21	2	1
2	111	1	19	0	0
2	108	0	21	1	0
2	95	0	19	2	1
2	99	0	17	0	1
2	103	1	19	0	0
2	94	0	15	0	1
2	101	1	17	1	0
2	114	0	21	2	0
2	97	0	20	1	0
2	99	1	18	0	1
2	113	0	18	0	1
2	89	0	19	1	0
2	98	0	20	0	0
2	102	0	17	0	0
2	105	0	19	1	1

*Group: 1 = experimental; 2 = control.
†Repeat pregnancy: 1 = yes; 0 = no.
‡Smoking status: 1 = smokes; 0 = does not smoke.

Suppose we were evaluating the effectiveness of an intervention for low-income pregnant adolescents. The intervention is a program of intensive health care, nutrition education, and contraceptive counseling. Thirty pregnant young women are randomly assigned to either the special program or routine care. Two key outcomes are infant birth weight and repeat pregnancy within 18 months of delivery. Fictitious data are presented in Table 21.10.

Figure 21.10 presents information from an SPSS frequency distribution printout for infant birth weight. Several descriptive statistics are shown first. The *Mean* is 104.7, the *Median* is 102.5, and the *Mode* is 99, suggesting a modestly skewed distribution. The SD (*Std Deviation*) is 10.9549, and the *Variance* is 120.0103 (10.9549^2). The *Range* is 52, which is equal to the *Maximum* of 128 minus the *Minimum* of 76.

The frequency distribution is shown in the second panel. Each birth weight is listed in the first column, from the low value of 76 to the high value of 128. The next column, *Frequency*, shows the number of occurrences of each birth weight. There was one 76-ounce baby, two 89-ounce babies, and so on. The next column, *Percent*, indicates the percentage of infants in each birth-weight category: 3.3% weighed 76 ounces, 6.7% weighed 89 ounces, and so on. The next column, *Valid Percent*, indicates the percentage in each category after removing any missing values. In this example, birth weights were obtained for all 30 infants, but if one birth weight had been missing, the valid percent for the 76-ounce baby would have been 3.4% (1 ÷ 29 rather than 30). The last column, *Cumulative Percent*, adds the percentage for a given birth-weight value to the percentage for all preceding values. Thus, we can tell by looking at the row for 99 ounces that, cumulatively, 33.3% of the babies weighed less than 100 ounces.

Many computer programs also produce graphs. Figure 21.11 shows a histogram for maternal age. The age values (ranging from 13 to 21) are on the horizontal axis, and frequencies are on the vertical axis. The histogram shows at a glance that the modal age is 19 ($f = 7$) and that age is negatively skewed (i.e., there are fewer very young mothers). Descriptive statistics to the left of the histogram indicate that the mean age for this group is 18.1667, with an SD of 2.0858.

If we wanted to compare the repeat-pregnancy rate of experimental versus control group mothers, we would instruct the computer to crosstabulate the two variables, as shown in the contingency table in Figure 21.12. This crosstabulation resulted in four main cells: (1) experimental subjects with no repeat pregnancy (upper left cell); (2) control subjects with no repeat pregnancy; (3) experimental subjects with a repeat pregnancy; and (4) control subjects with a repeat pregnancy. Each cell contains four pieces of information. The first is number of subjects in the cell (*Count*). In the first cell, 10 experimental subjects did not have a repeat pregnancy within 18 months of delivery. Below the 10 is the *row* percentage or *% within Repeat pregnancy*: 47.6% of the women who did not become pregnant again were experimental subjects (10 ÷ 21). The next entry is the *column* percentage or *% within GROUP*: 66.7% of the experimental subjects did not become pregnant (10 ÷ 15). Last is the *overall* percentage of the sample who were in that cell (10 ÷ 30 = 33.3%). Thus, Figure 21.12 indicates that a somewhat higher percentage of experimental (33.3%) than control subjects (26.7%) had an early repeat pregnancy. The row totals on the far right indicate that, overall, 30.0% of the sample ($N = 9$) had a subsequent pregnancy. The column totals at the bottom indicate that 50.0% of the subjects were in the experimental group, and 50.0% were in the control group.

CRITIQUING DESCRIPTIVE STATISTICS

Descriptive statistics help to set the stage for understanding quantitative research evidence. Descriptive statistics are particularly useful for communicating information about the study sample. Readers of a report cannot draw inferences about the external validity of the study without understanding who the participants were, especially with regard to key demographic characteristics and health-related attributes.

In addition to describing sample characteristics, descriptive statistics are useful in communicating information about the baseline values of key outcome variables in longitudinal or intervention studies, or correlations between a set of independent variables. Methodologic features that help readers with inferences about study quality also typically rely on descriptive statistics—for example, response rates and attrition rates are typically shown as percentages, and means are used to characterize such things as time elapsed between two interviews or average time

Frequencies

Statistics

Infant birth weight in ounces

N	Valid	30
	Missing	0
Mean		104.7000
Median		102.5000
Mode		99.00
Std. Deviation		10.9549
Variance		120.0103
Range		52.00
Minimum		76.00
Maximum		128.00
Percentiles	25	98.7500
	50	102.5000
	75	113.2500

Infant birth weight in ounces

		Frequency	Percent	Valid Percent	Cumulative Percent
Valid	76.00	1	3.3	3.3	3.3
	89.00	2	6.7	6.7	10.0
	94.00	1	3.3	3.3	13.3
	95.00	1	3.3	3.3	16.7
	97.00	1	3.3	3.3	20.0
	98.00	1	3.3	3.3	23.3
	99.00	3	10.0	10.0	33.3
	100.00	1	3.3	3.3	36.7
	101.00	2	6.7	6.7	43.3
	102.00	2	6.7	6.7	50.0
	103.00	1	3.3	3.3	53.3
	105.00	1	3.3	3.3	56.7
	107.00	1	3.3	3.3	60.0
	108.00	1	3.3	3.3	63.3
	111.00	2	6.7	6.7	70.0
	113.00	2	6.7	6.7	76.7
	114.00	1	3.3	3.3	80.0
	115.00	1	3.3	3.3	83.3
	116.00	1	3.3	3.3	86.7
	117.00	1	3.3	3.3	90.0
	119.00	1	3.3	3.3	93.3
	120.00	1	3.3	3.3	96.7
	128.00	1	3.3	3.3	100.0
	Total	30	100.0	100.0	

FIGURE 21.10 Frequency distribution printout for infant birth weight.

Frequencies

Statistics

Mother's age

N	Valid	30
	Missing	0
Mean		18.1667
Median		18.5000
Mode		19.00
Std. Deviation		2.0858
Variance		4.3506
Range		8.00
Minimum		13.00
Maximum		21.00

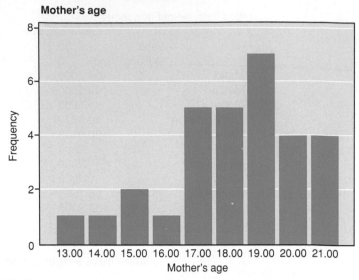

FIGURE 21.11 Histogram for maternal age.

to administer an interview. These purposes all require researchers to consider the readers' informational needs for drawing inferences about study validity.

Descriptive statistics are sometimes used to directly address research questions in studies that are primarily descriptive—as illustrated in the research example at the end of this chapter. However, when only descriptive statistics are presented, readers should think about whether the inclusion of inferential statistics would have been appropriate.

				GROUP	
			Experimental	Control	Total
Repeat pregnancy	No	Count	10	11	21
		% within Repeat pregnancy	47.6%	52.4%	100.0%
		% within GROUP	66.7%	73.3%	70.0%
		% of Total	33.3%	36.7%	70.0%
	Yes	Count	5	4	9
		% within Repeat pregnancy	55.6%	44.4%	100.0%
		% within GROUP	33.3%	26.7%	30.0%
		% of Total	16.7%	13.3%	30.0%
Total		Count	15	15	30
		% within Repeat pregnancy	50.0%	50.0%	100.0%
		% within GROUP	100.0%	100.0%	100.0%
		% of Total	50.0%	50.0%	100.0%

FIGURE 21.12 Crosstabulation of repeat pregnancy by group.

BOX 21.1 Guidelines for Critiquing Descriptive Statistics

1. Did the report include descriptive statistics? Do these statistics sufficiently describe the major characteristics of the data set?
2. Were descriptive statistics used appropriately—for example, were descriptive statistics used to describe the sample, the key variables, and methodologic features of the study, such as response rate or attrition rate? Were they used to answer research questions when inferential statistics would have been more appropriate?
3. Were the correct descriptive statistics used—for example, was a mean presented when percentages would have been more informative? Was the mean used without information about the median even though the distribution was severely skewed?
4. Was the descriptive information presented in a useful format—for example, were tables used effectively? Is information in the text and the tables redundant? Were the tables clear, with a good title and carefully labeled headings?
5. Were any risk indexes computed? If not, should they have been, to increase the clinical utility of the findings?

In critiquing the researcher's use of descriptive statistics, readers can consider whether the information was adequate, whether the correct statistical indexes were used, and whether the information was presented in a useful, efficient, and comprehensible manner. Box 21.1 ⊗ presents some guiding questions for critiquing the descriptive statistics in a research report.

RESEARCH EXAMPLE

Study: "Family caregiving in heart failure" (Bakas et al., 2006)

Statement of Purpose: The purpose of this study was to describe family caregiving in the context of heart failure. Specific aims included describing the tasks and outcomes caregivers perceived as most difficult, describing their perceptions of control over managing heart problems, and examining relationships among caregiver perceptions.

Methods: The study design was nonexperimental and cross-sectional. The researchers recruited a convenience sample of 21 caregivers, who were family members providing unpaid care to patients diagnosed as having heart failure. Data were collected from the family caregivers by means of a self-administered questionnaire completed during a regularly scheduled visit for the patients. The questionnaires included several scales designed to mea-

sure such constructs as perceived control, perceived difficulty with tasks, perceived outcomes, and perceived mental and general health.

Analysis and Findings: Because this study was primarily descriptive, a rich array of descriptive information was presented. Sample characteristics were described in the text. For example, it was reported that the mean age of caregivers was 59.6, with an SD of 9.1 years and a range from 45 to 76 years. A few caregivers (14%) were employed full time, and 24% said they had quit their job to provide care. One table (Table 4) listed 17 tasks that caregivers rated for perceived difficulty, and for each task, the table listed the mean rating, standard deviation, range of responses, and percentage who rated the difficulty greater than 2 on a 5-point scale (3 = moderately difficult, 4 = very difficult, 5 = extremely difficult). For example, household chores such as cleaning had a mean rating of 2.2 (1.3), and 47.6% of the sample rated this task higher than 2.

Another table presented a correlation matrix for correlations among various caregiver variables. Spearman rho coefficients were computed, perhaps reflecting the researchers' view that their scale scores were ordinal rather than interval measures—or perhaps because of their small sample size. An adapted version of this matrix is presented in Table 21.11.* This table lists, on the left, six variables: caregivers' age (variable 1), and their various perceptions (variables 2 through 6). The numbers in

*Although we present only descriptive information, Bakas and her colleagues also applied inferential statistics.

| TABLE 21.11 | Spearman Rho Correlation Matrix for Key Study Variables: Caregiver Age and Perceptions |

VARIABLE	1	2	3	4	5	6
1 Caregiver age	1.00					
2 Perceived control	−.07	1.00				
3 Perceived difficulty with tasks	−.60	−.25	1.00			
4 Perceived outcomes	.34	.21	−.46	1.00		
5 Perceived mental health	.43	.44	−.51	.66	1.00	
6 Perceived general health	.13	−.12	−.14	.15	.44	1.00

Adapted from Bakas, T., Pressler, S., Johnson, E., Nauser, J., & Shaneyfelt, T. (2006). Family caregiving in heart failure. *Nursing Research, 55*(3), 184, Table 2.

the top row, from 1 to 6, correspond to the six variables: 1 is the caregivers' age, and so on. The correlation matrix shows, in the first column, the correlation coefficient between age with all six variables. At the intersection of row 1 and column 1, we find the value 1.00, which simply indicates that age values are perfectly correlated with themselves. The next entry in the first column is the correlation between age and perceived control. The value of −.07 indicates a very modest negative relationship between these two variables, but the next entry (−.60) indicates a fairly strong negative relationship between age and perceived difficulty with tasks: the older the caregiver, the *less* difficult they perceived their caregiving tasks. The strongest relationship in the matrix is the negative correlation between caregivers' perceived mental health and perceived outcomes—that is, how much they believed their lives had changed since assuming the caregiving role. As the coefficient of −.66 indicates, the more the caregivers viewed their lives as having changed, the lower their scores on the mental health indicator. Older caregivers perceived their mental health to be better than younger ones (.43), but age was weakly related to perceived general health (.13).

SUMMARY POINTS

- There are four **levels of measurement**: (1) **nominal measurement**—the classification of

characteristics into mutually exclusive categories; (2) **ordinal measurement**—the ranking of objects based on their relative standing to each other on an attribute; (3) **interval measurement**—indicating not only the ranking of objects but also the amount of distance between them; and (4) **ratio measurement**—distinguished from interval measurement by having a rational zero point.

- **Descriptive statistics** enable researchers to summarize and describe quantitative data.

- In **frequency distributions**, which impose order on raw data, numeric values are ordered from lowest to highest, accompanied by a count of the number (or percentage) of times each value was obtained.

- **Histograms** and **frequency polygons** are two common methods of displaying frequency information graphically.

- Data for a variable can be completely described in terms of the shape of the distribution, central tendency, and variability.

- A distribution is **symmetric** if its two halves are mirror images of each other. A **skewed distribution**, by contrast, is asymmetric, with one tail longer than the other.

- In a **positively skewed distribution**, the long tail points to the right (e.g., personal income); in a **negatively skewed distribution**, the long tail points to the left (e.g., age at death).

- The **modality** of a distribution refers to the number of peaks present: A **unimodal distribution** has one peak, and a **multimodal distribution** has more than one peak.

- A **normal distribution** (or *Gaussian distribution, bell-shaped curve*) is symmetric, unimodal, and not too peaked.

- Measures of **central tendency** are indexes, expressed as a single number, that represent the average or typical value of a set of scores. The **mode** is the value that occurs most frequently in the distribution; the **median** is the point above which and below which 50% of the cases fall; and the **mean** is the arithmetic average of all scores. The mean is usually the preferred measure of central tendency because of its *stability*.

- Measures of **variability**—how spread out the data are—include the range and standard deviation. The **range** is the distance between the highest and lowest scores. The **standard deviation** indicates how much, on average, scores deviate from the mean.

- The standard deviation (SD) is calculated by first computing **deviation scores**, which represent the degree to which each person's score deviates from the mean. The **variance** is equal to the standard deviation squared. In a normal distribution, 95% of all scores fall within 2 SDs above and below the mean.

- **Bivariate descriptive statistics** describe relationships between two variables.

- A **contingency table** is a two-dimensional frequency distribution in which the frequencies of two nominal- or ordinal-level variables are crosstabulated.

- Correlation coefficients describe the direction and magnitude of a relationship between two variables, and range from −1.00 (perfect negative correlation) through .00 to +1.00 (perfect positive correlation).

- The most frequently used correlation coefficient is the **product–moment correlation coefficient** (**Pearson's** *r*), used with interval- or ratio-level variables. The **Spearman rho coefficient** is used with ordinal-level variables.

- Graphically, the relationship between two variables can be displayed on a **scatter plot** or scatter diagram.

- Statistical indexes have been developed to describe risks and the magnitude of intervention effects, including many that are appropriate for a two-group (e.g., experimental versus control) situation with dichotomous outcomes (e.g., alive/dead). These indexes have gained prominence as a result of the EBP movement because they provide useful information for making clinical decisions.

- The **absolute risk reduction (ARR)** expresses the estimated proportion of people who would be spared from an adverse outcome through exposure to an intervention. **Relative risk (RR)** is the estimated proportion of the original risk for an adverse outcome that persists among people exposed to the intervention. **Relative risk reduction (RRR)** is the estimated proportion of untreated risk that is reduced through exposure to the intervention. The **odds ratio (OR)** is the ratio of the odds for the treated versus untreated group, with the *odds* reflecting the proportion of people with the adverse outcome relative to those without it. Finally, the **number needed to treat (NNT)** is an estimate of how many people would need to receive the intervention to prevent one adverse outcome.

⬤◗◯◗◯◗◯◗◯◗◯◗◯◗◯◗◯◗◯◗◯

STUDY ACTIVITIES

Chapter 21 of the accompanying *Resource Manual for Nursing Research: Generating and Assessing Evidence for Nursing Practice, 8th edition*, offers various exercises and study suggestions for reinforcing concepts presented in this chapter. In addition, the following study questions can be addressed:

1. What are the mean, median, and mode for the following set of data?

13 12 9 15 7 10 16 9 6 10

Compute the range and standard deviation.

2. Suppose that 400 subjects (200 per group) were in the intervention study described in connection with Table 21.9, and that 60% of those in the experimental group and 90% of those in the control group continued smoking. Compute the various risk indexes for this scenario.

3. Apply relevant questions in Box 21.1 to the research example at the end of the chapter (Bakas et al., 2006), referring to the full journal article as necessary.

⬤⬤⬤⬤⬤⬤⬤⬤⬤⬤⬤⬤⬤⬤⬤⬤⬤⬤⬤⬤

STUDIES CITED IN CHAPTER 21

Methodologic or theoretical references cited in this chapter can be found in a separate section at the end of the book.

Bakas, T., Pressler, S., Johnson, E., Nauser, J., & Shaneyfelt, T. (2006). Family caregiving in heart failure. *Nursing Research, 55*(3), 180–188.

Bastani, F., Hidarnia, A., Montgomery, K., Aguilar-Vafaei, M., Kazamnejad, A. (2006). Does relaxation education in anxious primigravid Iranian women influence adverse pregnancy outcomes? A random-ized controlled trial. *Journal of Perinatal & Neonatal Nursing, 20*(2), 138–146.

Chen, Y., & Narsavage, G. (2006). Factors related to chronic obstructive pulmonary disease readmission in Taiwan. *Western Journal of Nursing Research, 28*(1), 105–124.

Downe, S., Gerrett, D., & Renfrew, M. (2004). A prospective randomized trial on the effect of position in the passive second stage of labour on birth outcomes in nulliparous women using epidural analgesia. *Midwifery, 20*(2), 157–168.

Jesse, D. E., Graham, M., & Swanson, M. (2006). Psychosocial and spiritual factors associated with smoking and substance use during pregnancy in African American and white low-income women. *Journal of Obstetric, Gynecologic, & Neonatal Nursing, 35*(1), 68–77.

Miller, A., Sorokin, O., Wang, E., Feetham, S., Choi, M., & Wilbur, J. (2006). Acculturation, social alienation, and depressed mood in midlife women from the former Soviet Union. *Research in Nursing & Health, 29*(2), 134–146.

Shin, Y., Yun, S., Jang, H., & Lim, J. (2006). A tailored program for the promotion of physical exercise among Korean adults with chronic diseases. *Applied Nursing Research, 19*(2), 88–94.

Voyer, P., McCubbin, M., Preville, M., & Boyer, R. (2003). Factors in duration of anxiolytic, sedative, and hypnotic drug use in the elderly. *Canadian Journal of Nursing Research, 35*(4), 126–149.

22

Using Inferential Statistics to Test Hypotheses

R esearchers usually want to do more than *describe* their data. **Inferential statistics,** which are based on the **laws of probability,** provide a means for drawing conclusions about a population, given data from a sample. Inferential statistics would help us with such questions as, "What do I know about 3-minute Apgar scores of premature babies (the population) after learning that the mean Apgar score in a sample of 300 premature babies was 7.5?"

Researchers use inferential statistics to estimate population parameters from sample statistics. Probabilistic estimates involve some error, but inferential statistics provide a framework for making objective judgments about their reliability. Different researchers applying inferential statistics to the same data are likely to draw the same conclusions.

SAMPLING DISTRIBUTIONS

To estimate population parameters, it is clearly advisable to use representative samples, and probability samples are the best way to get representative samples (see Chapter 13). Inferential statistics are based on the assumption of random sampling from populations, an assumption that is widely violated. The validity of statistical calculations does depend,

however, on the extent to which the results from the sample are similar to what you would have obtained had you been able to randomly select subjects from the population.

Even when random sampling *is* used, sample characteristics are seldom identical to population characteristics. Suppose we had a population of 50,000 nursing school applicants whose mean score on a standardized entrance exam was 500 with a standard deviation (SD) of 100. Suppose we had to estimate these parameters from the scores of a random sample of 25 students. Would we expect a mean of *exactly* 500 and an SD of 100 for this sample? Obtaining the exact population value is unlikely. Let us say the sample mean is 505. If a new random sample were drawn, we might obtain a mean value such as 497. The tendency for statistics to fluctuate from one sample to another reflects **sampling error**. The challenge for researchers is to determine whether sample values are good estimates of population parameters.

Researchers compute statistics with only *one* sample, but to understand inferential statistics, we must perform a mental exercise. Consider drawing a sample of 25 students from the population of 50,000, calculating a mean, replacing the students, and drawing a new sample. Each mean is considered one datum. If we drew 10,000 such samples, we would have 10,000 means (data points) that

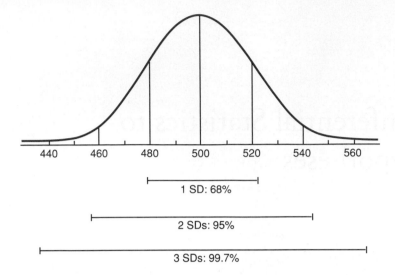

440   460   480   500   520   540   560

├─────── 1 SD: 68% ───────┤

├─────────────── 2 SDs: 95% ───────────────┤

├─────────────────────── 3 SDs: 99.7% ───────────────────────┤

FIGURE 22.1 Sampling distribution.

could be used to construct a frequency polygon (Fig. 22.1). This distribution is a **sampling distribution of the mean**. A sampling distribution is a theoretical rather than actual distribution because in practice no one draws consecutive samples from a population and plots their means. Theoretical distributions are the basis of inferential statistics.

Characteristics of Sampling Distributions

When an infinite number of samples is drawn from a population, the sampling distribution of the mean has certain characteristics. (Our example of 10,000 samples is large enough to approximate these characteristics.) Sampling distributions of means are normally distributed, and the mean of a sampling distribution with an infinite number of sample means always equals the population mean. In the example shown in Figure 22.1, the mean of the sampling distribution is 500, the same as the population mean.

Remember that when data are normally distributed, 68% of values fall within ±1 SD from the mean. Because a sampling distribution of means is normally distributed, we can say that the probability is 68 out of 100 that any randomly drawn sample mean lies between +1 SD and −1 SD of the population mean. Thus, if we knew the standard deviation of the sampling distribution, we could interpret the accuracy of a sample mean.

Standard Error of the Mean

The standard deviation of a sampling distribution of the mean is called the **standard error of the mean (SEM)**. The word *error* signifies that the various means in the sampling distribution have some error as estimates of the population mean. The smaller the SEM—that is, the less variable the sample means—the more accurate are the means as estimates of the population value.

Because no one actually constructs a sampling distribution, how can its standard deviation be computed? Fortunately, there is a formula for estimating the SEM from a single sample, using two pieces of information: the sample's standard deviation and sample size. The equation for the SEM is: $SD / \sqrt{N}$. In our example, if we use this formula to calculate the SEM for an SD of 100 with a sample of 25 students we obtain the following:

$$SEM = \frac{100}{\sqrt{25}} = 20.0$$

The standard deviation of the sampling distribution in our example is 20, as shown in Figure 22.1. This SEM is an estimate of how much sampling error there is from one sample mean to another when samples of 25 are randomly drawn.

Given that a sampling distribution of means follows a normal curve, we can estimate the probability of drawing a sample with a certain mean. With a sample size of 25 and a population mean of 500, the chances are about 95 out of 100 that any sample mean will fall between 460 and 540 (i.e., 2 SDs above and below the mean). Only 5 times out of 100 would the mean of a randomly selected sample exceed 540 or be less than 460. Only 5 times out of 100 would we get a sample whose mean deviated from the population mean by more than 40 points.

Because the SEM is partly a function of sample size, we need only increase sample size to increase the accuracy of our estimate. If we used a sample of 100 applicants, rather than 25, the SEM would be 10 (i.e., $100 / \sqrt{100} = 10.0$). In this situation, the chances are about 95 out of 100 that a sample mean will be between 480 and 520. The chances of drawing a sample with a mean very different from the population mean is reduced as sample size increases because large numbers promote the likelihood that extreme cases will cancel each other out.

ESTIMATION OF PARAMETERS

Statistical inference consists of two techniques: estimation of parameters and hypothesis testing. Parameter estimations are infrequently presented in nursing research reports, but that situation is changing. The emphasis on evidence-based practice has heightened interest among practitioners in learning not only whether a hypothesis was supported (through traditional hypothesis tests) but also the estimated value of a population parameter and the level of accuracy of the estimate (through parameter estimation). Many medical research journals *require* that estimation information be reported because it is more useful to clinicians, reflecting the view that this approach offers information about

both clinical and statistical significance (e.g., Braitman, 1991; Sackett et al., 2000). In this section, we present some general concepts relating to parameter estimation and offer some examples based on one-variable descriptive statistics. We expand on this discussion throughout the chapter within the context of specific bivariate statistical tests.

Confidence Intervals

Parameter estimation is used to estimate a parameter—for example, a mean, a proportion, or a mean difference between two groups (e.g., experimental and control subjects). Estimation can take two forms: point estimation or interval estimation. *Point estimation* involves calculating a single statistic to estimate the population parameter. To continue with the earlier example, if we calculated the mean entrance exam score for a sample of 25 nursing school applicants and found that it was 510, then this would be the point estimate of the population mean.

Point estimates that are simply descriptive statistics convey no information about margin of error, however, and so inferences about the accuracy of the parameter estimate cannot objectively be made. *Interval estimation* of a parameter is useful because it indicates a range of values within which the parameter has a specified probability of lying. With interval estimation, researchers construct a **confidence interval** (**CI**) around the estimate; the upper and lower limits are called **confidence limits**. Constructing a confidence interval around a sample mean establishes a range of values for the population value as well as the probability of being right—the estimate is made with a certain degree of confidence. Researchers usually use either a 95% or a 99% confidence interval, purely by convention.

➔ **TIP:** Confidence intervals address one of the key evidence-based practice (EBP) questions for appraising evidence presented in Box 2.1: How precise is the estimate of effects?

Confidence Intervals around a Mean

Calculating confidence limits around a mean involves the use of the SEM. As shown in Figure 22.1, 95% of the scores in a normal distribution lie within about 2 SDs (more precisely, 1.96 SDs) from the mean. In our example, suppose the point estimate for mean SAT scores is 510, and the SD is 100. The SEM for a sample of 25 would be 20. We can build a 95% confidence interval with the following formula:

$$CI\ 95\% = (\overline{X} \pm 1.96 \times SEM)$$

That is, the confidence is 95% that the population mean lies between the values equal to 1.96 times the SEM, above and below the sample mean. In the example at hand, we would obtain the following:

$$CI\ 95\% = (510 \pm (1.96 \times 20.0))$$
$$CI\ 95\% = (510 \pm (39.2))$$
$$CI\ 95\% = (470.8 \leq \mu \leq 549.2)$$

The final statement may be read as follows: the confidence is 95% that the population mean (symbolized by the Greek letter mu [μ] by convention) is between 470.8 and 549.2. This would be stated in a research report as 95% CI = 470.8 to 549.2, or 95% CI (470.8, 549.2).

Confidence intervals reflect how much risk researchers are willing to take of being wrong. With a 95% CI, researchers accept the probability that they will be wrong five times out of 100. A 99% CI sets the risk at only 1% by allowing a wider range of possible values. The formula is as follows:

$$CI\ 99\% = (\overline{X} \pm 2.58 \times SEM)$$

The 2.58 reflects the fact that 99% of all cases in a normal distribution lie within ±2.58 SD units from the mean. In the example, the 99% confidence interval would be as follows:

$$CI\ 99\% = . (510 \pm (2.58 \times 20.0))$$
$$CI\ 99\% = (510 \pm (51.6))$$
$$CI\ 99\% = (458.4 \leq \mu \leq 561.6)$$

In random samples with 25 subjects, 99 out of 100 confidence intervals so constructed would contain the population mean. The price of having a reduced risk of being wrong is reduced specificity. With a 95% interval, the range of the CI was only about 80 points; with a 99% interval, the range is more than 100 points. The acceptable risk for error depends on the nature of the problem. In research that could affect human health, a stringent 99% confidence interval might be used; for most studies, a 95% confidence interval is sufficient.

Confidence Intervals Around Proportions and Risk Indexes

Calculating confidence intervals around a proportion or percentage is extremely important in certain types of research, especially with regard to estimating risks. Consider, for example, this question: "What percentage of people exposed to a certain hazard will contract a disease?" This question calls for an estimated proportion (an absolute risk index, as described in Chapter 21) that will be more useful if it can be reported within a 95% confidence interval.

For proportions based on nominal-level dichotomous variables, as implied in the above question (positive/negative for a disease), the applicable theoretical distribution is not a normal distribution, but rather a **binomial distribution**. A binomial distribution is the probability distribution of the number of "successes" (e.g., heads) in a sequence of independent yes/no trials (e.g., a coin toss), each of which yields "success" with a specified probability.

Using binomial distributions to build confidence intervals around a proportion is computationally complex and is almost always done by computer, and so we do not provide any formulas here (see Motulsky, 1995). Certain features of confidence intervals around proportions are, however, worth noting. First, the CI is rarely symmetric around the sample proportion. For example, if 3 out of 30 sample members were "positive" for an outcome, such as hospital readmission, the estimated population proportion would be .10, and the 95% CI for the proportion would be from .021 to .265. Second, the width of the CI depends on both the value of the proportion and the sample size. The larger the sample, the smaller the CI. Also, the closer the sample proportion is to .50, the wider the CI. For example, with a sample size of 30, the range for a 95% CI for a proportion of .50 is .374 (.313, .687), whereas that for a proportion of .10 is only .188 (.021, .265). Finally, the CI for a proportion never extends below 0 or above 1.0, but a CI can be constructed around an *obtained* proportion of 0 or 1.0. For example, if 0 out of our 30 subjects were readmitted to the hospital, the estimated proportion would be 0.0, and the 95% CI would be from 0.0 to .116.

It is possible—and advisable—to construct confidence intervals around all of the indexes of risk described in the previous chapter, such as the ARR, RRR, OR, and NNT. The computed value of these indexes from study data represents a single "best estimate," but confidence intervals convey important information about the plausibility that the estimate is correct. Clearly, clinical inferences are enhanced when information about a plausible range of values for risk indexes is presented. Formulas for constructing CIs around the major risk indexes are presented in an appendix of DiCenso, Guyatt, and Ciliska (2005) and Sackett and colleagues (2000), but an easier method for constructing 95% CIs around major risk indexes is to use the University of British Columbia's "Clinical Significance Calculator" on the Internet (*http://www.healthcare.ubc.ca/calc/clinsig.html*).

Example of confidence intervals: Carruth and colleagues (2006) conducted a study in which they examined the proportion of farm women failing to obtain cervical cancer screening in three southern states. They presented failure rates (failure to obtain a Pap smear within the past 3 years) for women in different age, race, and education groups in the three states, along with 95% CI values. For example, for all women in Louisiana, the failure rate was 27.9 (24.5, 31.3), whereas in Texas the rate was 19.6 (15.6, 22.6).

HYPOTHESIS TESTING

Statistical hypothesis testing provides objective criteria for deciding whether hypotheses are supported by data. Suppose we hypothesized that participation of cancer patients in a stress management program would lower anxiety levels. The sample is 25 control group patients who do not participate in the program and 25 experimental subjects who do. The mean posttreatment anxiety score for experimental subjects is 15.8, and that for controls is 17.9. Should we conclude that the hypothesis was correct? Group differences are in the predicted direction, but the results might simply reflect sampling fluctuations. The two groups might *happen* to be different by chance, regardless of the intervention. Perhaps with a new sample, the group means would be nearly identical. Statistical hypothesis testing allows researchers to make objective decisions about whether study results likely reflect chance sample differences or true differences in a population.

The Null Hypothesis

Hypothesis testing is based on rules of negative inference. In our example, we found that subjects participating in the intervention had lower mean anxiety scores than control group subjects. There are two possible explanations: (1) the intervention was successful in reducing patients' anxiety; or (2) the differences resulted from chance factors, such as group differences in anxiety even before the treatment. The first explanation is our research hypothesis, and the second is the null hypothesis. The **null hypothesis**, it may be recalled, states that there is no relationship between variables. Statistical hypothesis testing is basically a process of rejection. It cannot be demonstrated directly that the research hypothesis is correct, but using theoretical sampling distributions, it can be shown that the null hypothesis has a high probability of being incorrect. Researchers seek to reject the null hypothesis through various **statistical tests**.

The null hypothesis in our example can be stated formally:

$$H_0: \mu_E = \mu_C$$

The null hypothesis (H_0) is that the mean population anxiety score for experimental subjects (μ_E)

is the same as that for controls (μ_C). The **alternative**, or research, **hypothesis** (H_A) claims the means are *not* the same:

$$H_A: \mu_E \neq \mu_C$$

Although null hypotheses are accepted or rejected based on sample data, hypothesis testing is used to make inferences about relationships within the population.

Type I and Type II Errors

Researchers decide whether to accept or reject a null hypothesis by determining how *probable* it is that observed results are due to chance. Researchers lack information about the population, and so cannot know with certainty whether a null hypothesis is or is not true. Researchers can only conclude that hypotheses are *probably* true or *probably* false, and there is always a risk for error.

Researchers can make two types of statistical error: rejecting a true null hypothesis or accepting a false null hypothesis. Figure 22.2 summarizes possible outcomes of researchers' decisions. Researchers make a **Type I error** by rejecting a null hypothesis that is, in fact, true. For instance, if we concluded that a drug was more effective than a placebo in reducing cholesterol, when in fact the observed differences in cholesterol levels resulted from sampling fluctuations, we would be making a Type I error—a false-positive conclusion. Con-

versely, if we concluded that group differences in cholesterol resulted by chance, when in fact the drug *did* reduce cholesterol, we would be committing a **Type II error**—a false-negative conclusion. In the context of drug testing, a good way to think about statistical error can be expressed as follows: A Type I error might allow an ineffective drug to come onto the market, but a Type II error might *prevent* an effective drug from coming onto the market.

Level of Significance

Researchers never know when they have made an error in statistical decision making. The validity of a null hypothesis could be known only by collecting data from the population. Researchers control the *risk* for a Type I error by selecting a **level of significance**, which signifies the probability of incorrectly rejecting a true null hypothesis.

The two most frequently used significance levels (referred to as **alpha** or α) are .05 and .01. With a .05 significance level, we accept the risk that out of 100 samples drawn from a population, a true null hypothesis would be rejected 5 times. With a .01 significance level, the risk for a Type I error is *lower*: In only 1 sample out of 100 would we erroneously reject the null hypothesis. The minimum acceptable level for α usually is .05. A stricter level (e.g., .01 or .001) may be needed when the decision has important consequences.

Naturally, researchers want to reduce the risk of committing both types of error, but unfortunately

The actual situation is that the null hypothesis is:

		True	False
The researcher calculates a test statistic and decides that the null hypothesis is:	True (Null accepted)	Correct decision	Type II error (False negative)
	False (Null rejected)	Type I error (False positive)	Correct decision

FIGURE 22.2 Outcomes of statistical decision making.

lowering the risk for a Type I error increases the risk for a Type II error. The stricter the criterion for rejecting a null hypothesis, the greater the probability of accepting a false null hypothesis. Researchers must deal with tradeoffs in establishing criteria for statistical decision making, but the simplest way of reducing the risk for a Type II error is to increase sample size. Type II errors are discussed later in this chapter.

➡ **TIP:** Levels of significance are analogous to the CI values describe earlier—an alpha of .05 is analogous to the 95% CI, and an alpha of .01 is analogous to the 99% CI.

Critical Regions

By selecting a significance level, researchers establish a decision rule. That rule is to reject the null hypothesis if the test statistic falls at or beyond the limits that establish a **critical region** on the applicable theoretical distribution, and to accept the null hypothesis otherwise. The critical region indicates whether the null hypothesis is *improbable*, given the results.

A simple (if contrived) example illustrates the statistical decision-making process. Suppose we measured attitudes toward *in vitro* fertilization (IVF) among infertile couples. We ask a sample of 100 patients with infertility to express their attitude toward IVF on a scale ranging from 0 (extremely negative) to 10 (extremely positive). We want to test the null hypothesis that the mean rating for the population is 5.0, the score reflecting a neutral attitude. The null hypothesis is $H_0: \mu = 5.0$, and the alternate hypothesis is $H_A: \mu \neq 5.0$.

Now suppose that data from the 100 patients result in a mean rating of 5.5 with an SD of 2.0. This mean is consistent with the alternative hypothesis that patients are not neutral, but can we reject the null hypothesis? Because of sampling fluctuation, there is a possibility that the mean of 5.5 occurred simply by chance and not because the population is moderately favorable toward IVF.

In hypothesis testing, researchers *assume* the null hypothesis is true and then gather evidence to

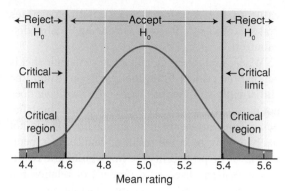

FIGURE 22.3 Critical regions in the sampling distribution for a two-tailed test: IVF attitudes example.

disprove it. In this example, we would assume the population mean is 5.0 and then estimate the SEM by dividing the actual standard deviation (2.0) by the square root of the sample size (100). In this example, the SEM is 0.2 ($2.0 \div \sqrt{100}$).

The resulting sampling distribution is shown in Figure 22.3. Based on the normal distribution, we can determine *probable* and *improbable* values of sample means drawn from the infertility population. If, as the null hypothesis assumes, the population mean is 5.0, then 95% of all sample means (for $N = 100$) would fall roughly between 4.6 and 5.4— that is, about 2 SDs above and below the mean. Only 5% of sample means would be less than 4.6 or greater than 5.4 if the null hypothesis were true. The obtained sample mean of 5.5 is improbable using a significance level of .05 as our criterion of improbability. We can reject the null hypothesis that the population mean equals 5.0. We cannot say we have *proved* the alternative hypothesis: There is a 5% possibility that we made a Type I error. But we can *accept* the alternative hypothesis that patients with infertility are not, on average, neutral about IVF.

Statistical Tests

In practice, researchers do not compute critical regions. They use research data to compute **test statistics**. For every test statistic, there is a related theoretical distribution. Researchers compare the value of the computed test statistic to values that specify critical limits for the applicable distribution.

When researchers calculate a test statistic that is beyond the critical limit, the results are said to be **statistically significant**. The word *significant* does not mean *important* or *clinically relevant*. In statistics, *significant* means that obtained results are not likely to have been the result of chance, at a specified level of probability. A **nonsignificant result** means that an observed difference or relationship could have resulted from chance fluctuations.

⬭ **TIP:** When the null hypothesis is retained (i.e., when results are nonsignificant), this is sometimes referred to as a **negative result**. Negative results are often disappointing to researchers and may lead to rejection of a manuscript by journal editors. Research reports with negative results are not rejected because editors are prejudiced against certain types of outcomes; they are rejected because negative results are usually inconclusive and difficult to interpret. A nonsignificant result indicates that the result *could* have occurred as a result of chance, and offers no evidence that the research hypothesis is or is *not* correct.

One-Tailed and Two-Tailed Tests

In most hypothesis-testing situations, researchers use **two-tailed tests**. This means that both ends, or tails, of the sampling distribution are used to determine improbable values. In Figure 22.3, for example, the critical region that contains 5% of the sampling distribution's area involves 2½% in one tail of the distribution and 2½% at the other. If the significance level were .01, the critical regions would involve ½% in each tail.

When researchers have a strong basis for a directional hypothesis (see Chapter 4), they sometimes use a **one-tailed test**. For example, if we did a randomized clinical trial (RCT) involving a program to improve prenatal practices among rural women, we would expect birth outcomes for the two groups not to just be *different*; we would expect program participants to *benefit*. It might make little sense to use the tail of the distribution signifying *worse* outcomes in the intervention group.

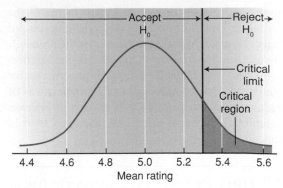

FIGURE 22.4 Critical region in the sampling distribution for a one-tailed test: IVF attitudes example.

In one-tailed tests, the critical region of improbable values is in only one tail of the distribution—the tail corresponding to the direction of the hypothesis, as illustrated in Figure 22.4. The research hypothesis being tested is not just that the population mean for IVF attitudes is different from 5.0; the hypothesis is that the population mean is *greater than* 5.0—that is, that patients with infertility are positive toward IVF, on average. When a one-tailed test is used, the critical 5% area of "improbability" covers a bigger area of the specified tail, so one-tailed tests are less conservative. This means it is easier to reject the null hypothesis with a one-tailed test than with a two-tailed test. In our example, with an alpha of .05, a sample mean of 5.3 or greater would result in rejecting the null hypothesis for a one-tailed test, rather than 5.4 for a two-tailed test.

One-tailed tests are controversial. Most researchers use a two-tailed test even if they have a directional hypothesis. In reading research reports, one can assume two-tailed tests were used unless one-tailed tests are specifically mentioned. When there is a strong theoretical reason for a directional hypothesis and for assuming that findings in the opposite direction are virtually impossible, however, a one-tailed test may be warranted. In the remainder of this chapter, the examples are for two-tailed tests.

⬭ **TIP:** You should choose a one-tailed test only if you state a directional hypothesis in advance of statistical testing. And, you must be prepared to attribute group differences in the "wrong" direction to chance, even if the group differences are large.

Parametric and Nonparametric Tests

There are two broad classes of statistical tests, parametric and nonparametric. **Parametric tests** are characterized by three attributes: (1) they involve the estimation of a parameter; (2) they require measurements on at least an interval scale; and (3) they involve several assumptions, such as the assumption that the variables are normally distributed in the population. **Nonparametric tests**, by contrast, do not estimate parameters. They involve less restrictive assumptions about the shape of the variables' distribution than do parametric tests. For this reason, nonparametric tests are sometimes called **distribution-free statistics**.

Parametric tests are more powerful than nonparametric tests and are usually preferred, but there is some disagreement about the use of nonparametric tests. Purists insist that if the requirements of parametric tests are not met, these tests are inappropriate. Statistical studies have shown, however, that statistical decision making is not affected when the assumptions for parametric tests are violated when sample sizes are large. Nonparametric tests are most useful when data cannot in any manner be construed as interval level, when the distribution is markedly nonnormal, or when the sample size is very small.

➲ **TIP:** Some statisticians advise that when *N* is 50 or greater, it may not be necessary to use nonparametric statistics, unless the population has a markedly unusual distribution. Such advice invokes the **central limit theorem**, which, briefly, concerns the fact that when samples are large, the theoretical distribution of sample *means* tends to follow a normal distribution — *even if* the variable itself is not normally distributed in the population. With small *Ns*, you cannot rely on the central limit theorem, so probability values could be wrong if a parametric test is used.

Between-Subjects Tests and Within-Subjects Tests

Another distinction in statistical tests concerns the nature of the comparisons. When comparisons involve different people (e.g., men versus women),

the study uses a between-subjects design, and the statistical test is a **test for independent groups**. Other designs involve one group of subjects—for example, with a crossover design, subjects are exposed to two or more treatments. In within-subjects designs, comparisons are not independent because the same subjects are used in all conditions, and the appropriate statistical tests are **tests for dependent groups**.

Overview of Hypothesis-Testing Procedures

This chapter describes several bivariate statistical tests. The discussion emphasizes applications rather than computations, but we urge you to consult other references (e.g., Polit, 1996; Munro, 2004; Gravetter & Wallnau, 2006; Motulsky, 1995) for fuller explanations if you are conducting a statistical analysis. In this research methods textbook, our main interest is to provide an overview of the use and interpretation of some common statistical tests.

Each statistical test described in this chapter has a particular application, but the process of testing hypotheses is basically the same. The steps are as follows:

1. *Select an appropriate test statistic.* Figure 22.5 provides a quick reference guide for selecting a bivariate statistical test. (Multivariate tests are discussed in the next chapter.) Researchers must consider such factors as which levels of measurement were used, whether a parametric test is justified, whether a dependent test is needed, and whether the focus is correlations or group comparisons—and how many groups are being compared.
2. *Establish the level of significance.* Researchers establish the criterion for accepting or rejecting the null hypothesis. An α of .05 is usually acceptable.
3. *Select a one-tailed or two-tailed test.* In most cases, a two-tailed test should be used.
4. *Compute a test statistic.* Using collected data, researchers calculate a test statistic using appropriate computational formulas, or instruct a computer to calculate the statistic.

Level of Measurement of Dependent Variable	Group Comparisons: Number of groups (the independent variable)				Correlational analyses (to examine relationship strength)
	2 Groups		3+ Groups		
	Independent Groups Tests	Dependent Groups Tests	Independent Groups Tests	Dependent Groups Tests	
Nominal (categorical)	χ^2 (or Fisher's exact test)	McNemar's test	χ^2	Cochran's Q	Phi coefficient (dichotomous) or Cramér's V (not restricted to dichotomous)
Ordinal (rank)	Mann-Whitney test (or Median test)	Wilcoxon signed ranks test	Kruskal-Wallis H test	Friedman's test	Spearman's rho (or Kendall's tau)
Interval or ratio (continuous)*	Independent group t-test	Paired t-test	ANOVA	RM-ANOVA	Pearson's r
	Multifactor ANOVA for 2+ independent variables				
	RM-ANOVA for 2+ groups x 2+ measurements over time				

$\chi^2 = 8.00$, $df = 1$, $\rho = .005$

FIGURE 22.5 Quick guide to bivariate statistical tests.

5. *Determine the degrees of freedom* (symbolized as *df*). **Degrees of freedom** refers to the number of observations free to vary about a parameter. The concept is too complex for full elaboration here, but *df* is easy to compute.

6. *Compare the test statistic with a tabled value.* The theoretical distributions for test statistics enable researchers to determine whether obtained values of the test statistic (step 4) are beyond the range of what is *probable* if the null hypothesis were true. Researchers compare the value of the computed test statistic to values in a table.* If the absolute value of the test statistic is larger than the tabled value, the results are statistically significant. If the computed value is smaller, the results are nonsignificant.

When a computer is used for analysis, as is usually the case, researchers follow only the first two steps and then give commands to the computer. The computer calculates the test statistic, the degrees of freedom, and the *actual* probability that the null hypothesis is true. For example, the computer may show that

the two-tailed probability (*p*) of an intervention group being different from a control group by chance alone is .025. This means that in only 25 times out of 1000 would a group difference as large as the one obtained reflect haphazard differences rather than true intervention effects. The computed probability level can then be compared with the desired significance level. If the significance level desired were .05, then the results would be significant because .025 is more stringent than .05. By convention, any computed probability greater than .05 (e.g., .20) indicates a nonsignificant relationship (sometimes abbreviated *NS*)—that is, one that could have occurred by chance in more than 5 out of 100 samples.

⮕ **TIP:** The reference guide in Figure 22.5 does not include every test you may need, but it does include the bivariate tests most often used by nurse researchers. There are many resources now available on the Internet to help with selecting an appropriate test, including interactive decision-tree tools. Useful websites include the following: http://graphpad.com/www/book/Choose.htm or http://www.socialresearchmethods.net/selstat/ssstart.htm. Links to these websites are included on the accompanying CD-ROM for you to click on directly.

*Tables for four frequently used statistics (*t*, *F*, *r*, and chi-square) are included in a file on the accompanying Student Resource CD-ROM.

In the sections that follow, several of the most common bivariate statistical tests and their applications are described. Computer examples are provided at the end of the chapter.

TESTING DIFFERENCES BETWEEN TWO GROUP MEANS

A common research situation involves comparing two groups of subjects on a continuous dependent variable. For instance, we might compare an experimental and control group of patients with regard to their blood pressure. Or, we might contrast men and women with regard to mean cholesterol levels.

The parametric procedure for testing differences in group means is the *t*-test (sometimes referred to as **Student's *t***). The *t*-test can be used when there are two independent groups (e.g., experimental versus control), and when the sample is paired or dependent (e.g., pretreatment and posttreatment scores for a single group).

t-Tests for Independent Groups

Suppose we wanted to test the effect of early discharge of maternity patients on perceived maternal competence. We administer a scale of perceived maternal competence at discharge to 20 primiparas who had a vaginal delivery: 10 who remained in the hospital 25 to 48 hours (regular discharge group) and 10 who were discharged 24 hours or less after delivery (early discharge group). Data for this example are presented in Table 22.1. The mean scores for these two groups are 25.0 and 19.0, respectively. Are these differences *reliable* (i.e., would they be found in the population of early-discharge and later-discharge mothers?), or do group differences reflect chance fluctuations?

Note that the 20 scores in Table 22.1—10 per group—vary from one person to another. Some variability reflects individual differences in perceived maternal competence. Some variability might be due to measurement error (e.g., the scale's low reliability), some could result from participants' moods on a particular day, and so forth. The research question is: Can a significant portion of the variability be attributed to the independent variable—time of discharge from the hospital? The *t*-test allows us to answer this question objectively. The hypotheses are:

$$H_{0: } \mu_A = \mu_B \qquad H_{A: } \mu_A \neq \mu_B$$

TABLE 22.1	Fictitious Data for *t*-Test Example: Scores on a Perceived Maternal Competence Scale for Two Groups of Mothers	
REGULAR-DISCHARGE MOTHERS		**EARLY-DISCHARGE MOTHERS**
30		23
27		17
25		22
20		18
24		20
32		26
17		16
18		13
28		21
29		14
Mean = 25.0		Mean = 19.0
	$t = 2.86$: $df = 18$; $p = .011$	

To test these hypotheses, a t-statistic would be computed. The formula for the t-statistic uses group means, variability, and sample size to calculate a value for t. When the data from Table 22.1 are used in the formula, the value of t is 2.86. Next, degrees of freedom are determined. In this situation, degrees of freedom equal the total sample size minus 2 ($df = 20 - 2 = 18$). For a two-tailed probability (p) of .05 and $df = 18$, the tabled value of t is 2.10. *This value establishes an upper limit to what is probable if the null hypothesis is true.* Thus, the calculated t of 2.86, which is larger than the tabled value of the statistic, is improbable (i.e., statistically significant). We can now say that the primiparas discharged early had significantly lower perceptions of maternal competence than those who were not discharged early. The group difference in perceived maternal competence is sufficiently large that it is unlikely to reflect merely chance fluctuations. In fewer than 5 out of 100 samples would a difference in means this great be found by chance alone. When a computer is used to analyze the data presented in Table 22.1, the computer would show the *exact* probability, which is .011. This means that in only 11 out of 1000 samples would one expect a group difference of 6.0 points by chance alone.

> **Example of independent *t*-tests:** Tsay and Hung (2004) tested the effectiveness of an empowerment intervention on the empowerment level and depression of Taiwanese patients with end-stage renal disease, using an experimental design. The results indicated that patients in the experimental group had significantly higher empowerment scores ($t = 6.54$, $df = 48$, $p < .001$) and significantly lower depression scores ($t = 2.49$, $df = 48$, $p < .05$) than those in the control group.

When multiple tests are run with the same data—that is, when there are multiple dependent variables—the risk for a Type I error increases. One t-test with $\alpha = .05$ has a 5% probability of a Type I error. Two t-tests with the same data set, however, have a probability of 9.75% of one spurious significant result; and with three tests, the risk goes up to 14.3%. Cautious researchers apply a **Bonferroni**

correction when multiple tests are being run to establish a more conservative alpha level. As an example, if the desired α is .05, and there are three separate t-tests (or other tests discussed in this chapter), the corrected alpha needed to reject the null hypothesis for *all* tests would be .017, not .05. The correction is computed by dividing the desired α by the number of tests—that is, .05/3 = .017. If we concluded that mean group differences were significant for three tests at or below $p = .017$, there would be only a 5% probability of wrongly rejecting the null across all three comparisons. Using the Bonferroni correction is a conservative approach that can be problematic in that it tends to increase the risk for making a Type II error—incorrectly concluding there is no statistical association when in fact there is one.

Confidence Intervals for Mean Differences

Confidence intervals can be constructed around the difference between two means, and the results provide information about both statistical significance (i.e., whether the null hypothesis should be rejected) and precision of the estimated difference. Because CI information is richer and more useful in clinical applications, it is increasingly preferred—although nursing journals have not yet required it, as some medical journals have.

In the example in Table 22.1, the mean maternal competence scores were 25.0 in the regular discharge group and 19.0 in the early discharge group. Using a formula to compute the *standard error of the difference,* CIs can be constructed around the mean difference of 6.0. For a 95% CI, the confidence limits in our example are 1.6 and 10.4. This means that we can be 95% confident that the true difference between population means for early- and regular-discharge mothers lies somewhere between these values.

In the t-test analysis, we obtained an estimate of mean group differences (6.0) and the probability that group differences were spurious ($p = .011$). With CI information, we learn the range within which the mean difference probably lies. We can see from the CI that the mean difference is significant at the .05 level *because the range does not include 0*. Given that there is a 95% probability that the mean difference is not lower than 1.6, this means that there is less than a 5% probability that there is no difference at all—thus, the null hypothesis can be rejected.

Because the CI does not give exact probabilities about the plausibility of the null hypothesis, it is often useful to present both parameter estimation and hypothesis testing information in reports. In the current example, the results could be reported as follows: "Mothers who were discharged early had significantly lower maternal competence scores (19.0) than mothers with a regular discharge (26.0) ($t = 2.86$, $df = 18$, $p = .011$); the mean difference of 6.0 had a 95% CI of 1.6 to 10.4." Such information is most conveniently displayed in tables when there are multiple dependent variables. The Toolkit section of the accompanying *Resource Manual* has some table templates that may be useful for presenting findings from analyses described in this chapter. ✖

Example of CIs for mean group differences: McFarlane and colleagues (2006) studied two alternative treatments for abused women. Many findings were reported with CI information. For example, 2 years after treatment, women in one treatment group (referral card) had experienced 9.6 threats of assault, whereas those in an RN case management group had experienced 8.9 threats. The mean difference of 0.7 threats (95% CI = −1.9, 3.3) was not significant—the CI range encompassed the value of 0.0.

Paired *t*-Tests

Researchers sometimes obtain two measures from the same subjects, or measures from paired sets of subjects (e.g., siblings). Whenever two sets of scores are not independent, researchers must use a **paired *t*-test**—a *t*-test for dependent groups.

Suppose we were studying the effect of a special diet on the cholesterol level of elderly men. A sample of 50 men is randomly selected, and their cholesterol levels are measured before and again after 2 months on the special diet. The hypotheses being tested are:

$$H_0: \mu_x = \mu_y \qquad\qquad H_A: \mu_x \neq \mu_y$$

where X = pretreatment cholesterol levels
Y = posttreatment cholesterol levels

A *t*-statistic then would be computed from pretest and posttest data, using a different formula than for the independent group *t*-test. The obtained *t* would be compared with tabled *t*-values. For this type of *t*-test, degrees of freedom equal the number of paired observations minus 1 ($df = N - 1$). Confidence intervals can be constructed around mean differences for paired as well as independent means. For example, in the study by McFarlane and associates (2006) described earlier, for the two groups of women combined, the mean decline in threats of assault from baseline to follow-up was 14.5, 95% CI (12.6, 16.4).

Example of paired *t*-tests: Chan and colleagues (2005) tested the effectiveness of a telemedicine program for elderly diabetic patients in Hong Kong using a one-group pretest–posttest design. Paired *t*-tests that compared baseline values with outcomes measured 8 weeks later revealed significant reductions in total calorie intake ($p < .001$) and body mass index ($p = .005$).

Nonparametric Two-Group Tests

In certain two-group situations a nonparametric test may be needed (e.g., the dependent variable is on an ordinal scale that cannot be construed as an interval scale, or the distribution is markedly non-normal). We mention a few such tests here.

The **median test** involves comparing two independent groups based on deviations from the median rather than the mean. Scores for both groups are combined, an overall median is calculated, and then the number of cases above and below this median is counted separately for each group. This results in a 2 × 2 contingency table: (above/below median) × (group A/group B). From the contingency table, a chi-square statistic (described in a subsequent section) can be computed to test the null hypothesis that the medians are the same for the two populations.

The **Mann-Whitney U test** is another nonparametric procedure for testing the difference between two independent groups. The test involves assigning ranks to the two groups of measures. The sum of the ranks for the two groups can be compared by calculating the U statistic. The Mann-Whitney U test is more powerful than the median tests because it throws away less information.

When ordinal-level data are paired (dependent), the Wilcoxon signed-rank test can be used. The **Wilcoxon signed-rank test** involves taking the difference between paired scores and ranking the absolute difference.

TESTING MEAN DIFFERENCES WITH THREE OR MORE GROUPS

Analysis of variance (ANOVA) is the parametric procedure for testing differences between means when there are three or more groups. The statistic computed in ANOVA is the **F-ratio**. ANOVA decomposes total variability in a dependent variable into two parts: (1) variability attributable to the independent variable; and (2) all other variability, such as individual differences, measurement error,

and so on. Variation *between* groups is contrasted with variation *within* groups to get an F-ratio. When differences between groups are large relative to fluctuations within groups, the probability is high that the independent variable is related to, or has resulted in, group differences.

One-Way ANOVA

Suppose we were comparing the effectiveness of different interventions to help people stop smoking. One group of smokers, at random, receives intensive nurse counseling (group A); a second group is treated by a nicotine patch (group B); and a third control group receives no special treatment (group C). The dependent variable is 1-day cigarette consumption measured 1 month after the intervention. Thirty smokers who wish to quit smoking are randomly assigned to one of the three conditions. **One-way ANOVA** tests the following hypotheses:

$$H_{0:}\ \mu_A = \mu_B = \mu_C \qquad H_{A:}\ \mu_A \neq \mu_B \neq \mu_C$$

The null hypothesis is that the population means for posttreatment cigarette smoking is the same for all three groups, and the alternative (research) hypothesis is inequality of means. Table 22.2 presents fictitious data for each subject. The mean numbers of posttreatment cigarettes consumed are 16.6, 19.2,

TABLE 22.2	Fictitious Data for a One-Way ANOVA: Posttreatment Smoking in Three Groups	
GROUP A **NURSE COUNSELING**	**GROUP B** **NICOTINE PATCH**	**GROUP C** **UNTREATED CONTROl**
28 19	0 27	33 35
0 24	31 0	54 0
17 0	26 3	19 43
20 21	30 24	40 39
35 2	24 27	41 36
$\bar{X}_A = 16.6$	$\bar{X}_B = 19.2$	$\bar{X}_C = 34.0$

$F = 4.98,\ df = 2, 27,\ p = .01$

and 34.0 for groups A, B, and C, respectively. These means are different, but are they significantly different—or do differences reflect random fluctuations?

In calculating an F-statistic, total variability in the data is broken down into two sources. The portion of the variance due to group membership (i.e., exposure to different treatments) is reflected in the **sum of squares between groups**, or SS_B. The SS_B represents the sum of squared deviations of individual group means from the overall **grand mean** for all subjects. SS_B reflects variability in scores attributable to group membership.

The second component is the **sum of squares within groups**, or SS_W. This index is the sum of the squared deviations of each individual score from its *own* group mean. SS_W indicates variability attributable to individual differences, measurement error, and so on. In using computer software to do an ANOVA analysis, you would not actually calculate SS_B or SS_W, but the terms appear in research reports, so you should become familiar with them.

Recall from Chapter 21 that the formula for calculating a variance is $\Sigma x^2 \div N$. The two sums of squares are like the numerator of this variance equation: both SS_B and SS_W are sums of squared deviations from means. So, to compute variance within and variance between groups, we must divide the sums of squares by something similar to N, which is the degrees of freedom for each sum of squares. For between groups, $df_B - G - 1$ (i.e., number of groups minus 1). For within groups, df_W is the number of subjects less 1, for each group.

In an ANOVA context, the variance is conventionally referred to as the **mean square (MS)**. The formulas for the mean square between groups and the mean square within groups are:

$$MS_B = \frac{SS_B}{df_B} \qquad MS_W = \frac{SS_W}{df_W}$$

The F-ratio statistic is the ratio of these mean squares, or:

$$F = \frac{MS_B}{MS_W}$$

The ANOVA summary table (Table 22.3) shows that the calculated F-statistic in our example is 4.98. For $df = 2$ and 27 and $\alpha = .05$, the tabled F value is 3.35. Because our obtained F-value of 4.98 exceeds 3.35, we reject the null hypothesis that the population means are equal. The *actual* probability, as calculated by a computer, is .014. Group differences in posttreatment cigarette smoking are beyond chance expectations. In only 14 samples out of 1000 would differences this great be obtained by chance alone.

The data support the research hypothesis that different treatments were associated with different cigarette smoking, but we cannot tell from the test whether treatment A was significantly more effective than treatment B. Statistical analyses known as **multiple comparison procedures** (or *post hoc tests*) are needed. Their function is to isolate the differences between group means that are responsible for rejecting the overall ANOVA null hypothesis. Note that it is *not* appropriate to use a series of t-tests (group A versus B, A versus C, and B versus C) because this would increase the risk for a Type I error. Multiple comparison methods are described in most intermediate statistical textbooks, such as that by Polit (1996).

TABLE 22.3	ANOVA Summary Table					
SOURCE OF VARIANCE		**SS**	**df**	**MEAN SQUARE**	**F**	**p**
Between groups		1761.9	2	880.9	4.98	.014
Within groups		4772.0	27	176.7		
TOTAL		6533.9	29			

Example of a one-way ANOVA: Meuhrer and co-researchers (2006) studied sexuality among women who simultaneously received a pancreas and kidney transplant. Based on scores on a measure of sexual function, the sample was divided into three groups: those with normal sexual functioning, those with some difficulty, and those with sexual dysfunction. Using ANOVA, they learned that the three groups differed significantly with regard to sexual self-esteem ($F[2, 59] = 3.77$, $p < .05$). *Post hoc* tests revealed that the "normal" group was significantly different from the other two groups, but the "some difficulty" and "dysfunctional" group were not significantly different from each other.

Two-Way ANOVA

One-way ANOVA is used to test the relationship between one categorical independent variable (e.g., different interventions) and a continuous dependent variable. Data from studies with multiple factors, as in a factorial design, are sometimes analyzed by a **multifactor ANOVA**. In this section, we describe some principles underlying a **two-way ANOVA**.

Suppose we wanted to determine whether the two smoking cessation treatments (intensive nurse counseling and a nicotine patch) were equally effective for men and women, without an untreated group. We randomly assign women and men, separately, to the two treatment conditions. One month after the intervention, subjects report the number of cigarettes they smoked the previous day. Fictitious data for this example are shown in Table 22.4.

With two independent variables, three hypotheses are tested. First, we are testing the effectiveness, for both men and women, of intensive nurse counseling versus the nicotine patch. Second, we are testing whether postintervention smoking differs for men and women, regardless of treatment

---

TABLE 22.4 Fictitious Data for a Two-Way (2 × 2) ANOVA

FACTOR A—TREATMENT

FACTOR B—GENDER	Nurse Counseling (1)		Nicotine Patch (2)		
Female (1)	24	25	27	23	
	28	38	0	18	
	2	21	45	20	
	19	0	29	12	Female
	27	36	22	4	
	$\bar{X}_{A1B1} = 22.0$		$\bar{X}_{A2B1} = 20.0$		$\bar{X}_{B1} = 21.0$
Male (2)	10	16	36	27	
	21	18	41	0	
	17	3	28	49	Male
	0	25	37	35	
	33	17	5	42	$\bar{X}_{B2} = 23.0$
	$\bar{X}_{A1B2} = 16.0$		$\bar{X}_{A2B2} = 30.0$		
Total	Treatment 1 $\bar{X}_{A1} = 19.0$		Treatment 2 $\bar{X}_{A2} = 25.0$		$\bar{X}_T = 22.0$

approach. These are tests for **main effects**. Third, we are testing for **interaction effects** (i.e., differential treatment effects on men and women). Interaction concerns whether the effect of one independent variable is consistent for all levels of a second independent variable.

The data in Table 22.4 reveal that subjects in the Nurse Counseling group smoked less, on average, than those in Nicotine Patch group (19.0 versus 25.0); that women smoked less than men after treatment (21.0 versus 23.0); and that men smoked less when exposed to Nurse Counseling, but women smoked less when exposed to the Nicotine Patch. By performing a two-way ANOVA on these data, we could learn whether the differences were statistically significant.

Multifactor ANOVA is not restricted to two-way analyses. In theory, any number of independent variables is possible, but in practice, studies with more than two factors are rare. Other statistical techniques typically are used with three or more independent variables, as we discuss in Chapter 23.

> **Example of a two-way ANOVA:** McCarthy and Graves (2006) conducted a factorial experiment with a murine sample. The two factors, fully crossed to yield four treatment conditions, were (1) diet (half had conjugated linoleic acid or CLA added to their diet) and (2) tumor injection (half were injected with tumor cells). Outcome variables included body weight and tumor necrosis factor-alpha. Two-way ANOVAs were performed. One finding was that, for B16 melanoma, there was a significant interaction of tumor and CLA on body weight ($p = .02$) and a main effect for tumor ($p < .05$). Body weight was highest in the tumor/CLA group and lowest in the no tumor/CLA group.

Repeated Measures ANOVA

Repeated measures ANOVA (RM-ANOVA) is used in several situations, one of which is when there are three or more measures of the same dependent variable for each subject. For instance, in some studies, physiologic measures such as blood pressure or heart rate might be collected before, during, and after a medical procedure. In this situation, an RM-ANOVA is an extension of a paired *t*-test. It can be used with a single group studied longitudinally, or in a crossover design with three or more different conditions.

In some applications of repeated measures ANOVA, there are two or more measurements of the dependent variables for subjects in two or more groups. For example, suppose we collected heart rate data at 2 hours (T1), 4 hours (T2), and 6 hours (T3) after surgery for subjects in an experimental group and a control group. Structurally, the ANOVA for analyzing these data would look similar to a 2×3 multifactor ANOVA, but calculations would differ. An *F*-statistic would be computed to test for a **between-subjects effect** (i.e., differences between experimental and control subjects). This statistic indicates whether, across all time periods, the mean heart rate differed in the two treatment groups. Another *F*-statistic is computed to test for a **within-subjects effect** or **time factor** (i.e., differences at T1, T2, and T3). This statistic indicates whether, across both groups, mean heart rates differed over time. Finally, an interaction effect would be tested to determine whether group differences varied across time.

> **Example of RM-ANOVA:** Barnason and colleagues (2006) studied patterns of recovery among patients who had a percutaneous coronary intervention (PCI). Various symptoms, and the impact of symptoms on functioning and life enjoyment, were studied at 2, 4, and 6 weeks after the PCI. RM-ANOVA was used to analyze trends over time. One significant finding, for example, was that the impact of fatigue on physical functioning was significantly higher at 4 weeks than at 2 weeks ($F[2, 26] = 3.6$, $p < .05$).

Nonparametric "Analysis of Variance"

Nonparametric tests do not, strictly speaking, analyze variance, but there are nonparametric analogues to ANOVA when a parametric test is inadvisable. The **Kruskal-Wallis test** is a generalized version of the Mann-Whitney *U* test, based on assigning ranks to the scores of various groups. This test is used when the number of groups is greater than two and a one-way test for independent samples is desired. When multiple measures are obtained from the same subjects, the **Friedman test** for "analysis of variance" by ranks can be used. Both tests are described by Polit (1996) and in other statistics textbooks.

TESTING DIFFERENCES IN PROPORTIONS

Tests discussed thus far involve dependent variables measured on an interval or ratio scale, when group means are being compared. In this section, we examine tests of group differences when the dependent variable is on a nominal scale.

The Chi-Square Test

The **chi-square (χ^2) test** is used to test hypotheses about the proportion of cases that fall into different categories, as when a contingency table has been created. Suppose we were studying the effect of nursing instruction on patients' compliance with a self-medication regimen. Nurses implement a new instructional strategy based on Orem's Self-Care Model with 100 randomly assigned experimental patients, whereas 100 control group patients are cared for using usual instruction. The research hypothesis is that a higher proportion of people in the treatment than in the control condition will be compliant.

The chi-square statistic is computed by comparing observed frequencies (i.e., values observed in the data) and expected frequencies. **Observed frequencies** for our example are shown in Table 22.5. As this table shows, 60 experimental subjects (60%), but only 40 controls (40%), reported self-medication compliance after the intervention. The chi-square test enables us to decide whether a difference in proportions of this magnitude is likely to reflect a real treatment effect or only chance fluctuations. **Expected frequencies** are the cell frequencies that would be found if there were *no* relationship between the two variables. In this example, if there were no relationship between the two groups, the expected frequency would be 50 subjects per cell because, overall, exactly half the subjects complied.

The chi-square statistic is computed by summarizing differences between observed and expected frequencies for each cell. In our example, $\chi^2 = 8.00$. For chi-square tests, *df* equals the number of rows minus 1 times the number of columns minus 1. In the current case, $df = 1 \times 1 = 1$. With 1 *df*, the tabled value from a theoretical chi-square distribution that must be exceeded to establish significance at the .05 level is 3.84. The obtained value of 8.00 is substantially larger than would be expected by chance (the actual $p = .005$). We can conclude that a significantly larger proportion of experimental patients than control patients were compliant.

TABLE 22.5	Observed Frequencies for Chi-Square Example		
	GROUP		
PATIENT COMPLIANCE	**EXPERIMENTAL**	**CONTROL**	**TOTAL**
Compliant	60	40	100
Noncompliant	40	60	100
TOTAL	100	100	200

$\chi^2 = 8.00$, *df* = 1, *p* = .005

Example of chi-square test: Nyamathi and colleagues (2006) examined the relationship between the background characteristics of homeless men and whether or not they were positive for hepatitis C virus (HCV) infection. They found that, for example, a significantly higher proportion of men who were veterans ($p < .01$), who were white or Latino ($p < .001$), and who had been in prison ($p < .001$) were HCV positive than men not in these categories.

Confidence Intervals for Differences in Proportion

As with means, it is possible to construct confidence intervals around the difference between two proportions. To do this, we would need to calculate (or, more likely, have the computer calculate) the *standard error (SE) of the difference of proportions*. In the example used to explain the chi square statistic, the difference in proportions was .20 (.60 − .40), and the SE of the difference is .069. The 95% CI in this example is .06 to .34. We can be 95% confident that the true population difference in compliance rates between those exposed to the intervention and those not exposed is between 6% and 34%. This interval does not include 0%, indicating that we can be 95% confident that group differences are "real." Motulsky (1995) provides formulas for computing the SE of the difference in proportions.

Example of CI for difference in proportions: Creedon (2006) tested compliance with hand-hygiene guidelines before and after implementation of a hand-hygiene program in an Irish ICU. The compliance rate among nurses improved from 56% before the intervention to 89% after it. The 33% difference had a 95% CI of 21% to 44%.

Other Tests of Proportions

Sometimes it is inappropriate to use a chi-square test. When the total sample size is small (total *N* of 30 or less) or when there are cells with small frequencies (5 or fewer), **Fisher's exact test** should be used to test the significance of differences in pro-

portions. When the proportions being compared are from two paired groups (e.g., when a pretest–posttest design is used to compare changes in proportions on a dichotomous variable), the appropriate test is the **McNemar's test**.

TESTING CORRELATIONS

The statistical tests discussed thus far are used to test differences between *groups*—they involve situations in which the independent variable is a nominal-level variable. In this section, we consider statistical tests used when the independent variable is on a higher level of measurement.

Pearson's *r*

In Chapter 21, we described the Pearson product–moment correlation coefficient. Pearson's *r*, calculated when two variables are measured on at least the interval scale, is both descriptive and inferential. Descriptively, the correlation coefficient summarizes the magnitude and direction of a relationship between two variables. As an inferential statistic, *r* tests hypotheses about population correlations, which are symbolized as ρ, the Greek letter rho. The null hypothesis is that there is no relationship between two variables. Stated formally:

$$H_0: \rho = 0 \qquad H_A: \rho \neq 0$$

For instance, suppose we studied the relationship between patients' self-reported level of stress and the pH level of their saliva. In a sample of 50 subjects, we find that $r = -.29$, indicating a modest tendency for people with high stress scores to have low pH levels. But can we generalize this finding to the population? Does the coefficient of $-.29$ reflect a random fluctuation, observable only for the subjects in our sample, or is the relationship *real*? We could compare our computed *r* to a tabled value from a theoretical distribution for *r*. Degrees of freedom for *r* equal the number of subjects minus 2, or ($N - 2$). With $df = 48$, the tabled value for *r* (for a two-tailed test with $\alpha = .05$) is .2803. Because the absolute value of the calculated r is .29, the null hypothesis can be rejected. We accept the research hypothesis that the correlation between stress and saliva acidity in the population is not zero.

Pearson's r can be used in both within-groups and between-groups situations. The example about the relationship between stress scores and the pH levels is a between-groups situation: The question is whether people with high stress scores tend to have significantly lower pH levels than *different* people with low stress scores. If stress scores were obtained both before and after surgery, however, the correlation between the two scores would be a within-groups situation.

Example of Pearson's r: Doran and co-researchers (2006) gathered data from charts in four acute-care Canadian hospitals and analyzed the relationship between key nursing interventions and patient outcomes. A correlation matrix summarized correlations among four patient characteristics (age, cognitive status, depression, and functional status at admission), three nursing interventions (positioning, exercise promotion, and oral hygiene self-care promotion), and two patient outcomes (discharge functional status and therapeutic self-care). As but one example, the correlation between positioning and discharge functional status was $r = .22$, $p < .01$.

➲ **TIP:** A CI can be constructed around Pearson's r. The formula is complex and would almost always be calculated by computer. In our example, the 95% CI around the r of .29 for stress levels and saliva pH, with a sample of 50 subjects, is (.01, .53).

Other Tests of Bivariate Relationships

Pearson's r is a parametric statistic. When the assumptions for a parametric test are violated, or when the data are ordinal level, then the appropriate coefficient of correlation is either **Spearman's rho** (r_S) or, less often, **Kendall's tau**. The values of these statistics range from -1.00 to $+1.00$, and their interpretation is similar to that of Pearson's r.

Measures of the magnitude of relationships can also be computed with nominal-level data. For example, the **phi coefficient** (ϕ) is an index

describing the relationship between two dichotomous variables. **Cramér's V** is an index of relationship applied to contingency tables larger than 2×2. Both statistics are based on the chi-square statistic and yield values that range between .00 and 1.00, with higher values indicating a stronger association between variables.

POWER ANALYSIS AND EFFECT SIZE

Many published nursing studies (and even more *un*published ones) result in nonsignificant findings—many of which could reflect Type II errors. As indicated earlier in this chapter, researchers set the probability of committing a Type I error (a false positive) as the level of significance, or alpha (α). The probability of a Type II error (a false negative) is **beta** (β). The complement of beta ($1 - \beta$) is the *probability of detecting a true relationship or group difference* and is referred to as the **power** of a statistical test. Polit and Sherman (1990) found that many published nursing studies have insufficient power, placing them at risk for Type II errors. Although many years have elapsed since their analysis was undertaken, a perusal of recent nursing research reports suggests that many studies continue to be underpowered.

Power analysis can be used to reduce the risk for Type II errors by estimating in advance how big a sample is needed. There are four components in a power analysis, three of which must be known or estimated; power analysis solves for the fourth. The four components are:

1. *The significance criterion*, α. Other things being equal, the more stringent this criterion, the lower the power.
2. *The sample size, N.* As sample size increases, power increases.
3. *The effect size* (ES). ES is an estimate of how wrong the null hypothesis is, that is, how strong the relationship between the independent variable and the dependent variable is in the population.
4. *Power, or $1 - \beta$.* This is the probability of rejecting a false null hypothesis.

Researchers typically use power analysis at the outset of a study to estimate the sample size needed to obtain significant results. To estimate needed sample size (N), researchers must specify α, ES, and $1 - \beta$. Researchers usually establish the risk for a Type I error (α) as .05, and the conventional standard for $1 - \beta$ is .80. With power equal to .80, there is a 20% risk for committing a Type II error. Although this risk may seem high, a stricter criterion requires sample sizes much larger than most researchers could afford.

With α and $1 - \beta$ specified, the information needed to solve for N is ES, the estimated population effect size. The **effect size** is the magnitude of the relationship between the research variables. When relationships (effects) are strong, they can be detected at statistically significant levels even with small research samples. When relationships are modest, large sample sizes are needed to avoid Type II errors.

In using power analysis to estimate sample size needs, the population effect size is not *known*; if it were known, there would be no need for a new study. Effect size must be estimated using available evidence. Sometimes evidence comes from a pilot study, which can be a good approach when the main study is costly. More often, an effect size is calculated based on findings from earlier studies on a similar problem. When there are *no* relevant earlier findings, researchers use conventions based on expectations of a *small, medium,* or *large* effect. In most nursing studies, effects are modest.

➲ TIP: One problem with using pilot data to estimate sample size needs for the main study is that pilots are small and sample values are thus unstable. One solution is to calculate the 95% CI around key effect size estimates from pilot data, and use the most conservative estimate of needed sample size. Another approach is to supplement the pilot ES information with estimates from other studies. Researchers can usually find more than one study from which the effect size can be estimated. In such a case, the estimate should be based on the study with the most reliable results or whose design most closely approximates that of the new study. Researchers can also estimate effect size by combining

information from multiple high-quality studies through averaging or weighted averaging. If you are fortunate enough to be studying a problem that has been the focus of a meta-analysis, ES estimates might be readily available in the report.

Procedures for estimating effects and sample size needs vary from one statistical situation to another. We focus mainly on a two-group situation for which we can estimate mean values, and provide more general information about other situations.

Sample Size Estimates for Testing Differences Between Two Means

Suppose we were testing the hypothesis that cranberry juice reduces the urinary pH of diet-controlled patients. We plan to assign some subjects randomly to a control condition (no cranberry juice) and others to an experimental condition in which they will be given 200 mL of cranberry juice with each meal for 5 days. How large a sample is needed for this study, given a desired α of .05 and power of .80?

To answer this, we must first estimate ES. In a two-group situation in which mean differences are of interest, ES is often designated as Cohen's *d,* the formula for which is:

$$d = \frac{\mu_1 - \mu_2}{\sigma}$$

That is, the effect size (d) is the difference between the two population means, divided by the population standard deviation. These values are not known in advance, but must be estimated based on available evidence. For example, suppose we found an earlier nonexperimental study that compared the urinary pH of subjects who had or had not ingested cranberry juice in the previous 24 hours. The earlier and current studies are different. In the nonexperimental study, the diets are uncontrolled, there likely are selection biases in who drinks or does not drink cranberry juice, the length of ingestion is only 1 day, and so on. This study is, however, a reasonable starting point. Suppose the results were as follows:

$\overline{X}_1$(no cranberry juice) $= 5.70$
$\overline{X}_2$(cranberry juice) $= 5.50$
SD $= .50$

Thus, the estimated value of d would be .40:

$$d = \frac{5.70 - 5.50}{.50} = .40$$

Table 22.6 presents approximate sample size requirements for various effect sizes and powers, for $\alpha = .05$ (for two-tailed tests), in a two-group mean-difference situation. We find in this table that the estimated n (number per group) to detect an effect size of .40 with power equal to .80 is 98 subjects. Assuming that the earlier study provided a good estimate of the population effect size, the total number of subjects needed in the new study would be about 200, with half assigned to the control group (no cranberry juice) and the other half assigned to the experimental group. With a sample size smaller than 200, there would be a greater than 20% chance of a false-negative conclusion, that is, a Type II error. For example, a sample size of 122 (61 per group) would result in an estimated 40% chance of incorrect nonsignificant results (power $= .60$).

If there is no prior research, researchers can, as a last resort, estimate whether the expected effect is small, medium, or large. By convention (Cohen, 1988), the value of ES in a two-group test of mean differences is estimated at .20 for small effects, .50 for medium effects, and .80 for large effects. With an α value of .05 and power of .80, the n (number of subjects per group) for studies with expected small, medium, and large effects would be 392, 63, and 25, respectively. Most nursing studies cannot expect effect sizes in excess of .50; those in the range of .20 to .40 are most common. In Polit and Sherman's (1990) analysis of effect sizes for all studies published in *Nursing Research* and *Research in Nursing & Health* in 1989, the average effect size for *t*-test situations was .35. Cohen (1988) noted that in new areas of research inquiry, effect sizes are likely to be small. A medium effect should be estimated only when the effect is so substantial that it can be detected by the naked eye (i.e., without formal research procedures).

➔ **TIP:** Performing a power analysis based on estimates of an effect size is an *evidence-based* approach to designing a new

| TABLE 22.6 | Approximate Sample Sizes* Necessary to Achieve Selected Levels of Power as a Function of Estimated Effect Size for Test of Difference of Two Means With $\alpha = .05$ |

ESTIMATED EFFECT SIZE (d)†

POWER	.10	.15	.20	.25	.30	.40	.50	.60	.70	.80
.60	977	434	244	156	109	61	39	27	20	15
.70	1230	547	308	197	137	77	49	34	25	19
.80	1568	697	392	251	174	98	63	44	32	25
.90	2100	933	525	336	233	131	84	58	43	33
.95	2592	1152	648	415	288	162	104	72	53	41

*Sample size requirements for each group; total sample size would be twice the number shown.

† Estimated effect size (d) is the estimated population mean group difference divided by the estimated population standard deviation -or $(\mu_1 - \mu_2)/\sigma$.

TABLE 22.7	Approximate Sample Sizes Necessary to Achieve Selected Levels of Power as a Function of Estimated Population Correlation With $\alpha = .05$									

ESTIMATED POPULATION CORRELATION COEFFICIENT (γ)

POWER	.10	.15	.20	.25	.30	.40	.50	.60	.70	.80
.60	489	218	123	79	55	32	21	15	11	9
.70	616	274	155	99	69	39	26	18	14	11
.80	785	349	197	126	88	50	32	23	17	13
.90	1050	468	263	169	118	67	43	30	22	17
.95	1297	577	325	208	145	82	53	37	27	21

study—that is, the new study uses evidence from earlier studies to estimate how many sample members will be needed to achieve an effect that seems plausible in light of what is already known. A useful supplementary approach is to ask, How big an effect would be needed to be clinically relevant? If effect-size estimates are both evidence based and clinically meaningful, the study will be stronger.

Sample Size Estimates for Other Bivariate Tests

🔵 Power analysis can be undertaken for the other statistical tests described in this chapter. It is relatively easy to do a power analysis online in this age of the Internet, and we provide several relevant websites on the free CD-ROM that accompanies this text. Here we discuss only a few basic features for situations in which ANOVA, Pearson's r, or a chi-square situation would be the basis for doing the power analysis.

There are alternative approaches to doing a power analysis in an ANOVA context. The simplest approach is to estimate **eta-squared** (η^2), which is an ES index indicating the proportion of variance explained in ANOVA. Eta-squared equals the sum of squares between (SS_B) divided by the total sum of squares (SS_T), and can be used directly as the estimate of effect size if sum of square information is available in a relevant research report. (For the

data in Table 22.2 and shown in an ANOVA summary table in Table 22.3, $\eta^2 = .27$, a large effect). When eta-squared cannot be estimated, researchers may be able to estimate whether effects are likely to be small, medium, or large. For ANOVA situations, the conventional estimates for small, medium, and large effects would be values of η^2 equal to .01, .06, and .14, respectively. Assuming $\alpha = .05$ and power $= .80$, this corresponds to sample size requirements of about 319, 53, or 22 subjects per group in a three-group study, and of about 272, 44, and 19 *per group* in a four-group study.*

When effect size estimates are expressed as the correlation between the independent and dependent variables, the estimated value of ES is ρ, the population correlation coefficient. Thus, the value of the correlation coefficient *(r)* from a relevant earlier study can be used directly as the estimated effect size. Table 22.7 shows sample size requirements in situations in which Pearson's r is used for various effect sizes and powers when $\alpha = .05$. For example, if our estimated population correlation was .25, we would need a sample size of 126 for power $= .80$. With a sample this size, we can expect that we would wrongly reject a true null hypothesis 5 times out of 100 and wrongly retain a

---

*When analysis of covariance (see Chapter 23) is used in lieu of *t*-tests or ANOVA, sample size requirements are smaller—sometimes appreciably so—because of reduced error variance.

false null hypothesis 20 times out of 100. When prior estimates of effect size are unavailable, the conventional values of small, medium, and large effect sizes in a bivariate correlation situation are .10, .30, and .50, respectively (i.e., samples of 785, 88, and 32 for a power of .80 and a significance level of .05). In Polit and Sherman's (1990) study, the average correlation in nursing studies was found to be around .20.

Estimating sample size requirements for testing differences in proportions between groups is complex. The effect size for contingency tables is influenced not only by expected differences in proportions (e.g., 60% in one group versus 40% in another, a 20-percentage point difference), but by the absolute values of the proportions. Effect sizes are *larger* (and thus sample size needs are *smaller*) at the extremes than near the midpoint. A 20-percentage point difference is easier to detect if the percentages are 10% and 30% than if they are near the middle, such as 60% and 40%. Because of this fact, it is difficult to offer information on values for small, medium, and large effects in this context. We can, however, give *examples* of differences in proportions that conform to the conventions in a 2 × 2 situation:

Small: .05 versus .10, .20 versus .29, .40 versus .50, .60 versus .70, .80 versus .87
Medium: .05 versus .21, .20 versus .43, .40 versus .65, .60 versus .82, .80 versus .96
Large: .05 versus .34, .20 versus .58, .40 versus .78, .60 versus .92, .80 versus .96

As an example, if the expected proportion for a control group were .40, the researcher would need about 385, 70, and 24 per group if higher values were expected for the experimental group and the effects were expected to be small, medium, and large, respectively. As in other situations, researchers are encouraged to avoid using the conventions, if possible, in favor of more precise estimates from prior empirical evidence. If the conventions cannot be avoided, conservative estimates should be used to minimize the risk for obtaining nonsignificant results.

Example of a power analysis: Hedges (2005) studied relationships among sleep, memory, and learning among off-pump coronary artery bypass patients. Power calculations to estimate sample size needs were based on an assumed medium effect ($r = .30$). With a power of .80 and $\alpha = .05$ for a one-tailed test, the power analysis indicated a need for 68 participants. A total of 96 patients were recruited, of whom 86 agreed to participate.

Effect Size Calculations in Completed Studies

Power analysis concepts are useful in after-the-fact descriptions of results. After analyses are completed, researchers can calculate estimated effects based on *actual N*s, and the effect size estimates are useful pieces of supplementary information (Owen, 2005). In this situation, power, alpha, and N are known, and so the task is to solve for ES.

Like the risk indexes described in Chapter 21, effect sizes provide readers and clinicians with estimates about the magnitude of effects within the research sample—an important issue in evidence-based practice (see Box 2.1). Effect size information can be crucial because, with large samples, even miniscule effects can be statistically significant at dramatic levels. The *p* values tell you whether results are likely to be *real,* but effect sizes can suggest whether they are important. Effect size estimates are needed in doing meta-analyses (see Chapter 25), and so when these values are presented directly in a report, they are helpful to meta-analysts.

Example of calculated effect size: Mackenzie, Poulin, and Seidman-Carlson (2006) tested a mindfulness-based stress reduction intervention for nurses and nurse aides. They presented a table of results that showed the values of *F*-ratio statistics, *p* values, and effect sizes (the values of η^2) for seven outcome variables.

THE COMPUTER AND BIVARIATE INFERENTIAL STATISTICS

We have stressed the logic and uses of various statistical tests rather than computational formulas.* Because computers are almost always used for statistical analysis, and because it is important to know how to read a computer printout, we include examples of computer analyses for two statistical tests. We return to the example described in Chapter 21, which involved an experiment to test the effects of a special prenatal program for young low-income women. The raw data for the 30 subjects in this example were presented in Table 21.10 in Chapter 21. Given these data, let us test some hypotheses.

Hypothesis One: *t*-Test

Our first research hypothesis is that the babies of experimental subjects have higher birth weights than babies of control subjects. The *t*-test for independent samples is used to test the hypothesis of mean group differences. The null and alternative hypotheses are:

$$H_0: \mu \text{ experimental} = \mu \text{ control}$$
$$H_A: \mu \text{ experimental} \neq \mu \text{ control}$$

Figure 22.6 presents the computer printout for the *t*-test. The top panel presents some descriptive statistics (mean, standard deviation, and standard error of the mean) for the birth weight variable, separately for the two groups. The mean birth weight of the babies in the experimental group is 107.5333 ounces, compared with 101.8667 ounces for those in the control group. The data are consistent with the research hypothesis; that is, the average weight of babies in the experimental group is higher than that of controls. But is the difference attributable to the intervention, or does it reflect random fluctuations?

The second panel of Figure 22.6 presents results of **Levene's test** for equality of variances. An assump-

tion underlying use of the *t*-test is that the population variances for the two groups are equal. The top panel shows that the standard deviations (and thus the variances) are quite different, with substantially more variability among experimental subjects than controls. Levene's test tells us that the two variances are, in fact, significantly different (Sig. = .046).

The third panel has two rows of information. The top row is for the **pooled variance *t*-test**, which is used when equality of variances can be assumed. Given the significantly different variances in this sample, however, we should use information in the second row, which uses a **separate variance *t*-test** formula. The value of the *t*-statistic is 1.443, and the two-tailed probability (Sig.) for the differences in group means is .163. This means that in about 16 samples out of 100, we could expect a mean difference in weights this large as a result of chance alone. Therefore, because $p > .05$ (a nonsignificant result), we cannot conclude that the intervention was effective in improving the birth weights of experimental group infants. Note that we cannot conclude that it was *not* effective, either. Failure to reject the null hypothesis does not mean that there is evidence that the null is true.

The last two columns of the bottom panel show the 95% CIs for the population mean difference. We can conclude with 95% confidence that the mean difference in birth weights for the population of young mothers exposed and not exposed to the intervention lies between -2.4885 ounces and $+13.8218$ ounces. Zero is within this interval, indicating the possibility that there are no group differences in the population. This is consistent with the fact that we could not reject the null hypothesis of equal means on the basis of the *t*-test.

It was noted earlier that power analysis can be used to estimate effect size. In our example, the effect size estimate (d) is as follows:

$$d = (107.5333 - 101.8667) \div 10.955 = .52$$

The estimated effect size is the experimental mean minus the control mean, divided by the overall (pooled) standard deviation, which is 10.955. The obtained effect size of .52 is moderate, but an

---

*Note that this introduction to inferential statistics has necessarily been superficial, and has neglected important issues such as specific assumptions that apply to various tests. We urge readers to undertake further exploration of statistical principles before undertaking quantitative analyses.

Group Statistics

	GROUP	N	Mean	Std. Deviation	Std. Error Mean
Infant birth weight in ounces	Experimental	15	107.5333	13.3784	3.4543
	Control	15	101.8667	7.2394	1.8692

Independent Samples Test

		Levene's Test for Equality of Variances	
		F	Sig.
Infant birth weight in ounces	Equal variances assumed	4.370	.046
	Equal variances not assumed		

		t-Test for Equality of Means					95% Confidence Interval of the Difference	
		t	df	Sig. (2-tailed)	Mean Difference	Std. Error Difference	Lower	Upper
Infant birth weight in ounces	Equal variances assumed	1.443	28	.160	5.6667	3.9276	–2.3787	13.7120
	Equal variances not assumed	1.443	21.552	.163	5.6667	3.9276	–2.4885	13.8218

FIGURE 22.6 t-Test printout: testing group differences in infant birth weight.

examination of Table 22.6 indicates that with a sample size of only 15 per group, our power to detect a true population difference is less (actually *far* less) than .60. This means that we had a very high risk for a Type II error. We can also see that with an effect size of .52, we would need about 60 subjects in each group to achieve a power of .80.

Hypothesis Two: Pearson Correlation

Our second research hypothesis is as follows: Older mothers have babies of higher birth weight than younger mothers. In this case, both birth weight and age are measured on the ratio scale, and the appropriate test statistic is the Pearson product-moment correlation. The hypotheses are:

$$H_0: \rho \text{ birth weight—age} = 0$$
$$H_A: \rho \text{ birth weight—age} \neq 0$$

The printout for the hypothesis test is presented in Figure 22.7. The correlation matrix shows, in row one, the correlation of infant birth weight with infant birth weight and of birth weight with mother's age; and in row two, the correlation of mother's age with infant birth weight and of age

Correlations

		Infant birth weight in ounces	Mother's age
Infant birth weight in ounces	Pearson correlation Sig. (2-tailed) N	1.000 . 30	.594* .001 30
Mother's age	Pearson correlation Sig. (2-tailed) N	.594* .001 30	1.000 . 30

*Correlation is significant at the 0.01 level (2-tailed)

FIGURE 22.7 Correlation matrix printout: testing the relationship between maternal age and infant birth weight.

with age. In the cell created at the intersection of age and birth weight, we find three numbers. The first is the correlation coefficient ($r = .594$), which indicates a moderately strong positive relationship: The older the mother, the higher the baby's weight tended to be, consistent with the research hypothesis. The second number in the cell shows the probability that the correlation occurred by chance: Sig. (for significance level) $= .001$ for a two-tailed test. In other words, a relationship this strong would be found by chance in fewer than 1 out of 1000 samples of 30 young mothers. Therefore, the research hypothesis is accepted. The final number in the cell is 30, the total sample size (N).

➡ **TIP:** You may find it helpful to consult the glossary of symbols in the inside back cover of this book to determine the meaning of statistical symbols that might be used in research reports. Note that not all symbols in this glossary are described in this book; therefore, it may be necessary to refer to a statistics textbook, such as Polit's (1996), for further information.

CRITIQUING INFERENTIAL STATISTICS

It is difficult to critique researchers' data analysis decisions without strong training in statistics and data analysis. Nevertheless, there are certain things you can do to critique the statistical analysis even if your background in statistics is modest.

You can begin by asking whether the report presents the results of statistical tests for all study hypotheses, and whether the researchers undertook analyses to address questions about the study's internal validity. For example, if groups were compared, were efforts made to examine their comparability with regard to factors other than the key independent variables (i.e., were analyses undertaken to test for selection biases)? Did key groups differ with regard to nonresponse or attrition? As we noted in Chapter 11, statistical analyses and design issues are sometimes intertwined, in the sense that both analytic and design decisions can affect statistical conclusion validity. When sample size is low, when an independent variable is weakly defined (or when participation in an intervention is low), and when a weak statistical procedure is used in lieu of a more powerful one, then the risk for drawing the wrong conclusion about the research hypotheses is heightened. You should pay particular attention to the possibility of statistical conclusion validity problems when research hypotheses are not supported.

Other issues important in a thorough critique concern whether the researcher used the right statistical tests, whether the statistical information

BOX 22.1 Guidelines for Critiquing Bivariate* Inferential Analyses

1. Does the report include any bivariate inferential statistics? Was a statistical test performed for each of the hypotheses or research questions? If inferential statistics were not used, should they have been?
2. Were statistical tests used appropriately to strengthen conclusions about the study's internal validity (e.g., to test for selection bias or attrition bias)?
3. Were the selected statistical tests appropriate, given the level of measurement of the variables and the nature of the hypotheses?
4. Were parametric tests used? Does it appear that the use of parametric tests was appropriate? If nonparametric tests were used, was a rationale provided, and does the rationale seem sound? Should more powerful parametric procedures have been used instead?
5. Was information provided about both hypothesis testing and estimation of parameters? Were effect sizes reported? Overall, did the statistical results provide readers and potential users of the study results with sufficient information about the evidence the study yields?
6. Were the results of any statistical tests significant? What do the tests tell you about the plausibility of the research hypotheses? Were effects sizable? What do the effects suggest about the clinical importance of the findings?
7. Were the results of any statistical tests nonsignificant? Is it plausible that these reflect Type II errors? What factors might have undermined the study's statistical conclusion validity?
8. In general, does the report provide a rationale for the use of the selected statistical tests? Does the report contain sufficient information for you to judge whether appropriate statistics were used?
9. Was there an appropriate amount of statistical information reported? Are the findings clearly and logically organized?
10. Were tables used judiciously to summarize large amounts of statistical information? Are the tables clearly presented, with good titles and carefully labeled column headings? Is the information presented in the text consistent with the information presented in the tables? Is the information totally redundant?

*Most of these questions are equally appropriate for critiquing the use of multivariate statistics, as described in Chapter 23.

reported is adequate to meet the information needs of clinicians, and whether the results were presented in a clear and thoughtful manner, with a judicious combination of information reported in the text and in well laid-out tables. Box 22.1 presents some guiding questions for critiquing the use of bivariate inferential statistics in a research report.

RESEARCH EXAMPLE

Study: "Effects of music therapy on physiological and psychological outcomes for patients undergoing cardiac surgery" (Sendelbach et al., 2006)

Statement of Purpose: The purpose of this study was to compare the effects of a relaxing music intervention, versus a quiet and uninterrupted rest period, on pain intensity, anxiety, physiologic indicators, and opioid consumption among patients who had undergone cardiac surgery.

Methods: Patients undergoing coronary artery bypass and/or valve replacement surgery in one of three Midwestern hospitals were recruited to participate in the study. A total of 86 patients were randomly assigned to a music/relaxation intervention group or to a control group. Patients in the intervention group were told to assume a comfortable position and were read a script that encouraged relaxation. Then they listened to a tape of relaxing music by headphones for 20 minutes. The intervention occurred each morning and afternoon on 3 postoperative days (POD). Those in the control group were advised to rest in bed in a comfortable position for 20 minutes. For both groups, measures for pain intensity, anxiety, heart rate, and blood pressure were obtained immediately before and after each intervention period. Medication usage was obtained from patients' charts.

Analysis and Findings: The researchers tested the preintervention comparability of the two groups to assess the risk for selection bias. The groups were similar for most of the characteristics examined. For example, the mean ages of the experimental and control group subjects were 62.3 and 64.7, respectively, and the t-test for this analysis was nonsignificant ($p = .43$). However, there was a nearly significantly difference with regard to type of procedure: those in the control group were more likely to have a joint coronary artery bypass and valve procedure (19.6%) than those in the intervention group (4.0%); the chi-square test yielded a $p = .051$.

The researchers used RM-ANOVA to compare group differences in pain, anxiety, blood pressure, and heart rate over time. Because of a high rate of missing data, the RM-ANOVA was done for only three time periods: the morning and afternoon of POD 1, and the morning of POD 2. The analysis indicated that those in the experimental group had significantly lower scores than those in the control group throughout the three time periods with respect to both anxiety ($p < .001$) and pain ($p = .009$). Group differences for heart rate and blood pressure were not significantly different. Differences in opioid consumption, measured in milligrams of parenteral morphine equivalents, were not significantly different as tested using t-tests. The researchers concluded that patients recovering from cardiac surgery may benefit from music therapy.

SUMMARY POINTS

- **Inferential statistics**, which are based on the **laws of probability**, allow researchers to make inferences about a population based on data from a sample; they offer a framework for deciding whether the **sampling error** that results from sampling fluctuation is too high to provide reliable population estimates.

- The **sampling distribution of the mean** is a theoretical distribution of the means of an infinite number of samples drawn from a popula-

tion. Because the sampling distribution of means follows a normal curve, it is possible to indicate the probability that a specified sample value will be obtained.

- The **standard error of the mean** (**SEM**)—the standard deviation of this theoretical distribution—indicates the degree of average error of a sample mean; the smaller the SEM, the more accurate are the estimates of the population mean based on a sample mean.

- Statistical inference consists of two major types of approaches: estimating parameters and testing hypotheses. **Parameter estimation** is used to estimate a population parameter.

- Point estimation provides a single descriptive value of the population estimate (e.g., a mean, proportion, or odds ratio). Interval estimation provides the upper and lower limits of a range of values—the **confidence interval** (**CI**)—between which the population value is expected to fall, at a specified probability level. Researchers establish the degree of confidence that the population value lies within this range. Most often, the 95% CI is reported, which indicates that there is a 95% probability that the true population value lies between the upper and lower **confidence limit**.

- Hypothesis testing through statistical procedures enables researchers to make objective decisions about the validity of their hypotheses.

- The **null hypothesis** states that no relationship exists between research variables, and that any observed relationship is due to chance. Rejection of the null hypothesis lends support to the research hypothesis; failure to reject it indicates that observed differences may be due to chance.

- If a null hypothesis is incorrectly rejected, this is a **Type I error** (a false positive). A **Type II error** occurs when a null hypothesis that should be rejected is accepted (a false negative).

- Researchers control the risk for making a Type I error by establishing a **level of significance** (or **alpha** level), which specifies the probability that such an error will occur. The .05 level means that in only 5 out of 100 samples would the null hypothesis be rejected when it should have been accepted.

- In testing hypotheses, researchers compute a **test statistic** and then determine whether the statistic falls at or beyond the **critical region** on the relevant theoretical distribution. If the value of the test statistic indicates that the null hypothesis is "improbable," the result is **statistically significant** (i.e., obtained results are not likely to result from chance fluctuations at the specified level of probability).

- Most hypothesis testing involves **two-tailed tests**, in which both ends of the sampling distribution are used to define the region of improbable values, but a **one-tailed test** may be appropriate if there is a strong rationale for an *a priori* directional hypothesis.

- **Parametric tests** involve the estimation of at least one parameter, the use of interval- or ratio-level data, and assumptions of normally distributed variables; **nonparametric tests** are used when the data are nominal or ordinal or when a normal distribution cannot be assumed—especially when samples are small.

- There are **tests for independent groups** for comparing separate groups of subjects, and **tests for dependent groups** for comparing the same group of subjects over time or conditions, as in within-subjects designs.

- Two common statistical tests are the *t*-test and **analysis of variance** (**ANOVA**), both of which are used to test the significance of the difference between group means; ANOVA is used when there are three or more groups (**one-way ANOVA**) or when there is more than one independent variable (e.g., **two-way ANOVA**). **Repeated measures ANOVA (RM-ANOVA)** is used when there are multiple means being compared over time.

- Nonparametric analogues of *t*-tests and ANOVA include the **median test**, the **Mann-Whitney *U* test,** the sign test and the **Wilcoxon signed-rank test** (two-group situations), and the **Kruskal-Wallis** and **Friedman tests** (three-group or more situations).

- The **chi-square test** is used to test hypotheses relating to group differences in proportions. For small samples or small cell sizes, **Fisher's exact test** should be used.

- Statistical tests to measure the magnitude of bivariate relationships and to test whether the relationship is significantly different from zero include Pearson's *r* for interval-level data, **Spearman's rho** and **Kendall's tau** for ordinal-level data, and the **phi coefficient** and **Cramér's *V*** for nominal-level data.

- Confidence intervals can be constructed around almost any computed statistic, including differences between means, differences between proportions, and correlation coefficients. CI information is valuable to clinical decision makers, who need to know more than whether differences are probably *real*.

- **Power analysis** is a method of estimating either the likelihood of committing a Type II error or sample size requirements. Power analysis involves four components: desired significance level (α), **power** ($1 - \beta$), sample size (N), and estimated **effect size** (ES). Effect size conveys important information about the magnitude of effects in a study and is a useful supplement to *p* values and CI values.

STUDY ACTIVITIES

Chapter 22 of the accompanying *Study Guide for Nursing Research: Principles and Methods, 8th edition*, offers various exercises and study suggestions for reinforcing the concepts presented in this chapter. In addition, the following study questions can be addressed:

1. What inferential statistic would you choose for the following sets of variables? Explain your answers (refer to Fig. 22.5).

   a. Variable 1 represents the weights of 100 patients; variable 2 is the patients' resting heart rate.

   b. Variable 1 is the patients' marital status; variable 2 is the patients' level of preoperative stress on a 10-item scale.

c. Variable 1 is whether an amputee has a leg removed above or below the knee; variable 2 is whether or not the amputee shows signs of aggressive behavior during rehabilitation.

2. Apply relevant questions in Box 22.1 to the research example at the end of the chapter (Sendelbach et al., 2006), referring to the full journal article as necessary.

● ● ● ● ● ● ● ● ● ● ● ● ● ● ● ● ●

STUDIES CITED IN CHAPTER 22

Methodologic or theoretical references cited in this chapter can be found in a separate section at the end of the book.

Barnason, S., Zimmerman, L., Brey, B., Catlin, S., & Nieveen, J. (2006). Patterns of recovery following percutaneous coronary intervention. *Applied Nursing Research, 19*(1), 31–37.

Carruth, A., Browning, S., Reed, D., Skarke, L., & Sealey, L. (2006). The impact of farm lifestyle and health characteristics. *Nursing Research, 55*(2), 121–127.

Chan, W., Woo, J., Hui, E., Lau, W., Lai, J., & Lee, D. (2005). A community model for care of elderly people with diabetes via telemedicine. *Applied Nursing Research, 18*(2), 77–81.

Creedon, S. (2006). Health care workers' hand decontamination practices. *Clinical Nursing Research, 15*(1), 6–26.

Doran, D., Harrison, M., Laschinger, H., Hirdes, J., Rukholm, E., Sidani, S., Hall, L. M., Tourangeau, A., & Cranley, L. (2006). Relationship between nursing interventions and outcome achievement in acute care settings. *Research in Nursing & Health, 29*(1), 61–70.

Hedges, C. (2005). Sleep, memory, and learning in off-pump coronary artery bypass patients. *Research in Nursing & Health, 28*(6), 462–473.

Mackenzie, C., Poulin, P., & Seidman-Carlson, R. (2006). A brief mindfulness-based stress reduction intervention for nurses and nurse aides. *Applied Nursing Research, 19*(2), 105–109.

McCarthy, D., & Graves, E. (2006). Conjugated linoleic acid preserves muscle mass in mice bearing the Lewis lung carcinoma, but not the B16 melanoma. *Research in Nursing & Health, 29*(2), 98–104.

McFarlane, J., Groff, J., O'Brien, J., & Watson, K. (2006). Secondary prevention of intimate partner violence. *Nursing Research, 55*(1), 52–61.

Muehrer, R., Keller, M., Powwattana, A., & Pornchaikate, A. (2006). Sexuality among women recipients of a pancreas and kidney transplant. *Western Journal of Nursing Research, 28*(2), 137–150.

Nyamathi, A., Dixon, E., Wiley, D., Christiani, A., & Lowe, A. (2006). Hepatitis C virus infection among homeless men referred from a community clinic. *Western Journal of Nursing Research, 28*(4), 475–488.

Sendelbach, S., Halm, M., Doran, K., Miller, E., & Gaillard, P. (2006). Effects of music therapy on physiological and psychological outcomes for patients undergoing cardiac surgery. *Journal of Cardiovascular Nursing, 21*(3), 194–200.

Tsay, S. L., & Hung, L. O. (2004). Empowerment of patients with end-stage renal disease: A randomized controlled trial. *International Journal of Nursing Studies, 41*, 59–65.

23

Using Multivariate Statistics to Analyze Complex Relationships

T he phenomena of interest to nurse researchers usually are complex. Patients' spirituality, nurses' effectiveness, or abrupt elevations of patients' temperature are phenomena that are multiply determined. Scientists, in efforts to explain or predict phenomena, have recognized that two-variable studies are often inadequate. The classic approach to data analysis and research design, which involved studying the effect of a single independent variable on a single dependent variable, is being replaced by more sophisticated **multivariate procedures**.*

Unlike the statistical methods reviewed in Chapters 21 and 22, multivariate statistics are computationally formidable. Our purpose is to provide a general understanding of how, when, and why multivariate statistics are used, without working out computations. Nevertheless, we must present more formulas than we did in the previous two chapters because, to read and produce tables with results from multivariate procedures, you must have some understanding of the underlying components. We note that this chapter introduces only a handful of multivariate techniques, albeit the most frequently used ones. Those needing more comprehensive coverage should

consult books such as those by Tabachnick and Fidell (2006) or Hair and colleagues (2005).

One of the mostly widely used multivariate procedures (and therefore the one we describe in greatest depth) is multiple regression analysis, which is used to understand the effects of two or more independent variables on a continuous dependent variable. The terms **multiple correlation** and **multiple regression** will be used almost interchangeably in reference to this technique, consistent with the strong bond between correlation and regression. To comprehend this bond, we first explain simple (i.e., bivariate) regression.

SIMPLE LINEAR REGRESSION

Regression analysis is used to make predictions. In simple (bivariate) regression, one independent variable (X) is used to predict a dependent variable (Y). For instance, we could use simple regression to predict stress from noise levels. An important feature of regression is that the higher the correlation between two variables, the more accurate the prediction. If the correlation between diastolic and systolic blood pressure were perfect (i.e., if $r = 1.00$), we would need to measure only one to know the value of the other. Because most variables are not perfectly correlated, predictions made through regression analysis usually are imperfect.

---

*We use the term *multivariate* in this chapter to refer to analyses with at least three variables.

614

| TABLE 23.1 | Example of Simple Linear Regression |

(1) X	(2) Y	(3) Y'	(4) e	(5) e^2
1	2	2.4	−.4	.16
3	6	4.2	1.8	3.24
5	4	6.0	−2.0	4.00
7	8	7.8	.2	.04
9	10	9.6	.4	.16
$\overline{X} = 5.0$	$\overline{Y} = 6.0$		0.0	$\Sigma e^2 = 7.60$

$r = .90 \quad Y' = a + bX = 1.5 + .9X$

The basic linear regression equation is

$$Y' = a + bX$$

where Y' = predicted value of variable Y
a = intercept constant
b = regression coefficient
X = actual value of independent variable X

Regression analysis solves for a and b, so for any value of X, a prediction about Y can be made. You may remember from high school algebra that the preceding equation is the algebraic equation for a straight line. **Linear regression** is used to determine a straight-line fit to the data that minimizes deviations from the line.

As an illustration, consider the data for five subjects on two variables, X and Y (Table 23.1) that are strongly related ($r = .90$). When we use the five pairs of X and Y values to solve for a and b in a regression equation, we will be able to predict Y values for a *new* group of people about whom we will have information on variable X only.

We do not illustrate the formulas for computing the values of a and b here, but suffice it to say they are fairly straightforward algebraic calculations involving deviation scores from the X and Y values. As shown at the bottom of Table 23.1, the solution to the regression equation is $Y' = 1.5 + .9X$. Now suppose for the moment that the X values in column 1 are the only data we have, and we want to predict values for Y.

For the first subject, $X = 1$; we would predict that $Y = 1.5 + (.9)(1)$, or 2.4. Column 3 shows Y' values for each X. These numbers show that Y' does not exactly equal the actual values obtained for Y (column 2). Most **errors of prediction** (e) are small, as shown in column 4. Errors of prediction occur because the correlation between X and Y is not perfect. Only when $r = 1.00$ or -1.00 does $Y' = Y$. The regression equation solves for a and b in a way that minimizes such errors. More precisely, the solution minimizes the sums of squares of prediction errors, which is why standard regression analysis is said to use a **least-squares** criterion. Indeed, standard regression is sometimes referred to as **ordinary least squares**, or **OLS**, regression. In column 5 of Table 23.1, the error terms—sometimes called **residuals**—have been squared and summed to yield a value of 7.60. Any values of a and b other than 1.5 and .9 would have yielded a larger sum of squared residuals.

Figure 23.1 displays the solution to this regression analysis graphically. The actual X and Y values are plotted on the graph with circles. The line running through these points represents the regression solution. The intercept (a) is the point at which the line crosses the Y axis, which in this case is 1.5. The slope (b) is the angle of the line. With $b = .90$, the line slopes so that for every 4 units on the X axis, we must go up 3.6 units ($.9 \times 4$) on the Y axis. The line, then, embodies the regression equation. To predict a value for Y, we would go to the point on the X

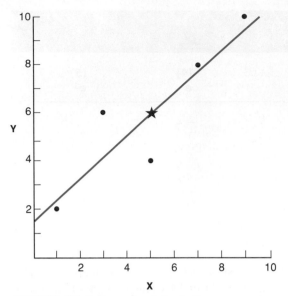

FIGURE 23.1 Example of simple linear regression.

axis for an obtained X value, go up to vertically to the point on the regression line directly above the X score, and then read the predicted Y' value horizontally on the Y axis. For example, for an X value of 5, we would predict a Y' of 6, indicated by the star.

Correlation coefficients show the degree to which variables are related. Statistically, correlations express how variation in one variable is associated with variation in another. The square of r (r^2) tells us the proportion of variance in Y that is accounted for by X. In our example, $r = .90$, so $r^2 = .81$. This means that 81% of the variability in Y values can be understood in terms of variability in X values. The remaining 19% is variability due to other factors.

In the regression problem, the sum of the squared residuals (e^2s) is 7.6. Although the calculations are not shown, the sum of the squared deviations of Y values from the mean of Y ($\sum y^2$) is 40; this represents total variability in Y. To demonstrate that the residuals are 19% of the unexplained variability in Y, we compute the following ratio:

$$\frac{7.6}{40} = .19 = 1 - r^2$$

These calculations reinforce a point made earlier: The stronger the correlation, the better the pre-

diction; the stronger the correlation, the greater the percentage of variance explained.

MULTIPLE LINEAR REGRESSION

Because the correlation between two variables is rarely perfect, researchers often try to improve predictions of Y by including multiple independent variables—which are often called **predictor variables** in a multiple regression context.

Basic Concepts for Multiple Regression

Suppose we wanted to predict graduate nursing students' grade-point averages (GPAs). Not all applicants can be accepted, so we want to select those with the greatest chance of success. Suppose we had previously found that students with high scores on the verbal portion of an entrance exam (EE-V) tended to get better grades than those with lower EE-V scores. The correlation between EE-V and graduate GPAs has been calculated as .50. With only 25% (.50²) of the variance of graduate GPAs accounted for, there will be many errors of prediction: Many admitted students will not perform as well as expected, and many rejected applicants would have made good students. It may be possible, by adding information, to make more accurate predictions through multiple regression. The basic multiple regression equation is

$$Y' = a + b_1 X_1 + b_2 X_2 + < \cdots b_k X_k$$

where Y' = predicted value for variable Y
$\quad a$ = intercept constant
$\quad k$ = number of predictor (independent) variables
$\quad b_1$ to b_k = regression coefficients for the k variables
$\quad X_1$ to X_k = scores or values on the k independent variables

In our example of predicting graduate nursing students' GPAs, suppose we hypothesized that undergraduate GPA (GPA-U) and scores on the quantitative portion of the entrance exam (EE-Q) would improve our ability to predict graduate GPA. Suppose the resulting equation were

$$Y' = .4 + .05(\text{GPA-U}) + .003(\text{EE-Q}) + .002(\text{EE-V})$$

For instance, suppose an applicant had an EE-V score of 600, an EE-Q score of 550, and a GPA-U of 3.2. The predicted graduate GPA would be

$$Y' = .4 + (.05)(3.2) + .003(550) + .002(600) = 3.41$$

We can assess the degree to which adding two independent variables improved our ability to predict graduate school performance through the multiple correlation coefficient. In bivariate correlation, the index is Pearson's r. With two or more independent variables, the correlation index is the **multiple correlation coefficient**, or R. Unlike r, R does not have negative values. R varies only from .00 to 1.00, showing the *strength* of the relationship between several independent variables and a dependent variable but not *direction*. The R statistic, when squared (R^2), indicates the proportion of variance in Y accounted for by the combined, simultaneous influence of the independent variables.

R^2 provides a way to evaluate the accuracy of a prediction equation. Suppose that with the three predictor variables in the current example, the value of $R = .71$. This means that 50% ($.71^2$) of the variability in graduate students' grades can be explained by their verbal and quantitative EE scores and their undergraduate grades. The addition of two predictors doubled the variance accounted for by EE-V alone, from .25 to .50.

The multiple correlation coefficient cannot be less than the highest bivariate correlation between an independent variable and the dependent variable. Table 23.2 presents a correlation matrix with the correlation coefficients for all pairs of variables in this example. The independent variable most strongly correlated with graduate performance is GPA-U, $r = .60$. The value of R could not have been less than .60.

Another important point is that R is more readily increased when the independent variables have low correlations among themselves. In the current case, the correlations range from .40 (between EE-Q and GPA-U) and .70 (EE-Q and EE-V). All correlations are fairly substantial, which helps to explain why R is not much higher than the r between the GPA-GRAD and GPA-U alone (.71 compared with .60). This somewhat puzzling phenomenon results from redundancy of information among predictors. When correlations among independent variables are high, they add little predictive power to each other. With low correlations among predictors, each one can contribute something unique to predicting the dependent variable. In our example, GPA-U predicts 36% of Y's variance ($.60^2$). The remaining two independent variables do not contribute as much as we would expect by considering their bivariate correlation with graduate GPA (r for EE-V = .50; r for EE-Q = .55). In fact, their *combined* additional contribution is only 14% (.50 − .36 = .14). The contribution is small because the two entrance exam scores have redundant information with undergraduate grades.

TABLE 23.2	Correlation Matrix			
	GPA-GRAD	**GPA-U**	**EE-Q**	**EE-V**
GPA-GRAD	1.00			
GPA-U	.60	1.00		
EE-Q	.55	.40	1.00	
EE-V	.50	.50	.70	1.00

GPA, grade point average; EE, entrance examination; GPA-GRAD, graduate GPA; GPA-U, undergraduate GPA; EE-Q, entrance examination quantitative score; EE-V, entrance examination verbal score.

A related point is that, as more independent variables are added to the regression equation, increments to R tend to decrease. It is rare to find predictor variables that correlate well with a criterion but modestly with one another. Redundancy is difficult to avoid as more and more variables are added to the equation. The inclusion of independent variables beyond the first four or five typically does little to improve the proportion of variance accounted for or the accuracy of prediction.

The dependent variable in multiple regression analysis, as in ANOVA, should be measured on an interval or ratio scale. Independent variables, on the other hand, can either be interval- or ratio-level variables *or* dichotomous variables. A text such as that by Cohen and colleagues (2002) should be consulted for information on how to use and interpret dichotomous **dummy variables**.

Tests of Significance

Multiple regression analysis is not used solely (or even primarily) to develop prediction equations. Researchers almost always ask inferential questions about relationships in the analysis (e.g., Is the calculated R the result of chance fluctuations, or does it reflect true relationships in the population?) There are several significance tests, each used to address different questions.

Tests of the Overall Equation and R

The most basic test in multiple regression is for the null hypothesis that the population multiple correlation coefficient equals zero. The test for the significance of R is based on principles analogous to those for ANOVA. With ANOVA, the F-ratio statistic is the ratio of the mean squares between divided by mean squares within. In multiple regression, the form is similar:

$$F = \frac{SS_{\text{due to regression}} / df_{\text{regression}}}{SS_{\text{of residuals}} / df_{\text{residuals}}}$$

$$= \frac{\text{Mean Square}_{\text{due to regression}}}{\text{Mean Square}_{\text{of residuals}}}$$

The basic principle is the same as in ANOVA: Variance from independent variables is contrasted with variance attributable to other factors, or error. In our example of predicting graduate GPAs, suppose a multiple correlation coefficient of .71 ($R^2 = .50$) was calculated for a sample of 100 graduate students. The computed value of the F-statistic in this example would be 32.05. The tabled value of F (with $df = 3$ and 96) for a significance level of .01 is about 4.0; thus, the probability that $R = .71$ resulted from chance fluctuations is considerably less than .01.

> **Example of multiple regression:** Anderson, Issel, and McDaniel (2003) examined the relationship between nursing home characteristics and management practices on the one hand, and nursing home residents' outcomes (e.g., restraint use) on the other. Using multiple regression, they found that communication openness and the nursing director's years of experience as director were significant predictors of restraint use. Overall, the R^2 between predictor variables and restraint use was .16, $p < .001$.

Tests for Adding Predictors

Another question researchers may want to answer is: Does *adding* X_k to the regression significantly improve the prediction of Y over that achieved with X_{k-1}? For example, does a third predictor increase our ability to predict Y after two predictors have been used? An F-statistic can be computed to answer this question.

Let us number each independent variable in the current example: $X_1 = $ GPA-U; $X_2 = $ EE-Q; and $X_3 = $ EE-V. We can then symbolize various correlation coefficients as follows:

$R_{y.1}$ = the correlation of Y with GPA-U = .60
$R_{y.12}$ = the correlation of Y with
    GPA-U *and* EE-Q =   .71
$R_{y.123}$ = the correlation of Y with
    all three predictors =   .71

These figures indicate that EE-V scores made no independent contribution to the multiple correlation coefficient. The value of $R_{y.12}$ is identical to the value of $R_{y.123}$. We cannot tell at a glance, however, whether adding X_2 to X_1 *significantly* increased the prediction of Y. What we want to know is whether

X_2 would improve predictions in the population, or if its added predictive power in this sample resulted from chance. In the current example, although we show no computations, the value of the F-statistic for testing whether adding EE-Q scores significantly improves our prediction of Y is 27.16. If we consulted a table for the theoretical distribution of F with $df = 1$ and 97 and a significance level of .01, we would find that the critical value is about 6.90. Therefore, adding EE-Q to the regression equation significantly improved the accuracy of predicting graduate GPA, beyond the .01 level.

Example of adding predictors in multiple regression: Carrère and colleagues (2005) used multiple regression analysis to study depressive symptoms in married men and women. They first studied marital satisfaction in relation to depressive symptoms. For the women, the initial r^2 between the two variables was .17, $p < .01$. Then they added a measure of *anger dysregulation* (problems with anger), and R^2 increased to .24; the increment was statistically significant.

Tests of the Regression Coefficients

Researchers often want to know the significance of individual predictors, which can be done by calculating t-statistics that test the unique contribution of each independent variable. A significant t indicates that the regression coefficient (b) is significantly different from zero.

In simple regression, the value of b indicates the amount of change in predicted values of Y, for a specified rate of change in X. In multiple regression, the coefficients represent the number of units the dependent variable is predicted to change for each unit change in a given independent variable *when the effects of other predictors are held constant*. "Holding constant" other variables means that they are statistically controlled, a feature that can enhance a study's internal validity. If a regression coefficient is significant and confounding variables are included in the regression equation, it means that the variable associated with the coefficient contributed significantly to the regression, even after confounding variables are taken into account.

Strategies for Handling Predictors in Multiple Regression

There are various strategies for entering predictor variables into regression equations. The three most common are simultaneous, hierarchical, and stepwise regression.

Simultaneous Multiple Regression

The most basic strategy, **simultaneous multiple regression**, enters all predictor variables into the regression equation at the same time. One regression equation is developed, and statistical tests indicate the significance of R and of individual regression coefficients. This strategy is most appropriate when there is no basis for considering any particular predictor as causally before another, and when the predictors are of comparable importance to the research problem.

Hierarchical Multiple Regression

Many researchers use **hierarchical multiple regression**, which involves entering predictors into the equation in a series of steps. Researchers control the order of entry, with the order typically based on theoretical considerations or logic. For example, some predictors may be thought of as causally or temporally before others, in which case they could be entered in an early step. Another reason for using hierarchical regression is to examine the effect of a key independent variable after first removing the effect of confounding variables.

Example of hierarchical multiple regression: Eller and colleagues (2006) studied factors that predicted quality of life among patients receiving treatment for prostate cancer. They used hierarchical regression to enter predictor variables in a series of steps. Demographic characteristics (e.g., age, income) were entered first, and then other variables in their theoretical model (e.g., physiologic factors, psychological factors) were entered according to a hypothesized sequence.

With hierarchical regression, researchers determine the number of steps and the number of predictors included in each step. When several variables are added as a block, as in the Eller example, the analysis is a simultaneous regression for those

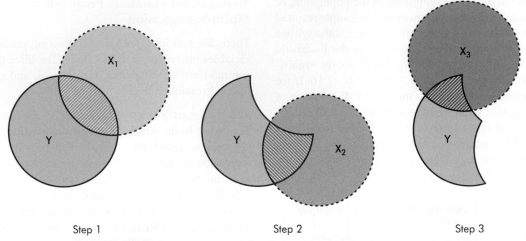

Step 1   **Step 2**   **Step 3**

FIGURE 23.2 Visual representation of stepwise multiple regression analysis.

variables at that stage. Thus, hierarchical regression can be considered a controlled sequence of simultaneous regressions.

Stepwise Multiple Regression

Stepwise multiple regression involves *empirically* selecting the combination of independent variables with the most predictive power. In stepwise multiple regression, predictors enter the regression equation in the order that produces the greatest increments to R^2. The first step selects the single best predictor of the dependent variable, that is, the independent variable with the highest bivariate correlation with Y. The second variable to enter the equation is the one that produces the largest increase to R^2 when used simultaneously with the variable selected in the first step. The procedure continues until no additional predictor significantly increases the value of R^2.

Figure 23.2 presents a simplified illustration of stepwise multiple regression. Suppose that the first variable (X_1) has a correlation of .60 with Y $(r^2 = .36)$ and that no other predictor is correlated more strongly with the dependent variable. The variable X_1 accounts for the portion of the variability of Y represented by the hatched area in step 1 of the figure. This hatched area is, in effect, removed from further consideration because this portion of Y's variability is explained or accounted for. Thus, the variable chosen in step 2 is not necessarily the X variable with the second largest

correlation with Y. The selected predictor is the one that explains the largest portion of what *remains* of Y's variability after X_1 has been taken into account. Variable X_2, in turn, removes a second part of Y so that the independent variable selected in step 3 is the one that accounts for the most variability in Y after *both* X_1 and X_2 are removed.

➡ **T I P :** Stepwise regression is a controversial procedure because variables are entered into the regression equation based solely on statistical rather than theoretical criteria. If stepwise regression is used, cross-validation is essential (e.g., by dividing the sample in half and running two independent regressions).

Relative Contribution of Predictors

Scientists want not only to predict phenomena, but also to explain them. Predictions can be made in the absence of understanding. For instance, in our graduate school example, we could predict performance moderately well without explaining *why* the factors contributed to students' success. For practical applications, it may be sufficient to make accurate predictions, but scientists typically want to understand phenomena.

In multiple regression, one approach to understanding a phenomenon is to explore the relative importance of independent variables. Unfortunately, the determination of the relative contributions of independent variables in predicting a dependent variable is a thorny issue. When independent variables are correlated, as they usually are, there is no ideal way to disentangle the effects of variables in the equation.

It may appear that the solution is to compare the contributions of the Xs to R^2. In our graduate school example, GPA-U accounted for 36% of Y's variance; EE-Q explained an additional 14%. Should we conclude that undergraduate grades are more than twice as important as EE-Q scores in explaining graduate school grades? This conclusion would be inaccurate because the order of entry of variables in a regression equation affects their apparent contribution. If these two predictor variables were entered in reverse order (i.e., EE-Q first), R^2 would remain unchanged at .50; however, EE-Q's contribution would be .30 (.55²), and GPA-U's contribution would be .20 (.50 − .30). This is because whatever variance the independent variables have in common is attributed to the first variable entered in the analysis.

Another approach to assessing the relative importance of the predictors is to compare regression coefficients. Earlier, we presented an equation for multiple regression that included a (the constant), and b's (regression coefficients) for each predictor. The b values cannot be directly compared because they are in the units of original scores, which differ from one X to another. X_1 might be in milliliters, X_2 in degrees Fahrenheit, and so forth. The use of **standard scores*** (or **z scores**) eliminates this problem by transforming all variables to scores with a mean of 0.0 and a standard deviation (SD) of 1.00. Transforming regular scores to z scores is easy—they are the difference between a score and the mean of that score divided by the standard deviation, or:

$$z_x = \frac{X - \overline{X}}{SD_x}$$

In standard score form, the regression equation simply uses standard scores (z's) instead of raw

scores (X's), and the regression coefficients for each z are standardized regression coefficients, called **beta [β] weights.** With all the β's in the same measurement units, can their relative size shed light on how much importance to attach to predictor variables? Many researchers have interpreted beta weights in this fashion, but there are problems in doing so. These regression coefficients will be the same no matter what the order of entry of the variables. The difficulty, however, is that regression weights are unstable. The values of β tend to fluctuate from sample to sample. Moreover, when a variable is added to or subtracted from the regression equation, the beta weights change. Because there is nothing absolute about the values of the regression coefficients, it is difficult to attach theoretical importance to them. (Another method of disentangling relationships is through causal modeling, described later in this chapter.)

Regression Results

Although there are no standard table formats for presenting multiple regression results, the most frequently reported elements are values of β, R^2, and significance levels. We illustrate tabular presentation of regression results using findings from the previously cited study by Anderson and her colleagues, who examined restraint use (and other outcomes) among nursing home residents in relation to nursing home and manager characteristics in 152 nursing homes.

The first column of Table 23.3 shows that the analysis used eight independent variables to predict average prevalence of restraint use. The next column shows the values for b, that is, the raw regression coefficients for each predictor. The next column shows the standard error (SE) of the regression coefficients. When b is divided by the SE, the result is a value for the t-statistic, which can be used to determine the significance of individual predictors. In this table, the t-values are not shown, but some regression tables *do* present them. We can compute them, though, from information in the table; for example, the value of t for the predictor *number of beds* would be −3.44 (−2.10 ÷ .61 = −3.44). This is highly significant, as shown in the last column: the probability (p) is less than 1 in 1000 that

---

*Consult a standard statistical textbook for a complete discussion of standard scores.

TABLE 23.3	Example of Multiple Regression Analysis: Average Prevalence of Restraint Use for Nursing Home Residents, Regressed on Nursing Home Characteristics, Manager Characteristics, and Management Practices			

PREDICTOR VARIABLE	b	SE	BETA (β)	p
Number of beds	−2.10	.61	−.29	<.001
Ownership type (profit vs. nonprofit)	1.29	.72	.14	NS
Director of nursing tenure in current position	−.41	.18	−.19	<.05
Years of experience as director of nursing	−.48	.22	−.18	<.05
Communication openness	−1.59	.61	−.23	<.05
RN participation in decision making	−.06	.24	−.02	NS
Relationship-oriented leadership	−.32	.53	−.05	NS
Formalization of rules and procedures	.21	.62	.03	NS

N = 152 nursing homes
F = 4.70 df = 8,143 p < .001 R^2 = .21   Adjusted R^2 = .16

Adapted from Anderson, R. A., Issel, L. M., & McDaniel, R. R. (2003). Nursing homes as complex adaptive systems: Relationship between management practice and resident outcomes (Table 3). *Nursing Research, 52,* 12–21.

the relationship between number of beds in a nursing home and the use of restraints is spurious. The table indicates that as the number of beds in a nursing home increases, the use of restraints *decreases*, as indicated by the negative regression coefficient. This relationship was found to be significant, even with the other seven predictors controlled. Three other predictor variables were significantly related to restraint use: the more experienced the director of nursing, the longer his or her tenure in the position, and the greater the communication openness in the nursing home, the lower the use of restraints. Other predictors in the analysis (e.g., whether the nursing home was for-profit or not-for-profit) were not related significantly to restraint use (shown as *NS*) once other factors were taken into consideration.

The fourth column of Table 23.3 shows the value of the beta (β) coefficients for each predictor. In this particular sample, and with these particular predictors, the variable *number of beds* was the best predictor of restraint use (β = −.29), and the variable *communication openness* was the second best predictor (β = −.23).

At the bottom of the table, we see that the F for the overall regression equation, with 8 and 143 df, was highly significant, p <.001. The value of R^2 is .21, but after adjusting for sample size and number of predictors, the value is reduced to .16. Thus, 16% of the variance in restraint use is explained by the combined effect of the eight predictors. The remaining 84% of variation is explained by other factors, including characteristics of the residents themselves.

➔ **TIP:** Knapp (1994) offered suggestions for reporting regression results. Also, some table templates for presenting multivariate results are included in the Toolkit of the accompanying *Resource Manual.*

Sample Size for Multiple Regression

Small samples are especially problematic in multiple regression and other multivariate procedures. Inadequate sample size can lead to Type II errors, and can also yield erratic and misleading regression coefficients.

One approach to estimating sample size needs concerns the ratio of predictor variables to total number of cases. Tabachnick and Fidell (2006) indicate that the barest minimum is to include 5 times as many cases as there are predictors in the regression. They *recommend*, however, a ratio of 20:1 for simultaneous and hierarchical regression and a ratio of 40:1 for stepwise. More cases are needed for stepwise regression because this procedure capitalizes on the idiosyncrasies of a specific data set.

A better way to estimate sample size needs is to perform a power analysis. The number of subjects needed to reject the null hypothesis that R equals zero is estimated as a function of effect size, number of predictors, desired power, and the significance criterion. For multiple regression, the estimated population effect size (γ) is R^2 divided by $1-R^2$. Researchers must either predict the value of R^2 on the basis of earlier research, or use the convention that the effect size will be small ($R^2 = .02$), moderate ($R^2 = .13$), or large ($R^2 = .30$). Next, the following formula is applied:

$$N = \frac{L}{\gamma} + k + 1$$

where N = estimated number of subjects needed
L = tabled value for the desired α and power
k = number of predictors
γ = estimated effect size

Table 23.4 presents values for L when $\alpha = .05$ and power is .50 to .90, in situations in which there are up to 15 predictor variables.

As an example, suppose we were planning a study to predict functional ability in nursing home residents using five predictor variables. We estimate a moderate effect size ($R^2 = .13$) and want to achieve a power of .80 and $\alpha = .05$. With $R^2 = .13$, the estimated population effect size (γ) is .149 ($.13 \div .87$). From Table 23.4, we find that the value of $L = 12.83$. Thus:

$$N = \frac{12.83}{.149} + 5 + 1 = 92.1$$

Thus, a sample of about 92 nursing home residents is needed to detect a population R^2 of .13 with five predictors, with a 5% chance of a Type I error and a 20% chance of a Type II error.

➔ **TIP:** Several websites (many of which are on the accompanying CD-ROM for you to click on) do instantaneous power calculations and sample size estimates for many of the multivariate procedures described in this chapter. An especially useful link, from which you can be directed to many others, is *http://statpages.org/*.

| TABLE 23.4 | Power Analysis Table for Multiple Regression: Values of L for α = .05 With k Predictor Variables |

| | POWER (1 − β) | | | | |
k	.50	.70	.80	.85	.90
2	4.96	7.70	9.84	10.92	12.65
3	5.76	8.79	10.90	12.30	14.17
4	6.42	9.68	11.94	13.42	15.41
5	6.99	10.45	12.83	14.39	16.47
6	7.50	11.14	13.62	15.26	17.42
7	7.97	11.77	14.35	16.04	18.28
8	8.41	12.35	15.02	16.77	19.08
9	8.81	12.89	15.65	17.45	19.83
10	9.19	13.40	16.24	18.09	20.53
15	10.86	15.63	18.81	20.87	23.58

ANALYSIS OF COVARIANCE

Analysis of covariance (**ANCOVA**) has much in common with multiple regression, but it also has features of ANOVA. Like ANOVA, ANCOVA is used to compare the means of two or more groups, and the central question for both is the same: Are mean group differences likely to be *real* or spurious? Like multiple regression, however, ANCOVA permits researchers to control confounding variables statistically.

Uses of Analysis of Covariance

ANCOVA is especially useful in certain situations. For example, if a nonequivalent control group design is used, researchers must consider whether obtained results are influenced by preexisting group differences. When experimental control through randomization is lacking, ANCOVA offers *post hoc* statistical control. Even in true experiments, ANCOVA can result in more precise estimates of group differences because, even with randomization, there are typically slight differences between groups. ANCOVA adjusts for initial differences so that the results more precisely reflect the effect of an intervention.

Strictly speaking, ANCOVA should not be used with preexisting groups because randomization is an underlying assumption of ANCOVA. This assumption is often violated, however. Random assignment should be done whenever possible, but when randomization is not feasible, ANCOVA can often improve the internal validity of a study.

ANCOVA Procedures

Suppose we were testing the effectiveness of biofeedback therapy on patients' anxiety. A group in one hospital is exposed to the treatment, and a comparison group in another hospital is not. Subjects' anxiety levels are measured both before and after the intervention, so pretest anxiety scores can be statistically controlled through ANCOVA. In such a situation, the dependent variable is the posttest anxiety scores, the independent variable is experimental/comparison group status, and the

covariate is pretest anxiety scores. Covariates can either be continuous variables (e.g., anxiety scores) or dichotomous variables (male/female); the independent variable is a nominal-level variable.

ANCOVA tests the significance of differences between group means after adjusting scores on the dependent variable to remove the effect of covariates. In essence, the first step in ANCOVA is the same as the first step in hierarchical multiple regression. Variability in the dependent measure that can be explained by the covariate is removed from further consideration. ANOVA is performed on what remains of Y's variability to see whether, once the covariate is controlled, significant differences between group means exist.

Let us consider another example to explore further aspects of ANCOVA. Suppose we were testing the effectiveness of weight-loss diets, and we randomly assigned 30 subjects to 1 of 3 groups. ANCOVA, using pretreatment weight as the covariate, permits a more sensitive analysis of weight change than simple ANOVA. Some hypothetical data for such a study are shown in Table 23.5. Two aspects of the weight values in this table are discernible. First, despite random assignment to treatment groups, initial group means are different. Subjects in diet B differ from those in diet C by an average of 10 pounds (175 versus 185 pounds). This difference, reflecting chance fluctuations, is not significant (calculations are not shown). Second, posttreatment means are also different by a maximum of only 10 pounds (160 to 170). However, the mean number of pounds *lost* ranged from 10 pounds for diets A and B to 25 pounds for diet C.

A summary table for ordinary ANOVA is presented in part A of Table 23.6. According to the results, group differences in posttreatment means result in a nonsignificant F-value. Based on ANOVA, we would conclude that all three diets had equal effects on weight loss.

Part B of Table 23.6 presents the summary table for ANCOVA. The first step of the analysis breaks total variability in posttreatment weights into two components: (1) variability explained by the covariate, pretreatment weights; and (2) residual variability. The table shows that the covariate

TABLE 23.5	Fictitious Data for ANCOVA Example

DIET A (X_A)		DIET B (X_B)		DIET C (X_C)	
X_A^*	Y_A	X_B^*	Y_B	X_C^*	Y_C
195	185	205	200	175	160
180	170	150	140	210	165
160	150	145	135	150	130
215	200	210	190	185	170
155	145	185	185	205	180
205	195	160	150	190	165
175	165	190	175	160	135
180	170	165	150	165	140
140	135	180	165	180	160
195	185	160	160	230	195

$\bar{X}_A^* = 180.0$ $\bar{Y}_A = 170.0$ $\bar{X}_B^* = 175.0$ $\bar{Y}_B = 165.0$ $\bar{X}_C^* = 185.0$ $\bar{Y}_C = 160.0$

Independent variable = diet; X^* = covariate (pretreatment weight); Y = dependent variable (posttreatment weight).

TABLE 23.6	Comparison of ANOVA and ANCOVA Results

SOURCE OF VARIATION		SUM OF SQUARES	df	MEAN SQUARE	f	p
A. Summary Table for ANOVA						
Between groups		500.0	2	250.0	0.55	>.05
Within groups		12,300.0	27	455.6		
TOTAL		12,800.0	29			
B. Summary Table for ANCOVA						
Step 1	Covariate	10,563.1	1	10,563.1	132.23	<.01
	Residual	2236.9	28	79.9		
	TOTAL	12,800.0	29			
Step 2	Between groups	1284.8	2	642.4	17.54	<.01
	Within groups	952.1	26	36.6		
	TOTAL	2236.9	28			

accounted for a significant amount of variance, which is not surprising given the strong relationship between pretreatment and posttreatment weights ($r = .91$). This merely indicates that people who started out especially heavy tended to stay that way, relative to others in the sample. In the second phase of the analysis, residual variance is broken down to reflect between-group and within-group contributions. With 2 and 26 degrees of freedom, the F of 17.54 is significant beyond the .01 level. The conclusion is that, after controlling for initial weight, there is a significant difference in weight attributable to exposure to different diets.

This fictitious example was contrived so that an ANOVA result of "no difference" would be altered by adding a covariate. Most actual results are less dramatic. Nonetheless, ANCOVA yields a more sensitive statistical test than ANOVA because the covariate reduces the error term (within-group variability) against which treatment effects are compared. In part A of Table 23.6, it can be seen that the within-group term is extremely large (12,300), masking the contribution of the experimental treatments.

Theoretically, it is possible to use any number of covariates. It is probably unwise, however, to use more than three or four. For one thing, including more covariates is often unnecessary because of the typically high degree of redundancy beyond the first few variables. Moreover, each covariate uses up a degree of freedom, and fewer degrees of freedom means that a higher computed F is required for significance. For instance, with 2 and 26 df, an F of 5.53 is required for significance at the .01 level, but with 2 and 23 df (i.e., adding three covariates), an F of 5.66 is needed.

Selection of Covariates

Useful covariates are almost always available. Background characteristics, such as age and gender, are good candidates, for example. Covariates should be variables that you suspect are correlated with the dependent variable. Background characteristics are especially important to control when there are significant differences on extraneous background characteristics between groups being compared. The literature is a good source of information about correlates of the dependent variable that should be controlled.

A pretest measure (i.e., a measure of the dependent variable before the occurrence of the independent variable) is another good covariate, although in such a situation, repeated measures ANOVA is an alternative when analyzing data from studies with before–after designs. Maxwell and colleagues (1991) have discussed the tradeoffs of these two approaches in terms of effects on power. Propensity scores, discussed briefly in Chapter 10, can be powerful covariates. Propensity scores capture group differences on a broad range of attributes because they represent an attempt to model group differences using available data. Rosenbaum (1995) provides a useful summary of using propensity scores as covariates.

In general, it is important to select covariates that have strong reliability. Measurement errors can lead to either overadjustments or underadjustments of the mean and can contribute to Type I or Type II errors.

⮕ TIP: In many situations, ANCOVA is preferable to ANOVA or *t*-tests, and is not appreciably more difficult to run on the computer. ANCOVA can enhance both statistical conclusion and internal validity in a study.

Adjusted Means

As shown in part B of Table 23.6, an ANCOVA summary table provides information about significance tests. The table indicates that at least one of the three groups had a posttreatment weight that is significantly different from the overall grand mean, after adjusting for pretreatment weights. It sometimes is useful to examine **adjusted means**, that is, group means on the dependent variable after adjusting for (i.e., removing the effect of) covariates. Adjusted means allow researchers to determine **net effects** (i.e., group differences on the dependent variable that are *net* of the effect of the covariate.) A subsequent section of this chapter, which presents computer examples of multivariate statistics, provides an illustration of adjusted means.

When ANCOVA results in a significant group F test, researchers can reject the null hypothesis that the adjusted group means are equal. As with ANOVA, further analysis is needed to determine which pairs of adjusted group means are significantly different from one another.

➡ **TIP:** For ANCOVA, an eta squared can be computed to summarize the magnitude of the *adjusted* relationship between the independent and dependent variables. Estimates of eta squared can be used in a power analysis to estimate sample size needs when planning a study. In general, when ANCOVA is used with carefully selected covariates, the analysis of group differences is more powerful with ANCOVA than with ANOVA because error variance is reduced.

Example of ANCOVA: Topp and co-researchers (2005) compared the efficacy of 16 weeks of either resistance training, aerobic walking, combined approaches, or a control condition on the performance of functional tasks among older adults with limited functional ability. Repeated measures ANCOVA was used to compare group means on functional tasks at two points in time (8 and 16 weeks after baseline), using preintervention outcome scores as the covariates.

OTHER LEAST-SQUARES MULTIVARIATE TECHNIQUES

In this section, methods called multivariate analysis of variance, discriminant function analysis, and canonical correlation are briefly introduced. The intent is to acquaint you with research situations for which these methods are appropriate.

Multivariate Analysis of Variance

Multivariate analysis of variance (MANOVA) is the extension of ANOVA to more than one dependent variable. MANOVA is used to test the significance of differences in group means for multiple dependent variables, considered simultaneously. For instance, if we wanted to examine the effect of two methods of exercise on diastolic *and* systolic blood pressure, MANOVA would be appropriate. Researchers often analyze such data by performing two separate ANOVAs. Strictly speaking, this practice is incorrect. Separate ANOVAs imply that the dependent variables have been obtained independently when, in fact, they have been obtained from the same subjects and are correlated. MANOVA takes the intercorrelations of dependent variables into account. ANOVA is, however, a more widely understood procedure than MANOVA, and thus its results may be more easily communicated to a broad audience.

MANOVA can be readily extended in ways analogous to ANOVA. For example, it is possible to perform **multivariate analysis of covariance (MANCOVA)**, which allows for the control of extraneous variables (covariates) when there are two or more dependent variables. MANOVA can also be used when there are repeated measures of the dependent variables.

➡ **TIP:** One problem with multivariate analyses is that findings are less accessible to statistically unsophisticated readers, such as practicing nurses. You may opt to use simpler analyses to enhance the utilizability of the evidence (e.g., three separate ANOVAs rather than a MANOVA). If the primary reason for *not* using appropriate multivariate tests is for communication purposes, you should run the analyses both ways. Then, you could present bivariate results (e.g., from an ANOVA) in the report, but indicate whether the more complex test (e.g. MANOVA) changed the conclusions.

Example of MANOVA: Amar and Gennaro (2005) studied factors associated with dating violence in college women. Using MANOVA, they compared victims and nonvictims of violence in terms of five mental health symptoms (somatization, interpersonal sensitivity, depression, anxiety, and hostility).

Discriminant Analysis

In multiple regression, the dependent variable is either an interval or ratio measure. The regression makes predictions about continuous scores, such as scores on a depression scale or heart rate. **Discriminant analysis**, in contrast, makes predictions about membership in groups. For instance, we may wish to predict membership in such groups as compliant versus noncompliant cancer patients, or patients who do or do not survive a medical treatment.

Discriminant analysis develops a regression equation—called a **discriminant function**—for a categorical dependent variable, with independent variables that are either dichotomous or continuous. Researchers begin with data from subjects whose group membership is known, and develop an equation to predict membership when only measures of the independent variables are available. The discriminant function indicates to which group each subject would likely belong.

Discriminant analysis for predicting membership into only two groups (e.g., survived versus died) can be interpreted in much the same way as multiple regression. When there are more than two groups, the calculations and interpretations are more complex. With three or more groups (e.g., very low–birth-weight, low-birth-weight, and normal-birth-weight infants), the number of discriminant functions is either the number of groups minus 1 or the number of independent variables, whichever is smaller. The first discriminant function is the linear combination of predictors that maximizes the ratio of between-group to within-group variance. The second function is the linear combination that maximizes this ratio, after the effect of the first function is removed. Because independent variables have different weights on the various functions, it is possible to develop theoretical interpretations based on the knowledge of which predictors are important in discriminating among different groups.

Discriminant analysis produces an index designating the proportion of variance in the dependent variable accounted for by predictor variables. The index is **Wilks' lambda** (λ), which actually indicates the proportion of variance *unaccounted for* by predictors, or $\lambda = 1 - R^2$.

Example of discriminant analysis: LePage and colleagues (2005) used discriminant function analysis to evaluate risk factors for violence in an inpatient psychiatric unit. The dependent variable was presence versus absence of at least one negative event (e.g., a patient injury) on a particular day. The predictors were case mix variables such as number of young adults and number of patients with mental retardation. The results suggested that when the combined number of young adults and patients with mental retardation exceeds 10, the unit is at high risk for the occurrence of aggressive behavior.

Canonical Correlation

Canonical correlation analyzes the relationship between two or more independent variables *and* two or more dependent variables. Conceptually, one can think of this technique as an extension of multiple regression to more than one dependent variable, but mathematically and interpretatively, the gap between multiple regression and canonical correlation is great.

Like other techniques described thus far, canonical correlation uses the least-squares principle to partition and analyze variance. Basically, two linear composites are developed, one of which is associated with the dependent variables, the other of which is for the independent variables. The relationship between the two linear composites is expressed by the **canonical correlation coefficient**, R_C, which, when squared, indicates the proportion of variance accounted for in the analysis. When there is more than one dimension of covariation in the two sets of variables, more than one canonical correlation can be found.

Example of canonical correlation: Walker and co-researchers (2006) studied the relationship between several cognitive-perceptual factors derived from the Health Promotion Model on the one hand and markers of physical activity on the other, in a sample of older rural women. They used canonical correlation to examine relationships between two sets of variables: *determinants* (e.g., self-efficacy for physical activity, barriers to physical activity) and *markers* of physical activity, such as VO_{2max} or weekly stretching minutes. One interpretable canonical variate was identified that explained 22% of the variance—that is, $R_C^2 = .22$.

Links Among Least-Squares Multivariate Techniques

We could state an analogy that canonical correlation is to multiple regression as MANOVA is to ANOVA. This analogy, although correct, obscures a point that astute readers have perhaps suspected: the close affinity between multiple regression and ANOVA.

In fact, ANOVA and multiple regression are virtually identical. Both techniques analyze total variability in a continuous dependent measure and contrast variability attributable to independent variables with that attributable to random error. Both multiple regression and ANOVA boil down to an F-ratio. By tradition, experimental data typically are analyzed by ANOVA, and correlational data are analyzed by regression. Nevertheless, *any data for which ANOVA is appropriate can be analyzed by multiple regression*, although the reverse is not true. Multiple regression may in some cases be preferable because it is more flexible and provides more information, such as a prediction equation and an index of association, *R*.

LOGISTIC REGRESSION

Logistic regression is being used with increasing frequency by nurse researchers. Like multiple regression, logistic regression analyzes the relationship between multiple independent variables and a dependent variable and yields a predictive equation. Like discriminant function analysis, logistic regression is used with categorical dependent variables. Logistic regression, however, is based on an estimation procedure that has less restrictive assumptions than multivariate procedures discussed thus far, which use least-squares estimation.

Basic Concepts for Logistic Regression

Logistic regression uses **maximum likelihood estimation**. Maximum likelihood estimators are ones that estimate the parameters most likely to have generated the observed data. Confirmatory factor analysis, discussed in Chapter 18 in relation to scale development, also uses maximum likelihood estimation.

Logistic regression is based on the assumption that the underlying relationships among variables is an S-shaped probabilistic function—an assumption that is usually more tenable than the least-squares assumptions of linearity and multivariate normality. Logistic regression thus is often more technically appropriate than discriminant analysis. Logistic regression is also well suited to many clinical questions because it models the probability of an outcome rather than predicting group membership. For example, we might be interested in modeling the probability of engaging in breast self-examination, or the probability of smoking cessation.

Logistic regression transforms the probability of an event occurring (e.g., that a woman will practice breast self-examination) into its odds. As discussed briefly in Chapter 21, **odds** reflect the ratio of two probabilities: the probability of an event occurring, to the probability that it will not occur. For example, if 40% of women practice breast self-examination, the odds would be .40 divided by .60, or .667.

Probabilities, which range between zero and one, are then transformed into continuous variables that range between zero and infinity. Because this range is still restricted, a further transformation is performed, namely calculating the logarithm of the odds. The range of this new variable (known as the **logit**, short for *log*istic probability un*it*) is from minus to plus infinity. Using the logit as the dependent variable, a maximum likelihood procedure estimates the coefficients of the independent variables, with the logit as a continuous dependent variable.

The solution yields an equation that predicts the logit from a weighted combination of independent variables, plus a constant, much like a multiple regression equation. The interpretation, however, is different because the equation does not predict *actual* values of the dependent variable. In logistic regression, a regression coefficient (*b*) can be interpreted as the change in the log odds associated with a one-unit change in the associated predictor variable.

The Odds Ratio

The meaning of the logistic regression equation is hard to comprehend because we do not think in terms of log odds. However, the equation can be transformed back to yield information in terms of odds rather than log odds. The factor by which the odds change is the odds ratio (OR).

For example, suppose that we used logistic regression to predict the probability of performing breast self-examination. One of the independent variables might be whether or not the woman has had a close family member (e.g., mother or sister) who had breast cancer. A logistic regression analysis might indicate that the OR was 12.1, with all other predictors in the equation held constant. As noted in Chapter 21, the odds ratio provides an estimate (around which confidence intervals can be built) of relative risk—the risk for an event occurring given one condition, versus the risk for it occurring given a different condition. In our example, we would estimate that the "risk" of performing breast self-examination is about 12 times greater if a woman has a family history of breast cancer than if she does not.

➔ **TIP :** Just as there is simple regression with least-squares estimation—that is, the prediction of a dependent variable based on a single independent variable—**bivariate logistic regression** is also possible. This is often done to produce estimates of unadjusted odds ratios—that is, odds ratios without controlling other variables. If, for example, marital status was a predictor of breast self-examination, a bivariate analysis could provide estimates of the relative risk of different marital statuses (e.g., never married, married, formerly married) on breast self-examination. In such an analysis, one group would be the reference group, with an OR of 1.0, and the other two groups would have ORs in relation to the reference group. As a hypothetical example, if the OR for never married was 1.0 and the OR for married was 1.23, this means that married women were 23% more likely to perform breast self-examination than never-married women.

Significance Tests in Logistic Regression

Several statistics help to assess the performance of the logistic regression analysis. One index is the **likelihood index**, which is the probability of the observed results, given parameters estimated in the analysis. If the model fits the data perfectly, the likelihood index is 1.0. Because the likelihood index is typically a small decimal, it is usually transformed by multiplying it by -2 times the log of the likelihood. The transformed index ($-2LL$) is a small number when the fit is good; in a perfect fit, the value is zero.

The chi square statistic is used to test the null hypothesis that the b regression coefficients are zero. The overall model chi-square test is the analog of the overall F test in multiple regression. A **goodness-of-fit statistic**, which also has a chi-square distribution, is based on the residuals for all cases in the analysis—which, in logistic regression, is the difference between the observed probability of an event and the predicted probability. This statistic is thus another mechanism for evaluating the fit of the predictive model.

It is also possible to test the significance of individual predictors in the model—just as the t-statistic is used in multiple regression. The most frequently used statistic for this purpose is the **Wald statistic**, which is distributed as a chi-square. Hosmer and Lemeshow (2000) and Pampel (2000) are good resources for learning more about logistic regression.

Example of logistic regression: Dunn and colleagues (2006) examined vulnerability factors in relation to whether or not mothers continued to breastfeed their infants at 6 weeks postpartum. Both bivariate and multiple logistic regression were performed. As an example of bivariate results, maternal age was categorized into three groups: younger than 25, 25 to 35, and older than 35 years, with older women being the reference group. The youngest women were found to be more than 3 times as likely (OR = 3.25) as the oldest mothers to have weaned (95% CI = 1.58–6.70). In the multiple logistic regression, maternal depression was significantly related to weaning even after controlling age and education. The OR of 0.28 (95% CI = .11–.71) indicated that women who were classified as depressed had a 28% higher probability of weaning.

➔ **TIP :** When a categorical dependent variable is not dichotomous (e.g., three different types of chronic illness), *multinomial logistic regression* can be used (Kwak & Clayton-Matthews, 2002).

SURVIVAL AND EVENT HISTORY ANALYSIS

Some dependent variables are time related. **Survival analysis** (or **life table analysis**) is widely used by epidemiologists when the dependent variable is a time interval between an initial event (e.g., onset of a disease) and a terminal event (e.g., death). Survival analysis calculates a survival score, which compares survival time for one subject with that for other subjects. When researchers are interested in group comparisons—e.g., comparing the survival function of subjects in an experimental group versus a control group—a statistic can be computed to test the null hypothesis that the groups are sampled from the same survival distribution.

Survival analysis can be applied to many situations unrelated to mortality. For example, survival analysis could be used to analyze such time-related phenomena as length of time in labor, or length of time elapsed between hospital release and readmission. Survival analysis is appropriate whenever time-related data are **censored**, that is, the observation period does not cover all possible events. As an example, if the outcome were readmission 2 years after release, the data are censored because there will be readmissions beyond the 2-year period, and some will never be readmitted. Further information about survival analysis can be found in Harrell (2001), Hosmer and Lemeshow (1999), and Kleinbaum and Klein (2005).

More recently, extensions of survival analysis have been developed that allow researchers to examine determinants of survival-type transitions in a multivariate framework. In these analyses, independent variables are used to model the risk (or hazard) of experiencing an event at a given point in time, given that one has not experienced the event before that time. The most common specification of the hazard is known as the **Cox proportional hazards model**. Further information may be found in Therneau and Grambsch (2000) and Hougaard (2000).

Example of a hazards model: Inglis and colleagues (2004) studied the effects of a nurse-led, home-based intervention (HBI) for patients with chronic atrial fibrillation. Discharged patients were randomly assigned to either HBI or usual care. Several outcomes were studied, including event-free survival time, with an event defined as death or rehospitalization. Cox proportional hazards models were used to compare the survival time of the two groups after adjustments were made for age, gender, comorbidity, treatment, and social status.

CAUSAL MODELING

Causal modeling involves testing a hypothesized causal explanation of a phenomenon, typically with data from nonexperimental studies. In a causal model, researchers posit causal linkages among three or more variables, and then test whether hypothesized pathways from the causes to the effect are consistent with the data. We briefly describe some features of two approaches to causal modeling without discussing analytic procedures.

Path Analysis

Path analysis, which relies on regression using least-squares estimation, is a method for studying causal patterns among variables. Path analysis is not a method for discovering causes; rather, it is a method applied to a prespecified model formulated on the basis of prior knowledge and theory.

In reports, path analytic results are usually displayed in a **path diagram**, and we use such a diagram (Fig. 23.3) to illustrate key concepts. This model postulates that the dependent variable, patients' length of hospitalization (V4), is the result of patients' capacity for self-care (V3); this, in turn, is affected by nursing actions (V1) and the severity of their illness (V2). This model is a **recursive model**, which means that the causal flow is unidirectional: it is assumed that variable 2 is a cause of variable 3, and that variable 3 is *not* a cause of variable 2.

Path analysis distinguishes exogenous and endogenous variables. An **exogenous variable** is a variable whose determinants lie outside the model. In Figure 23.3, nursing actions (V1) and illness severity (V2) are exogenous; no attempt is made in the model to elucidate what causes different nursing

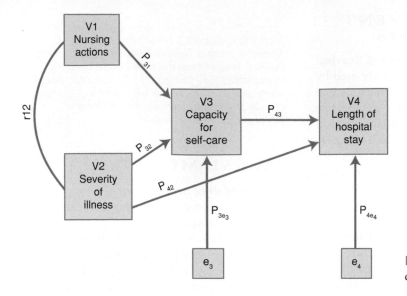

FIGURE 23.3 Example of a path diagram.

actions or different degrees of illness. An **endogenous variable**, by contrast, is one whose variation is hypothesized to be caused by other variables in the model. In our example, self-care capacity (V3) and length of stay (V4) are endogenous.

Causal linkages are shown on a path diagram by arrows drawn from presumed causes to presumed effects. In our illustration, severity of illness is hypothesized to affect length of hospitalization both directly (path P_{42}) and indirectly through the *mediating variable* self-care capacity (paths P_{32} and P_{43}). Correlated exogenous variables are indicated by curved lines, as shown by the curved line between nursing actions and illness severity.

Ideally, the model would totally explain the outcome (i.e., length of stay). In practice, this almost never happens because there are other determinants of the outcome, which are **residual variables**. The two boxes labeled *e* in Figure 23.3 denote a composite of all determinants of self-care capacity (e_3) and hospital stay (e_4) that are not in the model. If we could identify and measure additional causes and incorporate them into the theory, they should be in the model.

Path analysis solves for **path coefficients**, which are the weights representing the effect of one variable on another. In Figure 23.3, causal paths indicate that one variable (e.g., V3) is caused by

another (e.g., V2), yielding a path labeled P_{32}. In research reports, path symbols would be replaced by actual path coefficients, which are derived through regression procedures. Path coefficients are standardized partial regression slopes. For example, path P_{32} is equal to $\beta_{32.1}$—the beta weight between variables 2 and 3, holding variable 1 constant. Because path coefficients are in standard form, they indicate the proportion of a standard deviation difference in the caused variable that is directly attributable to a 1.00 SD difference in the specified causal variable. Thus, the path coefficients give us indication about the relative importance of various determinants.

Path analysis estimates path coefficients through the use of **structural equations**. The structural equations for Figure 23.3 are as follows:

$$z_1 = e_1$$
$$z_2 = e_2$$
$$z_3 = P_{31}z_1 + P_{32}z_2 + e_3$$
$$z_4 = P_{43}z_3 + P_{42}z_2 + e_4$$

These equations indicate that z_1 and z_2 (standard scores for variables 1 and 2) are determined by outside variables (*e*'s); that z_3 depends directly on z_1 and z_2 plus outside variables; and that z_4 (length of stay) depends directly on z_2, z_3, and outside variables. These structural equations could be solved to yield path coefficients by performing two multiple regressions: by regressing variable 3 on variables 1 and 2; and by regressing variable 4 on variables 2 and 3.

Path analysis involves a number of procedures for testing causal models and for determining effects. Kline (2005) offers further guidance on path analysis.

> **Example of path analysis:** Steele and Porche (2005) used path analysis to test the ability of the Theory of Planned Behavior to explain women's mammography screening. According to the theory, women's behavior is determined by their intentions, which in turn are caused by their attitudes, subjective norms, and perceived behavioral control. Overall, the model explained 24% of the variance in women's behavior. Perceived control was the strongest predictor of mammography intentions.

Structural Equations Modeling

A drawback of path analysis using OLS regression is that the method's validity is based on a set of restrictive assumptions, most of which are virtually impossible to meet. First, it is assumed that variables are measured without error, but (as discussed in Chapter 17) most measures contain error. Second, it is assumed that residuals (error terms) in the different regression equations are uncorrelated. This assumption is seldom tenable because error terms often represent unmeasured individual differences—differences that are not entirely random. Third, traditional path analysis assumes that the causal flow is unidirectional or recursive. In reality, causes and effects are often reciprocal or iterative.

Structural equations modeling (SEM) using maximum likelihood estimation (or a procedure called *full information maximum likelihood,* or *FIML*) is a more general and powerful approach that avoids these problems. Unlike path analysis, SEM can accommodate measurement errors, correlated residuals, and **nonrecursive models** that allow for reciprocal causation. Another attractive feature of SEM is that it can be used to analyze causal models involving latent variables. A *latent*

variable, as discussed in Chapter 18, is an unmeasured variable corresponding to an abstract construct. For example, factor analysis yields information about underlying, latent dimensions that are not measured directly. In SEM, latent variables are captured by two or more measured (manifest) variables that are indicators of the underlying construct.

SEM proceeds in two phases. In the first phase, which corresponds to a confirmatory factor analysis (CFA), a measurement model is tested. Measurement models were described in Chapter 18. When there is evidence of an adequate fit of the data to the hypothesized measurement model, the theoretical causal model is tested by structural equation modeling. In this part of the analysis, SEM yields information about the hypothesized causal parameters—that is, the path coefficients, which are presented as beta weights. The coefficients indicate the expected amount of change in the latent endogenous variable that is caused by a change in the latent causal variable. SEM programs provide information on the significance of individual paths. The residual terms—the amount of unexplained variance for the latent endogenous variables—can also be calculated from the SEM analysis. The overall fit of the causal model to the research data can be tested by means of several alternative statistics. Two such statistics are the **goodness-of-fit index (GFI)** and the **adjusted goodness-of-fit index (AGFI)**. For both indexes, a value of .90 or greater indicates a good fit of the model to the data.

SEM has gained considerable popularity among nurse researchers, but is a highly complex procedure that requires specialized software (e.g., AMOS, EQS, LISREL). Readers interested in further information on SEM are urged to consult Loehlin (2003) or Kline (2005).

> **Example of SEM:** Leiter and Laschinger (2006) used data from more than 8500 Canadian nurses to test a nursing work life model that examined relationships among work/practice environment and professional burnout. The SEM analysis provided support for a structural model that linked five factors (e.g., staffing, physician–nurse relationships) to quality of work life. The analysis supported a direct path (negatively weighted) between staffing and emotional exhaustion.

THE COMPUTER AND MULTIVARIATE STATISTICS

Multivariate analyses are invariably done by computer because computations are complex. To illustrate computer analyses for two multivariate techniques, we return to the example described in Chapters 21 and 22, involving the implementation of a special prenatal intervention for low-income young women. Data for these examples were presented in Table 21.10.

Example of Multiple Regression

In Chapter 22, we tested the hypothesis that older mothers in the sample had infants with higher birth weights than younger mothers, using Pearson's r. The calculated value of r (.594) was highly significant, thereby supporting the research hypothesis.

Suppose now that we want to test whether we can significantly *improve* our ability to predict infant birth weight by adding two predictor variables in a multiple regression analysis: whether the mother smoked while pregnant, and number of prior pregnancies. Figure 23.4 presents part of the Statistical Package for the Social Sciences (SPSS) printout for a multiple regression in which infant birth weight is the dependent variable and maternal age, smoking status, and number of prior pregnancies are predictor variables. We will explain some of the most noteworthy aspects of this printout.

The top panel of Figure 23.4 shows that we used hierarchical regression, in which mother's age was entered first (Model 1), and then smoking status and prior pregnancies were entered in a second block (Model 2).

The second panel (Model Summary) indicates that, in Model 1, $R = .594$—the same as the bivariate correlation shown in Figure 22.7. The value of R^2 is .353 ($.594^2$), which represents the proportion of variance in birth weight accounted for by mother's age. The *adjusted R^2* of .330 in Model 1 is the R^2 after it has been adjusted to reflect more closely the goodness of fit the regression model in the population, through a formula that involves

sample size and number on independent variables. Next, the standard error of the estimate (8.9702) is shown. The next few columns present information about changes to R^2. In Model 1, the change is from 0.0 to .353—which yields an F (15.252) that, with $df = 1$ and 28, is highly significant ($p = .001$). In Model 2, the value of R is higher (.598), but the F for change (.109) with 2 and 26 df is not remotely significant ($p = .897$).

The next panel (ANOVA) shows, for Model 1, the calculation of the F-ratio in which variability due to regression (i.e., to the relationship between birth weight and maternal age) is contrasted with residual variability. Again, it shows that the value of F (15.252) is significant at the .001 level. The information for Model 2 is for all *three* predictors that are in the model after variables in the second block are entered. Here, the value of F (4.834) with 3 and 26 df is statistically significant at $p = .008$.

The actual regression equations are presented in the next panel (Coefficients). If we wanted to predict new values of birth weight based on maternal age at birth, the equation (from Model 1) would be:

$$\text{Birth weight}' = (3.119 \times \text{age}) + 48.040$$

That is, predicted birth weight values for a new sample of young mothers would be equal to the regression coefficient ($b = 3.119$) times values of maternal age (X_1), plus the value of the intercept constant ($a = 48.040$). When values of b are divided by the standard error (.799 for maternal age in Model 1), the result is a t-statistic, which indicates the significance of each predictor. In Model 1, $t = 3.290$, which is significant ($p = .001$). The standardized beta weight for maternal age is .594. In the far right we see that the 95% CI for the regression coefficient b is 1.483 and 4.755—which indicates statistical significance because the interval does not include 0.0.

If we wanted to use all three predictors to predict infant birth weight, the equation for Model 2 shows the b coefficients for each of the three predictors. In model 2, neither number of prior pregnancies nor smoking status is significant: $p = .872$ and .653, respectively. The 95% CI for both these predictors *does* include 0.0. When we compare the standardized

Variables Entered/Removed[b]

Model	Variables Entered	Variables Removed	Method
1	Mother's age	.	Enter
2	Smoking status, No. of prior pregnancies[a]	.	Enter

[a]All requested variables entered.
[b]Dependent variable: Infant birth weight in ounces

Model Summary

Model	R	R^2	Adjusted R^2	Std. Error of the Estimate	R^2 Change	F Change	df1	df2	Sig. F Change
					Change Statistics				Sig. F
1	.594[a]	.353	.330	8.9702	.353	15.252	1	28	.001
2	598[b]	.358	.284	9.2700	.005	.109	2	26	.897

[a]Predictors: (Constant), mother's age
[b]Predictors: (Constant), mother's age, smoking status, no. of prior pregnancies

ANOVA[c]

Model		Sum of Squares	df	Mean Square	F	Sig.
1	Regression	1227.283	1	1227.283	15.252	.001[a]
	Residual	2253.017	28	80.465		
	Total	3480.300	29			
2	Regression	1246.061	3	415.354	4.834	.008[b]
	Residual	2234.239	26	85.932		
	Total	3480.300	29			

[a]Predictors: (Constant), mother's age
[b]Predictors: (Constant), mother's age, smoking status, no. of prior pregnancies
[c]Dependent variable: Infant birth weight in ounces

Coefficients[a]

Model		Unstandardized Coefficients B	Std. Error	Standardized Coefficients Beta	t	Sig.	95% Confidence Interval for B Lower Bound	Upper Bound
1	(Constant)	48.040	14.600		3.290	.003	18.133	77.947
	Mother's age	3.119	.799	.594	3.905	.001	1.483	4.755
2	(Constant)	52.170	18.398		2.836	.009	14.354	89.987
	Mother's age	2.916	1.021	.555	2.855	.008	.817	5.016
	No. of prior pregnancies	.394	2.410	.030	.163	.872	−4.561	5.349
	Smoking status	−1.643	3.610	−.076	−.455	.653	−9.064	5.778

[a]Dependent variable: Infant birth weight in ounces

Excluded Variables[b]

Model		Beta In	t	Sig.	Partial Correlation	Collinearity Statistics Tolerance
1	No. of prior pregnancies	.020[a]	.108	.915	.021	.727
	Smoking status	−.072	−.446	.659	−.086	.910

[a]Predictors in the model: (Constant), mother's age
[b]Dependent variable: Infant birth weight in ounces

FIGURE 23.4 Printout for hierarchical multiple regression of infant birthweight (from the Statistical Package for the Social Sciences).

coefficients (the betas) for the three variables, we see that the beta for maternal age is substantial, whereas the betas for the other two predictors are negligible.

The final panel (Excluded Variables) shows the two predictors not yet in the equation in Model 1, that is, number of prior pregnancies and smoking status. The printout shows that the t-values associated with the regression coefficients for the two predictors are both nonsignificant ($p = .915$ and .659, respectively), once variation due to maternal age is taken into account. This reinforces what we have already learned—that neither of the two predictors in block 2 would have significantly added to the prediction of birth weight, over and above what was already achieved with maternal age.

An additional piece of information shown in the "Excluded Variables" panel relates to the issue of **multicollinearity,** which is a problem that can occur when predictor variables are too highly intercorrelated. When multicollinearity is present, the computations required for the regression coefficients are seriously compromised, and results tend to be unstable. Multicollinearity can be diagnosed (and avoided) by computing an index of **tolerance**. If predictors are totally uncorrelated, tolerance is 1.0, and if they are perfectly intercorrelated, tolerance is 0.0. Thus, higher values are more desirable. The computer can be instructed to exclude predictors whose tolerance falls below a specified level (e.g., .10). In our example, tolerance values of .727 and .910 for the two variables not yet in the model are acceptable.

Example of Analysis of Covariance

In Chapter 22, we tested the hypothesis that infants in the experimental group would have higher birth weights than infants in the control group, using a t-test. The computer calculated t to be 1.44, which was nonsignificant with 28 df. The research hypothesis was therefore rejected.

Through ANCOVA, we can test the same hypothesis controlling for maternal age, which, as we have just seen, is significantly correlated with birth weight. Figure 23.5 presents the printout for ANCOVA for this analysis, with birth weight as the dependent vari-

able, maternal age (AGE) as the covariate, and GROUP (experimental versus control) as the independent variable. The first panel shows that the group variable involves 15 experimental subjects and 15 controls. In the next panel (Descriptive Statistics), means and SDs for the two groups and the overall sample of 30 mothers are presented.

In panel 3 (Tests of Between-Subjects Effects), the F-value for the overall model is highly significant (14.088, $p = .000$). The value of F for the covariate AGE is 24.358, significant at the .000 level (i.e., beyond the .001 level). The value of eta squared for age (i.e., the effect size) is .474, and the observed power to detect this effect, for $\alpha = .05$, is quite high, .997.

After controlling for AGE, the F-value for the independent variable GROUP is 8.719, which is significant at the .006 level. In other words, once AGE is controlled, the research hypothesis about experimental versus control differences in infant birth weight is supported rather than rejected. Moreover, the effect size for the intervention (.244) is fairly high. The unadjusted R^2 for predicting birth weight, based on both AGE and GROUP, is .511—substantially more than the R^2 between maternal age and birth weight alone (.352).

The next panel shows the overall mean (104.70) for the sample; the standard error (1.45); and the 95% CI for estimating the population mean (95% CI = 101.725, 107.675). The bottom panel shows the group means *after they are adjusted for maternal age.* The original, unadjusted means for the experimental and control groups were 107.53 and 101.87, respectively (panel 2). After adjusting for maternal age, however, the experimental mean is 109.08, and the control mean is 100.32, a much more sizable difference.

CRITIQUING MULTIVARIATE STATISTICS

As we advised in the previous chapter, it is difficult to critique researchers' statistical analysis without statistical skills. This caution is even more relevant when it comes to complex multivariate analyses.

Univariate Analysis of Variance

Between-Subjects Factors

		Value Label	N
Treatment group	1	Experimental	15
	2	Control	15

Descriptive Statistics

Dependent variable: Infant birth weight in ounces

Treatment group	Mean	Std.Deviation	N
Experimental	107.5333	13.3784	15
Control	101.8667	7.2394	15
TOTAL	104.7000	10.9549	30

Tests of Between-Subjects Effects

Dependent variable: Infant birth weight in ounces

Source	Type III Sum of Squares	df	Mean Square	F	Sig.	Eta Squared	Observed Power[a]
Corrected model	1777.228[b]	2	888.614	14.088	.000	.511	.997
Intercept	572.734	1	572.734	9.080	.006	.252	828
AGE	1536.395	1	1536.395	24.358	.000	.474	.997
GROUP	549.945	1	549.945	8.719	.006	.244	.812
Error	1703.072	27	63.077				
Corrected TOTAL	3480.300	29					

[a]Computed using alpha = .05
[b]R squared = .511 (adjusted R squared = .474)

Estimated Marginal Means

1. Grand Mean

Dependent variable: Infant birth weight in ounces

		95% Confidence Interval	
Mean	Std. Error	Lower Bound	Upper Bound
104.700[a]	1.450	101.725	107.675

[a]Evaluated at covariates appeared in the model: Mother's age = 18.1667.

2. Treatment group

Dependent variable: Infant birth weight in ounces

Treatment group	Mean	Std. Error	95% Confidence Interval	
			Lower Bound	Upper Bound
Experimental	109.080[a]	2.074	104.824	113.337
Control	100.320[a]	2.074	96.063	104.576

[a]Evaluated at covariates appeared in the model: Mother's age =18.1667.

FIGURE 23.5 Printout for ANCOVA (from the Statistical Package for the Social Sciences).

As with bivariate statistics, one issue is whether the researcher selected the right statistical tests. The selection of a multivariate procedure depends on several factors, including the nature of the research question and the measurement level of the variables. (It also depends on whether the data conformed to various assumptions underlying the tests—an issue we did not address in this brief chapter.) Table 23.7, which summarizes some of the major features of multivariate statistics discussed in this chapter, may

TABLE 23.7	Guide to Selected Multivariate Analyses

TEST NAME	PURPOSE	MEASUREMENT LEVEL OF VARIABLES*			NUMBER OF VARIABLES†		
		IV	DV	Cov	IVs	DVs	Cov
Multiple regression/ correlation	To test the relationship between 2+ IVs and 1 DV; to predict a DV from 2+ IVs	N, I, R	I, R	–	2+	1	–
Analysis of covariance (ANCOVA)	To test the difference between the means of 2+ groups, while controlling for 1+ covariate	N	I, R	N, I, R	1+	1	1+
Multivariate analysis of variance (MANOVA)	To test the difference between the means of 2+ groups for 2+ DVs simultaneously	N	I, R	–	1+	2+	–
Multivariate analysis of covariance (MANCOVA)	To test the difference between the means of 2+ groups for 2+ DVs simultaneously, while controlling for 1+ covariate	N	I,R	N, I, R	1+	2+	1+
Discriminant function analysis	To test the relationship between 2+ IVs and 1 DV; to predict group membership; to classify cases into groups	N, I, R	N	–	2+	1	–
Canonical correlation	To test the relationship between 2 sets of variables	N, I, R	N, I, R	–	2+	2+	–
Logistic regression	To test the relationship between 2+ IVs and 1 DV, to predict the probability of on event; to estimate relative risk	N, I, R	N	–	2+	1	–

*Variables: IV, independent variable; DV, dependent variable; Cov, covariate.

†Measurement levels: N, nominal; I, interval; R, ratio.

be helpful in determining the appropriateness of an analytic approach. It might also be noted that studies in which multivariate statistics were *not* used might well be critiqued in terms of whether or not they *should* have been used. As we illustrated, results from an ANOVA or *t*-test can sometimes be altered by controlling extraneous variables. Conversely, some researchers apply multivariate statistics when their sample size is too small to justify their use.

No specific critiquing guidelines for multivariate statistics are presented in this chapter, but most of the questions presented in Box 22.1 are also relevant for researchers' use of the statistics discussed in this chapter.

●●●●●●●●●●●●●●●●●●●●●●●●

RESEARCH EXAMPLE

Study: "Prevalence and correlates of perineal dermatitis in nursing home residents" (Bliss et al., 2006)

Statement of Purpose: The purpose of this study was to determine the prevalence of perineal dermatitis (inflammation or skin damage in the perineal area) in nursing home residents, and factors correlated with this adverse outcome in the nursing home population.

Methods: A secondary analysis was conducted, using a cross-sectional database with records from nearly 60,000 residents residing in 555 nursing homes located in 31 states. Assessment data in the Minimum Data Set were linked with nearly 3 million orders in the medical record, which enabled definition of variables related to perineal dermatitis (PD). Every case with PD ($N =$ 3405) was included in subsequent analyses. Two subsamples were created. Sample A contained the 3405 PD cases and a randomly selected set of 6810 of cases without PD. (The prevalence was thus estimated at 5.7%.) Sample B contained the same 3405 PD cases and a second randomly selected set of 6810 non-PD cases, which allowed for a cross-validation of correlational findings.

Analysis and Findings: The researchers first looked at bivariate relationships between PD status and a range of characteristics of the nursing home residents, using sample A data. Three broad categories of variables were examined: tissue tolerance (e.g., age, nutrition problems, perfusion problems); toileting ability (e.g., mobility deficits, restraint use, cognition problems); and perineal environment (e.g., urinary, fecal, or double incontinence). Depending on measurement level and distribution of the variable, either a t-test or chi-square or nonparametric test was used. Candidates for multivariate analysis were selected from the initial bivariate tests: variables with associations with PD at $p < .10$ were retained for use in logistic regression analysis, with PD as the dependent variable.

The logistic regression using sample A data yielded numerous statistically significant relationships at or beyond $p < .001$. For example, daily restraint use was associated with a 60% higher likelihood of PD (OR = 1.6, 95% CI = 1.4–1.8, $p < .001$), even after other factors were held constant in the analysis. Of particular interest was the link with incontinence. Urinary incontinence only was not correlated with PD (OR = .96, $p =$ .66), but fecal incontinence only was associated with a 70% increased likelihood of PD (OR = 1.7, 95% CI = 1.4–2.02, $p < .001$). Double incontinence was associated with a 20% greater risk for PD (OR = 1.2, 95% CI = 1.02–1.4, $p = .02$). Cross-validation of the results with sample B confirmed the vast majority of correlations, including the ones cited here.

●●●●●●●●●●●●●●●●●●●●●●●

SUMMARY POINTS

- **Multivariate procedures** are increasingly being used in nursing research to untangle complex relationships among three or more variables.

- Simple **linear regression** makes predictions about the values of one variable based on values of a second variable. **Multiple regression** is a method of predicting a continuous dependent variable on the basis of two or more independent (**predictor**) variables.

- The **multiple correlation coefficient** (R) can be squared (R^2) to estimate the proportion of variability in the dependent variable accounted for by the independent variables. The F-statistic is used to test the overall regression model, as well as changes to R^2 as new predictors are introduced.

- The regression equation yields regression coefficients (b's) for each predictor that, when standardized, are called **beta weights (βs).**

- **Simultaneous multiple regression** enters all predictor variables into the regression equation at the same time. **Hierarchical multiple regression** enters predictors into the equation in a series of steps controlled by researchers. **Stepwise multiple regression** enters predictors in steps using a statistical criterion for order of entry.

- **Analysis of covariance (ANCOVA)** extends ANOVA by removing the effect of confounding variables (**covariates**) before testing whether mean group differences are statistically significant.

- **Multivariate analysis of variance (MANOVA)** is the extension of ANOVA to situations in which there is more than one dependent variable.

- **Discriminant analysis** is used to make predictions about dependent variables that are categorical (i.e., predictions about membership in groups) on the basis of two or more predictor variables.

- **Canonical correlation** analyzes the relationship between two or more independent *and* two or more dependent variables; it yields a canonical correlation coefficient, R_C.

- Most multivariate procedures described in the chapter are based on **ordinary least-squares (OLS)** estimation, which minimizes the square of **errors of prediction** (the **residuals**). An alternative is **maximum likelihood estimation**, which estimates the parameters most likely to have generated observed data.

- **Logistic regression**, which is based on maximum likelihood estimation, is used to predict the probability of an outcome (categorical dependent variables). A useful feature of this technique is that it yields an odds ratio that is an index of relative risk, that is, the risk for an outcome occurring given one condition, versus the risk for it occurring given a different condition.

- The overall logistic regression model can be tested with a **goodness-of-fit statistic**. Individual predictors can be tested with the **Wald statistic**.

- **Survival analysis** and other related event history methods are used when the dependent variable of interest is a time interval (e.g., time from onset of a disease to death).

- **Causal modeling** involves the development and testing of a hypothesized causal explanation of a phenomenon.

- **Path analysis**, a regression-based method for testing causal models, involves the preparation of a **path diagram** that stipulates hypothesized causal links among variables. Path analysis tests **recursive models**, that is, ones in which causation is presumed to be unidirectional.

- Traditional path analysis applies ordinary least-squares regression to a series of **structural equations**, resulting in a series of **path coefficients**. The path coefficients represent weights associated with a causal path, in standard deviation units.

- **Structural equations modeling (SEM)**, another approach to causal modeling, does not have as many assumptions and restrictions as path analysis. SEM can accommodate measurement errors, **nonrecursive models** that allow for reciprocal causal paths, and correlated errors.

- SEM can analyze causal models involving latent variables, which are not directly measured but which are captured by two or more manifest variables (i.e., measured variables). SEM proceeds in two sequential phases: the measurement model phase and the structural equations modeling phase.

STUDY ACTIVITIES

Chapter 23 of the accompanying *Resource Manual for Nursing Research: Generating and Assessing Evidence for Nursing Practice, 8th edition*, offers various exercises and study suggestions for reinforcing the concepts presented in this chapter. In addition, the following study questions can be addressed:

1. A researcher has examined the relationship between preventive health care attitudes on the one hand and the person's educational level, age, and gender on the other. The multiple correlation coefficient is .62. Explain the meaning of this statistic. How much variation in attitudinal scores is explained by the three predictors? How much is *unexplained*? What other variables might improve the power of the prediction?

2. Using power analysis, determine the sample size needed to achieve power = .80 for $\alpha = .05$, when estimated $R^2 = .15$ and $k = 5$.

3. Which multivariate statistical procedures would you recommend using in the following situations?
   a. A researcher wants to test the effectiveness of a nursing intervention for reducing stress levels among surgical patients, using an experimental

group of patients from one hospital and a control group from another hospital.

b. A researcher wants to predict which college students are at risk for a sexually transmitted disease using background information such as gender, academic grades, socioeconomic status, religion, and attitudes toward sexual activity.

c. A researcher wants to test the effects of three different diets on blood sugar levels and blood pH.

STUDIES CITED IN CHAPTER 23

Methodologic or theoretical references cited in this chapter can be found in a separate section at the end of the book.

Amar, A., & Gennaro, S. (2005). Dating violence in college women. *Nursing Research, 54*(4), 235–242.

Anderson, R. A., Issel, L. M., & McDaniel, R. R. (2003). Nursing homes as complex adaptive systems: Relationship between management practice and resident outcomes. *Nursing Research, 52,* 12–21.

Bliss, D., Savik, K., Harms, S., Fan, Q., & Wyman, J. (2006). Prevalence and correlates of perineal dermatitis in nursing home residents. *Nursing Research, 55,* 243–251.

Carrère, S., Mittmann, A., Woodin, E., Tabares, A., & Yoshimoto, D. (2005). Anger dysregulation, depressive symptoms, and health in married men and women. *Nursing Research, 54*(3), 184–192.

Dunn, S., Davies, B., McCleary, L., Edwards, N., & Gaboury, I. (2006). The relationship between vulnerability factors and breastfeeding outcome. *Journal of Obstetric, Gynecologic, & Neonatal Nursing, 35*(1), 87–97.

Eller, L., Lev, E., Gejeman, G., Colella, J., Esposito, M., Lanteri, V., et al. (2006). Prospective study of quality of life of patients receiving treatment for prostate cancer. *Nursing Research, 55*(2S), S28–S36.

Inglis, S., McLennan, S., Dawson, A., Birchmore, L., Horowitz, J., Wilkinson, D., & Stewart, S. (2004). A new solution for an old problem? Effects of a nurse-led, multidisciplinary, home-based intervention on readmission and mortality in patients with chronic atrial fibrillation. *Journal of Cardiovascular Nursing, 19*(2), 118–127.

Leiter, M., & Laschinger, H. (2006). Relationships of work and practice environment to professional burnout. *Nursing Research, 55*(2), 137–146.

LePage, J., McGhee, M., Aboraya, A., Murphy, J., Van-Horn, L., Pollard, S., & Dean, P. (2005). Evaluating risk factors for violence at the inpatient unit level: Combining young adults with those with mental retardation. *Applied Nursing Research, 18*(2), 117–121.

Steele, S., & Porche, D. (2005). Testing the theory of planned behavior to predict mammography intention. *Nursing Research, 54*(5), 332–338.

Topp, R., Boardley, D., Morgan, A., Fahlman, M., & McNevin, N. (2005). Exercise and functional tasks among adults who are functionally limited. *Western Journal of Nursing Research, 27*(3), 252–270.

Walker, S., Pullen, C., Hertzog, M., Boekner, L., & Hageman, P. (2006). Determinants of older rural women's activity and eating. *Western Journal of Nursing Research, 28*(4), 449–468.

24

Designing a Quantitative Analysis Strategy: From Data Collection to Interpretation

T his chapter provides an overview of steps that are normally taken in designing and implementing a data analysis plan, including interpretation of the data. With small sets of data, analysis may be simple and straightforward. Often, however, a number of steps are necessary before analysis can begin. Figure 24.1 shows what the flow of tasks might look like, organized in phases. Progress in analyzing quantitative data is not always as linear as this figure suggests, but the figure provides a framework for discussing some key steps in the analytic process.

PREANALYSIS PHASE

The first (preanalysis) phase involves various clerical and administrative tasks, such as logging in forms, reviewing data for completeness and legibility, retrieving pieces of missing information, and assigning identification (ID) numbers. Another task involves selecting statistical software for doing the data analyses. Once these tasks have been performed, researchers typically must code the data and enter them onto computer files to create a **data set** (the total collection of data for all sample members) for analysis.

➲ **TIP:** Two of the most widely used statistical software packages are the Statistical Package for the Social Sciences (SPSS)

and the Statistical Analysis System (SAS). Both packages contain programs for a variety of descriptive, bivariate, and multivariate analyses.

Coding Quantitative Data

Coding is the process of transforming information into symbols—usually numbers. Certain variables are inherently quantitative (e.g., age, body temperature) and may not require coding, unless the information is gathered in categories (e.g., whether a person is younger than 30 years of age, or 30 years or older). Even with "naturally" quantitative data, researchers need to inspect and edit their data. All responses should be of the same form and precision. For example, for the variable *height*, researchers need to decide whether to record feet and inches or to convert the information entirely to inches. Whichever method is adopted, it must be used consistently for all subjects. There must also be consistency in handling information reported with different degrees of precision (e.g., coding a response such as 5 feet, 2½ inches).

Most data from structured instruments can be precoded, with codes assigned before data are collected. For example, questions with fixed response alternatives can be preassigned a numeric code that is printed on the data collection form, such as: under age 30 = 1 and 30 and older = 2. Codes are

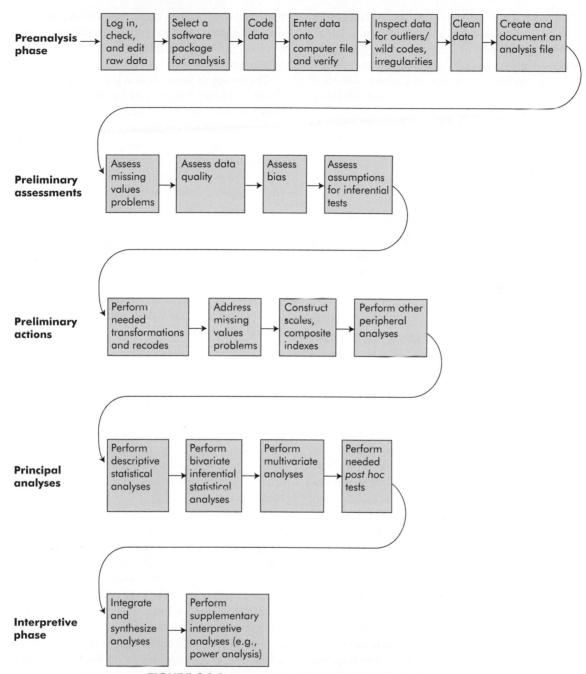

FIGURE 24.1 Flow of tasks in analyzing quantitative data.

often arbitrary, as in the case of the variable gender. Whether a female subject is coded 1 or 2 has no analytic importance as long as females are consistently assigned one code and males another code.

Respondents sometimes can check off more than one response to a question, as in the following:

To which of the following journals do you subscribe?
❏ *Journal of Advanced Nursing*
❏ *Nursing Research*
❏ *Qualitative Health Research*
❏ *Research in Nursing & Health*
❏ *Western Journal of Nursing Research*

With questions of this type, a 1-2-3-4-5 coding scheme cannot be used because respondents may check several, or none, of the responses. Responses must be coded as though the item were five separate questions: "Do you subscribe to the *Journal of Advanced Nursing?*" "Do you subscribe to *Nursing Research?*" and so on. Each check is treated as a "yes." The question yields five variables, with one code (e.g., 1) signifying "yes" and another code (e.g., 2) signifying "no."

Data from open-ended questions and other unstructured formats must be coded if they are going to be used in quantitative analysis. Sometimes researchers can develop codes ahead of time (e.g., occupational codes). Usually, however, unstructured data are collected specifically because responses cannot be anticipated. In such situations, codes are developed after data are collected. Researchers typically begin by reviewing a sizable portion of the data to understand content, and then develop a category scheme. The scheme should reflect both theoretical and analytic goals as well as the substance of the information. In developing such a coding scheme, categories should be both mutually exclusive and collectively exhaustive.

A code should be assigned to each variable for every sample member, even if there is no response. **Missing values** can be of various types. A person answering a question may be undecided, refuse to answer, or say, "Don't know." When skip patterns are used, there is missing information for those questions that are irrelevant to some respondents. A single missing values code may suffice, but it is sometimes important to distinguish different types of missing data using different codes (e.g., distinguishing refusals and *don't know*s).

The choice of what code to use for missing data is often arbitrary, but missing values codes must be ones that have not been used for actual pieces of information. Many researchers follow the convention of using 9 as the missing code because this value is out of the range of real codes for most variables. Others use blanks, periods, or negative values for missing information.

Precise coding instructions should be documented in a coding manual. Coders, like observers and interviewers, must be properly trained, and intercoder reliability checks are recommended.

➔ **TIP:** Some statistical software specifies how missing data should be coded, so you should decide what software to use before finalizing coding decisions.

Entering, Verifying, and Cleaning Data

Coded data typically are transferred onto a data file by keyboard entry, but other options (e.g., scanning of forms) are also available. Various programs can be used for data entry, including spreadsheets or databases. Major software packages for statistical analysis also have data editors that make data entry fairly easy.

Figure 24.2 presents a portion of a data file for SPSS, for data that we used in analytic examples in the preceding three chapters (see Table 21.10). The entire data file is a 30 × 10 matrix, with 30 rows (1 for each subject) and 10 columns for data on 7 variables. This figure displays data for only the first 5 subjects to conserve space. Each variable had to be named (group, birth weight, etc.). The subjects' unique ID should be entered along with actual data, which allows researchers to go back to original sources if need be. The ID number normally is entered as the first variable of the record, as in Figure 24.2.

Data entry is prone to error, and so it is essential to verify entries and correct mistakes. One method

	id	group	bweight	repeat	age	priors	smokstat
1	1	1	107	1	17	1	1
2	2	1	101	0	14	0	0
3	3	1	119	0	21	3	0
4	4	1	128	1	20	2	0
5	5	1	89	0	15	1	1

FIGURE 24.2 Portion of an SPSS data file.

is to compare visually the numbers on a printout of the data file with codes on the original source, and another is to double-enter data. There are also special verifying programs designed to perform comparisons during direct data entry.

Example of data verification: Santacroce and Lee (2006) studied uncertainty, posttraumatic stress, and health behavior in young adult childhood cancer survivors. Here is how they described data management: "Data were checked for completeness and then double-entered into separate computer files; inconsistencies were identified and addressed before data were analyzed using SPSS 12.0 statistical software" (p. 262).

Even verified data usually contain some errors, for example, from coding problems or misreported information. Entered data must thus be cleaned. **Data cleaning** involves two types of checks. The first is a check for outliers and wild codes. **Outliers** are values that lie outside the normal range of values. Outliers can be found by inspecting frequency distributions, paying special attention to the lowest and highest values. (Most researchers routinely begin data analysis by running **marginals**—constructing frequency distributions—for all variables in their data set.) In some cases, outliers are true, legitimate values (e.g., an income of $1 million in a distribution where the mean is below $100,000). In other cases, however, outliers indicate an error, as when there is a **wild code**—that is, a code that is not possible. For example, the variable gender might have the following three defined codes: 1 = female, 2 = male, and 9 = missing. If we discovered a code of 3 for gender

in our file, it would be clear that an error had been made. The computer could be instructed to list the ID number of the faulty record, and the correct code could then be tracked down. Some data entry programs automatically perform range checks.

Editing of this type will never reveal all errors. If the gender of a male subject is entered incorrectly as a 1, the mistake may never be detected. Because errors can have a big effect on the analysis and interpretation of data, it is naturally important to perform the coding, entering, verifying, and cleaning with great care.

A second data-cleaning procedure involves **consistency checks**, which focus on internal data consistency. In this task, researchers check for errors by testing compatibility of data within a case. For example, one question in a survey might ask current marital status, and another might ask number of marriages. If the data were internally consistent, respondents who answered "Single, never married" to the first question should have a zero (or a missing values code) for the second. As another example, if the respondent's gender were coded as *male* and the variable "Number of pregnancies" had a code of 2, then one of those two fields would contain an error. Researchers should search for opportunities to check the consistency of entered data.

Creating and Documenting the Analysis Files

The decisions that researchers make about coding and variable naming should be fully documented.

Memory should not be trusted; several weeks after coding, researchers may no longer remember if male subjects were coded 1 and female subjects 2, or *vice versa*. Moreover, colleagues may wish to borrow the data set to do a secondary analysis. Regardless of whether one anticipates a secondary analysis, documentation should be sufficiently thorough that a person unfamiliar with the original study could use the data.

Documentation primarily involves preparing a codebook. A **codebook** is essentially a listing of each variable together with information about placement in the file, codes associated with the values of the variable, and other basic information. Codebooks can be generated by statistical or data entry programs.

Example of data preparation: Scheetz (2005) studied relationships between injury severity, injury type, and survival among older motor vehicle trauma patients in a secondary analysis of data on nearly 1500 trauma cases. Here is what Scheetz said about checking her data: "Data were screened for errors by examining plausible ranges, missing values, normality, scatterplots, frequencies, descriptives, and outliers using SPSS . . ." (p. 203).

PRELIMINARY ASSESSMENTS AND ACTIONS

Researchers typically undertake several preanalytic activities before they test their hypotheses. Several preparatory activities are discussed next.

Assessing and Handling Missing Values Problems

Researchers strive for a **rectangular matrix** of data—data values for all subjects on all important variables—but they usually find that their data set has some missing values. Before they can deal with this problem, researchers must first explore the distribution and patterning of missing data. An appropriate solution depends on such factors as the extent of missing data, the role the variable with missing data plays in the analysis, and the extent to

which the missing data are *missing at random (MAR)*—that is, whether missing values are related systematically to key study variables. If the missing values disproportionately come from people with certain characteristics, there is likely to be bias.

The first step, then, is to assess the extent of the problem by examining the marginals on a variable-by-variable basis. Another step is to examine the cumulative extent of missing values by creating **flags** to count how many variables are missing for each subject. Once a missing values flag has been created, a frequency distribution can be computed for this new variable, which would show how many cases had no missing values, one missing value, and so on.

Another task is to evaluate the randomness of missing values. A simple procedure is to divide the sample into two groups—those with and without missing data on a specified variable. The two groups can then be compared in terms of subject characteristics to determine whether the two groups are comparable (e.g., were men more likely than women to leave certain questions blank?). Similarly, groups can be created based on the missing values flag (e.g., those with no missing data versus those with *any* missing data) and compared on other variables. Fox-Wasylyshyn and El-Masri (2005) discuss approaches to assessing *patterns* of missing data.

Once researchers have assessed the extent and patterning of missing values, decisions must be made about how to address the problem. There are two basic types of solutions: deletions and imputations.

Missing Data and Deletions

There are various deletion strategies, the simplest of which is to delete a subject entirely if there is missing information. When samples are small, the loss of cases can have a large impact on power. It is, however, advisable to delete cases for subjects with extensive missing information. This strategy is called **listwise deletion** of missing values.

Another option is to delete a variable for all subjects. This option may be suitable when a high percentage of cases have missing values on a variable. This may occur if, for example, a question was objectionable and was left blank, or if many respondents did not understand directions and inadvertently skipped it. Recommendations for how much missing data should drive this decision range from 15% to 40% of cases (Fox-Wasylyshyn & El-Masri, 2005).

Perhaps the most widely used (but often not the best) approach is to delete cases selectively, on a variable-by-variable basis. For example, in describing the characteristics of the sample, researchers might use whatever information is available for each characteristic, resulting in a fluctuating number of cases across descriptors. Mean age might be based on 95 cases, the gender distribution might be based on 102 cases, and so on. If the number of cases fluctuates widely across characteristics, the information is difficult to interpret because the sample is essentially a "moving target."

The same strategy is sometimes used to handle missing information for dependent variables. For example, in an evaluation of an intervention to reduce patient anxiety, the dependent variables might be blood pressure and self-reported anxiety. If 10 people out of a sample of 100 failed to complete the anxiety scale, we might base the analyses of anxiety data on the 90 subjects who completed the scale, but use the full sample of 100 subjects in the blood pressure analysis. This approach can, however, cause interpretive problems, especially if there are inconsistent findings. For example, if there were experimental versus control group differences on blood pressure but not anxiety, one possible explanation is that the anxiety scale sample was not representative of the full sample. In such a situation, we should, at a minimum, perform supplementary analyses using the rectangular matrix—that is, rerun the blood pressure analysis using the 90 subjects for whom complete data are available. If the results are different from when the full sample was used, we would at least be in a better position to interpret results.

In analyses involving a correlation matrix, researchers sometimes use **pairwise deletion** of cases with missing values. Figure 24.3 illustrates a 4-variable correlation matrix in which pairwise deletion was used. Correlations between pairs of variables are based on varying numbers of cases (shown in the row labeled N), ranging from 425 subjects (for the r between CES-D depression scores and total income), to 483 subjects (for the r between highest grade completed and number of

Correlations

		Highest school grade completed	Total # people in hh	Total household income	CES-D Score (Range 0 to 60)
Highest school grade completed	Pearson Correlation	1.000	−.127**	.068	−.081
	sig. (2-tailed)		.005	.154	.082
	N		484	483	437	460
Total # people in hh	Pearson Correlation	−.127**	1,000	.196**	−.021
	sig. (2-tailed)	.005		.000	.649
	N	483	492	446	467
Total household income	Pearson Correlation	.068	.196**	1.000	−.178**
	sig. (2-tailed)	.154	.000		.000
	N	437	446	446	425
CES-D score (Range 0 to 60)	Pearson Correlation	−.081	−.021	−.178**	1.000
	sig. (2-tailed)	.082	.649	.000	
	N	460	467	425	468

**Correlation is significant at the 0.01 level (2-tailed).

FIGURE 24.3 Correlation matrix for a nonrectangular data matrix.

household members). Pairwise deletion may be acceptable for descriptive purposes if data are missing at random and differences in *N*s are small. It is especially imprudent to use pairwise deletion for multivariate analyses such as multiple regression or factor analysis because the correlations are based on nonidentical subsets of subjects.

Missing Data and Imputations

A second and usually preferred approach to addressing missing values is through imputation, which involves calculating an estimate of the missing value and replacing it with the estimate. The simplest of these procedures is to use **mean substitution** or *median substitution*, which involves using "typical" sample values to replace missing data that are continuous. For example, if a subject's age were missing and if the average age of subjects in the sample were 45.2 years, we might substitute the value 45 in place of the missing values code.

A refinement on this strategy is to use subgroup means. For example, if the mean age for women in the sample were 41.8 years and the mean age for men were 48.9 years, we could substitute 42 for women with missing age data and 49 for men with missing age data. This likely would result in improved accuracy, compared with substituting the overall mean of 45 for everyone with missing age data.

Mean substitution can also be used to substitute missing values for items in multiple-item scales. Suppose, for example, we had a 20-item anxiety scale, and one person left two items blank. It would not be appropriate to score the scale by adding together responses on the 18 answered items, and it would be a waste of 18 pieces of information to score the entire scale as missing. Thus, for the two missing items, the researcher could substitute the most typical responses, such as the mean item value across subjects, so that a scale score could be computed. Another possibility is to use *case substitution*, which involves substituting, for each person with missing data, the mean item value for the other answered items of that individual on the scale. These approaches make sense only when a small proportion of scale items is missing.

Researchers are increasingly using imputation methods that make more extensive use of data in the data set. One example is to use regression analysis to "predict" the correct value of missing data. Suppose we found that subjects' age was correlated with gender, education, and health status. Based on data from subjects with complete data, age could be regressed on these three variables to predict age for subjects with missing age data, but whose values for the three other variables were not missing. Regression-based imputation can be used when up to about 40% of the data are missing, and is more accurate than previously discussed strategies.

Even more sophisticated solutions have been developed. Maximum likelihood estimation is useful because it uses all data points in a data set to construct estimated replacement values. **Expectation maximization** involves using an iterative procedure with a maximum likelihood–based algorithm to produce the best parameter estimates. Finally, **multiple imputation** is an approach that, unlike the single imputation procedures already described, creates more than one estimate for a single missing datum (McCleary, 2002; Patrician, 2002). The main advantage of multiple imputation is that it realistically reflects uncertainty about missing values.

Each missing values strategy is appropriate under varying conditions and offers different strengths and problems, so care should be taken in deciding how missing data are to be handled. Procedures for dealing with missing data are discussed at greater length by Allison (2000) and Little and Rubin (2002).

➡ **TIP:** Some statistical software packages (such as SPSS) have a special procedure for estimating the value of missing data. These procedures can also be used to examine the relationship between the missing values and other variables in the data set. ●

Example of handling missing values: Bennett and colleagues (2005) tested the effectiveness of nurse coaching in supporting healthy behavior change in older adults. Here is how they described their approach to missing data: "To reduce the impact of missing data on our sample size, scale scores for the health status outcomes were computed by taking the mean of the remaining items if 75% of the items comprising that scale were completed. No missing data were permitted in the General Health measure because it was a single item" (p. 192).

Assessing Data Quality

Assessing data quality is another key task in the early stage of analysis. For example, when psychosocial scales or composite indexes are used, researchers should usually assess their internal consistency reliability (see Chapter 17). The distribution of data values for key variables also should be examined to determine any anomalies, such as limited variability, extreme skewness, or the presence of ceiling or floor effects. For example, a vocabulary test for 10-year-olds likely would yield a clustering of high scores in a sample of 11-year-olds, creating a **ceiling effect** that would reduce correlations between test scores and other characteristics of the children. Conversely, there likely would be a clustering of low scores on the test with a sample of 9-year-olds, resulting in a **floor effect** with similar consequences. In such situations, data may need to be transformed to meet the requirements for certain statistical tests. (Note that, ideally, such problems would have been detected and addressed during the planning of the study.)

Assessing Bias

Researchers often undertake preliminary analyses to assess the direction and extent of any biases, including the following:

- *Nonresponse bias.* Whenever possible, researchers should assess whether a biased subset of people participated in a study. If there is information about the characteristics of all people who were asked to participate in a study (e.g., demographic information from hospital records), researchers should compare the characteristics of those who did and did not participate to determine the nature and direction of any biases.

- *Selection bias.* When nonrandomized comparison groups are used (e.g., in quasi-experimental or case-control studies), researchers should check for selection biases by comparing the groups' background characteristics. These variables should, if possible, be controlled—for example, through analysis of covariance or multiple regression. Even when an experimental design has been used, researchers should check the success of randomization.

- *Attrition bias.* In studies with multiple points of data collection, it is important to check for attrition biases, which involves comparing people who did and did not continue to participate in the study in later waves of data collection, based on characteristics of these groups at the initial wave.

In performing any of these analyses, significant group differences are an indication of bias, and such bias must be taken into consideration in interpreting and discussing the results. Whenever possible, the biases should be controlled in testing the main hypotheses.

Example of assessing bias: Keefe and co-researchers (2006) evaluated the effectiveness of a home-based nursing intervention for reducing parenting stress among parents with irritable infants. Infants were randomized to a treatment or control group. The groups were compared in terms of baseline demographic characteristics, and no significant differences were found. There were, however, group differences on a subscale of an outcome variable, and these differences were taken into account in subsequent analyses. The researchers also examined attrition bias. Study dropouts were found to be significantly less well educated than those who completed the study.

Testing Assumptions for Statistical Tests

Most statistical tests are based on a number of assumptions—conditions that are presumed to be true and, when violated, can lead to misleading or invalid results. For example, parametric tests assume that variables are distributed normally. Frequency distributions, scatter plots, and other assessment procedures provide researchers with information about whether or not underlying assumptions for statistical tests have been upheld.

Frequency distributions can reveal whether the normality assumption is tenable; graphic displays of data values indicate whether the distribution is severely skewed, multimodal, too peaked, or too flat. There are also statistical indexes of skewness or peakedness that programs can compute to determine whether the shape of the distribution deviates significantly from normality—although skewness may not be detected if the sample size is too small.

Example of testing assumptions: Gulick (2001) used multiple regression to explore the relationship of emotional distress, social support, and personal attributes *vis-à-vis* functional status in people with multiple sclerosis. She examined scatter plots and performed other analysis to determine whether the assumptions of linearity and normality were met.

Performing Data Transformations

Raw data often need to be modified or transformed before hypotheses can be tested. Various **data transformations** can easily be handled through commands to the computer. For example, as discussed in earlier chapters, the scoring of some items on multi-item scales might need to be reversed before the item scores can be summed. **Item reversals** can easily be accomplished by instructing the computer to create a new variable that is equal to the original value subtracted from the number of response options plus 1 (e.g., for a score of 1 on a 5-point Likert item [ITEM], the reversal would be NEWITEM = 6 – 1 = 5).

Another situation arises when researchers want a variable that is a cumulative **count** of the occurrence of an attribute. For example, suppose we asked people to indicate which types of illegal drug they had used in the past month, from a list of 10 options. Use of each drug would be answered independently in a yes (e.g., coded 1) or no (e.g., coded 2) fashion. We could then create a new variable that represented a count of all the "1" codes for the 10-drug items.

Other transformations involve **recodes** of original values. For example, in some analyses, an infant's original birth weight (entered in grams) might be used, whereas in others, we might want to compare low-birth-weight and normal-birth-weight infants. The computer could be instructed to create a new dichotomous variable (e.g., coded 1 for a low-birth-weight infant and 0 for a normal-birth-weight infant), based on whether the original birth-weight value was less than 2500 grams. Recoding is often used to create *dummy variables* for multivariate analyses.

Transformations also can be undertaken to render data appropriate for statistical tests. For example, if a distribution is markedly non-normal, a transformation can sometimes be done to make parametric procedures appropriate. A logarithmic transformation, for example, tends to normalize distributions. Discussions of the use of transformations for changing the characteristics of a distribution can be found in Ferketich and Verran (1994) and in many texts on statistical analysis.

Example of transforming variables: Jones (2004) examined interrelationships among sexual imposition (pressures to engage in sex), dyadic trust, and sensation seeking in young urban women. Jones noted the following: "As expected, sexual risk scores and sexual imposition scores were positively skewed and were transformed logarithmically to make them more symmetric. No substantive difference in results was found between logarithmically transformed and raw data; therefore, the results using the raw data are reported" (p. 190).

⊃ **TIP:** Whenever you create transformed variables, it is important to check that the transformations were done correctly by examining a sample of values for the original and transformed variables. This can be done by instructing the computer to list, for a sample of cases, the values of the newly created variables and the original variables used to create them.

Performing Additional Peripheral Analyses

Depending on the study, additional peripheral analyses may be needed before proceeding to substantive analyses. It is impossible to catalog all such analyses, but we offer a few examples to alert readers to the kinds of issues that need to be given some thought.

Data Pooling

Researchers sometimes obtain data from more than one source or about more than one type of subject. For example, researchers sometimes draw subjects from multiple sites, or may recruit subjects with different medical conditions. The risk in doing this is that subjects may not really be drawn from the same population, and so it is wise in such situations to determine whether **pooling** of data (combining data for all subjects) is warranted. This involves comparing the different subsets of subjects (i.e., subjects from the different sites, and so on) in terms of key research variables.

Example of testing for pooling: Fallis and colleagues (2006) tested the efficacy of a forced-air warming blanket, compared with the usual warmed cotton blanket, on the temperature and comfort of mothers and infants during cesarean delivery. Participants were recruited from two acute care sites in Winnipeg. There were no significant differences in the characteristics of women from the two sites at baseline, "justifying pooling of observations from the two hospitals" (p. 326).

Testing Cohort Effects

Nurse researchers sometimes need to gather data over an extended period of time to achieve adequate sample sizes. This can result in **cohort effects**, that is, differences in outcomes or subject characteristics over time. This might occur because sample characteristics evolve over time or because of changes in community characteristics, in health care services, and so on. If the research involves an experimental treatment, it may also be that the treatment itself changes—for example, if early program experience is used to improve the treatment or if those administering the treatment simply get better at doing it. Thus, researchers with a long period of *sample intake* should consider testing for cohort effects because such effects can confound the results or even mask existing relationships. This

activity usually involves examining correlations between entry dates and key research variables.

Example of testing for cohort effects: Polit, London, and Martinez (2001), in their study of health problems among low-income mothers, analyzed survey data from 4000 women that were collected over a 12-month period. They discovered that women interviewed later were significantly more disadvantaged than those interviewed early. In their multivariate analyses, a variable for timing of the interview was statistically controlled.

Testing Ordering Effects

When a crossover design is used (i.e., subjects are randomly assigned to different orderings of treatments), researchers should assess whether outcomes are different for people in the different treatment-order groups. That is, did getting A before B yield different outcomes than getting B before A? In essence, such tests offer evidence that it is legitimate to pool the data from the alternative orderings.

Example of testing for ordering effects: Cheng and Chang (2003) used a crossover design to test the efficacy of two alternative oral care protocols for addressing oral mucositis in pediatric patients undergoing chemotherapy. Each protocol was given to half the children at the onset of chemotherapy and continued for 21 days; then children got the other protocol for the next 21 days. There were differences relating to the treatments, with chlorhexidine found to be more effective than benzydamine in terms of outcomes such as mouth pain, but ordering of the conditions was unrelated to outcomes.

PRINCIPAL ANALYSES

At this point in the analysis process, researchers have a cleaned data set, with missing data problems resolved and transformations completed; they also have some understanding of data quality and biases. They can now proceed with more substantive data analyses.

The Substantive Data Analysis Plan

In many studies, researchers collect data on dozens of variables. They cannot analyze every variable in relation to all others, and so a plan to guide data analysis must be developed. One approach is to prepare a list of the analyses to be undertaken, specifying both the variables and the statistical test to be used. Another approach is to develop table shells. **Table shells** are layouts of how researchers envision presenting their findings, without numbers filled in. Once a table shell is prepared, researchers can do the analyses needed to complete the table. (The table templates in the Toolkit of the accompanying *Resource Manual*, for Chapters 21 to 23, can be used as a basis for table shells.) ⊗

Table 24.1 presents an example of a partial table shell created for an evaluation of an intervention for low-income women. This table guided a series of ANCOVAs that compared experimental and control groups in terms of several indicators of emotional well-being, after controlling for various characteristics measured at random assignment. The completed table that appeared in the research report was somewhat different than this table shell (e.g., other outcome variables were added). Researchers do not need to adhere rigidly to table shells, but they provide a good mechanism for organizing the analysis of large amounts of data.

Substantive Analyses

The next step is to perform the actual substantive analyses, typically beginning with descriptive analyses. For example, researchers usually develop a descriptive profile of the sample, and often look descriptively at correlations among variables. These initial analyses may suggest further analyses or further data transformations that were not originally envisioned. They also give researchers an opportunity to become familiar with their data.

➲ **TIP:** When you begin to acquaint yourself with the data, resist the temptation of going on a "fishing expedition," that is, hunting for *any* interesting relationships between variables. The facility with which computers can generate statistical information makes it easy to run analyses indiscriminately. The risk is that you will serendipitously find significant correlations between variables as a function of chance. For example, in a correlation matrix with 10 variables (which results in 45 nonredundant correlations), there are likely to be two to three *spurious* significant correlations when alpha $= .05$ (i.e., $.05 \times 45 = 2.25$).

TABLE 24.1	Example of a Table Shell: Program Impacts on Indicators of Emotional Well-Being at the Time of the 12-Month Follow-up Interview*				
	TREATMENT GROUP	**CONTROL GROUP**	**DIFFERENCE**		
OUTCOME	Mean (SD)	Mean (SD)	(95% CI)	*F*	*p*
CES-D (depression) Scale scores					
Mastery (self-efficacy) Scale scores					
Difficult Life Circumstances Scale scores					
Level of satisfaction with available social support					

*Analyses to be performed using ANCOVA, controlling for baseline characteristics.

Researchers then perform statistical analyses to test their hypotheses. Researchers whose data analysis plan calls for multivariate analyses (e.g., MANOVA) may proceed directly to their final analyses, but they may begin with various bivariate analyses (e.g., a series of ANOVAs). The primary statistical analyses are complete when all the research questions are addressed and when table shells have the applicable numbers in them.

INTERPRETATION OF RESULTS

The analysis of research data provides the **results** of the study. These results need to be evaluated and interpreted, giving thought to the aims of the project, its theoretical basis, the existing body of related research evidence, and limitations of the adopted research methods. The interpretive task involves attending to five aspects of the results: (1) their credibility, (2) their meaning, (3) their importance, (4) the extent to which they can be generalized, and (5) their implications.

Credibility of the Results

One of the first interpretive tasks is to assess whether the results are *right*. This corresponds to the first question we proposed in Chapter 2 (see Box 2.1) within an evidence-based practice (EBP) context: "What is the quality of the evidence—that is, how rigorous and reliable is it?" This type of assessment requires a careful analysis of the study's methodologic and conceptual limitations and strong points. Regardless of whether one's hypotheses are supported, the validity and meaning of the results depend on a full understanding of the study's strengths and shortcomings, and on a careful assessment of the *evidence* about study credibility.

Empirical studies inherently involve making inferences. We *infer* that scores on a depression scale are, in fact, capturing the depression construct. We *infer* that a sample can tell us something about a population. We use inferential statistics to make inferences about relationships observed in the data. Inference and validity are inextricably linked. As Shadish, Cook, and Campbell (2002) have stated, "We use the term *validity* to refer to the approximate truth of an inference" (p. 34). To be careful interpreters of their own results, researchers need to be skeptics about their inferences, and then look for ways to marshal evidence that those inferences are, in fact, valid. In essence, this is much like statistical hypothesis testing: if you begin by *assuming* that you "got it wrong" (the null hypothesis) but then look for evidence to support that you "got it right," you are likely to have a much more persuasive case to support your interpretation.

One type of evidence comes from prior research on the topic. Investigators should examine whether their results are consistent with those of other studies—and with theories that purport to explain phenomena examined in the study. If there are discrepancies, a careful analysis of plausible reasons for any differences should be undertaken.

Interpretation relies heavily on researchers' critical thinking skills and on their ability to be reasonably objective about their own decisions and how those decisions got implemented. Researchers should carefully evaluate (e.g., using criteria such as those presented at the end of each chapter in this book) the major methodologic decisions they made in planning and executing the study and consider whether different decisions might have yielded different results.

Researchers must continually ask such questions as, "Is it *plausible* that my results merely reflect selection biases? Is it *plausible* that if subjects had been blinded to the treatment, the results would have been different? Is it *plausible* that if I had used a different instrument, or had gotten a larger sample, or had less attrition, my results would change? Researchers hope that the answers to such questions are "no," but should start with the assumption that the answer is "yes" until they have satisfied themselves that this is not true.

Some questions may not be answerable, but many can be answered through scrutiny of the data. For example, if there is evidence of strong validity and reliability of an outcome measure, then it is unlikely that a different instrument would have yielded more accurate results. Evidence also can be developed through peripheral data analyses, some of which were discussed earlier in this chapter. For example, researchers can have greater confidence in the accuracy of their findings if they have ruled out (or controlled) biases.

Sometimes supplementary analyses can shed light on the tenability of inferences. For example, suppose our analyses revealed that an experimental exercise intervention was successful in lowering blood pressure levels in elderly hypertensive patients. In scrutinizing the sample characteristics, however, we find that women were underrepresented, which might lead critics to suggest that the evidence for effectiveness in the overall population is weak. In this situation, we might want to examine experimental and control group differences for just the women in the sample, to see if the evidence suggests that the under-representation of women affects the overall conclusions. If the results were similar for women and men (even if the smaller subsample size led to statistically nonsignificant results), they would make the inference about the potential benefits of the intervention for both genders more plausible.

Another strategy is to undertake what is referred to as **sensitivity analyses**. These are analyses that test key research hypotheses using different assumptions. For example, suppose we tested an intervention designed to help smokers quit smoking, and the key outcome is whether the sample members have smoked in the week following the intervention. We begin with a sample of 200 smokers, 100 of whom are assigned to the control group. After the intervention, we compare smoking in the two groups based on data from 170 subjects who provided follow-up data. If we tested for attrition biases and found no biases between those who completed the study and those who did not with regard to key baseline characteristics, we might assume that the 30 study dropouts were a random subset and therefore test our hypotheses using only 170 data points—an *on-protocol analysis*. To be conservative in drawing conclusions, however, we should also do an *intention-to-treat analysis*, which would assume that the 30 people who dropped out

of the study did *not* stop smoking. If the results suggested that the intervention was successful in reducing smoking in both analyses, our inferences about intervention efficacy would be greatly bolstered. Another example of sensitivity analyses is using different cut-points on a measure to establish "caseness."

A critical analysis of the research methods and a scrutiny of various types of external and internal evidence almost inevitably indicate some limitations. These limitations must be taken into account in interpreting and discussing the results.

Example of sensitivity analysis: Nachreiner and colleagues (2005) examined the effect of occupational violence training on work-related assault, using survey data from nearly 1300 nurses in Minnesota. In examining the relationship between self-reported receipt of training and an incidence of patient-perpetrated violence, the researchers undertook some sensitivity analyses. One such analysis focused on the issue of misclassification—that is, examining the effect of differences in risk estimates based on errors in reporting training and assault.

⊃ **TIP:** In evaluating whether the results are *real*, you should carefully evaluate the extent to which there is evidence of internal, statistical conclusion, and construct validity in your study.

Meaning of the Results

In qualitative studies, interpretation and analysis occur virtually simultaneously. In quantitative studies, however, results are in the form of test statistics, *p* levels, effect sizes, and confidence intervals, to which researchers need to attach meaning. This sometimes involves supplementary analyses—for example, if research findings are contrary to the hypotheses, other information in the data set sometimes can be examined to help researchers understand what the findings mean. In this section, we discuss the interpretation of various research outcomes within a hypothesis-testing context. Note, however, that you will be better armed to interpret the meaning of the findings if, in addition to having information about statistical significance, you have information about the precision of estimates (i.e., confidence intervals) and about the magnitude of effects (effect size estimates). These pieces of information address two other questions raised in connection with an EBP-based evaluation of research evidence: "What *is* the evidence—what is the magnitude of effects?" and "How precise is the estimate of effects?" (see Box 2.1).

Interpreting Hypothesized Results

Interpreting results is easiest when hypotheses are supported. Such interpretations have been partly accomplished beforehand because, in developing hypotheses, researchers have already brought together prior findings, a theoretical framework, and logical reasoning. This groundwork forms the context within which more specific interpretations are made.

Naturally, researchers are gratified when the results of many hours of effort support their predictions. There is a decided preference on the part of individual researchers, advisers, and journal reviewers for studies whose hypotheses have been supported. This preference is understandable, but it is important not to let personal preferences interfere with the critical appraisal appropriate to all interpretive situations. A few caveats should be kept in mind.

First, it is important to be conservative in drawing conclusions from the data. Although it may be tempting to go beyond the data to explain what results mean, this should be avoided. An example might help to explain what we mean by "going beyond" the data. Suppose we hypothesized that pregnant women's anxiety level about labor and delivery is correlated with the number of children they have already borne. The data reveal that a significant negative relationship between anxiety levels and parity ($r = -.40$) exists. We conclude that increased experience with childbirth results in decreased anxiety. Is this conclusion supported by the data? The conclusion appears to be logical, but in fact, there is nothing in the data that leads directly to this interpretation. An important, indeed critical, research precept is: *correlation does not prove causation*. The finding that two variables are related

offers no evidence suggesting which of the two variables—if either—caused the other. In our example, perhaps causality runs in the opposite direction, that is, that a woman's anxiety level influences how many children she bears. Or perhaps a third variable not examined in the study, such as the woman's relationship with her husband, causes or influences both anxiety and number of children. As discussed in Chapters 10 and 11, inferring causality is difficult in studies that have not used a true experimental design.

Alternative explanations for the findings should always be considered and, if possible, tested directly. If competing interpretations can be ruled out, so much the better, but every angle should be examined to see if one's own explanation has been given adequate competition.

Empirical evidence supporting research hypotheses never constitutes *proof* of their veracity. Hypothesis testing is probabilistic. There is always a possibility that observed relationships resulted from chance—that is, that there has been a Type I error. Researchers must be tentative about their results and about interpretations of them. Thus, even when the results are in line with expectations, researchers should draw conclusions with restraint and should give due consideration to limitations identified in assessing the accuracy of the results.

Example of corroboration of a hypothesis: Harrison and colleagues (2004) hypothesized that the stability of a marital relationship would influence the ability of people with multiple sclerosis to accept their disability. Consistent with the hypothesis, the researchers found in their longitudinal study of 399 participants (all of whom were married at the outset) that people who had remained married over a 6-year period had a higher acceptance of their disability at the end of the study than people whose marriages ended through separation, divorce, or widowhood.

This study is a good example of the challenges of interpreting findings in correlational studies. The researchers' interpretation was that marriage conferred psychosocial benefits, a conclusion that they supported with evidence from other studies. However, there is nothing in their data that would rule out the possibility that a person's difficulty accepting his or her disabilities *led to* marital discord.

Interpreting Nonsignificant Results

Nonsignificant results pose interpretative problems. Statistical procedures are geared toward disconfirmation of the null hypothesis. Failure to reject a null hypothesis can occur for many reasons, and researchers do not know which one applies. The null hypothesis *could* actually be true, for example. The nonsignificant result, in this case, accurately reflects the absence of a relationship among research variables. On the other hand, the null hypothesis could be false, in which case a Type II error has been committed.

Retaining a false null hypothesis can result from such problems as poor internal validity, an anomalous sample, a weak statistical procedure, unreliable measures, or too small a sample. Unless researchers have special justification for attributing the nonsignificant findings to one of these factors, interpreting such results is tricky. We suspect that failure to reject null hypotheses is often a consequence of insufficient power, usually reflecting too small a sample size.

In any event, researchers are never justified in interpreting a retained null hypothesis as proof of the *absence* of relationships among variables. *Nonsignificant results provide no evidence of the truth or the falsity of the hypothesis.* When significant results are not obtained, there may be a tendency to be overcritical of the research methods and undercritical of the theory or reasoning on which hypotheses were based. This is understandable: It is easier to say, "My ideas were sound, I just didn't use the right approach," than to admit to faulty reasoning. It is important to look for and identify flaws in the research methods, but it is equally important to search for theoretical shortcomings. The result of such endeavors should be recommendations for how the methods, the theory, or an experimental intervention could be improved.

Example of nonsignificant results: Griffin, Polit, and Byrnes (in press) hypothesized that pediatric nurses' stereotypes about children (based on children's gender, race, and physical attractiveness) would influence nurses' perceptions about children's pain and their recommendations for pain treatment. None of the hypotheses was supported—that is, there was no evidence of stereotyping. The conclusion that stereotyping was, in fact, essentially absent was bolstered by the fact that the randomly selected sample was rather large—334 nurses—and that nurses were blinded to the manipulation (child characteristics). Effect sizes were calculated in support of this conclusion. For example, the effect size (eta-squared) for the effect of children's race on nurses' perceptions of children's pain was an extremely low .006 (i.e., explaining less than 1% of variation in nurses' perceptions). Arguably, an effect this small could not be construed as clinically significant.

Because statistical procedures are designed to provide support for *rejecting* null hypotheses, these procedures are not well suited for testing actual research hypotheses about the absence of relationships between variables or about equivalence between groups. Yet sometimes this is exactly what researchers want to do—and this is especially true in clinical situations in which the goal is to determine whether one practice is just as effective as another. When the actual research hypothesis is null (i.e., a prediction of no group difference or no relationship), stringent additional strategies must be used to provide supporting evidence. For one thing, it is imperative to compute effect sizes and confidence intervals as a means of illustrating that the risk of a Type II error was small. There may also be clinical standards that can be used to corroborate that nonsignificant—but predicted—results can be accepted as consistent with the research hypothesis.

Example of support for a hypothesized nonsignificant result: Medves and O'Brien (2004) conducted a clinical trial to test the hypothesis that thermal stability would be comparable for infants bathed for the first time by a parent or by a nurse. As predicted, there was no difference in temperature change between newborns bathed by nurses or parents. The researchers provided additional support for concluding that heat loss was not associated with who bathed the newborn by indicating that a power analysis had been used to determine sample size needs and that parents for the two groups of infants were comparable demographically. Also, although the prebath temperatures of the infants in the two groups were significantly different, the researchers used initial temperature as a covariate to control these differences. Finally, they made an *a priori* determination that a change in temperature of 1°C would be clinically significant; at four points in time after the bath, the group differences in temperature were never this large; thus, the miniscule differences were judged clinically insignificant.

Interpreting Unhypothesized Significant Results

Unhypothesized significant results can occur in two situations. The first involves finding relationships that were not considered while designing the study. For example, in examining correlations among variables in the data set, we might notice that two variables that were not central to our research questions were nevertheless significantly correlated—and interesting. To interpret this finding, we would need to evaluate whether the relationship is real or spurious. There may be information in the data set that sheds light on this issue, but we might also need to consult the literature to determine whether other investigators have observed similar relationships.

Example of a serendipitous significant finding: Quinn (2005) studied delay in seeking care for symptoms of acute myocardial infarction (MI), guided by two theoretical frameworks. She noted that "the relationship of type of MI experienced with time to seek care was a serendipitous finding when correlations were performed examining the relationship of all clinical variables with time to seek care." She explored this unexpected finding in further analyses.

The second situation is more perplexing, although it does not happen often: obtaining results *opposite* to those hypothesized. For instance, we might hypothesize that individualized teaching about AIDS risks is more effective than group instruction, but the results might indicate that the group method was significantly better. It is, of course, unethical to alter a hypothesis after the results are "in." Some researchers view such situations as awkward or embarrassing, but there is little basis for such feelings. The purpose of research is not to corroborate researchers' predictions, but to arrive at truth and enhance understanding. There is no such thing as a study whose results "came out wrong" if they reflect the truth.

When significant findings are opposite to what was hypothesized, it is less likely that the methods are flawed than that the reasoning or theory is incorrect. As always, the interpretation of the findings should involve comparisons with other research, a consideration of alternate theories, and a critical scrutiny of data collection and analysis procedures. The result of such an examination should be a tentative explanation for the unexpected findings, together with suggestions for how such explanations could be tested in other studies.

Example of unhypothesized significant results: Provencher and co-researchers (2003) studied predictors of psychological distress in Canadian family caregivers of relatives with psychiatric disabilities. Contrary to their hypothesis that social support would be beneficial, the researchers found that caregivers who perceived more support from friends experienced a higher level of distress than those who perceived less support. Also contrary to their predictions, relatives who had more contact with their relatives' primary mental health providers were more distressed than those with less contact.

Interpreting Mixed Results

Interpretation is often complicated by *mixed results*: some hypotheses are supported by the data, but others are not. Or a hypothesis may be accepted with one measure of the dependent variable, but rejected with a different measure. When only some results run counter to a theoretical position or conceptual scheme, the research methods are the first aspect of the study deserving critical scrutiny. Differences in the validity and reliability of the various measures may account for such discrepancies, for example. On the other hand, mixed results may suggest that a theory needs to be qualified, or that certain constructs within the theory need to be reconceptualized. Mixed results sometimes present opportunities for making conceptual advances because efforts to make sense of disparate pieces of evidence may lead to a breakthrough.

Example of mixed results: Reishstein (2005) examined relationships between symptoms and functional performance in patients with chronic obstructive pulmonary disease (COPD). She hypothesized that dyspnea, fatigue, and sleep difficulty are related to functional performance. Dyspnea and fatigue had moderate negative correlations with functional performance, but sleep difficulty was not significantly related.

In summary, interpreting research results is a demanding task, but it offers the possibility of unique intellectual rewards. Researchers must in essence play the role of scientific detectives, trying to make pieces of the puzzle fit together so that a coherent picture emerges.

➲ **TIP:** In interpreting your data, remember that others will be reviewing your interpretation with a critical and perhaps even a skeptical eye. The job of consumers is to make decisions about the credibility and utility of the evidence, which is likely to be affected by how much support you offer for the validity and meaning of your results.

Importance of the Results

In quantitative studies, results that support the researcher's hypotheses are described as significant. A careful analysis of study results involves an evaluation of whether, in addition to being statistically significant, they are important.

Attaining statistical significance does not necessarily mean that the results are meaningful to nurses and clients. Statistical significance indicates that the results were unlikely to be due to chance. This means that observed group differences or relationships were probably real, but not necessarily important. With large samples, even modest relationships are statistically significant. For instance, with a sample of 500, a correlation coefficient of .10 is significant at the .05 level, but a relationship this weak may have little practical value. Researchers must pay attention to the numeric values, effect sizes, and confidence intervals obtained in an analysis, in addition to significance levels, when assessing the importance of the findings.

Conversely, the absence of statistically significant results does not mean that the results are unimportant—although because of the difficulty in interpreting nonsignificant results, the case is more complex. Suppose we compared two alternative procedures for making a clinical assessment (e.g., body temperature). Suppose further that we retained the null hypothesis, that is, found no statistically significant differences between the two methods. If an effect size analysis suggested a very small effect size for the differences *despite a large sample size*, we might be justified in concluding that the two procedures yield equally accurate assessments. If one of these procedures is more efficient or less painful than the other, nonsignificant findings could indeed be clinically important. Nevertheless, corroboration in replication studies would be needed before firm conclusions could be reached.

Generalizability of the Results

Researchers also should assess the generalizability and external validity of their results. Researchers are rarely interested in discovering relationships among variables for a specific group of people at a specific point in time. If a new nursing intervention is found to be successful, others will want to adopt it. Therefore, an important interpretive question is whether the intervention will "work" or whether the relationships will "hold" in other settings, with other people. Part of the interpretive process involves asking the question, "To what groups, environments, and conditions can the results of the study reasonably be applied?"

➲ **TIP:** Discussions about external validity can sometimes be enhanced by exploring *subgroup effects* within the data—that is, discovering whether observed relationships or impacts are true for different subsets of people, such as men and women, or older and younger people. Another way to explore this is by testing for *interaction effects*—that is, whether the independent variable, such as a treatment, interacts with subject or site characteristics.

Implications of the Results

Once researchers have drawn conclusions about the credibility, meaning, importance, and generalizability of the results, they are in a good position to make recommendations for using and building on the study findings. They should consider the implications with respect to future research, theory development, and nursing practice.

Study results are often used as a springboard for additional research, and researchers themselves often can readily recommend "next steps." Armed with an understanding of the study's limitations and strengths, researchers can pave the way for new studies that would avoid known pitfalls or capitalize on known strengths. Moreover, researchers are in a good position to assess how a new study might move a topic area forward. Is a replication needed, and, if so, with what groups? If observed relationships are significant, what do we need to know next for the information to be maximally useful?

> **TIP:** When a report is describing a pilot study, it is especially important for the Discussion section to include some "lessons learned" — that is, how the pilot might affect the parent study.

For studies based on a theoretical or conceptual model, researchers should also consider the study's theoretical implications. Research results should be used to document support for the theory, suggest ways in which the theory ought to be modified, or discredit the theory as a useful approach for studying the topic under investigation.

Finally, researchers should carefully consider the implications of the research evidence for nursing practice. How do the results contribute to a base of evidence to improve nursing? Specific suggestions for implementing the results of the study in a real nursing context are extremely valuable in the utilization process.

CRITIQUING INTERPRETATIONS

In the discussion section of research reports, researchers offer their interpretation of the findings and discuss what the findings might imply for nurs-ing. When critiquing a study, your own interpretation and inferences can be contrasted against those of the researchers.

As a reviewer, you should be wary if the discussion section fails to point out any limitations. Researchers are in the best position to detect and assess the impact of sampling deficiencies, practical constraints, data quality problems, and so on, and it is a professional responsibility to alert readers to these difficulties. Moreover, when researchers note methodologic shortcomings, readers know that these limitations were considered in interpreting the results. Of course, researchers are unlikely to note all relevant shortcomings of their own work. Thus, the inclusion of comments about study limitations in the discussion section, although important, does not relieve you of the responsibility of appraising methodologic and analytic decisions. Your task as reviewer is to develop your own interpretation and assessment of limitations, to challenge conclusions that do not appear to be warranted by the results, and to indicate how the study's evidence could have been enhanced.

In addition to comparing your interpretation with that of the researchers, your critique should draw conclusions about the stated implications of the study. Some researchers make grandiose claims or offer unfounded recommendations on the basis of modest results. Some guidelines for evaluating researchers' interpretation and implications are offered in Box 24.1. ✪

RESEARCH EXAMPLE

We conclude this chapter with an example of a study that involved interesting analyses to assist the researchers in interpreting their findings.

Study: "Relaxation and music reduce pain following intestinal surgery" (Good et al., 2005)

Statement of Purpose: The purpose of the study was to test the efficacy of three alternative interventions for pain relief following intestinal (INT) surgery: relaxation, chosen music, and both combined. Gate control theory of pain provided the theoretical context for the study.

BOX 24.1 Guidelines for Critiquing Interpretations in a Quantitative Research Report

Interpretation of the Findings

1. Are all important results discussed? If not, what is the likely explanation for omissions?
2. Does the report discuss the limitations of the study and possible effects of the limitations on the results?
3. Are interpretations consistent with results? Do the interpretations take limitations into account? Do the interpretations suggest distinct biases?
4. What types of evidence are offered in support of the interpretation, and is that evidence persuasive? Are results interpreted in light of findings from other studies? Are results interpreted in terms of the study hypotheses and the conceptual framework?
5. Are alternative explanations for the findings mentioned, and is the rationale for their rejection presented?
6. Does the interpretation distinguish between practical and statistical significance?
7. Are any unwarranted interpretations of causality made?
8. Are generalizations made that are not warranted on the basis of the sample used?

Implications of the Findings and Recommendations

9. Do the researchers discuss the study's implications for clinical practice, nursing education, nursing administration, or nursing theory, or make specific recommendations?
10. If yes, are the stated implications appropriate, given the study's limitations and given the body of evidence from other studies? Are there important implications that the report neglected to include?

Method: A sample of 217 patients from four hospitals who were undergoing INT surgery were randomly assigned to one of four conditions: a chosen music intervention, a jaw relaxation intervention, combined intervention, or a standard care control group. Fifty of the patients were lost to follow-up, leaving a final analysis sample of 167 patients. The primary outcome variables were patients' pain sensation and pain distress, both measured on a 100-mm visual analogue scale. Pain measurements were taken at multiple points, including preoperatively; before, during, and after ambulation for 2 days after surgery; and before and after a rest period for 2 days after surgery. Additional measures included pulse and respiratory rates and self-reported sleep quality. Patients in the treatment groups were also asked questions about their reactions to the treatment.

Analyses: The researchers analyzed potential selection biases by comparing the four groups on pretest pain measures. Although the groups were not significantly different, the baseline measures were used as covariates in the principal analyses to improve precision of estimated effects. Patients who completed the study were compared with those who dropped out on major demo-

graphic variables, and no significant differences were found. An intention-to-treat analysis approach was used with patients who completed at least one of the four posttest measurement sessions. Multiple analysis of covariance (MANCOVA) was used to analyze the pain data, controlling for baseline pain. The three treatment groups, taken together, had lower pain scores than those in the control group on both days at the postpreparatory and postrest phases, but not at postambulation. However, differences in pain among the three treatment groups were nonsignificant. There were no group differences on other outcome measures, such as respiratory or pulse rate or sleep quality.

The researchers did additional exploratory analyses, which they noted should be interpreted cautiously. They undertook subgroup analyses that explored whether the treatments had different effects for patients with different baseline pain levels. They found that, on day 2, the treatment effect was significant at postambulation for both those categorized as being in high and those in low pain before surgery. The researchers' analysis of impressionistic data also reinforced their conclusion that the effects of relaxation therapy or music were beneficial. For example,

96% of those in the three treatment groups reported that the treatment was helpful for pain, and 62% reported that it helped them feel more in control of their pain.

The researchers also presented information about clinical significance. For example, they computed effect sizes, and found most to be in the small to moderate range. Effect sizes were larger for those who were initially in greater pain. Clinical effects were also estimated by calculating the percentage decrease in pain sensation and distress between treatment and control group members. Differences were about 16% to 40% lower among those in intervention groups than among controls who used pain medication alone.

Discussion: Here are a few excerpts from the Discussion section of this report:

"In these INT surgery patients, relaxation, music, and the combination reduced pain at rest and at several ambulatory points on postoperative days 1 and 2. Subgroup analyses of those with high and low pain on day 2 showed further effects at post-ambulation and post-recovery, which suggests that the initial lack of effect may be related to the large variance in pain scores. Thus the interventions provided many patients with clinically significant relief, which was supported by exit reports of helpfulness . . ." (p. 248).

"It is recommended that researchers try longer listening times during the first 2 days to see if a larger dose improves pain, physiological measures, opioid uptake, side effects, sleep, recovery, and complications . . ." (p. 249).

"The results can be generalized to populations of INT surgery patients that are similar to this one: middle-aged Caucasian males and females undergoing specific surgeries in urban and suburban hospitals in the U.S. . . . with similar effects, it is recommended that nurses give patients choices among these interventions, encourage sequential use, and suggest using the music to relax or distract from pain" (p. 249).

SUMMARY POINTS

- Researchers who collect quantitative data typically progress through a series of steps in the analysis and interpretation of their data. Careful researchers lay out a data analysis plan in advance to guide that progress.

- Quantitative data must be converted to a form amenable to computer analysis through **coding**, which typically transforms all research data into numbers. Codes need to be developed to designate **missing values**.

- Researchers typically document decisions about coding, variable naming, and variable location in a **codebook**.

- Data entry is an error-prone process that requires verification and **data cleaning**. Cleaning involves (1) a check for **outliers** (values that lie outside the normal range of values) and **wild codes** (codes that are not legitimate), and (2) **consistency checks**.

- An important early task in analyzing data involves taking steps to evaluate and address missing data problems. Decisions on handling missing values must be based on the amount of missing data and how missing data are patterned (i.e., the extent to which it is random).

- Two basic missing values strategies involve *deletion* or *imputation*. Deletion strategies include deleting cases with missing values (i.e., **listwise deletion**), deleting variables with missing values, and selective **pairwise deletion** of cases. Imputation strategies include substitution of mean or median values, regression-based estimation of missing values, **expectation maximization**, and **multiple imputation**. Researchers strive to achieve a **rectangular matrix** of data (valid information on all variables for all cases), and these strategies help researchers to attain this goal.

- Raw data entered directly onto a computer file often need to be transformed for analysis. Examples of **data transformations** include reversing the coding of items, recoding the values of a variable (e.g., for dummy variables), and transforming data to meet statistical assumptions (e.g., through logarithmic transformations).

- Before the main analyses can proceed, researchers usually undertake additional steps to assess data quality and to maximize the value of the data. These steps include evaluating the reliability of measures, examining the distribution of values on key variables for any anomalies, and analyzing the magnitude and direction of any biases.

- Sometimes peripheral analyses involve tests to determine whether **pooling** of subjects is warranted, and tests for **cohort effects** or ordering effects.

- Once the data are fully prepared for substantive analysis, researchers should develop a formal analysis plan, to reduce the temptation to go on a "fishing expedition." One approach is to develop **table shells**, i.e., fully laid-out tables without numbers in them.

- The interpretation of research findings typically involves five subtasks: (1) analyzing the credibility of the results, (2) searching for underlying meaning, (3) considering the importance of the results, (4) analyzing the generalizability of the findings, and (5) assessing the implications of the study regarding future research, theory development, and nursing practice.

- Assessing the credibility and meaning of the results involves a consideration of the extent to which the study results are internally valid and reflect statistical conclusion and construct validity. Supplementary statistical analyses (e.g., testing competing hypotheses or doing **sensitivity analyses**) can sometimes facilitate interpretation.

STUDY ACTIVITIES

Chapter 24 of the accompanying *Resource Manual for Nursing Research: Generating and Assessing Evidence for Nursing Practice, 8th edition*, offers various exercises and study suggestions for reinforcing the concepts presented in this chapter. In addition, the following study questions can be addressed:

1. Read an article in a recent nursing research journal. Write out a brief interpretation of the results based on the report's "Results" section, and then compare your interpretation with that of the researchers.

2. Use the critiquing guidelines in Box 24.1 to critique the study used as the research example at the end of the chapter (Good et al., 2005), referring to the full study as necessary.

STUDIES CITED IN CHAPTER 24

Methodologic or theoretical references cited in this chapter can be found in a separate section at the end of the book.

Bennett, J., Perrin, N., Hanson, G., Bennett, D., Gaynor, W., Flaherty-Robb, M., et al. (2005). Health Aging Demonstration: Nurse coaching for behavior change in older adults. *Research in Nursing & Health, 28*(3), 187–197.

Cheng, K., & Chang, A. (2003). Palliation of oral mucosities in pediatric patients treated with cancer chemotherapy. *Cancer Nursing, 26*(6), 476–484.

Fallis, W., Hamelin, K., Symonds, J., & Wang, X. (2006). Maternal and newborn outcomes related to maternal warming during cesarean delivery. *Journal of Obstetric, Gynecologic, & Neonatal Nursing, 35*(3), 324–331.

Good, M., Anderson, G., Ahn, S., Cong, X., & Stanton-Hicks, M. (2005). Relaxation and music reduce pain following intestinal surgery. *Research in Nursing & Health, 28*, 240–251.

Griffin, R., Polit, D., & Byrnes, M. (in press). Stereotyping and nurses' recommendations for treating pain in hospitalized children. *Research in Nursing & Health, 30.*

Gulick, E. E. (2001). Emotional distress and activities of daily living functioning in persons with multiple sclerosis. *Nursing Research, 50*, 147–154.

Harrison, T., Stuifbergen, A., Adachi, E., & Becker, H. (2004). Marriage, impairment, and acceptance in persons with multiple sclerosis. *Western Journal of Nursing Research, 26*, 266–285.

Jones, R. (2004). Relationships of sexual imposition, dyadic trust, and sensation seeking with sexual risk behavior in young urban women. *Research in Nursing & Health, 27*(3), 185–197.

Keefe, M., Karlsen, K., Lobo, M., Kotzer, A., & Dudley, W. (2006). Reducing parenting stress in families with irritable infants. *Nursing Research, 55*(3), 198–205.

Medves, J. M., & O'Brien, B. (2004). The effect of bather and location of first bath on maintaining thermal stability in newborns. *Journal of Obstetric, Gynecologic, & Neonatal Nursing, 33*, 175–182.

Nachreiner, N., Gerberich, S., McGovern, P., Church, T., Hansen, H., Geisser, M., & Ryan, A. (2005). Impact of training on work-related assault. *Research in Nursing & Health, 28*(1), 67–78.

Polit, D. F., London, A. S., & Martinez, J. M. (2001). *The health of poor urban women*. New York: MDRC. (Available at *http://www.mdrc.org*)

Provencher, H. L., Perreault, M., St. Onge, M., & Rousseau, M. (2003). Predictors of psychological distress in family caregivers of persons with psychiatric disabilities. *Journal of Psychiatric and Mental Health Nursing, 10,* 592–607.

Quinn, J. (2005). Delay in seeking care for symptoms of acute myocardial infarction: Applying a theoretical model. *Research in Nursing & Health, 28*(4), 283–294.

Reishtein, J. (2005). Relationship between symptoms and functional performance in COPD. *Research in Nursing & Health, 28*(1), 39–47.

Santacroce, S., & Lee, Y. (2006). Uncertainty, posttraumatic stress, and health behavior in young adult childhood cancer survivors. *Nursing Research, 55*(4), 259–266.

Scheetz, L. (2005). Relationship of age, injury severity, injury type, comorbid conditions, level of care, and survival among older motor vehicle trauma patients. *Research in Nursing & Health, 28*(3), 198–209.

PART 6

BUILDING AN EVIDENCE BASE FOR NURSING PRACTICE

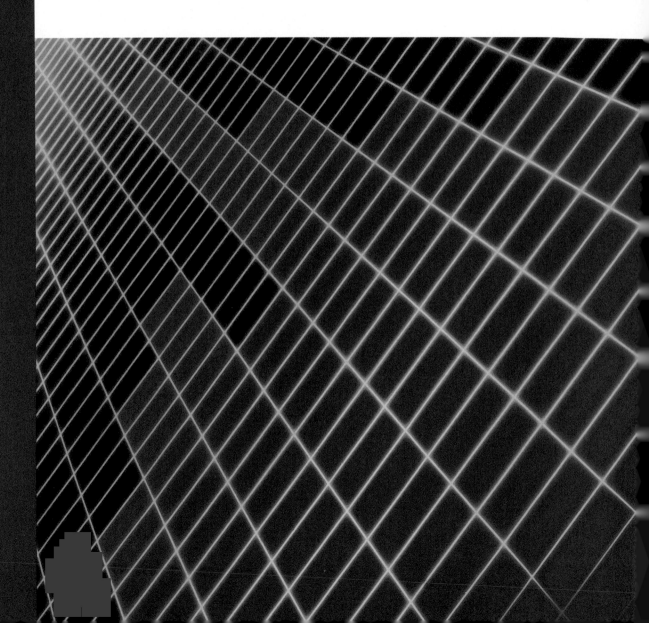

25 Integrating Research Evidence: Meta-Analysis and Metasynthesis

I n Chapter 5 we described major steps in conducting a literature review as an early step in designing and conducting a new study. This chapter also discusses reviews of existing evidence, but focuses on the conduct—and the evaluation—of integration projects that are in themselves considered research—**systematic reviews** and **meta-syntheses**.

RESEARCH INTEGRATION AND SYNTHESIS

Evidence-based practice (EBP) relies on meticulous integration of research evidence on a topic. If nurses are to glean best practices from research findings, they must take into account as much of the evidence as possible, organized and synthesized in a diligent manner. Indeed, many consider systematic reviews a cornerstone of EBP. This chapter provides some guidance in research integration. The type of integrative activities we discuss in this chapter are not just literature reviews, but rather systematic inquiries that follow many of the same rules as those described in this book for **primary studies**, that is, original empirical investigations.

Using systematic procedures to combine research evidence can take various forms, and sometimes different terms are used to distinguish

them. There are also different terms to distinguish the integration of quantitative and qualitative research findings. Whittemore (2005), for example, referred to an *integrative review* as a broad integration that can encompass theoretical or empirical literature—or both—and that uses a narrative approach to the integration of either qualitative or quantitative findings. She used the term *systematic review* to refer to rigorous and systematic syntheses of findings from quantitative studies on a common or strongly related research question.

Until fairly recently, the most common type of systematic review was narrative (qualitative) integration of quantitative findings, using nonstatistical methods to merge and synthesize research findings. More recently, meta-analytic techniques that use a common metric for combining study results statistically have been increasingly used to integrate quantitative evidence. Most of the reviews in the Cochrane Collaboration, for example, are meta-analyses. As we shall see, however, statistical integration is sometimes inappropriate, even when researchers start out with the intention of conducting a meta-analysis.

Qualitative researchers also are developing techniques to integrate findings across studies. Many terms exist for such endeavors (e.g., meta-study, meta-method, meta-summary, metaethnography, qualitative meta-analysis, formal grounded theory), but the one that appears to be emerging as the leading term among nurse researchers is *metasynthesis*.

In this chapter we focus primarily on meta-analysis as the form of synthesizing quantitative findings, and metasynthesis as the approach to integrating qualitative findings. The field of research integration is expanding at a rapid pace, in terms of both the number of integration studies being conducted and the techniques used to perform them. This chapter provides a brief introduction to this extremely important and complex topic—but our advice for those embarking on a review project is to keep abreast of recent developments in this emerging field and to pursue more extensive information in books devoted to the topic. Particularly good resources for further guidance on meta-analysis include the Cochrane Collaboration's (2005) *Handbook for Systematic Reviews of Interventions* and books by Cooper (1998) and Lipsey and Wilson (2001). For qualitative integration, we recommend Noblit and Hare (1988), Paterson and colleagues (2001), and various writings of Margarete Sandelowski and Julie Barroso (e.g., 2003a, 2003b, 2006).

UNDERTAKING A META-ANALYSIS

In most evidence hierarchies, meta-analyses of randomized clinical trials (RCTs) are at the pinnacle, and meta-analyses of all types of quantitative evidence rank high (see Fig. 2.1). The essence of a meta-analysis is that information from various studies is used to develop a common metric, often called the *effect size*. Effect sizes are averaged across studies, yielding not only information about the *existence* of a relationship between variables but also an estimate of its *magnitude*.

Advantages of Meta-Analyses

For systematic integration of quantitative evidence, meta-analysis offers a simple yet powerful advantage: *objectivity*. It is often difficult to draw objective conclusions about a body of evidence using narrative methods because reviewers almost inevitably use unidentified or subconscious criteria in pulling together disparate results. For example, narrative reviewers make subjective decisions about how much weight to give findings from different studies, and thus different reviewers could come to different conclusions about the state of the evidence. Meta-analysts also make decisions—sometimes based on personal preferences—but in a meta-analysis, these decisions are made explicit, and the impact of the decisions can be evaluated by readers of the synthesis report. Moreover, the integration itself is objective because it is statistical. Calculating the average efficacy of nurse-led interventions for smoking cessation across 20 studies is analogous to calculating the average efficacy of a single smoking cessation trial across 20 subjects. Readers of a meta-analysis can be confident that another analyst using the same data set would come to exactly the same conclusions.

Another advantage of meta-analysis concerns *power,* a statistical concept described in Chapter 22. Power, it may be recalled, refers to the probability of detecting a true relationship between the independent and dependent variables. By combining results across multiple studies, power is increased. Indeed, in a meta-analysis, it is possible to conclude with a given probability that a relationship is real (e.g., an intervention is effective), even when a series of small studies yielded ambiguous nonsignificant findings. In a narrative review, 10 nonsignificant findings would almost surely be interpreted as lack of evidence of a true relationship, which could be an erroneous conclusion.

Another benefit of meta-analysis concerns precision. Meta-analysts can draw conclusions about how big an effect an intervention has, with a specified probability that the results are accurate. Estimates of effect size across multiple studies yield smaller confidence intervals than individual studies, and thus precision is enhanced. Both power and precision are enticing qualities in EBP, as suggested by the EBP questions for appraising evidence described in Chapter 2 (see Box 2.1).

Despite these strengths, meta-analysis is not always appropriate. Indiscriminate use has led critics to warn against potential abuses, and so reviewers must carefully determine whether meta-analysis is justified.

Criteria for Using Meta-Analytic Techniques in a Systematic Review

At the outset of a synthesis project, reviewers can make preliminary decisions about whether it is prudent or desirable to use statistical integration. One basic criterion is that the research question being addressed or the hypothesis being tested across studies should be very similar, if not identical. This essentially means that the independent and the dependent variables, and the study populations, are sufficiently similar to merit integration. The variables may be operationalized differently, to be sure. A nurse-led intervention to promote exercise among diabetic patients could be a 4-week clinic-based program in one study and a 6-week home-based intervention in another, for example. Or the dependent variable (exercise) could be operationalized using different scales across studies. However, a study focusing on the effects of a 1-hour lecture to encourage exercise among overweight adolescents would be a poor candidate to include in this meta-analysis. This is frequently referred to as the "apples and oranges" or "fruit" problem. Meta-analyses should not be about *fruit*—that is, a broad and encompassing category—but rather about specific questions that have been addressed in multiple studies—that is, "apples," or, even better, "Granny Smith apples."

A second criterion concerns whether there is a sufficient base of knowledge for statistical integration. If there are only a few studies, or if all of the studies are weakly designed and harbor extensive bias, it usually would not make sense to compute an "average" effect. The amount and quality of the available evidence may not be known at the outset—but chances are a reviewer will have a preliminary sense of the evidence base.

One final issue concerns the consistency of the evidence. When the same hypothesis has been tested in multiple studies and the results are highly conflicting, meta-analysis is not appropriate. As an extreme example, if half the studies testing an intervention found benefits for those in the intervention group, but the other half found benefits for the controls, it would be misleading to compute an average effect. A more appropriate strategy would be to do an in-depth narrative analysis of why the results are conflicting. Sometimes reviewers learn early in the project that pooling of effects through meta-analysis is not warranted, but there are diagnostic techniques, described later, to test formally whether differences across studies are merely chance differences.

Example of inability to conduct a meta-analysis: Lee and Johnson (2005) did a systematic review of research on the effective management of central venous catheters and catheter sites in acute-care pediatric patients. Their intention "was to conduct a quantitative statistical pooling of results from similar studies. However, this was not possible due to the diversity of the reported interventions and outcome measures" (p. 7). A narrative systematic review was therefore conducted.

Steps in a Meta-Analysis

A systematic review, like a primary study, requires considerable upfront planning, including an evaluation of whether there are sufficient resources and personnel to complete the project. In this section we describe eight major steps in the conduct of a meta-analysis: formulating the research problem; designing the meta-analysis; searching for data; evaluating study quality; extracting and encoding the data; calculating effects; analyzing the data; and reporting results.

Formulating the Problem

Like any scientific endeavor, a systematic review begins with a problem statement and a research question or hypothesis. Data cannot be meaningfully collected and integrated until there is a clear sense of what question is being addressed and what types of information are needed to answer the question. Question templates such as those provided in Chapters 2 or 4 serve as a good starting place. ✪

As described in Chapter 4, the broadest question form for a research inquiry is: "In (population), what is the effect of (independent variable) on (dependent variable)?" This serves as an adequate starting place for many meta-analyses, although

variations as described in Chapter 4 may be preferred. As with a primary study, care should be
taken to develop a problem statement and questions
that are clearly worded and specific. Key constructs
should be conceptually defined, and the definitions
should indicate the boundaries of the inquiry. The
definitions will serve as an indispensable tool for
deciding whether a primary study qualifies for the
synthesis, and for extracting appropriate information from the studies.

**Example of a question from a systematic
review:** Hill-Westmoreland, Soeken, and Spellbring
(2002) conducted a meta-analysis that addressed
the following question: "What are the effects of fall
prevention programs on the proportion of falls in the
elderly? Falls were conceptually defined as coming
to rest on the ground, floor, or other lower level,
unintentionally" (p. 2). In this example, fall prevention
programs were the independent variable, falls were
the dependent variable, and elderly people
constituted the population.

As indicated previously, questions for a meta-
analysis are usually narrow, focusing, for example,
on a particular type of intervention and specific outcomes. Forbes (2003) described a systematic
review guided by the question, "What strategies,
within the scope of nursing, are effective in managing the behavioral symptoms associated with
Alzheimer's disease?" (p. 182). She noted that "in
retrospect, selecting specific interventions would
have made the review more manageable" (p. 182).
The broader the question, the more complex (and
costly) the meta-analysis becomes. And, the
broader the question, the less appropriate it is to
integrate studies through meta-analysis. In fact,
Forbes found it was not possible to use meta-analysis
in her systematic review.

Designing the Meta-Analysis Study

Meta-analysts, like other researchers, make many
decisions that affect the rigor and validity of the
study findings. Most decisions should be made in a
conscious, "planful" manner *before the study is
underway*, and should be fully documented so they
can be communicated to readers of the review. We
identify a few of the major design decisions in this

section, although some options of a technical
nature, although needing to be *addressed* during the
planning phase, can best be explained in our discussion of analytic procedures.

One up-front decision involves project organization. Systematic reviews are sometimes done by
individuals, but it is preferable to have at least two
reviewers. Multiple reviewers help not only in sharing the work load but also in minimizing subjectivity. Reviewers should have both substantive and
clinical knowledge of the problem, and sufficiently
strong methodologic skills to evaluate study quality
and guide the analysis. Even with a knowledgeable
team, clear guidelines and training in the use of the
guidelines are essential—just as they are in the collection of data for a primary study.

Sampling is another planning issue. In a systematic review, the sample consists of the primary studies that have addressed the research question.
Reviewers make many up-front decisions regarding
the sample, including a specification of the exclusion or inclusion criteria for the search. The sampling criteria typically cover substantive, methodologic, and practical elements. Substantively, the
criteria must stipulate specific variables. For example, if the review is integrating material about the
effectiveness of a nursing intervention, what outcomes (dependent variables) *must* the researchers
have studied? Another substantive issue concerns
the study population—for example, will certain age
groups of participants (e.g., children, the elderly)
be excluded? Methodologically, the criteria might
specify that (for example) only studies that used a
true experimental design will be included. From a
practical standpoint, the criteria might exclude, for
example, reports written in a language other than
English, or reports published before a certain date.
Of particular importance is the decision about
whether both published and unpublished reports
will be included in the review, a topic we discuss at
greater length in the next section.

Example of sampling criteria: Forbes (2003),
in the previously mentioned review of interventions
for Alzheimer's disease patients, stipulated
five criteria. The study must have (1) been

published or conducted between January 1985 and May 1997; (2) evaluated a nonpharmacologic intervention for individuals aged 65 years or older with Alzheimer's disease; (3) involved an intervention within the scope of nursing practice; (4) measured at least one outcome of a stipulated type (e.g., wandering, agitation); and (5) incorporated a control group or changes over time.

A related issue concerns the quality of the primary studies, a topic that has stirred some controversy. Researchers sometimes use quality as a sampling criterion, either directly or indirectly. Screening out studies of lower quality can occur indirectly if, for example, the meta-analyst decides to exclude studies that did not use a randomized design, or studies that were not published in a peer-reviewed journal. More directly, each potential primary study can be rated for quality, and excluded if the quality score falls below a certain threshold. Alternatives to handling study quality are discussed in a later section. Suffice it to say, however, that evaluations of study quality are inevitably part of the review process, and so before the project gets underway, the analysts need to decide how quality assessments will be made, and what will be done with the information from the assessments.

Another design issue concerns the **statistical heterogeneity** of results in primary studies. For each study, meta-analysts compute an index to summarize the strength and direction of relationship between an independent variable and a dependent variable. Just as there is inevitably variation *within* studies (not all people in a study have identical scores on the outcome measures), so too is there inevitably variation in effects *across* studies. If the results are highly variable (e.g., results are conflicting across studies), a meta-analysis may be inappropriate. But if the results are modestly variable, an important design decision concerns steps that will be take to explore the source of the variation. For example, the effects of an intervention might be systematically different for men and women (*clinical heterogeneity*). Or, the effects may be different if the period of follow-up is 6 months rather than 3 months (*methodologic heterogeneity*). If such subgroup effects are hypothesized, it is important to plan for subgroup analyses during the planning phase of the project.

Searching the Literature for Data

In Chapter 5, we discussed the importance of *owning* the research literature before preparing a written review. Ownership—becoming a leading authority on the research question under review—is even more important in a systematic review because of the pivotal role that such reviews play in EBP. Traditional strategies of searching for relevant studies, using electronic databases and ancestry/descendancy approaches that were described in Chapter 5, are rarely adequate without further retrieval efforts.

One of the design decisions that must be made before a search begins is whether the review will cover both published and unpublished study results. There is some disagreement about whether reviewers should limit their sample to published studies, or should cast as wide a net as possible and include **grey literature**—that is, studies with a more limited distribution, such as dissertations, unpublished reports, and so on. Some people restrict their sample to published reports in peer-reviewed journals, arguing that the peer-review system is an important, tried-and-true screen for findings worthy of consideration as evidence.

The limitations of excluding nonpublished findings, however, have increasingly been noted in the literature on systematic reviews (e.g., Conn et al., 2003; Ciliska & Guyatt, 2005). The primary issue concerns **publication bias**—the tendency for published studies to systematically over-represent statistically significant findings (this bias is sometimes referred to as the *bias against the null hypothesis*). Explorations of this bias have revealed that the bias is widespread: authors tend to refrain from submitting reports with negative findings, reviewers and editors tend to reject such reports when they are submitted, and users of evidence tend to ignore the findings when they are published. Studies have found that the exclusion of grey literature in a systematic review can lead to bias, particularly the overestimation of effects (Conn et al., 2003).

We advocate the retrieval of as many relevant studies as possible because methodologic weaknesses in unpublished reports can be dealt with later. Aggressive search strategies are essential and may include, in addition to methods noted in Chapter 5, the following:

- **Hand-searching** journals known to publish relevant content—that is, doing a manual search of the tables of contents or abstracts of key journals; hand-searching of the literature more than a decade old is especially valuable because computerized indexing systems were less sophisticated before the mid-1990s
- Identifying and contacting key researchers in the field to see if they have done studies that have not (yet) been published, or if they know of such studies—and asking them about other members of the *"invisible college"* and whether they participate in relevant listservs or newsgroups
- Doing an "author search" of key researchers in the field in bibliographic databases and on the Internet
- Reviewing abstracts from conference proceedings, and networking with researchers at conferences; conference abstracts are often available on the websites of the professional organizations sponsoring the conference
- Searching for unpublished reports, such as dissertations and theses, government reports (e.g. in the United States, *http://www.access.gpo.gov*), and registries of studies in progress (e.g., in the United States, through Computer Retrieval of Information on Scientific Projects or CRISP, *http://crisp.cit.nih.gov*)
- Searching Sigma Theta Tau International's registry of nursing research for unpublished studies
- Contacting foundations, government agencies, or corporate sponsors of the type of research under study to get leads on studies in progress or recently completed

---

→ TIP: It is especially important to carefully document and describe search strategy decisions and actions in a systematic review so that readers can understand the scope of the review. The Toolkit for Chapter 5 of the accompanying *Resource Manual* offers a template for documentation during a literature search.

Once relevant studies are identified, they must be retrieved, which can be a labor-intensive and expensive process. Retrieved studies need to be carefully screened to determine whether they do, in fact, meet the inclusion criteria. All decisions relating to exclusions (normally made by at least two reviewers to ensure objectivity) should be well documented and justified.

Example of a search strategy from a systematic review: Davenport (2004) did a systematic review to examine whether a standard (25-gauge, 16-mm) needle is more effective than a wider or longer needle in reducing local reactions in children receiving primary immunizations. Davenport's comprehensive search strategy included a search of electronic databases, hand-searching of journals, reference and citation searching, contacting researchers, and looking for unpublished reports. Screening to determine whether an identified study met the sampling criteria was independently completed by two people.

→ TIP: Reports of studies that meet the sampling criteria do not always provide sufficient information for computing effect sizes. Be prepared to devote time and resources to communicating with researchers to obtain supplementary information.

Evaluating Study Quality

In systematic reviews, the evidence from primary studies should be evaluated to determine how much confidence to place in the findings, using criteria similar to those we have presented throughout this book. Strong studies should be given more weight than weaker ones in coming to conclusions about a body of evidence.

In meta-analyses, evaluations of study quality often involve quantitative ratings of each study in terms of the strength of evidence it yields. The Agency for Healthcare Research and Quality, or AHRQ (2002), published a guide that describes and evaluates various systems and instruments to rate the strength of evidence in quantitative studies. Based on a comprehensive review of the literature, the authors identified 121 systems, including tools for evaluating randomized clinical trials, nonexperimental research, diagnostic test studies, and systematic reviews. The report offers some guidance to reviewers about which systems meet certain standards: 19 systems out of the 121 reviewed fully address essential quality domains.

Example of a quality assessment tool: One of the 19 systems that the AHRQ report considered to be of especially high quality was developed by a British team working at the Royal College of Nursing Institute at the University of Oxford (Sindhu, Carpenter, & Seers, 1997). The instrument, developed by an expert panel of researchers for assessing reports of randomized clinical trials, consists of 53 items on 15 dimensions (e.g., appropriateness of controls, measurement of outcomes, blinding of treatments). Those using the instrument assign scores for each dimension and then total the points, which can range from 0 to 100.

Despite the availability of many quality assessment instruments, there is little consensus about which ones are especially useful for nurse researchers. As Conn and Rantz (2003) have noted, one major obstacle is that there is no "gold standard" for determining the scientific rigor and validity of primary studies, and so it is difficult to validate the assessment instruments. Quality criteria vary widely from instrument to instrument, and the result is that study quality can be rated quite differently with two different assessment tools.

One other problem should be noted, and that is that assessment instruments that yield an overall quality rating typically involve at least some items that raters are unable to answer. For example, if an item asks whether data collectors were blinded to subjects' treatment condition, and a report does not specifically mention blinding, it *probably*, but not necessarily, means that blinding was not used. Space constraints in journals might make it impossible to include the level of methodologic detail needed to answer all questions on an assessment instrument with certainty. The question of how to compute an overall quality score when there is missing information is a difficult one, but two strategies are imputing values (see Chapter 24) and making consistently conservative assumptions (i.e.,

that a methodologic weakness was present) about the missing information.

Because of these complexities, some meta-analysts use an alternative—or supplementary—strategy of identifying those individual methodologic features that they judge to be of critical importance for the type of question begin addressed in the review—a *component approach,* as opposed to a *scale approach.* Each feature is given a separate rating or code for each study, and the relationship between these features and effect size estimates can be explored empirically. So, for example, a researcher might code for such design elements as whether randomization was used, whether subjects were blinded, the extent of attrition from the study, and so on. Decisions about such features clearly need to be made at the outset of the study so that the relevant information can be systematically extracted from the reports.

Quality assessments of primary studies, whether they are assessments of individual study features or overall ratings, should be done by at least two qualified individuals. If there are disagreements between the raters, there should be a discussion until a consensus has been reached or, if necessary, a third rater should be asked to help resolve the difference. Indexes of interrater reliability are often calculated to demonstrate to readers that rater agreement on study quality was adequate.

Extracting and Encoding Data for Analysis

The next step in a systematic review is to extract relevant information about study characteristics, methods, and findings, and to record the information in a form amenable to computer analysis. A data extraction protocol (either paper-and-pencil or computerized) must be developed, along with a coding manual to guide those who will be extracting and encoding information. The goal of this task is to produce a data set, and procedures similar to those used in creating a data set with raw data from individual subjects also apply.

Basic data source information should be recorded for all studies. This includes such features as year of publication, country where data were collected, type of report (journal article, dissertation, etc.), and language in which the report was published. Supplementary information that may also be of interest includes whether the report was peer-reviewed, the impact factor of the journal (see Chapter 26), whether the study was funded (and by whom), and the year in which data were collected.

In terms of methodologic information that should be encoded, the most critical element across all studies is sample size. Other important attributes that should be recorded vary by study question. Examples of features likely to be important—in terms of both exploring heterogeneity of effects and simply describing the nature of the body of evidence—include sampling method (e.g., by convenience); whether subjects were randomly assigned to treatments; whether blinding of subjects, agents, or data collectors was used; and the nature of any comparison group (e.g., "no treatment" versus alternative treatment controls). Measurement issues may also be important. For example, codes to designate the specific scales used to operationalize outcome variables could be developed, and scale reliability could be recorded. Information about the timing of the measurements (i.e., the period of follow-up) is also likely to be critical. In intervention studies, features of the intervention should be recorded, such as setting, length of intervention, and primary modality of the intervention. Information about attrition should be recorded, typically as a percentage for each group being compared, as well as how attrition was handled in the analysis (e.g., an intention-to-treat analysis or available-case analysis). Finally, if an assessment scale was used to rate methodologic quality, the overall score should be recorded.

Characteristics of the study participants must be encoded as well. A useful strategy is to record characteristics as percentages. For example, it is almost always possible to determine the percentage of the sample that was female. Other categorical characteristics that could be represented as percentages include race/ethnicity, educational level, and illness/treatment information (e.g., percentages of participants in different stages of cancer). Age should be recorded as mean age of sample members.

The final type of information that must be recorded concerns the findings. Either effect sizes (discussed in the next section) need to be calculated and entered, or the data extraction form needs to record sufficient statistical information that the computer program can compute the indexes. Effect size information is often recorded for multiple outcomes, and may also be recorded for different subgroups of study participants (e.g., effects for males versus females on the various outcomes).

Extraction and coding of information should be completed by two or more people, at least for a portion of the studies in the sample. This allows for an assessment of interrater agreement, which should be sufficiently high to persuade readers of the review that the recorded information is accurate.

Example of intercoder agreement: In Beck's (2001) meta-analysis of the predictors of postpartum depression, one fourth of the included studies (i.e., 20 of 84) were independently coded by Beck and a research assistant. Initial interrater agreement ranging from 85% to 100% was attained, and disagreements were resolved.

TIP: A very basic data extraction form is provided in the Toolkit of the accompanying *Resource Manual* as a Word document that can be easily adapted for use in simple meta-analyses. A paper-and-pencil form such as this one should usually be developed and pretested, but moving to a computerized platform is often attractive because data can be entered using pull-down menus and error-detection is usually possible by establishing out-of-range values (e.g., it would not be possible to enter a publication date of 1007 in lieu of 2007). Additional guidance on developing a coding scheme is offered by Brown, Upchard, and Acton (2003).

Calculating Effects

Meta-analyses depend on the calculation of an index that encapsulates the relationship between the independent and dependent variable in each study. Because effects are captured differently depending on the level of measurement of variables, there is no single formula for calculating an effect size. In nursing, the three most common scenarios for meta-analysis involve comparisons of two groups on a continuous outcome (e.g., the body mass index, or BMI), comparisons of two groups on a dichotomous outcome (e.g., continued smoking versus stopped smoking), or correlations between two continuous variables (e.g., the correlation between BMI and scores on a depression scale). Other scenarios are described by the Cochrane Collaboration (2005). For simplicity, most of our discussion will focus on the situation involving a comparison of two groups on a continuous variable.

The first scenario, comparison of group means, is especially common in nursing studies. When the outcomes across study are on identical scales (e.g., all outcomes are measures of weight in pounds), the effect is captured by simply subtracting the mean for one group from the mean for the other. For example, if the mean weight in an intervention group were 182.0 pounds and that for a control group were 194.0 pounds, the effect would be –8.0. More typically, however, outcomes are measured on different scales. For example, postpartum depression might be measured by Beck's Postpartum Depression Screening Scale in one study and by the CES-D in another. Mean differences across studies cannot in such situations be combined and averaged—we need an index that is neutral to the original metric employed in the primary study. Cohen's d, described in Chapter 22, is the effect size index most often used. It may be recalled that the formula for d is the group difference in means, divided by the pooled standard deviation, or:

$$d = \frac{\overline{X}_1 - \overline{X}_2}{SD_p}$$

This effect size index transforms all effects to standard deviation units. That is, if d were computed to be .50, the group mean for one group would be one half a standard deviation higher than the mean for the other group—regardless of the original measurement scale.

➲ **TIP:** The term *effect size* is widely used in the nursing literature, but the preferred term for Cochrane reviews is **standardized mean difference**, or SMD. Lipsey and Wilson (2001) refer to d, as described here, as ES_{SM}, that is, the effect size for standardized means. Cooper and Hedges (1994) refer to d as Hedges' g.

If meta-analysis software is used in the meta-analysis—as it usually would be—there is usually no need to calculate effect sizes manually. The relevant means and SDs would be entered. But what if this information is absent from the report, as is all too often the case? Fortunately, there are alternative formulas for calculating d from information in the primary study reports. For example, it is possible to derive the value of d when the research report gives such information as the value of t or F, an exact probability value, or a 95% confidence interval around the mean group difference. ⊗ (The Toolkit in the *Resource Manual* includes alternative formulas for computing d.) If none of this information is available in a research report, but the text suggests that relevant calculations were performed, it would be necessary to contact the researchers and request additional information.

When the outcomes in the primary studies are expressed as dichotomies, meta-analysts have a choice of effect index, but the most usual are ones we discussed in earlier chapters—the relative risk (RR) index, the odds ratio (OR), and absolute risk reduction (ARR). Details for how to compute these indexes were provided in Table 21.8. The selection of a summary effect index depends on several criteria, such as mathematical properties, ease of interpretation, and consistency. As noted in the Cochrane Collaboration's (2005) *Handbook,* no single index is uniformly best. The odds ratio is, unfortunately, difficult for many users of systematic reviews to interpret. Nevertheless, it appears to be the most frequently used effect index for dichotomous outcomes in the nursing literature.

Sometimes, especially for nonexperimental studies, the most common statistic used to express the relationship between independent and dependent variables in Pearson's r. If the primary studies in a meta-analysis provide statistical information in the form of a correlation coefficient, the r itself serves as the indicator of the magnitude and direction of effect.

Meta-analysts sometimes face a situation in which findings are not all reported using the same level of measurement. For example, if the variable *weight* (a continuous variable) was our key outcome variable, some studies might present findings for weight as a dichotomous outcome (e.g., *obese* versus *not obese*). One approach is to do separate meta-analyses for differently expressed effects. Another is to re-express some of the effect indicators so that all effects can be pooled. For example, an odds ratio can be converted to *d*, as can a value of *r*—and *vice versa*. A great many formulas for converting effect size information are presented in Appendix B of Lipsey and Wilson (2001).

> **➲ TIP:** Our discussion of calculating effect sizes glosses over a number of complexities. Alternative methods may be needed when, for some studies, the unit of analysis is not individual people, crossover designs were used, the data were severely skewed, an intention-to-treat analysis was used, and so on. Those embarking on a meta-analysis project should seek additional guidance from books on meta-analysis or from statisticians.

Analyzing the Data

Meta-analysis is often described as a two-step analytic process. In the first step, a summary statistic that captures an effect is computed for each study, as just described. In the second step, a pooled effect estimate is computed as a **weighted average** of the effects estimated for individual primary studies. A weighted average is defined as follows, with ES representing effect size estimates from each study:

$$\text{weighted average} = \frac{\text{sum of (ES} \times \text{weight for that ES)}}{\text{sum of the weights}}$$

The bigger the weight given to any study, the more that study will contribute to the weighted average. Thus, weights should reflect the amount of information that each study provides. One widely used approach in meta-analysis is called the **inverse variance method**, which uses the inverse of the variance of the effect estimate (i.e., 1 divided by the square of its standard error) as the weight. Thus, larger studies, which have smaller standard errors, are given greater weight than smaller ones. The basic data needed for this type of analysis is the estimate of the effect size and its standard error, for each study.

In formulating an analytic strategy, meta-analysts must grapple with many decisions. In this brief overview, we present some basic information about the following analytic issues: identifying heterogeneity; deciding whether to use a fixed effects or random effects meta-analysis; incorporating clinical and methodologic diversity into the analysis; handling study quality; and addressing possible publication biases.

> **➲ TIP:** A variety of software is available to perform meta-analyses. The Cochrane Collaboration has developed its own software—the Review Manager (RevMan) software—which is currently distributed as copyrighted freeware. Macros are also available for doing meta-analyses within the major software packages such as SPSS and SAS. Links to websites for other meta-analysis software are included on the accompanying CD-ROM.

Identifying Heterogeneity. As discussed earlier, heterogeneity across studies may rule out the possibility that a meta-analysis can be done, and remains an issue to be addressed within the analysis even when statistical pooling is justifiable. Unless it is obvious that effects are consistent in magnitude and direction based on a subjective perusal, heterogeneity should be formally tested.

Visual inspection of heterogeneity can most readily be accomplished by constructing a **forest plot**, which can typically be generated using meta-analytic software. A forest plot graphs the estimated effect size for each study, together with the 95% CI around each estimate. Figure 25.1 illustrates two forest plots for situations in which there is low heterogeneity (*A*) and high heterogeneity (*B*) for five studies in which the odds ratio was used as the effect size index. In the left panel (*A*), all effect size estimates favor the intervention group and are statistically significant for three of them (studies 2, 4, and 5), according to the 95% CI information. In the right panel, by contrast, the results are "all over the map," with two studies favoring controls at significant levels (studies 1 and 5) and two favoring the treatment group (studies 2 and 4). A meta-analysis is not appropriate for the five studies in *B*.

Heterogeneity can be evaluated using statistical procedures that test the null hypothesis that

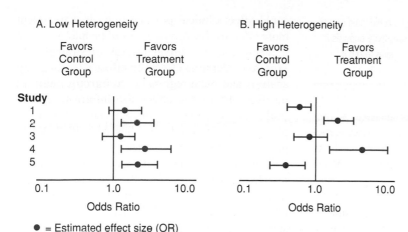

FIGURE 25.1 Two forest plots for five studies with low (*A*) and high (*B*) heterogeneity of effect size estimates.

heterogeneity across studies represents random fluctuations. The test—often a chi-square test—yields a *p* value that indicates the probability of obtaining effect size differences as large as those observed if the null hypothesis were true. A *p* value of .05 is usually used to determine significance, but because the test is underpowered when the meta-analysis involves a small number of studies, a *p* of .10 is sometimes considered an acceptable cut-off point.

Deciding on a Fixed Effect Versus Random Effects Analysis. There are two basic statistical models that can be applied in a meta-analysis, and the choice relates to heterogeneity. In a fixed effects model, the underlying assumption is that a single true effect size underlies all study results, and that observed estimates vary only as a function of chance. The error term in a fixed effects model represents only within-study variation, and between-study variation is ignored. Most fixed effects models use the inverse variance method of weighting studies.

A **random effects model**, by contrast, assumes that each study estimates *different*, yet related, true effects, and that the distribution of the various effects is normally distributed around a mean effect size value. A random effects model takes both within- and between-study variation into account.

When there is little heterogeneity, both models yield essentially identical results. When heterogeneity is extensive, however, the analyses will yield different estimates of the average effect size, and the confidence intervals around the estimates are of different widths. When there is heterogeneity across studies, the random effects model yields wider confidence intervals than the fixed effects model and is thus usually more conservative. But it is precisely when there *is* heterogeneity that the random effects model should be used.

Some argue that a random effects model is needed whenever the test for heterogeneity is statistically significant, whereas others argue that a random effects model is almost always more tenable. One approach that has been recommended is to perform a **sensitivity analysis**—which, in general, refers to an effort to test how sensitive the results of an analysis are to changes in the way the analysis was done. In this case, it would involve using both statistical models to determine how the results are affected. If the results differ substantially, it is usually more prudent to use estimates from the random effects model, and to urge readers of the review to be cautious in applying the results.

➲ TIP: In a set of studies with heterogeneous effects, a random effects model will award relatively more weight to small studies than such studies would receive in a fixed effects model. If effects from small studies are systematically different from those in larger ones, a random effects meta-analysis could yield biased results. One strategy is to perform another sensitivity analysis, running the analysis with and without small studies to see if results vary.

Examining Factors Affecting Heterogeneity. A random effects meta-analysis incorporates heterogeneity into the analysis, but is intended primarily to address variation that cannot be explained. Many meta-analysts seek to understand the determinants of effect size heterogeneity through formal analyses. Such analyses should always be considered exploratory because they are inherently nonexperimental (observational). Consequently, causal interpretations are necessarily speculative. To be considered scientifically appropriate, explorations of heterogeneity should be specified even before the review gets underway, to minimize the risk for spurious associations.

Heterogeneity across studies could reflect systematic differences with regard to clinical characteristics or methodologic characteristics, and both can be explored. Clinical heterogeneity can result from differences in study populations or in the way that the independent variable was operationalized. For example, in intervention studies, variation in effects could reflect who the agents were (e.g., nurses versus others), where the intervention occurred, how long the intervention lasted, whether the program components reflected one theoretical model versus another, and whether or not the intervention was individualized.

Methodologic heterogeneity could involve any number of study characteristics. Some could represent research design decisions, such as when the measurements were made (e.g., 3 months versus 6 months after an intervention) or what research design was used (true experimental or quasi-experimental). Other methodologic variables could be after-the-fact "outcomes," such as a high versus low attrition rates.

Explorations of methodologic diversity essentially examine the possibility that studies in the review suffer from different types and degrees of bias. Explorations of clinical diversity are more substantively relevant, in that they examine the possibility that effects differ because of factors that could affect clinical practice (e.g., is a treatment more effective for certain types of people?).

There are two broad classes of strategies to explore moderating effects on effect size: subgroup analysis and meta-regression. **Subgroup analyses** involve splitting the effect size information from studies into distinct categorical groups—for example, gender. Effects for studies with all-male (or predominantly male) samples could be compared with those for studies with all or predominantly female samples, using some threshold for "predominance" (e.g., 75% or more of study participants). Of course, if it is possible to derive separate effect size estimates for males and females directly from study data, it is advantageous to do so, but subgroup effects are seldom reported. The most straightforward procedure for comparing effects for different subgroups is to determine whether there is any overlap in the confidence intervals around the effect size estimates for the groups.

Example of a subgroup analysis: Smith and colleagues (2001) did a Cochrane review on the effectiveness of home care by outreach nurses for patients with chronic obstructive pulmonary disease. The meta-analysis indicated that such outreach programs were not effective in reducing mortality. However, a subgroup analysis indicated that the interventions *were* effective for patients with less severe disease.

When variables thought to influence study heterogeneity are continuous (e.g., "dose" of the intervention), or when there is a mix of continuous and categorical factors, then meta-regression might be appropriate. **Meta-regression** is similar in essence to multiple regression and involves predicting the effect size based on possible explanatory factors. As in ordinary regression, the statistical significance of regression coefficients indicates a nonrandom linear relationship between effect sizes and the associated explanatory variable.

TIP: Not all software can do meta-regression. The Cochrane Collaboration (2005) *Handbook* advises that meta-regression is best performed in the Stata statistical package.

Handling Study Quality. There are four basic strategies for dealing with the issue of study quality in a meta-analysis. One, as previously noted, is to establish a quality threshold for study inclusion. Exclusions could reflect requirements for certain methodologic features (e.g., only randomized studies) or for a sufficiently high score on a quality assessment scale. We prefer other alternatives because we think it is advantageous to summarize the full range of evidence in an area, but quality exclusions might in some cases be justified.

Example of excluding low-quality studies:
Peacock and Forbes (2003) did a systematic review of interventions for caregivers of persons with dementia. A total of 36 relevant studies were rated using various methodologic criteria, and then the scores were used to categorize the studies as strong, moderate, weak, or poor. Only the 11 studies in the strong category were included in the review.

A second strategy is to undertake sensitivity analyses to determine whether the exclusion of lower-quality studies changes the results of analyses based only on the most rigorous studies. Conn and colleagues (2003), for example, have described as one option beginning the meta-analysis with high-quality studies and then sequentially adding studies of progressively lower quality to evaluate how robust the effect size estimates are to variation in quality.

Another approach is to consider quality as the basis for exploring heterogeneity of effects, the issue discussed in the previous section. For example, do randomized designs yield different average effect size estimates than quasi-experimental designs? Do effects vary as a function of the study's score on a quality assessment scale? Both individual study components and overall study quality can be used in subgroup analyses and meta-regressions.

A fourth strategy is to weight studies according to quality criteria. Most meta-analyses routinely give more weight to larger studies, but effect sizes can also be weighted by quality scores, thereby placing more weight on the estimates from rigorous studies. One persistent problem, however, is the previously mentioned issue of the validity of quality

assessment scales and the unreliability of ratings. A mix of strategies, together with appropriate sensitivity analyses, is probably the most prudent approach to dealing with variation in study quality.

Addressing Publication Bias. Even a strong commitment to a comprehensive search for reports on a given research question is unlikely to result in the identification of all studies. Some researchers, therefore, use strategies to assess publication bias, and to make adjustments for them.

The most usual way to examine the possibility of publication bias among studies in the meta-analysis is to construct a **funnel plot**. In a funnel plot, effects from individual studies are plotted on the horizontal axis, and precision (e.g., the inverse of the standard error) is plotted on the vertical axis. Figure 25.2 illustrates two hypothetical funnel plots for a meta-analysis of a nursing intervention in which the pooled effect size estimate (d) for 20 studies (10 published and 10 unpublished) is 0.2. In the funnel plot on the left (A), the effects are fairly symmetric around the pooled effect size for both published and unpublished studies. In the asymmetric plot on the right (B), however, unpublished studies appear to have consistently lower effect size estimates, suggesting the possibility that the pooled effect size has been overestimated. More detailed guidance on detecting publication bias has been provided by Soeken and Sripusanapan (2003).

➲ TIP: Funnel plots can be created within many of the meta-analytic software packages. Often, sample size rather than type of publication is used to dichotomize studies in the plot — that is, small versus large study, with some cut-off point used to distinguish the two. It might be noted that biases and issues other than publication bias could be the cause of asymmetry in funnel plots, and this can often be explored in analyses of heterogeneity.

Strategies for *addressing* publication bias have been proposed in the meta-analytic literature. One is to compute a **fail-safe number** that estimates the number of studies reporting nonsignificant results that would be needed to reverse the conclusion of a significant effect in a meta-analysis. The fail-safe

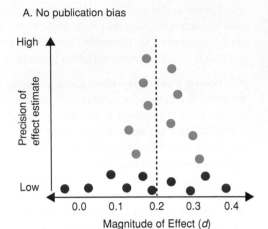
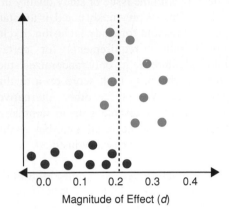

A. No publication bias

B. Possible publication bias

Precision of effect estimate

High

Low

0.0   0.1   0.2   0.3   0.4
Magnitude of Effect (d)

0.0   0.1   0.2   0.3   0.4
Magnitude of Effect (d)

- - - - Pooled estimate of effect

● = Effect for study published in a peer-review journal

● = Effect for study not published in a peer-review journal

FIGURE 25.2 Two funnel plots for studies suggesting no publication bias (*A*) or possible publication bias (*B*).

number is compared to a tolerance level ($5k + 10$), where k is the number of studies included in the analysis (Rosenthal, 1991). The Cochrane Collaboration *Handbook* advises that the best strategy involves comparison of published studies with prospectively registered studies whose results are not yet available (Langhorne, 1998).

> **Example of calculating a fail-safe number:**
> Fetzer (2002) conducted a meta-analysis of the effect of a eutectic mixture of local anesthetics (EMLA) on reducing pain during venipuncture. All nine studies in the review reported a significant positive effect. The fail-safe number was calculated to be 374, which far exceeded the reasonable tolerance level of 55.

Writing a Meta-Analytic Report

The final step in a systematic review project is to prepare a report to disseminate the findings. Typically such reports follow much the same format as for a research report for a primary study, with an Introduction, Method section, Results section, and Discussion.

Particular care should be taken in preparing the Method section. Readers of the review need to be able to assess the validity of the study, and so methodologic and statistical strategies, and their rationales, should be described. If the reviewers decided that a meta-analysis was not justified, the rationale for this decision must be made clear. The Cochrane Collaboration *Handbook* (2005) offers excellent suggestions for preparing reports for a systematic review, and our critiquing guidelines later in this chapter suggest the types of information to include.

A thorough Discussion section is also crucial in systematic reviews. The discussion should include an overall summary of the findings, the reviewers' assessment about the strength and limitations of the body of evidence, what further research should be undertaken to improve the evidence base, and what the implications of the review are for clinicians and patients. The review should also discuss the consistency of findings across studies and provide an interpretation of why there might be inconsistency. Did the samples, research designs, or data collection strategies in the studies differ in important ways? Or do differences reflect substantive differences, such as variation in the interventions or outcomes themselves?

➲ TIP: There are formal systems and scales for evaluating not only individual studies, but also a body of evidence. The report by AHRQ (2002) identified seven such systems as being especially useful for EBP, and noted that three domains are important in such systems: (1) *quality*—the aggregate of quality ratings for individual studies; (2) *quantity*—the magnitude of effect, number of studies, and sample size; and (3) *consistency*—the extent to which similar findings are reported using similar and different study designs. Meta-analysts do not typically apply such formal systems, but the discussion section should include comments about the three domains of quality, quantity, and consistency.

Tables and figures typically play a key role in reports of systematic reviews. Forest plots are often presented, showing effect size and 95% CI information for each study, as well as for the overall pooled result. Typically there is also a table showing the characteristics of studies included in the review. A template for such a table is included in the Toolkit of the accompanying *Resource Manual.* ✪

Finally, full citations for the entire sample of studies should be included in the bibliography of the review. Often these are identified separately from other citations—for example, by noting them with asterisks.

UNDERTAKING A METASYNTHESIS

Integration of qualitative findings is a burgeoning field—one that is rapidly evolving and for which there are no standard procedures. Indeed, five of the leading thinkers on qualitative integration noted the "terminological landmines" (p. 1343) that complicate the field, "the creeping use of the term *metasynthesis* to represent something more akin to 'metasoup'" (p. 1347), and the challenges of working in "an era of metamadness" (p. 1357) (Thorne et al., 2004).

Metasynthesis: Definition and Types

Terminology relating to qualitative integration is diverse and complex (see Finfgeld, 2003 for one

attempt at clarification). Thorne and colleagues (2004) acknowledged the diversity and used the term metasynthesis as an umbrella term, with metasynthesis broadly representing "a family of methodological approaches to developing new knowledge based on rigorous analysis of existing qualitative research findings" (p. 1343).

Many writers on this topic are fairly clear about what a metasynthesis is *not*. Metasynthesis is not a literature review—that is, not the collating or aggregation of research findings—nor is it a concept analysis. Schreiber, Crooks, and Stern (1997) offered a definition that has often been used for what metasynthesis *is*, ". . . the bringing together and breaking down of findings, examining them, discovering the essential features and, in some way, combining phenomena into a transformed whole" (p. 314). Consistent with this definition, Sandelowski (in Thorne et al., 2004) suggested that "Metasyntheses are integrations that are more than the sum of parts, in that they offer novel interpretations of findings" (p. 1358).

Schreiber and colleagues (1997), as well as Finfgeld (2003), described a typology of metasyntheses that puts the role of theory at center stage. This categorization includes three types linked to the overall purpose—theory building, theory explication, and description—although some overlapping occurs that may make it difficult to classify individual studies in one of the three categories. *Theory-building metasyntheses* are inquiries that extend the level of theory beyond what could be achieved in individual investigations. Grounded formal theory falls into this category, as do the **meta-study** methods proposed by Paterson and colleagues (2001). In *theory explication metasyntheses*, researchers "flesh out" and reconceptualize abstract concepts. Finally, *descriptive metasynthesis* involves a comprehensive analysis of a phenomenon based on a synthesis of qualitative findings; findings are not typically deconstructed and then reconstructed as they are in theory-related inquiries.

Metasynthesis has had its share of controversies, one of which concerns whether to integrate studies based on different research traditions and methods. Some researchers have argued against combining studies from different epistemologic perspectives, and have recommended separate analyses using groupings from different traditions. Others, however, advocate combining findings across traditions and methodologies. Which path to follow is likely to depend on several factors, including the focus of the inquiry, its intent *vis-à-vis* theory development, and the nature of the available evidence at the time the metasynthesis is undertaken.

Steps in a Metasynthesis

Many of the steps in a meta-synthesis are similar to ones we described in connection with a meta-analysis, and so many details will not be repeated here. However, we point out some distinctive issues relating to qualitative integration that are relevant in the various steps.

Formulating the Problem

In metasynthesis, researchers begin with a research question or a focus of investigation, and a key issue concerns the scope of the inquiry. Finfgeld (2003) recommended a strategy that balances breadth and utility. She advised that the scope be broad enough to fully capture the phenomenon of interest, but focused enough to yield findings that are meaningful to clinicians, other researchers, and public policy makers.

Example of a research question in a metaethnography: Varcoe, Rodney, and McCormick (2003) did a metaethnographic study that addressed the following question: How does organizational context shape relationships among patients, family members, and health care providers?

Designing a Metasynthesis Study

Like a quantitative systematic review, a metasynthesis requires considerable advance planning. Having a team of at least two researchers to design and implement the study is often advantageous, and this may be even more true for a metasynthesis than for a quantitative systematic review because of the highly subjective nature of interpretive efforts. Just as in a primary study, the design of a qualitative metasynthesis should involve efforts to enhance

integrity and rigor, and investigator triangulation is one such strategy.

⮕ **TIP:** Meta-analyses often are undertaken by researchers who did not do one of the primary studies in the review. Metasyntheses, by contrast, are often completed by researchers whose area of interest has led them to do both original studies and metasyntheses on the same topic. Prior work in an area offers obvious advantages in terms of researchers' ability to grasp subtle nuances and to think abstractly about a topic, but a disadvantage may be a certain degree of partiality about one's own work.

Like meta-analysts, metasynthesists must also make up-front decisions about sampling, and they face the same issue of deciding whether to include only findings from peer-reviewed journals in the analysis. One advantage of including alternative sources, in addition to wanting a more comprehensive analysis, is that journal articles tend to be highly constrained in what can be reported because of space limitations. Finfgeld (2003) noted that in her metasynthesis on *courage,* she used dissertations even when a peer-reviewed journal article was available from the same study because the dissertation offered much richer information. Another sampling decision, as previously noted, involves whether to search for qualitative studies about a phenomenon across traditions.

Example of up-front sampling decisions: Nelson (2002) conducted a metasynthesis of qualitative studies related to mothering other-than-normal children. She explained that "I made a deliberate decision to include studies that used various qualitative methodologies and represented a wide variety of children because I was unable to locate a sufficient number of studies using the same qualitative methodology and focusing on one group of children. . . . I believed that the potential significance of synthesizing qualitative knowledge in the broad area of mothering other-than-normal children outweighed the limitations of the endeavor and was philosophically consistent with the qualitative paradigm" (p. 517).

Decisions relating to study quality and how to assess it are also needed early in the project. Finfgeld

(2003), who did not advocate using peer review as a screen for quality, did, however, suggest two basic quality criteria. The first is that the report should provide sufficient assurance that the study used "widely accepted qualitative methods" (p. 899). The second is that the findings should be well supported by the raw data—that is, quotes from study participants.

Another related sampling issue concerns decisions about the *type* of findings to include. Sandelowski and Barroso (2003a) describe a continuum of qualitative findings that involves how close the analysis was to the original data—that is, the extent to which the researcher *transformed* the data to yield findings. The continuum ranges from a category closest to the data that they called "no finding" (meaning that the data themselves are presented, without judgments or integrated discoveries) to a category farthest from the data that they called "interpretive explanation." The category scheme is intended to be neutral to the underlying method and research tradition. Sandelowski and Barroso argued that "no finding" studies are not research, and so metasynthesists may choose not to include them.

Searching the Literature for Data

It is generally more difficult to find qualitative than quantitative studies using mainstream approaches such as searching electronic databases. One factor contributing to this difficulty is that the majority of databases do not index studies by methodology. For example, "qualitative" is not a MeSH (medical subject heading) term in MEDLINE—although "qualitative studies" *is* used in the controlled vocabulary of CINAHL. This means that a searcher typically has to try many different terms (e.g., "grounded theory," phenomenology*, ethnograph*, "case study," and so on) and hope that one of these terms was used in the abstract or title of relevant studies. Barroso and colleagues (2003) have discussed strategies for finding qualitative primary studies for integration purposes.

➲ **TIP:** Sample sizes in nursing metasyntheses are highly variable, ranging from a very small number—for example, three primary studies in the metaethnography of Varcoe and colleagues (2003)—to nearly 300 in Paterson's (2001) synthesis of

qualitative studies on chronic illness. Sample size is likely to vary as a function of scope of the inquiry, extent of prior research, and type of metasynthesis undertaken. As with primary studies, one guideline for sampling adequacy is whether categories in the metasynthesis are saturated (Finfgeld, 2003).

Evaluating Study Quality

Formal evaluations of primary study quality are not as common in metasynthesis as in meta-analysis, and developing quality criteria about which there would be widespread agreement is likely to prove challenging. One available instrument, developed by Paterson and colleagues (2001), is the Primary Research Appraisal Tool, which covers such aspects of a qualitative study as the sampling procedure, data gathering strategy, data analysis, researcher credentials, and researcher reflexivity. The tool was designed to be used to screen primary studies for inclusion in a meta-synthesis.

Not everyone agrees, however, that quality ought to be a criterion for eliminating studies for a metasynthesis. Sandelowski and Barroso (2003c), for example, advocated a certain degree of inclusiveness: "Excluding reports of qualitative studies because of inadequacies in reporting . . . , or because of what some reviewers might perceive as methodological mistakes, will result in the exclusion of reports with findings valuable to practice that are not necessarily invalidated by these errors" (p. 155).

Extracting and Encoding Data for Analysis

Information about various features of the study need to be abstracted and coded as part of the project. Just as in quantitative integration, the metasynthesist should abstract and record features of the data source (e.g., year of publication, country), characteristics of the sample (e.g., age, gender, number of participants), and methodologic features (e.g., research tradition).

Most important, of course, information about the study findings must be extracted and recorded. Sandelowski and Barroso (2003b) have defined *findings* as the "data-based and integrated discoveries, conclusions, judgments, or pronouncements researchers offered regarding the events, experiences, or cases under investigation (i.e., their interpretations, no matter the extent of the data transformation involved)" (p. 228). Others characterize findings as the key themes, metaphors, categories, concepts, or phrases from each study.

As Sandelowski and Barroso (2002, 2003a) have noted, however, *finding* the findings is not always easy. For example, qualitative researchers intermingle data with interpretation and findings from other studies with their own. Noblit and Hare (1988) advised that, just as primary study researchers must read and re-read their data before they can proceed with a meaningful analysis, metasynthesists must read the primary studies multiple times to fully grasp the categories or metaphors being explicated. In essence, a metasynthesis becomes "another 'reading' of data, an opportunity to reflect on the data in new ways" (McCormick, Rodney, & Varcoe, 2003, p. 936).

Analyzing and Interpreting the Data

It is at the analysis stage where strategies for metasynthesis diverge most markedly. We briefly describe three approaches, and advise you to consult more advanced resources for further guidance. No matter which approach researchers use, they need to understand that metasynthesis is a complex interpretive task that involves "carefully peeling away the surface layers of studies to find their hearts and souls in a way that does the least damage to them" (Sandelowski, Docherty, & Emden, 1997, p.370).

The Noblit and Hare Approach. Noblit and Hare's (1988) methods of integration have been highly influential among nurse researchers and, in Finfgeld's (2003) review of 17 metasynthesis studies since 1994, their approach was used with greatest frequency—although Noblit and Hare themselves referred to their approach as metaethnography. They argued that a metaethnography should be interpretive and not aggregative—that is, that the synthesis should focus on constructing interpretations rather than analyses. Their approach for synthesizing qualitative studies included seven phases that overlap and repeat as the metasynthesis progresses, the first three of which are preanalytic: (1) deciding on the phenomenon, (2) deciding which studies are relevant for the synthesis, and (3) reading and re-reading each study. Phases 4 through 6 concern the analysis:

Phase 4: Deciding how the studies are related to each other. In this phase the researcher makes a list of the key metaphors in each study and their relation to each other. Noblit and Hare used the term "metaphor" to refer to themes, perspectives, or concepts that emerged from the primary studies. Studies can be related in three ways: *reciprocal* (directly comparable), *refutational* (in opposition to each other), and in a line of argument rather than either reciprocal or refutational.

Phase 5: Translating the qualitative studies into one another. Noblit and Hare noted that "translations are especially unique syntheses because they protect the particular, respect holism, and enable comparison. An adequate translation maintains the central metaphors and/or concepts of each account in their relation to other key metaphors or concepts in that account" (p. 28).

Phase 6: Synthesizing translations. Here the challenge for the researcher is to make a whole into more than the individual parts imply.

The final phase (Phase 7) is to express the synthesis through the written word or alternatives.

> **Example of Noblit and Hare's approach:**
> Beck (2002) used Noblit and Hare's approach in her metasynthesis of 18 qualitative studies on postpartum depression. As part of the analysis, key metaphors were listed for each study and organized under four overarching themes, one being "spiraling downward." For instance, in one of the primary studies (Wood et al., 1997 [cited in study]), the key metaphors listed under this theme included "total isolation; façade of normalcy; obsessive thoughts; pervasive guilt; panic/overanxious/feels trapped; completely overwhelmed by infant demands; anger" (p. 459). Beck's paper presented an excellent table illustrating how the individual metaphors mapped onto the four themes.

The Paterson, Thorne, Canam, and Jillings Approach. Paterson and colleagues' (2001) method of metasynthesis involves three components: meta-data analysis, meta-method, and meta-theory. These components often are conducted concurrently, and the metasynthesis results from the integration of findings from these three analytic components. Paterson and colleagues define **meta-data analysis** as the study of results of reported research in a specific substantive area of investigation by means of analyzing the "processed data." **Meta-method** is the study of the methodologic rigor of the studies included in the metasynthesis. Lastly, **meta-theory** refers to the analysis of the theoretical underpinnings on which the studies are grounded. The end product is a metasynthesis that results from bringing back together the findings of these three meta-study components.

The Sandelowski and Barroso Approach. The strategies developed by Sandelowski and Barroso (2006) are likely to inspire metasynthesis efforts in the years ahead. In their multiple-year methodologic project, they developed the previously described continuum relating to how much data transformation had occurred in a primary study. Further, they dichotomized studies based on level of synthesis and interpretation. Reports can be described as *summaries* if the findings are descriptive synopses of the qualitative data, usually with lists and frequencies of topics and themes, without any conceptual reframing. *Syntheses*, by contrast, are findings that are more interpretive and explanatory, and that involve conceptual or metaphorical reframing. Sandelowski and Barroso have argued that only findings that are syntheses should be used in a metasynthesis.

Both summaries and syntheses can, however, be used in a **meta-summary**, which can lay a good foundation for a metasynthesis. Sandelowski and Barroso (2003b) provided an example of a meta-summary in which they used studies (including both summaries and syntheses) of mothering within the context of HIV infection. The first step, extracting findings, resulted in almost 800 complete sentences from the 45 reports they identified, which represented a comprehensive inventory of findings. The 800 sentences were then reduced to 93 thematic statements, or abstracted findings.

The next step in their meta-summary effort was to calculate **manifest effect sizes**, that is, effect sizes calculated from the manifest content pertaining to

motherhood within the context of HIV as represented in the 93 abstracted findings. Qualitative effect sizes are not to be confused with treatment effects, but the ". . . calculation of effect sizes constitutes a quantitative transformation of qualitative data in the service of extracting more meaning from those data and verifying the presence of a pattern or theme" (Sandelowski & Barroso, 2003b, p. 231). They argued that by calculating effect sizes, integration that avoids the possibility of overweighting or underweighting findings can be achieved.

Two types of effect size can be created from the abstracted findings. A **frequency effect size**, which indicates the magnitude of the findings, is the number of reports with unduplicated information that contain a given finding, divided by all unduplicated reports. For example, Sandelowski and Barroso (2003b) calculated an overall frequency effect size of 60% for the finding about a mother's struggle about whether or not to disclose her HIV status to her children. In other words, 60% of the 45 reports had a finding of this nature. Such effect size information can be calculated for subgroups of reports—for example, for published versus unpublished reports, for reports from different research traditions, and so on.

An **intensity effect size** indicates the concentration of findings *within* each report. It is calculated by dividing the number of different findings in a given report, divided by the total number of findings in all reports. As an example, one primary study had 29 out of the 93 total findings, for an intensity effect size of 31% (Sandelowski & Barroso, 2003b).

Metasyntheses can build upon meta-summaries, but require findings that are interpretive, that is, from reports that are characterized as syntheses. The purpose of a metasynthesis is not to summarize, but to offer novel interpretations of interpretive findings. Such interpretive integrations require metasynthesists to piece the individual syntheses together to craft a new coherent description or explanation of a target event or experience. An array of quantitative analytic methods can be used to achieve this goal, including, ". . . for example, constant comparison, taxonomic analysis, the reciprocal translation of in vivo concepts, and the use of imported concepts to frame data" (Sandelowski in Thorne et al., 2004, p. 1358).

Example of Sandelowski and Barroso's approach: Sandelowski and Barroso (2005) applied their procedures to an integration of findings from qualitative studies of expectant parents receiving positive prenatal diagnosis. Meta-summary techniques were used to aggregate findings from 17 reports, and metasynthesis techniques, including constant comparative analysis, were used to interpret the findings. A total of 39 meta-findings were abstracted, with frequency effect sizes ranging from 100% to 6%. The thematic emphasis was on the dilemmas of choice and decision making. Positive prenatal diagnosis was for couples an experience of chosen losses and lost choices.

Writing a Metasynthesis Report

Metasynthesis reports are similar in many respects to meta-analytic reports—except that the Results section contains the new interpretations rather than the quantitative findings. Of course, when a meta-summary has been done, the meta-findings would typically be presented in a table, a template for which is available in the Toolkit of the accompanying *Resource Manual*.

The Method section of a metasynthesis report should contain a detailed description of the sampling criteria, the search procedures, and efforts made to enhance the integrity and rigor of the integration. The sample of selected studies should also be described; key features are often summarized in a table.

As with primary studies, alternatives to written metasyntheses have been proposed. Noblit and Hare (1988) noted, for example, that when the qualitative synthesis' purpose is to inform clinicians or practitioners, other forms of expressing the synthesis may be preferred, such as through music, artwork, plays, or videos.

CRITIQUING SYSTEMATIC REVIEWS AND METASYNTHESES

Like all studies, systematic reviews should be thoroughly critiqued before the findings are deemed trustworthy and relevant to clinicians. Box 25.1 offers guidelines for evaluating systematic reviews.

Although these guidelines are fairly broad, not all questions apply equally well to all types of systematic reviews. In particular, we have distinguished questions about analysis separately for meta-analyses and metasyntheses. The list of questions in Box 25.1 is not necessarily comprehensive. Supplementary questions might be needed for particular types of review.

In drawing conclusions about a research integration, one issue is to evaluate whether reviewers did a good job in pulling together and summarizing the evidence. Another aspect, however, is drawing inferences about how you might use the evidence in clinical practice. It is not the reviewers' job, for example, to consider such issues as barriers to making use of the evidence, acceptability of an innovation, costs and benefits of change in various settings, and so on. These are issues for practicing nurses seeking to maximize the effectiveness of their actions and decisions.

RESEARCH EXAMPLES

We conclude this chapter with a description of two systematic reviews. We note also that two integration reports (a meta-analysis and a metasynthesis) appear in their entirety in the *Resource Manual* that accompanies this book.

Example 1: A Meta-Analysis

Study: "A meta-analysis of the effect of hospital-based case management on hospital length of stay and readmission" (Kim & Soeken, 2005)

Purpose: The purpose of the study was to integrate research evidence on the following research question: Is case management (CM) effective in reducing the length of hospitalization stay (LOS) and readmission rates of inpatients? LOS was defined as the average number of days hospitalized per patient, and readmission rate was defined as the proportion of patients readmitted at least once within the study's follow-up period.

BOX 25.1 Guidelines for Critiquing Systematic Reviews and Metasyntheses

THE PROBLEM

- Did the report clearly state the research problem and/or research question? Is the scope of the project appropriate?
- Is the topic of the integration important for nursing?
- Were concepts, variables, or phenomena adequately defined?
- Was the approach to integration adequately described, and was the approach appropriate?

SEARCH STRATEGY

- Did the report clearly describe criteria for selecting primary studies, and are those criteria reasonable?
- Were the databases used by the reviewers identified, and are they appropriate and comprehensive? Were key words identified, and are they exhaustive?
- Did the reviewers use adequate supplementary efforts to identify relevant studies?

THE SAMPLE

- Were inclusion and exclusion criteria clearly articulated, and were they defensible?
- Did the search strategy yield a strong and comprehensive sample of studies? Were strengths and limitations of the sample identified?
- If an original report was lacking key information, did reviewers attempt to contact the original researchers for additional information—or did the study have to be excluded?
- If studies were excluded for reasons other than insufficient information, did the reviewers provide a rationale for the decision?

QUALITY APPRAISAL

- Did the reviewers appraise the quality of the primary studies? Did they use a defensible and well-defined set of criteria, or a well-validated quality appraisal scale?
- Did two or more people do the appraisals, and was interrater agreement reported?
- Was the appraisal information used in an appropriate manner in the selection of studies, or in the analysis of results?

DATA EXTRACTION

- Was adequate information extracted about methodologic and administrative aspects of the study? Was adequate information about sample characteristics extracted?
- Was sufficient information extracted about study findings?
- Were steps taken to enhance the integrity of the dataset (e.g., were two or more people used to extract and record information for analysis)?

DATA ANALYSIS—GENERAL

- Did the reviewers explain their method of pooling and integrating the data?
- Was the analysis of data thorough and credible?
- Were tables, figures, and text used effectively to summarize findings?

BOX 25.1 (continued)

DATA ANALYSIS—QUANTITATIVE

- If a meta-analysis was not performed, was there adequate justification for using a narrative integration method? If a meta-analysis *was* performed, was this justifiable?
- For meta-analyses, were appropriate procedures followed for computing effect size estimates for all relevant outcomes?
- Was heterogeneity of effects adequately dealt with? Was the decision to use a random effects model versus a fixed effects model sound? Were appropriate subgroup analyses undertaken—or was the absence of subgroup analyses justified?
- Was the issue of publication bias adequately addressed?

DATA ANALYSIS—QUALITATIVE

- In a meta-synthesis, did the reviewers describe the techniques they used to compare the findings of each study, and did they explain their method of interpreting their data?
- If a meta-summary was undertaken, did the abstracted findings seem appropriate and convincing? Were appropriate methods used to compute effect sizes? Was information presented effectively?
- In a metasynthesis, did the synthesis achieve a fuller understanding of the phenomenon to advance knowledge? Do the interpretations seem well grounded? Was there a sufficient amount of data included to support the interpretations?

CONCLUSIONS

- Did the reviewers draw reasonable conclusions about the quality, quantity, and consistency of evidence relating to the research question?
- Are limitations of the review/synthesis noted?
- Are implications for nursing practice and further research clearly stated?

<table>
<tr><td>▭</td><td>All integrative reports</td></tr>
<tr><td>▭</td><td>Systematic reviews of quantitative studies</td></tr>
<tr><td>▭</td><td>Metasyntheses</td></tr>
</table>

Method: A meta-analytic method was used to integrate information about the effects of a CM intervention, versus care as usual, on LOS and readmission.

Eligibility Criteria: A study was included if it met the following criteria: (a) the sample included adults aged 18 years or older; (b) the intervention was a hospital-based CM for inpatients; (c) the research design was a randomized experiment; (d) the report provided data about at least one of the two outcomes for the experimental and control group; and (2) the sample size was reported. Only English-language reports were considered.

Search Strategy: The initial strategy involved a search of three databases: MEDLINE (1966–2003), CINAHL

(1982–2003), and HealthSTAR (1975–2003). Several keywords were used in the search, such as care management, CM, managed care, and disease management. A descendancy approach (footnote chasing) was then used, followed by communication with content experts.

Sample: A total of 129 abstracts were reviewed, and then the pool was narrowed to 25 studies. Based on agreement by both reviewers, 12 nonduplicative studies that met all study criteria were identified. The 12 studies in the meta-analysis involved a total of nearly 3000 study participants from the United States, Canada, Australia, and Sweden, with sample sizes ranging from 42 to 668.

Data Extraction: A wide array of administrative, methodologic, and substantive information was extracted from the 12 studies. Two coders independently extracted data, and initial coder agreement was 95%. Discrepancies were resolved through discussion.

Quality Assessments: The quality of both the study methods was assessed using a quality assessment scale that was adapted from an existing instrument. Total possible scores could range from 0 to 11. Studies with scores of 0 to 3 were considered low quality, those with scores of 4 to 7 were considered moderate quality, and those with scores of 8 or higher were considered high quality. Intervention quality was also rated. All ratings were completed by two judges who resolved any discrepancies. All studies in the analysis were of at least moderate quality.

Effect Size Calculation: The standardized mean difference (d) was used as the effect size for the LOS outcome, and the odds ratio was used for readmission. An OR less than 1.0 indicated that the CM group was less likely to have readmissions, and an OR greater than 1.0 indicated higher rates of readmission in the intervention group.

Statistical Analyses: Both fixed effects and random effects models were used to estimate pooled effect size. Random effects results were reported because the test for heterogeneity was significant. Sensitivity analyses and subgroup analyses were performed to examine whether the effect size results varied by study quality, components of the CM intervention, patient diagnoses, and country where the study was conducted. Publication bias was also assessed.

Key Findings: The overall average weighted effect size (d) of LOS was 0.09, with a 95% CI of −0.03 to 0.22, indicating that, across studies, the CM intervention could not be considered effective in reducing hospital LOS. The pooled OR for readmission of 0.87, with a 95% CI of 0.69 to 1.04, was also not statistically significant. Variation in effect size estimates was not found to be associated with study quality or intervention components. However, for studies conducted in the United States, CM *was* found to be effective in reducing readmission rates. Also, diagnosis played a role: the pooled effect of CM for LOS was significant for patients with heart failure, but not for those with stroke or for frail elders. Funnel plots suggested no publication bias for LOS, but the plot was somewhat asymmetric for readmission rates. However, the fail-safe N was calculated to be 153, substantially greater than the guideline value of 55, and thus publication bias was not considered to be problematic in this review.

Discussion: The researchers noted that one possible explanation for the nonsignificant findings is that "usual care" was typically not well described in the primary studies, and

that usual care could have included some CM components. Other weaknesses of the primary studies were noted, and the authors urged that other meta-analyses be conducted to examine the effectiveness of CM on other outcomes.

Example 2: A Meta-Synthesis

Study: "Adolescent motherhood: A meta-synthesis of qualitative studies" (Clemmens, 2003)

Purpose: The purpose of the study was to synthesize qualitative studies on the phenomenon of adolescent motherhood.

Eligibility Criteria: A study was included if the phenomenon under investigation was the experience of adolescent motherhood and if a qualitative approach was used, regardless of research tradition. Studies were excluded if the focus was on depression in adolescent mothers or if the study findings were not organized into themes or metaphors on the experience of adolescent motherhood.

Search Strategy: Clemmens searched the following databases for studies published between 1990 and 2001 with the keywords "adolescent motherhood" AND "Qualitative studies": CINAHL, Medline, PsychINFO, ERIC, Sociological Abstracts, and Dissertation Abstracts.

Sample: Of the 50 studies initially identified, 18 met the sample inclusion and exclusion criteria. The 18 studies included 7 descriptive studies, 5 interpretive/phenomenological studies, 3 grounded theory studies, and 3 ethnographies. Thirteen were from published journal articles, and 5 were from dissertations. The combined sample of participants included 257 adolescent mothers from the United States, Canada, Australia, England, and China.

Data Extraction and Analysis: Noblit and Hare's approach was used to compare study findings. The original metaphors, themes, concepts, and phrases from each of the 18 studies were organized into a grid and then reciprocally translated, one into the other, resulting in the construction of an initial list of metaphors. The complexity of experiences required a second level of analysis that revealed five overarching metaphors.

Key Findings: The five overarching metaphors were: (1) the reality of motherhood brings hardships; (2) living in the two worlds of adolescence and motherhood; (3) motherhood as positively transforming; (4) baby as a stabilizing influence; and (5) supportive context as turning point for future.

Discussion: Clemmens concluded that the meta-synthesis provides nurses with a comprehensive picture of adolescent motherhood. She argued that nurses working in hospital, home care, and school settings can use the results to help develop appropriate interventions, and she offered some examples. She noted that the regularity of the themes and metaphors was important considering the diversity of racial backgrounds and cultures in the original studies.

SUMMARY POINTS

- Evidence-based practice relies on rigorous integration of research evidence on a topic through **systematic reviews** of quantitative findings and **metasyntheses** of qualitative findings—both of which are rigorous, systematic inquiries with many similarities to original primary studies.
- Systematic reviews often involve statistical integration of findings through **meta-analysis**, a procedure whose advantages include objectivity, enhanced power, and precision; meta-analysis is not appropriate, however, for broad questions or when there is substantial inconsistency of findings.
- The steps in both quantitative and qualitative integration are similar and involve formulating the problem, designing the study (including establishing sampling criteria), searching the literature for a sample of **primary studies** to be included in the review, evaluating study quality, extracting and encoding data for analysis, analyzing the data, and reporting the findings.
- There is no consensus on whether integrations should include the **grey literature**—that is, unpublished reports; in quantitative studies, a concern is that there is a *bias against the null hypothesis,* a **publication bias** stemming from the under-representation of nonsignificant findings in the published literature.
- In meta-analysis, findings from primary studies are represented by an effect size index that quantifies the magnitude and direction of relationship between the independent and dependent variables. The most common effect size indexes in nursing are *d* (the **standardized mean difference**) and the odds ratio.

- Effects from individual studies are pooled to yield an estimate of the population effect size by calculating a **weighted average** of effects, often using the **inverse variance** as the weight—which gives greater weight to larger studies
- **Statistical heterogeneity** (diversity in effects across studies) is a major issue in meta-analysis and affects decisions about using a **fixed effects model** (which assumes a single true effect size) or a **random effects model** (which assumes a distribution of effects). Heterogeneity can be examined using a **forest plot**.
- Nonrandom heterogeneity can be explored through **subgroup analyses** or **meta-regression,** in which the purpose is to identify clinical or methodologic features systematically related to variation in effects.
- Quality assessments (which may involve formal quantitative ratings of overall methodologic rigor) are sometimes used to exclude weak studies from reviews, but they can also be used to differentially weight studies or in **sensitivity analyses** to determine whether including or excluding weaker studies changes conclusions.
- Publication bias can be examined by constructing a **funnel plot**, and can be partially addressed through a variety of strategies, including the calculation of a **fail-safe number** that estimates the number of studies with nonsignificant results that would be needed to reverse the conclusion of a significant effect.
- Metasyntheses are more than just summaries of prior qualitative findings, they involve a discovery of essential features of a body of findings and a transformation that yields new insights and interpretations. Metasyntheses have been classified with regard to the degree to which theory building and theory explication are achieved.
- Numerous approaches to meta-synthesis (and many terms related to qualitative integration) have been proposed. Issues with which metasynthesists have grappled include whether to combine findings from different research traditions and whether to use study quality as an eligibility criterion in sampling studies.

- One approach to qualitative integration, proposed by Noblit and Hare, involves listing key themes or metaphors across studies and then translating them into each other.
- Paterson and colleagues' meta-study method integrates three components: (1) **meta-data analysis**, the study of results in a specific substantive area through analysis of the "processed data"; (2) **meta-method**, the study of the studies' methodologic rigor; and (3) **meta-theory**, the analysis of the theoretical underpinnings on which the studies are grounded.
- Sandelowski and Barroso distinguish qualitative findings in terms of whether they are *summaries* (descriptive synopses) or *syntheses* (interpretive explanations of the data). Both summaries and syntheses can be used in a **meta-summary**, which can lay the foundation for a metasynthesis.
- A meta-summary involves developing a list of abstracted findings from the primary studies and calculating **manifest effect sizes**. A **frequency effect size** is the percentage of reports that contain a given finding. An **intensity effect size** indicates the percentage of all findings that are contained in any given report.
- In the Sandelowski and Barroso approach, only studies described as *syntheses* can be used in a meta-synthesis, which can use a variety of qualitative approaches to analysis and interpretations (e.g., constant comparison).

STUDY ACTIVITIES

Chapter 25 of the accompanying *Resource Manual for Nursing Research: Generating and Assessing Evidence for Nursing Practice, 8th edition*, offers various exercises and study suggestions for reinforcing the concepts taught in this chapter. In addition, the following study questions can be addressed:

1. Discuss the similarities and differences between the term "effect size" in qualitative and quantitative integration.

2. Apply relevant questions in Figure 25.3 to one of the research examples at the end of the chapter, referring to the full journal article as necessary.

STUDIES CITED IN CHAPTER 25

Methodologic or theoretical references cited in this chapter can be found in a separate section at the end of the book.

Beck, C. T. (2001). Predictors of postpartum depression: An update. *Nursing Research, 50,* 275–285.

Beck, C. T. (2002). Postpartum depression: A metasynthesis. *Qualitative Health Research, 12,* 453–472.

Clemmens, D. (2003). Adolescent motherhood: A metasynthesis of qualitative studies. *MCN: The American Journal of Maternal/Child Nursing, 28,* 93–99.

Davenport, J. (2004). A systematic review to ascertain whether the standard needle is more effective than a longer or wider needle in reducing the incidence of local reaction in children receiving primary immunization. *Journal of Advanced Nursing, 46*(1), 66–77.

Fetzer, S. J. (2002). Reducing venipuncture and intravenous insertion pain with eutectic mixture of local anesthetic. *Nursing Research, 51,* 119–124.

Forbes, D. A. (2003). An example of the use of systematic reviews to answer an effectiveness question. *Western Journal of Nursing Research, 25,* 179–192.

Hill-Westmoreland, E. E., Soeken, K., & Spellbring, A. M. (2002). A meta-analysis of fall prevention programs for the elderly: How effective are they? *Nursing Research, 51*(1), 1–8.

Kim, Y., & Soeken, K. (2005). A meta-analysis of the effect of hospital-based case management on hospital length of stay and readmission. *Nursing Research, 54*(4), 255–264.

Lee, O., & Johnson, L. (2005). A systematic review for effective management of central venous catheters and catheter sites in acute care paediatric patients. *Worldviews on Evidence-Based Nursing, 2*(1), 4–13.

Nelson, A. M. (2002). A metasynthesis: Mothering other-than-normal children. *Qualitative Health Research, 12,* 515–530.

Paterson, B. (2001). The shifting perspectives model of chronic illness. *Journal of Nursing Scholarship, 33,* 57–62.

Peacock, S. C., & Forbes, D. A. (2003). Interventions for caregivers of persons with dementia: A systematic review. *Canadian Journal of Nursing Research, 35,* 88–107.

Sandelowski, M., & Barroso, J. (2005). The travesty of choosing after positive prenatal diagnosis. *Journal of Obstetric, Gynecologic, & Neonatal Nursing, 34*(3), 307–318.

Smith, B., Appleton, S., Adams, R., Southcott, A., & Ruffin, R. (2001). Home care by outreach nursing for chronic obstructive pulmonary disease. *Cochrane Database of Systematic Reviews,* Issue 3, Art. No. CD000995.

Varcoe, C., Rodney, P., & McCormick, J. (2003). Health care relationships in context: An analysis of three ethnographies. *Qualitative Health Research, 13*(7), 957–973.

26

Disseminating Evidence: Reporting Research Findings

No study is complete until the findings have been shared with others. This chapter offers assistance on dissemination of research results.

GETTING STARTED ON DISSEMINATION

Researchers make several decisions in developing a dissemination plan, as we discuss in this section.

Selecting a Communication Outlet

Researchers who want to communicate their findings to other researchers or clinicians can present them orally or in writing. Oral presentations (typically at professional conferences) can be a formal talk in front of an audience or integrated with written material in a **poster session**. Major advantages of conference presentations are that they typically can be done soon after study completion, and offer opportunities for dialogue among people interested in the same topic. Written reports, in addition to theses or dissertations, can take the form of journal articles published in traditional professional journals, or in a variety of outlets on the Internet. The main advantage of journal articles is the ease with which they can be accessed worldwide.

Research reports for different outlets vary in a number of ways, as we discuss in a subsequent section. Nevertheless, our advice in this section is generally relevant for most types of dissemination.

Knowing the Audience

Good research communication depends on providing information that can be understood by consumers. Therefore, before researchers develop a dissemination strategy, they should consider the audience they are hoping to reach. Here are some questions to consider:

1. Will the audience be nurses only, or will it include professionals from other disciplines (e.g., physicians, psychologists)?
2. Will the audience be researchers, or will it include other professionals (clinicians, health care policymakers)?
3. Are clients (lay people) a possible audience?
4. Will the audience include people whose native language is not English?
5. Will reviewers, editors, and readers be experts in the field?

These questions underscore an important point—that researchers usually have to write with multiple audiences in mind, which means writing clearly and avoiding technical jargon to the extent possible.

It is also means that researchers sometimes must develop a multiprong strategy—for example, publishing a report for nurse researchers in a journal such as *Nursing Research*, and then publishing a summary for clinicians or clients in a hospital newsletter.

Although writing for a broad audience may be an important goal, it is also important to keep in mind the needs of the *main* intended audience. If consumers of a report are mostly clinical nurses, it is important to emphasize what the findings mean for nursing practice. If the audience is administrators or policymakers, explicit information should be included about how the findings relate to such outcomes as *cost*, *efficiency*, *accessibility*, and so on. If other researchers are the primary targets, explicit information about methods, study limitations, and implications for future research are important.

Developing a Plan

Before preparing a report, researchers should have a plan. Part of that plan involves how best to coordinate the actual tasks of preparing a **manuscript** (i.e., an unpublished paper or document).

Deciding on Authorship

When a study has been completed by a team, division of labor and authorship must be addressed. The International Committee of Medical Journal Editors (ICMJE, 2006) advises that authorship credit should be based on (1) having made a substantial contribution to the study's conception and design, to data acquisition, or to analysis and interpretation; (2) drafting or revising the manuscript; and (3) approving the final version of the manuscript.

The **lead author**, usually the first-named author, is the person with overall responsibility for the report. The lead author and co-authors should reach an agreement in advance about responsibilities for producing the manuscript. To avoid possible subsequent conflicts, they should also decide beforehand the order of authors' names. Ethically, it is most appropriate to list names in the order of authors'

contribution to the work, not according to status. When contributions of co-authors are comparable, an alphabetical listing is appropriate.

Deciding on Content

In many studies, more data are collected than can be presented in one report, and multiple publications are thus possible. In such situations, an early decision involves what part of the findings to present in a given paper. If there are multiple research questions, several papers may be required to communicate results adequately. Researchers who collect both qualitative and quantitative data often report on each separately.

It is, however, not appropriate to write several papers when one would suffice. Each paper from a study should independently make a contribution. Editors, reviewers, and readers expect original work, so unnecessary overlap should be avoided. It is also considered unethical to submit essentially the same or similar paper to two journals simultaneously. Oermann (2002) has offered excellent guidelines regarding duplicate and redundant publications.

Assembling Materials

Planning also involves assembling materials needed to begin a draft. One key ingredient is information about manuscript requirements. Traditional and online journals issue guidelines for authors, and these guidelines should be retrieved and understood.

Other materials also need to assembled, including notes about the relevant literature and references; instruments used in the study; descriptions of the study sample; output of computer analyses; relevant analytic memos or reflexive notes; figures or photographs that illustrate some aspect of the study; and permissions to use copyrighted materials. Other important tools are style manuals that provide information about both grammar and language use (e.g., Strunk, White, & Angell, 2000), as well as more specific information about writing professional and scientific papers (e.g., American Psychological Association, 2001; ICMJE, 2006).

Finally, there should be an outline and timeline. A written outline is essential if there are multiple co-authors who each have responsibility for different sections of the manuscript. The overall outline and individual assignments, together with "due dates," should be developed collaboratively.

Writing Effectively

Many people have a hard time putting their ideas down on paper. It is clearly beyond the scope of this book to teach good writing skills, but we can offer a few suggestions. One suggestion, quite simply, is: *do it*. Get in the habit of writing, even if it is only 15 minutes a day. "Writer's block" is probably responsible for thousands of unfinished (or never-started) manuscripts each year. So, just begin somewhere, and keep at it regularly—writing gets easier with practice.

Writing *well* is, of course, important, and there are resources that offer suggestions on how to write compelling sentences, select good words, and organize your ideas effectively (e.g., Matthews, Bowen, & Matthews, 2001). It is usually better to write a draft in its entirety, and then go back later to rewrite awkward sentences, correct errors, reorganize, and generally polish it up.

CONTENT OF RESEARCH REPORTS

Research reports can vary in terms of audience, purpose, and length. Theses or dissertations not only communicate research results but also document students' ability to perform scholarly work and therefore tend to be long. Journal articles, by contrast, are short because they compete for limited journal space and are read by busy professionals. Nevertheless, the general form and content of research reports are often similar. Chapter 3 summarized the content of major sections of research reports, and here we offer a few additional tips. Distinctions among various kinds of reports are described later in the chapter.

Quantitative Research Reports

Quantitative reports typically follow the **IMRAD format**, which involves organizing content into four sections—the **I**ntroduction, **M**ethod, **R**esults,

and **D**iscussion. These sections, respectively, address the following questions:

- Why was the study done? (I)
- How was the study done? (M)
- What was learned? (R)
- What does it mean? (D)

The Introduction

The introduction acquaints readers with the research problem, its significance, and the context in which it was developed. The introduction sets the stage by describing the existing literature; the study's conceptual framework; the problem, research questions, or hypotheses; and the study rationale. Although the introduction includes multiple components, it should be concise. A common critique of research manuscripts by reviewers is that the introduction is too long.

Introductions are often written in a funnel-shaped structure, beginning broadly to establish a framework for understanding the study, and then narrowing to the specifics of what researchers sought to learn. The end point of the introduction should be a concise delineation of the research questions or hypotheses, which provides a good transition to the method section.

> **➔ TIP:** Some researchers postpone stating the problem until late in the introduction, but readers profit from learning the general problem immediately. An up-front, clearly stated problem statement is of immense value in communicating the study's context. The first paragraph should be written with special care because the goal is to grab the readers' attention.

The introduction typically includes a summary of related research to provide a pertinent context. Except for dissertations, the literature review should be a brief summary and not an exhaustive review. The review should make clear what is already known, and what the deficiencies are, thus helping to clarify the contribution the new study can make to evidence.

The introduction also should describe the study's theoretical or conceptual framework, if relevant. The theoretical framework should be sufficiently explained so that readers who are unfamiliar with it can understand its main thrust. The introduction should include conceptual definitions of the concepts under investigation.

The various background strands need to be convincingly and cogently interwoven to persuade readers that, in fact, the new study holds promise for adding to evidence for nursing.

➲ TIP : Many journal articles begin without an explicit heading labeled *Introduction*. In general, all the material before the method section is considered the introduction. Some introductions include subheadings such as *Literature Review* or *Hypotheses*.

The Method Section

To evaluate the quality of a study's evidence, readers need to know exactly what methods were used to address the research problem. In dissertations, the method section should provide sufficient detail that another researcher could replicate the study. In journal articles and conference presentations, the method section needs to be condensed, but the degree of detail should permit readers to draw conclusions about the validity of the findings. Faulty method sections are a leading cause of manuscript rejection by journals. Your job in writing the method section of a quantitative report is to persuade readers that your study has sufficient internal, external, construct, and statistical conclusion validity to merit consideration.

➲ TIP : The method section is often subdivided into several parts, which helps readers to locate vital information. As an example, the method section might contain the following subsections: Research Design; Sample and Setting; Data Collection Instruments; Procedures; Data Analysis.

The method section usually begins with the description of the research design and its rationale. The design is often given detailed coverage in experimental studies, with information about what specific design was adopted, what variables were manipulated, how subjects were assigned to groups, and what type of blinding was used. Reports for studies with multiple points of data collection should indicate the number of times data were collected and the amount of time elapsed between those points. In all types of quantitative studies, it is important to identify steps taken to control the research situation in general and confounding variables in particular. The method section also addresses steps taken to protect the rights of study participants.

Readers also need to know about study participants. This subsection (which may be labeled *Research Sample*, *Subjects*, or *Study Participants*) normally includes a discussion of the population from which the sample was drawn, and a list of eligibility criteria, to clarify the group to whom results can be generalized. The method of sample selection and its rationale, recruitment techniques, and sample size should be indicated so readers can determine how representative subjects are of the target population. If a power analysis was undertaken to determine sample size needs, this should be clearly stated. There should also be information about response rates and, if possible, about response bias (or attrition bias, if this is relevant). Basic characteristics of study participants (e.g., age, gender, medical condition) should also be described.

Data collection methods are another critical component of the method section, and may be included in a subsection labeled *Instruments*, *Measures*, or *Data Collection*. A description of study instruments, and a rationale for their use, should be provided. If instruments were constructed specifically for the project, the report should describe their development. Any special equipment that was used (e.g., to gather biophysiologic or observational data) should be described, including information about the manufacturer. The report should also indicate who collected the data (e.g., the authors, research assistants, nurses) and how they were trained. The report must also convince readers that the data collection methods were sound. Any information relating to data quality, and the procedures used to evaluate that quality, should be described.

In experimental studies, there is usually a procedures subsection that includes information about the actual intervention. What exactly did the intervention entail? How was the intervention theory translated into components? How and by whom was the treatment administered, and how were they trained? What was done with subjects in the control group? How much time elapsed between the intervention and the measurement of the dependent variable? How was intervention fidelity monitored?

Analytic procedures are described either in the method or results section. It is usually sufficient to identify the statistical procedures used; computational formulas or references for commonly used statistics such as analysis of variance are not necessary. For unusual procedures, or unusual applications of a common procedure, a technical reference justifying the approach should be noted. If confounding variables were controlled statistically, the specific variables controlled should be mentioned. The level of significance is typically set at .05 for two-tailed tests, which may or may not be explicitly stated; however, if a different significance level or one-tailed tests were used, this must be specified.

A recent new development is that there are now explicit guidelines, called the Consolidated Standards of Reporting Trials or **CONSORT guidelines**, for reporting information about randomized clinical trials (RCTs), and these guidelines have been adopted by major medical and nursing journals, such as *Nursing Research* (Bennett, 2005). CONSORT guidelines include a checklist of 22 items to include in reports of RCTs, and a template for a flow chart to track participants through a trial, from eligibility assessment through analysis of outcomes. Although these materials were specifically designed for use with RCTs, many aspects can be productively applied to any quantitative study. However, efforts to develop analogous materials for nonexperimental (observational) studies are currently underway, and are referred to as Strengthening the Reporting of Observational studies in Epidemiology or STROBE (*http://www.strobe-statement.org/Checkliste.html*).

Example of a CONSORT flow chart: Hill, Weinert, & Cudney (2006) used an experimental design to test the efficacy of a computer intervention on the psychological well-being of chronically ill rural women. Figure 26.1 shows the progression of study participants through the study, from the 125 women originally recruited to the 100 who provided final data for analysis. (The full report is reprinted in full in Appendix A of the accompanying *Resource Manual*).

➲ **TIP:** The CONSORT checklist is included in the Toolkit of the *Resource Manual* that accompanies this book, together with a template for a CONSORT flow chart. Further information about the CONSORT guidelines is available at *http://www.consort-statement.org*, which includes an interactive checklist with detailed information about components in the checklist. Also, researchers who have promoted the RE-AIM schema (see Chapter 11) as a framework for addressing external validity issues have proposed additional guidelines and flow chart elements, which can be viewed at *http://www.re-aim.org.*

The Results Section

Readers scrutinize the method section to know if the study was done with rigor, but the results section is the heart of the report. In a quantitative study, the results of the statistical analyses are summarized in a factual manner. Descriptive statistics are ordinarily presented first, to provide an overview of study variables. If key research questions involve comparing groups with regard to dependent variables (e.g., in an experimental or case-control study), the early part of the results section usually provides information about the groups' comparability with regard to background or baseline variables, so readers can evaluate selection bias.

Research results are usually ordered in terms of overall importance. If, however, research questions or hypotheses have been numbered in the introduction, the analyses addressing them should be ordered in the same sequence.

When reporting the results of statistical tests, three pieces of information are typically reported—the value of the calculated statistic, degrees of

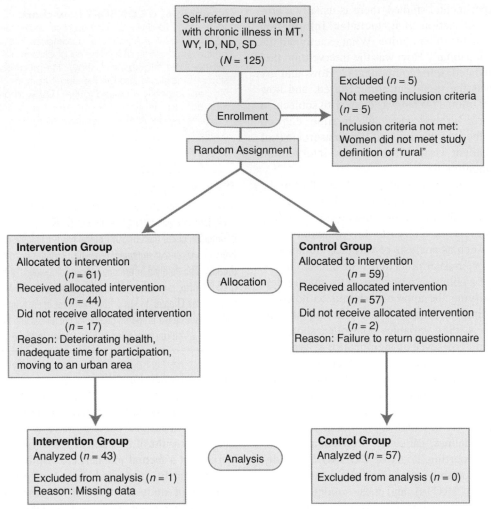

FIGURE 26.1 Example of CONSORT Guidelines Flowchart: Progression of Participants in an Intervention Study (From Hill, W., Weinert, C., & Cudney, S. [2006]. Influence of a computer intervention on the psychological status of chronically ill rural women. *Nursing Research, 55*[1], 34–42.)

freedom, and the *exact* probability level. For instance, it might be stated, "A chi-square test revealed that patients who were exposed to the experimental intervention were significantly less likely to develop decubitus ulcers than patients in the control group ($\chi^2 = 8.23$, $df = 1$, $p = .008$)." Increasingly, confidence intervals and effect sizes, as well as significance levels, are being reported. Beck (1999) has suggested further guidelines for

reporting quantitative results to facilitate the work of meta-analysts, who are often plagued with problems in retrieving data from the primary studies.

When results from several statistical analyses are reported, it is useful to summarize them in a **table**. Good tables, with precise headings and titles, are an important way to economize on space and to avoid dull, repetitive statements. When tables are used to present statistical information, the text

BOX 26.1 Guidelines for Preparing Statistical Tables

1. Number tables so they can be referenced in the text.
2. Give tables a clear, brief explanatory title.
3. Avoid both overly simple tables with information more efficiently presented in the text, and overly complex tables that intimidate and confuse readers.
4. Arrange data in such a way that patterns are obvious at a glance; take care to organize information in an intelligible way.
5. Give each column and row of data a heading that is succinct but clear; table headings should establish the logic of the table structure.
6. Express data values to the number of decimal places justified by the precision of the measurement. In general, it is preferable to report numbers to one decimal place (or to two decimal places for correlation coefficients) because rounded values are easier to absorb than more precise ones. Report all values in a table to the same level of precision.
7. Make each table a "stand-alone" presentation, capable of being understood without reference to the text.
8. Clearly indicate probability levels—usually the actual p values. In correlation matrixes, use the system of asterisks with a probability level footnote. The usual convention is to use one asterisk when $p < .05$, two when $p < .01$, and three when $p < .001$.
9. Indicate units of measurement for numbers in the table whenever appropriate (e.g., pounds, milligrams).
10. Use footnotes to explain abbreviations or special symbols used in the table, except commonly understood abbreviations such as N.

should refer to the table by number (e.g., "As shown in Table 2, patients in the experimental group . . ."). Box 26.1 presents some suggestions regarding the construction of effective statistical tables, and the table templates in the Toolkit (Chapters 21 to 23) can help you create clear and concise tables.

TIP: Do not repeat statistical information in text and in tables. Tables should display information that would be monotonous to present in the text—and to display it in such a way that patterns among the numbers are more evident. The text can be used to highlight major findings.

Figures may also be used to summarize results. Figures that display the results in graphic form are used less as an economy than as a means of dramatizing important findings and relationships. Figures are especially helpful for displaying information on some phenomenon over time, or for portraying conceptual or empirical models.

TIP: Research evidence does not constitute *proof* of anything, and so the report should never claim that the data proved, verified, confirmed, or demonstrated that hypotheses were correct or incorrect. Hypotheses are supported or unsupported, accepted or rejected.

The Discussion Section

The meaning that researchers give to the results plays a rightful and important role in the report. The discussion section is devoted to a thoughtful (and, it is hoped, insightful) analysis of the findings, leading to a discussion of their clinical and theoretical utility. A typical discussion section addresses the following questions: What were the main findings? What do the findings mean? What evidence is there that the results and the interpretations are valid? What limitations might threaten validity? How do the results compare with prior knowledge on the topic? What can be concluded about the findings *vis-à-vis* their use in nursing practice, in nursing theory, and in future nursing research?

TIP: The discussion is typically the most challenging section to write. It deserves your most intense intellectual and creative effort—and careful review by peers. The peers should be asked to comment on how persuasive your arguments are, how well organized the section is, and whether it is too long, which is a common flaw.

Typically, the discussion section begins with a summary of key findings. The summary should be brief, however, because the focus of the discussion is on making sense of (and not merely repeating) the results.

Interpretation of results is a global process, encompassing the findings themselves, methods and methodologic limitations, sample characteristics, related research findings, clinical dimensions, and theoretical issues. Researchers should justify their interpretations, explicitly stating why alternative explanations have been ruled out. Unsupported conclusions are among the most common problems in discussion sections. If the findings conflict with those of earlier studies, tentative explanations should be offered. A discussion of the generalizability of study findings should also be included.

Implications of study findings are speculative and, therefore, should be couched in tentative terms, as in the following example: "The results *suggest* that nurses' communication about advance directives is inconsistent and that nurses' years of experience affect the nature and amount of communication." The interpretation is, in essence, a hypothesis that can presumably be tested in another study. The discussion should include recommendations for studies that would help to test this hypothesis, as well as suggestions for other studies to answer questions raised by the findings.

Other Aspects of the Report

The materials covered in the four major IMRAD sections are found in some form in most quantitative research reports, although the organization might differ slightly. In addition to these major divisions, other aspects of the report deserve mention.

Title. Every research report should have a title indicating the nature of the study to prospective readers. Insofar as possible, the dependent and independent variables (or central phenomenon under study) should be named in the title. It is also desirable to indicate the study population. However, the title should be brief (no more than about 15 words), so writers must balance clarity with brevity. The length of titles can often be reduced by omitting unnecessary terms such as "A Study of . . . ," "Report of . . ." or "An Investigation to Examine the Effects of . . . ," and so forth. The title should communicate concisely what was studied—and stimulate interest in the research.

Abstract. Research reports usually include an abstract, that is, brief descriptions of the problem, methods, and findings of the study, written so readers can decide whether to read the entire report. As noted in Chapter 3, abstracts for journals can either be in a traditional (unstructured) paragraph of 100 to 200 words, or in a structured form with subheadings.

TIP: Take the time to write a compelling abstract. The abstract is your first main point of contact with reviewers and readers, so it deserves careful attention. It should demonstrate that your study is important clinically and that it was done with conceptual and methodologic rigor.

Key Words. It is often necessary to include key words that will be used in indexes to help others locate your study. Sometimes authors are given a list of key words from which to choose (often Medical Subject Headings or MeSH terms), but additional keywords can often be added. Substantive, methodologic, and theoretical terms can be used as key words.

References. Each report concludes with a list of references cited in the text, using a reference style required by those reviewing the manuscript or report. References can be cumbersome to prepare, but software programs are available to facilitate the preparation of reference lists (e.g., EndNote, ProCite, Reference Manager, Format Ease).

Acknowledgments. People who helped with the research but whose contribution does not qualify them for authorship are sometimes acknowledged at the end of the report. This might include statistical consultants, data collectors, or people who reviewed the manuscript. The acknowledgments should also give credit to organizations that made the project possible, such as funding agencies or organizations that helped with subject recruitment.

Qualitative Research Reports

As Sandelowski (1998) has noted, there is no single style for reporting qualitative findings. Qualitative research reports do, however, often follow the IMRAD format, or something akin to it. Thus, we present some issues of particular relevance for writing qualitative reports within the IMRAD structure.

Introduction

Qualitative reports usually begin with a statement of the problem, in a similar fashion to quantitative reports, but the focus is more squarely on the phenomenon under study. The way in which the problem is expressed and the types of questions the researchers sought to answer are usually tied to the research tradition underlying the study (e.g., grounded theory, ethnography), which is usually explicitly stated in the introduction. Prior research relating to the phenomenon under study may be summarized in the introduction, but sometimes this information is included in the discussion.

In many qualitative studies, but especially in ethnographic ones, it is critical to explain the study's cultural context. For studies with an ideological orientation (e.g., critical theory or feminist research), it is also important to describe the sociopolitical context. For studies using phenomenological or grounded theory designs, the philosophy of phenomenology or symbolic interaction, respectively, may be discussed.

As another aspect of explaining the study's background, qualitative researchers sometimes provide information about their personal experiences or qualifications relevant to the research. If a researcher who is studying decisions about long-term care placements is caring for two elderly parents and participates in a caregiver support group, this is relevant for readers' understanding of the study. In descriptive phenomenological studies, researchers may discuss their personal experiences in relation to the phenomenon being studied to communicate what they bracketed.

The concluding paragraph of the introduction usually offers a succinct summary of the purpose of the study or the research questions.

Method

Although the research tradition of the study is often noted in the introduction, the method section usually elaborates on specific methods used in conjunction with that tradition. Design features such as whether the study was longitudinal should also be noted.

The method section should provide a solid description of the research setting, so that readers can assess the transferability of findings. Study participants and methods by which they were selected should also be described. Even when samples are small, it is often useful to provide a table summarizing participants' key characteristics. If researchers have a personal connection to participants or to groups with which they are affiliated, this connection should be noted. At times, to disguise a group or institution, it may be necessary to omit or modify potentially identifying information.

Qualitative reports usually cannot provide much specific information about data collection, but some researchers provide a sample of questions, especially if a topic guide was used. The description of data collection methods should include how data were collected (e.g., interview or observation), who collected the data, how data collectors were trained, and what methods were used to record the data.

Information about quality and integrity is particularly important in qualitative studies. The more information included in the report about steps researchers took to enhance the trustworthiness of the data, the more confident readers can be that the findings are credible.

Quantitative reports typically have brief descriptions of data analysis techniques because standard statistical procedures are widely used and understood. By contrast, analytic procedures are often described in some detail in qualitative reports because readers need to understand how researchers organized, synthesized, and made sense of their data.

Results

In their results sections, qualitative researchers summarize their themes, categories, taxonomic structure, or the theory that emerged. This section can be organized in a number of ways. For example, if a process is being described, results may be presented chronologically, corresponding to the unfolding of the process. Key themes, metaphors, or domains are often used as subheadings, organized in order of salience to participants or to a theory.

Example of organization of qualitative results: Shambley-Ebron and Boyle (2006) did a critical ethnography to study the experiences of self-care and mothering among African-American women with HIV/AIDS. The overarching cultural theme was *creating a meaning of life*. The domains of *disabling relationships, strong mothering,* and *redefining self care* were used as subheadings to organize the results.

Sandelowski (1998) emphasized the importance of developing a story line before beginning to write the findings. Because of the richness of qualitative data, researchers have to decide which story, or how much of it, they want to tell. They must also make a decision about how best to balance description and interpretation. The results section in a qualitative paper, unlike that in a quantitative one, intertwines data and interpretations of those data. It is important, however, that sufficient emphasis be given to the voices, actions, and experiences of participants themselves so that readers can gain an appreciation of their lives and their worlds. Most often, this occurs through the inclusion of direct quotes to illustrate important points. Because of space constraints in journals, quotes cannot be extensive, and great care must be exercised in selecting the best possible exemplars. Gilgun (2005) has offered excellent guidance in writing up the results of qualitative research in a manner that has "grab."

➲ **TIP:** Using quotes is not only a skill but also a complex process. When inserting quotes in the results section, pay attention to how the quote is introduced and how it is put in context. Quotes should not be used haphazardly or listed one after the other in a string.

Figures, diagrams, and word tables that organize concepts are often useful in summarizing an overall conceptualization of the phenomena under study. Grounded theory studies are especially likely to benefit from a schematic presentation of the basic social process. Ethnographic and ethnoscience studies often present taxonomies in tabular form.

Discussion

In qualitative studies, findings and interpretation are typically interwoven in the results section because the task of integrating qualitative materials is essentially interpretive. The discussion section of a qualitative report, therefore, is not so much designed to give meaning to the results, but to summarize them, link them to other research, and suggest their implications for theory, practice, or future research. In some cases, researchers offer explicit recommendations about how their research can be corroborated (or how hypotheses can be tested) through quantitative studies.

Other Aspects of a Qualitative Report

Qualitative reports, like quantitative ones, include abstracts, key words, references, and acknowledgments. Abstracts for journals that feature qualitative reports (e.g., *Qualitative Health Research*) tend to be the traditional (single-paragraph) type, rather than structured abstracts with subheadings.

The titles of qualitative reports usually state the central phenomenon under scrutiny. Phenomenological studies often have titles that include such words as "the lived experience of . . ." or "the meaning of . . .". Grounded theory studies often indicate something about the *findings* in the title—for example, noting the core category or basic social process. Ethnographic titles usually indicate the culture being studied. Two-part titles are not uncommon, with substance and method, research tradition and findings, or theme and meaning, separated by a colon.

THE STYLE OF RESEARCH REPORTS

Research reports, especially for quantitative studies, are written in a distinctive style. Some style issues were discussed previously, but additional points are elaborated here.

A research report is not an essay. It is an account of how and why a problem was studied, and what was discovered as a result. The report should not include overtly subjective statements, emotionally laden statements, or exaggerations. This is not to say that the researchers' story should be told in a dreary manner. Indeed, in qualitative reports, there are ample opportunities to enliven the narration with rich description, direct quotes, and insightful interpretation. Authors of quantitative reports, although somewhat constrained by structure and the need to include numeric information, should strive to keep the presentation lively.

Quantitative researchers often avoid personal pronouns such as "I," "my," and "we" because impersonal pronouns, and use of the passive voice, suggest greater impartiality. Qualitative reports, by contrast, are often written in the first person and in an active voice. Even among quantitative researchers, however, there is a trend toward striking a greater balance between active and passive voice and first-person and third-person narration. If a direct presentation can be made without suggesting bias, a more readable product usually results.

It is not easy to write simply and clearly, but these are important goals of scientific writing. The use of technical jargon does little to enhance the communicative value of the report, and should especially be avoided in communicating findings to practicing nurses. The style should be concise and straightforward. If writers can add elegance to their reports without interfering with clarity and accuracy, so much the better, but the product is not expected to be a literary achievement.

A common flaw in reports of beginning researchers is inadequate organization. The overall structure is fairly standard, but the organization within sections and subsections needs careful attention. Sequences should be in an orderly progression with appropriate transitions. Continuity and logical thematic development are critical to good communication.

It may seem a trivial point, but methods and results should be described in the past tense. For example, it is inappropriate to say, "Nurses who receive special training perform triage functions significantly better than those without training." In this sentence, "receive" and "perform" should be changed to "received" and "performed" to reflect the fact that the statement pertains only to a particular sample whose behavior was observed in the past.

TYPES OF RESEARCH REPORTS

This section describes features of four major kinds of research reports: theses and dissertations, traditional journal articles, online reports, and presentations at professional meetings. Reports for class projects are excluded—not because they are unimportant but rather because they so closely resemble theses on a smaller scale.

Theses and Dissertations

Most doctoral degrees, and some master's degrees, are granted on the successful completion of an empirical research project. Most universities have a preferred format for their dissertations. Until recently, most schools used a traditional IMRAD format. The following organization for a traditional dissertation is typical:

- Front Matter: Title Page; Abstract; Copyright Page; Approval Page; Acknowledgment Page; Table of Contents; List of Tables; List of Figures; List of Appendices
- Main Body: Chapter I. Introduction; Chapter II. Review of the Literature; Chapter III. Methods; Chapter IV. Results; Chapter V. Discussion and Summary
- Supplementary Pages: Bibliography; Appendix

The **front matter** (preliminary pages) for dissertations is much the same as for a scholarly book. The title page indicates such information as the title of the study, the author's name, the degree requirement being fulfilled, and the name of the university awarding the degree. The acknowledgment page gives writers the opportunity to thank those who contributed to the project. The table of contents outlines major sections and subsections of the report, indicating on which page readers will find sections of interest. The lists of tables and figures identify by number, title, and page the tabular and graphic material in the text.

The main body of a traditionally formatted dissertation incorporates the IMRAD sections described earlier. The literature review often is so extensive that a separate chapter may be devoted to it. When a short review is sufficient, the first two chapters may be combined. In some cases, a separate chapter may also be required to elaborate the study's conceptual framework.

The supplementary pages include a bibliography or list of references used to prepare the report and one or more appendices. An appendix contains materials relevant to the study that are either too lengthy or too tangential to be incorporated into the body of the report. Data collection instruments, scoring instructions, codebooks, cover letters, permission letters, Institutional Review Board approval,

category schemes, and peripheral statistical tables are examples of the kinds of materials included in the appendix. Some universities also require *curriculum vitae* of the author.

A new approach to formatting dissertations or theses is the **paper format thesis**. The front matter and material at the end are similar to those in a traditionally formatted thesis, but the main sections differ. In a typical paper format thesis, there is an introduction, one or more publishable papers, and then a conclusion (Morris & Tipples, 1998). Such a format permits students to move directly from thesis to journal submission, but is more demanding than the traditional format. Morris and Tipples offered three possible scenarios for the papers to be included in the paper format thesis: (1) one paper focusing on a literature review followed by a second paper discussing study results; (2) two or more papers focusing on different findings from the project; and (3) one methodologic paper (e.g., describing the development of an instrument) and the second presenting findings.

If an academic institution does not use paper format theses, students will need to adapt their dissertations before submission to a journal. Johnson (1996) interviewed 15 journal editors for advice on converting a traditional dissertation to an acceptable manuscript format. Figure 26.2 summarizes sug-

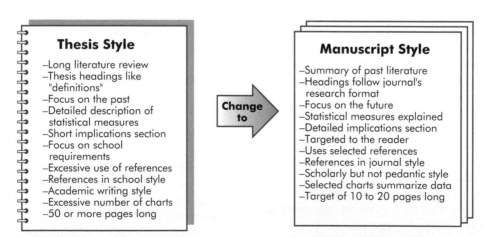

FIGURE 26.2 Suggested changes to convert theses to manuscripts. (Adapted with permission from Johnson, S. H. [1996]. Adapting a thesis to publication style: Meeting editor's expectations. *Dimensions of Critical Care Nursing, 15,* 160–167.)

gested changes to facilitate acceptance of a manuscript for publication in a nursing journal. Boyle (1997) has provided pointers to new recipients of doctoral degrees on how to publish their qualitative dissertations. This advice focuses on how to divide up or dissect the dissertation to generate two or more publications.

Journal Articles

Progress in evidence-based practice depends on researchers' efforts to share their work. Dissertations, which are too lengthy and inaccessible for widespread use, are read only by a handful of people. Publication in a professional journal ensures broad circulation of research findings, and it is professionally advantageous to publish. This section discusses issues relating to research reports in journals.

Selecting a Journal

Before writing begins, there should be a clear idea of the journal to which a manuscript will be submitted. Journals differ in their goals, types of manuscript sought, and readership; these factors need to be matched against personal interests and preferences. All journals issue goal statements, as well as guidelines for preparing and submitting a manuscript. This information is published in journals themselves and on their websites. Table 26.1 presents a list of nursing journals that have a high concentration of research articles.

➔ TIP: The websites of the journals shown in Table 26.1 are listed on the accompanying CD-ROM, for you to click on directly.

Example of statement of journal goal:
"Qualitative Health Research is an international, interdisciplinary, refereed journal for the enhancement of health care. It is designed to further the development and understanding of qualitative research methods in health care settings. We welcome manuscripts in the following areas: the description and analysis of the illness experience; health and health-seeking behaviors; the experiences of caregivers; the sociocultural organization of health care; health care policy; and related topics. We also seek critical reviews and commentaries addressing conceptual, theoretical, methodological, and ethical issues pertaining to qualitative inquiry. Letters of inquiry are not required."

Journals differ in prestige, acceptance rates, and circulation, and these may also need to be taken into account in selecting a journal. Prestige is most often assessed in terms of a journal's **impact factor**, which is an annual measure of citation frequency for an average article in a journal—that is, the ratio between citations and recent citable items published. For example, in 2005, the impact factor for *Nursing Research*, the second highest ranking nursing journal, was 1.528, whereas that for *Applied Nursing Research,* ranked 19th, was 0.580. Impact factor information can be found in Thompson's *Journal Citation Reports* (*http://scientific.thomson.com/products/ jcr/*), and some information (for 2005) is shown for the journals in Table 26.1. Not all nursing journals are included in the rankings, but prominent ones are, and the number included will soon expand (Freda, 2006).

Northam, Trubenbach, and Bentov (2000), in their article on publishing opportunities for nurses, offered information on editorial style, time for acceptance and publication, reasons for rejection, and acceptance rate for 83 U.S. journals in nursing and related health fields. As their survey showed, some journals are far more competitive than others. For example, *Nursing Research* accepted only 20% of submitted manuscripts, whereas the acceptance rates for many specialty journals was greater than 50%. Another resource is the Key Nursing Journals Chart, which can be accessed at the website of the Nursing and Allied Health Resource Section, Medical Library Association (*http:// nahrs.library.kent. edu/resource/index.html*). The chart indicates valuable information for numerous nursing journals, although some website information is now out of date. Also, McConnell (2000) has compiled information on 82 non-U.S. nursing journals.

TABLE 26.1 Peer-Reviewed Nursing Journals With High Concentration of Research Articles

NAME OF JOURNAL	Impact Factor in 2005[a]	Journal Rank, 2005[b]	APA Ref. Style?[c]
American Journal of Critical Care	1.343		
Applied Nursing Research	0.580	19	X
Archives of Psychiatric Nursing	0.527	21	X
Australian Journal of Advanced Nursing			
Birth	1.836	1	
Canadian Journal of Nursing Research			X
Cancer Nursing	0.823	11	
Clinical Nursing Research			X
Curationis			
Heart & Lung	0.863		X
International Journal of Nursing Practice			
International Journal of Nursing Studies	0.843	10	
Issues in Mental Health Nursing			X
Journal of Advanced Nursing	0.912	7	
Journal of Clinical Nursing	1.027	4	X
Journal of Family Nursing			X
Journal of National Black Nurses Association			X
Journal of Nursing Measurement			X
Journal of Nursing Scholarship	0.945	6	X
Journal of Pediatric Nursing			X
Midwifery	0.746	13	
Nursing History Review	0.105	28	
Nursing Research	1.528	2	X
Public Health Nursing	0.693	16	X
Qualitative Health Research	0.938		X
Research in Nursing & Health	1.077	3	X
Scandinavian Journal of Caring Sciences			
Western Journal of Nursing Research	0.745	14	X

[a]Impact factor information is from *Journal Citation Reports*, downloaded on August 18, 2006 from *http://jcrl.isiknowledge.com/JCR/JCR*. Journals without an entry were not rated in 2005. Highly ranked nursing journals are not listed if they are not primarily research focused (e.g., *Nursing Science Quarterly*, impact factor = 0.980 in 2005).

[b]The ranks shown are for rankings within the Nursing category of the *JCR Social Science Edition*; journals with an impact factor but no ranking were ranked in other categories—e.g., *Qualitative Health Research* ranked 23rd in the category "Health Policy & Services."

[c]APA, American Psychological Association (2001).

It may be useful to send a **query letter** to a journal to ask the editor whether there is interest in a manuscript. The query letter should briefly describe the topic and methods, a preliminary title, and a tentative submission date. Query letters are not essential if you have done a lot of homework about the journal's goals, but they might help to avoid problems that arise if editors have recently accepted several papers on a similar topic and do not wish to consider another. Indeed, the top three reasons cited by journal editors for rejecting manuscripts were an unsuitable topic for the journal, a noncurrent topic, and similarity to articles recently published (Northam et al., 2000). Query letters can be submitted by traditional mail or by e-mail using contact information provided at the journal's website.

Query letters can be sent to multiple journals simultaneously, but ultimately the manuscript can be submitted only to one—or rather, to one at a time. If several editors express interest in reviewing a manuscript, journals can be prioritized according to criteria previously described. The priority list should not be discarded because the manuscript can be resubmitted to the next journal on the list if the journal of first choice rejects it.

➔ **T I P :** One useful strategy in selecting a journal is to peruse your citation list. Journals that appear in your list have published related reports, and are strong candidates for publishing new studies on your topic.

Preparing the Manuscript

Once a journal has been selected, the information included in the journal's **Instructions to Authors** should be carefully reviewed. These instructions typically give authors such information as maximum page length; what font and margins are permissible; what type of abstract is desired; what reference style should be used; and how to submit the manuscript. Increasingly, manuscripts must be submitted online rather than sending hard copies to the journal. It is important to adhere to the journal's guidelines to avoid rejection for a nonsubstantive reason.

➔ **T I P :** Don't begin to write until you have identified a high-quality research report that you can use as a model. Select a journal article on a topic similar to your own, or one that used similar methods, in the journal you have selected as first choice. When you have written a draft, a review by colleagues or advisors can be invaluable in improving its quality.

Typically, a manuscript for journals must be no more than 15 to 20 pages, double-spaced (with 1-inch margins) in its entirety. In a typical article, the greatest space should be allocated to methods and results.

Care should be taken in using and preparing citations. Some nursing journals suggest that there be not more than 15 references. In general, only published work can be cited (e.g., not papers at a conference or manuscripts submitted but not accepted for publication). As shown in Table 26.1, most journals use the reference style of the American Psychological Association (APA, 2001), which is the style we use throughout this book.

➔ **T I P :** There is a wealth of online resources to assist you with the APA style, including an APA "cribsheet" (*http://www.docstyles.com*) and tutorials at university libraries. Several websites are listed on the accompanying CD-ROM for you to click on directly.

Submission of a Manuscript

When the manuscript is ready for journal submission, a cover letter should be drafted. The cover letter should include the following information: title of the paper, name and contact information of the **corresponding author** (the author with whom the journal communicates—usually, but not always, the lead author), and assurances that (1) the paper is original and has not been published or submitted elsewhere; (2) all authors have read and approved the manuscript; and (3) (in certain situations) there are no conflicts of interest. Many journals also require a signed copyright transfer form, which transfers all copyright ownership of the manuscript to the journal and warrants that all authors signing the form participated sufficiently in the research to justify authorship.

Manuscript Review

Most nursing journals that include research reports—including all those listed in Table 26.1—have a policy of independent, anonymous (**blind**) **peer reviews** by two or more experts in the field. By "anonymous," we mean that reviewers do not know the identity of the authors, and authors do not learn the identity of reviewers. Journals that have such a policy are **refereed journals**, and are in general more prestigious than nonrefereed journals. When submitting a manuscript to a refereed journal, authors' names should not appear anywhere except on the title page.

Peer reviewers make recommendations to the editors about whether to accept the manuscript for publication, accept it contingent on revisions, or reject it. Relatively few papers are accepted outright—both substantive and editorial revisions are the norm. Becker (2004) has described how the review process works at *Research in Nursing & Health*.

Example of reviewer recommendation categories: The journal *Research in Nursing & Health* asks reviewers to make one of six recommendations to the editorial staff: (1) Highly recommend; few revisions needed; (2) Publish if suggested revisions are satisfactorily completed; (3) Major revisions needed; revised version should be re-reviewed; (4) May have potential; encourage resubmission as a new manuscript; (5) Reject; do not encourage resubmission; and (6) Not appropriate for journal; send to another type of journal. Reviewers also complete a brief questionnaire that asks such questions as, "Are the interpretations and conclusions justified by the results?"

Authors are sent information about the editors' decision, together with reviewers' comments. When resubmitting a revised manuscript to the same journal, each reviewer recommendation should be addressed, either by making the requested change, or by explaining in the cover letter accompanying the resubmission the rationale for not revising. Defending some aspect of a paper against a reviewer's recommendation sometimes requires a

citation or other supporting information. If the manuscript is rejected, the reviewers' comments should be taken into consideration before submitting it to another journal. Competition for journal space is keen, and a rejection does not necessarily mean that a study is unworthy of publication. Manuscripts may need to be reviewed by several journals before final acceptance.

> **➲ TIP:** For some articles, the journal *Nursing Research* makes supplementary information available on the Internet, including information documenting the review process (e.g., Beck's 2006 study on the anniversary of birth trauma). These are posted at *http://www.nursing-research-editor.com*. The supplemental information is often a rich source of data for a meta-analysis.

Typically, many months go by between submission of the original manuscript and the publication of a journal article, especially if there are revisions, as there usually are. For example, according to information provided in the Northam and colleagues (2000) survey, an average of 7 months elapsed between submission and acceptance in *Western Journal of Nursing Research*, and an additional 18 months elapsed before publication.

Example of journal timeline: While working on this book, Polit and Beck (2006) discovered that nurse researchers were using alternative, but unspecified, methods to compute a content validity index for new scales. They developed a paper about this and submitted it to a journal with a high impact factor, *Research in Nursing & Health*. The timeline for acceptance and publication of this manuscript, which was relatively fast, is as follows:

December 12, 2005	Manuscript submitted to *Research in Nursing & Health (RINAH)* editor for review
February 6, 2006	Letter from editor informing of a revise-and-resubmit decision
February 19, 2006	Revised manuscript resubmitted
May 19, 2006	Revised manuscript accepted for publication
October, 2006	Publication in *RINAH*

Electronic Publication

Computers and the Internet have changed forever how information of all types is disseminated. Many nurse researchers are exploring opportunities to share their research findings through electronic publication. Most journals that publish in hard copy format (e.g., *Nursing Research*) now also have online capabilities. Such mechanisms, which serve as a document delivery system, expand a journal's circulation and make findings accessible worldwide, but they have little implications for authors. Such electronic publication is just a method of distributing reports already available in hard copy.

There are, however, other ways to disseminate research findings on the Internet. For example, some researchers or research teams develop their own web page with information about their studies. When there are hyperlinks embedded in the websites, consumers can navigate between files and websites to retrieve relevant information on a topic of interest. At the other extreme are peer-reviewed electronic journals (**ejournals**) that are exclusively in online format, such as the *Online Journal of Issues in Nursing*. In between are a variety of outlets of research communication, such as websites of nursing organizations and electronic magazines.

Electronic publication is advantageous in that dissemination can occur more rapidly, cutting down on publication lag time. Electronic research reports are accessible to a worldwide audience of potential consumers, typically without page limitations, thus enabling researchers to describe and discuss complex studies more fully. Qualitative researchers are able to use more extensive quotes from their raw data, for example. Research reports on the Internet can incorporate a variety of graphic material, including audio and video supplements not possible in hard copy journals. Raw data can also be appended to reports on the Internet for secondary analysis by other researchers.

Still, there are some potential drawbacks, one of which concerns peer review. Although many online journals perform peer reviews, there are many opportunities to "publish" results on the Internet without a peer review process. Although there are also non–peer-reviewed traditional journals, non-refereed journal articles are not as accessible worldwide as nonreviewed information on the Internet. There is a greater risk of having a glut of low-quality research available for consumption via the Internet than there was previously. Researchers who want their evidence to have an impact on nursing practice should seek publication in outlets that subject manuscripts to external review.

Presentations at Professional Conferences

Numerous international, national, and regional professional organizations sponsor meetings at which nursing studies are presented, either through the reading of a research report or through visual display in a poster session. Examples include the American Nurses Association and Sigma Theta Tau. Professional conferences are particularly good forums for presenting results to clinical audiences. Researchers also can take advantage of meeting and talking with others attending the conference who are working on similar problems in different parts of the country.

The mechanism for submitting a presentation to a conference is simpler than for journal submission. The association sponsoring the conference ordinarily publishes an announcement or **Call for Abstracts** in its newsletter, journal, or website 6 to 9 months before the meeting date. The notice indicates topics of interest, submission requirements, and deadlines for submitting a proposed paper or poster. Most universities and major health care agencies receive and post Call for Abstracts notices. The *Western Journal of Nursing Research* also publishes a calendar of national and international conferences at the beginning of each issue.

Oral Reports

Most conferences require prospective presenters to submit abstracts of 500 to 1000 words rather than complete papers. Abstracts are usually submitted online. Each conference has its own guidelines for abstract content and form. In some cases, abstracts are submitted to the organizer of a particular session; in other cases, conference sessions are organized after the fact, with related papers grouped together. Abstracts are evaluated based on the quality and originality of the research and the appropriateness of the paper for the conference audience. If abstracts are accepted, researchers are committed to appear at the conference to make a presentation.

Reports presented at professional meetings usually follow a traditional IMRAD format. The time allotted for presentation usually is about 10 to 15 minutes, with up to 5 minutes for questions from the audience. Thus, only the most important aspects of the study, with special emphasis on the results, can be included. It is especially challenging to condense a qualitative report to a brief oral summary without losing the rich, in-depth character of the data. A handy rule of thumb is that a page of double-spaced text requires 2½ to 3 minutes to read aloud. Although most presenters prepare a written paper or a script, presentations are most effective if they are delivered informally or conversationally, rather than if they are read verbatim. The presentation should be rehearsed to gain familiarity and comfort with the script, and to ensure that time limits are not exceeded.

TIP: Most conference presentations can be greatly enhanced by including visual materials, notably, Power Point materials. Visual materials should be kept simple for biggest impact. Tables are difficult to read on a slide but can be distributed to members of the audience in hard copy form. Make sure a sufficient number of copies is available.

The question-and-answer period can be a fruitful opportunity to expand on various aspects of the research and to get early feedback about the study. It is useful to make note of audience comments because these can be helpful in turning the conference presentation into a manuscript for journal submission.

Poster Presentations

Researchers sometimes present their findings in poster sessions. Abstracts, often similar to those required for oral presentations, must be submitted to conference organizers according to specific guidelines. In poster sessions, several researchers simultaneously present visual displays summarizing the highlights of their study, and conference attendees circulate around the exhibit area perusing displays. In this fashion, those interested in a particular topic can devote time to discussing the study with the researcher and bypass posters dealing with topics of less interest. Poster sessions are thus efficient and encourage one-on-one discussions. Poster sessions are typically 1 to 2 hours in length; researchers should stand near their posters throughout the session to ensure effective communication.

It is challenging to design an effective poster. The poster must convey essential information about the background, design, and results of a study, in a format that can be perused in minutes. Bullet points, graphs, and photos are especially useful devices on a poster for communicating a lot of information quickly. Large, bold fonts are essential because posters are often read from a distance of several feet. Another issue is that posters must be sturdily constructed for transport to the conference site. It is important to follow the conference guidelines in determining such matters as poster size (often 4 feet high $\times$ 6 or 8 feet wide), format, allowable display materials, and so on.

Several authors have offered advice on preparing for poster sessions (e.g., Keely, 2004; Gosling, 1999; Moore et al., 2001). Russell and colleagues (1996) have alerted qualitative researchers to the special challenges that await them in designing a poster. There is also software available for producing posters (*http://www.postersw.com*).

CRITIQUING WRITTEN RESEARCH REPORTS

Although the worth of the study itself can be evaluated using guidelines we have presented throughout this book, the manner in which study information is communicated in the research report can also be critiqued in a comprehensive critical appraisal. Box 26.2 summarizes major points to consider in evaluating the presentation of a research report.

BOX 26.2 Guidelines for Critiquing the Presentation of a Research Report

1. Does the report include a sufficient amount of detail to permit a thorough critique of the study's purpose, conceptual framework, design and methods, handling of ethical issues, analysis of data, and interpretation?
2. Is the report well written and grammatical? Are pretentious words or jargon used when a simpler wording would have been possible?
3. Is the report well organized? Is there an orderly, logical presentation of ideas? Is the report characterized by continuity of thought and expression?
4. Does the report effectively combine text with tables or figures?
5. Does the report suggest overt biases, exaggerations, or distortions?
6. Is the report written using appropriately tentative language?
7. Is sexist language avoided?
8. Does the title of the report adequately capture the key concepts and the population under investigation? Does the abstract (if any) adequately summarize the research problem, study methods, and important findings?

An important issue is whether the report provided sufficient information for a thoughtful critique of the other dimensions. When vital pieces of information are missing, researchers leave readers little choice but to assume the worst because this would lead to the most cautious interpretation of the results.

Styles of writing differ for qualitative and quantitative reports, and it is unreasonable to apply the standards considered appropriate for one paradigm to the other. Regardless of style, however, you should, in critiquing a report, be alert to indications of overt biases, unwarranted exaggerations, or melodramatic language.

In summary, the research report is meant to be an account of how and why a problem was studied and what results were obtained. The report should be clearly written, cogent, concise, and written in a manner that piques readers' interest and curiosity.

SUMMARY POINTS

- In developing a dissemination plan, researchers need to select a communication outlet (e.g., journal article versus conference presentation), identify the audience whom they wish to reach,

and decide on the content that can be effectively communicated in a single outlet.
- In the planning stage, researchers need to decide authorship credits (if there are multiple authors), who the **lead author** and **corresponding author** will be, and in what order authors' names will be listed.
- Quantitative reports (and many qualitative reports) typically follow the **IMRAD format**, with the following sections: introduction, method, results, and discussion.
- The *introduction* acquaints readers with the research problem. It includes the problem statement, the phenomenon under study, research hypotheses or questions, a summary of relevant related literature, identification of a framework, and definitions of the concepts being studied. In qualitative reports, the introduction also indicates the research tradition and, if relevant, the researchers' connection to the problem.
- The *method section* describes what researchers did to solve the research problem. It includes a description of the study design (or an elaboration of the research tradition); the study participants and how they were selected; instruments and procedures used to collect and evaluate the data; and techniques used to analyze the data.

- Researchers reporting on a clinical trial increasingly follow **CONSORT guidelines** (Consolidated Standards of Reporting Trials), including the use of a flow chart that shows the flow of subjects in and out of a study.
- In the *results section*, findings from the analyses are summarized. Qualitative reports summarize findings sequentially (if a process is being described) or in the order of salience of themes. Results sections in qualitative reports necessarily intertwine description and interpretation. Quotes from transcripts are essential for giving voice to study participants.
- Both qualitative and quantitative researchers include **figures** and **tables** that dramatize or succinctly summarize major findings or conceptual schema.
- The *discussion section* presents the interpretation of results, how the findings relate to earlier research, study limitations, and implications of the findings for nursing practice and future research.
- The major types of research reports are theses and dissertations, journal articles, online publications, and presentations at professional meetings.
- Theses and dissertations normally follow a standard IMRAD format, but some schools are now accepting **paper format theses**, which include an introduction, one or more papers ready to submit for publication, and a conclusion.
- In selecting a journal for publication, the following factors should be kept in mind: the journal's goals and audience, its prestige and acceptance rates, how often it publishes, and its circulation. One proxy for a journal's prestige is its **impact factor**, the ratio between citations to a journal and recent citable items published.
- Before beginning to prepare a **manuscript** for submission to a journal, researchers need to carefully review the journal's **Instructions to Authors**. Most journals limit manuscripts to 15 to 20 typed, double-spaced pages, for example.
- Most nursing journals that publish research reports are **refereed journals** with a policy of basing publication decisions on **peer reviews** that are usually **blind reviews** (identities of authors and reviewers are not divulged).
- There are many new opportunities for electronic publishing that nurse researchers can explore, including publications in **ejournals**. Electronic publishing offers the advantage of speedy dissemination to a worldwide audience. Peer-reviewed electronic publications are preferred for building a strong evidence base for nursing practice.
- Nurse researchers can also present their research at professional conferences, either through a 10- to 15-minute oral report to a seated audience, or in a **poster session** in which the "audience" moves around a room perusing research summaries attached to posters. Sponsoring organizations usually issue a **Call for Abstracts** for the conference 6 to 9 months before it is held.

STUDY ACTIVITIES

Chapter 26 of the accompanying *Resource Manual for Nursing Research: Generating and Assessing Evidence for Nursing Practice, 8th edition*, offers various exercises and study suggestions for reinforcing the concepts presented in this chapter. In addition, the following questions can be addressed:

1. Skim a qualitative and a quantitative research report. Make a bullet-point list of differences in style and organization between the two.
2. Read a research report. Write a two- to three-page summary of the report that communicates the major points of the report to a clinical audience with minimal research skills.

STUDIES CITED IN CHAPTER 26

Methodologic or theoretical references cited in this chapter can be found in a separate section at the end of the book.

Hill, W., Weinert, C., & Cudney, S. (2006). Influence of a computer intervention on the psychological status of chronically ill rural women. *Nursing Research, 55*(1), 34–42.

Polit, D., & Beck, C. T. (2006). The content validity index: Are you sure you know what's being reported?

Critique and recommendations. *Research in Nursing & Health, 29*(5), 489–497.

Shambley-Ebron, D., & Boyle, J. (2006). Self-care and mothering in African American women with HIV/AIDS. *Western Journal of Nursing Research, 28*(1), 42–60.

27

Writing Proposals to Generate Evidence

Research proposals are documents that communicate a research problem and proposed methods of solving it to an interested party. Research proposals are written both by students seeking faculty approval for projects, and by seasoned researchers seeking financial support. In this chapter, we offer tips on how to improve the quality of research proposals and how to develop proficiency in **grantsmanship**—the set of skills involved in securing project funding.

OVERVIEW OF RESEARCH PROPOSALS

In this section, we provide some general information regarding research proposals. Most of the information applies equally to dissertation proposals and grant applications.

Functions of a Proposal

Proposals are a means of opening communication between researchers and other parties. Those parties are typically either funding agencies or faculty advisors, whose job it is to accept or reject the proposed plan, or to demand modifications. An accepted proposal is a two-way contract: those accepting the proposal are effectively saying, "We are willing to offer our (emotional or financial) support, as long as the study proceeds as proposed," and those writing the proposal are saying, "If you offer support, then we will conduct the study as proposed."

Proposals often serve as the basis for negotiating with other parties as well. For example, a proposal may be used to secure institutional approval to conduct a study (e.g., for gaining access to participants or for using facilities). Proposals are often incorporated into submissions to human subjects committees or Institutional Review Boards.

Proposals usually help researchers to clarify their own thinking. By committing ideas to writing, ambiguities about how to proceed can be addressed at an early stage. Proposal reviewers also offer suggestions for conceptual and methodologic refinements.

When studies are undertaken collaboratively, proposals can help ensure that all researchers are "on the same page" about how the study is to proceed, and who is responsible for which tasks. Having a shared and agreed-upon document enhances communication among researchers and minimizes the possibility of friction.

Proposal Content

Proposal reviewers—faculty, sponsors, or peer reviewers—want a clear idea of what the researcher plans to study, why the study is needed, what specific methods will be used to achieve study goals, how and when tasks are to be accomplished, and whether the researcher has the skills to successfully complete the project. Proposals are usually evaluated on a number of criteria, including the importance of the research question, the adequacy of the research methods, the availability of appropriate personnel and facilities, and, if money is being requested, the reasonableness of the budget.

Proposal authors are usually given instructions about how to structure proposals. Funding agencies often supply an application kit that includes forms to be completed and specifies the format for organizing proposal contents. Universities usually issue guidelines for dissertation proposals.

Despite the fact that formats and the amount of detail required may vary widely, there is some similarity in the type of information that is expected in research proposals. The content and organization are broadly similar to those for a research report, but proposals are written in the future tense (i.e., indicating what the researcher *will* do) and obviously do not include results and conclusions. The description of proposed methods—what the researchers plan to do to develop evidence that is valid and trustworthy—is critically important to the success of the proposal.

Later in this chapter, we provide more detail about the contents for grant applications to the National Institutes of Health (NIH). Although the organization and mix of content vary for different funding agencies or proposal purposes, there is considerable overlap with other types of proposals.

Proposals for Qualitative Studies

Preparing proposals for qualitative research entails special challenges. Methodologic decisions typically evolve in the field, and therefore it is seldom possible to provide detailed, specific information about such matters as sample size, data collection strategies, data analysis, and so on. Enough detail needs to be provided, however, that reviewers will have confidence that the researcher will collect strong data and do justice to the data collected.

Qualitative researchers must persuade reviewers that the topic is important and worth studying, that they are sufficiently knowledgeable about the challenges of fieldwork and adequately skillful in eliciting rich data, and, in short, that the project would be a very good risk. Knafl and Deatrick (2005) offered 10 tips for successful qualitative proposals. The first tip was to make the case for the *idea*, not the method. They also advised qualitative researchers to avoid methodologic tutorials, to use examples to clarify the research design, and to write for both the experts and the skeptics.

Many resources have become available to help qualitative researchers with proposal development. For example, an entire issue of the journal *Qualitative Health Research* was devoted to writing proposals—the July 2003 issue (volume 13, number 6). Other useful information is available in Morse and Field (1995), Morse and Richards (2002), and Sandelowski, Davis, and Harris (1989).

Proposals for Theses and Dissertations

Dissertation proposals are sometimes a bigger hurdle than dissertations themselves. Many doctoral candidates flounder at the proposal development stage rather than while writing or defending the dissertation. Much of our advice—especially in our "Tips" section later in the chapter—applies equally to proposals for theses and dissertations and to grant applications, but some additional advice might prove helpful.

The Dissertation Committee

Choosing the right advisor (if an advisor is chosen rather than appointed) is almost as important as choosing the right topic to research. The ideal advisor is one who is a mentor, an expert with a strong reputation in the field, a good teacher, a patient and supportive coach and critic, and an advocate. The ideal advisor is also a person who has sufficient time and interest to devote to your research and someone who is likely to stick with your project until its completion. This means that it might matter whether the prospective advisor has plans for a sabbatical leave, or is nearing retirement. Having consistent guidance throughout the project may be more helpful than having brilliant mentoring for only part of the project and then having to switch horses in midstream.

Dissertation committees often involve three or more members. If the advisor lacks certain of the "ideal" characteristics, it is wise to balance those characteristics across committee members by seeking people with complementary talents. Putting together a group who will work well together and who have no personal antagonism toward each other can, however, be tricky. Advisors can usually make good suggestions about other committee members.

Once a committee has been chosen, it is important to develop a good working relationship with members and to learn about their viewpoints before and during the proposal development stage. This means, at a minimum, becoming familiar with their research and the methodologic strategies they have favored. It also means meeting with them and sounding them out with ideas about topics and methods. If the suggestions from two or more members are at odds, it is prudent to seek your advisor's counsel on how to resolve this.

⊃ TIP: When meeting with your advisor and committee members, take notes about their suggestions, and write them out in more detail after the meeting while they are still fresh in your mind. The notes should be reviewed while developing the proposal.

Practices vary from one institution to another and from advisor to advisor, but some faculty require a written prospectus before giving the go-ahead to prepare the full proposal. The prospectus is usually a three- to four-page paper outlining the research questions and the proposed methods.

Content of Dissertation Proposals
Specific requirements regarding the length and format of dissertation proposals vary in different settings, and it is important to know at the outset what is expected. Typically, dissertation proposals are 20 to 40 pages in length. In some cases, however, committees prefer what Sternberg (1981) described as a "mini-dissertation," that is, a document with fully developed sections that can be inserted with minor adaptation into the dissertation itself. For example, the review of the literature, theoretical framework, hypothesis formulation, and bibliography may be sufficiently refined at the proposal stage that they can be incorporated into the final product.

Literature reviews are often the most important section of a dissertation proposal (at least for quantitative studies) and thus merit special attention. Although not all committees want lengthy literature reviews, they certainly want to be assured that students are in command of knowledge in their field of inquiry.

Dissertation proposals sometimes include elements not normally found in proposals to funding agencies. One such element may be table shells (see Chapter 24), which are designed to demonstrate that the student knows how to analyze data and present results effectively. Another element is a draft of the table of contents for the dissertation. The table of contents serves as an outline for the final product, and shows that the student knows how to organize material.

Several books provide additional advice on writing a dissertation proposal, including those by Davis and Parker (1997) and Locke, Spirduso, and Silverman (2000).

FUNDING FOR RESEARCH PROPOSALS

Funding for research projects is becoming increasingly difficult to obtain because of keen and growing competition among researchers. As more nurses become prepared to do research, and as the push for evidence-based practice grows, so too will applications for research funds increase. Successful proposal writers need to have good research and proposal-writing skills, and they must also know from whom funding is available.

Federal Funding in the United States

The largest funder of research activities in the United States is the federal government. The two major types of federal disbursements are grants and contracts. **Grants** are awarded for studies conceived by researchers themselves, whereas **contracts** are for studies desired by the government.

Nurse researchers can seek federal funds for a research grant through a grant program of a government agency, such as NIH or the Agency for Healthcare Research and Quality (AHRQ). There are three basic mechanisms for federal grants, which can be awarded to researchers in both domestic and foreign institutions. One mechanism is for agencies and institutes to issue broad objectives relating to an overall mission, as the National Institute of Nursing Research (NINR) has done (see Chapter 1).

A second grant mechanism is for an agency to issue periodic **program announcements** (PAs) that describe new, continuing, or expanded program interests. For example, in June 2006, NINR issued a joint program announcement with two other NIH institutes titled "Behavioral and Social Research on Disasters and Health" (PA-06-454). The purpose of this PA, which expires in 2009, is "to stimulate research in the behavioral and social sciences on the consequences of natural and man-made disasters for the health of children, the elderly, and vulnerable groups, with an ultimate goal of preventing or mitigating harmful consequences. Examples of disasters include severe weather-related events, earthquakes, large-scale attacks on civilian populations, technological catastrophes or perceived catastrophes, and influenza pandemics." PAs are publicized on the websites of the relevant agencies, and *The Catalogue of Federal Domestic Assistance* publishes information about all federal programs that provide any kind of aid (*http://www.cfda.gov*).

The third grant mechanism allows federal agencies to identify a *specific* topic area in which they are interested in receiving proposals by a **Request for Applications (RFA)**. As an example, NINR issued an RFA entitled "Research on Research Integrity" in 2006. Unlike a PA, an RFA specifies a deadline for the receipt of proposals. General guidelines and goals for the competition are also specified, but researchers have considerable liberty to develop the specific research problem. Notices of such grant competitions are announced on the websites specific to each funding agency and are also published in *The Federal Register*, which is a daily publication of the Government Printing Office (*http://www.access.gpo. gov/su_docs*).

In addition to grants, government agencies also award contracts to do *specific* studies. Contract offers are announced in a **Request for Proposals (RFP)**, which details the *exact* study that the government wants done. Contracts, which are typically awarded to only one competitor, constrain researchers' activities, and so most nurse researchers compete for grants rather than contracts. Nevertheless, many interesting health-related RFPs have been issued. For example, NIH issued an RFP for a study of "Ethnic Differences in Life Style, Psychological Factors, and Medical Care during Pregnancy." A summary of federal RFPs is published in the *Commerce Business Daily* (*http://cbdnet.gpo.gov*). NIH also publishes the *NIH Guide for Grants and Contracts* weekly, available through the NIH website.

NIH and other agencies also offer career development support, including support for doctoral research. At NIH, there are two basic types of mentored career development grant programs, the Mentored Research Scientist Development Award (K01) and the Mentored Patient-Oriented Research Career Development Award (K23). These grants support research experience for doctorally prepared researchers who need a mentored research experience with an expert sponsor. In 2006, a new funding mechanism called Pathways to Independence Awards (K99) became available for postdoctoral research activity leading to the submission of an independent research project application.

Government funding for nursing research is, of course, also available in other countries. In Canada, for example, various types of health research are sponsored by the Canadian Institutes of Health

Research (CIHR). Information about CIHR's program of grants, training awards, and other funding opportunities is available at its website (*http://www.cihr.ca*).●

Private Funds

Health care research is supported by numerous philanthropic foundations, professional organizations, and corporations. Many researchers prefer private funding to government support because there is less "red tape" and fewer requirements. Not surprisingly, private organizations are besieged with proposed research projects.

Information about philanthropic foundations that support research is available through the Foundation Center (*http://www.fdncenter.org*).● The Foundation Center offers a wide variety of resources on foundation funding and how to secure it. The most comprehensive resource for identifying funding opportunities is the Center's *The Foundation Directory*, now available online for a fee. The directory lists the purposes and activities of the foundations and information for contacting them. The Foundation Center also offers seminars and training on grant writing and funding opportunities in locations around the United States, and has published two additional resources of relevance: *Guide to Grantseeking on the Web* and the *National Guide to Funding in Health*. Another resource for information on funding is the Community of Science, which maintains a database on funding opportunities (*http://www.cos.com*).●

Professional associations (e.g., the American Nurses Foundation, Sigma Theta Tau) offer funds for conducting research. Health organizations, such as the American Heart Association and the American Cancer Society, also support research activities.

Finally, research funding is sometimes donated by private corporations, particularly those dealing with health care products. The Foundation Center publishes a directory of corporate grantmakers and provides links through its website to a number of corporate philanthropic programs. Additional information concerning corporate requirements and interests should be obtained either from the organization directly or from staff in the research administration offices of the institution with which you are affiliated.

GRANT APPLICATIONS TO THE NATIONAL INSTITUTES OF HEALTH

NIH funds many nursing studies through NINR and through other institutes. Because of the importance of NINR as a funding source for nurse researchers, this section describes the process of proposal submission and review at NIH. (It should be noted that AHRQ, which also funds nurse-initiated studies, uses the same application kit and similar procedures.)

NIH Applications

Until recently, applications for NIH funding were made by completing and submitting a paper form (Public Health Service Grant Application Form PHS 398), but in 2006–2007, NIH transitioned to electronic submission using the SF424 (R&R) application through *Grants.gov*. Researchers require special software (PureEdge) to "fill in" and complete this new application. There is abundant information online about the new application process, and NIH offers training sessions on how to submit applications electronically. The application kit can be accessed from the NIH website at *http://www.nih.gov* under the "Grants and Opportunities" section.●

New grant applications are usually processed in three cycles annually. Different deadlines apply to different types of grants, but for most new grants (except for AIDS-related research applications) the deadline for receipt is 5 PM on February 1, June 1, and October 1. As shown in Table 27.1, the scientific merit review dates are about 4 to 5 months after each submission due date. For example, applications for the February 1 cycle are reviewed in June or July; the earliest project start date for applications in that cycle would be in December. Applicants

TABLE 27.1	Schedule for Processing New Research Project (R01) and Small Grant (R03) Applications, National Institutes of Health

APPLICATION DEADLINE	SCIENTIFIC MERIT REVIEW DATES	ADVISORY COUNCIL REVIEW DATES	EARLIEST POSSIBLE START DATES
February 1	June/July	September/October	December
June 1	October/November	January/February	April
October 1	February/March	May/June	July

All AIDS-related research applications are due January 2, May 1, and September 1.

should begin a registration process at least 2 to 4 weeks before the submission date.

Types of NIH Grants

NIH awards different types of research grants, and each has its own objectives and review criteria. The basic grant program—and the primary funding mechanism for independent research—is the **Research Project Grant** (R01). The objective of R01 grants is to support specific research projects in areas reflecting the interests and competencies of a Principal Investigator (PI). As of January 2007, the five explicitly stated review criteria were as follows:

1. *Significance*. Does this study address an important problem? If the aims of the application are achieved, how will scientific knowledge be advanced? What will be the effect of the study on the concepts or methods that drive this field?
2. *Approach*. Are the conceptual framework, design, methods, and analyses adequately developed and appropriate to the aims of the project? Does the applicant acknowledge potential problem areas and consider alternative tactics?
3. *Innovation*. Does the project employ novel concepts, approaches, or methods? Are the aims original and innovative? Does the project challenge existing paradigms or develop new methods or technologies?
4. *Investigator*. Is the investigator appropriately trained and well suited to carry out this work?

Is the work proposed appropriate to the experience level of the principal investigator and other researchers?

5. *Environment*. Does the scientific environment in which the work will be done contribute to the probability of success? Do the proposed experiments take advantage of unique features of the scientific environment or employ useful collaborative arrangements? Is there evidence of institutional support?

In addition to these five criteria, other factors are relevant in evaluating R01 proposals, including the reasonableness of the proposed budget, the adequacy of protections for human or animal subjects, and the appropriateness of the sampling plan in terms of including women, minorities, and children as participants.

Beside the R01 grant program, three others are worth noting. A special program (R15) has been established for researchers working in institutions that have not been major participants in NIH programs. These **Academic Research Enhancement Awards** (**AREA**) are designed to stimulate research in institutions that provide baccalaureate training for many individuals who go on to do health-related research. There is also a **Small Grant** Program (R03) that provides support for pilot or feasibility studies. R03 grants provide a maximum of $50,000 of direct support for up to 2 years. Finally, the R21 grant mechanism—the **Exploratory/Developmen-**

tal Research Grant Award—is intended to encourage new, exploratory and developmental research projects by providing support for the early stages of their development.

TIP: If you have an idea for a study and are not sure which type of grant program is suitable—or you are unsure whether NINR or another NIH institute might be interested—you should contact NINR directly (the telephone number is 301-594-6906). NINR staff can provide feedback about whether your proposed study matches NINR's program interests. Information about NINR's ongoing areas of research interests and areas of current opportunity is available at *http://www.nih.gov/ninr*. A one- to two-page concept paper can also be e-mailed to the address listed on the NINR website.

Preparing a Grant Application for NIH

Although the forms and procedures for NIH grant applications are changing, substantive aspects of the NIH grant application have not changed. Nevertheless, it is important to carefully review up-to-date instructions in preparing a grant application rather than relying on information in this chapter, inasmuch as many modifications are occurring during the transition period.

Forms: Screens and Uploaded Attachments
In the new SF424, the "front matter" consists of various forms that appear on a series of fillable screens. These forms help in processing the application and provide administrative information. Careful attention to detail with these forms is very important. Major forms include the following:

- *Cover Component.* On the cover form, researchers provide a descriptive title of the project (not to exceed 81 spaces), the name and affiliation of the PI, and other administrative information.

TIP: The project title should be given careful thought. It is the first thing that reviewers see, and should be crafted to create a good impression. The title should be concise and informative, but should also be compelling and interesting.

- *Project/Performance Site Location Component.* The next screen requests information about the primary site where the work will be performed.
- *Other Project Information Component.* This screen provides the mechanism for submitting key information. The form begins with questions about human subjects, and the last few items require attachments to be uploaded, including a project summary, a project narrative, bibliography, and facilities and equipment information. Attachments must be in PDF format and have strict size limitations. The *Project Summary* is intended to serve as a succinct, accurate description of the proposed study and must be no longer than 30 lines. For NIH applications, the *Project Narrative* is a brief (two or three sentences) description of the relevance of the research to public health. The *Bibliography* is a list of references cited in the research plan; any reference style is acceptable. The *Facilities* attachment is used to describe needed and available resources (e.g., laboratories).
- *Senior/Key Person Profile(s) Component.* For each key person proposed, the form requests basic identifying information and calls for two attachments: a biographical sketch and a description of current and pending support on other grants. The sketch must list education and training and a description of (a) positions and honors; (b) selected peer-reviewed publications or manuscripts in press; and (c) recently completed and ongoing research support. A maximum of four pages is permitted for each person.
- *Budget Component.* For NIH applications, researchers must choose between two budget options—the R&R Budget Component or the PHS398 Modular Budget Component. Detailed R&R budgets showing specific projected expenses are required if annual direct project costs exceed $250,000, but for smaller projects, budget information is obtained in another section.

These SF424 forms must be used to apply for funding in many federal agencies, but for grant applications to NIH and other public health service agencies, there are additional forms. These forms, referred to as PHS398 components, include the following:

- *Cover Letter Component.* Cover letters to the funding agency are encouraged. Information in the cover letter should include the application title, the name and number of the funding opportunity (the PA or RFA initiative), and a request to be assigned to a particular review group.
- *Cover Page Supplement Component.* This form supplements the SF424 cover page and requests mainly administrative information.

➲ **TIP:** One field on this Cover Page Supplement asks whether the PI is a *new* investigator (no prior R01 awards). NIH encourages new investigators to self-identify so they can be given special consideration. Peer reviewers are instructed to focus more on the proposed approach than on the PI's track record, and to expect less preliminary data than would be provided by an established investigator.

- *Modular Budget Component.* **Modular budgets**, paid in modules of $25,000, are appropriate for most applications requesting $250,000 or less per year of direct costs. (**Direct costs** include specific project-related costs such as staff and supplies; **indirect costs** are institutional **overhead** costs.) This form provides budget fields for annual summaries of projected costs for up to 5 years of support. There are also fields for cumulative summaries across all project years. A *budget justification* attachment, detailing primarily personnel costs, must be uploaded.

➲ **TIP:** Even though the modular budget form asks only for summaries of the funds needed to complete a study, you will have to prepare a more detailed budget for yourself to come up with a reasonable projection of needed funds. Beginning researchers are likely to need the assistance of a research administrator or an experienced, funded researcher in developing their first budget. Higdon and Topp (2004) have offered some advice on developing a budget.

- *Research Plan Component.* The PHS398 Research Plan form asks about application type (new, resubmission, revision, etc.) and then requires information, in the form of attachments, about the proposed study and the research plan. Research plan requirements are described in the next section.
- *Checklist Component.* The checklist includes various miscellaneous items, including organizational assurances and certifications.

Examples of all the forms for SF424 and PHS398 are presented in the Toolkit of the *Resource Manual* in nonfillable form—that is, they are included simply as illustrations, not to be used for submitting a grant application.✪

The Research Plan Component

The research plan component consists of 18 items, not all of which are relevant to every application—for example, several items are for revised applications or for continuation grants. Each item involves uploading separate PDF attachments. Items 2 through 5 are the core of the grant application, and, taken together, must not exceed 25 single-spaced pages, including any figures, charts, or tables. Applications that do not adhere to this page restriction are returned without review.

In this section, we briefly describe guidelines for items 2 through 18, with emphasis on items 2 through 5. We also present some advice based on an important study (Inouye & Fiellin, 2005) in which the researchers content-analyzed the criticisms articulated in the review sheets of 66 R01 applications submitted to a clinical research review group (not NINR). Thus, the advice relating to specific pitfalls can be considered "evidence-based," that is, based on issues identified as problematic in actual applications.

➲ **TIP:** Based on their analysis, Inouye and Fiellin (2005) created a grant-writing checklist designed as a self-assessment tool for proposal developers. We have included an adapted and expanded checklist in the Toolkit that is part of the accompanying *Resource Manual.*

Specific Aims (Item 2). In this section, researchers must provide a succinct summary of the research problem and the specific objectives to be undertaken, including any hypotheses to be tested. The aims statement should indicate the scope and importance of the problem. Care should be taken to be precise, and to identify a problem of manageable proportions—a broad and complex problem is unlikely to be solvable. The guidelines suggest that the Specific Aims be restricted to a single page.

Inouye and Fiellin (2005) found that the most frequent critique of the Specific Aims section was that the stated goals were overstated, overly ambitious, or unrealistic (18% of the review sheets). Other complaints were that the project was poorly conceptualized (15%) or that hypotheses were not clearly articulated (12%).

Background and Significance (Item 3). In this section, researchers must convince reviewers that the proposed study idea is sound and has clinical or theoretical relevance. Researchers provide the context for the study in this section, usually through a brief analysis of existing knowledge and gaps on the topic and through a discussion of a conceptual framework. Although researchers should demonstrate their command of current knowledge in a field, this section must be tightly written. NIH recommends restricting this section to two or three pages. This is challenging, but we urge you not to be tempted to exceed the three-page guideline so that space can be conserved for a full elaboration of the proposed research methods. Inouye and Fiellin (2005) found that the most frequent critique expressed by reviewers about this section was that the need for the study was not adequately justified (29%).

Preliminary Studies (Item 4). This section is used to describe previous work by members of the project team that is relevant to the proposed study. This section—although it is required only for renewal proposals—gives you an opportunity to persuade reviewers that you have the skills and background needed to do the research. The Preliminary Studies section provides a forum for describing any relevant work that key staff have either completed or are in the process of doing. Any pilot work that has served as a foundation for the proposed project should be described in full. If the only relevant research you have completed is your dissertation, here is an opportunity to describe that research. Other items that might be described include previous uses of an instrument or an experimental procedure that will be used in the new study, relevant clinical or teaching experience, and experience with and outreach to special relevant populations (e.g., homeless youth). The point is that this section allows you to demonstrate that the proposed work grew out of some ongoing commitment to, interest in, or experience with the topic. For new applications, no more than six to eight pages should be devoted to item 4; fewer pages are often sufficient.

Inouye and Fiellin's (2005) analysis is especially illuminating with regard to this section. They found that the single biggest criticism across the 66 review sheets was that more pilot work was needed, mentioned in 41% of the reviews.

➲ **T I P :** Novice researchers sometimes mistakenly believe that the Preliminary Studies section is designed for a literature review. If you make this mistake, it will indicate that you are a novice *and* unable to follow instructions.

Research Design and Methods (Item 5). In the Research Design attachment, you must describe the methods you will use to conduct the study. Although there are no specific page limitations for this attachment, you should remember that you have only 25 pages in total for items 2 through 5 combined.

The Research Design section is the heart of the proposal. It should be written with extreme care and reviewed with a self-critical eye. This section should be concise, but with sufficient detail to persuade reviewers that there is a sound rationale for methodologic decisions and that the study will yield evidence that is valid. A thorough method section describes the following:

1. The research design, including a discussion of comparison group strategies, methods of

controlling confounding variables, number of data collection points, and so on; in a qualitative study, the research tradition should be described.

2. The experimental intervention (if applicable), including a description of both the treatment and the control group condition, what protocols will be used, and how intervention fidelity will be maintained and monitored.

3. The sampling plan, including the eligibility criteria, specific sampling design, recruitment of study participants, sample size, power calculations (in quantitative studies), and expectations regarding attrition.

4. Data collection methods, operational definitions of key variables, and information about reliability and validity of measures (actual instruments are sometimes included in an appendix).

5. Procedures to be adopted, such as what equipment will be used to administer a treatment or collect data, how participants will be assigned to groups, and what type of blinding, if any, will be achieved.

6. Specific strategies for analyzing data, including how confounding variables will be controlled, how missing data will be handled, and (if appropriate) whether an intention-to-treat analysis will be performed.

The description of methods should include a discussion of the rationale for the proposed methods, potential methodologic problems, and intended strategies for handling such problems. In proposals for qualitative studies, special care should be given to steps that will be taken to enhance the integrity and trustworthiness of the study.

Inouye and Fiellin (2005) found that *all* of the reviews they analyzed had one or more criticism of the Research Design section, the most general of which was that the description of the methods was underdeveloped (15%). The most persistent complaints that reviewers noted for the 66 applications (which were primarily for clinical trials) were as follows:

- Inadequate blinding for outcome assessment (36%)

- Sample was flawed—biased or unrepresentative (36%)
- Important confounding variables inadequately controlled (32%)
- Inadequate sample size or inadequate power calculations (26%)
- Insufficient description of the approach to data analysis (24%)
- Outcome measures inadequately specified or described (23%)

Although some of these concerns relate to clinical trials (e.g., blinding), many are likely to be important issues in all reviews—small sample size, sample biases, uncontrolled confounding variables, and poorly described data collection and analysis plans can be problematic in any type of study. Other noteworthy complaints that are not specific to randomized clinical trials (RCTs) included lack of discussion about attrition (20%), poorly described samples (18%), exclusion criteria poorly justified (18%), insufficient information about reliability or validity of measures (14%), and poor description of study variables and instruments (14%).

Although the grant application kit does not specifically request a project timeline or work plan, it is often useful to develop and include one, unless the page limitation makes it impossible to do so. A timeline helps reviewers assess how realistic you have been in planning the project, and it should help you to develop an estimate of needed resources (i.e., your budget). Flow charts are often useful for highlighting the sequencing and interrelationships of project activities. (Figure 8.3 in Chapter 8 presents such a flow chart.)

Human Subjects Sections (Items 8–11). Researchers who plan to collect data from human subjects must complete items relating to the protection of subjects. An entire section of the application kit ("Part II, Supplemental Instructions for Preparing the Human Subjects Section of the Research Plan") provides guidance on the attachments needed for these items. Applicants must either address the involvement of human subjects and describe protections from research risks or provide a justification for exemption with enough information that reviewers can determine the appropriateness of requests for exemption. If no exemption is sought, the section must address various issues, as outlined in the application kit. The application must also include various types of information regarding the inclusion of women, minorities, and children. These sections often serve as the cornerstone of the document submitted to Institutional Review Boards (IRBs).

> **TIP:** NIH requires funded investigators to have specific training regarding protection of human study participants. Even researchers whose studies are exempt from an IRB review must demonstrate that they have had appropriate education.

Other Research Plan Sections (Items 13–17). Most remaining sections in the research plan component are not relevant to many applications. These include a description and justification of the use of vertebrate animals, a leadership plan if there are multiple principal investigators, a description of the use of hazardous biologic agents, and consortium or contractual arrangements for projects that involve the collaboration of two or more different institutions. One item that has relevance to many applications is item 16, Letters of Support. This item requires you to attach letters from individuals agreeing to provide services to the project, such as consultants.

Appendices (Item 18). Grant applications often include appended materials. A maximum of 10 PDF attachments is allowed, and a summary sheet listing all appended items is encouraged. Examples of appended materials include data collection instruments, detailed sample size calculations, scoring or coding instructions for instruments, letters from institutions that will provide access to subjects, complex statistical models, and other supplementary materials in support of the application. Researchers can also submit publications or manuscripts accepted for publication. Essential information should never be relegated to an appendix because only the primary reviewers receive appen-

dices. The guidelines warn that appendices should not be used to circumvent the 25-page limitation.

> **TIP:** In terms of content, the research plan for NIH applications is similar to what is required in most research proposals—although emphases and page restrictions may vary, and supplementary information may be required.

The Review Process

Grant applications submitted to NIH are reviewed for completeness and relevance by the NIH Center for Scientific Review. Acceptable applications are assigned to an appropriate Institute or Center, and to a peer review group.

As the schedule in Table 27.1 indicates, NIH uses a sequential, dual review system for making decisions about its grant applications. The first level involves a panel of peer reviewers (not NIH employees), who evaluate grant applications for their scientific merit. These review panels are called **scientific review groups** (SRGs) or, more commonly, **study sections**. Each panel consists of about 20 researchers with backgrounds appropriate to the specific study section for which they have been selected. Appointments to the review panels are usually for 4-year terms and are staggered so that about one fourth of each panel is new each year.

> **TIP:** Applications by nurse researchers usually are assigned to one of two Nursing Science study sections. One is the "Nursing Science: Adults and Older Adults Study Section" (NSAA), and the other is the "Nursing Science: Children and Families Study Section" (NSCF). Names of study section members are available at http://www.drg.nih.gov/Committees/rosterindex.asp#A. This information may be helpful in developing a grant application, *but* you should never contact a study section member directly.

The second level of review is by an Advisory Council, which includes both scientific and lay representatives. The Advisory Council considers not only the scientific merit of an application but also the relevance of the proposed study to the programs and priorities of the Center or Institute to which the application has been submitted, as well as budgetary considerations.

NIH has instituted a triage system for the first level of review. Study section members are sent applications and asked to evaluate whether they are in the upper half or lower half in terms of quality and likelihood for funding. Normally, each application is formally reviewed by at least two assigned reviewers, who prepare written critiques. If two reviewers agree that an application is not in the upper half, it is designated as "unscored" and is neither discussed at the study section meeting nor assigned a score.

Applications in the upper half are discussed in full at study section meetings and assigned a **priority score** that reflects each reviewer's opinion of the merit of the application. The ratings range from 1.0 (the best possible score) to 5.0 (the least favorable score), in increments of 0.1. Before the streamlined review procedures were instituted, priority scores typically ran the full range from 1.0 to 5.0. However, the full range is no longer routinely used because the only applications assigned a score are those previously designated as being in the upper half. Thus, priority scores tend to be between 1.0 and 3.0, but reviewers are free to "vote their conscience" and may therefore assign any priority score they think appropriate.

The individual scores from all study section members are then combined, averaged, and multiplied by 100 to yield scores that (technically) range from 100 to 500, with 100 being the best possible score. Among all scored applications, only those with the best priority scores actually obtain funding. Cut-off scores for funding vary from agency to agency and year to year, but a score of 200 or lower is often needed to get funding.

Within a few days after the study section meeting, applicants are able to learn their priority score and percentile ranking online via the NIH Commons (*https://commons.era.nih.gov/commons*). Within about 30 days, applicants can access a summary of the peer review panel's evaluation. These **summary sheets** (previously called *pink sheets* because

they were printed on pink paper) include the written critiques produced by the assigned reviewers, a summary of the study section's discussion, study section recommendations, and administrative notes of special consideration (e.g., human subjects issues). All applicants receive a summary sheet, even if their applications were unscored.

➲ TIP: Unless an unfunded proposal is criticized in some fundamental way (e.g., the problem area was not judged to be significant), applications should be resubmitted, with revisions that reflect the concerns of the peer reviewers. When a proposal is resubmitted, the next review panel members are given a copy of the original application and the summary sheet so that they can evaluate the degree to which concerns have been addressed. Applications can be resubmitted up to two times. Brown and her colleagues (1997) described how they responded to reviewers' critiques in their resubmission of a grant application that was not originally funded.

TIPS ON PROPOSAL DEVELOPMENT

Although it is impossible to tell you exactly what steps to follow to produce a successful proposal, we conclude this chapter with some advice that might help to improve the process and the product. Many of these tips are especially relevant for those preparing proposals for funding. Further suggestions for writing effective grant applications may be found in Beitz and Bliss (2005), Crain and Broome (2000), Grey (2000), Lusk (2004), and Inouye and Fiellin (2005).

Things to Do Before Writing Begins

Advance planning is essential to the development of a successful proposal. This section offers suggestions for things you can do to prepare for the actual writing.

Start Early
Writing a proposal, and attending to all of the details of a formal submission process, is time consuming, and almost always needs more time than

originally envisioned. Be sure to build in enough time that the product can be reviewed and re-reviewed, both by members of the team and by willing colleagues. Budget adequate time for administrative issues that can be protracted, such as securing permissions and getting budgets approved.

Having a proposal timeline is a good way to impose some discipline on the proposal development process. Figure 27.1 presents one example, but the list of tasks is merely suggestive. Ask a knowledgeable person to review your timeline before you get underway, and try to adhere to the timeline once you start. ⊗

TIP: It is tremendously advantageous to build pilot or preliminary work into your schedule. As noted earlier, a frequent NIH reviewer complaint is that inadequate pilot work had been completed. Incremental knowledge building is extremely attractive to reviewers. When you apply for funding, you are asking funders to make an *investment* in you; they will have the sense of being offered a better investment opportunity if some of the groundwork for a study has already been completed.

Select an Important Problem

There is probably nothing more critical to the success of a proposal than selecting a problem that has

Task	Timeline (Months Before Submission)												
	12+	12	11	10	9	8	7	6	5	4	3	2	1
Identify/conceptualize the problem	X												
Undertake a literature review	X												
Identify and approach possible data collection sites	X												
Initiate descriptive or pilot work	X												
Analyze pilot data, assess feasibility	XXXXX												
Develop a "brief," outlining significance & preliminary thoughts about overall study design		XX											
Identify methodologic and content experts; solicit input and possible collaboration		XXX											
Begin building a team of co-investigators and consultants		XXXX											
Identify contact funder/program officer (as needed)		XX											
Obtain all application forms and instructions		XX											
Review funding agencies' priorities; review recently funded grants		XXX											
Develop research plan, identify instruments, etc.; consult with statisticians, psychometricians, etc., as needed			XXXXXXX										
Collect site data for describing site, staff, clients			XXX										
Obtain written letters of agreement and/or support from data collection sites			XXX										
Prepare an outline of the proposal; develop writing assignments					XX								
Write draft of proposal						XXXXXXX							
Draft a budget							XX						
Draft other ancillary components (bio sketches, etc.)							XX						
Internal review by team members								XXX					
Make revisions based on review									XXX				
External review by colleagues/experts									XXX				
Team review of comments, make final revisions										XXX			
Write abstract/summary											XX		
Finalize budget and other ancillary components												X	
Prepare all final documents, get needed signatures													X

FIGURE 27.1 ⊗ Example of a grant-writing timeline.

clinical or theoretical significance, and that is viewed in a positive light by reviewers. The proposal must make a persuasive argument that the research could make a noteworthy contribution to evidence on a topic that is important and appealing to those making judgments.

Kuzel (2002), who shared some lessons about securing funding for a qualitative study, noted that researchers could profit by taking advantage of certain "hot topics" that have the special attention of the public and government officials—topics that have "sex appeal." Proposals can sometimes be cast in a way that links them to topics of national concern, and such a linkage can help to secure a favorable review. Kuzel used as an example his funded study of quality of care and medical errors in primary care practices, with emphasis on patient perspectives. The proposal was submitted at a time when the U.S. government was putting resources into research to enhance patient safety, and noted that "the reframing of 'quality' under the name of 'patient safety' has captured the stage and is likely to have an enduring effect on what work receives funding" (p. 141). This advice about being sensitive to political realities is equally true for quantitative research.

Know Your Audience

Learn as much as possible about the audience for your proposal. For dissertations, this means getting to know your committee members and learning about their expectations, interests, and schedules. If you are writing a proposal for funding, you should obtain information about the funding organization and, if possible, the reviewers. Information about funding priorities is crucial. It is also wise to examine recently funded projects. Funding agencies often publish the criteria that reviewers use to make funding decisions—such as the ones we described for NIH—and these criteria should be studied carefully.

Grey (2000), in her tips on grantsmanship, urged researchers to "talk it up" (p. 91), that is, to call program staff in agencies and foundations, or to send letters of inquiry about possible interest in a project. Grey also noted the importance of *listening* to what these people say and following their recommendations.

Another aspect to "knowing your audience" concerns understanding reviewers' perspective. Reviewers for funding agencies are busy professionals who are taking time away from their own work to consider the merits of proposed new research. They are likely to be methodologically sophisticated and experts in *their* field—but they probably have limited knowledge of your own area of research. They will be reviewing many (perhaps dozens) of other proposals. It is therefore imperative to realize the necessity of helping time-pressured reviewers to grasp the merits of your proposed study, and to do so without relying on jargon or specialized terminology.

Review a Successful Proposal

Although there is no substitute for actually writing a proposal as a learning experience, novice proposal writers can profit by examining a successful proposal. It is likely that some of your colleagues or fellow students have written a proposal that has been accepted (either by a funding sponsor or by a dissertation committee), and many people are glad to share their successful efforts with others. Also, proposals funded by the government are usually in the public domain—that is, you can ask to see a copy of funded proposals. To obtain a grant application funded by NIH, for example, you can contact the NIH Freedom of Information Coordinator for the appropriate NIH institute.

Several journals have published proposals in their entirety, except for administrative information such as budgets. Two early examples include a grant application entitled "Couvade: Patterns, Predictors, and Nursing Management" (Clinton, 1985), and a proposal for a study of comprehensive discharge planning for the elderly (Naylor, 1990). More recently, a proposal for a qualitative study of adolescent fathers was published, together with reviewers' comments (Dallas et al., 2005a, 2005b).

➲ **TIP:** The accompanying *Resource Manual* includes the entire successful grant application to NINR by Deborah Dillon McDonald entitled "Older adults response to health care practitioner pain communication," together with reviewers' comments and McDonald's response.

Create a Strong Research Team

For funded research, it is important to think strategically in putting together a team because reviewers often give considerable weight to researchers' qualifications. It is not enough to have a team of competent people; it is necessary to have the right *mix* of competence. A project team of three brilliant theorists without statistical skills for a study involving sophisticated analyses may be unable to convince reviewers that the project would be productive. Gaps and weaknesses can often be compensated for by the judicious use of consultants.

Another shortcoming of some project teams is that there are too many researchers with small time commitments. It is unwise to propose a staff with five or more top-level professionals who are able to contribute only 5% to 10% of their time to the project. Such projects often run into management difficulties because no one is in control of the work flow. Although collaborative efforts are commendable, you should be able to *justify* the inclusion of every person and to identify the unique contribution that each will make to the project.

Things to Do as You Write

If you have planned well and drafted a realistic schedule, the next step is to move forward with the development of the proposal. Some suggestions for the writing stage follow.

Build a Persuasive Case

Whether or not your proposal is a request for funding, you need to persuade reviewers that you are asking the right questions, that you are the right person to ask those questions, and that you will get valid and credible answers. You must also convince them that the answers will make a difference to nursing and its clients.

Beginning proposal writers sometimes forget that they are *selling* a product: themselves and their ideas. It is appropriate, therefore, to think of the proposal as a marketing opportunity. It is not enough to have a good idea and sound methods—you must have a persuasive presentation. When funding is at stake, the challenge is greater because *everyone is trying to persuade reviewers that their proposal is more meritorious than yours.* Grant competitions are analogous to a horse race with a field of champions, and so you must make every sentence, and every detail, count toward a finish that puts you "in the money."

Reviewers are aware that most of the applications they are reviewing will *not* get funded. For example, at NIH, only about one out of four applications gets support. The reviewers' job is to differentiate "winners" and "losers." In writing the proposal, you must consciously include features that will score you points and avoid problems that will cost you points—you must think of ways to gain a competitive edge. Be sure to give thought to issues persistently identified as problematic by reviewers (Inouye & Fiellin, 2005), and use a well-conceived checklist to ensure that you have not missed an opportunity to strengthen your study design and your proposal.

The proposal should be written in a positive, confident tone. If you do not sound convinced that the proposed study is important and will be rigorously done, then reviewers will not be persuaded either. There is no need to promise what cannot be achieved, but you should think about ways to put the proposed project in a positive light.

Justify Methodologic Decisions

Many proposals fail because they do not instill confidence that key decisions have a sound rationale. Almost every aspect of a research proposal involves a decision, and these decisions should be made carefully, keeping in mind the costs and benefits of alternatives. When you are confident that you have made the right decision, offer a compelling justification. To the extent possible, make your decisions evidence based—that is, *defend* your proposed methods with citations demonstrating their utility. Insufficient detail and scanty explanation of methodologic choices can be perilous, although page constraints often make full elaboration impossible.

Begin and End With a Flourish

The abstract or summary to the proposal should be written with extreme care. Because it is one of the first things that reviewers read, you need to be sure that it will create a favorable impression. (For NIH applications, the full review committee may read *only* the summary and not the entire application.) The ideal abstract is one that generates excitement and inspires confidence in the proposed study's rigor. Be sure to devote sufficient time to crafting a cogent and persuasive abstract. Although abstracts appear at the beginning of a proposal, they are often written last.

Proposals typically conclude with material that is somewhat unexciting, such as the data analysis section or the work plan. A brief, upbeat concluding paragraph that summarizes the significance and innovativeness of the proposed project can help to remind reviewers of its potential to contribute to nursing practice and nursing science.

Adhere to Instructions

Funding agencies (and universities) usually provide instructions on what is required in a research proposal. It is crucial to read these instructions carefully, and to follow them precisely. Proposals are sometimes rejected without review if they do not adhere to such guidelines as minimum font size or page limitations. For example, the instructions for grant applications to the NIH state the following about font size: "The height of the letters must not be smaller than 10 point; Helvetica or Arial 12-point is the NIH suggested font." It is wise to use the suggested font, and fatal to ignore the font limitations: "Deviations from the font size specifications . . . will be grounds for the Public Health Service to reject and return the entire application without peer review."

Pay Attention to Presentation

Reviewers are put in a better frame of mind if the proposals they are reading are attractive, well organized, grammatical, and easy to read. Glitzy figures are not needed, but the presentation should be professional and show respect for weary reviewers. In Inouye and Fiellin's (2005) study, 20% of the grant applications were criticized for such presentation issues as typographical or grammatical errors, poor layout, inconsistencies, and omitted tables.

Have the Proposal Critiqued

Before formal submission of a proposal, a draft should be reviewed by others. Reviewers should be selected for both substantive and methodologic expertise. If the proposal is being submitted for funding, one reviewer ideally would have first-hand knowledge of the funding source. If a consultant has been proposed because of specialized expertise that you believe will strengthen the study, he or she should be asked to participate by reviewing the draft and making recommendations for its improvement.

In universities, mock review panels are often held before submitting a proposal to the funding agency. Faculty and students are invited to these mock reviews and provide valuable feedback for enhancing a proposal.

⬤⬤⬤⬤⬤⬤⬤⬤⬤⬤⬤⬤⬤⬤⬤⬤⬤⬤

RESEARCH EXAMPLES

NIH makes available the abstracts of all funded projects through a database known as Computer Retrieval of Information on Scientific Projects (CRISP), which can be searched by subject or researcher name. Abstracts for two projects funded through NINR are presented here.

Example From a Funded Quantitative Project

Phyllis Sharps of Johns Hopkins University prepared the following abstract for a project entitled "Domestic Violence Enhanced Home Visitation Program." The application was reviewed by the Children and Families Study Section (NSCF), and received NINR funding in February 2006. The project is scheduled for completion in November 2011.

Abstract: Children witnessing the intimate partner violence (IPV) of their mothers are known to have serious long-term physical and mental health and behavioral consequences. While almost half of these children were less than 6 years old, little is known about appropriate interventions for very young children and their abused mothers. Building on the demonstrated positive effects of early home visitation models of providing care, this study proposes to incorporate routine screening for IPV and a structured IPV intervention into existing home visitation (HV) programs for young families expecting a child. Traditional home visitation and Olds' model of home visitation programs will be examined using a two-group quasi experimental design with nurses randomized to provide a structured IPV intervention to pregnant/postpartum women or to provide standard care or usual care to women who disclose IPV. Home visitors (nurses and trained lay visitors) in each home visitation program will be randomized to the intervention or a comparison condition. There will be four groups of 60 families from urban (2 groups) and rural (2 groups) home visitation settings. Mothers and infants plus one child less than 6 years (if there is one) in all families will be monitored at birth, 3 months, 6 months and then at 6-month intervals through 24 months. Maternal dependent measures include IPV, level of danger, and safety strategies as well as depression, parenting stress, high risk parenting, attachment, and perceived adaptability of the child. The infant plus one-index sibling dependent measures are physical and mental development (Bailey Infant Neurodevelopmental Screening) as well as physical and mental health problems. The study will provide intervention efficacy data as well as prospective information about patterns of IPV, maternal health, and infant and child development in homes where there is IPV. Analyses will include mixed linear models, ANCOVA and MANOVA procedures and logistic regression with generalized estimating equations (GEE).

Example From a Funded Qualitative Project

Elizabeth Davies of the University of California, San Francisco, submitted a successful application for a grounded theory study that was reviewed by the Children and Families study section (NSCF). The study was funded by NINR in February 2006 and is scheduled to end in November 2009. Davies prepared the following abstract for the study, which was entitled "Fathers' Experience With Pediatric End-of-Life Care":

Abstract: Despite the focus on providing care to all family members as a basic principle of pediatric palliative care, remarkably little attention has been paid to fathers when their child is seriously ill and dies. Findings from research team members' previous studies provide the basis for this application. The project's overall goal is to develop an empirically grounded and theoretical conceptualization of the experiences of fathers whose child has died following the receipt of end-of-life care for a life-limiting condition. Specific aims are to 1) describe fathers' understanding of themselves as fathers, men, spouse/partners, and workers/ community members in relation to their experiences of having a seriously ill child who died; 2) describe fathers' experiences with their ill child and other family members; 3) describe fathers' experiences with the health care system, particularly health care providers, and explore how the expectations of the health care system influence fathers' experiences; and 4) describe fathers' understanding of their ill child's and other family members' experiences with various health care providers. In addressing each specific aim, we will also examine how i) fathers' experience changed through the transitions from diagnosis to the final phase of the condition, to the time of death, and into bereavement with emphasis on the final phase of the illness; ii) fathers' ways of coping were affected and changed over time, and what factors influenced their coping; and iii) fathers' ethnic and cultural background influenced their overall experiences. Participants will include up to 70 fathers whose child received care at one of four types of settings or programs that provide pediatric end-of-life care (two children's hospitals, home care program, inpatient hospice) in three US geographic regions. Fathers will include various ethnic groups (Latino, Asian, African American, as well as Caucasian); concerted efforts will be made to include single, divorced, and gay fathers. Up to three semi-structured interviews will be conducted with each father by trained individuals. Translated and transcribed interviews, along with field notes, will be subjected to procedures of grounded theory analysis. Findings will offer insight, enhance understanding, and provide meaningful guidance for future family-level investigations and for clinical care in the area of pediatric end-of-life care.

SUMMARY POINTS

- A **research proposal** is a written document specifying what a researcher intends to study; proposals are written both by students seeking approval for dissertations and theses and by seasoned researchers seeking financial or institutional support. The set of skills associated with learning about funding opportunities and developing proposals that can be funded is referred to as **grantsmanship**.
- Preparing proposals for qualitative studies is especially challenging because methodologic decisions are made in the field; qualitative

proposals need to persuade reviewers that the proposed study is important and a good risk.

- Students preparing a proposal for a dissertation or thesis need to work closely with a well-chosen committee and advisor. Dissertation proposals are often "mini-dissertations" that include sections that can be incorporated into the dissertation.

- The federal government is the largest source of research funds for health researchers in the United States. In addition to regular grants programs, agencies of the federal government announce special funding programs in the form of **program announcements** and **Requests for Applications (RFAs)** for **grants** and **Requests for Proposals (RFPs)** for **contracts**.

- A major source of funding for nurse researchers is the National Institutes of Health (NIH), within which is housed the National Institute of Nursing Research (NINR). Nurses can apply for a variety of grants from NIH, the most common being **Research Project Grants** (R01 grants), **AREA Grants** (R15), **Small Grants** (R03), or **Exploratory/Developmental Grants** (R21).

- Grant applications to NIH are now submitted online using the SF424, which has a series of special forms (fillable screens) that require uploaded PDF attachments.

- The heart of an NIH grant application is the research plan component, which includes four major sections: Specific Aims, Background and Significance, Preliminary Studies, and Research Design and Methods. These four sections, combined, cannot exceed 25 single-spaced pages.

- NIH grant applications also require budgets, which can be an abbreviated **modular budget** if requested funds do not exceed $250,000 in direct costs per year.

- Grant applications to NIH are reviewed three times a year in a dual review process. The first phase involves a review by a peer review panel (or **study section**) that evaluates each proposal's scientific merit; the second phase is a review by an Advisory Council.

- In NIH's review procedure, the study section assigns **priority scores** only to applications judged to be in the top half of proposals based on their quality. A score of 100 is the most meritorious ranking, and a score of 500 is the lowest possible score.

- Applicants for NIH grants are sent a summary statement, which offers a detailed critique of the proposal, together with information on the priority score and percentile ranking.

- Some suggestions for writing a strong proposal include several for the planning stage (e.g., starting early, selecting an important topic, learning about the audience, reviewing a successful proposal, creating a strong team) and several for the writing stage (building a persuasive case, justifying methodologic decisions, beginning and ending with a flourish, adhering to proposal instructions, and having the draft proposal critiqued by reviewers).

STUDY ACTIVITIES

Chapter 27 of the accompanying *Resource Manual for Nursing Research: Generating and Assessing Evidence for Nursing Practice, 8th edition*, offers various exercises and study suggestions for reinforcing the concepts taught in this chapter. In addition, the following study questions can be addressed:

1. Suppose that you were planning to study the self-care behaviors of aging AIDS patients.
   a. Outline the methods you would recommend adopting.
   b. Develop a project timeline.
2. Suppose that you were interested in studying separation anxiety in hospitalized children. Using the funding mechanisms cited in this chapter, identify potential funding sources for your project.

REFERENCES CITED IN CHAPTER 27

All references cited in this chapter can be found in a separate section at the end of the book.

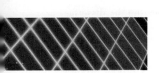# Methodologic and Theoretical References

AERA, APA, & NCME Joint Committee. (1985). *Standards for educational and psychological testing*. Washington, DC: American Psychological Association.

Agar, M. (1980). *The professional stranger: An informal introduction to ethnography*. New York: Academic Press.

Agency for Healthcare Research and Quality. (2002). *Systems to rate the strength of scientific evidence*. Washington, DC: Author.

AGREE Collaboration. (2001). *Appraisal of guidelines for research and evaluation (AGREE instrument)*. Retrieved January, 2006, from *http://www.agreecollaboration.org*.

Ahern, K. J. (1999). Ten tips for reflexive bracketing. *Qualitative Health Research, 9*, 407–411.

Ajzen, I. (2005). *Attitudes, personality, and behavior* (2nd ed.). Milton Keynes, UK: Open University Press/McGraw-Hill.

Ajzen, I., & Fishbein, M. (1980). *Understanding attitudes and predicting social behavior*. Englewood Cliffs, NJ: Prentice Hall.

Allen, F. M., & Warner, M. (2002). A developmental model of health and nursing. *Journal of Family Issues, 8*, 96–135.

Allison, P. D. (2000). *Missing data*. Thousand Oaks, CA: Sage Publications.

American Nurses' Association. (2001). *Code for nurses with interpretive statements*. Kansas City, MO: Author.

American Psychological Association. (2001). *Publication manual of the American Psychological Association* (5th ed.). Washington, DC: Author.

American Psychological Association. (2002). *Ethical principles of psychologists and code of conduct*. Washington, DC: Author.

American Sociological Association. (1997). *Code of ethics*. Washington, DC: Author.

Atwood, J. R., & Taylor, W. (1991). Regression discontinuity design: Alternative for nursing research. *Nursing Research, 40*(5), 312–315.

Bader, G., & Rossi, C. (2002). *Focus groups: A step-by-step guide* (3rd ed.). San Diego, CA : The Bader Group.

Baernholdt, M., & Clarke, S. P. (2006). Internet research in an international context. *Applied Nursing Research, 19*(1), 48–50.

Bakeman, R., & Gottman, J. (1997). *Observing interaction: An introduction to sequential analysis*. Cambridge, UK: Cambridge University Press.

Baker, C., Wuest, J., & Stern, P. N. (1992). Method slurring: The grounded theory/phenomenology example. *Journal of Advanced Nursing, 17*, 1355–1360.

Bandura, A. (1985). *Social foundations of thought and action: A social cognitive theory*. Englewood Cliffs, NJ: Prentice Hall.

Bandura, A. (1997). *Self-efficacy: The exercise of control*. New York: W. H. Freeman.

Barkauskas, V. H., Lusk, S. L., Eakin, B. L. (2005). Selecting control interventions for clinical outcome studies. *Western Journal of Nursing Research, 27*(3), 346–363.

Barroso, J., Gollop, C., Sandelowski, M., Meynell, J., Pearce, P., & Collins, L. (2003). The challenges of searching for and retrieving qualitative studies. *Western Journal of Nursing Research, 25*(2), 153–178.

Barry, C. A., Britten, N., Barber, N., Bradley, C., & Stevenson, F. (1999). Using reflexivity to optimize teamwork in qualitative research. *Qualitative Health Research, 9*(3), 26–44.

Beck, C. T. (1994). Replication strategies for nursing research. *Image: Journal of Nursing Scholarship, 26*, 191–194.

Beck, C. T. (1999). Facilitating the work of a meta-analyst. *Research in Nursing & Health, 22*, 523–530.

Beck, C. T. (2005). Benefits of participating in Internet interviews: Women helping women. *Qualitative Health Research, 15*, 411–422.

Beck, C. T., & Gable, R. K. (2001b). Item response theory in affective instrument development: An illustration. *Journal of Nursing Measurement, 9*, 5–22.

Beck, C. T., & Gable, R. K. (2001c). Ensuring content validity: An illustration of the process. *Journal of Nursing Measurement, 9*, 201–215.

Beck, C. T., Bernal, H., & Froman, R. D. (2003). Methods to document semantic equivalence of a translated scale. *Research in Nursing & Health, 26*, 64–73.

Becker, H. S. (1970). *Sociological work*. Chicago: Aldine.

Becker, M. (1976). *Health Belief Model and personal health behavior.* Thorofare, NJ: Slack.

Becker, M. (1978). The Health Belief Model and sick role behavior. *Nursing Digest, 6*, 35–40.

Becker, P. (2004). What happens to my manuscript when I send it to *Research in Nursing & Health. Research in Nursing & Health, 27*(6), 379–381.

Bellg, A., Borrelli, B., Resnick, B., Hecht, J., Minicucci, D., et al. (2004). Enhancing treatment fidelity in health behavior change studies: Best practices and recommendations from the NIH Behavior Change Consortium. *Health Psychology, 23*, 443–451.

Benner, P. (1994). The tradition and skill of interpretive phenomenology in studying health, illness, and caring practices. In P. Benner (Ed.), *Interpretive phenomenology* (pp. 99–127). Thousand Oaks, CA: Sage Publications.

Bennett, J. A. (2000). Mediator and moderator variables in nursing research: Conceptual and statistical differences. *Research in Nursing & Health, 23*, 415–420.

Bennett, J. A. (2005). The Consolidated Standards of Reporting Trials (CONSORT). *Nursing Research, 54*(2), 128–132.

Berk, R. A. (1990). Importance of expert judgment in content-related validity evidence. *Western Journal of Nursing Research, 12*, 659–671.

Best, S. J., & Krueger, B. S. (2004). *Internet data collection.* Thousand Oaks, CA: Sage Publications.

Blumer, H. (1986). *Symbolic interactionism: Perspective and method.* Berkeley: University of California Press.

Bogdan, R. C. (1972). *Participant observation in organizational settings.* Syracuse, NY: Syracuse University Press.

Boyle, J. S. (1997). Writing up: Dissecting the dissertation. In J. M. Morse (Ed.), *Completing a qualitative project: Details and dialogue* (pp. 9–37). Thousand Oaks, CA: Sage Publications.

Bradburn, N., Sudman, S., & Wansink, B. (2004). *Asking questions: The definitive guide for questionnaire design.* San Francisco: Jossey-Bass.

Bradford-Hill, A. (1971). *Principles of medical statistics* (9th ed.). New York: Oxford University Press.

Braitman, L. (1991). Confidence intervals assess both clinical significance and statistical significance. *Annals of Internal Medicine, 114*, 515–517.

Brewer, J. D. (2000). *Ethnography.* Philadelphia: Open University Press.

Brewer, J., & Hunter, A. (2006). *Foundations of multimethod research: Synthesizing styles.* Thousand Oaks, CA: Sage Publications.

Bringer, J. D., Johnston, L. H., & Brackenridge, C. H. (2004). Maximizing transparency in a doctoral thesis: The complexities of writing about the use of QRS*NVIVO within a grounded theory study. *Qualitative Research, 4*, 247–265.

Brislin, R. W. (1970). Back-translation for cross-cultural research. *Journal of Cross-Cultural Psychology, 1*, 185–216.

Broome, M. E. (1999). Consent (assent) for research with pediatric patients. *Seminars in Oncology Nursing, 15*, 96–103.

Brown, E. L. (1948). *Nursing for the future.* New York: Russell Sage Publications.

Brown, S., Upchurch, S., & Acton, G. (2003). A framework for developing a coding scheme for meta-analyses. *Western Journal of Nursing Research, 25*(2), 205–222.

Bruner, J. (1991). *Acts of meaning.* Cambridge, MA: Harvard University Press.

Burke, K. (1969). *A grammar of motives.* Berkley: University of California Press.

Campbell, D. T., & Fiske, D. W. (1959). Convergent and discriminant validation by the multitrait-multimethod matrix. *Psychological Bulletin, 56*, 81–105.

Campbell, D. T., & Stanley, J. C. (1963). *Experimental and quasi-experimental designs for research.* Chicago: Rand McNally.

Canadian Nurses Association. (2002). Ethical guidelines for nurses in research involving human subjects. Ottawa, ON: Author.

Carey, M. A., & Smith, M. W. (1994). Capturing the group effect in focus groups: A special concern in analysis. *Qualitative Health Research, 4*, 123–127.

Carroll, K., & Rounsaville, B. (2003). Bridging the gap: A hybrid model to link efficacy and effectiveness research in substance abuse treatment. *Psychiatric Services, 54*(3), 333–339.

Carspecken, P. F. (1996). *Critical ethnography in educational research.* New York: Routledge.

Chang, W., & Henry, B. M. (1999). Methodologic principles of cost analyses in the nursing, medical, and health services literature, 1990–1996. *Nursing Research, 48*, 94–104.

Chinn, P. L., & Kramer, M. K. (2004). *Theory and nursing: Integrated knowledge development* (6th ed.). St. Louis: C. V. Mosby.

Chiovitti, R., & Piran, N. (2003). Rigour and grounded theory research. *Journal of Advanced Nursing, 44*(4), 427–435.

Ciliska, D., & Guyatt, G. (2005). Publication bias. In DiCenso, A., Guyatt, G., & Ciliska, D. *Evidence-based nursing: A guide to clinical practice.* St. Louis, MO: Elsevier Mosby.

Clarke, S., & Cossette, S. (2000). Secondary analysis: Theoretical, methodological, and practical considerations. *Canadian Journal of Nursing Research, 32*(3), 109–129.

Closs, S. J., & Cheater, F. M. (1999). Evidence for nursing practice: A clarification of the issues. *Journal of Advanced Nursing, 30*, 10–17.

Cochrane Collaboration. (2005). *Cochrane handbook for systematic reviews of interventions.* Retrieved October 1, 2006, from *http://www.cochrane.org/resources/handbook/index.htm.*

Code of Federal Regulations. (2005). *Protection of human subjects: 45CFR46* (revised as of June 23, 2005). Washington, DC: U.S. Department of Health and Human Services.

Cohen, J. (1960). A coefficient of agreement for nominal scales. *Educational and Psychological Measurement, 20*, 37–46.

Cohen, J. (1988). *Statistical power analysis for the behavioral sciences* (2nd ed.). Hillsdale, NJ: Lawrence Erlbaum Associates.

Cohen, J., Cohen, P., West, S., & Aiken, L. (2002). *Applied multiple regression: Correlation analysis for behavioral sciences* (3rd ed.). Mahwah, NJ: Lawrence Erlbaum.

Colaizzi, P. F. (1973). *Reflection and research in psychology.* Dubuque, IA: Kendall/Hunt.

Colaizzi, P. F. (1978). Psychological research as the phenomenologist views it. In R. Valle & M. King (Eds.), *Existential phenomenological alternative for psychology* (pp. 48–71). New York: Oxford University Press.

Conn, V. S. (2004). Building a research trajectory. *Western Journal of Nursing Research, 26*(6), 592–594.

Conn, V. S., & Rantz, M. J. (2003). Research methods: Managing primary study quality in meta-analyses. *Research in Nursing & Health, 26*(4), 322–333.

Conn, V. S., Rantz, M. J., Wipke-Tevis, D. D., & Maas, M. L. (2001). Designing effective nursing interventions. *Research in Nursing & Health, 24*, 433–442.

Conn, V. S., Valentine, J., Cooper, H., & Rantz, M. J. (2003). Grey literature in meta-analyses. *Nursing Research, 52*(4), 256–261.

Cook, K. E. (2005). Using critical ethnography to explore issues in health promotion. *Qualitative Health Research, 15*(1), 129–138.

Cooper, H. (1998). *Synthesizing research* (3rd ed.). Thousand Oaks, CA: Sage Publications.

Cooper, H., & Hedges, L. (1994). *The handbook of research synthesis.* New York: Russell Sage Foundation.

Côté-Arsenault, D., & Morrison-Beedy, D. (1999). Practical advice for planning and conducting focus groups. *Nursing Research, 48*, 280–283.

Côté-Arsenault, D., & Morrison-Beedy, D. (2005). Maintaining your focus in focus groups: Avoiding common mistakes. *Research in Nursing & Health, 28*, 172–179.

Courtney, K., & Craven, C. (2005). Factors to weigh when considering electronic data collection. *Canadian Journal of Nursing Research, 37*(3), 150–159.

Cowling, W. R. (2004). Pattern, participation, praxis, and power in unitary appreciative inquiry. *Advances in Nursing Science, 27*(3), 202–214.

Crabtree, B. F., & Miller, W. L. (Eds.). (1999). *Doing qualitative research* (2nd ed.). Newbury Park, CA: Sage Publications.

Creswell, J. W. (1998). *Qualitative inquiry and research design: Choosing among five traditions.* Thousand Oaks, CA: Sage Publications.

Creswell, J. W. (2003). *Research design: Qualitative, quantitative, and mixed method approaches.* Thousand Oaks, CA: Sage Publications.

Cronbach, L. (1990). *Essentials of psychological testing* (5th ed.). New York: Harper & Row.

Davis, L. L. (1992). Instrument review: Getting the most from a panel of experts. *Applied Nursing Research, 5*, 194–197.

DeKeyser, F. G., & Pugh, L. C. (1990). Assessment of the reliability and validity of biochemical measures. *Nursing Research, 39*, 314–317.

Denzin, N. K. (1989). *The research act* (3rd ed.). New York: McGraw-Hill.

Denzin, N. K. (1997). *Interpretive ethnography: Ethnographic practices for the 21st century.* Thousand Oaks, CA: Sage Publications.

Denzin, N. K. (2000). The practices and politics of interpretation. In Denzin, N. K., & Lincoln, Y. S. (Eds.), *Handbook of qualitative research.* (2nd ed., pp. 897–922). Thousand Oaks, CA: Sage Publications.

Denzin, N. K., & Lincoln, Y. S. (Eds.). (2000). *Handbook of qualitative research.* (2nd ed.). Thousand Oaks, CA: Sage Publications.

DeSantis, L., & Ugarriza, D. N. (2000). The concept of theme as used in qualitative nursing research. *Western Journal of Nursing Research, 22*, 351–372.

DeVellis, R. F. (2003). *Scale development: Theory and application* (2nd ed.). Thousand Oaks, CA: Sage Publications.

DiCenso, A., Guyatt, G., & Ciliska, D. (2005). *Evidence-based nursing: A guide to clinical practice.* St. Louis, MO: Elsevier Mosby.

DiCenso, A., Virano, T., Bajnok, I., et al. (2002). A toolkit to facilitate the implementation of clinical practice guidelines in healthcare settings. *Hospital Quarterly, 5,* 55–60.

Diekelmann, N. L., Allen, D., & Tanner, C. (1989). *The NLN criteria for appraisal of baccalaureate programs: A critical hermeneutic analysis.* New York: NLN Press.

Dillman, D. (2000). *Mail and internet surveys: The tailored design method* (2nd ed.). New York: John Wiley & Sons.

Dochterman, J., & Bulecheck, G. (2004). *Nursing Interventions Classification (NIC)* (4th ed.). St. Louis: Mosby.

Dodd, M., Janson, S., Facione, N., Fawcett, J., Froelicher, E. S., Humphreys, J., et al. (2001). Advancing the science of symptom management. *Journal of Advanced Nursing, 33,* 668–676.

Donabedian, A. (1987). Some basic issues in evaluating the quality of health care. In L. T. Rinke (Ed.), *Outcome measures in home care* (Vol. I, pp. 3–28). New York: National League for Nursing.

Donaldson, S. K. (2000). Breakthroughs in scientific research: The discipline of nursing, 1960–1999. *Annual Review of Nursing Research, 18*, 247–311.

Donner, A., & Klar, N. (2004). Pitfalls and controversies in cluster randomization trials. *American Journal of Public Health, 94*(3), 416–422.

Drummond, M., O'Brien, B., Stoddart, G., & Torrance, G. (1997), *Methods for the economic evaluation of health care programs* (2nd ed.). Oxford: Oxford Medical Publications.

Duggleby, W. (2005). What about focus group interaction data? *Qualitative Health Research, 15*(6), 832–840.

Duren-Winfield, V., Berry, M. J., Jones, S. A., Clark, D. H., & Sevick, M. A. (2000). Cost-effectiveness analysis methods for the REACT study. *Western Journal of Nursing Research, 22*, 460–474.

Eder, C., Fullerton, J., Benroth, R., & Lindsay, S. (2005). Pragmatic strategies that enhance the reliability of data abstracted from medical records. *Applied Nursing Research, 18*(1), 50–54.

Ellis, C., & Bochner, A. P. (2000). Autoethnography, personal narrative, reflexivity. In N. K. Denzin & Y. S. Lincoln (Eds.). *Handbook of qualitative research* (2nd ed., pp. 733–768). Thousand Oaks, CA: Sage Publications.

Embretson, S. E., & Reise, S. P. (2000). *Item response theory for psychologists.* Mahwah, NJ: Lawrence Erlbaum.

Erlandson, D. A., Harris, E. L., Skipper, B. L., & Allen, S. (1993). *Doing naturalistic inquiry: A guide to methods.* Thousand Oaks, CA: Sage Publications.

Erwin, E., Meyer, A., & McClain, N. (2005). Use of an audit in violence prevention research. *Qualitative Health Research, 15*(5), 707–718.

Fahs, P., Morgan, L., & Kalman, M. (2003). A call for replication. *Image: Journal of Nursing Scholarship, 35*(1), 67–72.

Farmer, T., Robinson, K., Elliott, S., & Eyles, J. (2006). Developing and implementing a triangulation protocol for qualitative health research. *Qualitative Health Research, 16*(3), 377–394.

Fawcett, J. (1999). *The relationship between theory and research* (3rd ed.). Philadelphia: F. A. Davis.

Fawcett, J. (2005). *Contemporary nursing knowledge: Analysis and evaluation of nursing models and theories.* Philadelphia: F. A. Davis.

Ferketich, S. (1991). Focus on psychometrics: Aspects of item analysis. *Research in Nursing & Health, 14,* 165–168.

Ferketich, S. L., Figueredo, A., & Knapp, T. R. (1991). The multitrait-multimethod approach to construct validity. *Research in Nursing & Health, 14,* 315–319.

Ferketich, S., & Verran, J. (1994). An overview of data transformation. *Research in Nursing & Health, 17,* 393–396.

Fetterman, D. M. (1989). *Ethnography: Step by step.* Newbury Park, CA: Sage Publications.

Fetterman, D. M. (1997). *Ethnography: Step by step* (2nd ed.). Thousand Oaks, CA: Sage Publications.

Findorff, M., Wyman, J., Croghan, C., & Nyman, J. (2005). Use of time studies for determining intervention costs. *Nursing Research, 54*(4), 280–285.

Fineout-Overholt, E., & Johnston, L. (2005). Teaching EBP: Asking searchable, answerable clinical questions. *Worldviews on Evidence-Based Nursing, 2*(3), 157–160.

Finfgeld, D. (2003). Metasynthesis: The state of the art—so far. *Qualitative Health Research, 13*(7), 893–904.

Fink, A. (2005). *Conducting research literature reviews: From paper to the Internet* (2nd ed.). Thousand Oaks, CA: Sage Publications.

Fitzpatrick, J. J., & Montgomery, K. S. (2004). *Internet for nursing research: A guide to strategies, skills, and resources.* New York: Springer.

Fitzpatrick, M. L. (2001). Historical research: The method. In P. L. Munhall & C. J. Oiler (Eds.), *Nursing research: A qualitative perspective* (pp. 403–415). Norwalk, CT: Appleton-Century-Crofts.

Flanagan, J. C. (1954). The critical-incident technique. *Psychological Bulletin, 51*, 327–358.

Fleiss, J. (1971). Measuring nominal scale agreement among many raters. *Psychological Bulletin, 76*, 378–382.

Flesch, R. (1948). New readability yardstick. *Journal of Applied Psychology, 32*, 221–223.

Fletcher, R. H., Fletcher, S. W., & Wagner, E. H. (2005). *Clinical epidemiology: The essentials* (4th ed.). Philadelphia: Lippincott Williams & Wilkins.

Flicker, S., Haans, D., & Skinner, H. (2004). Ethical dilemmas in research on Internet communities. *Qualitative Health Research, 14,* 124–134.

Fogg, T., Wightman, C. W. (2000). Improving transcription of qualitative research interviews with speech recognition technology. Paper presented at Annual Meeting of American Educational Research Association, New Orleans, April, 2000.

Fontana, A., & Frey, J. H. (2003). The interview: From structured questions to negotiated text. In N. K. Denzin & Y. S. Lincoln (Eds.), *Collecting and interpreting qualitative materials* (pp. 61–106). Thousand Oaks, CA: Sage Publications.

Fonteyn, M. E., Kuipers, B., & Grober, S. J. (1993). A description of the think aloud method and protocol analysis. *Qualitative Health Research, 3*, 430–441.

Forbat, L., & Henderson, J. (2003). "Stuck in the middle with you": The ethics and process of qualitative research with two people in an intimate relationship. *Qualitative Health Research, 13*(10), 1453–1462.

Fowler, F. J. (1995). *Improving survey questions.* Thousand Oaks, CA: Sage Publications.

Fowler, F. J. (2001). *Survey research methods* (3rd ed.). Thousand Oaks, CA: Sage Publications.

Fowler, F. J., & Mangione, T. W. (1990). *Standardized survey interviewing.* Thousand Oaks, CA: Sage Publications.

Fox-Wasylyshyn, S., & El-Masri, M. (2005). Handling missing data in self-report measures. *Research in Nursing & Health, 28*(6), 488–495.

Freidman, L. M., Furberg, C. D., & DeMets, D. L. (1998). *Fundamentals of clinical trials* (3rd ed.). New York: Springer-Verlag.

Froman, R. D., & Schmitt, M. H. (2003). Thinking both inside and outside the box on measurement articles. *Research in Nursing & Health, 26*, 335–336.

Gable, R. K., & Wolf, M. B. (1993). *Instrument development in the affective domain* (2nd ed.). Boston: Kluwer Academic Publishers.

Gadamer, H. G. (1975). *Truth and method.* G. Borden & J. Cumming (Trans). London: Sheed and Ward.

Gadamer, H. G. (1976). *Philosophical hermeneutics.* (D. E. Linge, Ed., & Trans.) Berkeley: University of California Press.

Gaglio, B., Nelson, C., & King, D. (2006). The role of rapport: Lessons learned from conducting research in a primary care setting. *Qualitative Health Research, 16*(5), 723–734.

Galvan, J. L. (2003). *Writing literature reviews: A guide for students of the social and behavioral sciences* (2nd ed.). Los Angeles: Pyrczak Pub.

Gamel, C., Grypdonck, M., Hengeveld, M., & Davis, B. (2001). A method to develop a nursing intervention: The contribution of qualitative studies to the process. *Journal of Advanced Nursing, 33*(6), 806–819.

Garrard, J. (2004). *Health sciences literature review made easy: The matrix method.* Boston: Jones & Bartlett.

Gearing, R. E. (2004). Bracketing in research: A typology. *Qualitative Health Research, 14*(10), 1429–1452.

Gee, J. P. (1991). A linguistic approach to narrative. *Journal of Narrative and Life History, 1*, 15–39.

Gee, J. P. (1996). *Social linguistics and literacies: Ideology in discourses* (2nd ed.). London: Taylor & Francis.

Gennaro, S., Hodnett, E., & Kearney, M. (2001). Making evidence-based practice a reality in your institution. *MCN: The American Journal of Maternal/Child Nursing, 26*, 236–244.

Gibson, C. (1998). Semi-structured and unstructured interviewing: A comparison of methodologies in research with patients following discharge from an acute psychiatric hospital. *Journal of Psychiatric & Mental Health Nursing, 5,* 469–477.

Gilgun, J. F. (2004). Qualitative methods and the development of clinical assessment tools. *Qualitative Health Research, 14*(7), 1008–1019.

Gilgun, J. F. (2005). "Grab" and good science: Writing up the results of qualitative research. *Qualitative Health Research, 15*(2), 256–262.

Giorgi, A. (1985). *Phenomenology and psychological research.* Pittsburgh, PA: Duquesne University Press.

Giorgi, A. (1989). Some theoretical and practical issues regarding the psychological and phenomenological method. *Saybrook Review, 7,* 71–85.

Giorgi, A. (2005). The phenomenological movement and research in the human sciences. *Nursing Science Quarterly, 18,* 75–82.

Glaser, B. G. (1978). *Theoretical sensitivity.* Mill Valley, CA: Sociology Press.

Glaser, B. G. (1992). *Basics of grounded theory analysis.* Mill Valley, CA: Sociology Press.

Glaser, B. G. (1992). *Emergence versus forcing: Basics of grounded theory analysis.* Mill Valley, CA.: Sociology Press.

Glaser, B. G. (1998). *Doing grounded theory: Issues and discussions.* Mill Valley, CA: Sociology Press.

Glaser, B. G. (2001). *The grounded theory perspective: Conceptualization contrasted with description.* Mill Valley, CA: Sociology Press.

Glaser, B. G. (2003). *The grounded theory perspective II: Description's remodeling of grounded theory methodology.* Mill Valley, CA: Sociology Press.

Glaser, B. G. (2005). *The grounded theory perspective III: Theoretical coding.* Mill Valley, CA: Sociology Press.

Glaser, B. G., & Strauss, A. L. (1967). *The discovery of grounded theory: Strategies for qualitative research.* Chicago: Aldine.

Glaser, B. G., & Strauss, A. L. (1971). *Status passage: A formal theory.* Chicago: Aldine.

Glasgow, R. E. (2006). RE-AIMing research for application: Ways to improve evidence for family medicine. *Journal of the American Board of Family Medicine, 19*(1), 11–19.

Glasgow, R. E., Lichtenstein, E., & Marcus, A. (2003). Why don't we see more translation of health promotion research to practice? Rethinking the efficacy to effectiveness transition. *American Journal of Public Health, 93,* 1261–1267.

Glasgow, R. E., Magid, D., Beck, A., Ritzwoller, D., & Estabrooks, P. (2005). Practical clinical trials for translating research to practice: Design and measurement recommendations. *Medical Care, 43*(6), 551–557.

Godwin, M., Ruhland, L., Casson, I., MacDonald, S., Delva, D., Birtwhistle, R., Lam, M., & Seguin, R. (2003). Pragmatic controlled clinical trials in primary care: The struggle between external and internal validity. *BMC Medical Research Methodology, 3,* 28.

Goode, C. J. (2000). What constitutes "evidence" in evidence-based practice? *Applied Nursing Research, 13,* 222–225.

Goode, C., & Piedalue, F. (1999). Evidence based clinical practice. *Journal of Nursing Administration, 29*(6), 15–21.

Gosling, P. (1999). *Scientist's guide to poster presentations.* New York: Kluwer Academic.

Graham, I. D., Harrison, M. B., Brouwers, M., Davies, B. L., & Dunn, S. (2002). Facilitating the use of evidence in practice: Evaluating and adapting clinical practice guidelines for local use by health care organizations. *Journal of Obstetric, Gynecologic, & Neonatal Nursing, 31*(5), 599–611.

Grant, J. S., & Davis, L. T. (1997). Selection and use of content experts in instrument development. *Research in Nursing & Health, 20,* 269–274.

Gravetter, F., & Wallnau, L. (2006). *Statistics for the behavioral sciences.* (7th ed.). Belmont, CA: Wadsworth Publishing.

Green, J. C., & Caracelli, V. J. (Eds.). (1997). *Advances in mixed method evaluation: The challenges and benefits of integrating diverse paradigms.* San Francisco: Jossey-Bass.

Gross, D. (2005). On the merits of attention control groups. *Research in Nursing & Health, 28*(2), 93–94.

Gross, D., & Fogg, L. (2001). Clinical trials in the 21st century: The case for participant-centered research. *Research in Nursing & Health, 24*(6), 530–539.

Guadagno, L., VandeWeerd, C., Stevens, D., Abraham, I., Paveza, G., & Fulmer, T. (2004). Using PDAs in data collection. *Applied Nursing Research, 17*(4), 283–291.

Guba, E., & Lincoln, Y. (1981). *Effective evaluation.* San Francisco: Jossey-Bass.

Guba, E., & Lincoln, Y. (1994). Competing paradigms in qualitative research. In N. Denzin & Y. Lincoln (Eds.), *Handbook of qualitative research* (pp. 105–117). Thousand Oaks, CA: Sage Publications.

Gubrium, J. F., & Holstein, J. A. (Eds.). (2001). *Handbook of interview research: Context and method* (2nd ed.). Thousand Oaks, CA: Sage Publications.

Gunning, R. (1968). *The technique of clear writing* (rev. ed.). New York: McGraw-Hill.

Guyatt, G., & Rennie, D. (2002). *Users' guide to the medical literature: Essentials of evidence-based clinical practice.* Chicago: American Medical Association Press.

Hair, J., Black, W., Babin, B., Anderson, R., & Tatham, R. (2005). *Multivariate data analysis* (6th ed.). Upper Saddle River, NJ: Prentice Hall.

Hall, W. A., Long, B., Bermbach, N., Jordan, S., & Patterson, K. (2005). Qualitative teamwork issues and strategies: Coordination through mutual adjustment. *Qualitative Health Research, 15*(3), 394–410.

Hambleton, R. K., Swaminathan, H., & Rogers, H. J. (1991). *Fundamentals of item response theory.* Newbury Park, CA: Sage Publications.

Hammersley, M. (1992). *What's wrong with ethnography? Methodological explorations.* London: Routledge.

Hammersley, M., & Atkinson, P. (1995). *Ethnography: Principles in practice* (2nd ed.). London: Routledge.

Happ, M., Dabbs, A., Tate, J., Hricik, A., & Erlen, J. (2006). Exemplars of mixed methods data combination and analysis. *Nursing Research, 55*(2S), S43–S49.

Harper, D. (1994). On the authority of the image: Visual methods at the crossroads. In N. K. Denzin & Y. S. Lincoln (Eds.), *Handbook of qualitative research* (pp. 403–412). Thousand Oaks, CA: Sage Publications.

Harrell, F. E. (2001). *Regression modeling strategies: With applications to linear models, logistic regression, and survival analysis.* New York: Springer-Verlag.

Hauck, W. W., Gilliss, C. L., Donner, A., & Gortner, S. (1991). Randomization by cluster. *Nursing Research, 40,* 356–358.

Heidegger, M. (1962). *Being and time.* New York: Harper & Row.

Heidegger, M. (1971). *Poetry, language, thought.* New York: Harper & Row.

Higgins, P. A., & Daly, B. J. (1999). Research methodology issues related to interviewing the mechanically ventilated patient. *Western Journal of Nursing Research, 21,* 773–784.

Hilton, A., & Skrutkowski, M. (2002). Translating instrument into other language: Development and testing processes. *Cancer Nursing, 25,* 1–7.

Hinds, P. S., Vogel, R. J., & Clarke-Steffen, L. (1997). The possibilities and pitfalls of doing a secondary analysis of a qualitative data set. *Qualitative Health Research, 7,* 408–424.

Holden, R. R., Fekken, G. C., & Jackson, D. N. (1985). Structured personality test item characteristics and validity. *Journal of Research in Personality, 19,* 386–394.

Holtzclaw, B. J., & Hanneman, S. K. (2002). Use of nonhuman biobehavioral models in critical care nursing research. *Critical Care Nursing Quarterly, 24*(4), 30–40.

Homer, C. S. (2002). Using the Zelen design in randomized controlled trials: Debates and controversies. *Journal of Advanced Nursing, 38*(2), 200–207.

Horsley, J. A., Crane, J., & Bingle, J. D. (1978). Research utilization as an organizational process. *Journal of Nursing Administration, 8,* 4–6.

Hosmer, D., & Lemeshow, S. (1999). *Applied survival analysis: Regression modeling of time to event data.* New York: John Wiley.

Hosmer, D., & Lemeshow, S. (2000). *Applied logistic regression.* New York: John Wiley.

Hougaard, P. (2000). *Analysis of multivariate survival data.* New York: Springer-Verlag.

Hsieh, H., & Shannon, S. (2005). Three approaches to qualitative content analysis. *Qualitative Health Research, 15*(9), 1277–1288.

Hunter, A., Lusardi, P., Zucker, D., Jacelon, C., & Chandler, G. (2002). Making meaning: The creative component in qualitative research. *Qualitative Health Research, 12*(3), 388–398.

Husserl, E. (1962). *Ideas: General introduction to pure phenomenology.* New York: Macmillan.

Im, E., & Chee, W. (2002). Issues in protection of human subjects in Internet research. *Nursing Research, 51*(4), 266–270.

Ingersoll, G. L. (2005). Generating evidence through outcomes management. In B. Melnyk & E. Fineout-Overholt (Eds.), *Evidence-based practice in nursing and healthcare.* Philadelphia: Lippincott Williams & Wilkins.

International Committee of Medical Journal Editors. (2006). *Uniform requirements for manuscripts submitted to biomedical journals.* Retrieved October 5, 2006, from *http://www.icmje.org*.

Irwin, L., & Johnson, J. (2005). Interviewing young children: Explicating our practices and dilemmas. *Qualitative Health Research, 15*(6), 821–831.

Jack, S. (2005). Mothers with PTSD after traumatic childbirth struggled to survive and experienced nightmares, flashbacks, anger, anxiety, depression, and isolation. *Evidence-Based Nursing, 8,* 59.

Jacobson, G. A. (2005). Vulnerable research participants: Anyone may qualify. *Nursing Science Quarterly, 18*(4), 359–363.

Jadad, A. R., Cook, D. J., Jones, A., Klassen, T. P., Tugwell, P., Moher, M., & Moher, D. (1998). Methodology and reports of systematic reviews and meta-analyses: A comparison of Cochrane reviews with articles published in paper-based journals. *Journal of the American Medical Association, 280*, 278–280.

Jeffers, B. R. (2005). Research environments that promote integrity. *Nursing Research, 54*(1), 63–70.

Jennings, B. M. (2000). Evidence-based practice: The road best traveled. *Research in Nursing & Health, 23*, 343–345.

Joffe, M., & Rosenbaum, P. (1999). Invited commentary: Propensity scores. *American Journal of Epidemiology, 150*, 327–333.

Johnson, J. E. (1999). Self-Regulation Theory and coping with physical illness. *Research in Nursing & Health, 22*, 435–448.

Johnson, S. H. (1996). Adapting a thesis to publication style: Meeting editor's expectations. *Dimensions of Critical Care Nursing, 15*, 160–167.

Jones, P. S., Lee, J. W., Phillips, L. R., Zhang, X. E., & Jaceldo, K. B. (2001). An adaptation of Brislin's translation model for cross-cultural research. *Nursing Research, 50*, 300–304.

Jones, R. (2003). Survey data collection using audio computer assisted self-interview. *Western Journal of Nursing Research, 25*(3), 349–358.

Junker, B. H. (1960). *Field work: An introduction to the social sciences.* Chicago: University of Chicago Press.

Kahn, D. (1993). Ways of discussing validity in qualitative nursing research. *Western Journal of Nursing Research, 15*(1), 122–125.

Kahn, D. L. (2000). How to conduct research. In M. Z. Cohen, D. L. Kahn, & R. H. Steeves (Eds.), *Hermeneutic phenomenological research* (pp. 57–70). Thousand Oaks, CA: Sage Publications.

Kearney, M. H. (1998). Ready-to-wear: Discovering grounded formal theory. *Research in Nursing & Health, 21*, 179–186.

Kearney, M. H. (2001). New directions in grounded formal theory. In R. S. Schreiber & P. N. Stern (Eds.), *Using grounded theory in nursing* (pp. 227–246). New York: Springer.

Keely, B. (2004). Planning and creating effective scientific posters. *Journal of Continuing Education in Nursing, 35*(4), 182–185.

Keeney, S., Hasson, F., & McKenna, H. (2006). Consulting the oracle: Ten lessons from using the Delphi technique in nursing research. *Journal of Advanced Nursing, 53*(2), 205–212.

Kennedy, H. P. (2004). Enhancing Delphi research: Methods and results. *Journal of Advanced Nursing, 45*(5), 504–511.

Kerlinger, F. N., & Lee, H. B. (2000). *Foundations of behavioral research* (4th ed.). Orlando, FL: Harcourt College Publishers.

Kidd, P. S., & Parshall, M. B. (2000). Getting the focus and the group: Enhancing analytic rigor in focus group research. *Qualitative Health Research, 10*, 293–308.

Kimchi, J., Polivka, B., & Stevenson, J. S. (1991). Triangulation: Operational definitions. *Nursing Research, 40*, 364–366.

King, N. (1998). Template analysis. In C. Cassell & G. Symon (Eds.), *Qualitative methods and analysis in organizational research* (pp. 118–134). London: Sage Publications.

Kleinbaum, D., & Klein, M. (2005). *Survival analysis: A self-learning text* (2nd ed.). New York: Springer-Verlag.

Kline, R. (2005). *Principles and practice of structural equation modeling* (2nd ed.). New York: The Guilford Press.

Knapp, T. R. (1970). N vs. N − 1. *American Educational Research Journal, 7*, 625–626.

Knapp, T. R. (1994). Regression analysis: What to report. *Nursing Research, 43*, 187–189.

Knapp, T. R., & Brown, J. K. (1995). Ten measurement commandments that often should be broken. *Research in Nursing & Health, 18*, 495–469.

Knaus, W., Draper, E., Wagner, D., & Zimmerman, J. (1985). APACHE II: A severity of disease classification system. *Critical Care Medicine, 13*, 818–829.

Knaus, W., Wagner, D., Draper, E., Zimmerman, J., Bergner, M., et al. (1991). The APACHE III prognostic system. *Chest, 100*(6), 1619–1636.

Koch, T. (1994). Implementation of a hermeneutic inquiry in nursing: Philosophy, rigour, and representation. *Journal of Advanced Nursing, 24*, 174–184.

Kolcaba, K. (2003). *Comfort theory and practice.* New York: Springer.

Kralik, D., Proce, K., Warren, J., & Koch, T. (2006). Issues in data generation using email group conversations for nursing research. *Journal of Advanced Nursing, 53*(2), 213–220.

Krippendroff, K. (2005). *Content analysis: An introduction to its methodology.* Thousand Oaks, CA: Sage Publications.

Krueger, R., & Casey, M. (2000). *Focus groups: A practical guide for applied research* (3rd ed.). Thousand Oaks, CA: Sage Publications.

Kwak, C., & Clayton-Matthews, A. (2002). Multinomial logistic regression. *Nursing Research, 51*(6), 404–409.

Labov, W., & Waletzky, J. (1967). Narrative analysis: Oral versions of personal experience. In J. Helm (Ed.), *Essays on the verbal and visual arts* (pp. 12–44). Seattle: University of Washington Press.

Lambert, M. F., & Wood, J. (2000). Incorporating patient preferences into randomized trials. *Journal of Clinical Epidemiology, 53,* 163–166.

Lange, J. W. (2002). Methodological concerns for non-Hispanic investigators conducting research with Hispanic Americans. *Research in Nursing & Health, 25,* 411–419.

Langhorne, P. (1998). Bias in meta-analysis detected by a simple, graphical test: Prospectively identified trials could be used for comparison with meta-analyses. *British Medical Journal, 316,* 471.

Lapadat, J. C. (2000). Problematizing transcription: Purpose, paradigm and quality. *International Journal of Social Research Methodology, 3,* 203–219.

Lather, P. (1986). Issues of validity in openly ideological research: Between a rock and a hard place. *Interchange, 17,* 63–84.

Lather, P. (1991). *Getting smart: Feminist research and pedagogy with/in the postmodern.* New York: Routledge.

Lauver, D. R., Ward, S. E., Heidrich, S. M., Keller, M. L., Bowers, B. J., Brennan, P. F., Kirchhoff, K. T., & Wells, T. J. (2002). Patient-centered interventions. *Research in Nursing & Health, 25*(4), 246–255.

Lazarsfeld, P. (1955). Foreword. In H. Hyman (Ed.), *Survey design and analysis.* New York: The Free Press.

Lazarus, R. (1966). *Psychological stress and the coping response.* New York: McGraw-Hill.

Lazarus, R., & Folkman, S. (1984). *Stress, appraisal, and coping.* New York: Springer.

LeCompte, M., & Goetz, J. (1984). Problems of reliability and validity in ethnographic research. *Review of Educational Research, 52,* 31–60.

Leininger, M. M. (1985). Life-health-care history: Purposes, methods and techniques. In M. M. Leininger (Ed.), *Qualitative research methods in nursing* (pp. 119–132). New York: Grune & Stratton.

Leininger, M. M. (1991). *Culture care diversity and universality: A theory of nursing.* New York: NLN Press.

Leininger, M. M. (Ed.). (1985). *Qualitative research methods in nursing.* New York: Grune & Stratton.

Leininger, M. M., & McFarland, M. R. (2006). *Culture care diversity and universality: A worldwide nursing theory* (2nd ed.). Sudbury, MA: Jones & Bartlett.

Lenz, E. R., Pugh, L. C., Milligan, R. A., Gift, A., & Suppe, F. (1997). The middle-range theory of unpleasant symptoms. *Advances in Nursing Science, 19,* 14–27.

Levine, M. E. (1973). *Introduction to clinical nursing* (2nd ed.). Philadelphia: F. A. Davis.

Levy, P., & Lemeshow, S. (1999). *Sampling of populations: Methods and applications* (3rd ed.). New York: John Wiley & Sons.

Lewenson, S. B. (2003). Historical research approach. In Speziale, H. J., & D. R. Carpenter (Eds.), *Qualitative research in nursing: Advancing the humanistic perspective* (pp. 207–233). Philadelphia: Lippincott Williams & Wilkins.

Lewins, A., & Silver, C. (2006). Choosing a CAQDAS package: A working paper. Retrieved October 6, 2006, from *http://www.caqdas.soc.surrey.ac.uk/*.

Lewis, S. (2001). Further disquiet on the guidelines front. *Canadian Medical Association Journal, 154,* 180–181.

Lincoln, Y. S., & Guba, E. G. (1985). *Naturalistic inquiry.* Newbury Park, CA: Sage Publications.

Lindeke, L., Hauck, M. R., & Tanner, M. (2000). Practical issues in obtaining child assent for research. *Journal of Pediatric Nursing, 15,* 99–104.

Lindell, M. K., & Brandt, C. J. (1999). Assessing inter-rater agreement on the job relevance of a test: A comparison of the CVI, T, $r_{WG(J)}$, and $r^*_{WG(J)}$ indexes. *Journal of Applied Psychology, 84,* 640–647.

Lipsey, M. W. (1990). *Design sensitivity: Statistical power for experimental research.* Newbury Park, CA: Sage Publications.

Lipsey, M. W., & Wilson, D. B. (2001). *Practical meta-analysis.* Thousand Oaks, CA: Sage Publications.

Lipson, J. G. (1991). The use of self in ethnographic research. In J. M. Morse (Ed.), *Qualitative nursing research: A contemporary dialogue* (pp. 73–89). Newbury Park, CA: Sage Publications.

Little, R., & Rubin, D. (2002). *Statistical analysis with missing data.* (2nd ed.). New York: Wiley Interscience.

Loehlin, J. C. (2003). *Latent variable models: An introduction to factor, path, and structural equation analysis.* (4th ed.). Mahwah, NJ: Lawrence Erlbaum Associates.

Logan, J., & Graham, I. (1998). Toward a comprehensive interdisciplinary model of health care research use. *Science Communication, 20,* 227–246.

Lopez, K. A., & Willis, D. G. (2004). Descriptive versus interpretive phenomenology: Their contributions to nursing knowledge. *Qualitative Health Research, 14*(5), 726–735.

Lowe, N. K., & Ryan-Wenger, N. M. (1992). Beyond Campbell and Fiske: Assessment of convergent and discriminant validity. *Research in Nursing & Health, 15*, 67–75.

Lusk, B. (1997). Historical methodology for nursing research. *Image: Journal of Nursing Scholarship, 29*, 355–359.

Lusk, B., & Sacharski, S. (2005). Dead or alive: HIPAA's impact on nursing historical research. *Nursing History Review, 13*, 189–197.

Lutz, K. F., Shelton, K. C., Robrecht, L. C., Hatton, D. C., & Beckett, A. K. (2000). Use of Certificates of Confidentiality in nursing research. *Journal of Nursing Scholarship, 32*(2), 185–188.

Lynn, M. R. (1986). Determination and quantification of content validity. *Nursing Research, 35*, 382–385.

Lynn, M. R., & McMillen, B. J. (2004). The scale product technique as a means of enhancing the measurement of patient satisfaction. *Canadian Journal of Nursing Research, 36*, 66–81.

Mackey, S. (2005). Phenomenological nursing research: Methodologic insights derived from Heidigger's interpretive phenomenology. *International Journal of Nursing Studies, 42*(2), 179–186.

MacLean, L., Meyer, M., & Estable, A. (2004). Improving accuracy of transcripts in qualitative research. *Qualitative Health Research, 14*(1), 113–123.

MacMillan, K., & Koenig, T. (2004). The Wow factor: Preconceptions and expectations for data analysis software in qualitative research. *Social Science Computer Review, 22*, 179–186.

Magee, T., Lee, S., Giuliano, K., & Munro, B. (2006). Generating new knowledge from existing data. *Nursing Research, 55*(2S), S50–S56.

Magnani, R., Sabin, K., Saidel, T., & Heckathorn, D. (2005). Review of sampling hard-to-reach and hidden populations for HIV surveillance. *AIDS, 19*, S67–72.

Manderson, L., Kelaher, M., & Woelz-Stirling, N. (2001). Developing qualitative databases for multiple users. *Qualitative Health Research, 11*, 149–160.

Mann, C., & Steward, F. (2001). Internet interviewing. In J. F. Gubrium & J. A. Holstein (Eds.), *Handbook of interview research: Context and method* (pp. 603–627). Thousand Oaks, CA: Sage Publications.

Martyn, K., & Belli, R. (2002). Retrospective data collection using event history calendars. *Nursing Research, 51*(4), 270–274.

Matthews, J., Bowen, J., & Mathews, R. (2001). *Successful scientific writing: A step-by-step guide for the biological and medical sciences* (2nd ed.). Cambridge, UK: Cambridge University Press.

Maxwell, S., Cole, D., Arvey, R., & Salas, E. (1991). A comparison of methods for increasing power in randomized between-subjects designs. *Psychological Bulletin, 110*, 328–337.

McCain, N. L., Gray, D. P., Walter, J. M., & Robins, J. (2005). Implementing a comprehensive approach to the study of health dynamics using the psychoimmunology paradigm. *Advances in Nursing Science, 28*(4), 320–332.

McCleary, L. (2002). Using multiple imputation for analysis of incomplete data in clinical research. *Nursing Research, 51*(5), 339–343.

McConnell, E. A. (2000). Publishing opportunities outside the United States. *Journal of Nursing Scholarship, 32*, 87–92.

McCormick, J., Rodney, P., & Varcoe, C. (2003). Reinterpretations across studies: An approach to meta-analysis. *Qualitative Health Research, 13*(7), 933–944.

McGuire, D. B., DeLoney, V., Yeager, K., Owen, D., Peterson, D., Lin, L., & Webster, J. (2000). Maintaining study validity in a changing clinical environment. *Nursing Research, 49*, 231–235.

McGuire, D., DeLoney, V., Yeager, K., Owen, D., Peterson, D., Lin, L., & Webster, J. (2000). Maintaining study validity in a changing clinical environment. *Nursing Research, 49*(4), 231–236.

McLaughlin, G. H. (1969). SMOG grading: A new readability formula. *Journal of Reading, 12*, 639–646.

McNeill, P. (1993). *The ethics and politics of human experimentation.* Cambridge, UK: Cambridge University Press.

Meleis, A. I., Sawyer, L. M., Im, E., Hilfinger Messias, D., & Schumacher, K. (2000). Experiencing transitions: An emerging middle-range theory. *Advances in Nursing Science, 23*(1), 12–28.

Melnyk, B. M., & Fineout-Overhold, E. (2005). *Evidence-based practice in nursing and healthcare: A guide to best practice.* Philadelphia: Lippincott Williams & Wilkins.

Miles, M. B., & Huberman, A. M. (1994). *Qualitative data analysis: An expanded sourcebook* (2nd ed.). Thousand Oaks, CA: Sage Publications.

Millenson, M. L. (1997). *Demanding medical evidence.* Chicago: University of Chicago Press.

Milne, J., & Oberle, K. (2005). Enhancing rigor in qualitative description. *Journal of Wound, Ostomy, & Continence Nursing, 32*(6), 413–420.

Mishel, M. H. (1990). Reconceptualization of the Uncertainty in Illness Theory. *Image*: *Journal of Nursing Scholarship*, *22*(4), 256–262.

Mitchell, P., & Lang, N. (2004). Framing the problem of measuring and improving healthcare quality: Has the Quality Health Outcomes Model been useful? *Medical Care*, *42*(2 Supp), II4–11.

Mitchell, P., Ferketich, S., & Jennings, B. (1998). Quality health outcomes model. *Image: Journal of Nursing Scholarship*, *30*, 43–46.

Moffatt, S., White, M., Mackintosh, J., & Howel, D. (2006). Using quantitative and qualitative data in health services research—what happens when mixed method findings conflict? *BMC Health Services Research*, *6*, 28.

Moloney, M., Dietrich, A., Strickland, O., & Myerburg, S. (2003). Using Internet discussion boards as virtual focus groups. *Advances in Nursing Science*, *26*(4), 274–286.

Moore, L. W., Augspurger, P., King, M. O., & Proffitt, C. (2001). Insights on the poster presentation and presentation process. *Applied Nursing Research*, *14*, 100–104.

Moorhead, S., Johnson, M., & Maas, M. (2004). *Nursing Outcomes Classification (NOC)* (3rd ed.). St. Louis: Mosby.

Morgan, D. L. (2001). Focus group interviewing. In J. F. Gubrium & J. A. Holstein (Eds.), *Handbook of interview research: Context and method* (2nd ed., pp. 141–159). Thousand Oaks, CA: Sage Publications.

Morris, H. M., & Tipples, G. (1998). Choosing to write the paper format thesis. *Journal of Nursing Education*, *37*, 173–175.

Morris, S. M. (2001). Joint and individual interviewing in the context of cancer. *Qualitative Health Research*, *11*, 553–567.

Morrison, B., & Lilford, R. (2001). How can action research apply to health services? *Qualitative Health Research*, *11*, 436–449.

Morrison-Beedy, D., Côté-Arsenault, D., & Feinstein, N. (2001). Maximizing results with focus groups: Moderator and analysis issues. *Applied Nursing Research*, *14*(1), 48–53.

Morrow, R. A., & Brown, D. D. (1994). *Critical theory and methodology*. Thousand Oaks, CA: Sage Publications.

Morse, J. M. (1991a). Approaches to qualitative-quantitative methodological triangulation. *Nursing Research*, *40*(2), 120–123.

Morse, J. M. (1991b). Strategies for sampling. In J. M. Morse (Ed.), *Qualitative nursing research: A contemporary dialogue*. Newbury Park, CA: Sage Publications.

Morse, J. M. (1999). Myth # 93: Reliability and validity are not relevant to qualitative inquiry. *Qualitative Health Research*, *9*, 717–718.

Morse, J. M. (2000). Determining sample size. *Qualitative Health Research*, *10*, 3–5.

Morse, J.M. (2002a). Theory innocent or theory smart? *Qualitative Health Research*, *12*, 295–296.

Morse, J. M. (2002b). Where do interventions come from? *Qualitative Health Research*, *12*(4), 435–436.

Morse, J. M. (2003). Biasphobia. *Qualitative Health Research*, *13*(7), 891–892.

Morse, J. M. (2004a). Constructing qualitatively derived theory. *Qualitative Health Research*, *14*, 1387–1395.

Morse, J. M. (2004b). Qualitative comparison: Appropriateness, equivalence, and fit. *Qualitative Health Research*, *14*(10), 1323–1325.

Morse, J. M. (2005). Beyond the clinical trial: Expanding criteria for evidence. *Qualitative Health Research*, *15*(1), 3–4.

Morse, J. M. (2006a). The scope of qualitatively derived clinical interventions. *Qualitative Health Research*, *16*(5), 591–593.

Morse, J. M. (2006b). Insight, inference, evidence, and verification: Creating a legitimate discipline. *International Journal of Qualitative Methods*, *5*(1), Article 8. Retrieved January 12, 2007, from *http://www.ualberta.ca/ijqm/*.

Morse, J. M., & Field, P. A. (1995). *Qualitative research methods for health professionals*. (2nd ed.). Thousand Oaks, CA: Sage Publications.

Morse, J. M., Barrett, M., Mayan, M., Olson, K., & Spiers, J. (2002) Verification strategies for establishing reliability and validity in qualitative research. *International Journal of Qualitative Methods*, *1*(2), Article 2. Retrieved January 12, 2007, from *http://www.ualberta.ca/ijqm/*.

Morse, J. M., Solberg, S. M., Neander, W. L., Bottorff, J. L., & Johnson, J. L. (1990). Concepts of caring and caring as a concept. *Advances in Nursing Science*, *13*, 1–14.

Motulsky, H. (1995). *Intuitive biostatistics*. New York: Oxford University Press.

Munhall, P. L. (2001). Ethical considerations in qualitative research. In P. L. Munhall (Ed.), *Nursing research: A qualitative perspective* (pp. 537–549). Sudbury, MA: Jones & Bartlett.

Munhall, P. L. (2007). *Nursing research: A qualitative perspective* (4th ed.). Sudbury, MA: Jones & Bartlett.

Munro, B. H. (Ed.). (2004). *Statistical methods for healthcare research* (5th ed.). Philadelphia: Lippincott Williams & Wilkins.

NANDA International. (2005). *Nursing diagnoses: Definitions and classification, 2005–2006*. Philadelphia: Author.

National Commission for the Protection of Human Subjects of Biomedical and Behavioral Research. (1978). *Belmont report: Ethical principles and guidelines for research involving human subjects*. Washington, DC: U.S. Government Printing Office.

Naylor, M. D. (2003). Nursing intervention research and quality of care. *Nursing Research, 52*(5), 380–385.

Neuman, B., & Fawcett. J. (2001). *The Neuman Systems Model* (4th ed.). Englewood, NJ: Prentice Hall.

Newhouse, R., Dearholt, S., Poe, S., Pugh, L. C., & White, K. M. (2005). Evidence-based practice: A practical approach to implementation. *Journal of Nursing Administration, 35,* 35–40.

Newman, M. (1994). *Health as expanding consciousness* (2nd ed.). New York: National League for Nursing.

Newman, M. A. (1997). Evolution of the theory of health as expanding consciousness. *Nursing Science Quarterly, 10,* 22–25.

Nightingale, F. (1859). *Notes on nursing: What it is, and what it is not*. Philadelphia: J. B. Lippincott.

Noblit, G., & Hare, R. D. (1988). *Meta-ethnography: Synthesizing qualitative studies*. Newbury Park, CA: Sage Publications.

Northam, S., Trubenbach, M., & Bentov, L. (2000). Nursing journal survey: Information to help you publish. *Nurse Educator, 25,* 227–236.

Novak, J., & Canas, A. (2006). *The theory underlying concept maps and how to construct them* (IHMC CmapTools Technical Report 2006–01). Pensacola, FL: Institute for Human and Machine Cognition.

Nunnally, J. C., & Bernstein, I. H. (1994). *Psychometric theory* (3rd ed.). New York: McGraw-Hill.

Oermann, M. (2002). *Writing for publication in nursing*. Philadelphia: Lippincott Williams & Wilkins.

Olesen, V. (2000). Feminism and qualitative research at and into the millennium. In N. K. Denzin & Y. S. Lincoln (Eds.), *Handbook of qualitative research* (2nd ed., pp. 215–255). Thousand Oaks, CA: Sage Publications.

Olsen, D. P. (2003). HIPAA privacy regulations and nursing research. *Nursing Research, 52,* 344–348.

Orem, D. E., Taylor, S. G., Renpenning, K. M., & Eisenhandler, S. A. (2003). *Self-care theory in nursing: Selected papers of Dorothea Orem*. New York: Springer.

Ory, M. G., Jordan, P. J., & Bazzarre, T. (2002). The Behavior Change Consortium: Setting the stage for a new century of health behavior-change research. *Health Education Research, 17*(5), 500–511.

Owen, S. (2005). The significance of significance. *Research in Nursing & Health, 28,* 281–282.

Owen, S., & Froman, R. (2005). Why carve up your continuous data? *Research in Nursing & Health, 28*(6), 496–503.

Pampel, F. (2000). *Logistic regression: A primer*. Thousand Oaks, CA: Sage Publications.

Parse, R. R. (1999). *Illuminations: The human becoming theory in practice and research*. Sudbury, MA: Jones & Bartlett.

Paterson, B. L., Thorne, S. E., Canam, C., & Jillings, C. (2001). *Meta-study of qualitative health research*. Thousand Oaks, CA: Sage Publications.

Patrician, P. A. (2002). Multiple imputation for missing data. *Research in Nursing & Health, 25,* 76–84.

Patrician, P. A. (2004). Single-item graphic representational scales. *Nursing Research, 53*(5), 347–352.

Patton, M. (1999). Enhancing the quality and credibility of qualitative analysis. *Health Services Research, 34*(5 Pt. 2), 1189–1208.

Patton, M. Q. (2002). *Qualitative evaluation and research methods* (3rd ed.). Thousand Oaks, CA: Sage Publications.

Pender, N. J., Murdaugh, C., & Parsons, M. A. (2006). *Health promotion in nursing practice* (5th ed.). Upper Saddle River, NJ: Prentice Hall.

Pett, M. A., Lackey, N. R., & Sullivan, J. J. (2003). *Making sense of factor analysis: The use of factor analysis for instrument development in health care research*. Thousand Oaks, CA: Sage Publications.

Poland, B. D. (1995). Transcription quality as an aspect of rigor in qualitative research. *Qualitative Inquiry, 1,* 190–310.

Polit, D. F. (1996). *Data analysis and statistics for nursing research*. Stamford, CT: Appleton & Lange.

Polit, D. F., & Beck, C. T. (2006). The content validity index: Are you sure you know what's being reported? Critique and recommendations. *Research in Nursing & Health, 29*(5), 489–497.

Polit, D. F., & Sherman, R. (1990). Statistical power analysis in nursing research. *Nursing Research, 39,* 365–369.

Polit, D., Beck, C., & Owen, S. (in press). Is the CVI an acceptable indicator of content validity? *Research in Nursing & Health*.

Porter, E. J. (1999). Defining the eligible, accessible population for a phenomenological study. *Western Journal of Nursing Research, 21,* 796–804.

Portney, L. G., & Watkins, M. P. (2000). *Foundations of clinical research: Applications to practice* (2nd ed.). Upper Saddle River, NJ: Prentice Hall Heath.

Prochaska, J. O., & Velicer, W. F. (1997). The Transtheoretical Model of health behavior change. *American Journal of Health Promotion, 12*(1), 38–48.

Prochaska, J. O., Redding, C. A., & Evers, K. E. (2002). The Transtheoretical Model and stages of changes. In F. M. Lewis (Ed.), *Health behavior and health education: Theory, research and practice* (pp. 99–120). San Francisco: Jossey-Bass.

Punch, M. (1994). Politics and ethics in qualitative research. In N. K. Denzin & Y. S. Lincoln (Eds.), *Handbook of qualitative research*. Thousand Oaks, CA: Sage Publications.

Reason, O. (1981). Issues of validity in new paradigm research. In P. Reason & J. Rowan (Eds.), *Human inquiry* (pp. 239–250). New York: John Wiley.

Reed, P. G. (1991). Toward a nursing theory of self-transcendence. *Advances in Nursing Science, 13*(4), 64–77.

Reinharz, S. (1992). *Feminist methods in social research*. New York: Oxford University Press.

Reynolds, W. (1982). Development of reliable and valid short forms of the Marlow-Crowne Social Desirability Scale. *Journal of Clinical Psychology, 38,* 119–125.

Ricoeur, P. (1981). *Hermeneutics and the social sciences.* (J. Thompson, Trans., & Ed.). New York: Cambridge University Press.

Riessman, C. K. (1991). Beyond reductionism: Narrative genres in divorce accounts. *Journal of Narrative and Life History, 1,* 41 68.

Riessman, C. K. (1993). *Narrative analysis*. Newbury Park, CA: Sage Publications.

Robinson, K. M. (2001). Unsolicited narratives from the Internet: A rich source of qualitative data. *Qualitative Health Research, 11,* 706–714.

Rodgers, B. L., & Cowles, K. V. (1993). The qualitative research audit trail: A complex collection of documentation. *Research in Nursing and Health, 16,* 219–226.

Rogers, E. M. (1995). *Diffusion of innovations* (4th ed.). New York: Free Press.

Rogers, M. E. (1970). *An introduction to the theoretical basis of nursing*. Philadelphia: F. A. Davis.

Rogers, M. E. (1986). Science of unitary human beings. In V. Malinski (Ed.), *Explorations on Martha Rogers' science of unitary human beings*. Norwalk, CT: Appleton-Century-Crofts.

Rolfe, G. (2006). Validity, trustworthiness and rigour: Quality and the idea of qualitative research. *Journal of Advanced Nursing, 53*(3), 304–310.

Romazanoglu, C., & Holland, J. (2002). *Feminist methodology: Challenges and choices*. Thousand Oaks, CA: Sage Publications.

Rosenbaum. P. R. (1995). *Observational studies*. New York: Springer-Verlag.

Rosenfeld, P., Duthie, E., Bier, J., Bower-Ferres, S., Fulmer, T., Iervolino, L., McClure, M., McGivern, D., & Roncoli, M. (2000). Engaging staff nurses in evidence-based research to identify nursing practice problems and solutions. *Applied Nursing Research, 13,* 197–203.

Rosenthal, R. (1991). *Meta-analytic procedures for social research*. Newbury Park, CA: Sage Publications.

Rosswurm, M. A., & Larrabee, J. H. (1999). A model for change to evidence-based practice. *Image: Journal of Nursing Scholarship, 31,* 317–322.

Roy, C., & Zhan, L. (2006). Sister Callista Roy's Adaptation Model and its applications. In M. E. Parker (Ed.), *Nursing theories and nursing practice* (pp. 268–280). Philadelphia: F. A. Davis.

Roy, C., Sr., & Andrews, H. (1999). *The Roy Adaptation Model*. (2nd ed.). Norwalk, CT: Appleton & Lange.

Rubin, H., & Rubin, I. S. (2005). *Qualitative interviewing: The art of hearing data* (2nd ed.). Thousand Oaks, CA: Sage Publications.

Russell, C. K., Gregory, D. M., & Gates, M. F. (1996). Aesthetics and substance in qualitative research posters. *Qualitative Health Research, 6,* 542–553.

Rycroft-Malone, J., Seers, K., Titchen, A., Harvey, G., Kitson, A., & McCormack, B. (2004). Getting evidence into practice: Ingredients for change. *Nursing Standard, 16*(37), 38–43.

Sackett, D. L., Rosenberg, W., Muir Gray, J. A., Haynes, R., & Richardson, W. (1996). Evidence based medicine: What it is and what it isn't. *British Medical Journal, 312,* 71–72.

Sackett, D. L., Straus, S. E., Richardson, W. S., Rosenberg, W., & Haynes, R. B. (2000). *Evidence-based medicine: How to practice and teach EBM* (2nd ed.). Edinburgh: Churchill Livingstone.

Sandelowski, M. (1993a). Theory unmasked: The uses and guises of theory in qualitative research. *Research in Nursing & Health, 16,* 213–218.

Sandelowski, M. (1993b). Rigor or rigor mortis: The problem of rigor in qualitative research revisited. *Advances in Nursing Science, 16,* 1–8.

Sandelowski, M. (1996). Using qualitative methods in intervention studies. *Research in Nursing & Health, 19*, 359–364.

Sandelowski, M. (1998). Writing a good read: Strategies for re-presenting qualitative data. *Research in Nursing & Health, 21*, 375–382.

Sandelowski, M. (2000a). Whatever happened to qualitative description? *Research in Nursing & Health, 23*, 334–340.

Sandelowski, M. (2000b). Combining qualitative and quantitative sampling, data collection, and analysis techniques in mixed-method studies. *Research in Nursing & Health, 23*, 246–255.

Sandelowski, M. (2001). Real qualitative researchers do not count: The use of numbers in qualitative research. *Research in Nursing & Health, 24*, 230–240.

Sandelowski, M. (2004). Counting cats in Zanzibar. *Research in Nursing & Health, 27*(4), 215–216.

Sandelowski, M., & Barroso, J. (2002). Finding the findings in qualitative studies. *Journal of Nursing Scholarship, 34*, 213–219.

Sandelowski, M., & Barroso, J. (2003a). Classifying the findings in qualitative studies. *Qualitative Health Research, 13*(7), 905–923.

Sandelowski, M., & Barroso, J. (2003b). Creating meta-summaries of qualitative findings. *Nursing Research, 52*, 226–233.

Sandelowski, M., & Barroso, J. (2003c). Toward a meta-synthesis of qualitative findings on motherhood in HIV-positive women. *Research in Nursing & Health, 26*(2), 153–170.

Sandelowski, M., & Barroso, J. (2006). *Synthesizing qualitative research.* York: Springer Publishing Company.

Sandelowski, M., Docherty, S., & Emden, C. (1997). Qualitative metasynthesis: Issues and techniques. *Research in Nursing & Health, 20*, 365–377.

Santacroce, S. J., Maccarelli, L. M., & Grey, M. (2004). Intervention fidelity. *Nursing Research, 53*(1), 63–68.

Schreiber, R., Crooks, D., & Stern, P. N. (1997). Qualitative meta-analysis. In J. M. Morse (Ed.), *Completing a qualitative project* (pp. 311–326). Thousand Oaks, CA: Sage Publications.

Schrum, L. (1995). Framing the debate: Ethical research in the information age. *Qualitative Inquiry, 1*, 311–326.

Schultz, K. F., Chalmers, I., & Altman, D. G. (2002). The landscape and lexicon of blinding in randomized trials. *Annals of Internal Medicine, 136*(3), 254–259.

Schwandt, T. (1997). *Qualitative inquiry: A dictionary of terms.* Thousand Oaks, CA: Sage Publications.

Seidel, J. (1993). Method and madness in the application of computer technology to qualitative data analysis. In N. G. Fielding & R. M. Lee (Eds.), *Using computers in qualitative research* (pp. 107–116). Newbury Park, CA: Sage Publications.

Shadish, W. R., Cook, T. D., & Campbell, D. T. (2002). *Experimental and quasi-experimental designs for generalized causal inference.* Boston: Houghton Mifflin.

Shekelle, P. G., Woolf, S. H., Eccles, M., & Grimshaw, J. (1999). Clinical guidelines: Developing guidelines. *British Medical Journal, 318*(7183), 593–596.

Shrout, P., & Fleiss, J. (1979). Intraclass correlations: Uses in assessing rater reliability. *Psychological Bulletin, 86* (2), 420–428.

Sidani, S., & Braden, C. J. (1998). *Evaluating nursing interventions: A theory-driven approach.* Thousand Oaks, CA: Sage Publications.

Sigma Theta Tau International. (2005). Resource paper on global health and nursing research priorities. Retrieved November 22, 2005, from *http://www.nursingsociety.org/about/position_GHNRPRP.doc*.

Silva, M. C. (1986). Research testing nursing theory: State of the art. *Advances in Nursing Science, 9*, 1–11.

Silva, M. C. (1995). *Ethical guidelines in the conduct, dissemination, and implementation of nursing research.* Washington, DC: American Nurses Association.

Silva, M. C., & Sorrell, J. M. (1992). Testing of nursing theory: Critique and philosophical expansion. *Advances in Nursing Science, 14*, 12–23.

Silverman, D. (1993). *Interpreting qualitative data: Methods for analyzing talk, text, and interaction.* London: Sage Publications.

Sindhu, F., Carpenter, L., & Seers, K. (1997). Development of a tool to rate the quality assessment of randomized controlled trials using a Delphi technique. *Journal of Advanced Nursing, 25*, 1262–1268.

Sixsmith, J., & Murray, C. D. (2001). Ethical issues in the documentary data analysis of Internet posts and archives. *Qualitative Health Research, 11*, 423–432.

Smith, D. E. (1999). *Writing the social: Critique, theory, and investigation.* Toronto: University of Toronto Press.

Smith, J. (1993). *After the demise of empiricism: The problem of judging social and educational inquiry.* Norwood, NJ: Ablex.

Smith, M. J., & Liehr, P. (2003). *Middle-range theory for nursing.* New York: Springer.

Soeken, K., & Sripusanapan, A. (2003). Assessing publication bias in meta-analysis. *Nursing Research, 52*(1), 57–60.

Soukup, M., Sr. (2000). The Center for Advanced Nursing Practice evidence-based practice model: Promoting the scholarship of practice. *Nursing Clinics of North America, 35*, 301–309.

Sousa, V., Zausziewski, J., & Musil, C. (2004). How to determine whether a convenience sample represents the population. *Applied Nursing Research, 17*(2), 130–133.

Sparkes, A. (2001). Myth 94: Qualitative health researchers will agree about validity. *Qualitative Health Research, 11*(4), 538–552.

Spiegelberg, H. (1975). *Doing phenomenology.* The Hague: Nijhoff.

Spradley, J. (1979). *The ethnographic interview.* New York: Holt Rinehart & Winston.

Spradley, J. P. (1980). *Participant observation.* New York: Holt, Rinehart & Wilson.

Spradley, J. P., & McCurdy, D. W. (1972). *The cultural experience: Ethnography in complex society.* Prospect Heights, IL: Waveland Press.

Stake, R. (1995). *The art of case study research.* Thousand Oaks, CA: Sage Publications.

Stake, R. E. (2005). Qualitative case studies. In N. Denzin & Y. Lincoln (Eds.), *Handbook of qualitative research* (3rd ed., pp. 443–466). Thousand Oaks, CA: Sage Publications.

Stemler, S. (2004). A comparison of consensus, consistency, and measurement approaches to estimating interrater reliability. *Practical Assessment, Research, and Evaluation, 9*(4). Retrieved May 16, 2006, from *http://PARE online.net/getvn.asp?v=9&n=4.*

Stetler, C. B. (2001). Updating the Stetler model of research utilization to facilitate evidence-based practice. *Nursing Outlook, 49,* 272–279.

Stetler, C. B., & Marram, G. (1976). Evaluating research findings for applicability in practice. *Nursing Outlook, 24,* 559–563.

Stevens, K. R. (2001). Systematic reviews: The heart of evidence-based practice. *AACN Clinical Issues, 12,* 529–538.

Strahan, R., & Gerbasi, K. (1972). Short, homogeneous version of the Marlowe-Crown Social Desirability Scale. *Journal of Clinical Psychology, 28,* 191–193.

Strauss, A. L., & Corbin, J. M. (1998). *Basics of qualitative research: Techniques and procedures for developing grounded theory* (2nd ed.). Thousand Oaks, CA: Sage Publications.

Streiner, D. L., & Norman, G. R. (2003). *Health measurement scales: A practical guide to their development and use* (3rd ed.). Oxford, UK: Oxford University Press.

Strunk, W., Jr., White, E. B., & Angell, R. (2000). *The elements of style (*4th ed.). Boston: Allyn & Bacon.

Subcommittee on Measuring and Reporting the Quality of Survey Data. (2001). *Statistical working paper 31: Measuring and reporting sources of error in surveys.* Washington, DC: Office of Management and Budget. Retrieved September, 2005, from *http://www.fcsm.gov/01papers/SPWP31_final.pdf.*

Tabachnick, B. G., & Fidell, L. S. (2007). *Using multivariate statistics* (5th ed.). Boston: Allyn & Bacon.

Tashakkori, A., & Teddlie, C. (2003). *Handbook of mixed methods in social and behavioral research* (2nd ed.). Thousand Oaks, CA: Sage Publications.

Taylor, C. (2005). What packages are available? Retrieved October 6, 2006, from *http://www.caqdas.soc.surrey.ac.uk/.*

Therneau, T., & Grambsch, P. (2000). *Modeling survival data: Extending the Cox model.* New York: Springer-Verlag.

Thompson, A., Pickler, R., & Reyna, B. (2005). Clinical coordination of research. *Applied Nursing Research, 18*(2), 102–105.

Thorne, S. (1994). Secondary analysis in qualitative research: Issues and implications. In J. M. Morse (Ed.), *Critical issues in qualitative research methods.* Thousand Oaks, CA: Sage Publications.

Thorne, S., & Darbyshire, P. (2005). Land mines in the field: A modest proposal for improving the craft of qualitative health research. *Qualitative Health Research, 15*(8), 1105–1113.

Thorne, S., Jensen, L., Kearney, M., Noblit, G., & Sandelowski, M. (2004). Qualitative metasynthesis: Reflections on methodological orientation and ideological agenda. *Qualitative Health Research, 14*(10), 1342–1365.

Tilden, V. P., Nelson, C. A., & May, B. A. (1990). Use of qualitative methods to enhance content validity. *Nursing Research, 39,* 172–175.

Tilden, V., & Potempa, K. (2003). The impact of nursing science: A litmus test. *Nursing Research, 52*(5), 275.

Titler, M. G., & Everett, L. Q. (2001). Translating research into practice. Considerations for critical care investigators. *Critical Care Nursing Clinics of North America, 13*(4), 587–604.

Titler, M. G., Kleiber, C., Steelman, V., Rakel, B., Budreau, G., Everett, L., Buckwalter, K., Tripp-Reimer, T., & Goode, C. (2001). The Iowa model of evidence-based practice to promote quality care. *Critical Care Nursing Clinics of North America, 13,* 497–509.

Tobin, G., & Begley, C. (2004). Methodological rigour within a qualitative framework. *Journal of Advanced Nursing, 48*(4), 388–396.

Tomey, A., & Alligood, M. (2006). *Nursing theorists and their work.* (6th ed.). St. Louis, MO: C. V. Mosby.

Tuchman, G. (1994). Historical social science: Methodologies, methods, and meanings. In N. K. Denzin & Y. S. Lincoln (Eds.), *Handbook of qualitative research* (pp. 306–323). Thousand Oaks, CA: Sage Publications.

Tunis, S. R., Stryer, D., & Clancy, C. (2003). Practical clinical trials: Increasing the value of clinical research for decision making in clinical and health policy. *Journal of the American Medical Association, 290* (12) 1624–1632.

Turkel, M. C., Reidinger, G., Ferket, K., & Reno, K. (2005). An essential component of the magnet journey: Fostering an environment for evidence-based practice and nursing research. *Nursing Administration Quarterly, 29*(3), 254–262.

Van den Hoonaard, W. C. (2002). *Walking the tightrope: Ethical issues for qualitative researchers.* Toronto: University of Toronto Press.

Van Kaam, A. (1966). *Existential foundations of psychology.* Pittsburgh, PA: Duquesne University Press.

Van Manen, M. (1990). *Researching lived experience.* Albany, NY: State University of New York Press.

Van Manen, M. (1997a). From meaning to method. *Qualitative Health Research, 7,* 345–369.

Van Manen, M. (1997b). *Researching lived experience: Human science for an action sensitive pedagogy.* London, Ontario: Althouse.

Van Manen, M. (2002). *Writing in the dark: Phenomenological studies in interpretive inquiry.* Ontario: The Althouse Press.

Van Manen, M. (2006). Writing qualitatively or the demands of writing. *Qualitative Health Research, 16,* 713–722.

Van Meijel, B., Gamel, C., van Swieten-Duijfjes, B., & Grypdonck, M. (2004). The development of evidence-based nursing interventions. *Journal of Advanced Nursing, 48*(1), 84–92.

Vessey, J., & Gennarao, S. (1994). The ghost of Tuskegee. *Nursing Research, 43*(2), 67–68.

Walker, D., & Myrick, F. (2006). Grounded theory: An exploration of process and procedure. *Qualitative Health Research, 16*(4), 547–559.

Walker, L. O., & Avant, K. C. (2004). *Strategies for theory construction in nursing.* (4th ed.). Englewood Cliffs, NJ: Prentice Hall.

Walters, L. A., Wilczynski, N. L., & Haynes, R. B. (2006). Developing optimal search strategies for retrieving relevant qualitative studies in EMBASE. *Qualitative Health Research, 16*(1), 162–168.

Waltz, C. F., Strickland, O. L., & Lenz, E. R. (2005). *Measurement in nursing and health research.* (3rd ed.). New York: Springer.

Wang, W., Lee, H., & Fetzer, S. (2006). Challenges and strategies of instrument translation. *Western Journal of Nursing Research, 28*(3), 310–321.

Warnock, F. F., & Allen, M. (2003). Ethological methods to develop nursing knowledge. *Research in Nursing & Health, 26,* 74–84.

Warren, C. (2001). Qualitative interviewing (pp. 83–102). In J. F. Gubrium & J. A. Holstein (Eds.), *Handbook of interview research: Context and method* (2nd ed.). Thousand Oaks, CA: Sage Publications.

Watson, J. (2005). *Caring science as sacred science.* Philadelphia: F. A. Davis.

Watson, L., & Girard, F. (2004). Establishing integrity and avoiding methodological misunderstanding. *Qualitative Health Research, 14*(6), 875–881.

Weber, B., Yarandi, H., Rowe, M., & Weber, J. (2005). A comparison study: Paper-based versus web-based data collection and management. *Applied Nursing Research, 18,* 182–185.

Weitzman, E., & Miles, M. (1995). *Computer programs for qualitative data analysis: A software sourcebook.* Thousand Oaks, CA: Sage Publications.

Whitehead, L. (2004). Enhancing the quality of hermeneutic research. *Journal of Advanced Nursing, 45*(5), 512–518.

Whitmer, K., Sweeney, C., Slivjak, A., Sumner, C., & Barsevick, A. (2005). Strategies for maintaining integrity of a behavioral intervention. *Western Journal of Nursing Research, 27*(3), 338–345.

Whittemore, R. (2005). Combining evidence in nursing research: Methods and applications. *Nursing Research, 54*(1), 56–62.

Whittemore, R., & Grey, M. (2002). The systematic development of nursing interventions. *Journal of Nursing Scholarship, 34*(2), 115–120.

Whittemore, R., Chase, S. K., & Mandle, C. L. (2001). Validity in qualitative research. *Qualitative Health Research, 11*(4), 522–537.

Whyte, W. F. (Ed.). (1991). *Participatory action research.* Newbury Park, CA: Sage Publications.

Wolcott, H. (1994). *Transforming qualitative data.* London: Sage Publications.

Wolcott, H. (1995). *The art of fieldwork.* London: Sage Publications.

Wood, M. J. (2000). Influencing health policy through research. *Clinical Nursing Research, 9*(3), 213–216.

Yen, M., & Lo, L. (2002). Examining test–retest reliability: An intraclass correlation approach. *Nursing Research, 51,* 59–62.

Yin, R. (2003). *Case study research: Design and methods* (3rd ed.). Thousand Oaks, CA: Sage Publications.

Zelen, M. (1979). A new design for randomized controlled trials. *New England Journal of Medicine, 300,* 1242–1245.

Glossary

absolute risk The proportion of people in a group who experienced an undesirable outcome.

absolute risk reduction (ARR) The difference between the absolute risk in one group (e.g., those exposed to an intervention) and the absolute risk in another group (e.g., those not exposed); sometimes called the *risk difference* or *RD*.

abstract A brief description of a completed or proposed study, usually located at the beginning of a report or proposal.

accidental sampling Selection of the most readily available people as study participants; also called *convenience sampling.*

acquiescence response set A bias in self-report instruments, especially in psychosocial scales, created when participants characteristically agree with statements ("yea-say") independent of content.

adherence to treatment The degree to which those in an intervention group adhere to protocols or continue getting the treatment

after-only design An experimental design in which data are collected from subjects only after an intervention has been introduced.

allocation concealment The process used to ensure that those enrolling subjects into a clinical trial are unaware of upcoming assignments, that is, the treatment group to which new enrollees will be assigned.

alpha (α) (1) In tests of statistical significance, the level indicating the probability of a Type I error; (2) in assessments of internal consistency reliability, a reliability coefficient, Cronbach's alpha.

analysis The process of organizing and synthesizing data so as to answer research questions and test hypotheses.

analysis of covariance (ANCOVA) A statistical procedure used to test mean differences among groups on a dependent variable, while controlling for one or more covariates.

analysis of variance (ANOVA) A statistical procedure for testing mean differences among three or more groups by comparing variability between groups to variability within groups.

ancestry approach In literature searches, using citations from relevant studies to track down earlier research upon which the studies are based (the "ancestors").

anonymity Protection of participants' confidentiality such that even the researcher cannot link individuals with information provided.

applied research Research designed to find a solution to an immediate practical problem.

arm A group of participants allocated a particular treatment (e.g., the control *arm* or treatment *arm*).

assent The affirmative agreement of a vulnerable subject (e.g., a child) to participate in a study.

associative relationship An association between two variables that cannot be described as causal (i.e., one variable *causing* the other).

747

assumption A principle that is accepted as being true based on logic or reason, without proof.

asymmetric distribution A distribution of data values that is skewed, with two halves that are not mirror images of each other.

attention control group A control group that gets a similar amount of attention to those in the intervention group, without the "active ingredients" of the treatment.

attrition The loss of participants over the course of a study, which can create bias by changing the composition of the sample initially drawn.

audit trail The systematic documentation of material that allows an independent auditor of a qualitative study to draw conclusions about trustworthiness.

authenticity The extent to which qualitative researchers fairly and faithfully show a range of different realities in the analysis and interpretation of their data.

auto-ethnography Ethnographic studies in which researchers study their own culture or group.

axial coding The second level of coding in a grounded theory study using the Strauss and Corbin approach, involving the process of categorizing, recategorizing, and condensing first level codes by connecting a category and its subcategories.

back-translation The translation of a translated text back into the original language, so that a comparison of the original and back-translated versions can be made.

baseline data Data collected prior to an intervention, including pretreatment data measuring the dependent variables.

basic research Research designed to extend the base of knowledge in a discipline for the sake of knowledge production or theory construction, rather than for solving an immediate problem.

basic social process (BSP) The central social process emerging through an analysis of grounded theory data.

before–after design An experimental design in which data are collected from subjects both before and after the introduction of an intervention.

beneficence A fundamental ethical principle that seeks to maximize benefits for study participants, and prevent harm.

beta(β) (1) In multiple regression, the standardized coefficients indicating the relative weights of the predictor variables in the equation; (2) in statistical testing, the probability of a Type II error.

between-subjects design A research design in which there are separate groups of people being compared (e.g., smokers and nonsmokers).

bias Any influence that distorts the results of a study and undermines validity.

bimodal distribution A distribution of data values with two peaks (high frequencies).

binomial distribution A statistical distribution with known properties describing the number of occurrences of an event in a series of observations; forms the basis for analyzing dichotomous data.

bivariate statistics Statistics derived from analyzing two variables simultaneously to assess the empirical relationship between them.

blind review The review of a manuscript or proposal such that neither the author nor the reviewer is identified to the other party.

blinding The process of preventing those involved in a study (subjects, intervention agents, or data collectors) from having information that could lead to a bias, for example, knowledge of which treatment group a subject is in; also called *masking*.

Bonferroni correction An adjustment made to establish a more conservative alpha level when multiple statistical tests are being run from the same data set; the correction is computed by dividing the desired α by the number of tests—e.g., $.05/3 = .017$.

bracketing In phenomenological inquiries, the process of identifying and holding in abeyance any preconceived beliefs and opinions about the phenomena under study.

canonical analysis A statistical procedure for examining the relationship between two or more independent variables *and* two or more dependent variables.

carry-over effect The influence that one treatment can have on subsequent treatments.

case-control design A nonexperimental research design involving the comparison of a "case" (i.e., a person with the condition under scrutiny, such as lung cancer) and a matched control (a similar person without the condition).

case study A research method involving a thorough, in-depth analysis of an individual, group, or other social unit.

categorical variable A variable with discrete values (e.g., gender) rather than values along a continuum (e.g., weight).

category system In qualitative studies, the system used to sort and organize the data; in studies involving observation, the prespecified plan for recording the behaviors and events under observation.

causal modeling The development and statistical testing of an explanatory model of hypothesized causal relationships among phenomena.

causal (cause-and-effect) relationship A relationship between two variables such that the presence or absence of one variable (the "cause") determines the presence or absence (or value) of the other (the "effect").

cell (1) The intersection of a row and column in a table with two or more dimensions; (2) in an experimental design, the representation of an experimental condition in a schematic diagram.

census A survey covering an entire population.

central (core) category The main category or pattern of behavior in grounded theory analysis using the Strauss and Corbin approach.

central tendency A statistical index of the "typical-ness" of a set of scores, derived from the center of the score distribution; indices of central tendency include the mode, median, and mean.

chi-square test A statistical test used to assess differences in proportions; symbolized as χ^2.

clinical research Research designed to generate knowledge to guide nursing practice.

clinical trial A study designed to assess the safety, efficacy, and effectiveness of a new clinical intervention, sometimes involving several phases (e.g., Phase III is a *randomized clinical trial* using an experimental design).

closed-ended question A question that offers respondents a set of predetermined response options.

cluster randomization The random assignment of intact groups of subjects—rather than individual subjects—to treatment conditions.

cluster sampling A form of sampling in which large groupings ("clusters") are selected first (e.g., nursing schools), with successive subsampling of smaller units (e.g., nursing students).

Cochrane Collaboration An international organization that aims to facilitate well-informed decisions about health care by preparing and disseminating systematic reviews of the effects of health care interventions.

codebook A record documenting categorization and coding decisions.

coding The process of transforming raw data into standardized form for data processing and analysis; in quantitative research, the process of attaching numbers to categories; in qualitative research, the process of identifying recurring words, themes, or concepts within the data.

coefficient alpha (Cronbach's alpha) A reliability index that estimates the internal consistency or homogeneity of a measure composed of several items or subparts.

cognitive questioning A method sometimes used during a pretest of an instrument in which respondents are asked to verbalize what comes to mind when they hear a question.

cognitive test An instrument designed to assess intellectual skills or cognitive functioning (e.g., an IQ test).

Cohen's *d* An effect size for comparing two group means, computed by subtracting one mean from the other and dividing by the pooled standard deviation; also called *standardized mean difference.*

cohort design A nonexperimental design in which a defined group of people (a cohort) is followed over time to study outcomes for subsets of the cohorts; also called a *prospective design.*

cohort study A kind of trend study that focuses on a specific subpopulation (which is often an age-related subgroup) from which different samples are selected at different points in time (e.g., the cohort of nursing students who graduated between 1970 and 1974).

comparison group A group of subjects whose scores on a dependent variable are used to evaluate the outcomes of the group of primary interest (e.g., nonsmokers as a comparison group for smokers); term used in lieu of control group when the study design is not a true experiment.

computer-assisted personal interviewing (CAPI) In-person interviewing in which the interviewers read questions from, and enter responses onto, a laptop computer.

computer-assisted telephone interviewing (CATI) Interviewing done over the telephone in which the interviewers read questions from, and enter responses onto, a computer.

concept An abstraction based on observations of behaviors or characteristics (e.g., stress, pain).

conceptual definition The abstract or theoretical meaning of the concept being studied.

conceptual file A manual method of organizing qualitative data, by creating file folders for each category in the coding scheme, and inserting relevant excerpts from the data.

conceptual map A schematic representation of a theory or conceptual model that graphically represents key concepts and linkages among them.

conceptual model Interrelated concepts or abstractions assembled together in a rational scheme by virtue of their relevance to a common theme; sometimes called *conceptual framework.*

concurrent validity The degree to which scores on an instrument are correlated with an external criterion, measured at the same time.

confidence interval (CI) The range of values within which a population parameter is estimated to lie, at a specified probability (e.g., 95% CI).

confidence limit The upper (or lower) boundary of a confidence interval.

confidentiality Protection of study participants so that data provided are never publicly divulged.

confirmability A criterion for integrity in a qualitative inquiry, referring to the objectivity or neutrality of the data and interpretations.

confirmatory factor analysis (CFA) A factor analysis designed to confirm a hypothesized measurement model, using maximum likelihood estimation.

confounding variable An extraneous variable that confounds or obscures the relationship between the central variables of a study and that needs to be controlled.

consent form A written agreement signed by a study participant and a researcher concerning the terms and conditions of voluntary participation in a study.

CONSORT guidelines Guidelines (Consolidated Standards of Reporting Trials) for reporting information on clinical trials, including a checklist and flow chart for tracking participants through a trial.

constant comparison A procedure often used in a grounded theory analysis wherein newly collected data are compared in an ongoing fashion with data obtained earlier, to refine theoretically relevant categories.

construct An abstraction or concept that is deliberately invented (constructed) by researchers for a scientific purpose (e.g., health locus of control).

construct validity The validity of inferences from *observed* persons, settings, and interventions in a study to the constructs that these instances might represent; with an instrument, the degree to which it measures the construct under investigation.

contact information Information obtained from study participants in longitudinal studies, to facilitate their relocation at a future date.

contamination The inadvertent, undesirable influence of one treatment condition on another treatment condition.

content analysis The process of organizing and integrating narrative, qualitative information according to emerging themes and concepts.

content validity The degree to which the items in an instrument adequately represent the universe of content for the concept being measured.

content validity index (CVI) An index of the degree to which an instrument is content valid, based on aggregated ratings of a panel of experts; both items (I-CVI) and the overall scale content validity (S-CVI) can be assessed.

contingency table A two-dimensional table in which the frequencies of two categorical variables are cross-tabulated.

continuous variable A variable that can take on an infinite range of values along a specified continuum (e.g., height).

control The process of holding constant confounding influences on the dependent variable under study.

control group Subjects in an experiment who do not receive the experimental treatment and whose performance provides a baseline against which the effects of the treatment can be measured (see also *comparison group*).

controlled trial A trial that has a control group, with or without randomization.

convenience sampling Selection of the most readily available persons as participants in a study; also called *accidental sampling*.

convergent validity An approach to construct validation that involves assessing the degree to which two methods of measuring a construct are similar (i.e., converge).

core variable (category) In a grounded theory study, the central phenomenon that is used to integrate all categories of the data.

correlation An association or bond between variables, with variation in one variable systematically related to variation in another.

correlation coefficient An index summarizing the degree of relationship between variables, typically ranging from $+1.00$ (for a perfect positive relationship) through 0.0 (for no relationship) to -1.00 (for a perfect negative relationship).

correlation matrix A two-dimensional display showing the correlation coefficients between all pairs of a set of variables.

correlational research Research that explores the interrelationships among variables of interest without researcher intervention.

Cost/benefit analysis An economic analysis in which both costs and outcomes of a program or intervention are expressed in monetary terms, and compared.

cost-effectiveness analysis An economic analysis in which costs of an intervention are measured in monetary terms, but outcomes are expressed in natural units (e.g., the costs per added year of life).

cost-utility analysis An economic analysis that expresses the effects of an intervention as overall health improvement and describes costs for some additional utility gain—usually in relation to gains in quality-adjusted life years (QALY).

counterbalancing The process of systematically varying the order of presentation of stimuli or treatments to control for ordering effects, especially in a crossover design.

counterfactual The condition or group used as a basis of comparison in a study, embodying what would have happened *to the same people* exposed to a causal factor if they *simultaneously* were *not* exposed to the causal factor.

covariate A variable that is statistically controlled (held constant) in ANCOVA, typically an extraneous influence on, or a preintervention measure of, the dependent variable.

Cramér's *V* An index describing the magnitude of relationship between nominal-level data, used when the contingency table to which it is applied is larger than 2×2.

credibility A criterion for evaluating integrity and quality in qualitative studies, referring to confidence in the truth of the data; analogous to internal validity in quantitative research.

criterion-related validity The degree to which scores on an instrument are correlated with some external criterion.

critical ethnography An ethnography that focuses on raising consciousness in the group or culture under study in the hope of effecting social change.

critical incident technique A method of obtaining data from study participants by in-depth exploration of specific incidents and behaviors related to the topic under study.

critical region The area in the sampling distribution representing values that are "improbable" if the null hypothesis is true.

critical theory An approach to viewing the world that involves a critique of society, with the goal of envisioning new possibilities and effecting social change.

critically appraised topic (CAT) A quick summary of a clinical question and an appraisal of the best evidence that typically begins with a clinical bottom line (i.e., best-practice recommendation).

critique A critical, balanced appraisal of a research report or proposal.

Cronbach's alpha A widely used reliability index that estimates the internal consistency of a measure composed of several subparts; also called *coefficient alpha*.

crossover design An experimental design in which one group of subjects is exposed to more than one condition or treatment in random order.

cross-sectional design A study design in which data are collected at one point in time; sometimes used to infer change over time when data are collected from different age or developmental groups.

crosstabulation A calculation of frequencies for two variables considered simultaneously—e.g., gender (male/female) crosstabulated with smoking status (smoker/nonsmoker).

cutoff point The score on a screening or diagnostic instrument used to distinguish cases and noncases.

data The pieces of information obtained in a study (singular is *datum*).

data analysis The systematic organization and synthesis of research data and. in quantitative studies, the testing of hypotheses using those data.

data collection protocols The formal procedures researchers develop to guide the collection of data in a standardized fashion.

data saturation See *saturation.*

data set The total collection of data on all variables for all study participants.

data triangulation The use of multiple data sources for the purpose of validating conclusions.

deductive reasoning The process of developing specific predictions from general principles (see also *inductive reasoning*).

degrees of freedom (*df*) A statistical concept referring to the number of sample values free to vary (e.g., with a given sample mean, all but one value would be free to vary).

Delphi survey A technique for obtaining judgments from an expert panel about an issue of concern; experts are questioned individually in several rounds, with a summary of the panel's views circulated between rounds, to achieve some consensus.

dependability A criterion for evaluating integrity in qualitative studies, referring to the stability of data over time and over conditions; analogous to reliability in quantitative research.

dependent variable The variable hypothesized to depend on or be caused by another variable (the *independent variable*); the outcome variable of interest.

descendancy approach In literature searches, finding a pivotal early study and searching forward in citation indexes to find more recent studies ("descendants") that cited the key study.

descriptive research Research that has as its main objective the accurate portrayal of the characteristics of persons, situations, or groups, and/or the frequency with which certain phenomena occur.

descriptive statistics Statistics used to describe and summarize data (e.g., means, percentages).

determinism The belief that phenomena are not haphazard or random, but rather have antecedent causes; an assumption in the positivist paradigm.

deviation score A score computed by subtracting an individual score from the mean of all scores.

dichotomous variable A variable having only two values or categories (e.g., gender).

direct costs Specific project-related costs incurred during a study (e.g., for supplies, salaries of research staff, etc.).

directional hypothesis A hypothesis that makes a specific prediction about the direction of the relationship between two variables.

discrete variable A variable with a finite number of values between two points.

discriminant function analysis A statistical procedure used to predict group membership or status on a categorical (nominal level) variable on the basis of two or more independent variables.

discriminant validity An approach to construct validation that involves assessing the degree to which a single method of measuring two distinct constructs yields different results (i.e., discriminates the two).

disproportionate sample A sample in which the researcher samples varying proportions of subjects from different population strata to ensure adequate representation from smaller strata.

domain In ethnographic analysis, a unit or broad category of cultural knowledge.

domain sampling model The model used in developing a scale in the classical measurement theory framework, which involves the random sampling of a homogeneous set of items from a hypothetical universe of items relating to the construct

dose-response analysis An analysis to assess whether larger doses of an intervention are associated with greater benefits, usually in a quasi-experimental framework.

double-blind experiment An experiment in which neither the subjects nor those who administer the treatment know who is in the experimental or control group.

dummy variable Dichotomous variables created for use in many multivariate statistical analyses, typically using codes of 0 and 1 (e.g., female = 1, male = 0).

ecological validity The extent to which study designs and findings have relevance and meaning in a variety of real-world contexts.

economic analysis An analysis of the relationship between costs and outcomes of alternative health care interventions.

effect size A statistical expression of the magnitude of the relationship between two variables, or the magnitude of the difference between groups on an attribute of interest; also used in metasynthesis to characterize the salience of a theme or category.

effectiveness study A clinical trial designed to shed light on effectiveness of an intervention under ordinary conditions, with an intervention already found to be efficacious in an efficacy study.

efficacy study A tightly controlled clinical trial designed to establish the efficacy of an intervention under ideal conditions, using a design that stresses internal validity.

egocentric network analysis An ethnographic method that focuses on the pattern of relationships and networks of individuals; researchers develop lists of a person's network members (called *alters*) and seek to understand the scope and nature of interrelationships and social supports.

eigenvalue In factor analysis, the value equal to the sum of the squared weights for each factor.

element The most basic unit of a population for sampling purposes, typically a human being.

eligibility criteria The criteria designating the specific attributes of the target population, by which people are selected for inclusion in a study.

emergent design A design that unfolds in the course of a qualitative study as the researcher makes ongoing design decisions reflecting what has already been learned.

emergent fit A concept in grounded theory that involves comparing new data and new categories with previously existing conceptualizations.

emic perspective An ethnographic term referring to the way members of a culture themselves view their world; the "insider's view."

empirical evidence Evidence rooted in objective reality and gathered using one's senses as the basis for generating knowledge.

equivalence trial A trial designed to determine whether the outcomes of two or more treatments differ by an amount that is clinically unimportant.

error of measurement The deviation between true scores and obtained scores of a measured characteristic.

error term The mathematic expression (e.g., in a regression analysis) that represents all unknown or immeasurable attributes that can affect the dependent variable.

estimation procedures Statistical procedures that estimate population parameters based on sample statistics.

eta squared In ANOVA, a statistic calculated to indicate the proportion of variance in the dependent variable explained by the independent variables, analogous to R^2 in multiple regression.

ethics A system of moral values that is concerned with the degree to which research procedures adhere to professional, legal, and social obligations to the study participants.

ethnography A branch of human inquiry, associated with anthropology, that focuses on the culture of a group of people, with an effort to understand the world view of those under study.

ethnomethodology A branch of human inquiry, associated with sociology, that focuses on the way in which people make sense of their everyday activities and come to behave in socially acceptable ways.

ethnonursing research The study of human cultures, with a focus on a group's beliefs and practices relating to nursing care and related health behaviors.

etic perspective An ethnographic term referring to the "outsider's" view of the experiences of a cultural group.

evaluation research Research that investigates how well a program, practice, or policy is working.

event history calendar A data collection matrix that plots time on one dimension and events or activities of interest on the other.

event sampling A sampling plan that involves the selection of integral behaviors or events to be observed.

evidence-based practice A practice that involves making clinical decisions on the best available evidence, with an emphasis on evidence from disciplined research.

evidence hierarchy A ranked arrangement of the validity and dependability of evidence based on the rigor of the method that produced it; evidence hierarchies typically focus on evidence supporting causal influences.

exclusion criteria The criteria that specify characteristics that a population does *not* have.

exogenous variable In path analysis, a variable whose determinants lie outside the model.

experiment A study in which the researcher controls (manipulates) the independent variable and randomly assigns subjects to different conditions.

experimental group The subjects who receive the experimental treatment or intervention.

exploratory factor analysis (EFA) A factor analysis undertaken to explore the underlying dimensionality of a set of variables.

external criticism In historical research, the systematic evaluation of the authenticity and genuineness of data.

external validity The degree to which study results can be generalized to settings or samples other than the one studied.

extraneous variable A variable that confounds the relationship between the independent and dependent variables and that needs to be controlled either in the research design or through statistical procedures.

extreme response set A bias in psychosocial scales created when participants select extreme response alternatives (e.g., "strongly agree"), independent of the item's content.

F-ratio The statistic obtained in several statistical tests (e.g., ANOVA) in which variation attributable to different sources (e.g., between groups and within groups) is compared.

face validity The extent to which a measuring instrument looks as though it is measuring what it purports to measure.

factor analysis A statistical procedure for reducing a large set of variables into a smaller set of variables with common underlying dimensions.

factor extraction The first phase of a factor analysis, which involves the extraction of as much variance as possible through the successive creation of linear combinations of the variables in the data set.

factor loading In factor analysis, the weight associated with a variable on a given factor.

factor rotation The second phase of factor analysis, during which the reference axes for the factors are moved to more clearly align variables with a single factor.

factorial design An experimental design in which two or more independent variables are simultaneously manipulated, permitting a separate analysis of the main effects of the independent variables and their interaction.

fail-safe number In meta-analysis, an estimate of the number of studies with nonsignificant results that would be needed to reverse the conclusion of a significant effect.

feasibility study A small-scale test to determine the feasibility of a larger study (see also *pilot study*).

feminist research   Research that seeks to understand, typically through qualitative approaches, how gender and a gendered social order shape women's lives and their consciousness.

field diary   A daily record of events and conversations in the field; also called a log.

field notes   The notes taken by researchers to record the unstructured observations made in the field, and the interpretation of those observations.

field research   Research in which the data are collected "in the field" from individuals in their normal roles, with the aim of understanding the practices, behaviors, and beliefs of individuals or groups as they normally function in real life.

fieldwork   The activities undertaken by qualitative researchers to collect data out in the field, that is, in natural settings.

findings   The results of the analysis of research data.

Fisher's exact test   A statistical procedure used to test the significance of the difference in proportions, used when the sample size is small or cells in the contingency table have no observations.

fit   In grounded theory analysis, the process of identifying characteristics of one piece of data and comparing them with the characteristics of another datum to determine similarity.

fixed alternative question   A question that offers respondents a set of prespecified response options.

fixed effects model   In meta-analysis, a model in which studies are assumed to be measuring the same overall effect; a pooled effect estimate is calculated under the assumption that observed variation between studies is attributable to chance.

focus group interview   An interview with a group of individuals assembled to answer questions on a given topic.

focused interview   A loosely structured interview in which an interviewer guides the respondent through a set of questions using a topic guide.

follow-up study   A study undertaken to determine the outcomes of individuals with a specified condition or who have received a specified treatment.

forced-choice question   A question requiring respondents to choose between two statements that represent polar positions.

forest plot   A graphic representation of effects across studies in a meta-analysis, permitting an assessment of heterogeneity.

formal grounded theory   A theory developed at a more abstract level of theory by integrating several substantive grounded theories.

formative evaluation   An ongoing assessment of a product or program as it is being developed, to optimize its quality and effectiveness.

framework   The conceptual underpinnings of a study—for example, a *theoretical framework* in theory-based studies, or *conceptual framework* in studies based on a specific conceptual model.

frequency distribution   A systematic array of numeric values from the lowest to the highest, together with a count of the number of times each value was obtained.

frequency effect size   In a metasynthesis, the percentage of reports that contain a given thematic finding.

frequency polygon   Graphic display of a frequency distribution, in which dots connected by a straight line indicate the number of times score values occur in a data set.

Friedman test   A nonparametric analog of ANOVA, used with paired-groups or repeated measures situations.

full disclosure   The communication of complete, accurate information to potential study participants.

functional relationship   A relationship between two variables in which it cannot be assumed that one variable caused the other.

funnel plot   A graphical display of some measure of study precision (e.g., sample size) plotted against effect size that can be used to explore relationships that might reflect publication bias.

gaining entrée   The process of gaining access to study participants through the cooperation of key actors in the selected community or site.

generalizability   The degree to which the research methods justify the inference that the findings are true for a broader group than study participants; in particular, the inference that the findings can be generalized from the sample to the population.

"going native"   A pitfall in ethnographic research wherein a researcher becomes too emotionally involved with participants and therefore loses the ability to observe objectively.

grand tour question   A broad question asked in an unstructured interview to gain a general overview of a phenomenon, on the basis of which more focused questions are subsequently asked.

grant   A financial award made to a researcher to conduct a proposed study.

grantsmanship   The combined set of skills and knowledge needed to secure financial support for a research idea.

graphic rating scale A scale in which respondents are asked to rate a concept along an ordered bipolar continuum (e.g., "excellent" to "very poor").

grey literature Unpublished, and thus less readily accessible, research reports.

grounded theory An approach to collecting and analyzing qualitative data that aims to develop theories grounded in real-world observations.

hand searching The planned searching of a journal page by page (i.e., by hand), to identify all relevant reports that might be missed by electronic searching.

Hawthorne effect The effect on the dependent variable resulting from subjects' awareness that they are participants under study.

hermeneutics A qualitative research tradition, drawing on interpretive phenomenology, that focuses on the lived experiences of humans, and on how they interpret those experiences.

heterogeneity The degree to which objects are dissimilar (i.e., characterized by variability) on some attribute.

hierarchical multiple regression A multiple regression analysis in which predictor variables are entered into the equation in steps that are prespecified by the analyst.

histogram A graphic presentation of frequency distribution data.

historical research Systematic studies designed to discover facts and relationships about past events.

history threat The occurrence of events external to an intervention but concurrent with it, which can affect the dependent variable and threaten the study's internal validity.

homogeneity (1) In terms of the reliability of an instrument, the degree to which its subparts are internally consistent (i.e., are measuring the same critical attribute). (2) More generally, the degree to which objects are similar (i.e., characterized by low variability).

hypothesis A prediction, especially a statement of predicted relationships between variables.

impact analysis An evaluation of the effects of a program or intervention on outcomes of interest, net of other factors influencing those outcomes.

impact factor An annual measure of citation frequency for an average article in a given journal, that is, the ratio between citations and recent citable items published in the journal.

implementation analysis In evaluations, a description of the process by which a program or intervention was implemented in practice.

implementation potential The extent to which an innovation is amenable to implementation in a new setting, an assessment of which is usually made in an evidence-based practice project.

implied consent Consent to participate in a study that a researcher assumes has been given based on participants' actions, such as returning a completed questionnaire.

IMRAD format The organization of a research report into four sections: the Introduction, Method, Results, and Discussion sections.

incidence rate The rate of new cases with a specified condition, determined by dividing the number of new cases over a given period of time by the number at risk of becoming a new case (i.e., free of the condition at the outset of the time period).

independent variable The variable that is believed to cause or influence the dependent variable; in experimental research, the manipulated (treatment) variable.

indirect costs Administrative costs, over and above the specific (direct) costs of conducting the study; also called *overhead*.

inductive reasoning The process of reasoning from specific observations to more general rules (see also *deductive reasoning*).

inferential statistics Statistics that permit inferences on whether results observed in a sample are likely to occur in the larger population.

informant An individual who provides information to researchers about a phenomenon under study, usually in qualitative studies.

informed consent An ethical principle that requires researchers to obtain the voluntary participation of subjects, after informing them of possible risks and benefits.

inquiry audit An independent scrutiny of qualitative data and relevant supporting documents by an external reviewer, to determine the dependability and confirmability of qualitative data.

insider research Research on a group or culture—usually in an ethnography—by a member of the group or culture.

Institutional Review Board (IRB) In the United States, a group of individuals from an institution who convene to review proposed and ongoing studies with respect to ethical considerations.

instrument The device used to collect data (e.g., a questionnaire, test, observation schedule, etc.).

instrumentation threat The threat to the internal validity of the study that can arise if the researcher changes the measuring instrument between two points of data collection.

intensity effect size In a metasynthesis, the percentage of all thematic findings that are contained in any given report.

intensity sampling A sampling approach used by qualitative researchers involving the purposeful selection of intense (but not extreme) cases.

intention to treat A strategy for analyzing data in an intervention study that includes participants with the group to which they were assigned, whether or not they received or completed the treatment associated with the group.

interaction effect The effect of two or more independent variables acting in combination (interactively) on a dependent variable.

intercoder reliability The degree to which two coders, operating independently, agree on coding decisions.

internal consistency The degree to which the subparts of an instrument are all measuring the same attribute or dimension, as a measure of the instrument's reliability.

internal criticism In historical research, an evaluation of the worth of the historical evidence.

internal validity The degree to which it can be inferred that the experimental treatment (independent variable), rather than uncontrolled, extraneous factors, caused observed effects.

interrater (interobserver) reliability The degree to which two raters or observers, operating independently, assign the same ratings or values for an attribute being measured or observed.

interrupted time series design. See *time series design.*

interval estimation A statistical estimation approach in which the researcher establishes a range of values that are likely, within a given level of confidence, to contain the true population parameter.

interval measurement A measurement level in which an attribute of a variable is rank ordered on a scale that has equal distances between points on that scale (e.g., Fahrenheit degrees).

intervention fidelity The extent to which the implementation of a treatment is faithful to its plan.

intervention protocol The specification of exactly what an intervention and alternative treatment conditions will be, and how they are to be administered.

intervention research Research involving the development, implementation, and testing of an intervention.

intervention theory The conceptual underpinning of a health care intervention, which articulates the theoretical basis for what must be done to achieve desired outcomes.

interview A data collection method in which an interviewer asks questions of a respondent, either face-to-face or by telephone.

interview schedule The formal instrument that specifies the wording of all questions to be asked of respondents in structured self-report studies.

intuiting The second step in descriptive phenomenology, which occurs when researchers remain open to the meaning attributed to the phenomenon by those who experienced it.

inverse relationship A relationship characterized by the tendency of high values on one variable to be associated with low values on the second variable; also called a *negative relationship.*

inverse variance method In meta-analysis, a method that uses the inverse of the variance of the effect estimate (one divided by the square of its standard error) as the weight to calculate a weighted average of effects.

investigator triangulation The use of two or more researchers to analyze and interpret a data set, to enhance validity.

item A single question on an instrument, or a single statement on a scale.

item analysis A type of analysis used to assess whether items on a scale are tapping the same construct and are sufficiently discriminating.

journal article A report appearing in professional journals such as *Nursing Research.*

journal club A group that meets regularly in clinical settings to discuss and critique research reports appearing in journals.

kappa An index used to measure interrater agreement, which summarizes the extent of agreement beyond the level expected to occur by chance.

Kendall's tau A correlation coefficient used to indicate the magnitude of a relationship between ordinal-level variables.

key informant A person well-versed in the phenomenon of research interest and who is willing to share the information and insight with the researcher (often an ethnographer).

keyword An important term used to search for references on a topic in a bibliographic database.

known-groups technique A technique for estimating the construct validity of an instrument through an analysis of the degree to which the instrument separates groups predicted to differ based on known characteristics or theory.

Kruskal-Wallis test A nonparametric test used to test the difference between three or more independent groups, based on ranked scores.

latent trait scale A scale developed within an *item response theory* framework, an alternative psychometric theory to *classical measurement theory.*

latent variable An unmeasured variable that represents an underlying, abstract construct (usually in the context of a structural equations analysis).

law A theory that has accrued such persuasive empirical support that it is accepted as true (e.g., Boyle's law of gases).

least-squares estimation A method of statistical estimation in which the solution minimizes the sums of squares of error terms; also called OLS (ordinary least squares).

level of measurement A system of classifying measurements according to the nature of the measurement and the type of permissible mathematical operations; the levels are nominal, ordinal, interval, and ratio.

level of significance The risk of making a Type I error in a statistical analysis, established by the researcher beforehand (e.g., the .05 level).

life history A narrative self-report about a person's life experiences vis-à-vis a theme of interest.

likelihood ratio (LR) For a screening or diagnostic instrument, the relative likelihood that a given result is expected in a person with (as opposed to one without) the target attribute; LR indexes summarize the relationship between specificity and sensitivity in a single number.

Likert scale A composite measure of attitudes involving the summation of scores on a set of items that respondents rate for their degree of agreement or disagreement.

linear regression An analysis for predicting the value of a dependent variable from one or more predictors by determining a straight-line fit to the data that minimizes deviations from the line.

LISREL An acronym for linear structural relation analysis, used for testing causal models.

listwise deletion A method of dealing with missing values in a data set that involves the elimination of cases with missing data.

literature review A critical summary of research on a topic of interest, often prepared to put a research problem in context.

log In participant observation studies, the observer's daily record of events and conversations.

logical positivism The philosophy underlying the traditional scientific approach; see also *positivist paradigm.*

logistic regression A multivariate regression procedure that analyzes relationships between one or more independent variables and categorical dependent variables; also called *logit analysis.*

logit The natural log of the odds, used as the dependent variable in logistic regression; short for logistic probability unit.

longitudinal study A study designed to collect data at more than one point in time, in contrast to a cross-sectional study.

main effects In a study with multiple independent variables, the effects of each independent variable, taken separately, on the dependent variable.

manifest variable An observed, measured variable that serves as an indicator of an underlying construct, that is, a latent variable.

manipulation An intervention or treatment introduced by the researcher in an experimental or quasi-experimental study to assess its impact on the dependent variable.

manipulation check In experimental studies, a test to determine whether the manipulation was implemented as intended.

Mann-Whitney *U* test A nonparametric statistic used to test the difference between two independent groups, based on ranked scores.

MANOVA See *multivariate analysis of variance.*

marginals The distribution of grouped data in a crosstabulation, so called because they are found in the margins of a computer printout.

masking See *blinding.*

matching The pairing of subjects in one group with those in another group based on their similarity on one or more dimension, to enhance the overall comparability of groups.

maturation threat A threat to the internal validity of a study that results when changes to the outcome measure (dependent variable) result from the passage of time.

maximum likelihood estimation An estimation approach in which the estimators are ones that estimate the parameters most likely to have generated the observed measurements.

maximum variation sampling A sampling approach used by qualitative researchers involving the purposeful selection of cases with a wide range of variation.

McNemar test   A statistical test for comparing differences in proportions when values are derived from paired (nonindependent) groups.

mean   A measure of central tendency, computed by summing all scores and dividing by the number of subjects.

measurement   The assignment of numbers to objects according to specified rules to characterize quantities of some attribute.

measurement model   In structural equations modeling, the model that stipulates the hypothesized relationships among the manifest and latent variables.

median   A descriptive statistic that is a measure of central tendency, representing the exact middle value in a score distribution; the value above and below which 50 percent of the scores lie.

median test   A nonparametric statistical test involving the comparison of median values of two independent groups to determine if the groups are from populations with different medians.

mediating variable   A variable that mediates or acts like a "go-between" in a causal chain linking two other variables.

member check   A method of validating the credibility of qualitative data through debriefings and discussions with informants.

meta-analysis   A technique for quantitatively integrating the results of multiple similar studies addressing the same research question.

meta-matrix   A device sometimes used in a mixed method study that permits researchers to recognize important patterns and themes across data sources and to develop hypotheses.

meta-regression   In meta-analyses, an analytic approach for exploring clinical and methodologic factors contributing to heterogeneity of effects.

meta-summary   A process that lays the foundation for a metasynthesis, involving the development of a list of abstracted findings from primary studies and calculating manifest effect sizes (frequency and intensity effect size).

metasynthesis   The grand narratives or interpretive translations produced from the integration or comparison of findings from qualitative studies.

method triangulation   The use of multiple methods of data collection about the same phenomenon, to enhance validity.

methodologic research   Research designed to develop or refine methods of obtaining, organizing, or analyzing data.

methods (research)   The steps, procedures, and strategies for gathering and analyzing data in a study.

middle-range theory   A theory that focuses on only a piece of reality or human experience, involving a selected number of concepts (e.g., a theory of stress).

minimal risk   Anticipated risks that are no greater than those ordinarily encountered in daily life or during the performance of routine tests or procedures.

missing values   Values missing from a data set for some study participants, due, for example, to refusals, errors, or skip patterns.

mixed method research   Research in which both qualitative and quantitative data are collected and analyzed.

mixed-mode strategy   An approach to collecting survey data beginning with attempts at a telephone interview, followed by in-person interviewing only if necessary.

modality   A characteristic of a frequency distribution describing the number of peaks; that is, values with high frequencies.

mode   A measure of central tendency; the score value that occurs most frequently in a distribution of scores.

model   A symbolic representation of concepts or variables, and interrelationships among them.

moderator variable   A variable that affects (moderates) the relationship between the independent and dependent variables.

mortality threat   A threat to the internal validity of a study, referring to the differential loss of participants (attrition) from different groups.

multicollinearity   A problem that can occur in multiple regression when predictor variables are too highly intercorrelated, which can lead to unstable estimates of the regression coefficients.

multimodal distribution   A distribution of values with more than one peak (high frequency).

multiple comparison procedures   Statistical tests, normally applied after an ANOVA indicates statistically significant group differences, that compare different pairs of groups; also called *post hoc tests*.

multiple correlation coefficient   An index that summarizes the degree of relationship between two or more independent variables and a dependent variable; symbolized as R.

multiple regression analysis   A statistical procedure for understanding the effects of two or more independent (predictor) variables on a dependent variable.

multistage sampling   A sampling strategy that proceeds through a set of stages from larger to smaller sampling units (e.g., from states, to census tracts, to households).

multitrait–multimethod matrix method A method of assessing an instrument's construct validity using multiple measures for a set of subjects; the target instrument is valid to the extent that there is a strong relationship between it and other measures of the same attribute (convergence) and a weak relationship between it and measures purporting to measure a different attribute (discriminability).

multivariate analysis of variance (MANOVA) A statistical procedure used to test the significance of differences between the means of two or more groups on two or more dependent variables, considered simultaneously.

multivariate statistics Statistical procedures designed to analyze the relationships among three or more variables (e.g., multiple regression, ANCOVA).

N The symbol designating the total number of subjects (e.g., "the total *N* was 500").

n The symbol designating the number of subjects in a subgroup or cell of a study (e.g., "each of the four groups had an *n* of 125, for a total *N* of 500").

narrative analysis A type of qualitative approach that focuses on the story as the object of the inquiry.

natural experiment A nonexperimental study that takes advantage of a naturally occurring event (e.g., an earthquake) that is explored for its effect on people's behavior or condition, typically by comparing people exposed to the event with those not exposed.

naturalistic paradigm An alternative paradigm to the traditional positivist paradigm that holds that there are multiple interpretations of reality, and that the goal of research is to understand how individuals construct reality within their context; often associated with qualitative research.

naturalistic setting A setting for the collection of research data that is natural to those being studied (e.g., homes, places of work, and so on).

needs assessment A study designed to describe the needs of a group, community, or organization, usually as a guide to policy planning and resource allocation.

negative case analysis The refinement of a theory or description in a qualitative study through the inclusion of cases that appear to disconfirm earlier hypotheses.

negative predictive value (NPV) A measure of the usefulness of a screening/diagnostic test that can be interpreted as the probability that a negative test result is correct; calculated by dividing the number with a negative test who do not have disease by the number with a negative test.

negative relationship A relationship between two variables in which there is a tendency for high values on one variable to be associated with low values on the other (e.g., as stress increases, emotional well-being decreases); also called an *inverse relationship.*

negative results Results that fail to support the researcher's hypotheses.

negatively skewed distribution An asymmetric distribution of data values with a disproportionately high number of cases at the upper end; when displayed graphically, the tail points to the left.

net effect The effect of an independent variable on a dependent variable, after controlling for the effect of one or more covariates through multiple regression or ANCOVA.

network sampling The sampling of participants based on referrals from others already in the sample; also called *snowball sampling.*

nominal measurement The lowest level of measurement involving the assignment of characteristics into categories (e.g., males, category 1; females, category 2).

nominated sampling A sampling method in which researchers ask early informants to make referrals to other potential participants.

nondirectional hypothesis A research hypothesis that does not stipulate the expected direction of the relationship between variables.

nonequivalent control group design A quasi-experimental design involving a comparison group that was not created through random assignment.

nonexperimental research Studies in which the researcher collects data without introducing an intervention; also called *observational research.*

noninferiority trial A trial designed to determine whether the effect of a new treatment is not worse than a standard treatment by more than a pre-specified amount.

nonparametric tests A class of statistical tests that do not involve stringent assumptions about the distribution of critical variables.

nonprobability sampling The selection of sampling units (e.g., participants) from a population using non-random procedures (e.g., convenience and quota sampling).

nonrecursive model A causal model that predicts reciprocal effects (i.e., a variable can be both the cause of and an effect of another variable).

nonresponse bias A bias that can result when a non-random subset of people invited to participate in a study fail to participate.

nonsignificant result The result of a statistical test indicating that group differences or an observed relationship could have occurred by chance, at a given level of significance; sometimes abbreviated as NS.

normal distribution A theoretical distribution that is bell-shaped and symmetrical; also called a *normal curve* or a *Gaussian distribution.*

norms Test-performance standards, based on test score information from a large, representative sample.

null hypothesis A hypothesis stating no relationship between the variables under study; used primarily in statistical testing as the hypothesis to be rejected.

number needed to treat (NNT) An estimate of how many people would need to receive an intervention to prevent one undesirable outcome, computed by dividing 1 by the value of the absolute risk reduction.

nursing research Systematic inquiry designed to develop knowledge about issues of importance to the nursing profession.

objectivity The extent to which two independent researchers would arrive at similar judgments or conclusions (i.e., judgments not biased by personal values or beliefs).

oblique rotation In factor analysis, a rotation of factors such that the reference axes are allowed to move to acute or oblique angles and hence the factors are allowed to be correlated.

observational notes An observer's in-depth descriptions about events and conversations observed in naturalistic settings.

observational research Studies that do not involve an experimental intervention—that is, nonexperimental research; also, research in which data are collected through direct observation.

observed (obtained) score The actual score or numerical value assigned to a person on a measure.

odds A way of expressing the chance of an event—the probability of an event occurring to the probability that it will not occur, calculated by dividing the number of people who experienced an event by the number for whom it did not occur.

odds ratio (OR) The ratio of one odds to another odds, for example, the ratio of the odds of an event in one group to the odds of an event in another group; an odds ratio of one indicates no difference between groups.

on-protocol analysis A principle for analyzing data that includes data only from those members of a treatment group who actually received the treatment.

one-tailed test A statistical test in which only values in one tail of a distribution are considered in determining significance; sometimes used when the researcher states a directional hypothesis.

open coding The first level of coding in a grounded theory study, referring to the basic descriptive coding of the content of narrative materials.

open-ended question A question in an interview or questionnaire that does not restrict respondents' answers to preestablished alternatives.

operational definition The definition of a concept or variable in terms of the procedures by which it is to be measured.

operationalization The process of translating research concepts into measurable phenomena.

oral history An unstructured self-report technique used to gather personal recollections of events and their perceived causes and consequences.

ordinal measurement A measurement level that rank orders phenomena along some dimension.

ordinary least squares (OLS) regression Regression analysis that uses the least-squares criterion for estimating the parameters in the regression equation.

orthogonal rotation In factor analysis, a rotation of factors such that the reference axes are kept at right angles, and hence the factors remain uncorrelated.

outcome analysis An evaluation of what happens to outcomes of interest after implementing a program or intervention, typically using a one group before–after design.

outcome measure A term sometimes used to refer to the dependent variable, that is, the measure that captures the outcome of an intervention.

outcomes research Research designed to document the effectiveness of health care services and the end results of patient care.

outliers Values that lie outside the normal range of values for other cases in a data set.

***p* value** In statistical testing, the probability that the obtained results are due to chance alone; the probability of a Type I error.

pair matching See *matching.*

pairwise deletion A method of dealing with missing values in a data set involving the deletion of cases with missing data selectively (i.e., on a variable by variable basis).

panel study A longitudinal survey study in which data are collected from the same people (*a panel*) at two or more points in time.

paradigm A way of looking at natural phenomena that encompasses a set of philosophical assumptions and that guides one's approach to inquiry.

parameter A characteristic of a population (e.g., the mean age of all U.S. citizens).

parametric tests A class of statistical tests that involve assumptions about the distribution of the variables and the estimation of a parameter.

partially randomized patient preference (PRPP) design A design that involves randomizing only patients without a strong preference for a treatment condition, but observing outcomes for all.

participant See *study participant*.

participant observation A method of collecting data through the participation in and observation of a group or culture.

participatory action research (PAR) A research approach based on the premise that the use and production of knowledge can be political and used to exert power.

path analysis A regression-based procedure for testing causal models, typically using correlational data.

path coefficient The weight representing the impact of one variable on another in a path analytic model.

path diagram A graphic representation of the hypothesized interrelationships and causal flow among variables.

patient-centered intervention (PCI) An intervention tailored to meet individual needs or characteristics.

Pearson's *r* A correlation coefficient designating the magnitude of relationship between two variables measured on at least an interval scale; also called *the product-moment correlation*.

peer debriefing Sessions with peers to review and explore various aspects of a study, sometimes used to enhance trustworthiness in a qualitative study.

peer reviewer A researcher who reviews and critiques a research report or proposal, and who makes a recommendation about publishing or funding the research.

pentadic dramatism An approach for analyzing narratives, developed by Burke, that focuses on five key elements of a story: act (what was done), scene (when and where it was done), agent (who did it), agency (how it was done), and purpose (why it was done).

perfect relationship A correlation between two variables such that the values of one variable permit perfect prediction of the values of the other; designated as 1.00 or −1.00.

performance ethnography A scripted, staged reenactment of ethnographically derived notes that reflect an interpretation of the culture.

permuted block randomization Randomization that occurs for blocks of subjects of even size (e.g., 6 or 8 at a time), to ensure that, at any given time, roughly equal numbers of subjects have been allocated to all treatment groups.

persistent observation A qualitative researcher's intense focus on the aspects of a situation that are relevant to the phenomena being studied.

person triangulation The collection of data from different levels of persons, with the aim of validating data through multiple perspectives on the phenomenon.

personal interview A face-to-face interview between an interviewer and a respondent.

personal notes In field studies, written comments about the observer's own feelings during the research process.

phenomenology A qualitative research tradition, with roots in philosophy and psychology, that focuses on the lived experience of humans.

phenomenon The abstract concept under study, often used by qualitative researchers in lieu of the term *variable*.

phi coefficient A statistical index describing the magnitude of relationship between two dichotomous variables.

photo elicitation An interview stimulated and guided by photographic images.

pilot study A small-scale version, or trial run, done in preparation for a major study (the *parent study*).

placebo A sham or pseudo intervention, often used as a control group condition.

placebo effect Changes in the dependant variable attributable to the placebo.

point estimation A statistical procedure that uses information from a sample (a statistic) to estimate the single value that best represents the population parameter.

point prevalence rate The number of people with a condition or disease divided by the total number at risk, multiplied by the total number for whom the rate is being established (e.g., per 1000 population).

population The entire set of individuals or objects having some common characteristics (e.g., all RNs in Canada); sometimes called *universe*.

positive predictive value (PPV) A measure of the usefulness of a screening/diagnostic test that can be interpreted as the probability that a positive test result is correct; calculated by dividing the number with a positive test who have disease by the number with a positive test.

positive relationship A relationship between two variables in which high values on one variable tend to be associated with high values on the other (e.g., as physical activity increases, pulse rate increases).

positive results Research results that are consistent with the researcher's hypotheses.

positively skewed distribution An asymmetric distribution of values with a disproportionately high number of cases at the lower end; when displayed graphically, the tail points to the right.

positivist paradigm The paradigm underlying the traditional scientific approach, which assumes that there is a fixed, orderly reality that can be objectively studied; often associated with quantitative research.

post hoc test A test for comparing all possible pairs of groups following a significant test of overall group differences (e.g., in an ANOVA).

poster session A session at a professional conference in which several researchers simultaneously present visual displays summarizing their studies, while conference attendees circulate around the room perusing the displays.

posttest The collection of data after introducing an intervention.

posttest-only design An experimental design in which data are collected from subjects only after the intervention has been introduced; also called an *after-only design.*

power The ability of a design or analytic strategy to detect relationships that exist among variables.

power analysis A procedure for estimating either the likelihood of committing a Type II error or sample size requirements.

practical (pragmatic) clinical trial Trials that address practical questions about the benefits, risks, and costs of an intervention as they would unfold in routine clinical practice, using designs based on information needed for making clinical decisions.

precision In statistics, the extent to which random errors have been reduced, usually expressed in terms of the width of the confidence interval around an estimate.

prediction The use of empirical evidence to make forecasts about how variables will behave in a new setting and with different individuals.

predictive validity The degree to which an instrument can predict a criterion observed at a future time.

pretest (1) The collection of data prior to the experimental intervention; sometimes called baseline data; (2) The trial administration of a newly developed instrument to identify flaws or assess time requirements.

pretest-posttest design An experimental design in which data are collected from research subjects both before and after introducing an intervention; also called a *before–after design.*

prevalence study A cross-sectional study undertaken to estimate the proportion of a population having a particular condition (e.g., multiple sclerosis) at a given point in time.

primary source First-hand reports of facts or findings; in research, the original report prepared by the investigator who conducted the study.

principal investigator (PI) The person who is the lead researcher and who will have primary responsibility for overseeing the project.

probability sampling The selection of sampling units (e.g., participants) from a population using random procedures (e.g., simple random sampling, cluster sampling).

probing Eliciting more useful or detailed information from a respondent in an interview than was volunteered in the first reply.

problem statement An expression of a dilemma or disturbing situation that needs investigation.

process analysis A descriptive analysis of the process by which a program or intervention gets implemented and used in practice.

process consent In a qualitative study, an ongoing, transactional process of negotiating consent with study participants, allowing them to play a collaborative role in the decision-making regarding their continued participation.

product moment correlation coefficient (r) A correlation coefficient designating the magnitude of relationship between two variables measured on at least an interval scale; also called *Pearson's r.*

projective technique A method of measuring psychological attributes (values, attitudes, personality) by providing respondents with unstructured stimuli to which to respond.

prolonged engagement In qualitative research, the investment of sufficient time during data collection to have an in-depth understanding of the group under study, thereby enhancing credibility.

propensity score A score that captures the conditional probability of exposure to a treatment, given various preintervention characteristics; can be used to match comparison groups to enhance internal validity.

proportional hazards model A model in which independent variables are used to predict the risk (hazard) of experiencing an event at a given point in time.

proportionate sample A sample that results when the researcher samples from different strata of the population in proportion to their representation in the population.

proposal A document communicating a research problem, its significance, proposed procedures for solving the problem, and, when funding is sought, how much the study would cost.

prospective design A study design that begins with an examination of presumed causes (e.g., cigarette smoking) and then goes forward in time to observe presumed effects (e.g., lung cancer); also called a *cohort design.*

psychometric assessment An evaluation of the quality of an instrument, based primarily on evidence of its reliability and validity.

psychometrics The theory underlying principles of measurement and the application of the theory in the development of measuring tools.

publication bias The tendency for published studies to systematically over-represent statistically significant findings, reflecting the tendency of researchers, reviewers, and editors to not publish negative results; also called a *bias against the null hypothesis.*

purposive (purposeful) sampling A nonprobability sampling method in which the researcher selects participants based on personal judgment about which ones will be most informative; also called *judgmental sampling.*

Q sort A data collection method in which participants sort statements into a number of piles (usually 9 or 11) according to some bipolar dimension (e.g., most helpful/least helpful).

qualitative analysis The organization and interpretation of narrative data for the purpose of discovering important underlying themes, categories, and patterns of relationships.

qualitative data Information collected in narrative (nonnumeric) form, such as the transcript of an unstructured interview.

qualitative research The investigation of phenomena, typically in an in-depth and holistic fashion, through the collection of rich narrative materials using a flexible research design.

qualitizing The process of reading and interpreting quantitative data in a qualitative manner.

quantitative analysis The manipulation of numeric data through statistical procedures for the purpose of describing phenomena or assessing the magnitude and reliability of relationships among them.

quantitative data Information collected in a quantified (numeric) form.

quantitative research The investigation of phenomena that lend themselves to precise measurement and quantification, often involving a rigorous and controlled design.

quantitizing The process of coding and analyzing qualitative data quantitatively.

quasi-experimental design A design for an intervention study in which subjects are not randomly assigned to treatment conditions; also called a *nonrandomized trial* or a *controlled trial without randomization.*

quasi-statistics An "accounting" system used to assess the validity of conclusions derived from qualitative analysis.

query letter A letter written to a journal editor to ask whether there is interest in a proposed manuscript, or to a funding source to ask if there is interest in a proposed study.

questionnaire A document used to gather self-report data via self-administration of questions.

quota sampling A nonrandom sampling method in which "quotas" for certain sample characteristics are established to increase the representativeness of the sample.

r The symbol for a bivariate correlation coefficient, summarizing the magnitude and direction of a relationship between two variables measured on an interval or ratio scale.

R The symbol for the multiple correlation coefficient, indicating the magnitude (but not direction) of the relationship between the dependent variable and multiple independent variables, taken together.

R^2 The squared multiple correlation coefficient, indicating the proportion of variance in the dependent variable explained by a set of independent variables.

random assignment The assignment of subjects to treatment conditions in a random manner (i.e., in a manner determined by chance alone); also called *randomization.*

random effects model In meta-analysis, a model in which studies are not assumed to be measuring the same overall effect, but rather reflect a distribution of effects; often preferred to a fixed effect model when there is extensive heterogeneity of effects.

random number table A table displaying hundreds of digits (from 0 to 9) in random order; each number is equally likely to follow any other.

random sampling The selection of a sample such that each member of a population has an equal probability of being included.

randomization The assignment of subjects to treatment conditions in a random manner (i.e., in a manner determined by chance alone); also called *random assignment.*

randomized block design An experimental design involving two or more factors (independent variables), with only some experimentally manipulated.

randomized clinical trial (RCT) A full experimental test of an intervention, involving random assignment to treatment groups; phase III of a full clinical trial.

randomized consent design An experimental design in which subjects are randomized prior to informed consent; also called a *Zelen design.*

randomness An important concept in quantitative research, involving having certain features of the study established by chance rather than by design or personal preference.

range A measure of variability, computed by subtracting the lowest value from the highest value in a distribution of scores.

rating scale A scale that requires ratings of an object or concept along a continuum.

ratio measurement A measurement level with equal distances between scores and a true meaningful zero point (e.g., weight).

raw data Data in the form in which they were collected, without being coded or analyzed.

reactivity A measurement distortion arising from the study participant's awareness of being observed, or, more generally, from the effect of the measurement procedure itself.

readability The ease with which materials (e.g., a questionnaire) can be read by people with varying reading skills, often empirically determined through readability formulas.

RE-AIM framework (*Reach, Efficacy, Adoption, Implementation,* and *Maintenance*) A model for designing and evaluating intervention research that is strong on multiple forms of study validity.

receiver operating characteristic curve (ROC curve) A method used in developing and refining a screening instrument to determine the best cutoff point for "caseness."

rectangular matrix A matrix of data (variables × subjects) that contains no missing values for any variable.

recursive model A path model in which the causal flow is unidirectional, without any feedback loops; opposite of a nonrecursive model.

refereed journal A journal in which decisions about the acceptance of manuscripts are made based on recommendations from peer reviewers.

reflexive notes Notes that document a qualitative researcher's personal experiences, reflections, and progress in the field.

reflexivity In qualitative studies, critical self-reflection about one's own biases, preferences, and preconceptions.

regression analysis A statistical procedure for predicting values of a dependent variable based on one or more independent variables.

regression discontinuity design A quasi-experimental design that involves *systematic* assignment of subjects to groups based on cut-off scores on a preintervention measure.

relationship A bond or a connection between two or more variables.

relative risk (RR) An estimate of risk of "caseness" in one group compared to that in another, computed by dividing the absolute risk for one group (e.g., an exposed group) by the absolute risk for another (e.g., the nonexposed); also called the *risk ratio.*

relative risk reduction (RRR) The estimated proportion of baseline (untreated) risk that is reduced through exposure to the intervention, computed by dividing the absolute risk reduction (ARR) by the absolute risk for the control group.

reliability The degree of consistency or dependability with which an instrument measures an attribute.

reliability coefficient A quantitative index, usually ranging in value from .00 to 1.00, that provides an estimate of how reliable an instrument is (e.g., Cronbach's alpha).

repeated-measures ANOVA An analysis of variance used when there are multiple measures of the dependent variable over time (e.g., in a crossover design).

replication The deliberate repetition of research procedures in a second investigation for the purpose of determining if earlier results can be confirmed.

representative sample A sample whose characteristics are comparable to those of the population from which it is drawn.

research Systematic inquiry that uses orderly, disciplined methods to answer questions or solve problems.

research control See *control*.

research design The overall plan for addressing a research question, including specifications for enhancing the study's integrity.

research hypothesis The actual hypothesis a researcher wishes to test (as opposed to the *null hypothesis*), stating the anticipated relationship between two or more variables.

research methods The techniques used to structure a study and to gather and analyze information in a systematic fashion.

research misconduct Fabrication, falsification, plagiarism, or other practices that seriously deviate from those that are commonly accepted within the scientific community for conducting or reporting research.

research problem An enigmatic or perplexing condition that can be investigated through disciplined inquiry.

research proposal See *proposal*.

research question A statement of the specific query the researcher wants to answer to address a research problem.

research report A document summarizing the main features of a study, including the research question, the methods used to address it, the findings, and the interpretation of the findings.

research utilization The use of some aspect of a study in an application unrelated to the original research.

researcher credibility The faith that can be put in a researcher, based on his or her training, qualifications, and experience.

residuals In multiple regression, the error term or unexplained variance.

respondent In a self-report study, the study participant responding to questions posed by the researcher.

response rate The rate of participation in a study, calculated by dividing the number of persons participating by the number of persons sampled.

response set bias The measurement error resulting from the tendency of some individuals to respond to items in characteristic ways (e.g., always agreeing), independently of item content.

results The answers to research questions, obtained through an analysis of the collected data.

retrospective design A study design that begins with the manifestation of the dependent variable in the present (e.g., lung cancer), followed by a search for a presumed cause occurring in the past (e.g., cigarette smoking).

risk/benefit ratio The relative costs and benefits, to an individual subject and to society at large, of participation in a study; also, the relative costs and benefits of implementing an innovation.

risk ratio See *relative risk*

rival hypothesis An alternative explanation, competing with the researcher's hypothesis, for interpreting the results of a study.

sample A subset of a population, selected to participate in a study.

sampling The process of selecting a portion of the population to represent the entire population.

sampling bias Distortions that arise when a sample is not representative of the population from which it was drawn.

sampling distribution A theoretical distribution of a statistic, using the values of the statistic computed from an infinite number of samples as the data points in the distribution.

sampling error The fluctuation of the value of a statistic from one sample to another drawn from the same population.

sampling frame A list of all the elements in the population, from which the sample is drawn.

sampling plan The formal plan specifying a sampling method, a sample size, and procedures for recruiting subjects.

saturation The collection of qualitative data to the point where a sense of closure is attained because new data yield redundant information.

scale A composite measure of an attribute, involving the combination of several items that have a logical and empirical relationship to each other, resulting in the assignment of a score to place people on a continuum with respect to the attribute.

scatter plot A graphic representation of the relationship between two variables.

scientific merit The degree to which a study is methodologically and conceptually sound.

scientific method A set of orderly, systematic, controlled procedures for acquiring dependable, empirical—and typically quantitative—information; the methodologic approach associated with the positivist paradigm.

screening instrument An instrument used to determine whether potential subjects for a study meet eligibility criteria, or for determining whether a person tests positive for a specified condition.

secondary analysis A form of research in which the data collected by one researcher are reanalyzed by another investigator to answer new questions.

secondary source Secondhand accounts of events or facts; in research, a description of a study prepared by someone other than the original researcher.

selective coding A level of coding in a grounded theory study that involves selecting the core category, systematically integrating relationships between the core category and other categories, and validating those relationships.

selection threat (self-selection) A threat to the internal validity of the study resulting from preexisting differences between groups under study; the differences affect the dependent variable in ways extraneous to the effect of the independent variable.

self-determination A person's ability to voluntarily decide whether or not to participate in a study.

self-report A method of collecting data that involves a direct report of information by the person who is being studied (e.g., by interview or questionnaire).

semantic differential A technique used to measure attitudes in which respondents rate concepts of interest on a series of bipolar rating scales.

semi-structured interview An interview in which the researcher has a list of topics to cover rather than specific questions to ask.

sensitivity The ability of screening instruments to correctly identify a "case," that is, to correctly diagnose a condition.

sensitivity analysis An effort to test how sensitive the results of a statistical analysis are to changes in assumptions or in the way the analysis was done (e.g., in a meta-analysis, sometimes used to assess whether conclusions are sensitive to the quality of the studies included).

sequential clinical trial A trial in which data are continuously analyzed, and *stopping rules* are used to decide when the evidence about treatment efficacy is sufficiently strong that the trial can be stopped.

setting The physical location and conditions in which data collection takes place in a study.

significance level The probability that an observed relationship could be caused by chance; significance at the .05 level indicates the probability that a relationship of the observed magnitude would be found by chance only 5 times out of 100.

sign test A nonparametric test for comparing two paired groups based on the relative ranking of values between the pairs.

simple random sampling Basic probability sampling involving the selection of sample members from a sampling frame through completely random procedures.

simultaneous multiple regression A multiple regression analysis in which all predictor variables are entered into the equation simultaneously.

single-subject experiment An intervention study that tests the effectiveness of an intervention with a single subject, typically using a time series design.

site The overall location where a study is undertaken.

skewed distribution The asymmetric distribution of a set of data values around a central point.

snowball sampling The selection of participants through referrals from earlier participants; also called *network sampling*.

social desirability response set A bias in self-report instruments created when participants have a tendency to misrepresent their opinions in the direction of answers consistent with prevailing social norms.

space triangulation The collection of data on the same phenomenon in multiple sites, to enhance the validity of the findings.

Spearman's rank-order correlation (Spearman's rho) A correlation coefficient indicating the magnitude of a relationship between variables measured on the ordinal scale.

specificity The ability of a screening instrument to correctly identify noncases.

standard deviation The most frequently used statistic for measuring the degree of variability in a set of scores.

standard error The standard deviation of a sampling distribution, such as the sampling distribution of the mean.

standard scores Scores expressed in terms of standard deviations from the mean, with raw scores transformed to have a mean of zero and a standard deviation of one; also called *z* scores.

standardized mean difference (SMD) In meta-analysis, the effect size for comparing two group means, computed by subtracting one mean from the other and dividing by the pooled standard deviation; also called Cohen's *d*.

statement of purpose A broad declarative statement of the overall goals of a study.

statistic An estimate of a parameter, calculated from sample data.

statistical analysis The organization and analysis of quantitative data using statistical procedures, including both descriptive and inferential statistics.

statistical conclusion validity The degree to which inferences about relationships and differences from a statistical analysis of the data are accurate.

statistical control The use of statistical procedures to control extraneous, confounding influences on the dependent variable.

statistical inference The process of inferring attributes about the population based on information from a sample, using laws of probability.

statistical power The ability of the research design or analytic procedures to detect true relationships among variables.

statistical significance A term indicating that the results from an analysis of sample data are unlikely to have been caused by chance, at a specified level of probability.

statistical test An analytic tool that estimates the probability that obtained results from a sample reflect true population values.

stepwise multiple regression A multiple regression analysis in which predictor variables are entered into the equation in steps, in the order in which the increment to R is greatest.

strata Subdivisions of the population according to some characteristic (e.g., males and females); singular is *stratum*.

stratified random sampling The random selection of study participants from two or more strata of the population independently.

structural equations Equations representing the magnitude and nature of hypothesized relations among sets of variables in a theory.

structured data collection An approach to collecting data from participants, either through self-report or observations, in which response categories are specified in advance.

study participant An individual who participates and provides information in a study.

study section Within the National Institutes of Health, a group of peer reviewers that evaluates grant applications in the first phase of the review process.

subgroup effect The differential effect of the independent variable on the dependent variable for subsets of the sample.

subject An individual who participates and provides data in a study; term used primarily in quantitative research.

summated rating scale A composite measure of an attribute involving the summation of individual item scores.

survey research Nonexperimental research that obtains information about people's activities, beliefs, preferences, and attitudes via direct questioning.

survival analysis A statistical procedure used when the dependent variable represents a time interval between an initial event (e.g., onset of a disease) and an end event (e.g., death).

symmetric distribution A distribution of values with two halves that are mirror images of the each other.

systematic review A rigorous and systematic synthesis of research findings on a common or strongly related research question.

systematic sampling The selection of sample members such that every *kth* (e.g., every tenth) person or element in a sampling frame is chosen.

table shell A table without any numeric values, prepared in advance of data analysis as a guide to the analyses to be performed.

tacit knowledge Information about a culture that is so deeply embedded that members do not talk about it or may not even be consciously aware of it.

target population The entire population in which a researcher is interested and to which he or she would like to generalize the study results.

taxonomy In an ethnographic analysis, a system of classifying and organizing terms and concepts, developed to illuminate the internal organization of a domain and the relationship among the subcategories of the domain.

template analysis style An approach to qualitative analysis in which a preliminary template or coding scheme is used to sort the narrative data.

test statistic A statistic used to test for the statistical reliability of relationships between variables (e.g., chi-squared, *t*); the sampling distributions of test statistics are known for circumstances in which the null hypothesis is true.

test–retest reliability Assessment of the stability of an instrument by correlating the scores obtained on two administrations.

testing threat A threat to a study's internal validity that occurs when the administration of a pretest or baseline measure of a dependent variable results in changes on the variable, apart from the effect of the independent variable.

theme A recurring regularity emerging from an analysis of qualitative data.

theoretical notes In field studies, notes detailing the researcher's interpretations of observed behavior.

theoretical sampling In qualitative studies, the selection of sample members based on emerging findings to ensure adequate representation of important theoretical categories.

theory An abstract generalization that presents a systematic explanation about the relationships among phenomena.

theory triangulation The use of competing theories or hypotheses in the analysis and interpretation of data.

thick description A rich and thorough description of the research context in a qualitative study.

think aloud method A qualitative method used to collect data about cognitive processes (e.g., decision making), in which people's reflections on decisions or problem solving are captured as they are being made.

time sampling In structured observations, the sampling of time periods during which observations will take place.

time series design A quasi-experimental design involving the collection of data over an extended time period, with multiple data collection points both prior to and after an intervention.

time triangulation The collection of data on the same phenomenon or about the same people at different points in time, to enhance validity.

topic guide A list of broad question areas to be covered in a semistructured interview or focus group interview.

tracing Procedures used to relocate subjects to avoid attrition in a longitudinal study.

transferability The extent to which qualitative findings can be transferred to other settings or groups; analogous to generalizability.

treatment The experimental intervention under study; the condition being manipulated.

treatment group The group receiving the intervention being tested; the experimental group.

trend study A form of longitudinal study in which different samples from a population are studied over time with respect to some phenomenon (e.g., annual Gallup polls on abortion attitudes).

triangulation The use of multiple methods to collect and interpret data about a phenomenon, so as to converge on an accurate representation of reality.

true score A hypothetical score that would be obtained if a measuring instrument were infallible.

trustworthiness The degree of confidence qualitative researchers have in their data, assessed using the criteria of credibility, transferability, dependability, confirmability, and authenticity.

t-**test** A parametric statistical test for analyzing the difference between two means.

two-tailed tests Statistical tests in which both ends of the sampling distribution are used to determine improbable values.

Type I error An error created by rejecting the null hypothesis when it is true (i.e., the researcher concludes that a relationship exists when in fact it does not—a false positive).

Type II error An error created by accepting the null hypothesis when it is false (i.e., the researcher concludes that *no* relationship exists when in fact it does—a false negative).

unimodal distribution A distribution of values with one peak (high frequency).

unit of analysis The basic unit or focus of a researcher's analysis—typically individual study participants.

univariate statistics Statistical analysis of a single variable for purposes of description (e.g., computing a mean).

unstructured interview An interview in which the researcher asks respondents questions without having a predetermined plan regarding the content or flow of information to be gathered.

unstructured observation The collection of descriptive data through direct observation that is not guided by a formal, prespecified plan for observing, enumerating, or recording the information.

utilization See *research utilization.*

validity A quality criterion referring to the degree to which inferences made in a study are accurate and well-founded; in measurement, the degree to which an instrument measures what it is intended to measure.

validity coefficient An index, usually ranging from .00 to 1.00, yielding an estimate of how valid an instrument is.

variability The degree to which values on a set of scores are dispersed.

variable An attribute that varies, that is, takes on different values (e.g., body temperature, heart rate).

variance A measure of variability or dispersion, equal to the standard deviation squared.

vignette A brief description of an event, person, or situation to which respondents are asked to express their reactions.

visual analog scale (VAS) A scaling procedure used to measure certain clinical symptoms (e.g., pain, fatigue) by having people indicate on a straight line the intensity of the symptom.

vulnerable subjects Special groups of people whose rights in studies need special protection because of their inability to provide meaningful informed consent or because their circumstances place them at higher-than-average-risk of adverse effects (e.g., children, unconscious patients).

web-based survey   The administration of a self-administered questionnaire over the Internet on a dedicated survey website.

weighting   A correction procedure used to estimate population values when a disproportionate sampling design has been used.

Wilcoxon signed ranks test   A nonparametric statistical test for comparing two paired groups, based on the relative ranking of values between the pairs.

wild code   A coded value that is not legitimate within the coding scheme for that data set.

Wilk's lambda   An index used in discriminant function analysis to indicate the proportion of variance in the dependent variable *un*accounted for by predictors; $\lambda = 1 - R^2$.

within-subjects design   A research design in which a single group of subjects is compared under different conditions or at different points in time (e.g., before and after surgery).

z **score**   A standard score, expressed in terms of standard deviations from the mean.

Zelen design   An experimental design in which subjects are randomized prior to informed consent; also called *randomized consent design*.

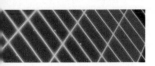

Index

Page numbers in bold indicate glossary entries.

GLOSSARY OF SELECTED STATISTICAL SYMBOLS

This list contains some commonly used symbols in statistics. The list is in approximate alphabetical order, with English and Greek letters intermixed. Nonletter symbols have been placed at the end.

a	Regression constant, the intercept
α	Greek alpha; significance level in hypothesis testing, probability of Type I error; also, a reliability coefficient
b	Regression coefficient, slope of the line
β	Greek beta, probability of a Type II error; also, a standardized regression coefficient (beta weight)
χ^2	Greek chi squared, a test statistic for several nonparametric tests
CI	Confidence interval around estimate of a population parameter
d	An effect size index, a standardized mean difference
df	Degrees of freedom
η^2	Greek eta squared, index of variance accounted for in ANOVA context
f	Frequency (count) for a score value
F	Test statistic used in ANOVA, ANCOVA, and other tests
H_O	Null hypothesis
H_A	Alternative hypothesis; research hypothesis
λ	Greek lambda, a test statistic used in several multivariate analyses (Wilks' lambda)
μ	Greek mu, the population mean
M	Sample mean (alternative symbol for $\bar{X}$)
MS	Mean square, variance estimate in ANOVA
n	Number of cases in a subgroup of the sample
N	Total number of cases or sample members
NNT	Number needed to treat
OR	Odds ratio
p	Probability that observed data are consistent with null hypothesis
r	Pearson's product–moment correlation coefficient for a sample
r_s	Spearman's rank-order correlation coefficient
R	Multiple correlation coefficient
R^2	Coefficient of determination, proportion of variance in *dependent variable* attributable to *independent variables*
R_c	Canonical correlation coefficient
RR	Relative risk
ρ	Greek rho, population correlation coefficient
SD	Sample standard deviation
SEM	Standard error of the mean
σ	Greek sigma (lowercase), population standard deviation
Σ	Greek sigma (uppercase), sum of
SS	Sum of squares
t	Test statistics used in t-tests (sometimes called Student's t)
U	Test statistic for the Mann-Whitney U-test
$\bar{X}$	Sample mean
x	Deviation score
Y'	Predicted value of Y, dependent variable in regression analysis
z	Standard score in a normal distribution
$\|\|$	Absolute value
$\leq$	Less than or equal to
$\geq$	Greater than or equal to
$\neq$	Not equal to